a LANGE medical book

CURRENT Critical Care Diagnosis & Treatment

second edition

Frederic S. Bongard, MD
Professor of Surgery
University of California, Los Angeles, School of Medicine
Chief, Division of Trauma and Critical Care
Director of Surgical Education
Harbor-UCLA Medical Center
Torrance, California.

Darryl Y. Sue, MD
Professor of Clinical Medicine
University of California, Los Angeles, School of Medicine
Director, Medical-Respiratory Intensive Care Unit,
Division of Respiratory and Critical Care Physiology and Medicine
Associate Chair, Department of Medicine
Harbor-UCLA Medical Center
Torrance, California.

Lange Medical Books/McGraw-Hill
Medical Publishing Division

New York Chicago San Francisco Lisbon London
Madrid Mexico City Milan Montreal New Delhi San Juan Seoul
Singapore Sydney Toronto

McGraw-Hill
A Division of The **McGraw-Hill** *Companies*

Current Critical Care Diagnosis & Treatment, Second Edition

ISBN: 0-8385-1454-5 (Domestic)

2 3 4 5 6 7 8 9 0 DOC/DOC 0 9 8 7 6 5 4 3

Notice

Medicine is an ever-changing science. As new research and clinical experience broaden our knowledge, changes in treatment and drug therapy are required. The authors and the publisher of this work have checked with sources believed to be reliable in their efforts to provide information that is complete and generally in accord with the standards accepted at the time of publication. However, in view of the possibility of human error or changes in medical sciences, neither the authors nor the publisher nor any other party who has been involved in the preparation or publication of this work warrants that the information contained herein is in every respect accurate or complete, and they disclaim all responsibility for any errors or omissions or for the results obtained from use of the information contained in this work. Readers are encouraged to confirm the information contained herein with other sources. For example and in particular, readers are advised to check the product information sheet included in the package of each drug they plan to administer to be certain that the information contained in this work is accurate and that changes have not been made in the recommended dose or in the contraindications for administration. This recommendation is of particular importance in connection with new or infrequently used drugs.

This book was set in Adobe Garamond by Pine Tree Composition, Inc.
The editors were Jack Farrell, Harriet Lebowitz, and Regina Y. Brown.
The production supervisor was Catherine H. Saggese.
The index was prepared by Edwin Durbin.
The book designer was Eve Siegel.
The cover designer was Mary McKeon.
RR Donnelley was printer and binder.

ISSN: 1071-3964

This book is printed on acid-free paper.

INTERNATIONAL EDITION ISBN: 0-07-121206-X

Contents

Preface

The second edition of *Current Critical Care Diagnosis & Treatment* is designed to serve as a single-source reference for the adult critical care practitioner. The diversity of illnesses encountered in the critical care population necessitates a well-rounded and thorough knowledge of the manifestations and mechanisms of disease. Unique to the discipline of critical care is the integration of an extensive body of medical knowledge that crosses traditional specialty boundaries. This approach is apparent to intensivists, whose primary background is in internal medicine, surgery, or anesthesiology. Thus, a central feature of this book is a unified and integrated approach to the problems encountered in critical care practice. Like other books in the Lange series, it emphasizes recall of major diagnostic features, concise descriptions of disease processes, and practical management strategies.

INTENDED AUDIENCE

Planned by a surgeon and an internist to meet the need for a concise, but thorough, source of information, *Current Critical Care Diagnosis & Treatment* is designed to facilitate critical care teaching and practice. Students will find its consideration of basic science and clinical application useful during clerkships on medicine, surgery, and intensive care unit electives. House officers will appreciate its concise descriptions of disease processes and organized approach to diagnosis and treatment. Fellows, and those preparing for critical care specialty examinations, will find those sections outside of their primary disciplines particularly useful. Clinicians will recognize this succinct reference on critical care as a valuable asset in their daily practice.

This book does *not* contain chapters on pediatric or neonatal critical care. These areas are highly specialized and require entire monographs of their own. Further, we have not included detailed information on the technical performance of bedside procedures such as central venous catheter or arterial line insertion. Multiple, well-illustrated pocket manuals are available for those readers who require basic technical information. Finally, we have chosen not to include a chapter on nursing or administrative topics. Details on nursing aspects of critical care can be found in a number of separate works.

ORGANIZATION

Current Critical Care Diagnosis & Treatment is conceptually organized into three major sections: 1) fundamentals of critical care applicable to all specialties; 2) topics related primarily to medical critical care; and 3) essentials of surgical intensive care. Early chapters provide information about the general physiology and pathophysiology of critical illness. The later chapters discuss pathophysiology using an organ or disease specific approach. Where appropriate, we have placed the medical and surgical chapters in succession to facilitate access to information.

OUTSTANDING FEATURES

- Concise, readable format, providing efficient use in a variety of clinical and academic settings.
- Edited by both a surgical and medical intensivist, with contributors from multiple specialties.
- Illustrations chosen to clarify basic and clinical concepts.
- Careful evaluation of new diagnostic procedures and their usefulness in specific diagnostic problems.
- Up-to-date drug selection and dosing guidelines.
- Carefully selected key references in *Index Medicus* format, which provide all information necessary to allow electronic retrieval.

ACKNOWLEDGMENTS

The editors and contributors wish to thank Dr. James Ransom for his tireless and precise editing of the manuscript. His understanding of medicine, education, literature, and syntax has resulted in a unique textbook. Additionally, we wish to thank Mr. Jack Farrell at McGraw-Hill for his motivation and encouragement in keeping us on track. We are also grateful to our families for their support.

Frederic S. Bongard, MD
Darryl Y. Sue, MD
September 2002

Authors

Jennifer H. Cupo Abbott, PharmD
Assistant Professor, Department of Clinical Pharmacy, University of Southern California School of Pharmacy, Los Angeles, California.

Tracey D. Arnell, MD
Assistant Professor of Surgery, Harbor-UCLA Medical Center, Torrance, California.

Lilly Barba, MD
Medical Director, Renal Transplant Program, Harbor-UCLA Medical Center
Associate Professor of Clinical Medicine, University of California, Los Angeles, School of Medicine.

Marie Beall, MD
Associate Professor of Obstetrics and Gynecology, University of California, Los Angeles, School of Medicine; Chief, Division of Obstetrics, Harbor-UCLA Medical Center, Torrance, California.

Howard Belzberg, MD
Associate Director, Surgical ICU, LAC & USC Medical Center, Los Angeles, California.

Shalender Bhasin, MD
Professor of Medicine, University of California, Los Angeles, School of Medicine
Chief, Division of Endocrinology, Metabolism, and Molecular Medicine, Charles Drew University, Los Angeles, California.

Diane Birnbaumer, MD
Professor of Clinical Medicine, University of California, Los Angeles, School of Medicine
Associate Residency Director, Department of Emergency Medicine, Harbor-UCLA Medical Center, Torrance, California.

Frederic S. Bongard, MD
Professor of Surgery
Chief, Division of Trauma and Critical Care,
Director of Surgical Education, University of California, Los Angeles, School of Medicine; Harbor-UCLA Medical Center, Torrance, California.

Kathleen Brown, MD
Professor of Radiology, University of California, Los Angeles, School of Medicine.

Leonard A. Cedars, MD
Director, Department of Maternal Fetal Medicine, Sierra Vista Regional Medical Center, San Luis Obispo, California.

John R. Chamberlain, MD
Fellow, Program in Psychiatry and the Law, Department of Psychiatry, University of California, San Francisco.

Linda Chang, MD
Scientist and Chair, Medical Department, Brookhaven National Laboratory, Upton, New York.

Laurie Anne Chu, MD
Southern California Permanente Medical Group, Kaiser Bellflower Medical Center, Bellflower, California.

William G. Cioffi, Jr., MD, FACS
J. Murray Beardsley Professor & Chairman, Department of Surgery, Brown Medical School
Surgeon-in-Chief, Department of Surgery, Rhode Island Hospital, Providence, Rhode Island.

Shawkat Dhanani, MD, MPH
Chief, Geriatric Evaluation & Management Unit, VA Greater Los Angeles Healthcare System
Associate Clinical Professor in Geriatric Medicine/Internal Medicine, University of California, Los Angeles, School of Medicine.

Curtis Doberstein, MD
Assistant Professor, Brown University School of Medicine; Director, Cerebrovascular Surgery, Rhode Island Hospital, Providence, Rhode Island.

Stuart J. Eisendrath, MD
Professor of Clinical Psychiatry, Director of Ambulatory Services, Langley Porter Psychiatric Hospital and Clinics, University of California, San Francisco.

Wilbert Fortson, MD
Resident, Obstetrics and Gynecology, Harbor-UCLA Medical Center, Torrance, California.

Arnold W. Gurevitch, MD†
Professor and Chief, Division of Dermatology, Keck School of Medicine, University of Southern California, Los Angeles, California.

Craig R. Hampton, MD
Senior Research Fellow, Cardiothoracic Surgery, The University of Washington, Seattle, Washington.

Darrell W. Harrington, MD
Assistant Professor of Medicine, University of California, Los Angeles, School of Medicine
Chief, Division of General Internal Medicine, Director of Inpatient Medical Consultation, Harbor-UCLA Medical Center, Torrance, California.

Eli Ipp, MB, BCh
Professor of Medicine, University of California, Los Angeles, School of Medicine
Head, Section of Diabetes and Metabolism, Harbor-UCLA Medical Center, Torrance, California.

Cindy Kallman, MD
Chief, Section of CT/Ultrasound, Cedars Sinai Imaging, Cedars Sinai Medical Center, Los Angeles, California.

Andre A. Kaplan, MD, FACP
Professor of Medicine, Division of Nephrology, University of Connecticut Health Center
Director, Dialysis Program, John Dempsey Hospital, Farmington, Connecticut.

James T. Lee, MD
Fellow in Peripheral Vascular and Endovascular Surgery, Division of Vascular Surgery, Harbor-UCLA Medical Center, Torrance, California.

Tai-Shion Lee, MD
Professor of Anesthesiology, University of California, Los Angeles, School of Medicine
Department of Anesthesiology, Harbor-UCLA Medical Center, Torrance, California.

†**Deceased.**

David A. Lewis, MD
Assistant Clinical Professor of Medicine, University of Washington
Associate Chief, Pulmonary, Critical Care, & Sleep Medicine, Group Health Permanente, Seattle, Washington.

Chris A. Lycette, MD
Chief Resident, Division of Neurosurgery, University of California, Los Angeles, School of Medicine.

Phong Mac, MD
Clinical Endocrinology Fellow, Division of Endocrinology, Metabolism and Molecular Medicine, Charles R. Drew University of Medicine and Science, Los Angeles, California.

James R. Macho, MD
Emeritus Professor of Surgery, University of California, San Francisco; Director, Bothin Burn Center
Chief, Critical Care Medicine, Saint Francis Memorial Hospital, San Francisco, California.

Duncan Q. McBride, MD
Associate Professor of Clinical Surgery, Division of Neurosurgery, University of California, Los Angeles, School of Medicine
Chief, Division of Neurosurgery, Harbor-UCLA Medical Center, Los Angeles, California.

Hugh B. McIntyre, MD, PhD
Professor of Neurology, University of California, Los Angeles, School of Medicine;
Harbor-UCLA Medical Center, Torrance, California.

Bruce L. Miller, MD
Clausen Distinguished Professor of Neurology, University of California, San Francisco Memory and Aging Center, San Francisco, California.

David W. Mozingo, MD, FACS
Professor, Department of Surgery and Anesthesiology
Director, Shands Burn Center, University of Florida, Gainesville, Florida.

James A. Murray, MD
Assistant Professor, Department of Surgery, LAC & USC Medical Center, Keck School of Medicine, University of Southern California.

Kenneth A. Narahara, MD
Professor of Medicine, University of California, Los Angeles, School of Medicine
Assistant Chair for Clinical Affairs, Department of Medicine
Director, Coronary Care, Division of Cardiology, Harbor-UCLA Medical Center, Torrance, California.

Gideon P. Naude, MD, FRCS, FACS
Chairman, Department of Surgery, Tuolumne General Hospital, Sonora, California.

Dean C. Norman, MD
Chief of Staff, VA Greater Los Angeles Healthcare System
Professor of Medicine, University of Southern California, Los Angeles, California.

Basil A. Pruitt, Jr., MD
Editor, The Journal of Trauma; Clinical Professor of Surgery, University of Texas Health Science Center at San Antonio, San Antonio, Texas.

Steven S. Raman, MD
Assistant Professor of Radiology, Division of Abdominal Imaging and Intervention, University of California, Los Angeles, Medical Center.

Gerald E. Rodts, Jr., MD
Associate Professor of Neurosurgery, Emory University, Atlanta, Georgia.

Maria I. Rudis, PharmD, FCCM, DABAT, BCPS
Assistant Professor, Departments of Clinical Pharmacy and Emergency Medicine, University of Southern California School of Pharmacy, Los Angeles, California.

William P. Schecter, MD
Chief of Surgery, San Francisco General Hospital, Professor of Clinical Surgery and Vice-Chairman, University of California, San Francisco.

Paul A. Selecky, MD, FACP, FCCP, FAARC
Clinical Professor of Medicine, University of California, Los Angeles, School of Medicine
Medical Director, Pulmonary Department, Hoag Memorial Hospital, Newport Beach, California.

Shelley Shapiro, MD, PhD
Professor of Clinical Medicine, University of Southern California, Keck School of Medicine, Division of Cardiovascular Diseases, Los Angeles, California.

Elizabeth D. Simmons, MD
Department of Hematology and Oncology, Kaiser Permanente, Southern California.

Michael J. Stamos, MD
Associate Professor of Surgery, University of California, Los Angeles, School of Medicine
Chief, Section of Colon & Rectal Surgery, Harbor-UCLA Medical Center, Torrance, California.

Samuel J. Stratton, MD, MPH
Associate Professor of Medicine, University of California, Los Angeles.

Darryl Y. Sue, MD
Professor of Clinical Medicine, University of California, Los Angeles, School of Medicine
Director, Medical-Respiratory Intensive Care Unit, Division of Respiratory and Critical Care Physiology and Medicine
Associate Chair, Department of Medicine, Harbor-UCLA Medical Center, Torrance, California.

Hassan J. Tabbarah, MD[†]
Professor of Medicine, University of California, Los Angeles, School of Medicine; Divisions of Oncology and General Internal Medicine;
Assistant Chairman, Department of Medicine, Harbor-UCLA Medical Center, Torrance, California.

[†]**Deceased.**

John A. Tayek, MD
Associate Professor of Medicine, University of California, Los Angeles, School of Medicine
Division of General Internal Medicine, Harbor-UCLA Medical Center, Torrance, California.
tayek@hume.edu

Laurie K.S. Tom, MD
Assistant Clinical Professor of Medicine, University of Hawaii, John A. Burns School of Medicine, Department of Medicine, Honolulu, Hawaii.

Hernan I. Vargas, MD
Assistant Professor of Surgery, University of California, Los Angeles, School of Medicine
Chief, Oncologic Surgery, Harbor-UCLA Medical Center, Torrance, California.

Edward D. Verrier, MD
Professor and Chief, Division of Cardiothoracic Surgery, University of Washington, School of Medicine Seattle, Washington.

Janine R.E. Vintch, MD
Assistant Clinical Professor of Medicine, University of California, Los Angeles, School of Medicine
Division of General Internal Medicine, Harbor-UCLA Medical Center, Torrance, California.

Kenneth Waxman, MD
Director of Trauma and Surgical Education, Santa Barbara Cottage Hospital, Santa Barbara, California.

Tricia L. Westhoff, MD
Clinical Endocrinology Fellow, Harbor-UCLA Medical Center, Torrance, California.

Mallory D. Witt, MD
Associate Professor of Medicine, University of California, Los Angeles, School of Medicine
Division of HIV Medicine, Harbor-UCLA Medical Center, Torrance, California.

Kory Zipperstein, MD
Chief, Department of Dermatology, Kaiser Medical Center, San Francisco, California.

Philosophy & Principles of Critical Care

1

Darryl Y. Sue, MD, & Frederic S. Bongard, MD

Critical care is unique among the specialties of medicine. While other specialties seek to narrow the focus of interest to a single body system, a particular therapy, or a particular age group, critical care is directed toward patients with a wide variety of illnesses. All have the common denominator of extreme severity of existing disease or the potential to develop severe complications from the disease or its treatment. The variety of illnesses seen in a critically ill population necessitates a well-rounded and thorough knowledge of the manifestations and mechanisms of disease. The severity of the disease requires an approach to the patient that is simultaneously global and focused, dependent on large accumulations of accurate data, and well integrated. Although practitioners of critical care medicine—sometimes called "intensivists"—are often specialists in pulmonary medicine, cardiology, nephrology, anesthesiology, surgery, or critical care itself, the ability to provide effective critical care is in all cases dependent on the principles of patient management in internal medicine and surgery. Therefore, critical care might be considered not a specialty but rather a philosophy of patient care.

Do the practitioners of critical care medicine make a difference in patient outcome? Several studies have shown that full-time intensivists do improve patient outcome. It can be argued, however, that local physician staffing practices, interactions between primary care clinicians, subspecialists, and intensivists, patient factors, and nursing and ancillary support might play a much larger role in determining outcomes. Nevertheless, it is clear that organization of the ICU, the use of protocols and guidelines, control of medications and procedures, policies for infection control, and continued feedback on the quality of care provided will be the focus of future studies.

The general principles of critical care are presented in this chapter as well as some guidelines for those who are responsible for leadership of ICUs.

GENERAL PRINCIPLES OF CRITICAL CARE

EARLY IDENTIFICATION OF PROBLEMS

Critical care involves taking care of patients with severe life-threatening illnesses. Therefore, it would be expected that such patients would manifest existing or imminent dysfunction of one or more organ systems. These individuals are not likely to have normal reserves of organ function and might be prone to develop—for example—renal failure, respiratory failure, or heart failure more easily than other classes of patients. Furthermore, there are definite causal relationships between failure of one organ system and failure of others, such as cardiac failure contributing to renal insufficiency, or renal failure associated with metabolic acidosis, platelet dysfunction, and hypocalcemia. Treatment of organ failure also plays a role in the complex interaction between organ systems. For example, mechanical ventilation of patients with respiratory failure contributes to decreased cardiac output and resultant impaired renal, central nervous system, or gastrointestinal dysfunction. Multiple medications are frequently prescribed, each one necessary for treatment of a specific aspect of the patient's problem, but the greater the number of drugs, the greater the potential for adverse drug interactions. Furthermore, it is clear that critically ill patients more frequently have drug toxicity and side effects, and the complications of drug reactions are more severe, prolonged, and associated with higher mortality rates.

Because of the high potential for complications in critically ill patients, the practitioner in the ICU must remain alert to early manifestations of other organ system dysfunction, the onset of complications of therapy, potential drug interactions, and other premonitory data (Table 1–1). This requires *frequent and regular review*

Table 1–1. Recommendations for routine patient care in the ICU.

- Assess current status, interval history, and examination.
- Review vital signs for interval period (since last review).
- Review medication record, including continuous infusions:
  - Duration and dose
  - Changes in dose or frequency based on changes in renal, hepatic, or other pharmacokinetic function
  - Changes in route of administration
  - Potential drug interactions
- Correlate changes in vital signs with medication administration and other changes by use of chronologic charting.
- Review, if indicated:
  - Respiratory therapy flow chart
  - Hemodynamics records
  - Laboratory flowsheets
  - Other continuous monitoring
- Integrate nursing, respiratory therapists, patient, family, and other observations.
- Review *all* problems, including adding, updating, consolidating or removing problems as indicated.
- Periodically, review supportive care:
  - Intravenous fluids
  - Nutritional status and support
  - Prophylactic treatment and support
  - Duration of catheters and other invasive devices
- Review and contrast risks and benefits of intensive care.

of all information available, including changes in symptoms, physical findings, laboratory data, and information obtained from monitoring modalities. Meticulous attention to detail is essential for prevention of or early intervention in a new problem.

EFFECTIVE USE OF THE PROBLEM-ORIENTED MEDICAL RECORD

Problem-oriented medical records have been in use for some time but are of special importance in the ICU. In order to define and follow "problems" effectively, each should be regularly reviewed and characterized. For example, if the general problem of "renal failure" has subsequently been determined to be due to aminoglycoside toxicity, it should be described in that way in an updated problem list. But even the satisfaction of identifying a cause of renal failure may be short-lived. The same patient may subsequently develop other related or unrelated renal problems, thereby forcing another reassessment and a new problem for the list.

Furthermore, problems must not be restricted to "diagnoses." An effective way to ensure that intraarterial catheters are not inadvertently left in place for too long is to list the placement of the line as a "problem" to be addressed daily. Other "nonproblems" may include nutritional support, prevention of deep vein thrombosis and decubitus ulcers, and drug allergies. It may be useful to include nonmedical issues as well so they can be discussed routinely. Examples are psychosocial difficulties, timely but unresolved end-of-life decisions, and other questions about patient comfort. Finally, the patient's current problem-oriented medical record should be shared appropriately with nonphysicians caring for the patient, a process that enhances communication, simplifies interactions between staff members, and furthers the ultimate goal of improved patient care.

MONITORING & DATA DISPLAY

A prominent characteristic of patient care in critical care units is continuous monitoring by trained personnel. Although such monitoring is often thought of as limited to electrocardiography, blood pressure measurements, pulse oximetry, and other automated procedures, any regular collection of relevant data constitutes monitoring. Serial blood glucose and electrolyte determinations, arterial blood gases, hourly or most frequent ventilator settings and airway pressure variables, and body temperature, among others, are part of ICU monitoring. While not frequently considered, daily weights may be invaluable in determining the net fluid balance of a patient. Flowcharts of laboratory data and mechanical ventilator activity, 24-hour vital signs records, graphs of hemodynamic data, and lists of medications are indispensable tools for good patient care, and efforts should be made to find the most effective and efficient ways of displaying such information. Methods that integrate the records of physicians, nurses, respiratory therapists, and others can be particularly useful.

Computerized data collection and display systems are increasingly found in ICUs. Some of these systems import data directly from bedside monitors, mechanical ventilators, intravenous infusion pumps, fluid collection devices, clinical laboratory instruments, and other devices. Physicians, nurses, and other caregivers may enter progress notes and information about medications administered and patient observations. Advantages of computerized data systems include decreased time and effort for data collection and the ability to display data in a variety of convenient formats, including flowcharts, graphs, and problem-oriented records. Such data can be sent to remote sites for consultation, if necessary. Computerized access to data facilitates research and quality assurance studies, including use of a variety of prognostic indicators, severity scores, and ICU decision-making tools. However, all data must be carefully reviewed before being accepted as accurate, and some time is needed to familiarize personnel with the use of these systems. Computerized information systems have the potential for improving patient care in the ICU, but their benefit to patient outcome has not yet been determined.

SUPPORTIVE & PREVENTIVE CARE

For many patients in the ICU, an important aspect of care is the prevention of secondary complications of disease and the side effects of treatment. Studies have pointed out the high prevalence of gastrointestinal hemorrhage, deep venous thrombosis, decubitus ulcers, inadequate nutritional support, nosocomial pneumonias, urinary tract infections, psychologic problems, sleep disorders, and other untoward effects of critical care. Efforts have been made to prevent, treat, or otherwise identify the risks for these complications. As outlined in subsequent chapters, highly effective prophylactic management is available for some of these risks (Table 1–2); for other complications, early identification and aggressive intervention may be of value. For example, aggressive nutritional support for critically ill patients is often indicated, both because of the presence of chronic illness and malnutrition and because of the rapid depletion of nutritional reserves in the presence of severe illness. Nutritional support; prevention of upper gastrointestinal bleeding with antacids, H_2 blockers, or sucralfate and deep venous thrombosis with unfractionated or low-molecular-heparin; aggressive skin care; and other supportive therapy should be included on the ICU patient's problem list. Furthermore, the importance of complications from indwelling vascular catheters suggests that these should be listed as "problems" so they can be addressed daily.

Because of expense and questions of effectiveness and safety, studies of preventive treatment of ICU patients are ongoing. For example, a multicenter study reported that clinically important gastrointestinal bleeding in critically ill patients was most often seen only in those with respiratory failure or coagulopathy (3.7% for one or both factors). Otherwise, the risk for significant bleeding was only 0.1%. The authors suggested that prophylaxis against stress ulcer could be safely withheld from critically ill patients unless they had one of these two risk factors. On the other hand, about half of the patients in this study were post-cardiac surgery patients, and the majority of patients in many ICUs have one of the identified risk factors. Thus, there may not be sufficient compelling evidence to discontinue the practice of providing routine prophylaxis for gastrointestinal bleeding in all ICU patients.

Other routine practices have been challenged. For example, an important study showed that routine transfusion of red blood cells in ICU patients who reached an arbitrary but physiologic hemoglobin level did not change outcome when compared with allowing hemoglobin to fall to a lower value. Outcome studies are ongoing for prevention of deep venous thrombosis in surgery patients, following hip or knee replacement, and for medical problems such as acute myocardial infarction or acute respiratory distress syndrome. Important findings include differences in the need for preventive therapy, critical differences in the intensity and type of therapy needed to prevent thrombosis, and the benefits to be expected for different problems. Further studies are needed to define the role of other preventive strategies.

ATTENTION TO PSYCHOSOCIAL & OTHER NEEDS OF THE PATIENT

Psychosocial needs of the patient are a major consideration in the ICU. The psychologic consequences of critical illness and its treatment have a profound impact on patient outcome. Leading factors include the patient's lack of control over the local environment, severe disruption of the sleep-wake cycle, inability to easily and quickly communicate with critical care providers, and pain and other types of physical discomfort. Inability to communicate with family members as well as concern about employment status, activities of daily living, finances, and other matters further inflate the emotional costs of being seriously ill. The intensivist and other staff members must pay close attention to these problems and issues and consider psychologic problems in the differential diagnosis of any patient's altered mental status.

There is increased awareness of the potential harm to patients and problems for caregivers of the ICU environment. The noise level is high (reported to exceed 60–84 dB, where a busy office might have 70 dB and a pneumatic drill at 50 feet might be as loud as 80 dB), notably from mechanical ventilators, conversations, and telephones, but especially from audio alarms on ICU equipment. One study found that caregivers were unable to discern and identify alarms accurately, including alarms that indicated critical patient or equipment conditions.

Sleep disruption deserves much more attention. Very disruptive sleep architecture has been identified in patients in the ICU. Frequent checking of vital signs and phlebotomy were most disruptive to patients, and environmental factors were less of a problem to patients surveyed.

UNDERSTAND THE LIMITS OF CRITICAL CARE

All physicians involved with critical care must become familiar with the limitations of such care. Interestingly, physicians and other care providers may have to be

Table 1–2. Things to think about and reminders for ICU patient care.

Things To Think About	Reminders
GENERAL ICU CARE	
1. Nosocomial infections, especially line- and catheter-related. 2. Stress gastritis. 3. Deep venous thrombosis and pulmonary embolism. 4. Exacerbation of malnourished state. 5. Decubitus ulcers. 6. Psychosocial needs and adjustments. 7. Toxicity of drugs (renal, pulmonary, hepatic, CNS). 8. Development of antibiotic-resistant organisms. 9. Complications of diagnostic tests. 10. Correct placement of catheters and tubes. 11. Need for vitamins (thiamine, C, K). 12. Tuberculosis, pericardial disease, adrenal insufficiency, fungal sepsis, rule out myocardial infarction, pneumothorax, volume overload or volume depletion, decreased renal function with normal serum creatinine, errors in drug administration or charting, pulmonary vascular disease, HIV-related disease.	1. Discontinue infected or possibly infected lines. 2. Need for H_2 blockers, antacids, or sucralfate. 3. Provide enteral or parenteral nutrition. 4. Change antibiotics? 5. Chest x-ray for line placement. 6. Review known drug allergies (including contrast agents). 7. Check for drug dosage adjustments (new liver failure or renal failure). 8. Need for deep venous thrombosis prophylaxis? 9. Pain medication and sedation. 10. Weigh patient. 11. Give medications orally, if possible. 12. Does patient really need an arterial catheter? 13. Give thiamine early.
NUTRITION	
1. Set goals for appropriate nutrition support. 2. Avoid or minimize catabolic state. 3. Acquired vitamin K deficiency while in ICU. 4. Avoidance of excessive fluid intake. 5. Diarrhea (lactose intolerance, low protein, hyperosmolarity, drug-induced, infectious). 6. Minimize and anticipate hyperglycemia during parenteral nutritional support. 7. Adjustment of support rate or formula in patients with renal failure or liver failure. 8. Early complications of refeeding. 9. Acute vitamin insufficiency.	1. Calculate estimated basic caloric and protein needs. Use 30 kcal/kg and 1.5 g protein/kg for starting amount. 2. Regular food preferred over enteral feeding; enteral feeding preferred over parenteral in most patients. 3. Increased caloric and protein requirements if febrile, infected, agitated, any inflammatory process ongoing, some drugs. 4. Adjust protein if renal or liver failure is present. Adjust again if dialysis is used. 5. Measure serum albumin as primary marker of nutritional status. 6. Give vitamin K, especially if malnourished and receiving antibiotics. 7. Consider volume restriction formulas (both enteral and parenteral). 8. Give phosphate early during refeeding. 9. Plan on giving insulin in TPN; control hyperglycemia (glucose < 110–120 mg/dL).
ACUTE RENAL FAILURE	
1. Volume depletion, hypoperfusion, low cardiac output, shock. 2. Nephrotoxic drugs. 3. Obstruction of urine outflow. 4. Interstitial nephritis. 5. Manifestation of systemic disease, multiorgan system failure. 6. Degree of preexisting chronic renal failure.	1. Measure urine Na^+, Cl^-, creatinine, and osmolality. 2. Volume challenge, if indicated. 3. Discontinue nephrotoxic drugs if possible. 4. Adjust all renally excreted drugs. 5. Renal medicine consultation for dialysis, other management. 6. Renal ultrasound if indicated. 7. Check catheter and replace if indicated. 8. Stop potassium supplementation if necessary. 9. Adjust diet (Na^+, protein, etc.). 10. If dialytic therapy is begun, adjust drugs if necessary. 11. Weigh patient daily.

(continued)

Table 1–2. Things to think about and reminders for ICU patient care. (continued)

Things To Think About	Reminders
ACUTE RESPIRATORY FAILURE, COPD	
1. Adequacy of oxygenation. 2. Exacerbation due to infection, malnutrition, congestive heart failure. 3. Airway secretions. 4. Other medical problems (coexisting heart failure). 5. Hypotension and low cardiac output response to positive-pressure ventilation. 6. Hyponatremia, SIADH. 7. Severe pulmonary hypertension. 8. Sleep deprivation. 9. Coexisting metabolic alkalosis.	1. Should patient be intubated or mechanically ventilated? Noninvasive mechanical ventilation? 2. Bronchodilators. 3. Consider corticosteriods, ipratropium. 4. Sufficient supplemental oxygen. 5. Antibiotic coverage for common bacterial causes of exacerbations. Evaluate for pneumonia as well as acute bronchitis. 6. Early nutrition support. 7. Check theophylline level, if indicated. 8. Ventilator management: low tidal volume, long expiratory time, high inspiratory flow, watch for auto-PEEP. 9. Think about weaning early.
ACUTE RESPIRATORY FAILURE, ARDS	
1. Sepsis as cause, from pulmonary or nonpulmonary site (abdominal, urinary). 2. Possible aspiration of gastric contents. 3. Fluid overload or contribution form congestive heart failure. 4. Anticipate potential multi-organ system failure. 5. Assess the risks of oxygen toxicity versus complications of PEEP. 6. Consider the complications of high airway pressure or large tidal volume in selection of type of mechanical ventilatory support. 7. Low serum albumin (contribution from hypo-oncotic pulmonary edema).	1. Early therapeutic goal of $F10_2 < 0.50$ and lowest PEEP (<5–10 cm H_2O), resulting in acceptable O_2 delivery. 2. Directed (if possible) or broad-spectrum antibiotics. 3. Evaluate for soft tissue or intra-abdominal infection source. 4. Diuretics, if necessary. Assess need for fluid intake to support O_2 delivery. 5. Evaluate intake and output daily; weigh patient daily. 6. Does patient really need a Swan-Ganz catheter? 7. Consider methods to restrict or lower airway pressure (pressure-control ventilation). 8. Follow renal function, electrolytes, liver function, mental status to assess organ system function.
ASTHMA	
1. Airway inflammation is the primary cause of status asthmaticus. 2. Auto-PEEP or hyperinflation dominates gas exchange when using mechanical ventilation. 3. Potentially increased complication rate of mechanical ventilation.	1. High-dose corticosteroids are primary treatment. 2. Aggressive inhaled aerosolized β_2 agonists (hourly, if needed). 3. Theophylline may be less helpful (check theophylline level). 4. Early intubation if necessary. 5. Adequate oxygen to inhibit respiratory drive. 6. Use low tidal volume, high inspiratory flow, low respiratory frequency with mechanical ventilation to avoid barotrauma and auto-PEEP. 7. May need to sedate or paralyze to reduce hyperinflation. 8. Measure peak flow or FEV, as a guide to therapeutic response.

(continued)

Table 1–2. Things to think about and reminders for ICU patient care. (continued)

Things To Think About	Reminders
DIABETIC KETOACIDOSIS	
1. Evaluate degree of volume depletion and relationship of water to solute balance (hyperosmolar component). 2. Avoid excessive volume replacement. 3. Look for a trigger for diabetic ketoacidosis (infection, poor compliance, mucormycosis, other). 4. Avoid hypoglycemia during correction phase. 5. Identify features of hyperosmolar complications. 6. Calculate water and volume deficits. 7. Evaluate presence of coexisting acid-base disturbances (lactic acidosis, metabolic alkalosis). 8. Avoid hypokalemia during correction phase.	1. Give adequate insulin to lower glucose at appropriate rate (increase aggressively if no response). Generally use continuous insulin infusion. 2. Give adequate volume replacement (normal saline) and water replacement, if needed (half normal saline, glucose in water). 3. Follow glucose and electrolytes frequently. 4. Consider stopping insulin infusion when glucose is about 250 mg/dL and HCO_3^- is > 18 meq/L. 5. Avoid hypoglycemia; if you continue insulin drip with glucose < 250mg/dL, then give D_5W. If glucose continues to fall, lower insulin drip rate. 6. Monitor serum potassium, phosphorus. 7. Calculate water deficit, if any. 8. Urine osmolality, glucose, etc. 9. Check sinuses, nose, mouth, soft tissue, urine, chest x-ray, abdomen for infection.
HYPONATREMIA	
1. Consider volume depletion (nonosmolar stimulus for ADH secretion). 2. Consider edematous state with hyponatremia (cirrhosis, nephrotic syndrome, congestive heart failure). 3. SIADH with nonsuppressed ADH. 4. Drugs (thiazide diuretics). 5. Adrenal insuffieiency, hypothyroidism.	1. Measure urine Na^+, Cl^-, creatinine, and osmolality. 2. Calculate or measure serum osmolality. 3. Volume depletion? Give volume challenge? 4. Ask if patient is thirsty (may be volume-depleted). 5. Review medication list. 6. Primary treatment may be water restriction. 7. Consider need for hypertonic saline (carefully calculate amount) and furosemide. 8. Other treatment (demeclocycline).
HYPERNATREMIA	
1. Diabetes insipidus. 2. Diabetes mellitus. 3. Has patient been water-depleted for a long-time? 4. Concomitant volume depletion? 5. Is the urine continuing to be poorly concentrated?	1. Calculate water deficit and ongoing water loss. 2. Replace with hypotonic fluids (0.45% NaCl, D_5W) at calculated rate. 3. Replace volume deficit, if any, with normal saline. 4. Measure urine osmolality, Na^+, Cl^-, creatinine. 5. Does patient need desmopressin acetate?
HYPOTENSION	
1. Volume depletion. 2. Sepsis. (Consider potential sources; may need to treat empirically.) 3. Cardiogenic. (Any reason to suspect?) 4. Drugs or medications (prescribed or not). 5. Adrenal insufficiency. 6. Pneumothorax, pericardial effusion or tamponade, fungal sepsis, tricyclic overdose, amyloidosis.	1. Volume challenge; decide how and what to give and how to monitor. 2. If volume-depleted, correct cause. 3. Gram-positive sepsis (or candidemia) may also cause hypotension and shock. 4. Give naloxone if clinically indicated. 5. Echocardiogram (left ventricular and right ventricular function, pericardial disease, acute valvular disease) may be helpful. 6. Does the patient need a Swan-Ganz catheter? 7. Cosyntropin stimulation test or empiric corticosteroids.

(*continued*)

Table 1–2. Things to think about and reminders for ICU patient care. (continued)

SWAN-GANZ CATHETERS

Things To Think About

1. Site of placement (safety, risk, experience of operator).
2. Coagulation times, platelet count, bleeding time, other bleeding risks.
3. Document in medical record.
4. Estimate need for monitoring therapy.
5. Predict whether interpretation of data may be difficult (mechanical ventilation, valvular insufficiency, pulmonary hypertension).

Reminders

1. Check for contraindications.
2. Write a procedure note.
3. Make measurements and document immediately after placement.
4. Obtain chest x-ray afterward.
5. Level transducer with patient before making measurement; eliminate bubbles in lines or transducer.
6. Discontinue as soon as possible.
7. Use Fick calculated cardiac output to confirm thermodilution measurements.
8. Send mixed venous blood for O_2 saturation.

UPPER GASTROINTESTINAL BLEEDING

Things To Think About

1. Rapid stabilization of patient (hemoglobin and hemodynamics).
2. Identification of bleeding site.
3. Does patient have a non-upper GI bleeding site?
4. Consider need for early operation.
5. Review for bleeding, coagulation problems.
6. Determine when "excessive" amounts of blood products given.
7. Do antacids, H_2 blockers, PPIs play a role?
8. Reversible causes or contributing causes.

Reminders

1. Monitor vital signs at frequent intervals.
2. Monitor hematocrit at frequent intervals.
3. Choose hematocrit to maintain.
4. Consider need and timing of endoscopy.
5. Consult surgery.
6. Patients with abnormally long coagulation time may benefit from fresh-frozen plasma (calculate volume of replacement needed).
7. Platelet transfusions needed?
8. Desmopressin acetate (renal failure).

FEVER, RECURRENT OR PERSISTENT

Things To Think About

1. New, unidentified source of infection.
2. Lack of response of identified or presumed source of infection.
3. Opportunistic organism (drug-resistant, fungus, virus, parasite, acid-fast bacillus).
4. Drug fever.
5. Systemic noninfectious disease.
6. Incorrect empiric antibiotics.
7. Slow resolution of fever (deep-seated infection: endocarditis, osteomyelitis).
8. Infected catheter site or foreign body (medical appliance).
9. Consider infections of sinuses, CNS, decubitus ulcers; septic arthritis.

Reminders

1. Examine catheter sites (old and new), surgical wounds, sinuses, back and buttocks, large joints, pelvic organs, catheters and tubes, skin rashes, hands and feet.
2. Consider pleural, pericardial, subphrenic spaces; perinephric infection; spleen, prostate, intra-abdominal abscess; bowel infarction or necrosis.
3. Abscess in area of previous known infection.
4. Review prior culture results and antibiotic use.
5. Consider change in empiric antibiotics.
6. Culture usual locations plus any specific areas.
7. Discontinue or change catheters.
8. Consider candidemia or disseminated candidiasis.
9. Discontinued antibiotics?
10. Abdominal ultrasound, CT scan, gallium, leukocyte scans.

PANCYTOPENIA (AFTER CHEMOTHERAPY)

Things To Think About

1. Fever, presumed infection, response to antimicrobials.
2. Thrombocytopenia and spontaneous bleeding.
3. Drug fever.
4. Transfusion reactions.
5. Staphylococcus, candida, other opportunistic infections.
6. Infection sites in patient without granulocytes may have induration, erythema, without fluctuance.
7. Pulmonary infiltrates and opportunistic infection.

Reminders

1. Fever workup; see above.
2. Special sites: soft tissues, perirectal abscess, urine fungal cultures, lungs.
3. Bronchoscopy with bronchoalveolar lavage.
4. Empiric antibiotics, continue until afebrile, doing well, granulocytes > 1000/μL.
5. Empiric or directed vancomycin, amphotericin B, antiviral drugs, antituberculous drugs.
6. Check intravascular catheters, bladder, catheter.
7. Platelet transfusions, prophylaxis for spontaneous bleeding (or if already bleeding).

reminded that critical illness is and always will be associated with high mortality and morbidity rates. The outcome of some disease processes simply cannot be altered despite the availability of modern comprehensive treatment methods. On the basis of medical decisions and after consultation with the patient and family, some patients will continue to receive aggressive treatment; for others, withdrawal of care may be the most appropriate decision.

It is not surprising that critical care physicians, together with medical ethicists, have played a major role in developing a body of ethical constructs concerned with such issues as withholding or withdrawal of life support, determination of brain death, and feeding and hydration. The critical care physician must become familiar with concepts of patient autonomy, informed consent and refusal, application of advanced directives for health care, surrogate decision makers, and the legal consequences of decisions made in this context. It is also anticipated that the cost of care in the ICU will be increasingly scrutinized because of economic constraints on health care.

There is evidence that care in the ICU improves outcome in only a small subgroup of patients admitted. Some patients may be so critically ill with a combination of chronic and acute disorders that no intervention will reverse or even ameliorate the course of disease. Others may be admitted with very mild illness, and in such cases admission to the ICU rather than a non-ICU area does not improve the outcome. On the other hand, two other subgroups emerge from this analysis of ICU patients. First, a small subgroup with a predictably poor outcome may have an unexpectedly successful result from ICU care. A patient with cardiogenic shock with a predicted mortality rate of over 90% who survives because of aggressive management and reversal of myocardial dysfunction would fall into this group. The other small group consists of patients admitted for monitoring purposes only or for minor therapeutic interventions who develop severe complications of treatment. In these patients with predicted favorable outcomes, unanticipated adverse effects of care may result in severe morbidity or death.

Areas of critical care outcome research have, for example, focused on the elderly, those with hematologic and other malignancies, patients with complications of AIDS, and those with very poor lung function from chronic obstructive pulmonary disease, acute respiratory distress syndrome, multiorgan failure, and pancreatitis. Much more needs to be learned about prognosis and factors that determine prognosis, but it is essential that data be used appropriately and not applied indiscriminately for individual patient decisions.

Alternatives to current care should be periodically reviewed and considered in every patient in the ICU. Some patients may no longer require the type of care available in the ICU; transfer to a lower level of care may benefit the patient medically and emotionally and may decrease the risk of complications and the costs of treatment. Admission criteria should be reviewed regularly by the medical staff. Similarly, ongoing resource utilization efforts should be directed at determining which types of patients are best served by continued ICU care.

ROLE OF THE MEDICAL DIRECTOR OF THE INTENSIVE CARE UNIT

The medical director of the ICU has traditional administrative and regulatory responsibilities for this patient care area. A leadership role is vital in establishing policies and procedures for patient care, maintaining communication across health care disciplines, developing and ensuring quality care, and helping to provide education in a rapidly and constantly changing medical field. The medical director and the ICU staff may choose to coordinate care in a number of areas.

PROTOCOLS & PRACTICE GUIDELINES

A survey of outcomes from ICUs concluded that established protocols for management of specific critical illnesses can contribute to improved results. The medical director and medical staff, nursing staff, and other health care practitioners may choose to develop protocols that define uniformity of care or ensure that complete orders are written. Some protocols may be highly detailed, complete, and focused on a single clinical condition. An example might be a protocol for treatment of patients with suspected acute myocardial infarction—the protocol could specify the frequency, timing, and types of cardiac enzyme determination and the timing for ECGs and other diagnostic tests. Certain standardized medications such as aspirin, heparin, angiotensin-converting enzyme inhibitors, beta-adrenergic blockers, and agents used for conscious sedation might be recommended in such a protocol, and the physician could choose to give these or not depending on the particular clinical situation.

Another type of protocol can be "driven" by critical care nurses or respiratory therapists. In these protocols, nurses or therapists are given orders to assess the effectiveness and side effects of therapy and given freedom to adjust therapy based on these results. A protocol for aerosolized bronchodilator treatment might specify administration of albuterol by metered-dose inhaler, but the respiratory therapist would determine the optimal frequency and dose on the basis of how much improvement in peak flow or FEV_1 was obtained and how much excessive tachycardia was encountered. The ICU medical director may consider limiting the use of certain medications based on established protocols. For example, some antibiotics may be limited in use because of cost, toxicity, or potential for development of microbial resistance. Neuromuscular blocking agents may be restricted to use only by certain qualified physicians because of the need for special expertise in dosing or patient support. Protocols can take several different forms, and patient care in the ICU may benefit from their development.

Physician practice guidelines are being developed for many aspects of medical practice. Although some critics of guidelines argue that these are unnecessarily restrictive and that elements of medical practice cannot be rigidly defined, practice guidelines may be useful for diagnosing and treating patients in the ICU. Guidelines may vary from recommendations for dose and adjustment of heparin infusion for anticoagulation to specific minimum standards of care for status asthmaticus, unstable angina, heart failure, or malignant hypertension. Practice guidelines will be found commonly in the ICU of the near future, and ICU directors will be called upon to develop, review, accept, or modify guidelines for individual ICUs.

QUALITY ASSURANCE

The medical director of critical care is obliged to participate in activities that evaluate the quality of care provided in the ICU. Quality of care may be assessed by measurement of patient satisfaction, analyzing frequency of delivery of care, monitoring of complications, duration of hospitalization, analysis of mortality data, and in other ways. Patient outcome may eventually emerge as the most effective global determination of the quality of care, but such measures suffer from the difficulty in stratifying severity in very complex patients with multiple medical problems. The development of protocols and programs to measure and enhance the quality of care is beyond the scope of this presentation. However, the medical and nursing leadership of the ICU must play key roles in any such projects.

The medical director also plays an important role in granting privileges to practice in the ICU. Competence in and experience with medical procedures must be investigated, documented, and maintained for all physicians who use the service. While this is especially important for invasive procedures such as placement of pulmonary artery catheters and endotracheal intubation, consideration should be given also to developing and granting privileges for mechanical ventilator management, management of shock, and other nonprocedural care. Similarly, the skills and knowledge of nurses, respiratory therapists, and other professionals in the ICU should be determined, documented, and matched to their duties. For both physicians and nonphysicians, the ICU medical director has the responsibility to develop standards for those who care for the patients in that unit.

It should be stressed that effective quality improvement activities go far beyond simple data collection and reporting. A dedicated group of health care providers should meet regularly to review the data, establish trends, and suggest methods for improvement. The importance of "closing the loop" in the quality improvement process cannot be overstated. Monitoring of outcomes after instituting change is an important part of this activity and is mandatory if patient care is to be effectively and expeditiously improved.

INFECTION CONTROL

Nosocomial infections are important problems in the ICU, and their prevention and management can provide insight into the effectiveness of protocols and quality assurance functions. As described elsewhere, nosocomial infections are often preventable by adherence to procedures and policies designed to limit spread of infection between patients and between ICU staff and patients. The ICU medical director must take the lead in establishing infection control protocols, including procedures for aseptic technique for invasive procedures, standards for universal precautions, duration of invasive catheter placement, suctioning of endotracheal tubes, appropriate use of antibiotics, procedures in the event of finding antibiotic-resistant microorganisms, and the need for isolation of patients with communicable diseases. Consequently, an important measure of the quality of care being provided is the nosocomial infection rate in the ICU, especially intravascular infections secondary to indwelling catheters. The ICU medical director should work closely with the nursing staff and hospital epidemiologist and infection control personnel in the event of excessive nosocomial infections. Often a breach in procedures can be identified and corrected.

EDUCATION

The ICU medical director is required to provide educational resources for the staff of the ICU, including critical care nurses, respiratory therapists, occupational therapists, and other physicians. This may be in the form of lectures, small group discussions, audiovisual presentations, or prepared handouts or directed readings. An effective strategy is to focus presentations on problems recently or commonly encountered; the recent experience may help to clarify and amplify the more didactic portion. Very often in critical care areas, there is a need for personnel to develop skills for using new equipment such as monitors, catheters, and ventilators. Appropriate time and feedback should be planned with the introduction of such equipment before it can be assumed that it can be used for patient care.

In the teaching hospital, the faculty and attending staff must not only convey the principles of critical care practice but must foster an attitude of rigorous critical review of data, cooperation between medical and other personnel, and attention to detail. For individual study, many fine World Wide Web sites now exist that provide abundant information. The sites should be reviewed in advance by the medical or nursing director to make certain that the material they contain is both accurate and applicable as well as appropriately updated from time to time.

COMMUNICATION

The ICU medical director serves as a communication link between physician staff, including primary care and consulting physicians, and the nursing and other health care professional staff in the ICU. Most of this communication will occur naturally as a result of interaction during patient care, quality assurance activities, and other administrative meetings. On occasion, further communication is needed to address specific complaints, procedures, or policies. Depending on the organization of the hospital, the ICU may also be served by a multidisciplinary committee that can participate in development of protocols and policies. This committee may function with respect to a single ICU in a hospital or may have responsibility for standardization of activities in several ICUs in the area.

OUTCOMES & ALTERNATIVES

In many facilities, ICU beds are limited in number, and incoming patients with varying degrees of morbidity must often be evaluated and compared to determine who might best be treated in the ICU. A number of published studies have confirmed that a good proportion of patients admitted to ICUs receive diagnostic studies and monitoring of physiologic variables *only*—ie, no therapy that could not be given outside the ICU. On the other hand, other patients admitted to the ICU do receive such "intensive" therapy, and some of these have better outcomes. Because ICU beds are a limited resource in all hospitals, ICU medical directors must develop familiarity with the overall outcomes and results of patients admitted to their ICU beds. They will be called upon not infrequently to make decisions about admissions, discharge, and transfer from the ICU, and these decisions may at times be painfully arrived at. As with all decisions impacting patient care, the medical director must weigh the body of medical knowledge available, the wishes of patients, families, and physicians, and the likelihood or not that intensive care will benefit the patient. At times these decisions will involve only "medical judgment"; at other times, the choice will reflect an ethical, legal, or philosophical perspective.

Specific practice guidelines for individual diseases have been developed for the purpose of identifying particular patients. For example, some patients with chest pain who may have myocardial infarction but were deemed low-risk were discharged from the coronary care unit after 2 days with no adverse effects. There was a considerable reduction in hospitalization time and some cost savings.

Recognition that many patients previously admitted to ICUs did not require or receive major diagnostic or therapeutic interventions led to the design of progressive care, "step-down," or noninvasive monitoring units in some hospitals. Equipped and staffed generally for electrocardiography, pulse oximetry, and sometimes for noninvasive respiratory impedance plethysmography—but not for intravascular instrumentation—these units have potential as highly effective, less costly alternatives to ICUs. A number of studies have provided justification for intermediate care units either as an area for patients leaving the ICU or as an area devoted to care of certain kinds of medical problems—primarily mild respiratory failure, cardiac arrhythmias, or moderately severe electrolyte disorders.

CRITICAL CARE SCORING

The combination of an increasing patient population and diminished funding for hospital services is creating a need for optimized distribution of medical resources. This challenge is being met in a number of ways, including regionalization of care, specialization of critical care facilities (both between and within hospitals), and better allocation of available personnel and equipment. To this end, the intensivist must be prepared to make both administrative and medical decisions about which patients will benefit most from admission to a critical care unit. Data released by the United States General Administration Office in 1987 indicate that up to 40% of patients in ICUs were inappropriately admitted, either because they would probably have died regardless of the care provided or because their illnesses were not

Table 1–3. The Glasgow Coma Scale.

Eye	Motor	Verbal
4 = Spontaneous	6 = Obedient	5 = Oriented
3 = To Voice	5 = Purposeful	4 = Confused
2 = To pain	4 = Withdrawal	3 = Inappropriate
1 = None	3 = Flexion	2 = Incomprehensible
	2 = Extension	1 = None
	1 = None	

life-threatening enough to require ICU care. Indeed, a substantial portion of patients treated in critical care units at teaching hospitals are admitted for "observation and monitoring" only.

Illness scoring has become a popular method for triage within and between hospitals. Many such scores have been introduced over the past two decades in an attempt to prioritize illness and injury for ICU admission purposes. Such scores must be used with full appreciation of their limitations. While they are useful for comparing institutional performances and outcomes in studies of certain groups of patients, great caution must be exercised when applying these protocols to individual patients.

The most commonly used trauma and critical care scores are discussed below and illustrated in the accompanying tables.

Glasgow Coma Scale

The Glasgow Coma Scale assesses the extent of coma in patients with head injuries (Table 1–3). The scale is based on eye opening, verbal response, and motor response. The total is the sum of each of the individual responses and varies between 3 points and 15 points. Mortality risk is correlated with the total score and with a similar Glasgow Outcome Scale. Examination of the patient and calculation of the score can all be accomplished in less than 1 minute. The scale is easy to use and highly reproducible between observers. It has been incorporated into several other scoring systems. The Coma Scale is useful for prehospital trauma triage as well as assessment of patient progress after arrival and during critical care admission.

Trauma Score & Revised Trauma Score

Because of the increasing number of trauma patients admitted to critical care facilities, familiarity with trauma scales is important. The Trauma Score is based on the Glasgow Coma Scale and on the status of the cardiovascular and respiratory systems. Weighted values are assigned to each parameter and summed to obtain the total Trauma Score, which ranges from 1 to 16 (Table 1–4). Mortality risk varies inversely with this score.

After extensive use and evaluation of the Trauma Score, it was found to underestimate the importance of head injuries. In response to this, the Revised Trauma Score (RTS) was introduced and is now the most widely used physiologic trauma scoring tool. It is based

Table 1–4. Trauma Score.

A. Systolic blood pressure		**B. Respiratory rate**		**C. Respiratory effort**		**D. Capillary refill**	
> 90	**4**	10–24	**4**	Normal	**1**	Normal	**2**
70–90	**3**	25–35	**3**	Shallow or retractions	**0**	Delay	**1**
59–69	**2**	> 35	**2**			None	**0**
< 50	**1**	10	**1**				
0	**0**	0	**0**				
E. 4 GCS points							
1. Eye opening		2. Motor response		3. Verbal response		(1 + 2 + 3)	
Spontaneous	**4**	Obedient	**6**	Oriented	**5**	14–15	**5**
To voice	**3**	Purposeful	**5**	Confused	**4**	11–13	**4**
To pain	**2**	Withdrawal	**4**	Inappropriate	**3**	8–10	**3**
None	**1**	Flexion	**3**	Incomprehensible	**2**	5–7	**2**
		Extension	**2**	None	**1**	3–4	**1**
		None	**1**				

TRAUMA SCORE (A + B + C + D + E) _________

Table 1–5. Revised Trauma Score.[1]

Glasgow Coma Scale (GCS)	Systolic Blood Pressure (SPB) (mmHg)	Respiratory Rate (RR) (Breaths/min)	Coded Value
13–15	> 89	10–29	4
9–12	76–89	> 29	3
6–8	50–75	6–9	2
4–5	1–49	1–5	1
3	0	0	0

[1]RTS = 0.9368 GCSc + 0.7326 SBPc + 0.2908 RRc, where the subscript c refers to coded value.

on the Glasgow Coma Scale, systolic blood pressure, and respiratory rate. For evaluation of in-hospital outcome, coded values of the coma scale, blood pressure, and respiratory rate are weighted and summed (Table 1–5). Better prognosis is associated with higher values.

CRAMS Scale

The Circulation, Respiration, Abdomen, Motor, Speech (CRAMS) scale is another trauma triage scale that has found regional acceptance (Table 1–6). It is frequently used to decide which patients require triage to a trauma center. Patients with lower CRAMS scores would be expected to require critical care unit admission.

Injury Severity Score (ISS)

The ISS attempts to quantitate the extent of multiple injuries by assignment of numerical scores to different body regions (head and neck, face, thorax, abdomen, pelvic contents, extremities, and external). A book of codes is available that provides information on the scoring of each injury. The worst injury in each region is assigned a numerical value, which is then squared and added to those from each of the other areas. The total score ranges from 1 to 75 and correlates with mortality risk. The major limitation of the ISS is that it considers only the highest score from any body region and considers injuries with equal scores to be of equal importance irrespective of body region. Similarly, since the ISS is an anatomic score, a small injury with a significant potential for deleterious outcome (closed head injury), may lead to the false impression of a minimally injured patient. ISS is the most commonly used measure of the severity of anatomic injury and provides a rough survival estimate for the severely injured patient.

Acute Physiology, Age, Chronic Health Evaluation (APACHE III)

The APACHE scoring system (APACHE II) is probably the most widely used critical care scale. It permits comparisons between groups of patients and between facilities. It was not designed to evaluate individual patient outcomes. To this end, APACHE III was introduced to objectively estimate patient risk for mortality and other important outcomes related to patient stratification. While some centers have adopted the APACHE III score, it is not widely used.

CURRENT CONTROVERSIES & UNRESOLVED ISSUES

The usefulness of scales such as APACHE III scoring modalities remains to be determined long after its introduction. Furthermore, the ability of the experienced physician to make such management decisions may be as good as such scales and perhaps often better. Some authors have concluded that ICU scoring systems can be used to compare outcomes within and between ICUs, and can provide adequate adjustment of mortality rates based on pre-admission severity for the purpose of assessing quality of care.

Table 1–6. The CRAMS Scale.[1]

Circulation	
Normal capillary refilll and BP > 100 mm Hg	2
Delayed capillary refill or 85 < BP < 100	1
No capillary refill or BP < 85 mm Hg	0
Respiration	
Normal	2
Abnormal	1
Absent	0
Abdomen	
Abdomen and thorax nontender	2
Abdomen or thorax tender	1
Abdomen rigid or flail chest	0
Motor	
Normal	2
Responds only to pain (other than decerebrate)	1
No response (or decerebrate)	0
Speech	
Normal	2
Confused	1
No intelligible words	0

[1]Score ≤ 8 indicates major trauma; score ≥ 9 indicates minor trauma.

Baker SP, O'Neill B: The injury severity score: An update. J Trauma 1976;16:822–5.

Champion HR et al: A revision of the trauma score. J Trauma 1989;29:623–9.

Champion HR et al: Trauma score. Crit Care Med 1981;9:672–6.

Gormican SP:CRAMS Scale: Field triage of trauma victim. Ann Emerg Med 1982;11:132–5.

Jennett B et al: Predicting outcome in individual patients after severe head injury. Lancet 1976;1:1031–4.

Knaus WA et al: The APACHE III prognostic system: Risk prediction of hospital mortality for critically ill hospitalized adults. Chest 1991;100:1619–36.

Knaus WA et al: Variations in mortality and length of stay in intensive care units. Ann Intern Med 1993;118:753–61.

Schuster DP. Predicting outcome after ICU admission. The art and science of assessing risk. Chest 1992;102:1861–70.

REFERENCES

Cropp AJ et al: Name that tone. The proliferation of alarms in the intensive care unit. Chest 1994;105:1217–20.

Freedman NS, Kotzer N, Schwab RJ: Patient perception of sleep quality and etiology of sleep disruption in the intensive care unit. Am J Respir Crit Care Med 1999;159;1155–62.

Hamel MB et al: Older age, aggressiveness of care, and survival for seriously ill, hospitalized adults. SUPPORT Investigators. Study to Understand Prognoses and Preferences for Outcomes and Risks of Treatments. Ann Intern Med 1999; 131:721–8.

Hebert PC et al: The Transfusion Requirements in Critical Care Investigators for the Canadian Critical Care Trials Group. A multicenter, randomized, controlled clinical trial of transfusion requirements in critical care. N Engl J Med 1999; 340:409–17.

Knaus WA et al: The SUPPORT prognostic model. Objective estimates of survival for seriously ill hospitalized adults. Study to understand prognoses and preferences for outcomes and risks of treatments. Ann Intern Med 1995;122:191–3.

Mayer TJ et al: Adverse environmental conditions in the respiratory and medical ICU settings. Chest 1994;105:1211–6.

Simini B: Patients' perceptions of intensive care. Lancet 1999; 354:571–2.

Spivack D: The high cost of acute health care: A review of escalating costs and limitations of such exposure in intensive care units. Am Rev Respir Dis 1987;136:1007–11.

Fluids, Electrolytes, & Acid-Base 2

Frederic S. Bongard, MD, & Darryl Y. Sue, MD

DISORDERS OF FLUID VOLUME

In normal persons, 50–60% of total body weight is made up of water distributed between the intracellular and extracellular spaces. Critical illness can not only result from abnormalities in the amount and distribution of water but can also cause strikingly abnormal disorders of water and solutes.

Distribution of Body Water

Total body water is distributed freely throughout the body except for a very few areas in which movement of water is limited (eg, parts of the renal tubules and collecting ducts). Water diffuses freely between the intracellular space and the extracellular space in response to solute concentration gradients. Therefore, the concentration of solute everywhere in the body is made equal by water movement, and the amount of water in different compartments of the body depends on the quantity of solute present in that compartment.

The two major fluid compartments of the body are the intracellular space, in which the major solute is potassium and various anions; and the extracellular space, for which sodium and various anions are the major solutes. Sodium will move into and potassium out of cells passively along concentration gradients. Thus, active transport of sodium out of and potassium into cells by Na^+-K^+ ATP-dependent transport pumps on the cell membranes determines the relative quantities of these cations on the inside and outside of each cell. The distribution of Na^+ and K^+ between the two compartments determines their relative volumes. In normal individuals, about two-thirds of total body water is intracellular and one-third is extracellular.

Addition of any solute to either compartment without concomitant addition of water will increase the volume of that compartment by redistribution of water from the compartment of lower solute (higher water) concentration into the compartment to which the solute was added. The solute concentration in both compartments will increase (see Water Balance, p. 23). To restore normal volume and distribution of water within the compartments, the body will then seek to eliminate or redistribute the added solute and correct the increased solute concentration (stimulation of thirst, conservation of water). Similarly, the loss of solute from a compartment results in a shrinkage of that compartment as water leaves. The body then tries to restore the lost solute to reestablish the original volume and distribution of solute and water.

Distribution of Extracellular Volume

Extracellular volume is divided into the interstitial space and the intravascular space. The distribution of water between these two compartments is complex in normal subjects and more so during disease states in which edema (increase in interstitial volume) or accumulation of fluid in normally nearly dry spaces (peritoneal cavity, pleural space) is present. Normally, intravascular volume is maintained by the oncotic pressure of large molecules that are confined to the intravascular space; by movement of lymph from the interstitial to the intravascular space; and by forces that maintain extracellular volume. Countering these forces are the hydrostatic pressure developed by the heart and circulation, which tends to push fluid from the intravascular space into the interstitial space; and interstitial fluid oncotic pressure, which tends to pull fluid out of the vasculature. The volume of the intravascular compartment directly determines the adequacy of the circulation; this in turn determines the adequacy of delivery of oxygen, nutrients, and other substances needed for organ system function.

Hypovolemia & Hypervolemia

Because sodium is the predominant extracellular solute, extracellular volume is determined primarily by the sodium content of the body and the mechanisms responsible for maintaining sodium content (Table 2–1). However, the term "hypovolemia" generally refers only to decreased intravascular volume and not decreased extracellular volume, and this disorder results from insufficient function of the normal mechanisms of intravascular volume maintenance. On the other hand, the term "hypervolemia" generally denotes increased extracellular volume with or without increased intravascular volume. Thus, patients with edema or ascites have hypervolemia (often with decreased intravascular volume),

Table 2–1. Factors affecting body sodium balance.

Increased body sodium content (increased extracellular volume)
- Increased sodium intake (in absence of increased sodium excretion)
- Decreased sodium excretion by kidneys
    - Decreased glomerular filtration
    - Increased renal tubular sodium reabsorption
    - Increased renin, angiotensin, aldosterone
    - Excessive mineralocorticoid activity

Decreased body sodium content (decreased extracellular volume)
- Decreased sodium intake (in presence of normal sodium excretion)
- Increased sodium excretion
    - Renal:
        - Renal failure
        - Salt-losing nephropathy
        - Osmotic diuresis
        - Diuretic drugs
        - Atrial natriuretic peptide
        - Decreased renin, angiotensin, aldosterone, or cortisol
    - Extrarenal:
        - Diarrhea
        - Vomiting
        - Sweating
        - Surgical drainage

but so do patients with congestive heart failure (who have increased intravascular volume).

Normally, daily sodium excretion equals sodium intake, indicating that sodium excretion varies with dietary or other intake. The average diet contains 4–8 g of sodium daily, and this quantity must be excreted daily. With severe limitation of dietary sodium, normal kidneys can vigorously reabsorb sodium, so that as little as 1–5 meq Na^+/L of urine appears and only 1–2 meq of Na^+ is excreted daily. A daily sodium intake and excretion of approximately 40–65 meq (about 1–1.5 g) is adequate in normal individuals.

HYPOVOLEMIA

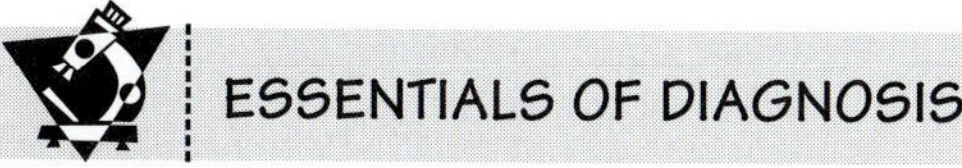
ESSENTIALS OF DIAGNOSIS

- *Evidence of decreased effective intravascular volume: hypotension, low central venous or pulmonary artery wedge pressure.*
- *Indirect evidence of decreased effective intravascular volume: tachycardia, oliguria, avid renal sodium reabsorption.*
- *Circumstantial evidence of depleted effective intravascular volume: end-organ dysfunction, peripheral vasoconstriction.*
- *Potential source of loss of extracellular volume or evidence of inadequate repletion.*

General Considerations

A. Definition

Hypovolemia is decreased volume of the effective intravascular space. Although extracellular volume, of which the intravascular space is a part, is often diminished, hypovolemia can occur even in the presence of normal or increased extracellular volume (Table 2–2). The assessment of adequacy of intravascular volume in the presence of normal or increased extracellular volume is often difficult, especially in critically ill patients. It is central to the concept of hypovolemia that *total* intravascular volume need not be diminished but that *effective* intravascular volume is low. Normal effective intravascular volume consists of having sufficient volume in the appropriate part of the circulation to provide circulatory adequacy. The term "effective arterial volume" is sometimes used to characterize the physiologically effective part of the intravascular volume.

Table 2–2. Hypovolemia (decreased effective intravascular volume).

With decreased extracellular volume
- Increased fluid losses
    - GI tract (diarrhea, vomiting, fistulas, nasogastric suction)
    - Renal (polyuria with renal sodium wasting, osmotic diuresis)
    - Skin or wound losses (sweating, burns)
    - Hemorrhage (trauma, other bleeding site)
- Decreased intake of sodium and water
- Impaired normal capacity to retain sodium and water
    - Renal sodium wasting (polycystic kidneys, diuretics)
    - Adrenal insufficiency
    - Osmotic diuresis (hyperglycemia)

With increased or normal extracellular volume
- Congestive heart failure
- Cirrhosis with ascites
- Protein-losing enteropathy
- Increased vascular permeability (sepsis, shock, trauma, burns)

Many clinicians use the term "dehydration" as a substitute for hypovolemia. This is incorrect, and the term should be reserved to denote a lack of water relative to total body solute (see below).

B. Pathophysiology

Decreased effective intravascular volume can occur in the presence of decreased, normal, or increased extracellular volume. Decreased extracellular volume leading to depletion of intravascular volume is most common and can arise from increased loss of extracellular fluid, failure to replete normal losses, or a combination of both. Bleeding, diarrhea, vomiting, and excessive skin loss of fluid (sweating, burns) can quickly deplete extracellular and intravascular volume. Abnormally large urinary losses of sodium and water from renal diseases, adrenal insufficiency, diuretics, and hyperglycemia (osmotic diuresis) should also be considered as sources of volume depletion. Decreased extracellular volume can also arise from normal losses if they are inadequately replaced; this is particularly likely to occur in ill patients who do not eat or drink appropriately or who do not have access to adequate amounts of water and solutes.

Hypovolemia with normal extracellular volume occurs as a result of any disorder that alters the balance between intravascular and extravascular fluid compartments. Intravascular oncotic pressure and intact vascular integrity largely maintain intravascular volume, while hydrostatic pressure tends to push fluid out of the circulation. Sepsis, ARDS, shock, and other critical illnesses alter this balance by increasing permeability of the vasculature. The result is an increase in the nonintravascular fluid volume (interstitial compartment, pleural effusions, ascites) at the acute expense of the intravascular volume. Although decreased vascular oncotic pressure and increased hydrostatic pressure should also shift fluid balance in this direction, these rarely develop rapidly enough to allow total extracellular fluid volume to remain constant.

Disorders that increase hydrostatic pressure in certain vascular beds or reduce intravascular oncotic pressure can deplete intravascular volume. The reduced intravascular volume stimulates chronically increased renal sodium reabsorption that causes an increase in total extracellular volume. Thus, cirrhosis with hypoalbuminemia results in ascites from a combination of portal hypertension and decreased oncotic pressure; heart failure leads to edema from increased hydrostatic pressure; and edema in nephrotic syndrome results from severely reduced oncotic pressure. The paradox in these clinical situations is that effective intravascular volume may be severely reduced though extracellular volume is greatly increased.

Clinical Features

The diagnosis of volume depletion in the critically ill patient is often difficult, largely because of the confounding effects of organ system dysfunction and the frequency with which drugs, edematous states, altered cardiovascular and renal function, and other factors interfere with assessment of volume status.

A. Symptoms and Signs

Symptoms and signs suggesting hypovolemia in the critically ill patient may or may not be helpful. Volume depletion causing inadequate systemic perfusion can lead to altered mental status, confusion, lethargy, and coma; cold skin and extremities from vasoconstriction; cardiac ischemia and dysfunction; and liver and kidney failure. None of these are specific for hypovolemia, but all are common to hypotension and shock from any cause. A potentially important sympton is thirst in a patient with hyponatremia; lack of an osmotic stimulus leaves volume depletion as the only physiologic reason for thirst. In the patient with hypovolemia with increased extracellular fluid volume, edema and ascites make determination of effective intravascular volume more difficult.

Sensitivity and specificity for a variety of symptoms and signs of acute and subacute volume depletion have been reported. None have sufficiently high sensitivity and high specificity to be of definite clinical value. Postural lightheadedness increases the likelihood of volume depletion, but an increase in heart rate from supine to standing must be greater than 30/min to be specific for hypovolemia. Orthostatic blood pressure changes lack sensitivity and specificity, but these should be part of the evaluation of potential hypovolemia. Dry axillae, longitudinal furrow on the tongue, and sunken eyes have some slight diagnostic value for hypovolemia if they are present.

An identified source of volume loss or an explanation for inadequate volume repletion strongly supports the diagnosis of hypovolemia. In the ICU patient, blood loss, diarrhea, and polyuria are usually obvious; less easily identified are heavy sweating during fever, fluid losses from extensive burns, volume changes during hemodialysis or ultrafiltration, and drainage from surgical incisions or wounds. Review of intravenous and enteral fluid intake is often helpful, along with comparison of patient weights on a daily basis or more often.

Indirect evidence of hypovolemia can come from the response of the cardiovascular and renal systems. Depleted intravascular volume leads to decreased venous return to the heart; the normal response is a lower stroke volume and, as compensation, sinus tachycardia to maintain cardiac output.

B. Laboratory Findings

Intravascular volume depletion may lead to avid retention of water because of increased ADH release and, if there is sufficient water intake, hyponatremia. Decreased intravascular volume results in prerenal azotemia with elevation of serum creatinine and urea nitrogen.

Except in the case of a primary renal cause of hypovolemia, decreased renal blood flow, even if glomerular filtration is maintained, leads to increased renal tubular sodium reabsorption. Urine volume diminishes, and urine becomes highly concentrated under the influence of antidiuretic hormone and other factors. Urine sodium and chloride concentration may become very low (often < 5–10 meq/L) with correspondingly low fractional excretion of sodium and chloride. Because of decreased renal tubular flow, urea is reabsorbed more readily, and the serum urea nitrogen:serum creatinine ratio increases, often > 30:1. In some patients, avid sodium reabsorption comes at the expense of increased potassium losses in the urine and hypokalemia. Potassium depletion and increased sodium reabsorption in the distal tubule enhance hydrogen ion excretion, with resultant metabolic alkalosis (contraction alkalosis); this is especially common in volume depletion due to vomiting.

On the other hand, if there is a primary renal-mediated mechanism of hypovolemia, urine sodium concentration and FE_{Na} do not decrease in the face of decreased intravascular volume. Urinary indices of volume depletion will be misleading, and paradoxical polyuria and high urine sodium may be found. Some patients will have mild to severe renal insufficiency. Excessive and inappropriate renal sodium loss is also seen in adrenal insufficiency; these patients may also have hyponatremia, hyperkalemia, hyperchloremic metabolic acidosis, and other features of inadequate adrenocortical hormone production. Osmotic diuresis (eg, from hyperglycemia or administration of mannitol) and diuretic drugs also result in hypovolemia with increased urine sodium and water.

C. ICU Monitoring

Venous pressure measurements provide evidence of volume depletion but must be interpreted with caution. The volume of the intravascular space determines "pressure" as a function of the physical properties, size, and character of the vessels—whether arteries or veins—along with the amount of propulsive force imparted to the blood by the heart. In a patient with "normal" vessels and a normal heart, hypotension indicates that the volume of fluid is insufficient to fill the arterial vessels. Hypotension of the venous system can be assessed in the same way, whether the pressure measured is central venous pressure (CVP) or pulmonary capillary wedge pressure (PCWP).

Differential Diagnosis

Because ICU patients frequently have disorders of the heart and circulation, the diagnosis of hypovolemia cannot always be made when hypotension is present. Hypotension from cardiogenic shock results from decreased systolic function of the heart, and septic shock arises largely from extreme dilation of the vascular space. Orthostatic changes in blood pressure in the absence of hypovolemia may be seen with autonomic dysfunction, peripheral neuropathy, diabetes mellitus, or hypokalemia and in response to antihypertensive medications. Nevertheless, it may be worth considering that hypotension (low systemic pressure, low CVP, or low PCWP) should be viewed as at least a relative state of hypovolemia in most patients.

Treatment

A. Estimate Magnitude of Hypovolemia

The amount of volume depletion in the hypovolemic patient in the ICU cannot be easily estimated. In a normal-sized adult, extracellular volume depletion of 15–25% or 2–4 L is needed before orthostatic blood pressure and pulse changes occur. During acute blood loss, changes in blood pressure and heart rate are seen only when more than 2 units of blood (about 1 L) are lost. This is about 20% of normal blood volume.

Central venous pressure and PCWP measurements are most useful for identifying volume depletion, but the magnitude of pressure provides only a rough guide to the degree of hypovolemia. The response to a trial of fluid administration is often the best evidence of hypovolemia and gives a useful (albeit retrospective) measure of the amount of volume depletion originally present. Acutely, such as during hemodialysis or ultrafiltration, the change in weight is an accurate measure of extracellular fluid change, but this may not be true in other circumstances. Further confounding the assessment of hypovolemia is the highly variable speed of mobilization of interstitial fluid (edema) or pleural or peritoneal fluid as intravascular volume decreases. In general, an adult ICU patient in whom hypovolemia is strongly suspected is likely to be depleted by about 1–4 L of extracellular volume, but correction of severe volume depletion may require considerably more.

B. Determine Rate of Correction of Hypovolemia

Hypovolemic shock with severe organ dysfunction, hypotension, and oliguria requires immediate and rapid correction of hypovolemia. Under less severe circumstances, repletion of extracellular and intravascular volume can be undertaken more slowly and carefully to avoid overcorrection with subsequent pulmonary and peripheral edema. In all cases, the volume of replacement should be estimated and some proportion of this quantity given over a defined period of time. Evidence of volume depletion should be reviewed at regular intervals, and vigorous volume repletion should be halted as soon as there is no longer evidence of hypovolemia or when complications of therapy (pulmonary edema) are discovered.

About 50–80% of the estimated fluid replacement volume should be given over 12–24 hours if the patient is not acutely hypotensive. This generally puts the rate of fluid intake in the range of 50–150 mL/h above maintenance fluid administration, depending on the estimated degree of volume depletion. In other patients—especially those in whom the diagnosis of hypovolemia is less certain or those who have known or suspected heart disease—a "fluid challenge" may be more appropriate, ie, giving 100–300 mL (less in smaller persons) of intravenous fluid over 1–2 hours and then making a careful reassessment and checking urine output, CVP or PCWP, blood pressure, and other signs. At this point, a decision can be made about whether to repeat the challenge, start a continuous infusion, or consider other issues. Patients with severe volume depletion and organ dysfunction should be given fluid rapidly (200–300 mL/h) for short periods and reassessed frequently.

C. Type of Fluid Replacement

Because hypovolemia is depletion of the volume of the intravascular space, replacement fluid should predominantly fill and remain in the intravascular space. In practice, replacement fluids given intravenously consist of crystalloid solutions, made of water and small solutes; and colloid solutions, consisting of water, electrolytes, and higher-molecular-weight proteins or polymers (Table 2–3).

At first glance, crystalloid solutions would appear to be inefficient for intravascular fluid repletion because the small solutes (sodium and chloride) and water move quickly into the interstitial space and out of the vasculature. Nevertheless, repletion of the total extracellular volume is essential in patients with hypovolemia and extracellular fluid depletion (blood loss, gastrointestinal tract losses, polyuria, sweating), and intravascular volume will be corrected along with correction of extracellular volume. In theory, large volumes of crystalloid would be undesirable in patients with hypovolemia and increased extracellular volume (ascites, edema), but this does not present serious problems in most patients. Solutions containing only dextrose and water (eg, 5% dextrose in water) without other solutes are poor volume replacement solutions because the glucose is rapidly taken up by cells (with water subsequently distributed freely into both the intracellular and extracellular compartments). Although sometimes used to replace extracellular volume deficits, Ringer's lactate (containing Na^+, K^+, Cl^-, Ca^{2+}, and lactate) is no more effective than 0.9% NaCl.

Colloid solutions have been advocated for more efficient repletion of intravascular volume, especially in states of normal or elevated extracellular volume and in hypovolemic shock. In theory, colloids are restricted at least transiently to the intravascular space and thereby exert an intravascular oncotic pressure that draws fluid out of the interstitial space and expands the intravascular space by an amount out of proportion to the volume of colloid solution actually administered. A theoretic

Table 2–3. Fluids for intravenous replacement of extracellular volume or water deficit.

	$[Na^+]$ (meq/L)	$[Cl^-]$ (meq/L)	[osm] (mosm/L)	Other
Crystalloids				
0.9% NaCl (normal saline)	154	154	308	
5% dextrose in 0.9% NaCl	154	154	560	Glucose, 50 g/L
Ringer's lactate	130	109	273	K^+, Ca^{2+}, lactate[1]
5% dextrose in water[2]	0	0	252	Glucose, 50 g/L
0.45% NaCl	77	77	154	
5% dextrose in 0.45% NaCl	77	77	406	Glucose, 50 g/L
Colloids				
Albumin (5%)				
Albumin (25%)				
6% hetastarch in 0.9% NaCl				

[1]K^+ 4 meq/L, Ca^{2+} 3 meq/L, lactate 28 meq/L.
[2]Not recommended for rapid correction of intravascular or extracellular volume deficit.

disadvantage is that the interstitial space would be depleted of water, leading to an increase in interstitial oncotic pressure that would draw water back out. Numerous studies have failed to identify a clear-cut advantage of colloid-containing solutions over crystalloid solutions in critically ill patients. This is probably because increased capillary permeability in patients with sepsis, shock, and other problems negates the potential benefit of retaining colloid within the vascular space. Furthermore, some investigators have suspected that leakage of colloid into the interstitial space of the lungs and other organs can contribute to persistent organ system dysfunction and edematous states. In hypovolemia associated with ascites, rapid movement of colloid into the ascitic fluid may occur, resulting in only a transient increase in intravascular volume. In patients with nephrotic syndrome or protein-losing enteropathies, albumin and other colloids may be lost fairly rapidly. A large review of studies in which albumin solutions were given for hypovolemia, burns, or hypoalbuminemia did not find any benefit, and there was a trend toward increased mortality for patients given albumin.

Colloid solutions for intravenous replacement include human albumin (5% and 25% serum albumin, heat-treated to reduce infectious risk) and hetastarch (6% hydroxyethyl starch). Albumin is considered nonimmunogenic, but it is expensive, offers few advantages over other solutions, and has not been shown to improve outcome. Only a few clinical situations have been shown to benefit from albumin infusions. Patients with cirrhosis and spontaneous bacterial peritonitis given antibiotics and intravenous albumin, 1.5 g/kg on day 1 and 1 g/kg on day 3, had a significant reduction in mortality and renal failure. Albumin may be helpful after large-volume paracentesis. Hetastarch is a synthetic colloid solution used for volume expansion. Clinical benefit of the use of this solution is unclear. Fresh frozen plasma is an expensive and inefficient volume expander and should be reserved for correction of coagulation factor deficiencies. There is little rationale for the use of whole blood; red cells and other blood components should be given for specific indications, along with crystalloid or colloid supplements as needed.

D. Complications

Complications of fluid replacement include primarily excessive fluid repletion due to overestimation of the hypovolemia or inadvertent excessive fluid administration. Patients with renal and cardiac dysfunction are especially prone to fluid overload, and pulmonary edema may be the first manifestation. Pulmonary edema is also likely—and may occur without excessive fluid repletion—in patients who have increased lung permeability or ARDS. During fluid repletion, worsening of peripheral edema or ascites may occur. Large amounts of isotonic saline may contribute to expansion acidosis—a hyperchloremic metabolic acidosis due largely to dilution of serum bicarbonate—but this is uncommon.

E. Maintenance Fluid Requirements

Normal maintenance fluids to prevent hypovolemia should provide 1.5–2.5 L of water per day for normal-sized adults, adjusted to account for other sources of water intake (medications, food intake) and the ability of the kidneys to concentrate and dilute the urine. Sodium intake in the intensive care unit should generally be limited to a total of 50–70 meq/d, but many critically ill patients avidly retain sodium, and they may have net positive sodium balance on even a smaller sodium intake. Patients are frequently given much more sodium than needed. For example, 0.9% NaCl has 154 meq/L of sodium and chloride, and some patients are inadvertently given as much as 3–4 L/d. Al-

Table 2–4. Replacement guidelines for gastrointestinal fluid loss.[1]

	Volume Replacement, mL (per L lost)			
	Normal Saline	**D_5W**	**KCl[2] (meq/L)**	**$NaHCO_3$ (meq/L)**
Salivary	250	750	20	45 (1 amp)[3]
Gastric	250	750	20	…
Small bowel	750	250	5	22 (1/2 amp)
Pancreatic	500	…	5	90 (2 amps)
Biliary	750	250	5	45 (1 amp)
Diarrheal	500	500	40	45 (1 amp)

[1]Modified with permission, from Cogan MG: *Fluid and Electrolytes: Physiology and Pathophysiology.* Appleton & Lange, 1991.
[2]Increase supplement if K^+ depleted; add urinary K^+ loss.
[3]Standard ampule (some, 7.5% $NaHCO^3$, 44.6 me/q Na^+)

though it is sometimes necessary, it is difficult to rationalize giving diuretics to a patient simply to enhance removal of sodium given as part of replacement fluid. On the other hand, diuretics are useful when needed to facilitate excretion of the sodium ingested from an appropriate diet. In states of ongoing losses of extracellular volume, appropriate fluid replacement in addition to maintenance water and electrolytes should be given as needed (Table 2–4).

Human albumin administration in critically ill patients: systemic review of randomized controlled trials. Cochrane Injuries Group Albumin Reviews BMJ 1998;317:235–40.

McGee S, Abernethy WB, Simel DL: Is this patient hypovolemic? JAMA 1999;281:1022–9.

Mange K et al: Language guiding therapy: the case of dehydration versus volume depletion. Ann Intern Med 1997;127:848–53.

Rosenthal MH: Intraoperative fluid management—what and how much? Chest 1999;115(5 Suppl):106S–112S.

Schierhout G, Roberts I: Fluid resuscitation with colloid or crystalloid solutions in critically ill patients: a systematic review of randomized trials. BMJ 1998;316:961–4.

Sort P et al: Effect of intravenous albumin on renal impairment and mortality in patients with cirrhosis and spontaneous bacterial peritonitis. N Engl J Med 1999;341:403–9.

HYPERVOLEMIA

ESSENTIALS OF DIAGNOSIS

- *Edema, ascites, or other evidence of increased extracellular volume.*
- *Intravascular volume may be judged to be normal, low (hypovolemia), or high.*
- *Potential causes of increased extracellular volume: renal insufficiency, congestive heart failure, liver disease, or some other mechanism of sodium retention, or excessive sodium administration.*

General Considerations

In contrast to hypovolemia, in which there is decreased volume of the intravascular space, hypervolemia is almost always an increase of extracellular volume with peripheral edema, ascites, or other fluid collection. The intravascular volume may be low, normal, or high. Increased extracellular volume by itself is usually not an emergency situation in ICU patients, but it depends on how much and where the excess fluid accumulates. If associated with decreased *effective* intravascular volume (hypovolemia) or increased intravascular volume (eg, congestive heart failure with pulmonary edema), rapid intervention may be required.

A. Hypervolemia With Decreased Intravascular Volume

Because sodium—along with anions—is the predominant solute in the extracellular space, increased extracellular volume indicates an abnormally increased quantity of sodium and water. The body normally determines whether sodium and water should be retained by sensing the adequacy of intravascular volume, and it appears that the nonvascular component of extracellular volume does not play a direct role in stimulating or inhibiting sodium and water retention. In other words, the body increases sodium and water retention in response to inadequate circulation regardless of whether the total extracellular volume is increased, decreased, or normal. Thus, excessive sodium retention or hypervolemia may occur appropriately in states of inadequate effective circulation, such as heart failure, or suboptimal filling of the vascular space resulting from loss of fluid into other compartments, as occurs with hypoalbuminemia, portal hypertension, or increased vascular permeability to solute and water.

Ascites due to liver disease arises from a combination of portal hypertension and hypoalbuminemia, as seen usually in severe hepatic parenchymal disease but occasionally as a result of pre- or posthepatic portal obstruction. Decreased serum albumin by itself, though it is a cause of edema, is an unusual cause of severe ascites or pleural effusions. Ascites may also be a marker of local inflammatory or infectious disorders. Pleural effusion may indicate hypervolemia if associated with heart failure or hypoalbuminemia, but it may also be associated with pneumonia or other local causes.

B. Hypervolemia With Primary Increased Sodium Retention

The other major mechanism of hypervolemia is primary excessive function of the normal mechanisms that ensure sodium and water balance. Normal extracellular volume is maintained by a complex interactive system that includes renin, angiotensin, aldosterone, glomerular filtration, renal tubular handling of sodium and water, atrial natriuretic factor, and antidiuretic hormone along with the intake of sodium and water in the diet. Hyperfunction of some of these mechanisms, such as hyperaldosteronism or excessive intake of sodium, or dysfunction of others, such as renal dysfunction or decreased glomerular filtration, causes net positive sodium balance with inevitable expansion of the extracellular volume. Although due in some degree to hypoalbuminemia with decreased effective intravascular volume, nephrotic syndrome with renal dysfunction is considered a state in which there is also impaired renal sodium excretion. While not technically a dysfunction of normal mechanisms of sodium and water balance, excessive administration of sodium, especially from hypertonic fluid or dietary sources, may expand the extracellular volume. Administration of drugs that impair sodium excretion may also contribute, including corticosteroids (eg, prednisone, methylprednisolone) and some antihypertensive agents.

Clinical Features

A. Symptoms and Signs

Increased extracellular volume may be localized to certain compartments (eg, ascites) or generalized. Edema is often a major feature of increased extracellular volume. Edema collects in dependent areas of the body, and the lower back and sacral areas may demonstrate edema in the absence of edema of the lower extremities in ICU patients. Edema always indicates increased extracellular volume except when there is a localized mechanism of fluid transudation or exudation, eg, local venous insufficiency, cellulitis, lymphatic obstruction, or trauma. The presence of edema may or may not signify that the intravascular volume is increased.

Abdominal distention and other findings consistent with ascites may be present. Pleural effusions indicate hypervolemia when associated with congestive heart failure.

Other clinical findings depend on the mechanism of hypervolemia. Intravascular volume may be low, high, or normal in the face of increased extracellular volume. If low, evidence of inadequate circulation may be found, including tachycardia, peripheral cyanosis, and altered mental status. If extracellular volume is high, rales and wheezes consistent with pulmonary edema may be present. Patients with hypervolemia due to endocrine disorders or renal failure may have findings specific to the underlying cause. As shown in Table 2–5, the associated conditions leading to hypervolemia can be divided according to the presumed pathogenesis into those associated with decreased effective intravascular volume (heart failure, liver disease, increased vascular permeability) and those associated with increased or normal intravascular volume (primary disorder of sodium excretion or excessive administration of sodium).

B. Laboratory Findings

Except in a few instances, laboratory findings in hypervolemia are nonspecific. Hypoalbuminemia is seen in patients with nephrotic syndrome, protein-losing enteropathy, malnutrition, and liver disease. Urine sodium is usually very low in the face of avid sodium retention in the untreated patient. Nephrotic syndrome patients have moderate to severe proteinuria. Decreased glomerular filtration (increased serum creatinine and urea nitrogen) is seen in patients with severely decreased intravascular volume.

Table 2–5. Hypervolemia (increased extracellular volume).

With decreased effective intravascular volume
- Cirrhosis with ascites
- Pre- and posthepatic portal hypertension with ascites
- Hypoalbuminemia from protein-losing enteropathy, malnutrition, nephrotic syndrome
- Congestive heart failure

With increased intravascular volume
- Excess sodium intake
- Increased sodium retention
  - Renal insufficiency (especially glomerular disease)
  - Hyperaldosteronism, hypercortisolism
  - Increased renin and angiostensin
  - Drugs (corticosteroids, some antihypertensives)

Despite the increased extracellular quantity of sodium, plasma sodium concentrations are often low (120–135 meq/L) in patients with decreased effective intravascular volume because of stimulation of ADH secretion. Plasma potassium is often low as well. Patients with excess endogenous or administered corticosteroids (Cushing's syndrome) or mineralocorticoids may have hypokalemic metabolic alkalosis; those with cirrhosis often have respiratory alkalosis.

Treatment

The need for treatment and the treatment approach depend on the mechanism of hypervolemia. Although not always a critical problem, hypervolemia associated with severely decreased or markedly increased intravascular volume requires rapid and aggressive treatment.

A. Hypervolemia With Decreased Intravascular Volume

The critically ill patient with decreased intravascular volume and increased extracellular volume may have an acute increase in permeability of the vascular system with leakage of fluid into the interstitial space (eg, sepsis). More commonly, the patient may have a chronic condition leading to edema or ascites accompanied by subtle and gradual decrease in intravascular volume. Diuretic treatment should be delayed until the intravascular fluid deficit is corrected to avoid further deterioration. Treatment of decreased intravascular volume is described above (in the section on hypovolemia), but with preexisting hypervolemia, necessary fluid replacement may worsen edema, ascites, or other fluid accumulations. In most patients, some worsening of hypervolemia (edema) must be accepted for a time until intravascular volume is repleted. However, by improving renal perfusion, there may be appropriate natriuresis with mobilization of edema fluid. A special situation is the patient with cor pulmonale who develops edema secondary to impaired right ventricular function and who may have low effective intravascular volume. These patients may benefit from reduction of pulmonary hypertension with administration of oxygen with decreased edema and increased intravascular volume.

B. Hypervolemia With Increased Intravascular Volume

In these patients, severely increased intravascular volume will be manifested by pulmonary edema, hypoxemia, and respiratory distress.

If intravenous fluids are being administered, these should be discontinued unless blood transfusions are necessary for severe anemia. Intravenous furosemide (10–80 mg) is given, with repeated doses every 30 minutes depending on the diuretic response. Supportive care includes oxygen, changes in the patient's position, and mechanical ventilation if necessary. Cardiogenic pulmonary edema may also benefit from morphine, vasodilators (nitroprusside, ACE inhibitors), or venoodilators (nitrates). Mechanical ventilatory support, either intubation or noninvasive positive-pressure ventilation may be necessary.

In some critically ill patients, sodium excretion is impaired, and diuretics must be given in larger than usual doses. Patients with previous diuretic use, those with severe cardiac failure, and those with renal insufficiency may require furosemide in doses up to 400 mg given slowly. Metolazone, which acts in the distal renal tubule, may facilitate the response to furosemide. There is no role for osmotic diuretics such as mannitol because these will further expand the intravascular volume, especially if ineffective in producing diuresis. Potassium-sparing collecting tubule diuretics, such as triamterene, amiloride, and spironolactone, usually have little acute effect in these patients. Failure to induce appropriate diuresis in the situation of expanded intravascular volume may require acute hemodialysis or ultrafiltration.

For critically ill patients, rapid decreases in intravascular volume may be particularly hazardous in those with chronic hypertension (associated with hypertrophic, poorly compliant ventricles), pulmonary hypertension, pericardial effusion, sepsis, diabetes mellitus, autonomic instability, electrolyte disturbances, or recent blood loss. Patients receiving alpha- or beta-adrenergic blockers, arterial or venous dilators (including hydralazine, nitroprusside, and nitroglycerin), and mechanical ventilation may be very sensitive to rapid depletion of intravascular volume. Severe hypotension and hypovolemic shock may be induced by diuretics or other fluid removal.

C. Increased Extracellular Volume Without Change in Intravascular Volume

These are usually chronic conditions. Edema and ascites do not by themselves cause immediate problems, but edema may impair skin care and lead to immobility, while ascites may become uncomfortable, may cause respiratory distress and hypoxemia, and may become infected (spontaneous bacterial peritonitis).

1. Sodium restriction—Treatment centers around creating net negative sodium balance. Urine sodium concentration can provide a guide to the degree of sodium intake restriction and diuretics needed. In severe states of sodium retention, urine sodium concentration may be as low as 1–2 meq/L, but more often it is 5–20 meq/L. With daily urine volumes of 1–2 L, only a total of 1–40 meq of Na^+ may be excreted daily. In contrast, moderate dietary sodium restriction is often considered to be 2 g (87 meq) of sodium per day. Thus, moderate sodium restriction alone is unlikely to be successful in resolving severe hypervolemia associated with avid sodium reabsorption, and strict limitation of dietary sodium often is associated with decreased nutrient intake. Nevertheless, most patients should be restricted to 1–2 g of sodium daily, though only 10–15% of patients with severe fluid retention will respond.

2. Diuretics—Ascites and edema without increased or decreased intravascular volume will often respond best to a combination of furosemide and spironolactone. Furosemide is usually started at 40 mg; spironolactone's starting dose is 100 mg, with both given once daily. If needed, furosemide can be increased to 160 mg/d and spironolactone up to 400 mg/d.

Diuretics should be used cautiously in patients with increased extracellular volume if there is concomitant marginal or decreased effective intravascular volume (ascites, heart failure, nephrotic syndrome). Too-rapid depletion of extracellular volume will not only worsen circulatory dysfunction but will often lead to further enhanced sodium retention, perhaps inducing a state of "escape" from diuretic responsiveness. Concern has been expressed about the possibility of an increased incidence of hepatorenal syndrome in patients with severe liver disease who are given large doses of diuretics.

Complications of diuretics depend somewhat on their effectiveness in inducing natriuresis and volume depletion. Furosemide may cause severe hypokalemia and contributes to metabolic alkalosis, and hypomagnesemia and hypernatremia are occasionally significant problems. Spironolactone and triamterene should not be used in patients with hyperkalemia, and patients receiving potassium supplementation should be carefully monitored when these agents are given. Patients may have allergic or other unpredictable reactions to any of these drugs.

3. Increased elimination of extracellular fluid—Removal of ascites by paracentesis in patients with chronic liver disease has some advocates. Although earlier studies found an association of excessive depletion of intravascular volume following removal of more than 800–1500 mL of ascitic fluid, recent investigations have suggested that large-volume paracentesis (> 1500 mL) may be safe—sometimes if intravenous albumin is given to maintain intravascular volume immediately after fluid removal. Paracentesis is indicated in patients with severe respiratory distress or discomfort from their ascites, but the exact amount of fluid that can be safely removed remains unclear.

Patients with congestive heart failure with hypervolemia are often treated with a combination of diuretics, inotropic agents such as digitalis, and systemic vasodilators. Systemic vasodilators that reduce left ventricular afterload and improve cardiac output may be very effective in decreasing hypervolemia without compromising organ system perfusion. These agents, primarily ACE inhibitors, have been particularly useful in reversing consequences of decreased effective intravascular volume.

Extracellular volume can be readily removed in most ICU patients by ultrafiltration. This can be accomplished rapidly or slowly depending upon the method chosen. Hypotension may accompany too rapid intravascular fluid removal.

Daniels BS, Ferris TF: The use of diuretics in nonedematous disorders. Semin Nephrol 1988;8:342–53.

Hura CE, Kunau RT Jr, Stein JH: Use of diuretics in salt-retaining states. Semin Nephrol 1988;8:318–32.

Runyon BA: Care of patients with ascites. N Engl J Med 1994;330:337–42.

Schrier RW: Pathogenesis of sodium and water retention in high-output and low-output cardiac failure, nephrotic syndrome, cirrhosis, and pregnancy. (Two parts.) N Engl J Med 1988;319:1065–72, 1127–34.

DISORDERS OF WATER BALANCE

The term "water balance" denotes the normally closely regulated relationship between total body water and total body solute that determines solute concentration throughout the body. With the exception of a few special areas such as the renal medulla and collecting ducts, water moves freely into and out of all body compartments—intracellular and extracellular—as a result of osmotic gradients. Therefore, while solute concentration is equal everywhere, the amount of water in a given body space is determined by the quantity of solute contained within that space.

Clinical disorders of water balance are estimated from serum sodium $[Na^+]$, because the concentration of that predominantly extracellular cation is inversely proportionate to the quantity of total body water relative to total solute. There is one caveat, however. Hypernatremia always denotes hypertonicity (increased solute relative to total body water), but hyponatremia may be seen with hypotonicity, normotonicity, or hypertonicity. This is because solutes other than sodium may be present in high enough quantity to exert an osmotic effect.

Total Body Water & Serum Sodium Concentration

If total body exchangeable solute is dissolved hypothetically in a volume equal to total body water (TBW), the osmolality of the solution will be as shown in the following equation:

$$\text{Body osmolality (mosm/kg)} = \frac{\text{Total solute (mosm)}}{\text{TBW (kg)}}$$

If water is allowed to move freely between all compartments, then water will move out of any body compartment with a low osmolality into any compartment with a high osmolality, thus equalizing solute concentration everywhere. Therefore, for the serum compartment:

$$\text{Serum osmolality (mosm/kg)} = \frac{\text{Total solute (mosm)}}{\text{TBW (kg)}}$$

Serum osmolality is approximately the sum of cation plus anion concentrations, usually approximated as meq/L rather than mosm/kg for monovalent solutes. Since sodium is the most abundant extracellular cation, the sum of cation and anion concentrations is approximately $2 \times [Na^+]$. Therefore,

$$2 \times [Na^+] = \frac{\text{Total solute (mosm)}}{\text{TBW (L)}}$$

or

$$[Na^+] \propto \frac{1}{\text{TBW (L)}}$$

A useful form of this equation relates TBW and [Na⁺] under abnormal conditions to normal TBW and [Na⁺], assuming that total body solute does not change:

$$\text{TBW (L)} = \text{Normal TBW (L)} \times \frac{\text{Normal }[\text{Na}^+]}{[\text{Na}^+]}$$

This equation allows estimation of TBW when [Na⁺] is measured, and the difference between TBW and normal TBW represents the water deficit or water excess. Normal TBW is approximately 60% of body weight in men and 50% of body weight in women who are at or near ideal body weight. The proportion of body weight that is made up of water decreases with obesity and in the elderly to 45–50% of body weight.

Regulation of Water Balance

Normal water balance is maintained primarily by water intake (water consumption mediated by thirst plus water produced from metabolism) and water excretion by the kidneys. Other sources of water loss such as from intestinal secretions and sweating are unregulated but must be taken into account by the mechanisms that do regulate water balance. Normally, enough excess water is taken in to allow the kidneys to control total body osmolality by increasing or decreasing water excretion as necessary. Although normal subjects filter as much as 150 L/d through the glomeruli, about 99% of the water is reabsorbed in the renal tubules. The range of water volume that can be excreted in 24 hours depends on minimum and maximum urine concentrations (dependent on renal function) and the daily urinary excretion of solute, mostly in the form of urea (Table 2–6), that can vary in quantity dependent on dietary intake of protein and catabolic rate. Healthy normal subjects are theoretically able to maintain normal water balance with as little as 670 mL or as much as 12,000 mL water intake per day. This wide range depends on normal glomerular filtration rate, normal urinary concentrating or diluting ability, and normal solute excretion rate. Patients with abnormal renal function are consequently much more limited in their ability to tolerate and correct water imbalances.

A. Urine Concentration

The urine concentration depends largely on the amount of the posterior pituitary peptide antidiuretic hormone (ADH) present. ADH, also known as arginine vasopressin (AVP), is secreted by the posterior pituitary in response to plasma osmolal changes sensed by the hypothalamic supraoptic and paraventricular nuclei. Increased plasma osmolality increases ADH secretion; decreased osmolality inhibits ADH secretion. ADH also is released in response to decreased extracellular volume, sensed by receptors in the atria. Extracellular volume status and osmolality interact to determine serum ADH levels. For example, in the presence of hypovolemia plus hyponatremia, ADH release may continue despite an inhibitory influence of decreased plasma osmolality.

Maximum urine concentrating capacity depends on sufficient solute load to the distal nephron, maintenance of a high solute concentration in the renal medulla, and high levels of ADH. Active transport of sodium out of the ascending limb of the loop of Henle generates high solute concentration in the renal medullary interstitium while tubular fluid becomes progressively more dilute as solute is removed but water is allowed to remain in the tubules. In the collecting ducts, the tubular fluid is exposed to the medullary concentration gradient, and—in the presence of ADH—water moves freely out of the lumen, thereby concentrating the urine. Maximum urine concentration, when needed to conserve water excretion, may not be reached if there is insufficient sodium presented to the loop of Henle (renal insufficiency), inhibition of active transport in the thick ascending limb (furosemide), inadequate response to ADH (nephrogenic diabetes insipidus due to drugs or renal disease), or absence of ADH (central diabetes insipidus).

Table 2–6. Range of urinary water excretion with normal solute load.

- Minimum urine concentration: 50 mosm/L
- Maximum urine concentration: 1200 mosm/L
- Normal urine solute excretion: 800 mosm/d
- Minimum urine volume (water excretion) per day $= \frac{800 \text{ mosm/d}}{1200 \text{ mosm/L}} = 0.67 \text{ L/d}$
- Maximum urine volume (water excretion) per day $= \frac{800 \text{ mosm/d}}{50 \text{ mosm/L}} = 16 \text{ L/d}$

Maximum urine diluting capacity depends on function of the diluting segments of the ascending loop of Henle and the distal convoluted tubule as well as maintenance of an impermeable collecting duct and suppression of ADH release. The presence of excess water in the body is countered by increased volume of maximally diluted urine. Failure to dilute urine maximally may result from renal insufficiency, especially with tubulointerstitial diseases, inappropriate secretion of ADH, and abnormally increased permeability of the collecting ducts to water (adrenal insufficiency). In addition, sedative-hypnotic drugs, analgesics, opioids, and antipsychotic drugs may interfere with renal diluting ability.

B. Solute Excretion and Water Excretion Rate

The quantity of solute excreted also determines the maximum and minimum water excretion rates. There is an obligate solute loss of about 800 mosm/d in normal subjects, including sodium, potassium, anions, ammonium, and urea. Urea, from breakdown of amino acids, makes up about 50% of the solute excreted. In the presence of severely limited protein intake, 24-hour urine urea excretion is reduced. The decrease in urine solute excretion causes a decrease in maximum water excretion, even if urine is maximally diluted. A fall in the total 24-hour urine solute excretion to 300 mosm/d, for example, means that even if urine concentration is 50 mosm/kg, only 6 L of water can be excreted per day. In contrast, if there is 800 mosm/d of solute to excrete, 16 L of water per day could have been excreted with maximum urinary dilution.

HYPONATREMIA

ESSENTIALS OF DIAGNOSIS

- *Serum sodium < 135 meq/L.*
- *Altered mental status or new onset of seizure disorder.*
- *Most cases discovered by review of routinely obtained serum electrolytes.*

General Considerations

Hyponatremia is a commonly encountered electrolyte problem in the ICU. It has been estimated that 2.5% of hospitalized patients have hyponatremia. Low serum sodium is associated with a variety of endocrine, renal, neurologic, and respiratory disorders; medications and other treatment; and other medical conditions. When serum sodium is extremely low, hyponatremia is manifested by altered mental status (hyponatremic encephalopathy), seizures, and high mortality. Correction of severe hyponatremia must be done carefully and in a controlled fashion to avoid further complications.

In the absence of hyponatremia associated with normal or increased tonicity (see below), low serum sodium indicates excess total body water for the amount of solute (dilutional hyponatremia). In normal subjects, this condition would initiate compensatory mechanisms that would facilitate rapid excretion of water and correct the imbalance. Therefore, in states of persistent hyponatremia, there is physiologic or pathologic inability to excrete water normally.

Hyponatremia is seen in three distinct clinical situations in which extracellular volume is low, high, or normal (Table 2–7).

A. Hyponatremia With Decreased Extracellular Volume

Decreased extracellular volume leads to vigorous water conservation, primarily mediated by increased ADH release stimulated by atrial receptors, and increased thirst

Table 2–7. Disorders of water balance: Hyponatremia.

Normal plasma osmolality
- Pseudohyponatremia (hyperlipidemia); rare if measured with ion-specific Na^+ electrode

Elevated plasma osmolality
- Hyperglycemia
- Mannitol, glycerol, radiocontrast agents

Decreased plasma osmolality

Urine maximally diluted:
1. Decreased solute excretion (low protein intake)
2. Excessive water ingestion or intake

Urine not maximally diluted:
1. Normal extracellular volume
    - a. SIADH
        - Lung disease
        - CNS disease
        - Drugs
        - Anxiety
    - b. Adrenal insufficiency (may also have volume depletion)
    - c. Hypothyroidism
2. Low extracellular volume
    - a. Extrarenal loss
    - b. Renal loss: diuretics, sodium-losing nephropathy
3. Increased extracellular volume
    - a. Congestive heart failure
    - b. Cirrhosis
    - c. Nephrotic syndrome

leading to increased water intake. Generally, urinary sodium excretion is very low and water intake and retention lead to relatively increased TBW despite the reduced amount of solute. But in conditions in which the hypovolemic state is due to sodium and water loss in the urine, such as adrenal insufficiency, diuretic use, and salt-losing nephropathy, urine sodium excretion may be normal or high. Hyponatremia is facilitated in adrenal insufficiency because lack of cortisol causes collecting ducts to be excessively permeable to water movement, leading to impaired maximum water excretion. Furthermore, ADH levels in adrenal insufficiency may remain elevated despite hyponatremia, suggesting that there is an abnormal ADH response to decreased serum osmolality.

A common form of hypovolemic hyponatremia is seen with thiazide diuretics (less commonly with furosemide). Chronic volume depletion leading to stimulation of ADH release is an important factor. In addition, thiazides impair urinary dilution by blocking sodium and chloride transport in the diluting segment of the distal nephron and potentiate the effect of ADH. Finally, thiazide-induced renal potassium excretion further reduces total body solute content, also contributing to hyponatremia.

B. Hyponatremia With Increased Extracellular Volume

Hyponatremia in the presence of increased extracellular volume is seen in congestive heart failure, nephrotic syndrome, cirrhosis, protein-losing enteropathy, and pregnancy. These disorders have in common edema, ascites, pulmonary edema, or other evidence of increased extracellular volume. However, these patients appear to have inability to maintain normal effective intravascular volume because of forces generating excessive venous and extravascular volume. Hyponatremia is a consequence of ADH release in response to decreased intravascular volume, even though total extracellular volume is increased and total body water is high. Some patients with hypothyroidism have hyponatremia due primarily to heart failure, but hypothyroidism also interferes directly with the ability to maximally dilute urine.

C. Hyponatremia With Normal Extracellular Volume

Hyponatremia in association with normal extracellular volume is seen with psychogenic water ingestion, decreased solute intake, and, most commonly, the syndrome of inappropriate secretion of ADH (SIADH). Massive intake of water rarely results in severe hyponatremia if ability to excrete water is unimpaired. However, decreased solute intake as described above limits the maximum volume of water that can be excreted even when urine is maximally diluted. The syndrome of "beer-drinker's hyponatremia" results from heavy consumption of beer and other low-solute fluids that limit the quantity of solute available for excretion. A very low protein diet also generates very little solute in the form of urea. However, the majority of patients with normovolemic hyponatremia have SIADH.

SIADH results from release of ADH in response to a variety of systemic disorders but primarily in response to lung and central nervous system problems. Lung diseases include lung cancer, tuberculosis, pneumonia, COPD, asthma, respiratory failure due to any cause, and use of mechanical ventilation. SIADH is also associated with encephalitis, status epilepticus, brain tumors, meningitis, head trauma, and strokes. The mechanism of ADH release in these disorders is unclear. Some cancer chemotherapeutic drugs, chlorpropamide, nicotine, tricyclics, serotonin reuptake inhibitors, and some opioids are associated with SIADH.

D. Hyponatremia Without Hypotonicity

Hyponatremia without hypotonicity was commonly seen in patients with severe hypertriglyceridemia or hyperproteinemia (> 10 g/dL) when serum sodium was measured by flame photometry. This is no longer a problem with the use of ion-specific sodium electrodes.

E. Hyponatremia With Hyperglycemia (Hypertonic Hyponatremia)

Hyperglycemia with hyponatremia is associated with decreased TBW rather than with increased TBW relative to total solute. Enhanced gluconeogenesis or glycogenolysis in diabetics—or exogenous glucose administration—adds a large quantity of osmotically active molecules to the extracellular compartment. Water moves from the intracellular space to the extracellular space to equalize osmotic gradients. The result is increased osmolality throughout the body but dilution of plasma sodium by the additional water moving out of the cells and into the extracellular space. The hyponatremia may be mistakenly thought to be evidence for excessive TBW relative to solute content when instead there is a TBW deficit.

Hyponatremia in the presence of hyperglycemia can be addressed in several ways. First, laboratory measurement of serum osmolality will give a correct assessment of water balance; serum osmolality will be higher than estimated from serum sodium. Another way is to "correct" the serum sodium for the degree of hyperglycemia. One empiric correction is to add to the measured serum sodium 1 meq/L for every 60 mg/dL the serum glucose is increased above 100 mg/dL. For example, if measured serum sodium is 130 meq/L and serum glucose is 1300 mg/dL (1200 mg/dL above 100 mg/dL), the "corrected" serum sodium will be 130 + 20

= 150 meq/L. The corrected serum sodium then can be used to give a valid estimate of increase or decrease of TBW relative to solute. Although glucose is the most commonly encountered solute that causes this phenomenon, other extracellular solutes such as mannitol and radiopaque contrast agents can cause hyponatremia with hypertonicity.

Clinical Features

Figure 2–1 shows a clinical and laboratory approach to diagnosis of hyponatremia and identification of the cause of low serum sodium.

A. Symptoms and Signs

Hyponatremia associated with decreased osmolality is often asymptomatic until serum sodium falls below 125 meq/L, but the rate of change is clearly important. Rapid development is associated with more severe acute changes. Subtle neurologic findings can sometimes be identified, such as decreased ability to concentrate or perform mental arithmetic. Severe symptoms—including altered mental status, seizures, nausea, vomiting, stupor, and coma—occur when serum sodium is < 115 meq/L when hyponatremia develops acutely or when it is < 105–110 meq/L during chronic hyponatremia. A

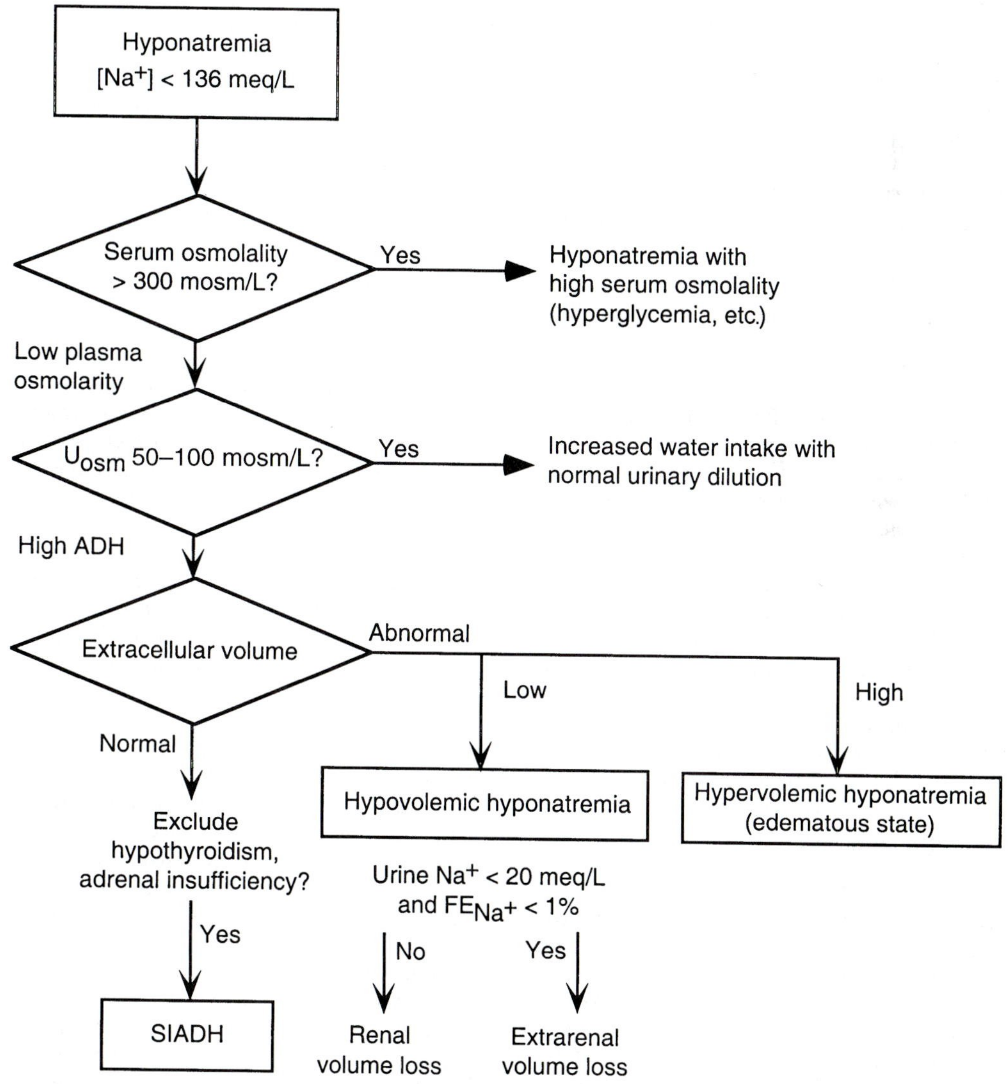

Figure 2–1. Clinical and laboratory approach to the diagnosis of hyponatremia.

syndrome of opisthotonos, respiratory depression, impaired responsiveness, incontinence, hallucinations, decorticate posturing, and seizures has been termed hyponatremic encephalopathy. Occasionally, patients with chronic hyponatremia may be awake, alert, and oriented even with serum sodium as low as 100 meq/L; these patients are almost always found to have slowly developed hyponatremia.

Symptoms and signs of any underlying disorder should be sought. Medications that can affect urinary water excretion should be identified and discontinued. These include thiazide diuretics and drugs that impair renal function. Thiazide-induced hyponatremia has been reported to be more common in women, but advanced age was not a risk factor. Enalapril given to elderly patients is reported to cause hyponatremia. Excessive water drinking can be identified from the history and the presence of polyuria, but large volumes of water may be inadvertently given in the ICU. Adrenal insufficiency and hypothyroidism should be considered if there are features suggesting these disorders. Hyponatremia has been associated with hospitalized AIDS patients. Volume depletion from gastrointestinal fluid losses and SIADH were the most common causes and there was an increase in morbidity and mortality of those with hyponatremia. For unclear reasons, young women recovering from surgery can have particularly severe symptoms and a poor prognosis from hyponatremia. Although previously thought to be caused by excessive hypotonic fluid replacement, the hyponatremia results from generation of inappropriately concentrated urine.

Patients with hypovolemia may have evidence of volume depletion such as hypotension, tachycardia, decreased skin turgor, or documented weight loss, but these findings may be subtle or absent; those with hypervolemia have edema and weight gain. SIADH is confirmed by lack of evidence of high or low extracellular volume and is sometimes accompanied by clinical findings suggesting pulmonary or central nervous system disease.

Hyponatremic encephalopathy is thought to be due to cerebral edema from water shift into the brain and increased intracranial pressure. Decreased cerebral blood flow plays a role. Movement of solute out of brain cells—given sufficient time—minimizes the effects, probably explaining the lack of symptoms of slowly evolving hyponatremia. On the other hand, evidence has linked a specific neurologic syndrome, osmotic demyelination syndrome (central pontine and extrapontine myelinolysis), with both severe hyponatremia and rapid correction of hyponatremia. It is speculated that adaptation to hyponatremia may be the cause of demyelination in susceptible regions of the brain. A firm conclusion cannot be made about whether osmotic demyelination syndrome is due to severity of hyponatremia or to excessively fast correction. Osmotic demyelination syndrome is reported to occur about 3 days after the start of correction of hyponatremia, but findings may be seen before, during, or after serum sodium has been corrected. Corticospinal and corticobulbar signs are most often reported, including weakness, spastic quadriparesis, dysphonia, and dysphagia, but impaired level of consciousness is common. Radiolucent areas on CT scan or decreased T1-weighted MRI intensity provides evidence of myelinolysis in the central pons (central pontine myelinolysis) and elsewhere.

B. Laboratory Findings

Serum electrolytes, glucose, creatinine, and urea nitrogen, serum osmolality, urine osmolality, urine Na^+, and urine creatinine (to calculate fractional excretion of Na^+) should be measured. Low serum osmolality (< 280 mosm/kg) confirms hyponatremia due to increased water relative to solute. The corrected serum sodium value should be used if there is hyperglycemia. An association has been found between hyponatremia with hypokalemia and severe body potassium depletion. Hypokalemia may also predispose patients with hyponatremia to osmotic demyelination syndromes and encephalopathy.

In patients with excessive water intake as the cause of hyponatremia, urine osmolality will be low (< 300 mosm/kg). Patients with hypovolemia will have low urine sodium (< 20 meq/L) and fractional excretion of sodium (< 1%), and this may also be seen in patients with increased extracellular volume and low intravascular volume. If, however, hypovolemia is caused by a renal mechanism, urine sodium may not be appropriately conserved.

The diagnosis of SIADH is made by the finding of inappropriately high urine osmolality (usually 300–500 mosm/kg) in the presence of low serum osmolality and the absence of low urinary sodium concentration. It should be noted that in SIADH, urine osmolality may be less than serum osmolality but not as low as it should be, because urine should be maximally diluted in the presence of severe hyponatremia. For example, in SIADH serum osmolality may be 240 mosm/kg, indicating severe water excess, while urine osmolality is 200 mosm/kg. Because maximally dilute urine can be as low as 50 mosm/kg in young healthy persons, these findings are consistent with SIADH. Patients with renal disease may be limited in their maximum urinary diluting ability to 100–200 mosm/kg.

Treatment

Severity of hyponatremia ($[Na^+]$ < 120 meq/L), acuteness of onset, and the presence of neurologic symptoms (confusion, stupor, coma, or seizures) determine how quickly treatment should be instituted and how aggressively it should pursued. If the patient is asymptomatic and hyponatremia is mild and chronic, the need to treat is less emergent, and aggressive treatment is contraindicated.

A. Estimation of Water Excess

Water excess can be estimated by relating current measured [Na^+] to TBW and substituting 140 meq/L for normal [Na^+]:

$$\text{TBW (L)} = \text{Normal TBW (L)} \times \frac{140}{[\text{Na}^+]}$$

For a 70-kg man with a normal TBW of 0.6 L/kg, normal TBW would be 42 L. If [Na^+] is 110 meq/L, TBW would be estimated as 42 × 140 ÷ 110 = 53.5 L. The water excess would be 53.5 L – 42 L = 11.5 L. If it is desired to correct [Na^+] to 125 meq/L because of concern about too-rapid correction to normal in a patient with chronic hyponatremia, the estimated water excess to be corrected would be 53.5 L – (42 × 125 ÷ 110) = 5.8 L.

B. Determine Need for Rapid or Aggressive Correction

Patients with hyponatremia who have altered mental status or seizures attributed to hyponatremia require rapid treatment. Most patients with severely reduced [Na^+] (< 105 meq/L) are also a concern even if asymptomatic. Symptomatic hyponatremia is usually associated with severely reduced [Na^+], and only rarely do these patients have water intoxication from psychogenic water ingestion, thiazide diuretics, decreased solute excretion, or conditions of hypo- or hypervolemia. SIADH is the most commonly encountered problem requiring aggressive and rapid correction of hyponatremia.

C. Correct the Underlying Problem

Of the underlying problems leading to hyponatremia, the most straightforward and easily corrected is hypovolemia. Administration of normal saline repletes the intravascular volume and inhibits ADH release by reducing the hypovolemic stimulus. Water excretion is enhanced by the increased glomerular filtration rate, and urine should become quickly and near maximally dilute, facilitating water excretion. Patients with psychogenic water intoxication and those being given large volumes of intravenous fluid should be already maximally excreting water; removing the intake of water leads to rapid restoration of normal [Na^+] if there are no other medical problems. Discontinuation of thiazide diuretics results in rapid restoration of maximum urinary dilution in most patients. Hypokalemia should be corrected, as this has been associated with complications of hyponatremia and its treatment.

Hypervolemia (edematous states) with hyponatremia represents a more difficult problem of management, but severe hyponatremia is unusual. It is especially important to avoid "correcting" a low serum [Na^+] in congestive heart failure by giving more sodium and chloride. Although effective arterial volume is diminished, additional volume expansion will have only a transient effect on ADH release and can worsen peripheral edema, ascites, or pulmonary edema. In patients with congestive heart failure, improvement of hyponatremia has followed successful treatment with afterload reduction. Patients with nephrotic syndrome and cirrhosis have a temporary response to albumin infusions, but longer-term therapy depends on improving the underlying disease.

Adrenal insufficiency, hypothyroidism, and other specific causes of hyponatremia will respond to correction of the underlying problem. SIADH occasionally responds to treatment of the condition leading to this syndrome, but therapy is usually directed toward correction of the hyponatremia itself.

D. Specific Treatment of Hypotonic Hyponatremia

The following discussion applies primarily to hyponatremia in the face of normal volume status (SIADH). There is not yet agreement on the rate of correction of hyponatremia that minimizes the risk from low serum tonicity or the risk of excessively rapid correction with osmotic demyelination syndrome. Because symptomatic hyponatremia will almost always respond to a small increase in [Na^+] (about 5 meq/L) and the risk of osmotic demyelination appears to be minimal when [Na^+] increases at < 12 meq/L per day, a compromise target of about 8 meq/L per day is recommended. In general, rapid correction of hyponatremia is not indicated after the patient's [Na^+] is > 125 meq/L or symptoms have abated.

The specific treatment of hypotonic hyponatremia is a combination of water restriction and efforts to enhance water excretion. Water restriction is usually sufficient for asymptomatic or mild hyponatremia; hypertonic saline and furosemide are indicated for symptomatic hyponatremia and asymptomatic hyponatremia in which serum [Na^+] is < 105 meq/L.

1. Restriction of water intake—Restriction of water intake, both oral and parenteral, will improve hyponatremia from any cause and should be considered in all patients except those with hypovolemia. Most patients with hyponatremia have decreased ability to excrete water, but water restriction to a volume the kidneys can adequately eliminate will lead to net water loss and correction of hyponatremia. Water restriction to < 1000–1500 mL/d is usually successful in reversing hyponatremia when $[Na^+]$ is between 125 meq/L and 135 meq/L and patients are asymptomatic. More severe water restriction may be useful in some patients. It is a mistaken belief that only electrolyte-free water must be restricted and that normal saline can be given safely. Normal saline (osmolality 300 mosm/kg) may be hypertonic to the serum but is frequently hypotonic relative to the urine of patients with SIADH. Administration of normal saline may result in a net gain of water and worsening of hyponatremia.

2. Hypertonic saline and furosemide—The most potent combination therapy for treating symptomatic hyponatremia is hypertonic saline (usually 3% NaCl) and furosemide. Furosemide alone (40–80 mg given frequently enough to maintain a brisk diuresis) will increase sodium and chloride excretion and, by inhibiting solute transport from the ascending loop of Henle, produce urinary dilution. Although this will promote water loss, sodium and chloride will be lost. Therefore, the goal is to replace solute losses but in a smaller amount of water, so that there is a net loss of water from the body.

Ideally, the amount of sodium in the urine can be measured hourly, and the exact amount of sodium and chloride can be replaced using hypertonic saline. However, a more practical approach assumes that urine osmolarity will be about 280–300 mosm/L in the presence of furosemide. Furosemide should be given to achieve a urine output of 200–300 mL/h. If the urine contains approximately 280 mosm/L, then about 70 mosm/h is lost if urine output is 250 mL/h. Replacing 70 mosm/h using 3% NaCl (1026 mosm/L) requires only 68 mL/h, and a net water excretion rate of 182 mL/h (250 mL/h – 68 mL/h) with a rise in serum $[Na^+]$ of about 1 meq/L per hour. In practice, replacing about 25–30% of urine volume each hour with 3% NaCl will approximate the solute replacement required. As recommended above, furosemide and 3% NaCl solution should be discontinued when $[Na^+]$ is above 120–125 meq/L. Furthermore, $[Na^+]$ must not exceed 130 meq/L in the first 48 hours. Excessive volume or rate of hypertonic saline should not be given, because acute volume overload and pulmonary edema may occur. Calculation of the amount of hypertonic saline needed should be double-checked, and it is unlikely that the total amount of hypertonic saline will exceed 1000 mL or a rate > 60–75 mL/h. Serum sodium should be followed closely and appropriate adjustments made in the rate of correction.

A very useful formula can be derived from the above relationship between serum $[Na^+]$ and total body water. This formula estimates the amount of change in serum $[Na^+]$ when 1 L of any fluid is administered:

$$\Delta \text{ Serum Na}^+ = \frac{\text{Fluid Na}^+ - \text{Serum Na}^+}{\text{TBW} + 1}$$

where TBW is the calculated estimate of total body water (see above). This formula is useful for determining how much the serum $[Na^+]$ will change in response to administration of 1 L of hypertonic or normal saline. It does not take into account fluid losses, however. To calculate the change for more than 1 L of fluid administration, you must calculate for each liter incrementally—ie, calculate the change in serum $[Na^+]$ for the first liter, then enter the new value into the formula to calculate the change for the next liter.

E. Other Treatment for Chronic Hyponatremia

Patients with reversible central nervous system or lung disease will generally respond after correction or resolution of the underlying problem. Mild to moderate water restriction may be necessary. A few patients will need additional help to facilitate water excretion; demeclocycline induces a mild nephrogenic diabetes insipidus-like condition and may be useful in management of chronic hypotonic hyponatremia.

Adrogue HJ, Madias NE: Aiding fluid prescription for the dysnatremias. Intensive Care Med 1997;23:309–16.

Adrogue HJ, Madias NE: Hyponatremia. N Engl J Med 2000;342:1581–9.

Arieff AI: Hyponatremia, convulsions, respiratory arrest, and permanent brain damage after elective surgery in healthy women. N Engl J Med 1986;314:1529–35.

Karp BI, Laureno R: Pontine and extrapontine myelinolysis: a neurologic disorder following rapid correction of hyponatremia. Medicine 1993;72:359–73.

Katz MA: Hyperglycemia-induced hyponatremia: Calculation of expected serum sodium depression. N Engl J Med 1973; 289:843–4.

Steele A et al: Postoperative hyponatremia despite near-isotonic saline infusion: a phenomenon of desalination. Ann Intern Med 1997;126:20–5.

Tang WW et al: Hyponatremia in hospitalized patients with the acquired immunodeficiency syndrome (AIDS) and the AIDS-related complex. Am J Med 1993;94:169–74.

HYPERNATREMIA

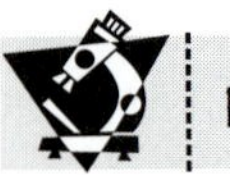

ESSENTIALS OF DIAGNOSIS

- *Serum sodium > 145 meq/L.*
- *Serum osmolality > 300 mosm/kg.*

- *Evidence of increased solute administration, polyuria with dilute urine (diabetes insipidus), or inadequate water intake.*
- *Altered mental status.*

General Considerations

In contrast to hyponatremia, for which hypotonicity is often but not always present, hypernatremia, defined as $[Na^+]$ > 145 meq/L, is always associated with hypertonicity, defined as serum osmolality > 300 mosm/kg with potential for shifts of water between different fluid compartments. Severe hypernatremia must be treated vigorously but carefully to avoid excessively rapid correction and further complications.

Hypernatremia indicates a deficit of total body water relative to total body solute (Table 2–8). This condition occasionally develops when a large amount of solute is given in concentrated form (such as administration of hypertonic sodium chloride or hypertonic sodium bicarbonate) but hypernatremia is much more commonly associated with either insufficient water intake or excessive water loss.

Table 2–8. Disorders of water balance: Hypernatremia.

Increased sodium load
  Hypertonic sodium chloride infusion
  Hypertonic sodium bicarbonate infusion
Increased net water loss (nonrenal)
  Sweating
  Diarrhea
  Exertion during hot weather
Associated with polyuria
  Osmotic diuresis:
  1. Sodium diuresis
     Loop Diuretics
  2. Nonsodium diuresis
     a. Mannitol
     b. Glucose
     c. Urea (postobstructive diuresis)

  Water diuresis:
  1. Decreased ADH release (central diabetes insipidus)
     a. Head trauma
     b. Surgery
     c. Pituitary tumor
     b. Infection, granulomatous diseases
     c. Vascular (aneurysms)
  2. Decreased ADH effectiveness (nephrogenic diabetes insipidus)
     a. Tubulointerstitial disease
     b. Lithium
     c. Demeclocycline
     d. Hypokalemia
     e. Hypercalcemia

A. Addition of Solute

Net addition of solute to the body without a corresponding addition of water to TBW results in an increase in serum osmolality. The source of solute may be exogenous, such as administration of hypertonic saline or sodium bicarbonate, glucose, mannitol, or other solutes. The only common endogenous mechanism of additional solute production is gluconeogenesis and glycogenolysis causing hyperglycemia. As discussed above, hyperglycemia increases serum osmolality without causing hypernatremia. In the case of addition of solute to the body, increased serum osmolality stimulates maximum ADH release to minimize water excretion (urine osmolality increases). Correction of the hyperosmolal state results when the excess solute is disposed of or, in the case of glucose, excreted or taken into the cells as glycogen. However, the obligate loss of water needed to excrete solute requires that water be given to the patient to achieve appropriate correction.

B. Inadequate Water Intake

Insufficient water intake results in hypernatremia because of obligatory renal and nonrenal water losses. Daily insensible loss of water accounts for the loss of about 500 mL of water, increasing somewhat with body temperature and sweating. Because most insensible loss is through the airways, intubation and mechanical ventilation with humidified air decrease insensible losses to minimal amounts.

Minimum urine volume is determined primarily by maximum potential urine concentration and obligate solute excretion. As calculated in Table 2–6, the normal urinary solute excretion of 800 mosm/d necessitates a mandatory loss of 670 mL of water per day if urine is maximally concentrated (to 1200 mosm/L). Thus, minimal water loss in adults of normal size is approximately 1170 mL/d (670 mL urine plus 500 mL insensible loss). Because metabolism generates about 500–600 mL water per day, there is a mandatory intake of 600–700 mL water per day. Failure to take in at least this much water predictably results in hypernatremia.

C. Excessive Water Loss

The final major mechanism of hypernatremia is excessive water loss with inadequate replacement. Some patients are unable to concentrate urine maximally, thereby making mandatory an increased intake of water to avoid development of hyperosmolality. Maximum urine concentration in normal subjects is 1200 mosm/L but depends on having normal renal tubular function, normal solute load, and normal ADH release and response. Renal tubulointerstitial disease such as seen in sickle cell anemia, urate nephropathy, and renal cystic disease, use of loop diuretics such as furosemide, and drugs such as demeclocycline and lithium interfere with urine concentrating ability. An increase in nonsodium solute load forces the renal tubules to produce a urine that is isosmotic (isosthenuria) with plasma. Glucose, mannitol, and urea are the most likely encountered poorly reabsorbable solutes that contribute to such an "osmotic diuresis," resulting in net water loss from the body.

Patients who lack appropriate ADH release from the posterior pituitary or whose kidneys do not respond properly to ADH have impaired urine concentrating ability and polyuria and will develop hypernatremia in the absence of increased water intake. Lack of ADH production is termed central diabetes insipidus and can result from head trauma, pituitary tumors, tumors adjacent to the pituitary, granulomatous diseases such as tuberculosis and sarcoidosis, meningitis, and vascular anomalies near the hypothalamus. Occasionally, diabetes insipidus is idiopathic. If ADH is present but the patient does not respond by increasing urine concentration, a diagnosis of nephrogenic diabetes insipidus is made. This relative or absolute resistance to ADH is seen in a familial form, may be due to drugs such as demeclocycline or lithium, or may be found in conjunction with tubulointerstitial diseases of the kidneys.

Sweating increases water loss greatly, especially during exertion in hot weather, and gastrointestinal tract losses may be marked in patients with diarrhea or vomiting.

Clinical Features

Hypernatremia and hyperosmolality should be suspected in patients with decreased access to water, especially with altered mental status, or those with a history of polyuria. The elderly patient living in a chronic care facility is especially susceptible. However, many patients are identified through routine electrolyte determinations. The severity of water deficit is estimated from the serum electrolytes and body weight. Figure 2–2 shows a clinical and laboratory approach to patients with hypernatremia.

A. Symptoms and Signs

As with hyponatremia, hypernatremia and hypertonicity affect primarily the brain. Both the addition of solute to the extracellular compartment (sodium chloride, sodium bicarbonate, glucose, or mannitol) and the net loss of water from the body cause water to move out of cells and into the extracellular space. Acute decrease in the size of brain cells can lead to altered mental status, impaired thinking, and loss of consciousness. There is an association of cerebral hemorrhage and hypertonicity and hypernatremia, thought to be due to tearing of blood vessels due to brain shrinkage. In patients who can respond, thirst is an important clue to both hypovolemia and hypertonicity. A history of polyuria and nocturia is important in establishing the cause of hypernatremia as diabetes insipidus of some kind.

The clinical situation and the symptoms and signs may provide clues to the cause of hypernatremia. Addition of large quantities of solute is a rare cause. Salt water near-drowning is said to cause hypernatremia by absorption of Na^+ and Cl^- through the lungs, but this is rare in those who survive asphyxiation. Others will have a history of receiving hypertonic saline, mannitol, glucose, or sodium bicarbonate. Volume overload may cause pulmonary and peripheral edema in these patients, especially when water is given to correct hypernatremia.

A history of decreased water intake may be obtained in patients who have not had access to water at home or in the hospital (acute illness, altered mental status, trauma) or who have had increased normal losses of water from extrarenal mechanisms (exertion in hot weather, diarrhea). Features suggestive of decreased extracellular volume status include hypotension, tachycardia, and oliguria.

Polyuria due to excessive water ingestion is associated with hyponatremia and dilute urine. If the patient has hypernatremia, polyuria with dilute urine suggests that the excessive water loss is due to inability to concentrate the urine appropriately (central or nephrogenic diabetes insipidus).

B. Laboratory Findings

Laboratory studies are needed to make the diagnosis of hypernatremia, confirm serum hyperosmolality, and determine the cause. In general, serum electrolytes and osmolality, glucose, creatinine, and urea nitrogen, urine osmolality, urine Na^+ and creatinine, and urine volume should be measured. Serum sodium > 145 meq/L makes the diagnosis of hypernatremia, and this will be accompanied by serum osmolality > 300 mosm/kg. Special tests to determine the exact mechanism of hypernatremia are performed as needed.

1. Hypernatremia without polyuria—In the absence of renal disease and with normal ADH response, patients in whom addition of solute is the cause of hypernatremia will excrete small amounts of concentrated urine. Urine osmolality is > 300 mosm/kg and usually much higher (up to 1200 mosm/kg in normal young adults). Patients with decreased water intake relative to nonrenal water losses with normal renal function will

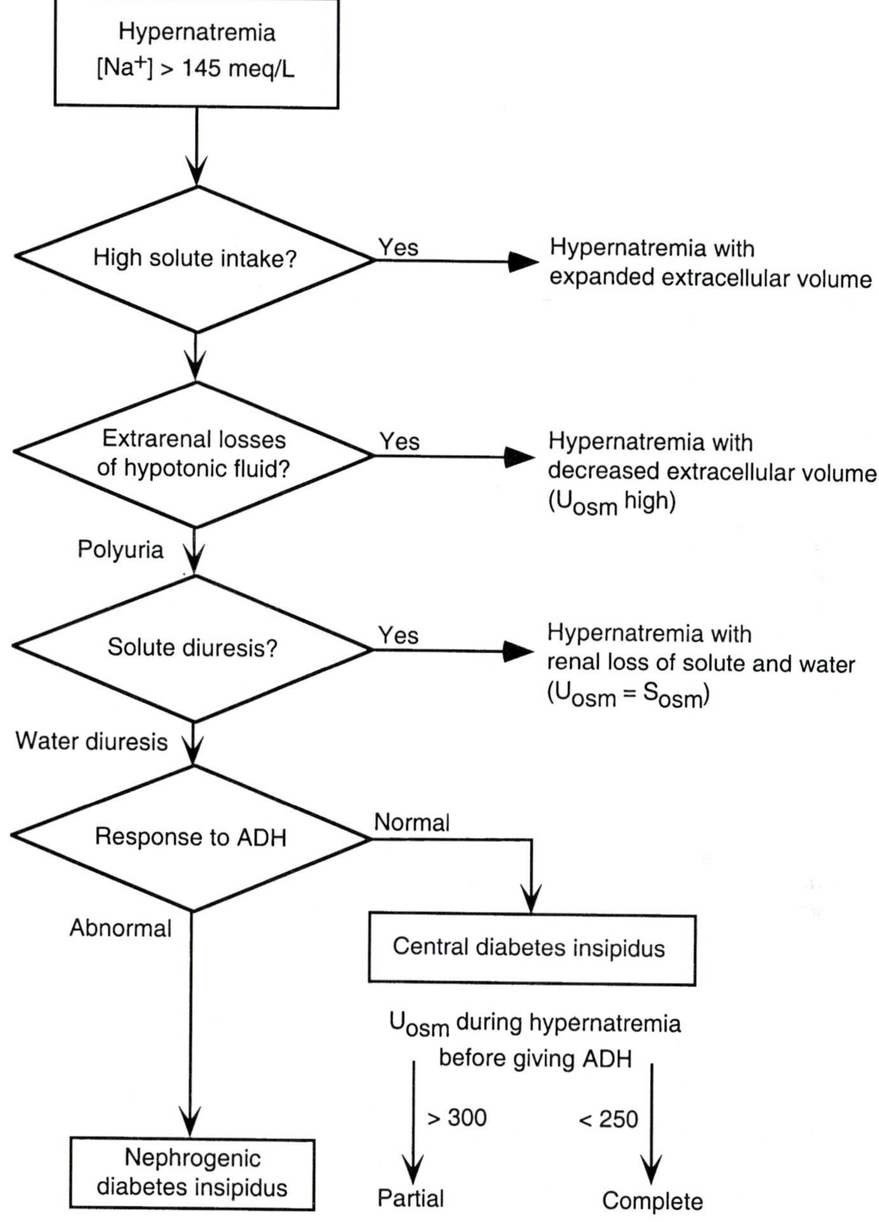

Figure 2–2. Clinical and laboratory approach to the diagnosis of hypernatremia.

also have maximum conservation of urine volume with oliguria, high urine osmolality, serum urea nitrogen: creatinine ratio > 30, low urine Na^+, and low fractional excretion of Na^+.

2. Hypernatremia with polyuria—In the presence of hypernatremia, polyuria with dilute urine suggests that the mechanism of water loss is inability to concentrate the urine appropriately, but the driving force for polyuria may be either solute (osmotic) diuresis or water diuresis.

Water diuresis and solute diuresis can be distinguished by the ratio of urine to serum osmolality (U_{osm}/P_{osm}). U_{osm}/P_{osm} in solute diuresis (osmotic diuresis) is > 0.9; U_{osm}/P_{osm} in water diuresis is < 0.9. This is another way of indicating that solute or osmotic diuresis generally is associated with isosthenuria whereas water diuresis is associated with excretion of dilute urine. Solute diuresis can be further subdivided into that demonstrating electrolyte diuresis and that demonstrating nonelectrolyte diuresis. If $2 \times (U[Na^+] + U[K^+]) > 0.6 \times U_{osm}$, then the majority of solute in the urine consists of electrolytes such as sodium and potassium; if $< 0.6 \times U_{osm}$, then urea, glucose, mannitol, or other nonelectrolyte solute is the cause of the diuresis. Electrolyte diuresis is seen with administration of diuretics and is the normal response to correction of increased extracellular volume. Patients in the ICU who are receiving excessive amounts of normal saline have increased urine output and NaCl diuresis. Urea-induced diuresis occurs after relief of obstructive nephropathy and in the diuretic phase of acute tubular necrosis.

The presence of polyuria with water diuresis may be normal (if the patient has hyponatremia, for example) but is abnormal during hypernatremia, suggesting some form of diabetes insipidus.

3. Diabetes insipidus—Although diabetes insipidus is usually characterized by hypernatremia, polyuria, and decreased ability to concentrate urine maximally, some mild cases may be difficult to identify, and in other cases earlier treatment may confuse the diagnosis. A water deprivation test may be necessary. In this test, a patient with normal or near-normal serum osmolality is deprived of water for a scheduled interval while body weight, serum sodium and osmolality, and urine volume and osmolality are measured. With diabetes insipidus, the patient's polyuria contin–ues despite loss of water, and urine concentration fails to increase into an appropriately high range (> 800 mosm/kg) despite serum osmolality > 290–300 mosm/kg.

Water deprivation is allowed to continue until the patient loses 3–5% of body weight. For safety when designing the water deprivation test, patients should be anticipated to continue to maintain urine output at the starting rate. Thus, for example, if urine volume is initially 600 mL/h, a 60-kg patient could be expected to lose 3% of body weight in just 3 hours; if this urine was maximally dilute (severe central diabetes insipidus), the expected increase in serum osmolality can also be calculated. This does not mean that the test should be stopped at 3 hours. Actual weight loss and urine volume should be used to make the decision. Five units of aqueous vasopressin is administered at the end of the test to see if urine concentration increases. Failure to increase in the presence of diabetes insipidus indicates that the cause is nephrogenic rather than failure of release of ADH. Lack of ADH or of response to ADH can be complete or partial. Identification of intermediate response may be important in deciding treatment, and this can usually be concluded from the degree of urine concentration achieved during the water deprivation test.

Treatment

A. Calculation of Water Deficit

All patients with hypernatremia have increased serum osmolality, and the amount of water needed to correct this state can be calculated from the following equation:

$$\text{TBW (L)} = \text{Normal TBW (L)} \times \frac{140}{[Na^+]}$$

If $[Na^+]$ is 170 meq/L and normal TBW is 0.6 L/kg, the TBW for a man whose customary weight is 70 kg is approximately 42 L × 140 ÷ 170 = 35 kg (L), and the water deficit is 42 − 35 = 7 L. Note that this is the amount of water needed to correct $[Na^+]$ to 140 meq/L. In practice, the patient's normal body weight may not be known but only the current body weight. Using current weight is acceptable as an estimate, but it is potentially misleading because there is a deficit of water contributing to the weight difference.

B. Rate of Correction of Hypernatremia

Just as with hyponatremia, too rapid correction of hypernatremia may be harmful. Cerebral edema with neurologic complications has occurred during correction as a result of a compensatory mechanism intended to maintain normal brain cell volume. In response to development of hypertonicity, brain cells fairly rapidly increase the amount of inorganic ions; this restores cell volume to near-normal but at the expense of disrupted cellular function. With persistence of hypertonicity, brain cells generate and take up idiogenic osmoles, sometimes called organic osmolytes. As cell volume is determined from the amount of solute contained within the cell, organic osmolytes resist the movement of water out of the cells and maintain brain volume close to normal. Many of the organic osmolytes are taken up from the extracellular space by the formation of specific membrane channels. These channels do not quickly disappear or reverse function when hypernatremia is corrected. Therefore, rapid restoration of water to the body may theoretically cause overexpansion of these cells, resulting in cerebral edema. Although mild controversy exists, conservative recommendations are to correct hypernatremia by no more than 10 meq/L per day to allow elimination of organic osmolytes and avoid cerebral edema. This slow rate of correction may not be necessary in patients who develop hypernatremia over the course of a few hours, however.

The following formula is very helpful in calculating the anticipated changes in serum [Na^+] in the hypernatremic patient given intravenous fluids. The rate of correction of serum [Na^+] can be estimated. This formula estimates the amount of change in serum [Na^+] when 1 L of any fluid is administered:

$$\Delta \text{ Serum Na}^+ = \frac{\text{Fluid [Na}^+\text{]} - \text{Serum [Na}^+\text{]}}{\text{TBW} + 1}$$

where TBW is the calculated estimate of total body water (see above). This formula demonstrates how little the serum [Na^+] changes when normal saline ([Na^+] = 154 meq/L) is given to a hypernatremic patient. In order to determine how much hypotonic fluid is needed to achieve a 10 meq/L decrease in serum [Na^+] in 24 hours, begin by calculating the change for 1 L of fluid administered, then calculate for the next liter, etc, until the desired change is reached. The total number of liters of fluid divided by 24 hours will be the hourly infusion rate. Serial measurements of serum [Na^+] are essential because the formula does not account for other fluid sources, urinary losses, or insensible water loss.

C. Hypernatremia Associated With Increased Solute

These patients should have facilitation of solute excretion—if possible, with diuretics and administration of water or 5% dextrose in water. Diuretics will speed removal of sodium and chloride, but the obligate loss of water with the solute will increase the amount of water that must be given. If patients have renal insufficiency, removal of solute may require hemodialysis or ultrafiltration with replacement of water. A few patients have been treated by hemodialysis with dialysate containing hypotonic solution, facilitating water replacement. Peritoneal dialysis using hypotonic solutions should be efficacious in removing extracellular solute and increasing water replenishment.

Patients with hyperosmolality due to severe hyperglycemia are treated with intravenous insulin to lower blood glucose, but normal saline (0.9% NaCl) is the preferred initial fluid replacement. Movement of blood glucose into cells is accompanied by rapid movement of water out of the intravascular space, resulting in severe volume depletion. After adequate normal saline is given, hypotonic fluids (5% dextrose in water) is used to correct net water deficits.

D. Hypernatremia With Diminished Extracellular Volume

These patients have either an extrarenal or renal loss of hypotonic fluid. Therefore, both solute and water have to be replaced. Extracellular volume should be replaced with normal saline first, but it should be remembered that even large volumes of normal saline, despite being hypotonic to plasma in most hypernatremic patients, only very slightly corrects the water deficit. For example, if [Na^+] = 170 meq/L for a normally 70-kg patient, 1 L of 0.9% NaCl will add 308 mosm of solute and 1 L of water, predictably decreasing [Na^+] to only about 169.5 meq/L. Therefore, if more rapid correction of hypernatremia is desired, hypotonic fluid (5% dextrose in water or 0.45% NaCl) should be given as well. In practice, volume repletion is generally a higher priority, but after some correction of the volume deficit, the water deficit should be addressed directly.

E. Hypernatremia Associated With Diabetes Insipidus

Hypernatremia in diabetes insipidus will respond to administration of water orally or 5% dextrose in water intravenously, but correction of hypernatremia depends on giving enough water both to overcome the water deficit and to compensate for continued urine water losses. In severe diabetes insipidus, urine volume can exceed 500 mL/h, and with a severe water deficit, water may have to be given at rates exceeding 600–700 mL/h.

Central diabetes insipidus should respond to synthetic ADH compounds. Aqueous vasopressin (5–10 units two or three times daily) can be given subcutaneously, or desmopressin acetate, which lacks vasopressor effects but retains ADH activity, can be given intravenously or subcutaneously (2–4 μg/d) or by nasal spray. The dose should be adjusted on the basis of serum sodium, urine output, and urine osmolality. Ideally, urine output should be reduced to 3–4 L/d, an amount that can be replaced readily by oral or intravenous administration.

Nephrogenic diabetes insipidus is rarely as severe as complete central diabetes insipidus, and during water deprivation urine osmolality is sometimes as high as 300–400 mosm/kg. Administration of enough water to maintain normal serum [Na^+] can usually be achieved. If a reversible cause such as lithium toxicity is found, the offending agent can be discontinued, though the effect on renal concentrating ability may persist for days. Patients have been given thiazide diuretics to induce a state of mild volume depletion. This leads to increased proximal tubular sodium reabsorption and decreased delivery of sodium and water to the distal diluting segment so that less water is lost thereby.

Adrogue HJ, Madias NE: Aiding fluid prescription for the dysnatremias. Intensive Care Med 1997;23:309–16.

Adrogue HJ, Madias NE: Hypernatremia. N Engl J Med 2000;342:1493–9.

McManus ML, Churchwell KB, Strange K: Regulation of cell volume in health and disease. N Engl J Med 1995;333:1260–6.

Narins RG, Riley LJ: Polyuria: Simple and mixed disorders. Am J Kidney Dis 1991;17:237–41.

Palevsky PM, Bhagrath R, Greenberg A: Hypernatremia in hospitalized patients. Ann Intern Med 1996;124:197–203.

Pazmino PA, Pazmino BP: Treatment of acute hypernatremia with hemodialysis. Am J Nephrol 1993;13:260–5.

DISORDERS OF POTASSIUM BALANCE

Potassium is the most abundant intracellular cation and the second most common cation in the body. The ratio of intracellular to extracellular potassium concentration is normally about 35:1, while sodium is much higher in the extracellular space; and the importance of these distributions is reflected in the ubiquitous Na^+-K^+ ATPase pumps at the cell membranes that continuously move K^+ into and Na^+ out of the cells to maintain these gradients. The intracellular:extracellular ratios for Na^+ and K^+ determine the electrical potential across the cell membrane and are responsible for initiating and transmitting electrical signals in nerves, skeletal muscle, and myocardium. The two major mechanisms that determine potassium balance and serum [K^+] are renal potassium handling and the distribution of potassium between the intracellular and extracellular compartments.

Serum Potassium & Total Body Potassium

Laboratory determinations of potassium are made on either serum or plasma. There is no appreciable difference between the two in the absence of thrombocytosis (which can cause elevated serum potassium but has minimal effect on plasma potassium), and serum potassium will be used in this discussion. Serum potassium [K^+] is closely regulated, but hyper- and hypokalemia do not necessarily indicate increased and decreased total body potassium because of the high proportion of unmeasurable intracellular potassium. For example, movement of K^+ out of the cells into the extracellular space can mask severe depletion of total body K^+; similarly, hypokalemia may be seen despite increase in total body K^+. The use of serum [K^+] to estimate the need to administer or remove potassium from a patient must always take into account factors that alter the intracellular:extracellular distribution of potassium.

Renal Potassium Handling

In the normal steady state, dietary potassium intake is excreted almost entirely by the kidneys, though small amounts of potassium are lost in sweat and gastrointestinal fluids. Large amounts of potassium can be excreted by the kidneys as long as sufficient time to adapt is given, and potassium can be conserved with moderate efficiency in normal individuals, though not to the same extent as sodium.

Almost all potassium in the glomerular filtrate is reabsorbed. Therefore, potassium appearing in the urine comes from secretion of potassium into the tubular fluid through potassium channels on distal renal tubular cells, especially those of the cortical collecting tubules. The rate of potassium secretion is determined by the concentration of tubular cell potassium and the degree of electronegativity of adjacent tubular fluid. Any factors that favor an increase in intracellular potassium or make the tubular fluid more electronegative will increase potassium secretion and urinary potassium excretion. But the strongest impetus to potassium secretion is sodium reabsorption. The aldosterone-regulated Na^+-K^+ ATPase pump on the blood side of the tubular cell transfers potassium from blood into the cell against its concentration gradient and moves Na^+ out of the cell into the blood. This creates a sodium gradient from the tubular lumen into the cell, causing passive movement of sodium through epithelial sodium channels (enhanced by aldosterone) and generating an electronegative luminal fluid as anions such as chloride and bicarbonate follow more slowly than Na^+. In turn, potassium moves from a high concentration inside the cell into the tubule, both because of the lower tubular potassium concentration and because of the more electronegative fluid. It can be seen that potassium excretion would be facilitated by increased aldosterone (increased Na^+-K^+ ATPase pump activity), increased tubular Na^+ delivery (larger quantity of Na^+ to draw out of tubule), the presence of poorly reabsorbable tubular anions (larger negative gradient), and increased intracellular potassium concentration. Clinical correlates of each of these factors can be seen in Table 2–9, by which normal and abnormally excessive potassium excretion can be explained. It follows that failure of these mechanisms for potassium excretion potentially leads to increased total body potassium in the face of continued potassium intake.

Distribution of Total Body Potassium

The other major mechanism determining potassium balance and serum [K^+] is the intracellular:extracellular distribution of potassium. Only a small quantity of

Table 2–9. Serum and total body potassium regulation by renal excretion and extracellular: intracellular distribution.

Mechanism of Regulation	Examples
Renal potassium excretion	
Facilitated by:	
Increased Na^+ reabsorption in distal nephron	Volume depletion, aldosterone
Increased Na^+ delivery to distal nephron	Loop diuretics, thiazides
Increase in poorly reabsorbable anions	Carbenicillin, bicarbonate, keto acids, inorganic anions
Increased intracellular K^+ concentration	Increased intracellular K^+ distribution
Magnesium depletion	Amphotericin B, cisplatin, aminoglycosides
Impaired by:	
Decreased K^+ filtration	Renal insufficiency
Decreased Na^+ delivery to distal nephron	Volume depletion with proximal Na^+ reabsorption
Inhibition of K^+ secretion	Amiloride, spironolactone, triamterene, trimethoprim, decreased aldosterone
Decreased extracellular:intracellular K^+ ratio (hypokalemia)	
Increased plasma insulin level	Exogenous insulin, hyperalimentation
Catecholamines (beta-adrenergic agonists)	Bronchodilators, decongestants, theophylline
Metabolic alkalosis	Vomiting, volume depletion
Increased extracellular:intracellular K^+ ratio (hyperkalemia)	
Decreased plasma insulin level	Diabetes mellitus
Beta-adrenergic blockade	Propranolol
Metabolic acidosis (hyperchloremic)	Ammonium chloride, lysine hydrochloride, arginine hydrochloride, parenteral nutrition
Depolarizing neuromuscular blockade	Succinylcholine

potassium is found in the extracellular space in normals. If serum [K^+] is 4 meq/L and potassium is freely distributed throughout the estimated 12 L of extracellular water in a normal 60-kg subject, then only 48 meq of K^+ is present in this space. The intracellular compartment has a concentration of 130 meq K^+/L × 24 L intracellular volume, or 3120 meq K^+ within cells. The main mechanisms for maintaining this distribution are the Na^+-K^+ ATPase membrane pumps that draw K^+ into the cells and move Na^+ out of cells. These pumps are subject to control by insulin and epinephrine, each stimulating increased Na^+ and K^+ exchange by different mechanisms. Insulin has in fact been considered by some to have serum potassium regulation as its major role. Clinically, exogenous insulin administration is associated with potential for hypokalemia despite no change in total body potassium. In addition, insulin-dependent diabetics with renal insufficiency (inability to excrete potassium readily) are prone to severe hyperkalemia unless adequate insulin therapy is given. Beta-adrenergic agonists also can cause hypokalemia by an epinephrine-like effect, and beta-adrenergic antagonists prolong and amplify the rise in serum potassium after administration of oral or intravenous potassium.

Arterial pH also has an effect on the intracellular: extracellular potassium distribution but does not act through the Na^+-K^+ ATPase pump. However, acid-base disturbances have less effect on serum [K^+] than is generally assumed. Of the acid-base disturbances, metabolic acidosis in which the acid is predominantly extracellular and inorganic—ie, hyperchloremic acidosis–causes the largest change in serum potassium, potentially with severe life-threatening hyperkalemia. The mechanism is thought to be exchange of extracellular hydrogen ion for intracellular potassium in the absence of simultaneous movement of chloride into the cell. Metabolic acidosis in which an organic anion is intracellular—eg, lactic acidosis or ketoacidosis—results in little or no change in serum [K^+]. Metabolic alkalosis often has profound effects on serum [K^+], but the major effect of metabolic alkalosis is to increase the quantity of poorly reabsorbable anion in the distal tubule (bicarbonate) and cause severe renal potassium losses, leading to hypokalemia.

HYPOKALEMIA

ESSENTIALS OF DIAGNOSIS

- *Serum [K⁺] < 3.5 meq/L.*
- *Usually asymptomatic, but there may be muscular weakness.*
- *Severe hypokalemia affects neuromuscular function and electrical activity of the heart: arrhythmias, ventricular tachycardia, increased likelihood of digitalis toxicity.*

General Considerations

Hypokalemia is a potentially hazardous electrolyte disturbance in many critically ill patients. Because the intracellular potassium concentration is so much larger and because it is the ratio of intracellular to extracellular potassium that determines cell membrane potential, small changes in extracellular potassium can have serious effects on cardiac rhythm, nerve conduction, skeletal muscles, and metabolic function. Patients in the ICU may have a variety of disorders that are associated with hypokalemia, including diarrhea, osmotic diuresis, vomiting, metabolic alkalosis, and malnutrition. Treatment with insulin, beta-adrenergic agonists, diuretics, some antibiotics, and other drugs increase the likelihood of potassium depletion and hypokalemia.

Hypokalemia may or may not be associated with depletion of total body potassium. Thus, mechanisms of hypokalemia can be divided into those in which total body potassium is low (decreased intake, increased loss) or those in which total body potassium is normal or high (redistribution of extracellular potassium into cells).

A. Depletion of Body Potassium

Normal subjects require at least 30–40 meq/d to replace obligate losses of potassium, but decreased intake of potassium alone is very rarely a cause of hypokalemia except in critically ill patients who are not being fed or given potassium. More commonly, potassium depletion results from increased potassium loss without adequate replacement. One classification is to divide potassium loss into nonrenal and renal sources (Table 2–9).

Nonrenal potassium losses can occur during severe diarrhea and excessive sweating (although vomiting and nasogastric suction stimulate renal potassium excretion), but renal potassium loss, which results from increased secretion of potassium, is more commonly found in ICU patients. Almost all filtered potassium is reabsorbed, and renal tubular dysfunction rarely leads to impaired reabsorption.

Several factors facilitate renal potassium secretion. First, any cause of increased mineralocorticoids contributes to renal loss of potassium—including volume depletion, in which aldosterone increase is compensatory, and primary hyperaldosteronism. Cushing's syndrome and pharmacologic administration of hydrocortisone, prednisone, or methylprednisolone often lead to decreased [K⁺] due to the mineralocorticoid activity of these corticosteroids. Unusual causes of increased mineralocorticoid activity include licorice ingestion and excess administration of potent synthetic mineralocorticoids such as fludrocortisone. Second, increased delivery of sodium to the distal nephron enhances potassium secretion. Osmotic diuresis from glucose, mannitol, or urea increases distal sodium delivery by interfering with proximal sodium reabsorption. Furosemide, which also increases potassium loss because of volume depletion, increases distal tubular sodium delivery by inhibiting sodium reabsorption in the ascending loop of Henle. Thiazide diuretics increase potassium exchange for sodium in the distal tubules.

Any increased quantity of poorly reabsorbed anions in the tubular lumen increases the electronegative gradient, drawing potassium out of the distal tubular cells. Bicarbonate is less easily absorbed than chloride, and increased distal tubular bicarbonate is found in renal tubular acidosis (proximal type), during compensation for respiratory alkalosis, and in metabolic alkalosis. Other anions include those of organic acids such as keto acids and antibiotics such as sodium penicillin. Hypomagnesemia reduces Na⁺-K⁺ ATPase pump activity, impairing intracellular potassium movement and preventing repletion of total body potassium. Hypokalemia is seen in about 40% of patients with magnesium deficiency; and renal potassium loss paradoxically increases during repletion of potassium in this condition because of failure of cellular uptake. The antifungal agent amphotericin B can cause renal potassium wasting by acting as a potassium channel in the distal tubular cell. Aminoglycosides have been said to be associated with hypokalemia by a similar mechanism, but clinically significant hypokalemia attributed to aminoglycosides is uncommon.

B. Abnormal Distribution of Potassium

Hypokalemia in the face of normal or increased total body potassium must be due to abnormal distribution of potassium between the extracellular and intracellular space. Common causes of decreased [K⁺] from potassium redistribution in ICU patients include drugs and acid-base disturbances. Insulin has a major role in transmembrane potassium transport. Either endogenous insulin, increased after glucose administration, or the combination of exogenous insulin and glucose can lead to hypokalemia by this mechanism. Beta-agonists increase the activity of Na^+-K^+ ATPase pumps, so that beta-adrenergic bronchodilators, sympathomimetic vasopressors, and theophylline are causes of decreased [K^+]. Metabolic and respiratory alkalosis do result in some shift of potassium into cells in exchange for hydrogen ion; the major effect of metabolic alkalosis, however, is to increase renal potassium secretion.

Clinical Features

Figure 2–3 shows a clinical and laboratory approach to the diagnosis of hypokalemia.

A. Symptoms and Signs

Most hypokalemic patients are asymptomatic, but mild muscle weakness may be missed in critically ill patients. More severe degrees of hypokalemia may result in skeletal muscle paralysis, and respiratory failure has been reported due to weakness of respiratory muscles. Cardiovascular complications include electrocardiographic changes, arrhythmias, and postural hypotension. Cardiac arrhythmias include premature ventricular beats, ventricular tachycardia, and ventricular fibrillation. Rhythm disturbances are more commonly seen in association with myocardial ischemia, hypomagnesemia, or when drugs such as digitalis and theophylline have been given. Hypokalemia may exacerbate hepatic encephalopathy by stimulating ammonia generation. The combination of severe hypokalemia, metabolic alkalosis, and hyponatremia is often seen in patients with evidence of volume depletion such as tachycardia, hypotension, and mild renal insufficiency.

Although hypokalemia is most often a laboratory diagnosis, it should be suspected in patients at risk. In the ICU, hypokalemia is commonly found because many critical illnesses and their treatment contribute to renal and nonrenal potassium wasting. Patients being given diuretics (thiazides, loop diuretics, acetazolamide, or osmotic diuretics), beta-adrenergic bronchodilators, theophylline, corticosteroids, insulin, large amounts of glucose, total parenteral nutrition, aminoglycosides, high-dose sodium penicillin, and amphotericin B are among those who should have particular attention paid to monitoring serum [K^+]. Toxic levels of theophylline in particular can cause profoundly reduced serum [K^+]. Patients with volume depletion, especially from diarrhea, vomiting, or nasogastric suctioning (which induces both volume depletion and metabolic alkalosis), and osmotic diuresis should be carefully watched for development of hypokalemia. In patients with renal failure undergoing dialysis, excessive potassium losses are unusual, though they may occur.

B. Laboratory Findings

A serum potassium < 3.5 meq/L makes the diagnosis of hypokalemia. However, there is some evidence that complications of hypokalemia may occur even when serum potassium is in the low end of the normal range. The electrocardiogram may show nonspecific ST and T wave changes, although flattening of the T wave with development of a U wave is considered characteristic with more severe hypokalemia. Serum [Na^+] may be low as a consequence of total body potassium depletion.

Other laboratory findings are helpful for identifying the cause of hypokalemia. Finding the mechanism of hypokalemia is important because inappropriate replacement with large amounts of potassium may lead to hyperkalemia if redistribution rather than depletion of potassium is the cause of hypokalemia. Confirmation of renal potassium wasting can be useful. In the presence of hypokalemia, urinary potassium concentration < 20 meq/L suggests nonrenal potassium wasting, whereas urinary potassium > 20 meq/L enhances the likelihood of renal potassium wasting as the cause of hypokalemia.

The transtubular potassium gradient (or ratio) can be helpful in diagnosing renal potassium wasting:

$$\text{TTKG} = \frac{\text{Urine }[K^+]}{\text{Plasma }[K^+]} \times \frac{P_{osm}}{U_{osm}}$$

where [U_{osm}] is urine osmolality and [P_{osm}] is plasma osmolality. This formula estimates the potassium concentration in the distal nephron by multiplying the urine [K^+] concentration by the ratio of urine osmolality to plasma osmolality to account for the change in water concentration through the collecting ducts. A ratio of distal tubular [K^+] (numerator) to serum [K^+] (denominator) < 2 indicates appropriate renal conservation of potassium in the face of hypokalemia. A ratio > 4 suggests renal tubular potassium wasting. Even if it is known that the mechanism of hypokalemia is excessive urinary loss (diuretics, metabolic alkalosis), urinary potassium determination can be a useful guide to the amount of potassium replacement needed to maintain normal levels or to correct hypokalemia.

Identification of a large quantity of poorly-absorbable anion in the urine is usually not feasible, but an increased quantity of unmeasured anions can be inferred if the sum of urine sodium and potassium exceeds urine chloride concentration by > 40 meq/L.

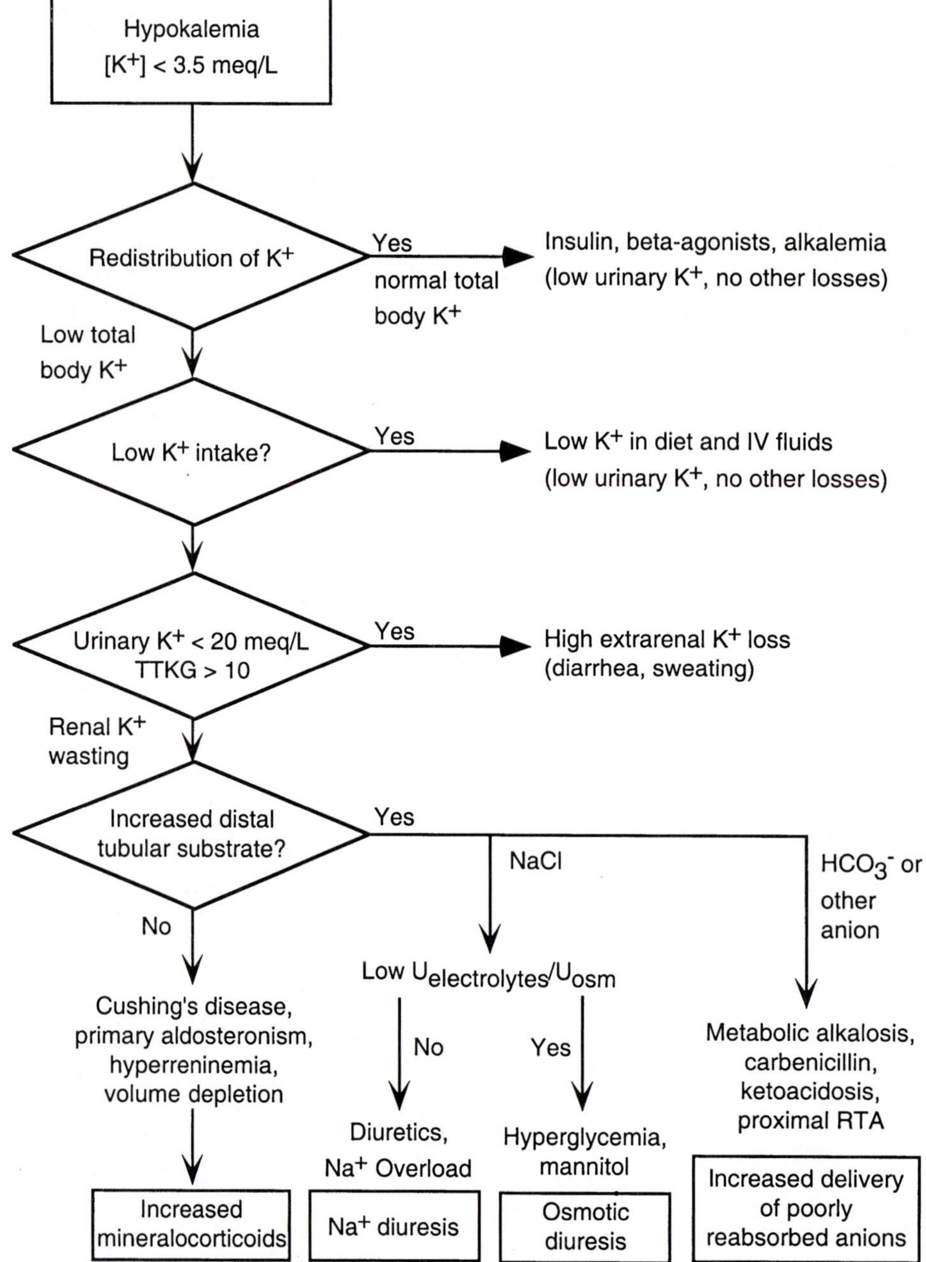

Figure 2–3. Clinical and laboratory approach to the diagnosis of hypokalemia.

Redistribution of potassium leading to hypokalemia cannot be definitely diagnosed by laboratory studies, though metabolic or respiratory alkalosis can be identified by arterial blood gases. Measurement of drug level may confirm theophylline toxicity as a factor contributing to hypokalemia.

Treatment

A. Estimating Total Body Potassium Deficit

Serum $[K^+]$ reflects only the extracellular potassium. Although normal intracellular potassium concentration is 35 times extracellular and normal intracellular volume is twice extracellular, there is no simple relationship between serum [K^+] and total body potassium deficit. Nomograms and formulas for estimating total body potassium deficit based on serum [K^+], pH, and serum osmolality are available, but these should not be relied on heavily. However, in general, patients with severe hypokalemia ([K^+] < 2.5 meq/L) and severe metabolic alkalosis have the largest potassium deficits—up to 400 or 500 meq—while those with hyperchloremic acidosis and mild hypokalemia have milder deficits.

The magnitude of the potassium deficit has implications for the amount of potassium needed to correct the deficit but not necessarily for the urgency or amount immediately needed. Because the clinical manifestations of hypokalemia are determined by the ratio of extracellular and intracellular [K^+], any degree of moderate to severe hypokalemia, regardless of the size of the deficit, may impose the same risk on the patient.

B. Severe Hypokalemia

The oral route is preferred for potassium replacement except in those patients whose oral intake is restricted or whose hypokalemia is life threatening. The rate of administration and the amount of potassium that can be given are limited by local complications (irritation at the intravenous site) and because potassium is initially distributed only into the extracellular space. Too-rapid administration can result in large and dangerous increases in extracellular and serum [K^+] before potassium can be taken into cells. Special care should be taken in patients receiving beta-adrenergic blockers, in type 1 diabetics, and patients with oliguric acute or chronic renal failure.

Potassium chloride and potassium phosphate are available for intravenous use. Potassium chloride should be given unless there is hypophosphatemia (see Hypophosphatemia, on page 46). Intravenous potassium chloride can be given in concentrations as high as 60 meq/L. The total amount of potassium in a single intravenous bag should be restricted, however, to 20–40 meq to avoid the risk of inadvertent rapid administration of excessive amounts, and these amounts should be administered over at least 1 hour into a peripheral vein. Because of the size of the extracellular space into which potassium is initially distributed, 20–40 meq of potassium can cause the potassium to rise as much as of 2–4 meq/L if not quickly distributed to the intracellular compartment.

Intravenous potassium into central venous catheters must be given cautiously and only when absolutely necessary. Very high serum [K^+] levels can be achieved within the heart, resulting in conduction system disturbances. However, the large volume of blood into which the potassium mixes generally dilutes [K^+] rapidly. Large quantities of potassium may be needed in special circumstances to counteract hypokalemia, such as after open heart surgery. It is recommended that each ICU develop a protocol to ensure safety in giving potassium into central venous sites. In any patient receiving intravenous potassium, frequent (every 1–2 hours) serial monitoring of serum [K^+] is mandatory.

C. Potassium Replacement

Potassium needs should be anticipated in ICU patients to avoid hypo- and hyperkalemia. Patients receiving potent diuretics, those on continuous nasogastric suction, those starting intravenous glucose for parenteral nutrition, and those receiving digitalis should be considered for increased potassium supplementation.

Patients with acute myocardial ischemia and infarction may be more prone to arrhythmias, which can be prevented by careful attention to serum potassium levels. Other patients with a potential for hypokalemia include those prescribed beta-adrenergic agonists (bronchodilators) or theophylline and patients with hypomagnesemia. A special case is the treatment of diabetic ketoacidosis. Insulin is expected to drive potassium into cells along with glucose. Although potassium should be withheld in those presenting with hyperkalemia, patients with normal serum [K^+] can generally be expected to require potassium supplementation during insulin treatment because most patients have moderate to severe potassium deficits from earlier osmotic diuresis. In many patients with diabetic ketoacidosis, moderate to severe hypophosphatemia develops, and potassium phosphate is often given.

D. Correct Underlying Disease

The underlying disorder contributing to hypokalemia may or may not be correctable. Correction of magnesium deficiency may correct a state of refractory potassium deficiency. Efforts should be made to control extrarenal losses of potassium and fluid. Diuretics causing hypokalemia generally must be continued for treatment of volume overload states, but benefit can sometimes obtained from potassium-sparing diuretics such as spironolactone, triamterene, or amiloride, though these are less potent natriuretic agents than furosemide. In critically ill patients, potassium replacement plus furosemide is generally preferred over potassium-sparing diuretics, especially if there is renal insufficiency, hypokalemia requiring simultaneous potassium supplementation, and a severe edematous state. Similarly, amphotericin B, aminoglycosides, corticosteroids, and other drugs associated with hypokalemia used in critically ill patients may not be avoidable and must be continued.

Gennari FJ: Hypokalemia. N Engl J Med 1998;339:451–8.

Halperin ML, Kamel KS: Potassium. Lancet 1998;352:135–40.

Kruse JA, Carlson RW: Rapid correction of hypokalemia using concentrated intravenous potassium chloride infusions. Arch Intern Med 1990;150:613–7.

Whang R, Whang DD, Ryan MP: Refractory potassium repletion: A consequence of magnesium deficiency. Arch Intern Med 1992;152:40–5.

HYPERKALEMIA

ESSENTIALS OF DIAGNOSIS

- *Serum [K^+] > 5 meq/L.*
- *Severe hyperkalemia affects neuromuscular function and electrical activity of the heart, with abnormal ECG. May develop heart block, ventricular fibrillation, or asystole.*

General Considerations

While hypokalemia is more common in ICU patients, renal failure, metabolic acidosis, potassium-sparing diuretics, adrenal insufficiency, drugs, and iatrogenic administration of potassium may lead to hyperkalemia. Hyperkalemia has serious effects on myocardial conduction, and most life-threatening emergencies from hyperkalemia involve the heart.

The mechanisms of hyperkalemia can be divided into those in which increased addition of potassium to the extracellular space overwhelms the normal mechanisms of potassium disposal, and those in which the capacity for potassium disposal is impaired. Because hyperkalemia reflects serum [K^+] and not total body potassium, impaired disposal may be due to impaired redistribution of potassium into the cell or impaired excretion of potassium.

A. Addition of Potassium to Extracellular Space

Both exogenous and endogenous sources are causes of hyperkalemia. Exogenous potassium can lead to hyperkalemia if enough potassium is given rapidly enough to raise potassium concentration in the extracellular space. Impaired insulin release or beta-adrenergic blockade facilitates hyperkalemia, but, because the normal extracellular potassium store is only as little as 40–60 meq, rapid potassium administration can easily overwhelm normal redistribution mechanisms. If potassium is given more slowly, however, normal renal excretion makes development of hyperkalemia much less likely. Endogenous sources of large potassium loads are not infrequent in the ICU from rhabdomyolysis due to infection, trauma, or drugs; tumor lysis of lymphoma or leukemia; or severe hemolysis.

A special case of endogenous potassium leading to a false diagnosis of hyperkalemia results from hemolysis of red blood cells after blood has been drawn. Pseudohyperkalemia can also be seen in patients with extreme thrombocytosis or leukocytosis.

B. Impaired Disposal of Potassium

Hyperkalemia can occur if there is redistribution of potassium from the intracellular to the extracellular space or if normal mechanisms of potassium disposal are impaired.

Metabolic acidosis, insulin deficiency, and beta-adrenergic blockade may redistribute potassium out of cells and cause hyperkalemia. Administration of acids with chloride anion (hydrochloric acid, lysine hydrochloride, arginine hydrochloride) is associated with hyperkalemia because of exchange of hydrogen ion for potassium inside the cell. Organic acidoses affect serum potassium much less. Muscle paralysis with succinylcholine, a depolarizing muscle relaxant, releases potassium from muscle cells and prevents reuptake. Type 1 diabetic patients are prone to hyperkalemia because they lack the ability to increase insulin secretion in the face of increased potassium appearance.

1. Renal insufficiency—The kidneys are largely responsible for excretion of potassium and can greatly increase potassium excretion in response to hyperkalemia. Potassium is filtered and then almost completely reabsorbed; this is true even in the face of hyperkalemia. However, in contrast to hypokalemia, in which increased filtration does not cause potassium depletion, decreased filtration does contribute to hyperkalemia. As with hypokalemia, aldosterone plays an important role in renal potassium handling.

Acute renal insufficiency more commonly causes hyperkalemia than chronic renal insufficiency in the absence of increased intake of potassium. Chronically, aldosterone is released in direct response to hyperkalemia (even in anephric patients) and facilitates secretion of potassium in the distal nephron. Decreased glomerular filtrate affects potassium secretion primarily by decreasing the amount of sodium available for lumen-tubular cell exchange, thereby limiting generation of the electronegative gradient that drives potassium secretion.

2. Aldosterone deficiency—Deficiency of aldosterone predictably causes hyperkalemia. Diseases that destroy the adrenal glands result in loss of endogenous glucocorticoids and aldosterone (Addison's disease), but isolated cases of hypoaldosteronism are also seen. In longstanding diabetes, hyporeninemic hypoaldosteronism causes hyperkalemia and hyperchloremic metabolic acidosis (type IV renal tubular acidosis). Spironolactone, an aldosterone antagonist, causes hyperkalemia in susceptible patients.

C. Drugs Associated With Hyperkalemia

Drugs associated with hyperkalemia are classified according to their mechanism of hyperkalemia. Those that impair intracellular potassium distribution include beta-adrenergic blockers, succinylcholine, hydrochloric acid, and other acidifying agents. Some earlier formulations of total parenteral nutrition solutions contained excess chloride salts of amino acids that contributed to hyperkalemia. Drugs that interfere with renal potassium secretion include aldosterone antagonists (spironolactone), potassium-sparing diuretics (triamterene, amiloride), angiotensin-converting enzyme inhibitors, and drugs that decrease renal function (NSAIDs). Patients with heart failure are at risk for both hypokalemia and hyperkalemia because they may be prescribed potent loop diuretics, aldosterone, beta-adrenergic blockers, and angiotensin-converting enzyme inhibitors simultaneously.

A significant number of patients receiving high doses of trimethoprim-sulfamethoxazole have been found to have hyperkalemia. Trimethoprim has been shown to have an amiloride-like effect, blocking distal tubular sodium channels and inhibiting potassium secretion because of decreased tubular electronegativity. Small amounts of potassium in potassium penicillin G (1.7 meq per million units) and transfused blood can cause hyperkalemia, but usually only in patients with impaired potassium handling.

Clinical Features

A clinical and laboratory approach to the diagnosis of hyperkalemia is shown in Figure 2–4.

A. Symptoms and Signs

Hyperkalemia is generally identified by routine measurement of electrolytes in the ICU. In critically ill patients, hyperkalemia may present acutely without warning. The most serious concern is cardiac rhythm disturbances, but weakness may also be present.

The medical history should be reviewed for medications that cause hyperkalemia, recently transfused blood, potential for tumor lysis syndrome, diabetes, renal failure, and other disorders. Intravenous lines should be checked for inadvertent potassium administration. For critically ill patients, consideration of acute adrenal insufficiency is mandatory, especially if the patient had been receiving corticosteroids or has hypotension and hyponatremia.

Those at high risk for development of hyperkalemia include any patient receiving potassium supplementation or who is receiving potassium-sparing diuretics, digitalis, beta-adrenergic blockers, trimethoprim, or angiotensin-converting enzyme inhibitors. Patients with renal insufficiency (especially acute renal failure) or diabetes mellitus (especially type 2 diabetes) may develop hyperkalemia. Hyperkalemia can sometimes occur in patients who are sodium-restricted if they are allowed to use salt substitutes that contain primarily potassium chloride.

The most common associations of hyperkalemia in hospitalized patients were reported to be renal failure, drugs, and hyperglycemia. In one study, administration of potassium to correct hypokalemia was the most frequent cause of subsequent hyperkalemia.

B. Laboratory Findings

Hyperkalemia is diagnosed when serum potassium is > 5 meq/L. The ECG is an important indicator of severity of hyperkalemia, but ECG abnormalities were seen in only 14% of hospitalized patients with hyperkalemia in one study. Asymptomatic electrocardiographic changes occur as serum $[K^+]$ rises, with increased height and sharper peaks of T waves seen first. The QRS duration then lengthens, and the P wave decreases in amplitude before disappearing as serum $[K^+]$ rises. At very high serum $[K^+]$, electrical activity becomes a broad sine-like wave preceding ventricular fibrillation or asystole.

Serum sodium, chloride, glucose, creatinine, and urea nitrogen, arterial blood pH, Pa_{CO_2}, hematocrit, and platelet count should be determined to aid in establishing the cause of hyperkalemia. If the platelet count exceeds 1,000,000/μL, serum potassium may be falsely elevated as the blood clots and potassium is released from platelets; in such cases, plasma potassium will reflect the true value in the body. In renal insufficiency, serum creatinine and urea nitrogen are elevated. Urine potassium may be helpful in determining whether renal potassium elimination is appropriate. The transtubular potassium gradient (see Hypokalemia, on page 38) can determine if the kidneys are contributing to hyperkalemia; a nonrenal cause is more likely if > 10. Serum sodium and chloride may provide evidence of adrenal insufficiency, but other tests of adrenocortical function should be performed. A very low serum cortisol, for example, in the presence of hyperkalemia can be diagnostic of adrenal insufficiency. Arterial blood pH and serum glucose are helpful in deciding on the approach to treatment of hyperkalemia.

Treatment

Arrhythmias suspected of being due to hyperkalemia or electrocardiographic changes with serum $[K^+]$ above the normal range (ie, > 5 meq/L) should be aggressively treated, and the same is true if serum $[K^+]$ is > 6 meq/L even if the ECG shows no evidence of hyperkalemia.

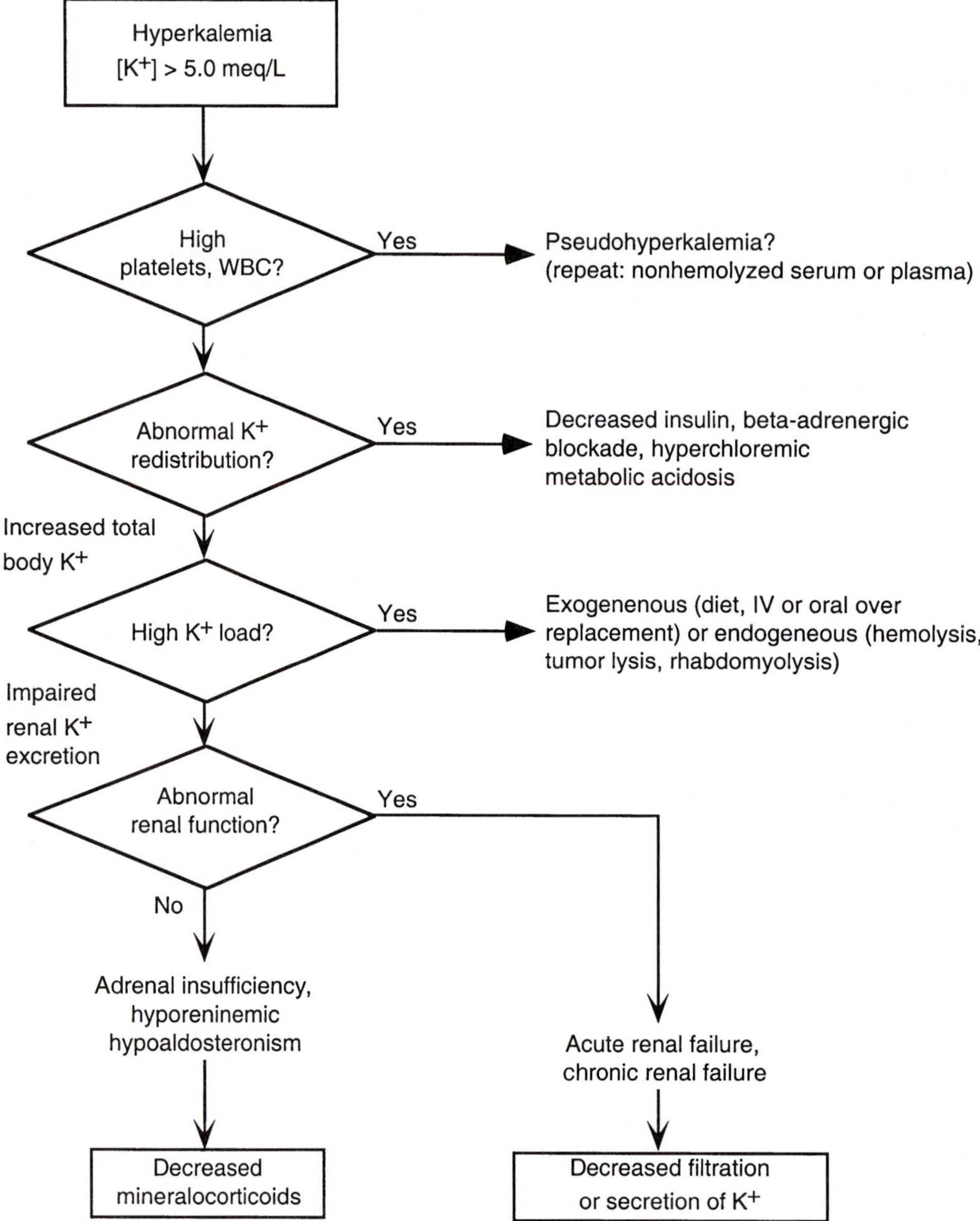

Figure 2–4. Clinical and laboratory approach to the diagnosis of hyperkalemia.

A. Calcium

Combination therapy is usually given to counter the effects of hyperkalemia on the heart and redistribute potassium into cells. Calcium directly reverses the effects of potassium on the cardiac conduction system, though intravenous calcium chloride or calcium gluconate does not affect serum potassium levels. One recommendation is to give 10 mL of 5% calcium chloride intravenously every 1–2 hours as long as [K^+] exceeds 6 meq/L and there are electrocardiographic abnormalities, but the number of doses should not exceed two or three. Calcium should be given cautiously in the presence of digitalis toxicity.

B. Redistribution of Potassium

Insulin has an immediate serum [K^+] lowering effect, but hypoglycemia ensues unless glucose is given simultaneously. Insulin can be given subcutaneously or by intravenous bolus or continuous infusion; a reasonable method for severe hyperkalemia is to administer regular insulin intravenously at a rate of 1–2 units/h while 5% dextrose in water is given at a rate of 125 mL/h (8–10 units insulin in each liter of 5% dextrose in water). One should monitor electrolytes and glucose hourly and watch closely for hypoglycemia. The rate of administration of insulin and glucose can be adjusted accordingly.

Metabolic acidosis contributing to hyperkalemia, if present, can be ameliorated with sodium bicarbonate given intravenously. This treatment is not without hazard, with volume overload and hyperosmolality possible complications. Only enough $NaHCO_3$ should be given to reverse hyperkalemia, not completely correct acidemia. Treatment should begin with one ampule, usually containing 44 meq $NaHCO_3$, given over several minutes. Another ampule can be given if needed in 15–30 minutes. Alternatively, two ampules can be added to 1 L of 5% dextrose in water for continuous intravenous administration (final sodium concentration about 90 meq/L) at 50–150 mL/h. This infusion can be stopped as soon as serum potassium normalizes or in the event of fluid overload.

A few patients with hyperkalemia and renal failure have been reportedly treated with the beta-adrenergic agonist albuterol by nebulization. Modest transient reduction in serum [K^+] can be achieved even with standard bronchodilator doses, but the risks of arrhythmias and other potential problems suggest that this form of therapy should be used only when conventional therapy has failed.

C. Increased Excretion of Potassium

Facilitation of renal excretion mechanisms can help rid the body of excess potassium, but this route of excretion is usable only in patients whose renal potassium excretion is unimpaired. Furosemide increases distal tubule sodium delivery and promotes potassium secretion. Volume replacement with normal saline may be necessary if the patient begins with normal extracellular fluid volume. Mineralocorticoids increase renal potassium excretion, but in patients with a normal adrenal response, aldosterone levels are maximal. Therefore, mineralocorticoids such as fludrocortisone are useful only in patients with adrenal insufficiency or some other cause of depressed aldosterone.

In patients with impaired renal potassium excretion or to increase potassium elimination in any patient with hyperkalemia, increased nonrenal potassium excretion is indicated. A cation exchange resin designed for oral or rectal administration (sodium polystyrene sulfonate) binds potassium in exchange for sodium. If the gastrointestinal tract is functional, 15–60 g mixed in 20–100 mL of water or sorbitol solution can be given orally; the dose can be repeated every 4–6 hours. The suspension can also be given as a retention enema.

Hemodialysis is an effective way of decreasing serum potassium, but hyperkalemia may return rapidly after dialysis as potassium diffuses back out of the cells. Therefore, as much potassium removal as possible is indicated during hemodialysis if it is concluded that a large increase in total body potassium is present. Serum potassium should be carefully monitored during dialysis. Continuous dialysis is very effective, and peritoneal dialysis with dialysate containing no potassium can be used.

D. Other Treatment

Dietary potassium intake should be restricted. In practice, the diet should avoid high-potassium foods, but in ICU patients in whom sparing of body protein is a goal, at least 2.5 g (64 meq) of potassium daily is usually necessary to maintain acceptable protein intake. All intravenous infusions should be double-checked to make sure potassium (sometimes in the form of phosphate as well as chloride) is not being given inadvertently. Potassium penicillin should be switched to sodium penicillin. The need for drugs contributing to potassium maldistribution, impaired excretion, metabolic acidosis, and renal insufficiency should be re-evaluated and the drugs discontinued if possible. These include angiotensin-converting enzyme inhibitors, beta-adrenergic blockers, and potassium-sparing diuretics.

Acker CG et al: Hyperkalemia in hospitalized patients. Arch Intern Med 1998;158:917–24.

Allon M, Dansby L, Shanklin N: Glucose modulation of the disposal of an acute potassium load in patients with end-stage renal disease. Am J Med 1993;94:475–82.

Greenberg S et al: Trimethoprim-sulfamethoxazole induces reversible hyperkalemia. Ann Intern Med 1993;119:291–5.

Halperin ML, Kamel KS: Potassium. Lancet 1998;352:135–40.

Velazquez H et al: Renal mechanism of trimethoprim-induced hyperkalemia. Ann Intern Med 1993;119:296–301.

DISORDERS OF PHOSPHORUS BALANCE

Phosphorus is found in both inorganic (phosphate) and organic forms. Most of the body's store of phosphorus is in the bones (80%), and the vast majority of the remainder is, like potassium, distributed inside cells (muscles, 10%) as organic phosphates. Only 1% is in the blood, and serum phosphorus does not reflect the total body phosphorus. Organic phosphates play a major role in metabolic functions, especially in energy-producing reactions, as part of ATP and other cofactors. In the erythrocyte, 2,3-diphosphoglycerate (2,3-DPG) levels decrease with decreased serum phosphorus concentration, and hypophosphatemia leads to impaired tissue oxygen delivery. In the ICU, hypophosphatemia is associated with dysfunction of red cells, respiratory muscles, the heart, platelets, and white cells and is often due to acute ICU interventions in susceptible patients. Patients with hypophosphatemia may have heart failure, hemolysis, respiratory failure, and impaired oxygen delivery.

Serum phosphorus is reported by the laboratory in milligrams of elemental phosphorus per deciliter but is largely in the form of inorganic phosphate in the divalent (HPO_4^{2-}) and monovalent forms ($H_2PO_4^-$). There are two major determinants of phosphorus balance in the body: the distribution of phosphorus compounds between intracellular and extracellular spaces and the daily intake compared with excretion. The total body store of phosphorus is great, and only a small proportion of total body phosphorus participates in intracellular reactions and shifts between cells and extracellular spaces.

The intracellular phosphorus concentration is considerably larger than the extracellular concentration. Factors that determine the distribution of phosphorus between the two compartments include the rate of glucose entry into cells and the presence of respiratory alkalosis. Glucose movement into cells, facilitated by insulin, traps phosphate intracellularly through generation of ATP for phosphorylation of intermediates of glycolysis. Acute respiratory alkalosis facilitates glycolysis, thereby reducing extracellular phosphorus concentration.

Phosphate intake depends on the type of diet ingested and the presence of active 1,25$(OH)_2$-vitamin D_3, which facilitates both calcium and phosphorus absorption in the gastrointestinal tract. Corticosteroids, dietary magnesium, hypothyroidism, and intestinal phosphate-binding drugs (aluminum hydroxide, calcium carbonate) decrease phosphorus absorption. Net phosphate excretion is primarily through the kidneys by filtration and reabsorption. Normally, reabsorption in the proximal tubules determines phosphorus excretion, and this mechanism is driven and controlled by factors that determine proximal tubular sodium reabsorption. Thus, there is enhanced phosphorus reabsorption in the face of increased proximal sodium reabsorption in volume-depleted states. However, proximal phosphorus reabsorption is also independently regulated by the parathyroid hormone level. This can lead to dissociation between sodium reabsorption and phosphorus reabsorption, as in hyperparathyroidism.

HYPOPHOSPHATEMIA

ESSENTIALS OF DIAGNOSIS

- *Serum phosphorus < 2.5 mg/dL; severe, < 1.5 mg/dL.*
- *May have muscle weakness, including respiratory muscle weakness (failure to wean from respirator) and myocardial dysfunction.*
- *Evidence of impaired oxygen transport.*
- *Impaired platelet and leukocyte function. Hemolysis and rhabdomyolysis may occur with serum phosphorus < 1 mg/dL.*

General Considerations

Hypophosphatemia is associated in the ICU mostly with shift of extracellular phosphorus into cells and is seen as a consequence of acid-base disturbances and as a complication of drugs and nutritional support more often than as a primary problem. Acute hypophosphatemia should be anticipated in postoperative patients; in patients with chronic or acute alcoholism, diabetic ketoacidosis, or head trauma; and in patients receiving total parenteral nutrition or mechanical ventilation.

In theory, hypophosphatemia always results from a problem of maldistribution of total body phosphorus. This is because of the very large quantity of phosphorus in the intracellular space plus the amount of phosphorus in bone even in those with hypophosphatemia (decreased serum phosphorous and extracellular phosphorus). Thus, even states of "phosphate depletion" from increased losses and decreased intake represent a problem of distribution because there must also be decreased ability to mobilize and transfer phosphorus to the extracellular space coincident with depletion. Nevertheless, it is helpful to think of the pathophysiology of hypophosphatemia as being due primarily to redistribution, decreased intake, or increased excretion of phosphorus.

A. Redistribution of Phosphorus

In the ICU, the most common causes of hypophosphatemia are administration of insulin and glucose or acute hyperventilation. Glucose movement into cells (facilitated by insulin) and subsequent glycolysis produce phosphorylated intermediates that are trapped intracellularly. The most striking examples of rapid, severe falls in serum phosphorus are seen in the treatment of diabetic ketoacidosis and in the refeeding syndrome. Diabetic ketoacidosis is associated with pretreatment extracellular phosphate loss from osmotic diuresis and high serum glucose concentrations. The administration of insulin results predictably in hypophosphatemia as glucose and phosphate move into cells. The marked fall in serum phosphate during enteral or parenteral refeeding of chronically malnourished individuals, including alcoholics, reflects low extracellular phosphorus from decreased intake, followed by rapid movement of phosphate and glucose intracellularly. Hypophosphatemia is even more severe if parenteral nutrition formulas lack sufficient phosphorus.

Respiratory alkalosis also causes a shift of extracellular phosphorus into cells. This has been attributed to enhanced activity of the glycolytic enzyme phosphofructokinase at high pH, but this mechanism has been called into question because metabolic alkalosis of comparable degree has little effect on serum phosphorus. Hypophosphatemia seen in salicylate toxicity, sepsis, and hepatic encephalopathy is probably secondary to hyperventilation.

B. Decreased Phosphorus Intake

Decreased intake of phosphorus is usually a chronic problem and is seen in ICU patients with preexisting diseases leading to decreased dietary intake of calcium, phosphorus, and vitamin D. However, binding of phosphate in the gastrointestinal tract by magnesium- and aluminum-containing antacids prevents absorption and can lead to hypophosphatemia, especially when the diet is limited in phosphate content. Because most diets contain adequate phosphorus, low dietary intake of phosphorus is seen only in patients who are not being fed at all.

C. Increased Excretion of Phosphorus

Among all patients, increased renal tubular excretion of phosphate is the most common cause of hypophosphatemia, primarily from subclinical hyperparathyroidism. This mechanism is less common in critically ill patients in whom renal phosphate excretion increases with osmotic diuresis and with the use of acetazolamide, a carbonic anhydrase inhibitor. Metabolic acidosis increases the release of inorganic phosphate into the extracellular space, resulting in increased renal excretion of phosphate, but this is not usually a cause of hypophosphatemia because phosphorus can be easily mobilized from the intracellular stores.

D. Physiologic Effects of Hypophosphatemia

Phosphorus in the form of phosphate plays an important role in intermediary metabolism, especially in intracellular energy production. Clinical consequences of hypophosphatemia relate to decreased production of ATP and erythrocyte 2,3-DPG. Erythrocyte inorganic phosphate concentration is directly related to serum phosphorus, and inorganic phosphate is required for the conversion of glyceraldehyde 3-phosphate to 1,3-diphosphoglyceric acid, a key step in glycolysis. In hypophosphatemia, glycolytic intermediates preceding this enzymatic step accumulate and those following, including ATP and 2,3-DPG, decrease in concentration. Low 2,3-DPG increases the O_2 affinity of hemoglobin ("left-shifted" oxyhemoglobin curve), potentially impairing O_2 delivery to the tissues. Hemolysis is due to impaired ATP generation, probably in a way similar to erythrocyte glycolytic enzyme deficiencies such as pyruvate kinase deficiency. Impaired function of skeletal muscles, including respiratory muscles, and myocardium have been related to both decreased 2,3-DPG and decreased availability of phosphorus to the muscles. In one study, decreased respiratory and peripheral muscle phosphate concentrations were found in 50% of patients with COPD and respiratory failure compared with normal controls.

Clinical Features

Although most patients with hypophosphatemia are identified by routine monitoring of electrolytes, hypophosphatemia should be suspected in certain high-risk ICU patients, ie, those with preexisting total body or extracellular phosphorus depletion or a severe acute disorder causing redistribution of extracellular phosphorus (Table 2–10). The most likely candidates for symptomatic hypophosphatemia are those with combinations of mechanisms, such as patients with diabetic ketoacidosis with osmotic diuresis and insulin administration, and malnourished alcoholics given glucose, insulin, and phosphate-binding antacids. Severely burned patients may have a combination of respiratory alkalosis, pain, sepsis, and increased tissue uptake of phosphate. Patients with severe head injury are reported to have hypophosphatemia and hypomagnesemia due to excessive urinary losses.

A. Symptoms and Signs

Mild to moderate hypophosphatemia is usually asymptomatic. When hypophosphatemia is severe (serum phosphorus < 1.5 mg/dL), patients may complain of muscle weakness. Skeletal and cardiac muscles are involved primarily, and signs of weakness may be present in the respiratory muscles. Patients may be found to have difficulty weaning from mechanical ventilation or may present with symptoms and signs of reversible congestive heart failure. Rhabdomyolysis and hemolysis are uncommon features of severe hypophosphatemia. Al-

Table 2–10. ICU patients at risk for hypophosphatemia.

Preexisting total body or extracellular phosphorus depletion
Malnutrition
Chronic increased renal phosphate loss
Diabetic ketoacidosis (osmotic diuresis)
Alcoholism
Vitamin D deficiency
Fat malabsorption
Chronic antacid use
Acute redistribution of extracellular phosphorus
Respiratory alkalosis
Sepsis
Salicylate toxicity
Hepatic encephalopathy
Toxic shock syndrome
Glucose-insulin administration
Diabetic ketoacidosis
Refeeding syndrome
Hyperalimentation
Treatment of hyperkalemia

though unusual, leukocyte dysfunction may result in an increased tendency to infection, and platelet dysfunction may contribute to bleeding.

Central nervous system dysfunction has been attributed to hypophosphatemia, but consistent features have not been found. Findings have included changes in mental status, seizures, and neuropathy. Changes may be related to direct effects or may occur because of reduced central nervous system oxygen delivery.

B. Laboratory Findings

The diagnosis of hypophosphatemia is made when serum phosphorus is < 2.5 mg/dL, but symptoms are not likely to appear until the serum phosphorus is < 1.5 mg/dL. Other laboratory findings may include features of hemolysis, elevated creatine kinase, and qualitative platelet dysfunction (prolonged bleeding time) when serum phosphorus is 0.5–1 mg/dL. For determining the specific cause of hypophosphatemia, the clinical history is most useful; arterial blood gases, serum glucose, and serum electrolytes and calcium may be helpful. Although useful in evaluation of chronic hypophosphatemia, urinary phosphorus measurement is seldom necessary in ICU patients.

Treatment

A. Assess Urgency of Treatment

In critically ill patients, development of severe hypophosphatemia may require immediate treatment if weakness involving the respiratory muscles precipitates respiratory failure. Generally, serum phosphorus < 1–1.5 mg/dL should be treated immediately. This is especially important when further decrease in phosphorus is anticipated, as in the treatment of diabetic ketoacidosis. Supportive care is essential while severe hypophosphatemia is corrected.

B. Phosphorus Replacement

Recommendations for phosphorus repletion are often confusing because of the way elemental phosphorus and phosphate concentrations and amounts are expressed. At physiologic pH, inorganic phosphate anion exists almost entirely in the monovalent ($H_2PO_4^-$) and divalent (HPO_4^{2-}) forms (about 1:4 monovalent:divalent). This means that the use of milliequivalents is potentially misleading. Laboratories report serum phosphorus as milligrams of elemental phosphorus per deciliter. To avoid confusion, calculations for repletion should be based on milligrams of elemental phosphorus or millimoles of phosphorus or phosphate (these are the same because there is one phosphorus atom for each phosphate regardless of valence). One millimole of phosphate or phosphorus is the same as 31 mg of phosphorus.

Intravenous phosphate is given as sodium or potassium phosphate, available usually at a concentration of 93 mg phosphorus/mL (3 mmol/mL). The amount of phosphorus to be given is difficult to estimate because total body phosphorus may not be decreased (redistribution), and rapid phosphate shifts during treatment may resolve or worsen the problem. Therefore, close monitoring of serum phosphorus and other electrolytes is necessary during repletion, especially if phosphate is given as the potassium salt.

In severe cases (serum phosphorus < 1.5 mg/dL), give 5–7 mg phosphorus/kg intravenously in 1 L of D_5W over 4–6 hours. For a 60-kg adult, this would be approximately 400 mg phosphorus, or about 4 mL of sodium or potassium phosphate solution (3 mmol/mL) in the 1 L infusion. Alternatively, 1 g of phosphorus (about 10 mL of sodium or potassium phosphate [3 mmol/mL]) is added to 1 L D_5W and infused over 12–24 hours or until the serum phosphorus is > 1.5 mg/dL. In less severe hypophosphatemia, an appropriate starting dose would be 2–4 mg/kg intravenously over 8 hours. Oral supplementation can be provided using potassium phosphate or mixtures of sodium and potassium phosphate.

Prevention of hypophosphatemia is important. In patients receiving intravenous glucose, phosphorus supplementation should be considered. Adult patients receiving parenteral hyperalimentation generally require about 1 g of phosphorus daily, or approximately 12 mmol (372 mg) for every 1000 kcal provided.

Routine repletion of phosphorus in patients with diabetic ketoacidosis has been recommended because of the high frequency of hypophosphatemia reported during treatment with insulin infusions. It has been proposed that hypophosphatemia contributes to decreased oxygen delivery, insulin resistance, hyperchloremic acidosis, and other complications of diabetic ketoacidosis. However, routine phosphate replacement has not demonstrated any improvement in intermediate or final outcome.

C. Complications of Treatment

Complications of excessive phosphate repletion include volume overload from sodium phosphate, hyperkalemia from potassium phosphate, precipitation of calcium phosphate in the face of hypercalcemia, and hypocalcemia. In older patients with renal insufficiency and small children, especially with fluid restriction, phosphate salts given for bowel preparation are associated with severe hyperphosphatemia, marked anion gap metabolic acidosis, and hypocalcemia.

Brown GR, Greenwood JK: Drug- and nutrition-induced hypophosphatemia: mechanisms and relevance in the critically ill. Ann Pharmacother 1994;28:626–32.

Fiaccadori E et al: Hypophosphatemia and phosphorus depletion in respiratory and peripheral muscles of patients with respiratory failure due to COPD. Chest 1994;105:1392–8.

Miller DW, Slovis CM: Hypophosphatemia in the emergency department therapeutics. Am J Emerg Med 2000;18:457–61.

Polderman KH et al: Hypomagnesemia and hypophosphatemia at admission in patients with severe head injury. Crit Care Med 2000;28:2022–5.

Subramanian R, Khardori R: Severe hypophosphatemia. Pathophysiologic implications, clinical presentations, and treatment. Medicine 2000;79:1–8.

Weisinger JR, Bellorin-Font E: Magnesium and phosphorus. Lancet 1998;352:391–6.

HYPERPHOSPHATEMIA

ESSENTIALS OF DIAGNOSIS

- *Serum phosphorus > 5 mg/dL.*
- *Usually no symptoms.*
- *Cardiac conduction system disturbances and features of hypocalcemia may occur.*

General Considerations

Hyperphosphatemia as a clinical problem is most often the result of long-standing elevation of serum phosphorus > 5 mg/dL, but acute elevation can have consequences due to precipitation of calcium phosphate salts in the heart, kidneys, and lungs; rarely, acute cardiac conduction disturbances can occur. In addition, calcium phosphate precipitation results in acute hypocalcemia and its consequences.

Severe hyperphosphatemia is associated in the ICU with a shift of intracellular phosphorus out of cells and is seen when there is massive tissue breakdown. Rarely, in patients inadvertently given large amounts of phosphate salts as a bowel preparation, severe anion gap metabolic acidosis may result. Patients in whom this has been reported are elderly or very young, and often have renal insufficiency. More commonly, hyperphosphatemia is seen in chronic renal failure, where there is decreased ability to excrete phosphorus.

Hyperphosphatemia results from impaired excretion of phosphorus or increased addition of phosphorus to the extracellular space.

A. Impaired Phosphate Excretion

There is a large quantity of phosphorus in the intracellular space as well as the phosphorus stored in bone, but the quantity of extracellular phosphorus is small. Normal cell turnover releases a steady quantity of phosphorus into the extracellular space that is taken back up into the cells or bone or excreted by the kidney. Impaired excretion primarily results from chronic renal insufficiency, and—because parathyroid hormone facilitates renal phosphate excretion—hypoparathyroidism impairs renal phosphorus excretion even with normal renal function.

B. Redistribution of Phosphorus

A cause of hyperphosphatemia unique to critically ill patients is massive tissue breakdown, a form of "redistribution" of a large amount of intracellular phosphorus into the extracellular space. The most common form of tissue injury seen in the ICU is rhabdomyolysis from trauma or other muscle injury from infection, drugs, seizures, or metabolic problems. Tumor lysis syndrome, seen after chemo- or radiotherapy of highly responsive tumors (eg, lymphoma), releases large quantities of phosphorus as well as purines (to become uric acid) and potassium. Tumor lysis syndrome is very uncommonly seen in patients with solid tumors except with extensive necrosis. Bowel necrosis may also be associated with hyperphosphatemia. Renal insufficiency exacerbates hyperphosphatemia caused by redistribution of phosphorus. Because insulin and glucose drive phosphorus into cells, diabetics with insulin deficiency might also be more prone to hyperphosphatemia, but this is rarely significant.

C. Excessive Replacement of Phosphorus

Excessive replacement of phosphorus in patients with hypophosphatemia may cause hyperphosphatemia. Factors that may lead to this situation include renal insufficiency and continued replacement of phosphorus after reversal of the cause of hypophosphatemia (correction of respiratory alkalosis). Patients receiving total parenteral nutrition should be monitored closely because standard solutions may contain 300–500 mg of phosphorus per liter. Enemas or oral bowel preparation products used prior to radiographic procedures or colonoscopy may contain a large quantity of sodium phosphate as an osmotic agent. If patients absorb phosphate, severe hyperphosphatemia (serum phosphorus > 20 mg/dL) and anion gap metabolic acidosis have been reported.

Clinical Features

Patients at high risk for development of hyperphosphatemia are those with tissue injury and renal insufficiency (Table 2–11), especially in combination. Other patients in the ICU who may develop hyperphosphatemia include those receiving intravenous or oral phosphorus supplementation for treatment of hypophosphatemia, patients with decreased glomerular filtration because of extracellular volume depletion, those with chronic renal failure, and those given large amounts of oral phosphate salts.

A. Symptoms and Signs

Most patients with hyperphosphatemia of mild to moderate degree are asymptomatic. In more severe cases, if the calcium × phosphorus product is > 60 the risk of ectopic calcification in various organs increases, including the heart, lungs, and kidneys. Acute problems from precipitation of calcium phosphate are mainly restricted to the development of cardiac conduction system disturbances such as heart block.

Table 2–11. ICU patients at risk for hyperphosphatemia.

Impaired excretion of phosphate
Chronic renal failure
Acute renal failure
Extracellular volume depletion
Hypoparathyroidism
Acute redistribution of intracellular phosphorus
Massive tissue breakdown
Rhabdomyolysis
Tumor lysis syndrome (lymphoma)
Hemolysis
Exogenous phosphorus intake
Excessive treatment of hypophosphatemia
Increased dietary phosphorus (with renal insufficiency)
Excessive sodium phosphate enema or laxative use

Acute hyperphosphatemia also can lead to hypocalcemia with development of tetany, seizures, cardiac arrhythmias, and hypotension. Serum calcium should be monitored during treatment of both hypo- and hyperphosphatemia. Hypocalcemia results both from precipitation of calcium phosphate and because of inhibition of renal 1α-hydroxylase necessary for vitamin D activation.

B. Laboratory Findings

The diagnosis of hyperphosphatemia is most often made only by the laboratory finding of serum phosphorus > 5 mg/dL. The specific cause of hyperphosphatemia can usually be determined from the clinical history, but serum creatinine and electrolytes should be obtained. Serum uric acid and potassium are expected to be elevated in tumor lysis syndrome. In rhabdomyolysis, serum creatine kinase and aldolase are elevated and myoglobinuria may be present. In patients who have hyperphosphatemia from administration of phosphate salts, metabolic acidosis with a large anion gap can be found.

Treatment

A. Assess Urgency of Treatment

There is no absolute elevated serum concentration of phosphorus that requires immediate treatment. Rapid treatment should be considered if there is evidence of a cardiac conduction disturbance such as heart block or evidence of symptomatic or severe hypocalcemia. Hypocalcemia in the presence of hyperphosphatemia should be treated by lowering the serum phosphorus rather than by administration of calcium, because the latter action may worsen ectopic calcification.

B. Remove Phosphorus From the Body

Renal excretion of phosphorus depends upon having an adequate glomerular filtration rate. Because phosphate reabsorption is dependent on proximal tubular sodium reabsorption, normal saline infusion in patients who can tolerate this treatment will enhance phosphate excretion. This should be avoided in patients with preexisting increased extracellular volume, congestive heart failure, and renal insufficiency.

Hemodialysis is effective in removing extracellular phosphate but has only a transient effect because of the small proportion of phosphorus in the extracellular fluid. Phosphate binders in the gastrointestinal tract contain calcium, magnesium, or aluminum. Acute administration of these agents has only a mild effect, especially if patients are not being fed enterally. Chronic administration of calcium-containing agents is preferred because of toxicity from magnesium and aluminum in chronic renal failure. However, calcium carbonate should be avoided in acute hyperphosphatemia because of the potential for raising the calcium × phosphorus product. Therefore, aluminum hydroxide is the phosphate binder of choice until the serum phosphorus is returned closer to normal—calcium carbonate is then preferred.

C. Minimize Phosphorus Intake

Exogenous sources of phosphate should be discontinued, largely from total parenteral nutrition solutions and supplemental phosphorus given orally or intravenously. Dietary phosphorus can be minimized by prescribing a low-protein diet and avoiding dairy products that contain both calcium and phosphorus, but this may conflict with nutritional goals.

Kirschbaum B: The acidosis of exogenous phosphate intoxication. Arch Intern Med 1998;158:405–8.

Sutters M, Gaboury CL, Bennett WM: Severe hyperphosphatemia and hypocalcemia: a dilemma in patient management. J Am Soc Nephrol 1996;7:2056–61.

Thatte L et al: Review of the literature: severe hyperphosphatemia. Am J Med Sci 1995;310:167–74.

Weisinger JR, Bellorin-Font E: Magnesium and phosphorus. Lancet 1998;352:391–6.

DISORDERS OF MAGNESIUM BALANCE

Magnesium is the most abundant intracellular divalent cation and, after calcium, the most common divalent cation in the body. The distribution of magnesium is similar to that of potassium, with the vast majority (99%) of magnesium residing inside cells. Consequently, serum magnesium concentration does not reflect total body magnesium. Magnesium plays an important role in neuromuscular coupling, largely through its interaction with calcium. In the ICU, disorders of magnesium primarily reflect hypomagnesemia, with cardiac arrhythmias and other features similar to those of hypocalcemia. Among the causes of hypomagnesemia are drugs frequently used in critically ill patients such as amphotericin B, diuretics, and aminoglycoside antibiotics, but hypomagnesemia is also seen in malnutrition, chronic alcoholism, and malabsorption. In contrast, hypermagnesemia in ICU patients is relatively uncommon and almost always results from a combination of renal insufficiency and increased magnesium intake. On occasion, hypermagnesemia results from overzealous repletion of hypomagnesemia.

Magnesium Intake & Distribution

Magnesium is found in many foods, including green vegetables and meat products, and the normal diet is usually more than ample. Approximately 5 mg/kg/d of magnesium is required for normal magnesium balance. Magnesium is supplied as part of enteral feedings and is added to parenteral nutrition formulations. Factors that control gastrointestinal magnesium absorption are unclear, but about one-third of ingested magnesium is absorbed. The absorbed fraction decreases with increased ingestion, suggesting an active transport mechanism. Magnesium binds to fatty acids and oxalate in the gut, decreasing absorption. Like potassium, magnesium is distributed largely within cells, but the mechanisms controlling distribution do not seem to be controlled by circulating levels of hormones such as insulin or epinephrine or by acid-base status. About 25% of plasma magnesium is protein-bound.

Magnesium Excretion

Free magnesium is filtered and largely reabsorbed under steady state conditions in the proximal nephron (a minor role), ascending loop of Henle (accounting for about 60–70% of reabsorption), and the distal nephron (about 10%). The distal nephron, however, is the major site of fine regulation of magnesium excretion. Only about 100 mg of magnesium is excreted per day even though as much as 2400 mg is filtered by the glomeruli, and reabsorption is increased in the face of magnesium deficiency. The driving force for magnesium reabsorption is the reabsorption of Na^+ and K^+, causing an electropositive gradient from lumen to extracellular space. As would be expected, drugs that interfere with sodium reabsorption interfere with magnesium reabsorption. Because the ascending portion of the loop of Henle accounts for a large fraction of magnesium reabsorption, loop-acting diuretics predictably have a potent magnesium-wasting effect.

Disposal of excess magnesium appears to be due to decreased reabsorption. When serum magnesium levels are elevated—as happens, for example, shortly after intravenous administration of a large quantity of magnesium salt—renal magnesium excretion increases. This is partly because a lower proportion is protein-bound and partly because only a fixed amount rather than a fixed proportion of the larger filtered load is excreted. Maximum magnesium excretion is essentially limited by glomerular filtration, as would be expected from its renal handling.

Role of Magnesium

A major role of magnesium is that of a cofactor for hundreds of identified enzymes that produce or require ATP, such as kinases, ATPase, and adenylyl cyclase. Disorders of magnesium may lead to impaired energy production, substrate utilization, and synthetic processes.

HYPOMAGNESEMIA

ESSENTIALS OF DIAGNOSIS

- *Serum [Mg^{2+}] < 1.7 mg/dL.*
- *Cardiac arrhythmias, refractory potassium deficiency.*
- *Features suggestive of hypocalcemia: tetany, weakness, increased deep tendon reflexes, altered mental status, and seizures.*

General Considerations

Decreased serum magnesium has serious consequences in critically ill patients, potentiating arrhythmias, interfering with potassium repletion, and causing neuromuscular weakness. However, hypomagnesemia is frequently unrecognized because routine serum [Mg^{2+}] levels are not always obtained. Some investigators have recommended that this test be included as part of daily electrolyte determinations whenever these are deemed necessary for patient care. The prevalence of hypomagnesemia in ICU patients has been estimated to be about 20–65%, and most of these patients are on the medical rather than surgical services. Hypomagnesemia is defined as a serum magnesium concentration < 1.7 mg/dL, but about 25% of plasma magnesium is bound to albumin. While the serum level does reflect both bound and unbound magnesium, the clinical effects of magnesium, like those of calcium, are due to the unbound ion.

The mechanisms of hypomagnesemia can be divided into decreased intake and increased losses of magnesium, both renal and extrarenal in nature (Table 2–12).

A. Decreased Magnesium Intake

Decreased intake is an unusual cause of decreased [Mg^{2+}], but patients with no oral intake who receive parenteral nutrition without magnesium supplementation can develop hypomagnesemia. More commonly, the diet contains sufficient magnesium, but intestinal causes of malnutrition interfere with its absorption. Alcoholism is often associated with hypomagnesemia, but it is likely that factors in addition to malnutrition play roles in causing low [Mg^{2+}] in these patients, such as increased renal losses, vomiting, and diarrhea. In malabsorption syndromes, increased levels of free fatty acids in the intestinal lumen may bind magnesium in a poorly absorbable state.

Table 2–12. Risks for hypomagnesemia in ICU patients.

Increased loss of magnesium
Renal loss
Volume expansion
Osmotic diuresis
Diuretics
Amphotericin B
Aminoglycosides
Cyclosporine
Diuretic phase of acute tubular necrosis
Extrarenal loss
Diarrhea
Nasogastric suction or vomiting
Pancreatitis
Intestinal fistulas with external drainage

B. Increased Loss of Magnesium

Increased losses of magnesium are most commonly due to renal magnesium wasting. Intrinsic renal parenchymal diseases primarily lead to hypermagnesemia, but relief of acute obstructive nephropathy (postobstructive diuresis), osmotic diuresis, and the diuretic phase of acute tubular necrosis sometimes lead to large amounts of magnesium excretion. In the ICU, renal magnesium wasting is most commonly secondary to drugs, including loop diuretics, cyclosporine, cisplatin, aminoglycosides, amphotericin B, pentamidine, and poorly absorbable anionic antibiotics such as ticarcillin and carbenicillin in large doses. These drugs, along with ethanol, decrease tubular magnesium reabsorption. Nonrenal losses of magnesium occur in association with intestinal bypass, sprue, malabsorption, severe diarrhea, short bowel syndrome, biliary fistulas, and other mechanisms of fluid loss from the gastrointestinal tract. Hypomagnesemia is also found in association with diabetes mellitus, phosphate depletion, hyperparathyroidism, and thyrotoxicosis.

Two specific primary renal magnesium wasting disorders are described. Gitelman's syndrome is due to a defect in the thiazide-sensitive sodium/chloride cotransporter and presents with hypocalciuria and hypomagnesemia. The other is a syndrome of hypercalciuria, nephrocalcinosis, and renal tubular acidification defect.

Whether abnormally low serum [Mg^{2+}] can result from maldistribution of this cation between extracellular and intracellular spaces is debated. One possible cause of hypomagnesemia is vigorous refeeding after starvation. Both hypomagnesemia and hypocalcemia may be seen during acute pancreatitis, primarily from deposition of these cations into the tissue.

C. Hypomagnesemia and Acute Myocardial Infarction

There is an association between hypomagnesemia and acute myocardial infarction that is not explicable by renal or other increased excretion of magnesium. Hypomagnesemia occurring with acute myocardial infarction persists for 5–12 days, and $[Mg^{2+}]$ then generally returns to normal. Whatever the mechanism, the association is strengthened by the finding that treatment with magnesium has a beneficial effect in such patients found to have decreased $[Mg^{2+}]$ by reducing the frequency and consequences of ventricular arrhythmias.

Clinical Features

A. Symptoms and Signs

Hypomagnesemia has individual effects, but because it may be accompanied by hypokalemia, hypocalcemia, and metabolic alkalosis, clinical features may result from a composite of abnormalities. Cardiac arrhythmias are the most important complications of hypomagnesemia. Ventricular rhythms such as torsade de pointes, ventricular tachycardia, and ventricular fibrillation as well as atrial tachycardia and atrial premature beats can be seen. There is an association of increased arrhythmias with digitalis toxicity and hypomagnesemia. Acute myocardial infarction imposes a further arrhythmia risk when decreased serum $[Mg^{2+}]$ is found. Hypocalcemia is strongly associated with hypomagnesemia. Tetany, a positive Chvostek and Trousseau sign, seizures, weakness, and altered mental status may be seen.

Most patients with hypomagnesemia are identified by routine serum $[Mg^{2+}]$ determinations, but the disorder should be anticipated in certain high-risk groups, ie, patients with hypocalcemia, acute myocardial infarction, congestive heart failure, alcoholism, acute pancreatitis, malnutrition, diarrhea, or seizures and those receiving diuretics, amphotericin B, or aminoglycosides.

B. Laboratory Findings

Hypomagnesemia is diagnosed when serum $[Mg^{2+}]$ is < 1.7 mg/dL. In critically ill patients, $[Mg^{2+}]$ levels should be obtained when routine serum electrolytes are needed. This probably means at least daily for most high-risk patients. In patients with hypomagnesemia, other electrolytes, serum calcium, phosphorus, and urinary magnesium may be helpful for diagnostic purposes.

Because magnesium is largely intracellular, serum $[Mg^{2+}]$ may not reflect magnesium depletion. Red cell and leukocyte $[Mg^{2+}]$ concentrations do not offer much better sensitivity or specificity. Some studies have shown that a functional magnesium loading test can identify patients who may benefit from supplemental magnesium, including those with normal $[Mg^{2+}]$ levels. These patients may be identified by greater retention of magnesium (> 70% of a loading dose of 30 mmol of magnesium sulfate).

Two electrolyte disturbances are closely tied to hypomagnesemia and total body magnesium depletion: hypokalemia and hypocalcemia. Hypomagnesemia is seen in a large percentage of those with hypokalemia (40%). Although this may be due to similar renal handling of these cations or coincidental gastrointestinal losses, refractory potassium deficiency may be due to magnesium deficiency. Hypomagnesemia interferes with potassium movement into cells, leading to net potassium leakage out of cells (enhancing total body potassium depletion), by inhibiting Na^+-K^+ ATPase pumps. Intracellular potassium falls while intracellular sodium concentration rises. Refractory potassium deficiency occurs because administered potassium is unable to enter cells readily and is therefore excreted in the urine. Hypomagnesemia also stimulates renin release and thereby increases aldosterone, further enhancing potassium excretion.

Hypomagnesemia is also strongly associated with hypocalcemia and inappropriately low levels of parathyroid hormone. Parathyroid hormone release is impaired by hypomagnesemia, and the hormone has a reduced effect in the presence of hypomagnesemia. In fact, serum $[Ca^{2+}]$ has been used to estimate the effective $[Mg^{2+}]$ concentration. Clinical findings of severe hypocalcemia, including Chvostek's sign and tetany, can be due both to hypomagnesemia and to the resultant hypocalcemia.

The electrocardiogram may show arrhythmias, but flattened T waves, widening of the QRS, PR prolongation, and U waves may be seen in moderate to severe magnesium deficiency.

Treatment

Serum magnesium measures both protein-bound and unbound magnesium, but more than 95% of magnesium in the body is found in the bones and intracellularly. In contrast to potassium, however, rarely are there instances of normal or high serum $[Mg^{2+}]$ in patients with depletion of total body magnesium. These considerations suggest that serum $[Mg^{2+}]$ is a reasonable guide to deciding that total body magnesium is low but perhaps not ideal for determining the degree of depletion. Fortunately, in the absence of a decreased glomerular filtration, administered magnesium is readily excreted when serum $[Mg^{2+}]$ is > 2 mg/dL, suggesting that repletion of magnesium is apt to be indicated and safe in almost all patients with $[Mg^{2+}]$ < 1.5–1.7 mg/dL.

A. Assess Urgency of Treatment

Therapy is indicated in patients having or anticipated to have serious cardiac arrhythmias due to or contributed to by hypomagnesemia. Seizures, especially if not responsive to seizure medications, should receive immediate treatment with magnesium if hypomagnesemia is suspected. In high-risk groups, serum [Mg^{2+}] should be used as a guide, but even a mildly reduced serum [Mg^{2+}] may call for aggressive magnesium replacement therapy, especially for patients with myocardial infarction, digitalis toxicity, or congestive heart failure. If hypocalcemia is symptomatic and due to hypomagnesemia, repletion of magnesium may be more effective and safer than administration of calcium. Hypokalemia refractory to potassium administration may respond to magnesium replacement; an arrhythmia due to hypokalemia or hypomagnesemia is an indication for urgent magnesium therapy.

B. Estimate Replacement Requirements

Estimation of total body magnesium deficiency is often inaccurate. In magnesium deficiency, the deficit ranges between 6 mg/kg and 24 mg/kg body weight. For a 60-kg adult with moderate magnesium deficiency (12 mg/kg), the deficit is about 720 mg. Because serum levels may not reflect the magnitude of the deficit, replacement is usually initiated and serum [Mg^{2+}] is followed with repeated measurements.

C. Magnesium Replacement

Intravenous magnesium sulfate ($MgSO_4$) can be given as 50% solution added to 5% dextrose in water or normal saline. Each 1 mL of 50% solution contains 500 mg of $MgSO_4$, or about 2 mmol (48 mg) of elemental magnesium.

In severe hypomagnesemia, 1–2 g of $MgSO_4$ (4–8 mmol) can be given over 20–30 minutes (2–4 mL of 50% solution of $MgSO_4$ in 50–100 mL of 5% dextrose in water). This can be followed by 4–8 mmol of magnesium over 6–8 hours and repeated as needed. It is not uncommon to find that patients need 25–50 mmol in 24 hours. It has been recommended that one should limit intravenous magnesium replenishment to 50 mmol in 24 hours except in severe life-threatening hypomagnesemia, though about 50% of intravenous magnesium will be excreted into the urine even in the presence of magnesium deficiency. Although serum levels of Mg^{2+}, Ca^{2+}, and K^+ are useful for following replacement, some clinicians recommend following deep tendon reflexes. These reflexes disappear with hypermagnesemia but usually only at very high toxic levels. Replacement doses of magnesium in patients with renal insufficiency should be reduced, and [Mg^{2+}] must be carefully watched.

Dietary intake of approximately 5 mg/kg/d (about 300 mg) of magnesium is required for normal magnesium balance. Magnesium supplementation is not usually required in patients eating a reasonable diet or who are receiving enteral feeding formulas. Parenteral nutrition solutions should provide about 12 mmol/d (about 300 mg/d) of magnesium.

D. Correction of Cause of Hypomagnesemia

Patients with self-limited gastrointestinal tract losses will not require continued magnesium therapy, but renal magnesium wasting may be caused by required medications such as antibiotics, amphotericin B, and diuretics. In these patients, continued magnesium supplementation may be necessary.

Dacey MJ: Hypomagnesemic disorders. Crit Care Clin 2001;17:155–73.

Hebert P et al: Functional magnesium deficiency in critically ill patients identified using a magnesium-loading test. Crit Care Med 1997;25:749–55.

Oster JR, Epstein M: Management of magnesium depletion. Am J Nephrol 1988;8:349–54.

Weisinger JR, Bellorin-Font E: Magnesium and phosphorus. Lancet 1998;352:391–6.

Whang R, Whang DD, Ryan MP: Refractory potassium repletion: A consequence of magnesium deficiency. Arch Intern Med 1992;152:40–5.

HYPERMAGNESEMIA

ESSENTIALS OF DIAGNOSIS

- *Serum [Mg^{2+}] > 2.7 mg/dL.*
- *Serum [Mg^{2+}] > 7 mg/dL: weakness, loss of deep tendon reflexes, and paralysis.*
- *Serum [Mg^{2+}] > 10 mg/dL: hypotension and cardiac arrhythmias.*

General Considerations

In contrast to hypomagnesemia, increased [Mg^{2+}] is seen in a limited number of disorders. The normal kidney's generous magnesium excretion capacity suggests that both increased intake of magnesium and decreased glomerular filtration rate are necessary for hypermagnesemia to develop. Hypermagnesemia in critically ill patients occasionally occurs, and impaired neuromuscular and cardiac function may result.

A. Increased Magnesium Intake

Increased intake alone is a very rare cause of increased serum [Mg^{2+}]. High intake of magnesium by the oral route is unusual and is almost never from dietary sources. Magnesium-containing antacids (magnesium hydroxide) and laxatives (magnesium citrate) provide the only likely sources of increased oral magnesium ingestion. Excessive amounts of intravenous magnesium sulfate can be given inadvertently in the course of parenteral nutrition or during replacement therapy, making close monitoring of serum [Mg^{2+}] mandatory. In the treatment of preeclampsia-eclampsia, large amounts of intravenous magnesium sulfate are sometimes given, with the goal of achieving serum [Mg^{2+}] well above the usual normal range.

B. Decreased Magnesium Excretion

Unbound magnesium is filtered, and the amount appearing in the urine represents what is not reabsorbed. In the presence of increased serum [Mg^{2+}], a larger quantity is non-protein-bound, increasing the amount filtered compared with the glomerular filtration rate. Magnesium is reabsorbed as a result of sodium reabsorption in proximal, loop of Henle, and distal sites. In the absence of enhanced sodium reabsorption, there is no change in the quantity of reabsorbed magnesium, and the net result in hypermagnesemia is increased renal excretion. However, any disorder impairing glomerular filtration has the potential for causing hypermagnesemia, including acute and chronic renal failure. An increase in sodium reabsorption, such as seen in volume-depleted states, may impair renal magnesium excretion by facilitating magnesium reabsorption.

Clinical Features

A. Symptoms and Signs

Effects of hypermagnesemia are nonspecific and include lethargy, weakness, and hyporeflexia. More severely increased [Mg^{2+}] levels are associated with loss of deep tendon reflexes, hypotension (from interference with membrane calcium transport), cardiac arrhythmias, respiratory depression, and drowsiness.

Hypermagnesemia should be suspected in patients with renal insufficiency who are receiving magnesium-containing medications or oral or parenteral magnesium supplementation or replacement. Other high-risk critically ill patients include those receiving nephrotoxic drugs, those with hypotension or hypovolemia and oliguria, and those with preeclampsia-eclampsia who are receiving large doses of intravenous magnesium. Patients with chronic renal failure should have antacids containing magnesium restricted. Elderly patients with diminished renal function who use magnesium-containing antacids and laxatives or vitamins containing magnesium salts may have an increased incidence of hypermagnesemia.

B. Laboratory Findings

A serum magnesium level over 2.7 mg/dL makes the diagnosis of hypermagnesemia. Other laboratory studies that should be obtained include other serum electrolytes and serum creatinine and urea nitrogen. Urinary magnesium may of value in confirming that hypermagnesemia is due to increased intake of magnesium rather than decreased renal excretion.

Treatment

A. Hypermagnesemia Requiring Urgent Treatment

Patients who are symptomatic and who have serum [Mg^{2+}] > 8–10 mg/dL should be urgently treated. Most commonly they will have muscle weakness or paralysis and hypotension, prompting evaluation and treatment. Intravenous calcium gluconate or calcium chloride will counter the effects of excessively high [Mg^{2+}]. The amount of calcium should be limited in the presence of renal failure if serum phosphorus is elevated.

B. Decrease Intake of Magnesium

Magnesium-containing antacids and other agents should be identified and discontinued. Intravenous fluids, especially parenteral nutrition fluids, should have magnesium sulfate removed.

C. Increase Magnesium Excretion

In patients with normal renal function who develop hypermagnesemia, even a large excess of magnesium will be excreted rapidly without intervention. The majority of patients with decreased glomerular filtration will not be able to increase excretion appreciably, as they are limited by decreased filtration. Nevertheless, inhibition of ascending loop of Henle sodium reabsorption with furosemide may impair magnesium reabsorption somewhat. Patients who can tolerate volume expansion should also be given normal saline to facilitate magnesium excretion. In patients who have severe hypermagnesemia, greatly enhanced magnesium removal requires hemodialysis.

Clarck BA, Brown RS: Unsuspected morbid hypermagnesemia in elderly patients. Am J Nephrol 1992;12:336–43.

Fassler CA et al: Magnesium toxicity as a cause of hypotension and hypoventilation. Arch Intern Med 1985;145:1604–6.

Weisinger JR, Bellorin-Font E: Magnesium and phosphorus. Lancet 1998;352:391–6.

DISORDERS OF CALCIUM BALANCE

Calcium is the most abundant divalent cation in the body. The vast majority (98%) of calcium is in the form of hydroxyapatite in the bone, and only a very small amount is in the extracellular fluid. Nevertheless, plasma and extracellular calcium has a major role in the control of neuromuscular coupling and contraction. Serum calcium is regulated by a very complex system of hormones, vitamins, and organ function and is closely tied to phosphorus and magnesium regulation. In the ICU, both hyper- and hypocalcemia are seen. Severe hypercalcemia is due primarily to malignant disorders; there are fewer patients who have severe hypercalcemia from hyperparathyroidism, vitamin D toxicity, sarcoidosis, and other disorders. Hypocalcemia is seen in patients with chronic or acute renal failure, hyperphosphatemia, hypomagnesemia, and drug treatment.

Physiologic Considerations

A. Calcium Intake

Dietary calcium has a wide range in adult patients. Calcium absorption from the intestinal tract is influenced by 1,25-dihydroxyvitamin D, but calcium uptake is also proportionate to calcium intake. Calcium is primarily taken up in the duodenum and jejunum. Binding of calcium in the lumen to form insoluble salts (phosphate and free fatty acids) will interfere with absorption.

B. Plasma Calcium

Plasma calcium is about 40% protein-bound to albumin and other plasma proteins, and a smaller fraction (10%) is attached to various anions. Total calcium is normally about 9–10 mg/dL; therefore ionized calcium is normally about 4.5–5 mg/dL. An important cause of decreased total plasma calcium is hypoalbuminemia, but ionized calcium, the component important in symptomatic hypocalcemia, may not be reduced. One approximation is that for each decrease of 1 g/dL of albumin from normal, 0.2 mmol/L (0.8 mg/dL) is added to the serum calcium as a correction factor. A change in plasma pH will affect the degree of protein binding of calcium to plasma proteins; acidosis increases and alkalosis decreases ionized calcium.

C. Renal Calcium Excretion

Free calcium is filtered and largely reabsorbed (> 95%) under steady state conditions in the proximal nephron (accounting for about 60% of reabsorption), the ascending loop of Henle, and the distal nephron. Although passive movement of calcium is largely responsible for calcium uptake in the proximal tubule, there is some active transport. In the loop of Henle, the driving force for calcium reabsorption is the reabsorption of Na^+ and K^+, causing an electropositive gradient from lumen to extracellular space. Drugs that interfere with sodium reabsorption here (loop-acting diuretics) interfere with calcium reabsorption and lead to increased calcium excretion. On the other hand, the action of thiazide diuretics in the distal tubule favors calcium reabsorption, increasing serum calcium and decreasing calciuria. Under physiologic conditions, the normal kidneys can conserve calcium extremely well (< 100 mg/d) and can increase excretion to very high levels in the face of hypercalcemia.

D. Regulation of Plasma Calcium

In contrast to magnesium, which does not appear to be under hormonal control, plasma calcium is regulated primarily by two interacting hormones: parathyroid hormone (PTH) and vitamin D ($1,25[OH]_2$ D_3). These two hormones serve to control the complex cycle of calcium between the intestinal lumen (dietary calcium), the large reserve of calcium in the bone, and renal excretion. They also play important roles in the control of phosphorus distribution, absorption, and excretion.

1. Parathyroid hormone—Hypocalcemia stimulates release of PTH from the parathyroid glands. PTH binds to receptors in bone and renal tubular cells and stimulates adenylyl cyclase, resulting in increased intracellular cAMP levels. The effect of PTH is to mobilize calcium by bone resorption and, in the kidneys, to decrease calcium excretion, increase phosphate excretion, and stimulate increased synthesis of active vitamin D ($1,25[OH]_2$ D_3). In the absence of PTH, patients can have severe hypocalcemia and hyperphosphatemia; in states of excess PTH from hyperplasia of the parathyroid glands, hypercalcemia and hypophosphatemia are noted.

2. Vitamin D—Vitamin D_3 is a fat-soluble vitamin that is found in various amounts in the diet. Ultraviolet light also results in some conversion of precursor substances to vitamin D_3 in the skin. The most active vitamin D compound is $1,25(OH)_2$ D_3, which is synthesized by conversion of vitamin D_3 in two stages to $25(OH)D_3$ by the liver and to $1,25(OH)_2$ D_3 by the kidneys. The rate of conversion of $25(OH)D_3$ to $1,25(OH)_2$ D_3 is indirectly accelerated by hypocalcemia through the action of PTH on the kidneys. Active $1,25(OH)_2$ D_3 has as its major actions increases in calcium and phosphorus absorption from the gastrointestinal tract and helps PTH mobilize calcium from the bone.

HYPOCALCEMIA (Table 2–13)

ESSENTIALS OF DIAGNOSIS

- *Serum Ca^{2+} < 8.5 mg/dL.*
- *Nervous system irritability, including altered mental status, focal and grand mal seizures, paresthesias, tetany, hyperreflexia, muscle weakness.*
- *Prolonged QT interval, cardiac arrhythmias.*

General Considerations

Decreased plasma calcium can have serious consequences in critically ill patients, potentiating arrhythmias and seizures. However, most patients in the ICU with hypocalcemia (total Ca^{2+} < 8.5 mg/dL) are asymptomatic. This is because most of these patients have low serum albumin levels, and the non-albumin bound or ionized fraction of Ca^{2+} that participates in neuromuscular coupling is normal. Total serum Ca^{2+} can be "corrected" for hypoalbuminemia by adding 0.8 mg/dL to the measured total Ca^{2+} for every 1 g/dL decrease in albumin below 3.5 g/dL. If the value is above 8.5 mg/dL, ionized calcium is likely to be normal except with extreme changes in pH. Ionized serum calcium measurements can confirm this correction, if indicated.

There is an abundance of calcium in the body, but much of it is in poorly mobilized forms. Therefore, when hypocalcemia occurs, there must be a failure of the normal regulatory mechanisms for serum calcium. Calcium can leave the extracellular space when driven by reactions that deposit calcium in the bones and soft tissues or when there is insufficient PTH to mobilize calcium from the bone. In the ICU, a few other factors may also lead to hypocalcemia—notably drugs and hyperphosphatemia.

Table 2–13. Risks for hypocalcemia in ICU patients.

Decreased intake of calcium
Malabsorption of calcium or vitamin D
Steatorrhea
Decreased PTH or decreased PTH effectiveness
Hypoparathyroidism, parathyroidectomy
Hypomagnesemia
Acute pancreatitis
Vitamin D deficiency
Chronic renal insufficiency
Other
Septic shock
Rhabdomyolysis
Acute hyperphosphatemia
Treatment of hypercalcemia
Hypoalbuminemia

A. Calcium Deposition

In critically ill patients, hypocalcemia may be seen in acute pancreatitis and rhabdomyolysis. Calcium is deposited in the form of calcium soaps (poorly soluble salts of Ca^{2+} and fatty acids) in the case of pancreatitis or in other forms in damaged skeletal muscle. Rarely—less commonly than at one time believed—large amounts of blood transfusions have been associated with hypocalcemia, probably from chelation of Ca^{2+} by citrate used as an anticoagulant. Most other patients with hypocalcemia from deposition have hyperphosphatemia. In these patients, when the product of calcium × phosphorus > 60, there is a tendency to form calcium phosphate in soft tissues. An important cause of hypocalcemia is the tumor lysis syndrome, in which there is sometimes massive release of phosphorus into the blood. Hyperphosphatemia may also be seen in ICU patients in whom excessive phosphorus repletion is given to correct hypophosphatemia or from bowel preparation solutions containing sodium phosphate. Most patients with chronic renal failure will have some degree of hyperphosphatemia that facilitates hypocalcemia unless they are effectively treated with oral phosphate-binding agents and vitamin D supplementation.

B. Decreased PTH or PTH Effect

Hypoparathyroidism is occasionally seen in the ICU but is rarely undiagnosed or unsuspected prior to admission. It is still occasionally seen after thyroid surgery when parathyroid glands are not adequately preserved. On the other hand, hypomagnesemia has an important effect of decreasing PTH release from parathyroids, contributing to hypocalcemia. There are rare congenital forms of PTH resistance.

In critically ill patients, hypocalcemia may also be due to a decreased effect of PTH action. Hypomagnesemia decreases the action of PTH on bone. Pancreatitis is usually thought to cause hypocalcemia from soft tissue deposition, but there may also be resistance to PTH in this disease. Vitamin D deficiency also interferes with the action of PTH.

C. Other Causes

Loop-acting diuretics such as furosemide may cause excessive calcium excretion by the kidneys, but this is rarely a cause of hypocalcemia alone because of effective counterregulatory mechanisms. Treatment of hypercalcemia with plicamycin and calcitonin may lead to excessively low Ca^{2+}—but again, this is rarely seen. Finally, patients with renal failure have hypocalcemia from a combination of mechanisms, including hyperphosphatemia and decreased vitamin D conversion.

Clinical Features

A. Symptoms and Signs

Central nervous system and peripheral nervous system effects are the most common features of hypocalcemia. Altered mental status, including lethargy and coma, may be present. Seizures may be focal or generalized, and hypocalcemia may complicate a known seizure disorder. More often, hypocalcemia is manifested by tetany, paresthesias, and hyperreflexia. The Chvostek and Trousseau signs may be positive. When severe, hypocalcemia may result in muscle weakness. Hypocalcemia prolongs the QT interval on the ECG. Ventricular arrhythmias may be seen, including ventricular fibrillation.

Patients with chronic hypocalcemia may have manifestations of bone resorption of calcium and have features of the underlying disease leading to decreased serum Ca^{2+}.

For ICU patients, review of medications and recent conditions that may affect serum Ca^{2+} should be undertaken. Medications that may play a role include furosemide, phenytoin, calcium-lowering drugs such as plicamycin and bisphosphonates, blood transfusions, and phosphate therapy. Patients with renal failure (acute or chronic), rhabdomyolysis, pancreatitis, tumors, malnutrition, and gastrointestinal disorders should be considered at risk for hypocalcemia.

B. Laboratory Findings

Hypocalcemia is diagnosed when serum Ca^{2+} is < 8.5 mg/dL after appropriate correction for low serum albumin levels. In critically ill patients, Ca^{2+} should be measured when routine serum electrolytes are needed. This probably means at least daily for most high-risk patients. In patients with hypocalcemia, serum sodium, potassium, chloride, magnesium, phosphorus, amylase, and creatine kinase may be helpful for making a specific diagnosis.

Vitamin D levels in the blood can be measured, including $1,25(OH)_2\ D_3$ if necessary. PTH can also be assayed and the value compared with the normal range for the Ca^{2+} concentration. In most cases of hypocalcemia in the ICU, these measurements are not necessary.

Treatment

A. Need for Treatment

Low serum Ca^{2+} calls for treatment if the patient is symptomatic, especially with very low Ca^{2+} and tetany, arrhythmias, or seizures. Hypomagnesemia, because of multiple effects leading to hypocalcemia, is also a treatment priority and can usually be corrected with little risk of complications except in patients with renal insufficiency.

Patients with decreased total serum calcium but with hypoalbuminemia or pH changes sufficient to maintain a normal estimated ionized calcium do not require calcium replacement.

Patients with both acute severe hyperphosphatemia and hypocalcemia represent a treatment problem. Raising serum calcium in the face of hyperphosphatemia may precipitate widespread calcium phosphate deposition. Only enough calcium to prevent or reverse cardiovascular complications should be given. It may be advisable to determine serum ionized calcium in this situation for guidance. Acute hemodialysis to lower serum phosphorus could be helpful.

B. Treatment of Severe Hypocalcemia

Treatment with intravenous calcium gluconate or calcium chloride is indicated. Calcium chloride may be less well tolerated than calcium gluconate, but this is often not an important consideration. Each compound is available in ampules containing 10 mL of 10% solution containing 93 mg of Ca^{2+} for calcium gluconate and 273 mg of Ca^{2+} for calcium chloride. For rapid intravenous infusion, give one ampule over 10–30 minutes. For persistent hypocalcemia, intravenous calcium gluconate can be given as 8–12 mg/kg (about 6–8 ampules of calcium gluconate) of Ca^{2+} over 6–8 hours.

During treatment, serum Ca^{2+} should be rechecked, along with phosphorus and magnesium. Following the physical examination and the ECG may be helpful in deciding when treatment should be slowed or changed to oral supplementation.

C. Correction of Cause of Hypocalcemia

Patients with pancreatitis and rhabdomyolysis may have transient hypocalcemia of varying duration followed by release of Ca^{2+} back into the extracellular space. Therefore, these patients should be monitored closely for development of normocalcemia or even hypercalcemia. In other patients, treatment of the underlying cause of hypocalcemia may be effective. Patients with chronic renal failure with hypocalcemia may respond to vitamin D and dialysis.

Bushinsky DA, Monk RD: Calcium. Lancet 1998;352:305–11.

Desai TK, Carlson RW, Geheb MA: Hypocalcemia and hypophosphatemia in acutely ill patients. Crit Care Clin 1987;3:927–41.

Tohme JF, Bilezikian JP: Hypocalcemic emergencies. Endocrinol Metab Clin North Am 1993;22:363–75.

Zaloga GP, Chernow B: Hypocalcemia in critical illness. JAMA 1986;256:1924–9.

HYPERCALCEMIA (Table 2–14)

ESSENTIALS OF DIAGNOSIS

- *Serum Ca^{2+} > 10.5 mg/dL.*
- *Altered mental status with confusion, lethargy, psychosis, and coma.*
- *Hyporeflexia and muscle weakness.*
- *Constipation, shortening of QT interval, pancreatitis.*
- *Features of chronic hypercalcemia may be seen: bone changes, band keratopathy.*
- *May have features of underlying disease: hyperparathyroidism, malignancy, sarcoidosis, vitamin A toxicity.*

General Considerations

Hypercalcemia is frequently a cause of admission to the ICU as well as a complication of a variety of disorders. Most often, hypercalcemia is identified by a routine serum calcium level (Ca^{2+} > 10.5 mg/dL), but severe hypercalcemia with altered mental status is a medical emergency. Patients may be admitted to the ICU for management, especially for close monitoring of intravascular fluid therapy but also for treatment with a variety of medications. Hypercalcemia of severe degree is almost always due to malignant disease, including solid tumors, lymphoma, and multiple myeloma. Causes of more mild hypercalcemia include granulomatous diseases such as sarcoidosis, tuberculosis, and fungal diseases, and hyperparathyroidism.

The mechanisms of hypercalcemia, like hypocalcemia, reflect the large amount of Ca^{2+} flux between the gastrointestinal tract, bone, kidneys, and extracellular space. Hypercalcemia is the result of failure of the regulatory mechanisms for calcium, including inability to suppress PTH, or the presence of an abnormal amount of mobilization of calcium by an abnormally produced PTH-like compound or active vitamin D. PTH activates or stimulates osteoclasts that mobilize calcium from bone. Vitamin D primarily increases calcium absorption from the gastrointestinal tract. A few other miscellaneous causes of hypercalcemia are occasionally seen in the ICU.

Table 2–14. Risks for hypercalcemia in ICU patients.

Increased intake of calcium
Calcium-containing antacids
Milk-alkali syndrome
Increased PTH or PTH effectiveness
Hyperparathyroidism
Vitamin D intoxication
Hypercalcemia of malignancy
PTH-related peptide
Increased vitamin D conversion
Bone destruction
Cytokines
Others
Thiazide diuretics
Immobilization
Thyrotoxicosis
Granulomatous diseases (vitamin D conversion)

A. Failure of Normal Calcium Regulation by Parathyroid Hormone

Hypercalcemia is seen in primary hyperparathyroidism from adenoma or hyperplasia. In the past, patients were identified when symptomatic from renal stones, bone pain, or symptoms of hypercalcemia. Most often, these patients are now identified from routine screening laboratory tests that include serum Ca^{2+}. A diagnosis can be easily made by the finding of PTH levels that are high in the presence of elevated serum Ca^{2+}.

B. Abnormal PTH-Like Substance

The most frequent cause of severe hypercalcemia is malignancy. Although a variety of mechanisms of hypercalcemia have been identified, the most important is release by the tumor of a peptide that has homology with PTH. This has been called parathyroid hormone-related peptide (PTHrP). The effects of PTHrP are similar to those of PTH, causing increased serum calcium and decreased serum phosphorus. Hypercalcemia from this substance is seen in bronchogenic carcinoma and many other malignancies. Hypercalcemia in malignant disease is also caused by other factors, including bony metastases with bone destruction, and the effects of cytokines, including interleukins and TGF-β.

C. Abnormally Produced Vitamin D

Excessive administration or ingestion of vitamin D can cause hypercalcemia, but this does not occur immediately. Toxic doses of vitamin A may also cause hypercalcemia. Granulomatous diseases are associated with increased production of $1,25(OH)_2\ D_3$ by macrophages within the granulomas. Although sarcoidosis is the best-known entity that is associated with hypercalcemia, tuberculosis, berylliosis, and fungal diseases behave similarly. In some patients with granulomatous diseases, hypercalciuria is more common than hypercalcemia. This is probably because both elevated Ca^{2+} and vitamin D inhibit PTH release. In the absence of elevated PTH, renal calcium excretion is high, resulting in hypercalciuria without hypercalcemia.

D. Other Causes

Patients recovering from acute pancreatitis or rhabdomyolysis can have a rebound of serum Ca^{2+} levels as Ca^{2+} is released back into the extracellular space. Milk-alkali syndrome results from ingestion of calcium and antacids by a patient with renal failure. Milk-alkali syndrome is associated with the unusual combination of hypercalcemia and hyperphosphatemia. Hypercalcemia can rarely be seen as a manifestation of hyperthyroidism. Thiazide diuretics decrease renal calcium excretion. Immobilization does not cause hypercalcemia but exacerbates other mechanisms.

Clinical Features

Most patients with hypercalcemia of mild degree are identified by routine serum Ca^{2+} determinations on screening laboratory tests. On occasion, patients are symptomatic, and hypercalcemia is detected during workup.

A. Symptoms and Signs

Hypercalcemia has effects on mental status, including lethargy and psychosis. Patients may develop absent deep tendon reflexes and muscle weakness. A major complaint may be constipation, and bowel sounds are usually decreased. Polyuria and impaired urinary concentrating ability (nephrogenic diabetes insipidus) are consequences of hypercalcemia. The ECG may show a shortened QT interval. Arrhythmias may be precipitated in patients receiving digitalis. Hypercalcemia is associated with and may be a causal factor in peptic ulcer disease and pancreatitis.

Hypercalcemia should be suspected in patients with malignancies of the breast, prostate, lung, kidney, liver, and head and neck. Patients with multiple myeloma may have hypercalcemia as well. Sarcoidosis, tuberculosis, fungal infections, and other granulomatous diseases may be associated with significant hypercalcemia, but rarely is serum [Ca^{2+}] high enough to cause severe symptoms.

Other symptoms and signs are related to the underlying disease, especially with long-standing hyperparathyroidism (renal stones, fractures, bony deformities, band keratopathy, and conjunctivitis). Patients with hypercalcemia of malignancy usually do not have evidence of long-term hypercalcemia but may have findings related to the primary or metastatic tumor.

B. Laboratory Findings

A serum calcium level over 10.5 mg/dL makes the diagnosis of hypercalcemia. Other laboratory studies that should be obtained include serum phosphorus, other electrolytes, and creatinine and urea nitrogen. In hypercalcemia, polyuria may result from inability to concentrate the urine. Renal calcification and obstructive uropathy from renal stones may lead to renal insufficiency.

For severe hypercalcemia, treatment can be initiated without knowledge of the underlying cause. However, specific diagnosis may be helped by obtaining a PTH level. Assays for PTH and PTHrP are available to distinguish primary hyperparathyroidism from hypercalcemia of malignancy mediated by PTHrP. Vitamin D levels are rarely needed for workup of hypercalcemia.

Treatment

A. Need for Treatment

Patients with mild hypercalcemia need not be treated immediately or aggressively unless symptomatic. Severe hypercalcemia ([Ca^{2+}] > 12–13 mg/dL) should be treated even if asymptomatic, and hypercalcemia of any degree with symptoms, especially altered mental status or seizures, should be vigorously treated. Treatment is directed at lowering serum Ca^{2+} by increased renal excretion and by decreasing mobilization from the bone stores.

In patients with symptomatic or severe hypercalcemia, a four-pronged approach is used: expansion of extracellular volume, furosemide, calcitonin, and pamidronate.

B. Increased Excretion of Calcium

As discussed above, unbound plasma calcium is filtered and largely reabsorbed. Calcium reabsorption is closely tied to sodium reabsorption in the proximal nephron and loop of Henle. Expansion of extracellular volume with 0.9% NaCl decreases passive proximal reabsorption of calcium. Loop diuretics are given both to prevent volume overload and to inhibit active sodium and passive calcium reabsorption in the loop of Henle. In severe hypercalcemia, intravenous 0.9% NaCl should be given at a rate of 200–300 mL/h or more. Patients with cardiac disease and the elderly may be unable to tolerate these large volumes, and pulmonary edema may develop. In such patients, central venous pressure or pulmonary artery wedge pressure measurements may be necessary.

Because calcium absorption is coupled to sodium reabsorption in the ascending loop of Henle, furosemide will increase calcium excretion. Furosemide can be given in a dosage of 20–60 mg every 2–6 hours as needed to maintain urine output. Furosemide is also useful to maintain natriuresis in patients given large volumes of intravenous NaCl. Thiazide diuretics should not be given, since these drugs have a tendency to cause hypercalcemia by inhibiting renal calcium excretion in the distal tubule. In patients given large doses of furosemide, hypokalemia and hypomagnesemia may be problems.

Serum magnesium will predictably fall with the combination of furosemide and saline. Serum calcium will usually begin to decline within a few hours as long as 0.9% NaCl is given at a sufficient rate.

C. Decreased Bone Mobilization of Calcium

Bisphosphonates are very effective agents used for management of hypercalcemia and have low toxicity. These drugs bind to bone hydroxyapatite and inhibit osteoclast activity for a prolonged period. Their action is moderately rapid, with onset of effect within 2 days and maximum effect at about 1 week. The effect of these drugs is evidenced by a fall in serum Ca^{2+} while urinary Ca^{2+} decreases. With use of bisphosphonates, a large proportion of patients will have return of Ca^{2+} to normal range regardless of the cause of hypercalcemia.

Pamidronate is more effective than etidronate because of its longer duration of action and effect on hypercalcemia. Pamidronate is given as a single dose of 60 or 90 mg intravenously over 24 hours, with 60–100% of patients having normal serum Ca^{2+} 10–13 days later. The higher dose is given for more severe hypercalcemia (> 13.5 mg/dL). Patients with renal insufficiency should be given a smaller dose of pamidronate. Side effects of pamidronate are minor, and the effect may last for up to 2 weeks, though the calcium-lowering effect may be shorter and less pronounced in patients with hypercalcemia of malignancy. Newer bisphosphonates, including oral agents, are used mostly for mild hypercalcemia or to prevent osteoporosis or hypercalcemia.

Calcitonin (calcitonin-salmon, 4 IU/kg intramuscularly as a starting dosage) has a slight and short-term effect but can be used in the initial phase of therapy. It is nontoxic and acts most quickly of all of these agents. Calcitonin promotes renal excretion of calcium, inhibits bone resorption, and inhibits gut absorption of calcium. The effect of calcitonin diminishes within a few days, but other treatments are likely to be effective by then.

Plicamycin blocks bone resorption of calcium. It can be given to any patient with hypercalcemia but is used most often in hypercalcemia of malignancy. The usual dose is 25 μg/kg in 50 mL D_5W intravenously over 3–6 hours. Ca^{2+} begins to decline at about 24 hours and normalizes in about 60% of patients. Plicamycin should not be used in the presence of severe renal or liver failure or thrombocytopenia. It is much less used since the advent of bisphosphonates.

D. Other Therapy

Hemodialysis is effective in lowering serum Ca^{2+} in patients who have inadequate renal function or who cannot tolerate forced diuresis. Corticosteroids have a role in hypercalcemia mediated by elevated vitamin D (in granulomatous disorders) and in multiple myeloma. The effect is not immediate, as corticosteroids probably decrease absorption of calcium from the gut by interfering with vitamin D activation. Gallium nitrate works by inhibiting bone resorption but without affecting osteoclast activity directly. While intravenous sodium phosphate has a predictable calcium-lowering effect, this treatment is rarely used at present because of the precipitation of calcium phosphate in soft tissues. On the other hand, oral sodium phosphate therapy is effective in forming insoluble calcium phosphate deposits in the gut.

Bilezikian JP: Management of acute hypercalcemia. J Clin Endocrinol Metab 1993;77:1445–9.

Bushinsky DA, Monk RD: Calcium. Lancet 1998;352:305–11.

Mundy GR, Guise TA: Hypercalcemia of malignancy. Am J Med 1997;103:134–45.

Nussbaum SR et al: Single-dose intravenous therapy with pamidronate for the treatment of hypercalcemia of malignancy: comparison of 30-, 60-, and 90-mg dosages. Am J Med 1993;95:297–304.

Ralston SH et al: Cancer-associated hypercalcemia: Morbidity and mortality. Clinical experience in 126 treated patients. Ann Intern Med 1990;112:499–504.

ACID-BASE HOMEOSTASIS & DISORDERS

PATHOPHYSIOLOGY

Arterial pH is largely determined by the relative concentrations of bicarbonate (HCO_3^-) and carbon dioxide (CO_2) in the blood. The former is controlled principally by renal conservation or excretion of bicarbonate and hydrogen ion, the latter largely by pulmonary ventilation. Decreased arterial pH is called **acidemia** and increased arterial pH **alkalemia.** The disturbances responsible for these changes are **acidosis** and **alkalosis,** respectively, and these changes are defined as "metabolic" (not due to an increase or decrease in CO_2) or "respiratory" (due to primary increase or decrease in CO_2).

Acid-Base Buffering Systems

The major acid-base buffering system in the blood involves carbon dioxide and bicarbonate anion. Carbon dioxide, bicarbonate, and carbonic acid are interconverted according to the following reaction:

$$H^+ + HCO_3^- \Leftrightarrow H_2CO_3 \Leftrightarrow CO_2 + H_2O$$

The relationship between the species that define pH is known as the Henderson-Hasselbalch equation:

$$pH = 6.1 + \log\frac{[HCO_3^-]}{0.03 \times Paco_2}$$

Under normal conditions, the balance between these components is tightly controlled. Within 95% confidence limits, the pH of the arterial blood is between 7.35 and 7.43. For $Paco_2$, the limits are 37 mm Hg and 45 mm Hg. Bicarbonate concentration normally varies between 22 meq/L and 26 meq/L. If hydrogen ions are added to the blood, the reaction shifts rightward, with production of CO_2 and water. Normally, the CO_2 so produced is rapidly eliminated by the lungs.

The bicarbonate-carbon dioxide buffering system is the major extracellular buffer. Other minor extracellular buffer systems also contribute to stabilization of the pH. After extracellular buffering occurs, a second intracellular phase takes place over the next several hours. The main intracellular buffer systems include hemoglobin, protein, dibasic phosphate, and carbonate in bone. The ratio of extracellular to intracellular buffering is approximately 1:1 unless the acid load is very large or continues over a long period of time. Contribution by both the extracellular and intracellular buffers means that an exogenous acid load (or deficit) has a volume of distribution approximately equal to that of the total body water (50–60% of ideal body weight).

Finally, both bicarbonate and CO_2 act as a "dynamic" buffering system. For usual buffers, the addition or removal of hydrogen ion, for example, is countered by corresponding opposite effects of the buffer components. This minimizes pH change at the expense of consumption of some of the buffer components, limiting the maximum buffering capacity. For the bicarbonate-CO_2 system, however, physiologic mechanisms greatly increase the buffer capacity. For example, metabolic acidosis can be countered by decreased arterial $Paco_2$ whereas a respiratory acidosis is countered by increased serum bicarbonate. Because the lungs can eliminate a vast amount of CO_2 per day, this serves as a very powerful buffering system. Similarly, the kidneys can eliminate bicarbonate if necessary or can regenerate bicarbonate.

Renal Handling of Bicarbonate

The kidneys perform two major functions in acid-base homeostasis. First, they reclaim filtered bicarbonate by secreting hydrogen ions. Within the cells of the proximal tubule, carbonic anhydrase converts CO_2 and water into protons and bicarbonate ions. The bicarbonate is returned to the blood while the hydrogen is secreted into the proximal tubule, where it combines with tubular bicarbonate to reform CO_2 and water. The result is a net reclamation of bicarbonate; 80–85% is reabsorbed in the proximal convoluted tubule, with lesser amounts in the loop of Henle (5%), the distal tubule (5%), and the collecting system (5%).

In addition to bicarbonate, the salts of other acids are filtered by the glomeruli. The formation of these acids in the body, along with their hydrogen ions, results in an equimolar decrease in bicarbonate. The most important of these salts is monohydrogen phosphate. When hydrogen ion, secreted by the proximal tubules, combines with monohydrogen phosphate, it forms dihydrogen phosphate ($H_2 PO_4^-$), which is a weak acid with a pK_a of 6.8. The lowest pH attainable in the proximal tubule is approximately 4.5. Because the pK_a of this acid is within the tubular physiologic range, it can be reformed and excreted. When acids can be excreted by this process, they are referred to as titratable acids. The net effect is the regeneration of a bicarbonate anion.

On the other hand, acids with pK_a's lower than 4.5 (such as sulfuric acid, which is formed as a metabolic product of some proteins) cannot be regenerated in this way. Therefore, excess hydrogen ions secreted into the proximal tubule must be excreted in conjunction with another buffer to permit the continued formation of bicarbonate by the tubular cells. The tubular cells deaminate glutamine, and ammonia diffuses into the proximal tubules. Ammonia can react with hydrogen ion produced in the distal tubule to form ammonium ion. Ammonium excretion can increase from its normal level of 35 meq/d to over 300 meq/d in the face of severe acidemia. Hydrogen ion secretion in the proximal and collecting tubules is directly proportionate to luminal buffer concentration and $Paco_2$ and inversely proportionate to blood pH. Three to 5 days are required before maximum excretion of ammonium is achieved. As ammonium excretion increases, plasma bicarbonate concentration rises, as does urinary pH. Because a greater absolute quantity of hydrogen ions can be excreted in buffered (ammonium-rich) urine, urinary pH does not always reflect the extent of renal acidification.

Both ammonia production and proton secretion in the proximal tubules are increased by acidemia and decreased by alkalemia.

Loss of acidic fluids (e.g., in vomiting) or increase in alkali (e.g., antacid ingestion) in the body results in a reduction in hydrogen ion concentration and an increase in bicarbonate and pH. About two-thirds of the alkaline load is buffered in the extracellular space, while only one-third enters the intracellular compartment. At the same time, there is a modest shift of potassium into the cells, resulting in a decline in potassium concentration of approximately 0.4–0.5 meq/L for each 0.1 unit increase in pH. The acute response to an infusion of bicarbonate is an increase in $Paco_2$, which results from combination with H^+, and the release of CO_2. The pulmonary response to chronic alkalemia is inhibition of the respiratory drive. This causes a rise in $Paco_2$ of about 0.5 mm Hg for each 1 meq/L increase in the plasma bicarbonate concentration.

The kidney is able to excrete large amounts of excess bicarbonate under normal physiologic conditions. Increased concentration of bicarbonate in the glomerular ultrafiltrate, in combination with elevated pH of the blood perfusing the cells of the proximal tubules, decreases renal reabsorption and creates alkaline urine. Titratable acid and ammonia excretion are rapidly reduced. Both hypovolemia (volume contraction alkalosis) and hypokalemia can compromise the kidney's ability to excrete bicarbonate. Three mechanisms may be responsible: (1) Decreased GFR caused by hypovolemia, in conjunction with an elevated bicarbonate concentration, produces a normal amount of filtered bicarbonate, resulting in normal reabsorption; (2) proximal tubular reabsorption of HCO_3^- may be stimulated by hypovolemia and hypokalemia; and (3) increased aldosterone concentration, produced by hypovolemia, may generate and sustain increased bicarbonate reabsorption.

Respiratory Acid-Base Changes

Chemoreceptors normally maintain the $Paco_2$ between 37 mm Hg and 45 mm Hg. Lung disease, chest wall abnormalities, neurologic disease, or trauma may interfere with pulmonary excretion of CO_2 and cause hypercapnia. An acute rise in $Paco_2$ produces a fall in blood pH within several minutes. Initial control is by nonbicarbonate buffering of the resultant hydrogen ion, but bicarbonate falls because of a "mass action" effect. The concentration falls by about 0.25 meq/L for each 1 mm Hg decrease in $Paco_2$ and increases by 0.1 meq/L for each 1 mm Hg increase in $Paco_2$ during acute respiratory acidosis. Eventually, the kidneys respond to the rise in CO_2 concentration by increasing bicarbonate reabsorption from the proximal tubules, compensating for the rise in $Paco_2$. Plasma bicarbonate concentration increases by an average of 0.5 meq/L for each mm Hg increase in $Paco_2$ during chronic hypercapnia. Chronic hypercapnia stimulates ammonia production and increases urinary ammonium excretion. Occasionally, pH becomes slightly alkaline due to excessive renal bicarbonate production and retention.

Hypocapnia appropriately increases urinary bicarbonate excretion and transiently reduces urinary net acid secretion. The increased excretion of bicarbonate also results in kaliuresis and a decline in serum potassium concentration. In the steady state, the plasma bicarbonate concentration falls by about 0.5 meq/L for each mm Hg decrease in $Paco_2$.

Classification of Acid-Base Disorders

Acid-base disorders are classified according to whether there is a primary abnormality in plasma bicarbonate concentration, plasma $Paco_2$, or both. Abnormal pH due to altered bicarbonate concentration with $Paco_2$ changes in response to the primary disorder is referred to as either **metabolic acidosis** or **metabolic alkalosis.** When the defect in pH is due primarily to altered $Paco_2$, the condition is referred to as either **respiratory acidosis** or **respiratory alkalosis.** A change in HCO_3^- brings about a compensatory change in $Paco_2$, and a primary change in $Paco_2$ stimulates a compensatory adjustment in serum HCO_3^-. The compensatory changes may take minutes ($Paco_2$) or hours to days (HCO_3^-) to reach a steady-state.

Simple acid-base disorders occur when there is a primary change either in the bicarbonate concentration or in the $Paco_2$, with an appropriate (normal) secondary change in the other parameter (Table 2–15 and Figure 2–5). When values do not follow these rules, a **complex (mixed) acid-base disorder** exists. Mixed acid-base disorders include all possible combinations. For example, a patient may develop metabolic acidosis and respiratory acidosis simultaneously. Another patient may have a combination of respiratory alkalosis and metabolic acidosis. Some patients who have toxicity from

Table 2–15. Identification of acid-base disorders.

I. Confirm that pH, $Paco_2$, and [HCO_3^-] are compatible:
    Henderson-Hasselbalch equation
    Acid-based nomogram
II. Identify the primary disturbance:
    Arterial pH and $Paco_2$ + [HCO_3^-] to identify acidema or alkalemia
III. Determine whether the disorder is simple or complex:
    Acid-base nomogram
    Anion gap

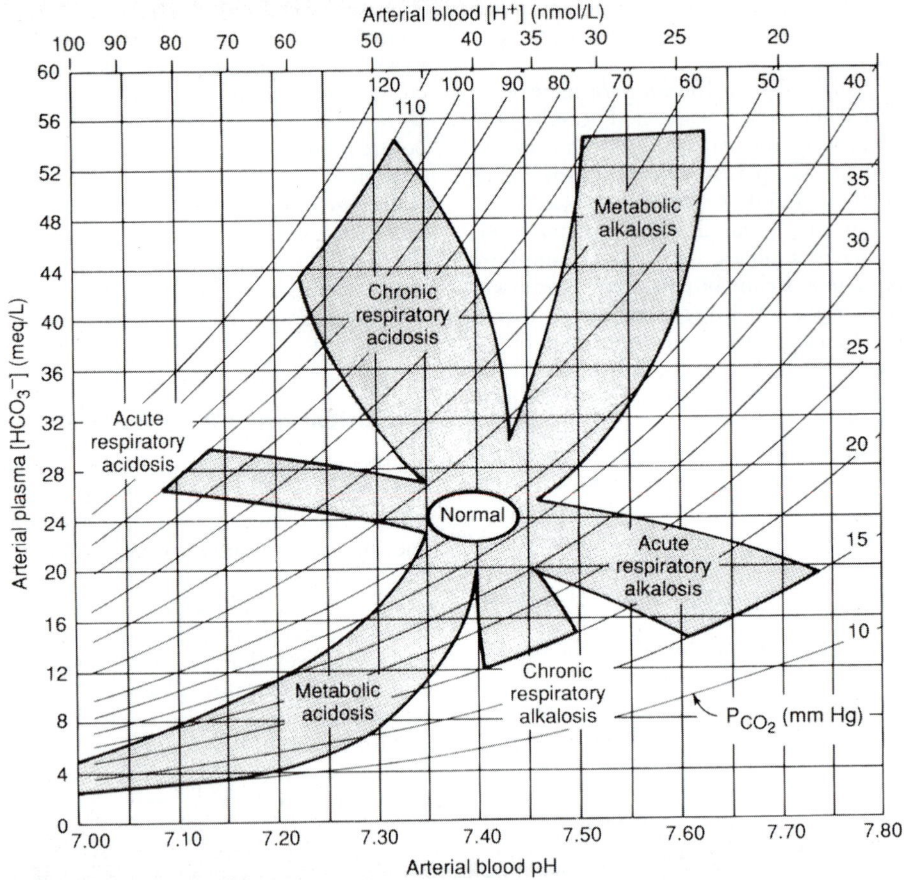

Figure 2–5. Acid-base nomogram. Shown are the 95% confidence limits of the normal respiratory and metabolic compensations for primary acid-base disturbances. (Reproduced, with permission, from Cogan MG, Rector FC Jr: Acid-base disorders. In: ***The Kidney,*** 3rd ed. Brenner BM, Rector FC Jr [editors]. Saunders, 1986.)

excessive salicylates will develop metabolic acidosis along with respiratory alkalosis.

It is helpful in evaluating acid-base disorders to follow some general rules. First, simple disorders are identified by the direction of the pH change. That is, any patient with a low pH (acidemia) must have at least metabolic acidosis, respiratory acidosis, or both. If both $PaCO_2$ and HCO_3^- contribute to either acidemia or alkalemia, then the patient must have two (or more) problems. Third, because compensatory mechanisms are never sufficient to restore the pH to normal, any patient with a normal pH (about 7.40) and appreciably abnormal $PaCO_2$ and HCO_3^- must have at least two primary acid-base disturbances. For example, acidemia with a decreased HCO_3^- concentration and a reduced $PaCO_2$ is most often a simple metabolic acidosis with respiratory compensation. However, if the pH is very close to 7.40, then respiratory compensation is abnormally excessive and a second primary disturbance, respiratory alkalosis, should be suspected.

Figure 2–5 will help in determining whether appropriate compensation is present. Location of a patient's position on the diagram will help suggest if a mixed acid-base problem is present. The areas shown represent 95% confidence intervals for single acid-base problems (labeled). If a point falls outside an area, then it is unlikely to be a single acid-base problem, and a mixed acid-base disturbance (two or more processes) should be suspected. General rules for the identification and verification of disorders are listed in Tables 2–15 and 2–16.

The next several sections will discuss both primary and compensated disorders.

Table 2–16. Physiologic response of pH, Pco_2, and HCO_3^- in acid-base disorders.[1]

Respiratory alterations
- Acute:
  - Acidosis
    - ↑1 mm Hg Pco_2
      - ↑$[HCO_3^-]$ = 0.1 meq/L
      - ↑$[H^+]$ = 0.8 nmol/L; ↓pH = 0.008 pH unit
  - Alkalosis
    - ↓1 mm Hg Pco_2
      - ↓$[HCO_3^-]$ = 0.25 meq/L
      - ↓$[H^+]$ = 0.7 nmol/L; ↑pH = 0.007 pH unit
- Chronic:
  - Acidosis
    - ↑1 mm Hg Pco_2
      - ↑$[HCO_3^-]$ = 0.5 meq/L
      - ↑$[H^+]$ = 0.25 nmol/L; ↓pH = 0.0025 pH unit
  - Alkalosis
    - ↓1 mm Hg Pco_2
      - ↓$[HCO_3^-]$ = 0.5 meq/L
      - ↓$[H^+]$ = 0.3 nmol/L; ↑pH = 0.003 pH unit

Metabolic alterations
- Acidosis
  - ↓1 meq/L $[HCO_3^-]$
  - ↓Pco_2 = 1.25 mm Hg
  - ↑$[H^+]$ = 1.2 nmol/L; ↓pH = 0.012 pH unit
- Alkalosis
  - ↑1 meq/L $[HCO_3^-]$
  - ↑Pco_2 = 0.5 (0.2–0.9) mm Hg
  - ↓$[H^+]$ = 0.3–0.8 nmol/L; ↑pH = 0.003–0.008 pH unit

[1]Adapted from Cogan MG, Rector FD Jr: Acid-based disorders. Pages 457–517 in: *The Kidney,* 3rd ed. Brenner BM, Rector FC (editors). Saunders, 1986.

Rose BD, Post TW: *Clinical Physiology of Acid-Base and Electrolyte Disorders,* 5th ed. McGraw-Hill, 2001.

Schoolwerth AC: Regulation of renal ammoniagenesis in metabolic acidosis. Kidney Int 1991;40:961–73.

Ventriglia WJ: Arterial blood gases. Emerg Med Clin North Am 1986;4:235–51.

METABOLIC ACIDOSIS

ESSENTIALS OF DIAGNOSIS

- *Decreased serum HCO_3^- with appropriately decreased $Paco_2$ (simple metabolic acidosis).*
- *Evidence that low serum HCO_3^- is primary problem (and not due to compensation for hypocapnia)*
- *May present with peripheral vasodilation; depressed cardiac contractility in severe acidosis; fatigue, weakness, stupor, coma.*

General Considerations

Metabolic acidosis occurs when there is a primary reduction in serum bicarbonate concentration, often accompanied by a compensatory decrease in $Paco_2$. The degree of $Paco_2$ depression depends slightly upon whether the condition is acute or chronic with more complete respiratory compensation. The kidneys' response is to increase reabsorption of bicarbonate, unless the cause of the low bicarbonate is a renal tubular defect leading to bicarbonate wasting or inability to reabsorb bicarbonate (renal tubular acidosis).

A useful classification scheme for metabolic acidosis involves calculation of the "anion gap." The anion gap is calculated as:

$$\text{Anion gap} = [Na^+] - ([HCO_3^-] + [Cl^-])$$

The normal value for the anion gap is 12 ± 4 meq/L. It can be shown that the anion gap is equal to the difference between "unmeasured" anions and "unmeasured" cations. In normal subjects, unmeasured anions include albumin (2 meq/L), phosphate (2 meq/L), sulfate (1 meq/L), lactate (1–2 meq/L), and the salts of weak acids (3–4 meq/L). The predominant unmeasured cations include calcium (5 meq/L), magnesium (2 meq/L), and certain cationic immunoglobulins.

The anion gap widens with either a reduction in unmeasured cations or, more commonly, when there is an increase in unmeasured anions. In patients with metabolic acidosis, an increase in the anion gap suggests that there are strong acids present which dissociate into hydrogen ion and an anion. The hydrogen ion reacts with bicarbonate to form CO_2 and water. The former is eliminated in the expired gas. The result is an increase in unmeasured anion and an increase in the anion gap. On the other hand, failure to generate sufficient bicarbonate is often associated with an increase in chloride concentration as the predominant anion. In these patients, the metabolic acidosis does not generate an unmeasured anion; therefore, the anion gap does not widen. This classification scheme divides states of metabolic acidosis, therefore, into those with an increased anion gap and those without an increase in the anion gap. The latter are often called hyperchloremic metabolic acidosis.

While challenged by some investigators, an additional calculation may be helpful as well. Because the increase in the anion gap must be due to the addition of a highly dissociated anion to the plasma (a strong acid), the increase in the anion gap must be equal to the fall in serum bicarbonate. Thus, adding the numerical increase in anion gap to the measured serum bicarbonate estimates the serum bicarbonate "before" the anion gap acidosis occurred. If the result is lower than normal (22–26 meq/L), then a preexisting low serum bicarbonate can be assumed (metabolic acidosis or chronic respiratory alkalosis). On the other hand, if the calculated value is > 26 meq/L, then the preexisting serum bicarbonate can be assumed to be high (chronic respiratory acidosis or metabolic alkalosis). This estimate is not perfect, but if the clinical situation fits it may allow the identification of mixed acid-base disturbances that might otherwise be missed.

Normal Anion Gap Metabolic Acidosis

Hyperchloremic metabolic acidosis occurs from one of four mechanisms: (1) dilution of extracellular buffer (bicarbonate) by bicarbonate-free solutions; (2) addition of net hydrochloric acid; (3) a defect in mechanisms of renal acidification; or (4) renal excretion of large quantities of nonchloride anions with reabsorption of chloride.

Dilutional acidosis occurs when patients are rapidly infused with solutions devoid of buffer. A common scenario is the use of normal saline to resuscitate a trauma victim or patient with hypovolemic shock. This produces a reduction in the concentration of bicarbonate by dilution. Dilutional acidosis is usually mild and does not produce a plasma bicarbonate concentration < 15 meq/L. Renal mechanisms usually correct the situation by excreting excess acid or by natriuresis and diuresis to normalize the extracellular volume and plasma bicarbonate concentration.

Administration of dilute hydrochloric acid for treatment of severe metabolic alkalosis is rarely needed, but excess hydrochloric acid will result in hyperchloremic metabolic acidosis. More commonly, bicarbonate is lost as a result of gastrointestinal losses in the form of diarrhea or alkaline fluid from fistulas. Regeneration of bicarbonate in the gut accounts for the net addition of hydrogen ion to the blood without adding an unmeasured anion. When such losses of bicarbonate are severe, extracellular volume depletion, electrolyte imbalances, and stimulation of aldosterone and renin ensue. In response to such conditions, renal net acid excretion increases, with a tendency for urine pH to rise because of ammonium production.

Failure of the normal mechanisms of urinary acidification results in increased bicarbonate loss. This condition, renal tubular acidosis, produces metabolic acidosis because the kidneys are unable to compensate for normal acid production or because of failure to reabsorb normal amounts of filtered bicarbonate. At least four types of renal tubular acidosis exist, differentiated on the basis of the primary tubular abnormality. The major features of each type are summarized in Table 2–17. Similar results can be seen when the carbonic anhydrase inhibitor and diuretic acetazolamide is given. With this drug, proximal tubular bicarbonate reabsorption is inhibited; the net result is metabolic acidosis with inappropriate loss of renal tubular bicarbonate, a drug-induced renal tubular acidosis.

Patients with diabetic ketoacidosis will almost always present with anion gap metabolic acidosis (see below). Because, however, the anions of the keto acids β-hydroxybutyrate and acetoacetate are readily excreted in the urine, the anion gap may not persist in patients who are able to maintain adequate glomerular filtration. Thus, a small fraction of those with diabetic ketoacidosis will present with an anion gap increase that is smaller than the decrease in serum bicarbonate, evidence for both an anion gap and non-anion gap metabolic acidosis. This observation is much more common during the treatment and correction of diabetic ketoacidosis, in which as many as 80% of such patients will have a non-anion gap metabolic acidosis. The mechanism is the urinary loss of anions of the keto acids while bicarbonate regeneration is too slow to correct for the earlier loss of bicarbonate. Several days are sometimes required for the bicarbonate to return to normal.

Anion Gap Metabolic Acidosis

The major causes of high anion gap metabolic acidosis are listed in Tables 2–18 and 2–19. Except for uremia, they all occur acutely and are due to overproduction of an acid that dissociates into a hydrogen ion and an "unmeasured" anion. Unlike the situation in renal tubular acidosis, renal mechanisms for acid handling are intact unless otherwise impaired but are unable to keep pace with the extent of acid production.

A. Lactic Acidosis

Lactic acidosis may occur in a number of situations among critically ill patients, including shock, diabetes, renal failure, liver disease, sepsis, drug intoxication, severe volume depletion, and hereditary metabolic abnormalities (such as G6PD deficiency). Transient lactic acidosis is a feature of grand mal seizures. Patients with liver disease will have difficulty removing lactate. Thiamin deficiency has been reported as an association. Metformin may cause lactic acidosis rarely. Identification and correction of the underlying process is essential to the management of this disorder. Specific therapy of this and other causes of metabolic acidosis will be discussed subsequently.

Table 2–17. Hyperchloremic, normal anion gap metabolic acidoses.[1]

	Renal Defect	GFR	Serum [K^+]	Proximal H+ Secretion[2]	Distal H^+ Secretion: Minimal Urine pH	Distal H^+ Secretion: Urinary NH_4^++ Titratable Acid	Urinary Anion Gap	Treatment
Renal tubular acidosis I. Proximal	Proximal H^+ secretion	Normal	↓	↓[3]	<5.5	Normal	Zero or positive	$NaHCO_3$ or $KHCO_3$ (10–15 meq/kg/d), thiazide
II. Classical distal	Distal H^+ secretion	Normal	↓	Normal	>5.5	↓	Zero or positive	$NaHCO_3$ (1–3 meq/kg/d)
III. Buffer deficiency distal	Distal NH_3 delivery	↓	Normal	Normal	<5.5	↓	Zero or positive	$NaHCO_3$ (1–3 meq/kg/d)
IV. Generalized distal	Distal Na^+ reabsorption, K^+ secretion, and H^+ secretion	↓	↑	Normal	<5.5	↓	Zero or positive	Fludrocortisone (0.1–0.5 mg/d), dietary K^+ restriction, furosemide (40–160 mg/d), $NaHCO_3$ (1–3 meq/kg/d)

[1]Adapted from Cogan MG: *Fluid and Electrolytes,* 1st ed. Appleton & Lange, 1991.
[2]HCO_3^- reabsorption during HCO_3^- loading.
[3]Fractional excretion of bicarbonate >15% during bicarbonate loading; usually associated with Fanconi's syndrome.

Table 2–18. Normochloremic, high anion gap metabolic acidoses.[1]

Type	Acid	Unmeasured Plasma Anion	Treatment[2]
Lactic acidosis	Lactic acid	Lactate	Treat underlying disorder
Ketoacidosis Diabetic	β-Hydroxybutyric acid, acetpacetoc acid	β-Hydroxybutyrate, acetoacetate	Insulin, saline (K^+, phosphate, Mg^{2+} repletion)
Alcoholic			Glucose and saline (K^+, phosphate, Mg^{2+} repletion)
Starvation			Carbohydrate
Toxins[3] Salicylate	Salicylate acid	Salicylate, lactate	Alkaline diuresis, hemodialysis
Ethylene glycol	Glycolic acid	Glycolate	Ethanol, thiamine and pyridoxine, ECV expansion, hemodialysis
Methanol	Formic Acid	Formate	Ethanol, ECV expansion, hemodialysis
Uremia	Organic acids	Organic anions	$NaHCO_3$ (1–3 mg/kg/d)

[1]Adapted from Cogan MG: *Fluid and Electrolytes,* 1st ed. Appleton & Lange, 1991.
[2]$NaHCO_3$ for severe symptomatic acidemia.
[3]Also generate lactic acidosis and ketoacidosis.

Table 2–19. Causes of normochloremic, high anion gap metabolic acidosis.[1]

Lactic acidosis
- Overproduction
  - Severe exercise
  - Seizures
  - Sepsis
  - Leukemias
- Underutilization
  - Type A: Poor tissue perfusion or oxygenation
    - Shock
    - Cardiogenic
    - Hemorrhagic
    - Septic
  - Type B: Various common disorders
    - Diabetes mellitus
    - Renal failure
    - Liver disease
    - Infection
  - Drugs or other toxic substances
    - Metformin
    - Ethanol
    - Methanol
    - Salicylates
    - Sorbitol
    - Xylitol
    - Dithiazinine iodide
    - Streptozocin
    - Isoniazid
    - Cyanide
    - Nitroprusside
  - Hereditary forms
    - Glucose-6-phosphate deficiency (type 1 glycogenosis)
    - Fructose-1, 6-diphosphatase deficiency
    - Pyruvate carboxylase deficiency
    - Pyruvate dehydrogenase deficiencies
    - Methylmalonic aciduria
  - Miscellaneous
    - Ingestion of "lactic acid milk"
    - D-Lactic acidosis in short bowel syndrome

Ketoacidosis
- Diabetic
- Ethanol intoxication
- Starvation
- Inborn errors of metabolism

Intoxications
- Salicylates
- Ethylene glycol
- Methanol
- Paraldehyde

Uremia (late)

[1]Adapted from Cogan MG, Rector FD Jr: Acid-based disorders. Pages 457–517 in: *The Kidney,* 3rd ed. Brenner BM, Rector FC (editors). Saunders, 1986.

B. Ketoacidosis

Ketoacidosis occurs most commonly as a result of poorly controlled diabetes mellitus, occasionally in those with heavy ethanol consumption in the absence of food intake, and during starvation. In all cases, keto acids (β-hydroxybutyrate and acetoacetate) accumulate. With diabetic ketoacidosis, glycosuria, osmotic diuresis, extracellular volume contraction, hyperreninemic hyperaldosteronism, kaliuresis, magnesuria, and phosphaturia occur. When a patient has discontinued food intake but continues to drink ethanol, β-hydroxybutyrate and lactate accumulate more than acetoacetate. Glucose metabolism usually remains normal, and blood glucose concentrations are usually only minimally elevated. Starvation produces mild ketoacidosis accompanied by mild renal wasting of sodium, chloride, potassium, calcium, phosphate, and magnesium. In all three conditions, unmeasured anions accumulate and cause elevation of the anion gap.

C. Uremia

When the glomerular filtration rate falls below 20 mL/min, filtration of organic acids is impaired. Plasma bicarbonate concentration falls to about 15 meq/L, producing an excess anion gap of approximately 10 meq/L. When chronic renal deficiency develops, hyperchloremic metabolic acidosis may occur initially due to impaired ammonia generation, followed eventually by a high anion gap acidosis from inability to excrete fixed acids. A mixed metabolic acidosis is not uncommon with renal failure.

D. Poisons

Ingestion of ethylene glycol (radiator antifreeze), methanol (wood alcohol), and excessive salicylic acid may give rise to anion gap metabolic acidosis. Ethylene glycol is oxidized by alcohol dehydrogenase to glycolic acid, which is the major acid anion found in the blood. Further oxidation produces oxalic acid with resultant sodium oxalate crystals precipitating in the urine. Lactic acid may be present if circulatory shock develops. Methanol is oxidized to formaldehyde and formic acid. Although salicylate is itself a weak acid, it probably produces its major effect by inducing simultaneous lactic acidosis. The management of poisoning is discussed in greater detail in Chapter 37.

Clinical Features

A. Symptoms and Signs

The physical findings associated with mild acidemia are nonspecific and may reflect the underlying disease or associated conditions. As acidosis worsens, increased tidal volumes (Kussmaul respiration) provide partial respiratory compensation. Peripheral vasodilation occurs and produces palpable cutaneous warmth. Paradoxical venoconstriction increases central pooling and may result in pulmonary edema. Cardiac contractility decreases below a pH of 7.10 and may result in reduced blood pressure. Central nervous system depression produces fatigue, weakness, lethargy, and ultimately stupor and coma. Nonspecific complaints of abdominal pain are common.

B. Laboratory Findings

Laboratory abnormalities vary depending upon the cause of the acidosis and the degree of compensation.

When hyperchloremic acidosis is secondary to gastrointestinal bicarbonate loss, hypovolemia-induced renin and aldosterone secretion causes an associated hyperkalemia. Findings associated with each of the renal tubular acidosis (RTA) syndromes are detailed in Table 2–17. The distinction between gastrointestinal causes and RTA may be based on the presence of increased urinary ammonium excretion in the former. Because tests for urinary ammonium are not always available, calculation of the urine anion gap ($[Na^+]$ + $[K^+]$ − $[Cl^-]$) may be helpful. The normal urine anion gap is negative because of the presence of an unmeasured cation, ammonium. The urine anion gap becomes more negative as the ammonium concentration increases, which should be the case if the hyperchloremic metabolic acidosis is caused by diarrhea or some other extrarenal mechanism. On the other hand, the urine gap remains close to zero or becomes positive when there is no ammonium excretion, which occurs in all types of RTA.

In patients with an increased anion gap metabolic acidosis, the unmeasured anion can sometimes be identified. Serum lactate levels are elevated (> 2–3 meq/L) when lactic acidosis is the cause of a high anion gap acidosis. Diabetic ketoacidosis is associated with hypokalemia, hypomagnesemia, hypophosphatemia, and hyperglycemia. The ratio of keto acids present depends on the plasma redox potential (NADH:NAD ratio). Because the commonly used nitroprusside reaction measures only the acetoacetate concentration, tests for ketones may be falsely negative if the β-hydroxybutyrate:acetoacetate ratio is very high. Alcoholic ketoacidosis presents with similar laboratory findings with the exception that glucose concentration is only minimally elevated. Because β-hydroxybutyrate is the predominant keto acid in this situation, routine testing for ketones may yield a negative result. Following starvation, decreased serum concentrations of sodium, chloride, potassium, calcium, phosphate, and magnesium may be present.

Findings associated with ingestions are specific to the toxin and are discussed in Chapter 37. The specific anion is usually not measured when, for example, one of the commonly ingested toxic alcohols is present. Of note, isopropyl alcohol ingestion is associated with ketonemia but does not cause metabolic acidosis. When uremia is the cause, increases in serum potassium, serum urea nitrogen, and serum creatinine are typically observed.

Differential Diagnosis

The history of the present illness and careful questioning regarding drug intake and use are essential in determining the cause of the acidosis. When ingestion is suspected, microscopic examination of the urine looking for oxalate crystals may aid in the diagnosis of ethylene glycol ingestion. Similarly, visual impairment, nausea and vomiting, and disordered central nervous system functioning are characteristic of methanol ingestion. A history of insulin requirement and use—along with the blood glucose concentration—aids in the diagnosis of diabetic ketoacidosis. Differentiation between hyperchloremic acidosis and renal tubular acidosis is aided by calculation of the urine anion gap and the presence or absence of diarrhea.

Treatment

A. Assessment of the Need for Therapy

Whenever metabolic acidosis is present, a diligent search should be made for its underlying cause. Therapy directed toward treatment of the primary disorder should always be instituted. Correction of fluid and electrolyte disturbances is key in patients with diabetic ketoacidosis or with lactic acidosis due to hypovolemic, septic, or cardiogenic shock and in patients with various toxic ingestions.

There are few data supporting improved patient outcome with treatment directed specifically at the metabolic acidosis in patients with anion gap acidosis, including diabetic ketoacidosis and lactic acidosis. However, there are few or no randomized trials in patients with very severe acidemia. Thus, when acidemia is acute and the pH falls below 7.00, therapy should be considered. For pH values between 7.00 and 7.20, the need to treat should be individualized based on such considerations as the patient's basic physical state and the presumed cause of the disturbance. There is experimental evidence that bicarbonate therapy of acute lactic acidosis may promote further lactate production and actually worsen the situation. Furthermore, bicarbonate buffering yields considerable carbon dioxide that produces local respiratory acidosis. However, because severe acidosis acts as a myocardial and circulatory depressant, treatment should be considered if there is evidence of circulatory impairment and other factors have been addressed.

When acidosis is chronic, as with uremia or the renal tubular acidosis syndromes, the need for treatment should be based on the patient's overall status and the presence of signs and symptoms related to the acidosis rather than upon the absolute arterial pH itself.

B. Treatment

Intravenous sodium bicarbonate is the preferred agent for treatment of severe acute metabolic acidosis. It is most commonly supplied in 50 mL ampules containing 44.6 meq of HCO_3^-. The amount of bicarbonate required is based upon the degree of acidemia. Because the administered base will partition equally between intracellular and extracellular spaces, dosing is based on total body water (approximately one-half the total body weight) and the extent of the acidemia. Typically, one-half of the bicarbonate required to completely correct the deficit is administered acutely, with the rest given by slow intravenous infusion over the ensuing 8–12 hours. For example, if a 70-kg patient has a bicarbonate concentration of 14 meq/L, the amount of bicarbonate administered acutely can be calculated as follows:

$$[HCO_3^-]\ \text{deficit} = \text{Normal concentration} - \text{Present concentration} = (24-14) = 10\ \text{meq/L}$$

$$\text{Distribution volume} = \text{Total body weight} \times 0.5 = 70 \times 0.5 = 35\ \text{L}$$

$$\text{Dose} = \text{Deficit} \times \text{Distribution} \times 0.5\ (\text{to correct half the deficit}) = 10 \times 35 \times 0.5 = 175\ \text{meq}$$

Some laboratories routinely calculate base deficit from blood gas values. The base deficit is an approximation of base depletion secondary to metabolic causes. The base deficit is usually reported as a positive number. It is negative when a **base excess** is present. The base deficit can be used to calculate the amount of bicarbonate required according to the following equation:

$$[HCO_3^-]\ \text{required} = \text{Base deficit} \times 0.4 \times \text{Body weight (kg)}$$

The amount required to completely correct the deficit is then halved to arrive at an appropriate acute bolus dose.

Because of the considerable intracellular buffering of hydrogen ion in severe acidosis, the bicarbonate volume of distribution can be underestimated. Thus, the improvement in pH may be less than expected. However, because of the risks of excessive bicarbonate therapy and the greatest benefit seen in correcting severe acidosis, the goal is to correct pH to more than 7.20, and often to much less than that (see below)

Bicarbonate must be administered with extreme care in patients with potentially compromised respiratory status because the combination of HCO_3^- with H^+ will yield H_2O and CO_2. If hypoventilation is present, acute respiratory acidosis may occur. Furthermore, if the acidosis is chronic or well compensated by respiratory mechanisms, rebound alkalosis can follow bicarbonate administration. Because bicarbonate is administered as the sodium salt and given in high concentration, both volume overloading and hyperosmolality can result.

Current Controversies & Unresolved Issues

No issue in critical care medicine is currently more controversial and less resolved than the administration of bicarbonate in acute metabolic acidosis. Animal studies support both a benefit of bicarbonate in severe acidosis and numerous complications of such therapy. Human studies are limited because, although inconclusive, they fail to randomize patients with severe acidosis. It is very likely that the outcome of patients with metabolic acidosis is more closely linked to the underlying disease than to the severity of acidemia. In the words of some investigators, there is no evidence that bicarbonate therapy improves the outcome for any patient with an acute anion gap metabolic acidosis (diabetic ketoacidosis or lactic acidosis).

A small increase in pH in patients with severe metabolic acidosis can be associated with significant improvement in the function of physiologic systems. Because a patient with a very low serum bicarbonate (2–4 meq/L) will have a substantial increase in pH when the bicarbonate reaches 6–8 meq/L, one approach is to treat only those who have very severe metabolic acidosis with only a relatively small amount of sodium bicarbonate. In theory, this patient will have the greatest potential benefit with the least generation of carbon dioxide and risks of volume overload and osmotic excess.

Another approach has been to use non-CO_2-generating buffering agents. A mixture of carbonate and bicarbonate has been given experimentally. This product, called carbicarb, generates less CO_2 for the degree of buffering, but clinical experience is limited. There are studies using THAM—tris(hydroxymethyl) aminomethane—as a buffering agent. This compound, which also does not produce CO_2 during use, may be a useful alkalizing agent if further studies demonstrate its value.

Androgue HJ, Madias NE: Management of life-threatening acid-base disorders. Part 1. N Engl J Med 1998;338:26–34.

Kushner RF: Total parenteral nutrition-associated metabolic acidosis. JPEN J Parenter Enteral Nutr 1986;10:306–10.

Luft FC: Lactic acidosis update for critical care clinicians. J Am Soc Nephrol 2001;12:S15–S19.

Narins FG, Cohen JJ: Bicarbonate therapy for organic acidosis: the case for its continued use. Ann Intern Med 1987;106:615–8.

Rose BD, Post TW: *Clinical Physiology of Acid-Base and Electrolyte Disorders,* 5th ed. McGraw-Hill, 2001.

Stackpoole PW: Lactic acidosis: the case against bicarbonate therapy. Ann Intern Med 1986;105:276–8.

Warnock DG: Uremic acidosis. Kidney Int 1988;34:278–87.

METABOLIC ALKALOSIS

ESSENTIALS OF DIAGNOSIS

- *Alkalemia with increased serum [HCO_3^-].*
- *Lethargy and confusion progressing to seizures in severe cases.*
- *Ventricular and supraventricular arrhythmias.*
- *Altered oxyhemoglobin binding increases $Paco_2$ and decreases PaO_2.*

General Considerations

Metabolic alkalosis consists of the triad of increased [HCO_3^-], increased pH, and decreased serum chloride concentration. Because the decline in chloride does not equal the rise in bicarbonate, the anion gap always increases. The principal causes of metabolic alkalosis include (1) addition of bicarbonate to the plasma, (2) loss of hydrogen ion, (3) volume depletion, (4) chronic use of chloruretic diuretics, and (5) potassium depletion.

Pathophysiology

A. Addition of Bicarbonate

Addition of bicarbonate is an unusual cause of metabolic alkalosis but may occur with prolonged administration of high amounts of alkali (milk-alkali syndrome) or after therapy with solutions that contain bicarbonate, carbonate, acetate, lactate, or citrate. In normal adults, up to 20 meq/kg/d of bicarbonate may be administered without significantly altering serum pH. When calcium and vitamin D intakes are high, as in the milk-alkali syndrome, nephrocalcinosis causes renal insufficiency and diminishes GFR. This reduced renal capacity permits the retention of bicarbonate and increases pH. High concentrations of acetate in hyperalimentation fluids may be an unsuspected cause in critically ill patients. When the GFR is normal, elevated serum bicarbonate results in the presentation of increased bicarbonate to the proximal tubules, which reduces bicarbonate reabsorption and causes bicarbonaturia.

B. Vomiting

The most common cause of loss of hydrogen ion is vomiting. Prolonged emesis is one of the most common causes of metabolic alkalosis among critically ill patients. Nasogastric suction will result in the same syndrome. Parietal cells produce hydrochloric acid from carbonic acid. For each proton secreted into the gastric lumen, one molecule of bicarbonate is returned to the blood. Chloride accompanies H^+ secretion to form hydrochloric acid. Both hydrogen and chloride are lost in the vomitus, resulting in both alkalosis and volume contraction. Reduction in blood volume causes the secretion of renin, which produces kaliuresis in an attempt to retain sodium and chloride. Both the hypovolemia and the hypokalemia cause GFR to fall. Decreased GFR and hypokalemia allow complete conservation of the filtered bicarbonate rather than the appropriate excretion of bicarbonate as a result of alkalemia. Thus, urine may be paradoxically acid when it should be alkaline. The defect is best repaired by expanding the extracellular volume and by providing potassium. When sodium chloride and potassium are given, GFR increases and appropriate renal excretion of bicarbonate begins.

C. Volume Depletion

Many cases of chronic metabolic alkalosis are accompanied by extracellular volume depletion, and volume depletion may generate and certainly maintains metabolic alkalosis. In response to volume depletion, renin and aldosterone production are increased and result in kaliuresis and hypokalemia. Furthermore, because hydrogen ion secretion by the α-intercalated cells of the collecting tubules is sensitive to the concentration of aldosterone, hyperreninemia also increases bicarbonate reabsorption in the distal tubules. Thiazide and loop diuretics are important causes of volume depletion and metabolic alkalosis, but there are important additional factors with these drugs. Sodium delivery to the distal tubule is increased, resulting in increased hydrogen and potassium secretion. As circulating volume falls, renin secretion further enhances renal hydrogen and potassium losses. Hypokalemia stimulates ammoniagenesis and increases ammonium excretion. Thus, new bicarbonate is generated and metabolic alkalosis is created and sustained by the combined effects of increased distal tubular sodium delivery, elevated aldosterone levels, and hypokalemia. Administration of saline and potassium increases GFR and repairs the hypokalemia, permitting excretion of the accumulated bicarbonate.

There has been an ongoing debate about the specific role of chloride ion compared with volume repletion (regardless of the exact solution). Earlier experiments seemed to demonstrate that replacement of volume deficit with non-chloride-containing solutions led to prompt bicarbonaturia and resolution of the metabolic alkalosis. However, more recently, administration of chloride-containing solutions corrected the alkalosis (bicarbonaturia) despite insufficient volume, suggesting a key role for chloride. This is why some patients with metabolic alkalosis who have volume depletion and hypokalemia are variably termed "volume-responsive" or "chloride-responsive."

D. Potassium Depletion

Potassium depletion results in a shift of hydrogen ions into the cells, raising pH. However, potassium depletion increases renal ammonia generation, stimulating bicarbonate generation and reabsorption. The combination of potassium depletion and mineralocorticoid excess appears to amplify the metabolic alkalosis effect.

E. Other Causes

Some nonreabsorbable anions (salts of penicillin and carbenicillin) promote tubular secretion of hydrogen and potassium by increasing luminal electronegativity. The metabolic alkalosis produced can be repaired readily by administering saline and potassium. A related cause is particularly common in the intensive care unit and follows carbohydrate refeeding after starvation ketoacidosis. During the period of starvation, renal production of bicarbonate in response to the acidemia helps to maintain pH. However, when refeeding is instituted, ketones are converted into bicarbonate, thereby producing metabolic alkalosis. Coexisting potassium and volume depletion will maintain the alkalosis unless sodium chloride and potassium are provided.

Other common causes of metabolic alkalosis, categorized by physiology and response to NaCl or KCl infusion, are listed in Table 2–20. On rare occasions, a patient requiring critical care will present with hypervolemia, potassium deficiency, and primary hypersecretion of aldosterone. The increased mineralocorticoid level serves to cause sodium retention with volume expansion, produce kaliuresis, and increase hydrogen ion secretion, which generates metabolic alkalosis and subsequently enhances bicarbonate reabsorptive capacity. A phenomenon known as "mineralocorticoid escape" occurs and leads to an equilibrium state of hypertension, hypokalemia, and metabolic alkalosis. Because aldosterone levels are high and the plasma volume is expanded, this disorder is not responsive to saline administration. Management is best directed toward determining the cause of the increased aldosterone secretion. Rarely, adult patients with undiagnosed Gitelman's syndrome will be seen in the intensive care unit. The defect is located in the thiazide-sensitive NaCl cotransporter in the distal tubule, resulting in a thiazide diuretic-like syndrome of hypokalemia, metabolic alkalosis, hypocalciuria, and hypomagnesemia.

Table 2–20. Causes of metabolic alkalosis.

I. Exogenous bicarbonate administration:
   Bicarbonate, citrate, acetate, lactate
   Milk-alkali syndrome
II. Volume contraction + potassium depletion (saline-responsive)
   Gastrointestinal loss (emesis, gastric suction, villous adenoma)
   Renal loss (loop and thiazide diuretics)
   Posthypercapric states
   Nonreabsorbable anions (ketones, penicillin, carbenicillin)
   After treatment for lactic acidosis or ketoacidosis
   Carbohydrate refeeding after starvation
   Hypokalemia, hypomagnesemia
III. Volume expansion + potassium deficiency (not saline-responsive)
   High renin (malignant hypertension, renin-secreting tumor)
   Low renin (primary hyperaldosteronism, adrenal enzymatic defects, Cushing's disease)

Clinical Features

A. Symptoms and Signs

Symptoms and physical findings associated with mild metabolic alkalosis are nonspecific and are usually related more closely to the underlying disorder than to the acid-base disturbance itself. Review of the patient's medical record with particular attention to medications received and net negative fluid balances reported will often aid in determining the origin of alkalemia. On physical examination, a difference between supine and sitting blood pressures may reveal hypovolemia. Hypertension suggests hypervolemia. When both hypertension and metabolic alkalosis are present, a history of glucocorticoid or mineralocorticoid use or endogenous aldosterone production should be considered.

A decrease in minute ventilation is usually noted in moderate cases of metabolic alkalosis. If preexisting pulmonary disease is present, CO_2 retention may result in severe hypercapnia. As alkalemia progresses, the ionized calcium concentration decreases and produces neuromuscular findings similar to those of hypocalcemia. Initial lethargy and confusion give way to obtundation and seizures as the alkalemia worsens. Patients may complain of paresthesias and muscle cramps. The Chvostek and Trousseau signs may be present. In severe cases, respiratory muscle paralysis may develop.

Alkalemia acts as a negative inotropic substance, with the change in blood pressure dependent upon the degree of hypo- or hypervolemia. Furthermore, the increase in pH lowers the arrhythmia threshold, with supraventricular and ventricular arrhythmias predominating. There are no electrocardiographic abnormalities specific for alkalemia, though the presence of arrhythmias should alert the clinician to the potential severity of the acid-base disturbance.

B. Laboratory Findings

Review of arterial blood gases is the critical step in the laboratory diagnosis of metabolic alkalosis. An increase in serum [HCO_3^-] may be present with either chronic respiratory acidosis or metabolic alkalosis. Comparison of the $Pa{CO_2}$ with the nomogram in Figure 2–5 will aid in determining whether respiratory compensation is appropriate or whether a mixed acid-base disorder is present.

Once it has been determined that a simple metabolic alkalosis is present, further evaluation will determine the cause of the disorder. Serum potassium is almost always decreased. The magnitude of total body potassium depletion cannot be estimated precisely from the serum potassium. Hyponatremia is common in hypovolemic disorders, which are ultimately responsive to saline infusion.

A useful distinction can be made be separating metabolic alkalosis into those that are "chloride-sensitive" (sometimes called volume- or saline-responsive) and those that are "non-chloride-sensitive." Chloride- or volume-sensitive patients are volume-depleted, hypokalemic, and will respond to chloride or volume administration (see above). The latter group is usually volume-overloaded and will worsen or fail to improve with chloride-containing solutions or volume repletion.

These groups can be distinguished by measurement of urine chloride. Volume contraction usually results in concentrated urine with a low sodium concentration. However, if metabolic alkalosis develops, high renal tubular bicarbonate concentrations may carry sodium out in the urine. Thus, there is a paradoxically high urine sodium and fractional excretion of sodium despite volume depletion. However, urine chloride concentrations can be relied upon in this situation. A low urine [Cl^-] (< 10 meq/L) indicates potential volume-responsive or chloride-responsive metabolic alkalosis. On the other hand, diuretics will confuse this picture because both urine sodium and urine chloride will be increased in spite of hypovolemia. Hypomagnesemia from gastrointestinal and renal losses is occasionally observed in this situation.

When primary hyperaldosteronism is the cause of metabolic alkalosis, urinary sodium and chloride output are approximately equal to intake and in the range of 100–200 meq/L. Volume expansion and hypertension are usually present.

Differential Diagnosis

Once a high serum bicarbonate is identified, the most important distinction must be made between metabolic alkalosis and chronic respiratory acidosis with renal compensation. Diuretic therapy may superimpose additional metabolic alkalosis on top of chronic respiratory acidosis, which further increases the [HCO_3^-] and may actually result in an alkaline pH. Consideration of the patient's history and diuretic use will aid in the differential. Noting increased concentrations of sodium and chloride in the urine prior to discontinuation of diuretic therapy is another useful tool. When simple metabolic alkalosis is present, the distinction between chloride-responsive and chloride-unresponsive disorders must be made.

Treatment

It has become clear that alkalemia in critically ill patients is associated with poor outcome, just as acidemia is linked to decreased survival. The underlying disease in all situations must be addressed to slow or reverse the cause of metabolic alkalosis. The decision to treat is based both on the severity of alkalemia and the risks of complications.

A. Saline-Responsive Metabolic Alkalosis

Mild alkalemia (pH 7.40–7.50) is well tolerated and does not require treatment unless preexistent cardiac or pulmonary disease complicates the situation. If the alkalemia worsens (pH > 7.60) or if findings consistent with cardiac, pulmonary, or neuromuscular complications appear, treatment is indicated.

The key to therapy is restoration of normal circulating blood volume and repair of the associated hypokalemia. Potassium replacement can be estimated from the extent of the potassium deficit. The volume of normal saline required should be infused so that one-half of the deficit is replaced within 8 hours and the remainder within the ensuing 16 hours. As discussed above, there is evidence that chloride-containing solutions stimulate a more marked bicarbonaturia, leading to more rapid correction of the alkalosis. Therefore, volume repletion should be preferentially with NaCl and KCl solutions.

In unusual situations, acetazolamide, an inhibitor of carbonic anhydrase, can be used to correct metabolic alkalosis as long as the patient is not volume-depleted. This situation is rarely encountered, and the drug will exacerbate both volume depletion and hypokalemia. Acetazolamide, 250–500 mg, can be given orally and repeated if necessary with close monitoring of serum potassium. Very rarely, if alkalemia is extremely severe, dilute hydrochloric acid (0.1 mol/L) can be infused into a central vein. The quantity required can be calculated from the serum bicarbonate concentration. Assuming that the volume of distribution of bicarbonate is that of total body water (one-half of body weight), the amount of HCl required is calculated as follows:

$$\text{HCl required (meq)} = ([HCO_3^-] - 24) \times 0.5 \times \text{Weight (kg)}$$

One-half the calculated dose should be given over the first 4–8 hours, with the remainder infused over the next day. Several other acidifying agents have been used, including ammonium chloride, arginine monohydrochloride, and lysine monohydrochloride. The latter two should not be given because of the very high risk of hyperkalemia, sometimes fatal, associated with large and rapid shifts of potassium out of the cells.

B. Saline-Resistant Metabolic Alkalosis

These disorders are rarely encountered and may result from reversible (drug-induced) causes or unchecked endogenous secretion of aldosterone. In both cases, mineralocorticoids lead to sodium retention and potassium excretion despite high extracellular volume and hypokalemia. Retention of bicarbonate is due to the combination of potassium depletion and increased generation of hydrogen ion in the renal tubules.

Therapy of these disorders should be aimed at identifying the source of the aldosterone or other mineralocorticoid. When the condition follows excessive administration of mineralocorticoids, their use should be stopped. If the patient has excessive aldosterone secretion from an adrenal adenoma, medical management with an inhibitor of aldosterone (spironolactone) may play a role until more definitive therapy can be planned.

Androgue HJ, Madias NE: Management of life-threatening acid-base disorders. Part 2. N Engl J Med 1998;338:107–11.

Fine A: Application of principles of physiology and biochemistry to the bedside: Metabolic alkalosis and hypokalemia. Clin Invest Med 1990;13:47–52.

Galla JH: Metabolic alkalosis. J Am Soc Nephrol 2000;11:369–75.

RESPIRATORY ACIDOSIS

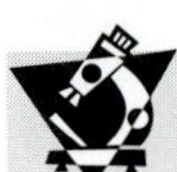

ESSENTIALS OF DIAGNOSIS

- *Acidemia with increased $Paco_2$ and near-normal (acute) or appropriately elevated $[HCO_3^-]$ (chronic)*
- *Fatigue, weakness, confusion, and headaches.*
- *Decreased cardiac contractility, pulmonary artery hypertension.*
- *Splanchnic vasodilation.*

General Considerations

Respiratory acidosis results from an increase in the blood level of dissolved CO_2 that, after solution, dissociates into hydrogen ion and bicarbonate. The major problem in acute hypercapnic states is that increased quantities of dissolved CO_2 rapidly produce tissue acidosis because CO_2 diffuses easily into tissues and cells. This is of particular importance at the blood-brain barrier, where pH of cerebrospinal fluid falls rapidly after an acute increase in $Paco_2$.

Hypercapnia is usually attributed to lung disease, such as chronic obstructive pulmonary disease. However, hypercapnia can be produced either by an increase in the production of CO_2 without a compensatory rise in elimination or by constant production with decreased elimination. The second mechanism is usually operative in patients with chronic obstructive or restrictive pulmonary disease, in those with a severely deformed chest wall or neuromuscular weakness, after trauma, and following anesthesia, where either the respiratory mechanics or the drive for CO_2 elimination are compromised.

Increased CO_2 production is not uncommon because CO_2 output follows metabolic rate and patients in the critical care unit are frequently hypermetabolic. What is unusual, however, is failure of the ventilatory control mechanisms to respond to the increase in CO_2 production by stimulating ventilation and maintaining $Paco_2$ at a constant value. When sepsis intervenes, continued metabolism of mixed fuel substrates elevates the respiratory quotient and results in further enhancement of CO_2 production relative to oxygen consumption.

Common causes of respiratory acidosis among critically ill patients are listed in Table 2–21, and there is additional discussion of hypercapnic respiratory failure in Chapter 12.

Table 2–21. Causes of respiratory acidosis.

Acute	Chronic
Airway obstruction Emesis with aspiration Bronchospasm Laryngospasm	**Airway obstruction** Chronic obstructive pulmonary disease
Respiratory center depression General anesthesia Sedative or narcotic overdose Head injury	**Respiratory center depression** Chronic sedative overdose Obesity (Picwickian syndrome) Brain tumor
Circulatory collapse Cardiac arrest Pulmonary edema	
Neurogenic causes Cervical spine injury Guillain-Barré syndrome Myasthenic crisis Drugs (paralytic agents, organophosphates)	**Neurogenic causes** Multiple sclerosis Muscular dystrophy Amyotrophic lateral sclerosis Myxedema Posttraumatic diaphragmatic paralysis Phrenic nerve injury
Restrictive defects Hemothorax or pneumothorax Flail chest ARDS	**Restrictive defects** Hydrothorax or fibrothorax Ascites Obesity

An acute change in $PaCO_2$ produces a blood pH change within approximately 10 minutes. There is a small rise in serum bicarbonate concentration due to "mass action" shifts. The predicted response of $[HCO_3^-]$ is a fall of approximately 0.25 meq/L for each 1 mm Hg increase in $PaCO_2$. More marked changes in serum bicarbonate concentration suggest than an additional or mixed acid-base disturbance is present.

Chronic hypercapnia (beginning at about 30 minutes) stimulates renal ammonia production, increases urinary ammonium excretion, and causes chloruresis, both because of an increase in local $PaCO_2$ and because of the fall in pH. Urine pH decreases appropriately as newly generated bicarbonate is added to the blood. An increase in bicarbonate absorptive capacity also occurs, so that increased quantities of filtered bicarbonate are completely reabsorbed. Once equilibrium has been reached (after several days), the plasma bicarbonate concentration should increase by about 0.5 meq/L for each 1 mm Hg increase in $PaCO_2$. Arterial pH may actually become slightly alkalemic because of the avid retention of bicarbonate; this is one situation in which "complete" correction may occur and might not represent a mixed acid-base disturbance.

Clinical Features

A. Symptoms and Signs

There are no symptoms or signs specific to mild respiratory acidosis. Findings are usually related to the underlying cause. When airway obstruction is the cause, patients may present with shortness of breath and labored breathing. If respiratory center depression is the cause, slow and shallow or even apneustic breathing may be noted. If there is a history of chronic obstructive pulmonary disease, an acute exacerbation with wheezing or dyspnea is often present. As discussed in Chapter 12, patients may have tachypnea or hyperpnea (increased minute ventilation) despite hypercapnia (alveolar hypoventilation).

In cases of marked respiratory acidosis, fatigue, weakness, and confusion are present. In milder cases, patients may complain of headache. Physical findings are nonspecific and include tremor, asterixis, weakness, incoordination, cranial nerve signs, papilledema, retinal hemorrhages, and pyramidal tract findings. The syndrome of pseudotumor cerebri (increased cerebrospinal fluid pressure and papilledema) may be reproduced by respiratory acidosis. Coma begins at levels of CO_2 that vary from 70 mm Hg to 100 mm Hg depending on arterial pH (pH < 7.25) and the rate of increase of $PaCO_2$. It is critical to remember that almost all patients with hypercapnia will have concomitant hypoxemia unless they receive supplemental oxygen.

B. Laboratory Findings

Respiratory acidosis is manifested by acidemia and elevated $PaCO_2$ in the presence of an appropriate $[HCO_3^-]$ (Figure 2–5). Acutely, because renal ammonia production and hydrogen ion secretion are stimulated, urine pH falls paradoxically. In chronic respiratory acidosis, serum pH may be very close to normal as bicarbonate concentration rises in compensation. A mild increase in potassium secretion occurs, though hypokalemia is not inevitable.

Treatment

The key to management of respiratory acidosis is correction of its primary cause (see also Chapter 12). For some patients, this will require endotracheal intubation and mechanical ventilation or noninvasive positive-pressure ventilation.

Restoration of pH and $PaCO_2$ should take place over several hours if the respiratory acidosis is chronic to prevent alkalemia. The compensatory increase in serum bicarbonate in response to hypercapnia may take hours to days to be eliminated if the $PaCO_2$ is immediately corrected to normal. This results in a form of "metabolic alkalosis" that requires renal elimination of bicarbonate to a normal value. In many patients, overcorrection of chronic hypercapnia to normal is not advised because these patients have poor lung or ventilatory function. When mechanical ventilation is removed, they will be unable to maintain sufficient ventilation to keep the $PaCO_2$ at the lower level, resulting in recurrence of severe acute respiratory acidosis.

Current Controversies & Unresolved Issues

Acute hypercapnia and respiratory acidosis can almost always be effectively reversed by increasing minute ventilation until the underlying disorder can be treated (COPD, neuromuscular weakness, etc.). It is now recognized that excessively high tidal volume, respiratory rate, or both may be associated with damage to the lungs, prolonged hospitalization, and increased mortality. Therefore, low tidal volume and low pressure strategies are recommended (Chapter 12). The consequence is mild to moderate hypercapnia in some of these patients. The bulk of the evidence from large studies suggests that hypercapnia is well tolerated and rarely associated with complications. In fact, recent studies have suggested that hypercapnia is not merely a consequence that must be tolerated but that it may actually be instrumental in improving outcomes of patients with acute lung injury (ARDS).

Therefore, while there have been limited studies of the effects of ameliorating the fall in pH during so-called permissive hypercapnia, it remains to be seen if preventing the fall in pH with bicarbonate or other buffers is beneficial, hazardous, or neither.

Kallet RH et al: The treatment of acidosis in acute lung injury with tris-hydroxymethyl aminomethane (THAM). Am J Respir Crit Care Med 2000;161:1149–53.

Laffey JG, Engelberts D, Kavanagh BP: Buffering hypercapnic acidosis worsens acute lung injury. Am J Respir Crit Care Med 2000;161:141–6.

Potkin RT, Swenson ER: Resuscitation from severe acute hypercapnia: Determinants of tolerance and survival. Chest 1992; 102:1742–5.

RESPIRATORY ALKALOSIS

ESSENTIALS OF DIAGNOSIS

- *Alkalemia with decreased $PaCO_2$ and normal or appropriately decreased HCO_3^-.*
- *Anxiety, irritability, vertigo, and syncope.*
- *Flattened ST segments or T waves.*
- *Tetany in severe cases.*

General Considerations

Because of normal regulation of carbon dioxide in the blood, a primary decrease in the concentration of dissolved CO_2 indicates respiratory alkalosis. By definition, alveolar hyperventilation is synonymous with hypocapnia. The most common causes of hyperventilation include hypoxemia, central nervous system disorders, pulmonary disease, and excessive mechanical ventilation. Patients who are anxious, pregnant, have liver failure, or are toxic from salicylates will often hyperventilate. In the intensive care unit, hyperventilation may be an early feature of sepsis. Primary hyperventilation must be distinguished from compensation for metabolic acidosis. In both situations, $PaCO_2$ is reduced and serum HCO_3^- is low. The difference is that in respiratory alkalosis, low $PaCO_2$ is primary and pH is above normal, whereas in metabolic acidosis pH is in the acidic range and low HCO_3^- represents the primary disturbance.

The principal compensatory response is renal elimination of bicarbonate. It takes several hours to days to complete the response. Hypocapnia itself reduces bicarbonate reabsorption from the proximal tubule. Hydrogen ion secretion in the collecting tubule is also decreased. The increased delivery of sodium bicarbonate from the proximal tubule produces a marked kaliuresis with some degree of sodium excretion and chloruresis. In the steady state, plasma bicarbonate concentration falls by about 0.5 meq/L for each mm Hg decrease in $PaCO_2$ during chronic respiratory alkalosis. The arterial pH is therefore corrected *toward normal but not to normal.*

Clinical Features

A. Symptoms and Signs

Severe hyperventilation may result in tetany clinically indistinguishable from the hypocalcemic variety except that total serum calcium and the ionized fraction of calcium are normal. Hyperventilation may also decrease blood pressure and cerebral perfusion, which can cause increased irritability, anxiety, and an inability to concentrate. Occasionally, awake patients will complain of vertigo and experience syncope. Other features are those of the underlying disorder leading to respiratory alkalosis. Patients with severe damage to the mid brain may have central neurogenic hyperventilation. Prolonged respiratory alkalosis may have adverse effects on patients with head injury, despite transient reduction in intracranial pressure acutely.

B. Laboratory Findings

The hallmark of respiratory alkalosis is the presence of alkalemia (pH > 7.44) and decreased $Pa{CO_2}$ in the presence of normal or decreased HCO_3^-. The extent of serum bicarbonate reduction depends on the duration of the respiratory disorder and the effectiveness of the kidneys. The nomogram in Figure 2–5 may aid in determining whether the respiratory alkalosis is simple or combined with other disorders (mixed). Most patients with compensated or chronic respiratory alkalosis will have a decline in serum bicarbonate of 0.5 meq/L for each 1 mm Hg decrease in $Pa{CO_2}$. Mild hyponatremia and hypochloremia are often present. Hypophosphatemia due to excess renal phosphate wasting seems to be more marked with respiratory alkalosis than in metabolic alkalosis.

For patients with central neurogenic hyperventilation, evaluation may include CT or MRI of the head. Drug ingestions (particularly salicylates) can be investigated with a toxicology screen or blood measurements.

C. Electrocardiography and Electroencephalography

Electrocardiographic changes may include ST segment or T wave flattening or inversion. Alterations in the QRS complex have also been reported. Electroencephalographic studies are usually normal but may show an increase in the number of slow high-voltage waves.

Differential Diagnosis

The most important differential is metabolic acidosis with respiratory compensation. As described above, in metabolic acidosis the blood pH is less than 7.38, while respiratory alkalosis is associated with alkalemia. Mixed or combined disturbances are often seen with respiratory alkalosis—notably salicylate overdose, which may cause primary metabolic acidosis and primary respiratory alkalosis simultaneously.

Treatment

A. Correction of Underlying Disorder

The key to treatment is identification and management of underlying disorders such as sepsis or liver failure. If the patient is hypoxemic, the inspired oxygen concentration may need to be increased. Anemia may also be contributory and may be helped by blood transfusion. Other potentially reversible causes include sepsis and liver failure.

B. Mechanical Ventilation

Probably the most common cause of respiratory alkalosis among critically ill patients is iatrogenic mechanical hyperventilation. Strict attention to routine blood gases and examination of trends over several days will usually disclose this problem. If the ventilator has been set to deliver excessive minute ventilation and the patient is not triggering the machine, reducing the respiratory rate and tidal volume will cause a marked and predictable fall in pH. One reasonable goal is to reduce minute ventilation just until the patient begins to develop adequate spontaneous ventilation. At this point, pH is likely to be near normal.

On the other hand, if the patient is triggering the mechanical ventilator, ie, choosing the respiratory rate, then he or she is generating the primary drive for hyperventilation. In most of these cases, changing the settings on the ventilator will not affect the patient's spontaneous respiratory rate. Hyperventilation can sometimes be moderated by increasing paradoxically the inspiratory flow rate or tidal volume. Clinicians often select an intermittent mandatory ventilation mode, thinking that respiratory alkalosis will be minimized; controlled trials have shown that this does not work. Lengthening the ventilator circuit tubing to add dead space should not be done because of the risk of increasing work of breathing. In rare circumstances, severe respiratory alkalosis that cannot be managed in any other way may require paralyzing the patient and controlling the $Pa{CO_2}$ and pH precisely.

Laffey JG, Kavanagh BP: Carbon dioxide and the critically ill—too little of a good thing? Lancet 1999;354:1283–6.

Muizelaar JP et al: Adverse effects of prolonged hyperventilation in patients with severe head injury: a randomized trial. J Neurosurg 1991;75:731–9.

Rose BD, Post TW: *Clinical Physiology of Acid-Base and Electrolyte Disorders,* 5th ed. McGraw-Hill, 2001.

Transfusion Therapy 3

Elizabeth D. Simmons, MD

The discovery of the ABO and Rh blood groups and the development of nontoxic anticoagulant-preservative solutions for blood storage during the first half of the 20th century made it possible for human blood to be widely used as lifesaving therapy in critically ill patients. Subsequent refinements in cross-matching and the development of sophisticated screening tests for transmissible diseases have made blood transfusion a safe and often lifesaving form of therapy. Because of the wide range of potential adverse effects of transfusion therapy, however, the clinician must have a clear understanding of the indications, efficacy, and complications of blood component therapy.

BLOOD COMPONENTS

In modern transfusion practice, blood is separated into various components (Table 3–1), and individual components are selected for transfusion based on the needs of the patient. Blood component therapy is superior to whole blood replacement because it concentrates those portions of blood a patient needs, thereby increasing efficiency and minimizing volume and subsequent transfusion requirements—as well as increasing the efficiency of blood banking by putting donated blood to maximal and optimal use.

RED BLOOD CELLS

The products available for replacement of red blood cells are listed in Table 3–1. Homologous packed red blood cells from volunteer donors are transfused most often. Leukocyte-poor red cells are prepared by a variety of techniques to remove at least 70% of leukocytes. Washing red cells in saline removes most plasma proteins and some leukocytes and platelets. Red blood cells frozen in liquid nitrogen with glycerol as a cryoprotective agent can be stored for up to 10 years. Extensive washing after thawing removes most plasma proteins and cellular debris. Neocytes (young red blood cells) can be prepared by differential centrifugation or cell separators and have a longer circulating life span than standard red cells, but they are rarely used. Directed donations of red blood cells from ABO- and Rh-compatible individuals who are appropriately screened may be substituted for homologous red cells at the patient's request. Autologous red blood cells may be collected preoperatively, by perioperative blood salvage, or by acute normovolemic hemodilution to decrease homologous red cell use.

Indications

Red blood cell transfusions are indicated to promote oxygen delivery in patients who are actively bleeding, for symptomatic anemia unresponsive to conservative management, or when time does not permit alternative treatment. Red blood cell transfusions may also be useful for improving the bleeding tendency of a severely anemic patient with platelet dysfunction (eg, uremia) or severe thrombocytopenia.

The decision to transfuse red blood cells should be made only after consideration of several factors. The age and general condition of the patient and the presence of coexisting cardiac, pulmonary, or vascular conditions will influence the patient's ability to tolerate acute blood loss or chronic anemia. The degree and chronicity of the anemia are also important determinants of the physiologic responses to anemia. Finally, the cause of the anemia must be considered, as alternative therapy (eg, iron sulfate, vitamin B_{12}, folate, or epoetin alfa [erythropoietin] may eliminate the need for transfusions altogether.

A. Chronic Hypoproliferative Anemia

Chronic anemia is accompanied by several physiologic adaptations that enhance oxygen delivery despite a reduced red cell oxygen-carrying capacity. Increased cardiac output, increased intravascular volume, and redistribution of blood flow to vital organs maintain organ function. Tissue extraction of oxygen occurs over a wide range of hemoglobin concentrations and is enhanced by a rightward shift in the oxyhemoglobin dissociation curve (due to increased erythrocyte 2,3-DPG production and the Bohr effect). Additional responses to anemia include increased erythropoietin production and early release of young red blood cells into the circulation. These adaptive responses allow most individuals to tolerate severe decreases in oxygen-carrying capacity. Therefore, red blood cell transfusions are rarely necessary for patients with chronic anemia who have hemo-

Table 3–1. Blood component therapy.

Products Available	Indications for Transfusion
Red blood cells (RBC)	
Homologous packed RBC	Promote oxygen delivery for patients with active bleeding or severe anemia; improve bleeding tendency in severely anemic patients with platelet dysfunction.
Leukocyte-poor RBC (filtered or irradiated)	Prevent nonhemolytic transfusion reactions due to platelet or white blood cell antigens in previously sensitized patients; prevent HLA sensitization in potential transplant recipients or those requiring chronic platelet transfusions; may reduce risk of CMV transmission.
Washed RBC	Substitute for homologous RBC in patients sensitive to a plasma component; avoid transfusion of anti-A and anti-B antibodies when O-negative blood is used in patients who are type A, B, or AB.
Frozen RBC	Preserve autologous RBC; maintain store of rare blood types.
Neocytes	Increase efficacy of individual transfusion for patients with transfusion-dependent anemia.
Directed donor RBC	After screening and informed consent, may be substituted for volunteer RBC at patient request.
Autologous RBC	Decrease or eliminate need for homologous RBC in patients undergoing elective surgical procedures or obstetric delivery.
Platelets	
Random donor platelets	Treat or prevent bleeding associated with severe thrombocytopenia or platelet dysfunction; replace platelets lost with massive bleeding; treat excessive bleeding associated with cardiopulmonary bypass.
Single-donor platelets	Decrease exposure to infectious agents.
Leukocyte-poor platelets (filtered or irradiated)	Prevent alloimmunization to HLA antigens in patients requiring repeated platelet transfusions.
HLA-matched platelets	Treat bleeding associated with thrombocytopenia in patients who are refractory to platelet transfusions due to HLA sensitization.
Plasma and derivatives	
Fresh frozen plasma (FFP)	Correct coagulation factor deficiencies in bleeding patients or those who require invasive procedures if concentrated or recombinant product not available; treat TTP/HUS, protein-losing enteropathy in infants; antithrombin III deficiency; C-1 esterase inhibitor deficiency.
Cryoprecipitate-poor plasma	Correct coagulation factor deficiencies other than VIII, XIII, fibrinogen, vWF; may be indicated for treatment of refractory TTP.
Cryoprecipitate	Correct severe hypofibrogenemia; may be useful for treatment of bleeding associated with uremia.
Granulocytes	
Stimulated leukapheresis	Treat severe bacterial infections unresponsive to antibiotics in patients with prolonged, severe neutropenia or congenital neutrophil dysfunction; may be indicated in the management of neonatal sepsis.

globin concentrations above 7 g/dL, and transfusions may result in circulatory overload if given rapidly or in excessive quantity.

B. Acute Blood Loss

In contrast, physiologic responses may be inadequate to maintain organ function and hemodynamic stability when faced with acute blood loss, even with apparently normal hemoglobin concentration, since it takes time for mobilization of extracellular fluid into the intravascular space and for increased production of erythrocyte 2,3-DPG. However, a healthy young person generally tolerates 500–1000 mL of acute blood loss without red blood cell transfusion, and intravascular volume can be repleted with crystalloid solutions. Acute blood loss of 1000–2000 mL usually can be managed with volume replacement alone, but red cell transfusions are occasionally necessary. More than 2 L of acute blood loss will usually require red blood cell transfusion. Other clinical factors are important. For example, because of the vasodilatory effects of anesthesia, intraoperative blood loss of more than 500 mL may require red cell transfusion to maintain hemodynamic stability, and burn patients often require vigorous blood product support because of volume depletion through denuded body surfaces.

C. High-Risk Patients

Any condition that impairs the patient's ability to increase intravascular volume, heart rate, stroke volume, or blood flow will result in poor tolerance of chronic anemia or acute blood loss. Older patients or those with impaired cardiac function may not be able to generate the necessary increase in cardiac output to maintain tissue perfusion. Patients with coronary artery disease especially may not tolerate a decrease in oxygen-carrying capacity because the rise in myocardial oxygen demand accompanying increased cardiac output may exceed the supply. Vascular disease may impair the ability to increase blood flow to vital organs, such as the brain. Diuretic use, gastrointestinal losses, or redistribution of extracellular fluid volume will decrease intravascular volume, resulting in decreased blood flow and thus decreased tissue oxygenation. In these circumstances, transfusion may be necessary in a symptomatic patient at higher hemoglobin concentrations than in a normal individual with adequate physiologic reserves. The use of objective scoring systems (such as the APACHE II—Acute Physiologic and Chronic Health Evaluation II—and the multiorgan dysfunction scores) to stratify patients according to severity of illness may be useful for determining which critically ill patients may benefit from a restrictive transfusion approach.

Studies have demonstrated that patients younger than 55 years of age with less severe illness may have improved outcomes using a lower hemoglobin threshold (< 7 g/dL) for transfusion compared with more liberal use of transfusion (< 10 g/dL). Exceptions include those with acute myocardial ischemia or acute bleeding. This lower threshold for transfusion also appears to be at least as safe even in older patients and those with more severe disease.

D. Hemolytic Anemia

Red cell transfusions are indicated in the management of some patients with a variety of severe and symptomatic hemolytic anemias. Patients with markedly symptomatic antibody-mediated hemolytic anemias may require red cell transfusion until definitive therapy can become effective. Autoantibodies are often reactive with all donor red cells in vitro, such that cross-matching is impossible. Transfusion of ABO- and Rh-compatible red cells is usually safe in these patients; the blood bank can perform an extended cross-match to identify units with the least degree of in vitro hemolysis. Patients with cold-reacting antibodies (usually IgM) should receive blood through a blood warmer if transfusion is necessary.

E. Sickle Cell Anemia

Patients with sickle cell anemia may require red cell transfusion (and, in selected cases, partial or complete exchange transfusion) for management of specific complications, including splenic sequestration and aplastic crises (with rapidly falling hemoglobin concentration), recurrent priapism, chronic unremitting osteomyelitis, severe leg ulcers, pneumonia, or pulmonary sequestration crises. Red cell transfusion is also indicated for such patients undergoing major surgery, particularly those undergoing orthopedic procedures. Simple preoperative transfusion to achieve hematocrit levels of about 30% appears to be as effective as regimens aimed at reducing the fraction of hemoglobin S to 30% of total hemoglobin (by exchange transfusion or multiple transfusions over time) and is associated with fewer transfusion-related complications. Patients with sickle cell anemia are not candidates for autologous donation and transfusion.

Exchange transfusion is also indicated in the management of acute central nervous system infarction or hemorrhage (followed by chronic transfusion therapy to prevent recurrent strokes). Chronic prophylactic transfusion reduces the risk of initial stroke in children with sickle cell disease who have abnormal cerebrovascular blood flow on Doppler ultrasonography; however, alloimmunization (even with phenotypically-matched, leukodepleted red blood cells), iron overload, and infections complicating chronic transfusion programs have limited the acceptance of this approach. Furthermore, the duration of transfusion required to prevent stroke is unclear.

Routine transfusion during pregnancy should be avoided. Patients with severe, symptomatic sickle cell anemia or those suffering recurrent painful crises may require periodic transfusion during pregnancy. Likewise, routine transfusion is not indicated in the management of painful vaso-occlusive sickle cell crises, and should be reserved for those patients with symptomatic anemia. Patients with sickle cell anemia appear to be unusually susceptible to the development of alloantibodies (see Complications of Transfusion, on page 87), which limits the utility of chronic transfusion programs. The use of blood from racially matched donors that has been screened for selected minor blood group antigens may prevent alloimmunization in patients requiring chronic transfusion therapy, but this approach awaits confirmation.

E. Perioperative Transfusion

Transfusion is rarely indicated for patients undergoing noncardiac surgery who have hemoglobin values > 7–8 g/dL and no risk factors for myocardial ischemia. However, elderly patients with hematocrits < 28% (hemoglobin of approximately 9 g/dL) may be at risk for myocardial ischemia during surgery, especially if tachycardia is present. In these patients—and others at risk for myocardial ischemia—a hemoglobin < 10 g/dL probably warrants transfusion.

F. Unacceptable Indications

Red blood cell transfusions should not be used to enhance a patient's general sense of well being, to promote wound healing, or to expand vascular volume when oxygen-carrying capacity is adequate.

RED BLOOD CELL TRANSFUSION REQUIREMENTS

There is no single hemoglobin threshold that is universally appropriate for determining transfusion requirements. The amount of red blood cells to be transfused should be determined by the clinical status of the patient rather than by the hemoglobin concentration. In patients who are actively bleeding, crystalloid volume repletion is essential. Hemodynamic instability, symptoms and signs of impaired organ function, rate of blood loss, and response to transfusion should be used to determine how much blood should be transfused. Patients with chronic anemia should receive only the amount of red blood cells necessary to reverse symptoms and signs. Patients with self-limited anemia (eg, transient blood loss, hemolysis, or marrow suppression) or those for whom alternative therapy is available (eg, nutritional deficiencies, anemia of renal failure) should receive red blood cells only when an immediate need for increased oxygen-carrying capacity is present such as during myocardial ischemia, heart failure, impaired central nervous system oxygenation, hypotension, or other evidence of tissue hypoxia. The patient should be reevaluated after each unit of red blood cells is transfused rather than given an arbitrary or predetermined number of units. Volume overload following red blood cell transfusion in patients with chronic severe anemia may eliminate any benefit of increasing the oxygen-carrying capacity and must be monitored carefully.

When untreatable chronic anemia is present (eg, bone marrow failure or chronic severe hemolytic anemia), red blood cell transfusions must be given conservatively to delay long-term treatment complications such as alloimmunization, infections, and iron overload. Red blood cell transfusions may be administered more liberally in the treatment of anemia associated with severe thrombocytopenia or platelet dysfunction (eg, acute leukemia or uremic bleeding episodes), because the salutary effect of increased hematocrit on platelet function may decrease platelet transfusion requirements and lessen clinical bleeding.

PLATELETS

Platelet products available are listed in Table 3–1. The choice of platelet product depends on the underlying condition of the patient (eg, acute, reversible thrombocytopenia versus chronic thrombocytopenia) as well as the local availability of supplies. Pooled random donor platelets or single-donor platelets obtained by apheresis are the usual products transfused for correction of severe thrombocytopenia. Filtration or irradiation with ultraviolet B of pooled donor platelets depletes them of donor leukocytes, and these are equally effective strategies for preventing alloantibody-mediated refractoriness to platelet transfusions. This leukodepletion is appropriate for patients likely to require repeated platelet transfusions (eg, acute leukemia, aplastic anemia, and other bone marrow failure states). Leukocyte depletion performed shortly after collection of platelets may also decrease the risk of febrile reactions by preventing in vitro accumulation of cytokines, which are released during storage. Single donor platelets decrease the total number of donor exposures and may reduce the risk of transfusion-transmitted infections but do not appear to offer additional benefit over filtration or irradiation for prevention of alloimmunization.

Product availability will often determine whether pooled platelets or single donor platelets are transfused. Whenever possible, ABO type-specific platelets should be used; however, because platelets have a limited storage period, they are not always available. A decreased response to platelet transfusion may result from the use of ABO-incompatible platelets, but the most significant risk occurs when ABO-incompatible plasma is infused (ie, type O donor, type A or B recipient), resulting in hemolysis (estimated risk 1:9000–1:6600). Apheresis units may increase this risk by increasing the dose of incompatible plasma. If type-specific platelets are not available, pooled platelets are preferable to single-donor platelets. Washing the platelets to remove plasma may help to minimize exposure to incompatible plasma. Although platelets do not carry Rh antigens, platelets from Rh-negative donors should be used for transfusion in Rh-negative women of childbearing years to prevent sensitization from contaminating red blood cells.

Indications

Platelet transfusions are indicated for treatment of bleeding associated with thrombocytopenia or intrinsic platelet dysfunction. Platelet transfusions are also indicated in the management of massive bleeding if severe thrombocytopenia develops. Patients undergoing cardiopulmonary bypass may require platelet transfusions if excessive bleeding occurs because of thrombocytopenia and decreased platelet function induced by the bypass procedure. Other surgical procedures in thrombocytopenic patients generally require prophylactic platelet transfusions to maintain adequate perioperative platelet counts for at least 3 days (> 50,000/μL for major procedures; > 30,000/μL for minor procedures). Prophylactic platelet transfusions are also indicated for severely thrombocytopenic (eg, < 5000–10,000/μL platelets) patients undergoing intensive chemotherapy for acute leukemia; the threshold for transfusion may be higher in the presence of fever, infection, or drugs that cause platelet dysfunction.

Factors that determine the risk of serious bleeding due to thrombocytopenia include the cause and severity of thrombocytopenia, the presence of vascular defects, the functional status of the patient's platelets, and the presence of other hemostatic defects. Severe anemia may also contribute to bleeding in patients with thrombocytopenia or platelet dysfunction. Because of the increased functional capacity of younger platelets in patients with decreased platelet survival, decreased production of platelets carries a higher risk of serious bleeding at any given platelet count than thrombocytopenia due to destruction, consumption, or hypersplenism. Typical bleeding manifestations related to the level of thrombocytopenia are shown in Table 17–8. If bleeding is out of proportion to a given platelet count, other contributing factors to bleeding should be investigated.

The risk of bleeding in patients with disorders of platelet function likewise depends on the cause and severity of the disorder and whether vascular defects, other hemostatic abnormalities, or severe anemia is present. Bleeding time is the most widely used test of platelet function, and, although it is useful in the diagnosis of certain disorders (eg, von Willebrand's disease, hereditary platelet disorders), prolonged bleeding time in the absence of a history of bleeding is not a reliable predictor of subsequent bleeding. A prolonged bleeding time in the absence of thrombocytopenia or severe anemia in a bleeding patient, however, may indicate the presence of platelet dysfunction.

The efficacy of platelet transfusions can be assessed by observing a sustained rise in platelet count in a patient who has stopped bleeding. Patients with thrombocytopenia due to decreased production of platelets are most likely to experience a significant, sustained increase in platelet count following platelet transfusion. Patients with increased destruction of platelets and those who have hypersplenism usually do not achieve a significant increase in platelet count after transfusion, and any increase that occurs is usually transient. Similarly, patients with massive platelet consumption due to bleeding will have a suboptimal increase in platelet count following transfusion. Hemorrhage due to platelet dysfunction can be controlled with platelet transfusions only if the defect is intrinsic to the platelet (aspirin ingestion, cardiopulmonary bypass, inherited platelet disorders), rather than extrinsic (eg, von Willebrand's disease or uremia).

Platelet transfusions are minimally useful in the treatment of thrombocytopenia due to decreased platelet survival and should not be given unless severe life-threatening bleeding occurs. They are also ineffective in the treatment of bleeding due to platelet dysfunction caused by extrinsic factors such as von Willebrand's disease or uremia. Platelet transfusions may be harmful in patients with thrombotic thrombocytopenic purpura-hemolytic uremic syndrome (TTP-HUS) despite the presence of thrombocytopenia, presumably due to accelerated thrombosis in vital organs. Because platelet survival is short in this disorder, platelet transfusions are usually ineffective for controlling hemorrhage. The diagnosis of TTP-HUS should be suspected in a patient with severe thrombocytopenia and hemolysis with schistocytes on peripheral blood smear (microangiopathic hemolytic anemia), with or without associated central nervous system dysfunction, renal dysfunction, or fever. Patients with heparin-associated thrombocytopenia may also suffer increased thrombotic complications if platelets are transfused. Platelet transfusions should be administered to these patients only when the risk of death from bleeding outweighs the potential risk of clinical deterioration from transfusion.

Platelet Transfusion Requirements

The quantity of platelets to be transfused depends on the source of the platelets, the cause and degree of thrombocytopenia, and the observed response to transfusions. The usual initial amount transfused is six to eight units of random donor platelets or one single-donor apheresis product. Platelet packs should contain a minimum of 5.5×10^9 platelets per unit.

The response to platelet transfusions should be determined by obtaining a platelet count 1 hour after transfusion and daily thereafter and by observing the effect on control of bleeding. The 1-hour count should increase by about 5000–10,000 per unit of random donor platelets, or 30,000–50,000 per unit of single-donor platelets. Stored homologous platelets survive about 3 days in thrombocytopenic patients. The 1-hour count and subsequent platelet survival will be reduced in patients with increased destruction or hypersplenism. These measurements will help determine the magnitude of the benefit to be expected from subsequent transfusions. If only a minimal response occurs or if the platelet rise is short-lived, subsequent prophylactic transfusions should be withheld. However, in patients with severe thrombocytopenia due to destruction or hypersplenism who have serious bleeding, platelet transfusions may be warranted. In any patient, if clinical bleeding does not improve despite platelet transfusion, other causes of bleeding should be evaluated and the utility of subsequent platelet transfusions in such patients reassessed.

The underlying cause of thrombocytopenia or platelet dysfunction should be determined so that specific therapy to reverse the process can be given if available. Alternatives to platelet transfusions in bleeding patients with thrombocytopenia or platelet dysfunction are set forth in Table 3–2.

Table 3–2. Alternatives to platelet transfusions.

Alternative	Possible Indications
High-dose IgG	Life-threatening bleeding in immune-mediated thrombocytopenia (ITP).
Anti-D immune globulin	Treatment of bleeding in ITP in Rh-positive patients.
Desmopressin (DDAVP)	Bleeding associated with platelet dysfunction, uremia, von Willebrand disease.
Antifibrinolytic agents (eg, aminocaproic acid)	Excessive bleeding without evidence of thrombotic diathesis or hematuria.
Estrogens	Bleeding associated with uremic platelet dysfunction.
Red cell transfusions	Severe anemia associated with thrombocytopenia or platelet dysfunction.
Erythropoietin	Bleeding in anemic, uremic patients
Corticosteroids	ITP, possibly thrombotic thrombocytopenic purpura-hemolytic uremic syndrome (TTP-HUS)
Splenectomy	Refractory ITP, severe hypersplenism, possibly TTP
Immunosuppressives or chemotherapy	Refractory ITP
Danazol	Refractory ITP
Vinca alkaloids	Refractory ITP
Alpha-interferon	Refractory ITP
Protein-A immunoadsorption	Refractory ITP
Plasma infusion or exchange	TTP-HUS
Thrombopoietin	Severe thrombocytopenia following chemotherapy

PLASMA

Plasma products available are listed in Table 3–1. Fresh frozen plasma (FFP) is prepared by separating plasma from red blood cells (after collection of whole blood or during plasmapheresis) and freezing it within 6 hours after collection at −18 °C or colder. It can be stored for up to 1 year and is thawed over 20–30 minutes prior to administration. Activities of coagulation factors are adequate for 24 hours after thawing. Fresh plasma and plasma recovered from outdated blood products are used for preparation of plasma derivatives (immunoglobulin, cryoprecipitate, albumin, coagulation factor concentrates) and are otherwise not usually available for patient use.

Cryoprecipitate-poor plasma is the supernatant plasma remaining after preparation of cryoprecipitate and contains adequate quantities of all coagulation factors except fibrinogen, factors VIII and XIII, and von Willebrand factor. Solvent-detergent treatment of plasma (S/D plasma) inactivates lipid-enveloped viruses and has been recently licensed by the FDA to minimize the risk of transfusion-transmitted infections in the management of coagulopathies and thrombotic thrombocytopenic purpura. Numerous other derivatives of plasma are now available; Table 3–3 outlines some of these products and their therapeutic uses.

Indications

The major indication for FFP is correction of coagulation factor deficiencies in patients with active bleeding or who require invasive procedures. Isolated congenital factor deficiencies (eg, factors II, V, VII, X, XI, or XIII) may be treated with FFP if no specific concentrate is available. Multiple acquired factor deficiencies complicate severe liver disease and disseminated intravascular coagulation and, if associated with significant bleeding, may be treated with FFP. However, excessive volume expansion or decreased survival of coagulation factors may decrease the usefulness of FFP in these conditions. Vitamin K deficiency and warfarin therapy result in a functional deficiency of factors II, VII, IX, and X, and parenteral vitamin K administration will reverse these

Table 3–3. Therapeutic products derived from plasma.

Plasma Derivative	Therapeutic Use
Fibrin glue (human fibrinogen combined with bovine thrombin)	Prevent surgical oozing with topical use
Albumin (heat-treated)	Hypoalbuminemia in nephrotic syndrome
Factor VIII concentrate	Hemophilia A
Humate: P	Von Willebrand's disease
Prothrombin complex concentrate	Coagulation inhibitors
Activated factor IX concentrates (Autoplex, FEIBA)	Factor VIII inhibitors
Factor IX complex concentrate with high factor IX-specific activity	Hemophilia B
Factor XIII concentrate	Factor XIII deficiency
Antithrombin III concentrate	Thrombosis in AT III deficiency
C1 esterase inhibitor concentrate	Angioedema
α_1-Antitrypsin concentrate	Prevent lung damage in α_1-antitrypsin deficiency
Protein C and S concentrate	Severe protein C or S deficiency
Intravenous immunoglobulin	Immunodeficiency states; immune cytopenias, Kawasaki syndrome, Guillain-Barre syndrome, dermatomyositis
Immune serum globulin	Passive immunization against hepatitis A, measles, poliomyelitis, chickenpox, rubella

deficiencies within about 24 hours. If immediate correction is necessary because of active bleeding, FFP can be given. Massively bleeding patients requiring transfusion of red blood cells greater than 100% of normal blood volume in less than 24 hours may become deficient in multiple coagulation factors, and FFP is indicated if a demonstrable coagulopathy develops following massive transfusion and bleeding continues. However, bleeding in such patients is more often due to thrombocytopenia than coagulation factor deficiencies, so prophylactic administration of FFP is not usually indicated.

Other indications for treatment with FFP include antithrombin III deficiency in patients at high risk for thrombosis or who are unresponsive to heparin therapy; severe protein-losing enteropathy in infants; severe C1 esterase inhibitor deficiency with life-threatening angioedema; and TTP-HUS.

Plasma exchange therapy, with removal of undesirable plasma substances and reinfusion of normal plasma, appears to be effective alone or as an adjunct in the management of cryoglobulinemia, Goodpasture's syndrome, Guillain-Barré syndrome, homozygous familial hypercholesterolemia, and posttransfusion purpura. Plasma exchange may be of value in some patients with chronic inflammatory demyelinating polyneuropathy, cold agglutinin disease, autoimmune thrombocytopenia, rapidly progressive glomerulonephritis, and systemic vasculitis. Rarely, patients with alloantibodies, pure red cell aplasia, warm autoimmune hemolytic anemia, multiple sclerosis, or maternal-fetal incompatibility may benefit from therapeutic plasma exchange.

Fresh frozen plasma should not be administered for reversal of volume depletion or to counteract nutritional deficiencies (except severe protein-losing enteropathy in infants) because effective alternatives are available. Purified human immunoglobulin has replaced FFP in the treatment of humoral immunodeficiency. Patients with coagulation factor deficiencies who are not bleeding or not in need of invasive procedures should likewise not be treated with FFP. Patients with mild coagulation factor deficiencies (ie, prothrombin time < 16–18 seconds, partial thromboplastin time < 55–60 seconds) are unlikely to have bleeding in the absence of an anatomic lesion, and even with surgery or other invasive procedures these patients may not have excessive bleeding. Therefore, prophylactic administration of FFP should be discouraged in such cases.

Plasma Transfusion Requirements

ABO type-specific FFP should be used to prevent transfusion of anti-A or anti-B antibodies. Rh-negative donor plasma should be administered to Rh-negative patients to prevent Rh sensitization from contaminating red blood cells (particularly important for women of childbearing years).

The amount of FFP must be individualized. In the treatment of coagulation factor deficiencies, the appropriate dose of FFP must take into account the plasma volume of the patient, the desired increase in factor activity, and the expected half-life of the factors being replaced. The average adult patient with multiple factor deficiencies requires two to nine units (about 400–1800 mL) of FFP acutely to control bleeding, with smaller quantities given at periodic intervals as necessary to maintain adequate hemostasis. Control of bleeding and measurement of coagulation times (prothrombin time and partial thromboplastin time) should be used to determine when and if to give repeated doses of FFP. Smaller amounts of FFP are usually sufficient for treatment of isolated coagulation factor deficiencies.

Plasma infusion and plasma exchange for treatment of TTP-HUS usually necessitate very large quantities of FFP—up to ten units per day (or even more)—for several days until the desired clinical response is achieved. The precise dose of FFP required to treat hereditary angioedema is unknown; two units is probably adequate, and a concentrate is now available to treat C1 esterase inhibitor deficiency.

CRYOPRECIPITATE

Preparation

When fresh frozen plasma is thawed at 4 °C, a precipitate is formed. This cryoprecipitate is separated from the supernatant plasma and resuspended in a small volume of plasma. It is then refrozen at −18 °C and kept for up to 1 year. The supernatant plasma is used for preparation of other plasma fractions (coagulation factor concentrates, albumin, and immunoglobulin). Each bag of cryoprecipitate (about 50 mL) contains approximately 100–250 mg of fibrinogen, 80–100 units of factor VIII, 40–70% of the plasma von Willebrand factor concentration, 50–60 mg of fibronectin, and factor XIII at one and one-half to four times the concentration in FFP.

Indications

Cryoprecipitate is indicated in patients with severe hypofibrinogenemia (< 100 mg/dL) for treatment of bleeding episodes or as prophylaxis for invasive procedures. It may be useful in the treatment of severe bleeding in uremic patients unresponsive to desmopressin and dialysis. Cryoprecipitate can also be used to make a topical fibrin glue for use intraoperatively to control local bleeding and has been used in the removal of renal stones when combined with thrombin and calcium.

Purified factor VIII concentrates or recombinant factor VIII products are preferred over cryoprecipitate in the management of hemophilia A because of the lower risk of infectious disease transmission as well as fewer other complications (eg, allergic reactions to other plasma or cryoprecipitate constituents). Antihemophilic factor/von Willebrand factor complex (human), dried, pasteurized (Humate-P), a concentrate rich in von Willebrand factor, is now preferred over cryoprecipitate in the treatment of von Willebrand's disease when treatment with desmopressin is inadequate or unsuitable. Likewise, factor XIII concentrate is available for treatment of bleeding due to factor XIII deficiency.

Cryoprecipitate is not indicated for bleeding due to thrombocytopenia; for bleeding due to multiple coagulation factor deficiencies unless severe hypofibrinogenemia is present; or for bleeding due to unknown cause. It is not indicated for treatment of patients with deficiencies of factors VIII, XIII, or von Willebrand factor in the absence of bleeding or the need for invasive procedures.

Administration

ABO type-specific cryoprecipitate is thawed and pooled into the desired quantity and administered intravenously by infusion or syringe. In treatment of bleeding due to hypofibrinogenemia, the goal of therapy is to maintain the fibrinogen concentration above 100 mg/dL. Two to three bags per 10 kg body weight will increase the fibrinogen concentration by about 100 mg/dL. Maintenance doses of one bag per 15 kg body weight can be given daily until adequate hemostasis is achieved. When hypofibrinogenemia is due to increased consumption (eg, DIC), larger and more frequent doses may be required to control bleeding.

GRANULOCYTES

Granulocyte concentrates (Table 3–1) are prepared by automated leukapheresis from ABO-compatible donors stimulated several hours before collection with corticosteroids. Granulocytes have decreased function if refrigerated or agitated, so these concentrates should be given as soon as possible after collection (preferably within 6 hours; never after 24 hours). Granulocytes do not survive prolonged storage and so must be prepared before each transfusion.

Indications

The indications for granulocyte transfusions are controversial. Severe neutropenia (< 500/μL) is associated with a marked increase in the risk of bacterial and fungal infections. Most authorities agree that granulocyte transfusions are most likely to be helpful in patients with documented bacterial infections unresponsive to antibiotics accompanied by prolonged severe neutropenia when bone marrow recovery is expected in 7–10 days or in patients with congenital severe granulocyte dysfunction complicated by life-threatening fungal infections. Granulocyte transfusions may also be of value in the treatment of neonatal sepsis, though this remains controversial.

Granulocyte transfusions are not helpful for preventing infections in neutropenic patients, in treating infections associated with transient neutropenia, or in treating fevers and neutropenia not associated with documented infection. Patients who are unlikely to recover bone marrow function (aplastic anemia or refractory acute leukemia) appear to derive less benefit than patients who will ultimately recover (eg, acute leukemia following successful chemotherapy). Granulocyte transfusions should be used with caution in patients receiving amphotericin B or in those with pulmonary infiltrates because of the potential for adverse pulmonary events.

Administration

Granulocytes should be administered as soon as possible after collection from a corticosteroid-stimulated ABO-compatible donor. The minimal dose recommended is 2–3 × 10^{10} granulocytes per transfusion, infused slowly under constant supervision. Daily transfusions should be administered for at least 4 days and perhaps longer until the infection is controlled.

Complications

Granulocyte transfusions are associated with numerous adverse effects, including febrile reactions (25–50%), alloantibodies (HLA and neutrophil-specific), CMV infections if granulocytes from seropositive donors are given to seronegative patients, pulmonary reactions, and graft-versus-host disease (preventable with irradiation of the product). These complications—as well as the development of more effective antibiotics and more effective antileukemic therapy—have diminished the occasions for use of granulocyte transfusions over the last decade. Human recombinant cytokines, such as granulocyte colony-stimulating factor (filgrastim; G-CSF) and granulocyte macrophage colony-stimulating factor (sargramostim; GM-CSF) can be used to decrease the severity and duration of neutropenia in patients receiving chemotherapy for nonmyeloid malignancies and even in selected patients with myeloid malignancies.

COAGULATION FACTORS

Available coagulation factor products, indications, dosing, alternatives, and complications are discussed in Chapter 17.

BLOOD COMPONENT ADMINISTRATION

INFORMED CONSENT

Before elective transfusion of any blood component is undertaken, the patient should be informed of the benefits of transfusion, the potential risks of transfusion, and the alternatives to transfusion. The patient should be given the opportunity to ask questions about the recommended transfusion, and consent should be obtained before proceeding. Informed consent should also be obtained from competent patients in emergency situations. Many states have passed laws requiring informed consent prior to elective transfusion, including providing the patient with the option of autologous donation where appropriate (usually for elective surgical procedures).

PATIENT IDENTIFICATION

The identity of the patient should be verified when obtaining specimens for cross-match, and blood collected should be immediately labeled with the patient's name and hospital identification number, dated, and signed by the phlebotomist. At the time of transfusion, the label on the unit should be compared with the name and identification number on the patient's bracelet. There should be no discrepancies in spelling or medical record number. Rigid adherence to these practices eliminates the great majority of major acute hemolytic transfusion reactions.

PREPARATION OF BLOOD COMPONENTS

Potential donors are screened with a questionnaire prior to donation to eliminate donors with identifiable risk factors for complications in both the donor and the recipient. After collection, donor blood is screened for the presence of infectious diseases or their markers, including VDRL, hepatitis B surface antigen and core antibody, hepatitis C, HIV-1 and 2 antibodies, HIV-1 p24 antigen, HTLV-1 and -2, and occasionally cytomegalovirus. The ABO and Rh types of donor and recipient red blood cells are determined, and the sera of both donor and recipient are screened for clinically significant alloantibodies to the major red cell antigens. If donor red blood cells appear to be Rh-negative, they are typed further to exclude a weakly reactive Rh-positive variant (weak D, D^u). Recipient serum is incubated with donor red blood cells to detect antibodies that may react with donor red cells (the "cross-match"). Some patients have autoantibodies that react with virtually all red blood cells. In these situations, the in vitro cross-match should be performed with multiple type-specific donor samples to find red cells with the least in vitro incompatibility.

ADMINISTRATION

All blood components should be administered through a standard blood filter to trap clots and other large particles into any accessible vein or central venous catheter. When leukocyte-depleted red blood cells or platelets are desired, third-generation leukoreduction filters may be used if filtration has not been performed in the laboratory. Red blood cells should not be administered by syringe or by automatic infusion pump because forcible administration may cause mechanical hemolysis, but other cellular components and plasma derivatives may be administered by pumps. Nothing should be added to the blood component (eg, medications, hyperalimentation) or administered through the same line as the component. Only physiologic saline solution should be administered through the same line and may be used to dilute red blood cells and thus promote easier flow. Hypotonic solutions (5% dextrose in water) may cause hemolysis, and solutions containing calcium (Ringer's lactate) may initiate coagulation. These should not be administered through the same line with blood components.

Blood components should be administered slowly for the first 5–10 minutes while the patient is under observation, and the patient should be periodically reassessed throughout the transfusion process for adverse effects. Blood components should not be kept at room temperature for more than 4 hours after the blood bag has been opened. If a slower infusion rate is necessary to avoid circulatory overload, the unit may be divided into smaller portions. Each portion should be refrigerated until used, and each can then be administered over 4 hours. Catheter size should be sufficiently large to allow blood to be administered within the 4-hour time period (generally 20 gauge or larger). Use of very small gauge catheters will impede flow, especially of packed red blood cells, and should be reserved for pediatric patients, who require much smaller volumes of blood. A blood warmer should be used for transfusion of patients with cold-reacting antibodies to prevent acute hemolysis.

COMPLICATIONS OF TRANSFUSION

RED CELL ANTIBODY-MEDIATED REACTIONS

Acute Reactions

Acute hemolytic transfusion reactions are almost always due to human error, resulting in transfusion of incompatible blood, and are preventable by rigid adherence to a standardized protocol for collection, labeling, storage, and release of all blood involved in transfusion. When incompatible red blood cells are transfused, recipient antibodies directed against donor red cells may cause acute intravascular hemolysis. ABO incompatibility is most common, because anti-A and anti-B antibodies are naturally occurring, but other antibodies due to prior sensitization can cause acute hemolytic reactions.

Acute hemolytic transfusion reactions range in severity from mild, clinically undetected hemolysis to fulminant, fatal events. Back pain, chest tightness, chills, and fever are the most common complaints in conscious patients. If the patient is unconscious (eg, under general anesthesia), hypotension, tachycardia, or fever may be the first clues, followed by generalized oozing from venipuncture and surgical sites. Since the severity of acute hemolytic transfusion reactions is related to the amount of incompatible blood given, it is vital to recognize early warning symptoms and signs to minimize sequelae of such a transfusion.

Complications of acute hemolytic transfusion reactions include cardiovascular collapse, oliguric renal failure, and disseminated intravascular coagulation. Massive immune complex deposition, stimulation of the coagulation cascade, and activation of vasoactive substances are the main pathophysiologic mechanisms underlying these complications, with subsequent decreased perfusion and hypoxia resulting in tissue damage. The degree of damage is related to the dose of incompatible blood received.

Any transfusion complicated by even apparently mild findings such as fever or allergic symptoms, should be stopped. The identity of the patient and the label on the unit should be verified quickly. If the patient has never been transfused or has never had any adverse reaction to prior transfusions, even a minor febrile reaction should prompt an evaluation for incompatibility. The remainder of the unit of blood and additional samples (anticoagulated and coagulated) from the patient should be sent to the blood bank for repeat crossmatch and direct antiglobulin testing. Patient plasma and urine should be examined for hemoglobin. It may be useful to check serum bilirubin and haptoglobin levels for evidence of hemolysis.

If acute hemolysis has occurred, the patient should be managed with aggressive supportive care. Vital signs should be monitored and intravenous volume support provided to maintain adequate blood pressure and renal perfusion for at least 24 hours following acute hemolysis. Loop or osmotic diuretics may be used in combination with intravenous fluids to maintain renal perfusion and urine output over 100 mL/h. Renal and coagulation status should be monitored clinically and with appropriate laboratory tests. Disseminated intravascular coagulation may occur and occasionally requires treatment with factor replacement. It is important to remember that an adverse reaction to an incompatible unit of red blood cells does not obviate the initial need for the transfusion. Therefore, transfusion with compatible red cells should be undertaken to provide the oxygen-carrying capacity the patient required prior to the transfusion.

In a patient who had been previously transfused and has had prior febrile reactions, the decision to evaluate each subsequent febrile reaction may be difficult. At a minimum, verification of the identity of the unit and the patient should always be performed. Whether to initiate the entire evaluation for hemolysis will depend upon the clinical circumstances. When in doubt, it is safer to stop the transfusion and perform a complete evaluation before continuing. Alternatively, if judged safe to continue without further evaluation, antipyretics may be used to lessen or prevent subsequent reactions.

Delayed Reactions

Hemolysis occurring about 1 week after red blood cell transfusion may occur when the initial cross-match fails to detect recipient antibodies to donor red cell antigens. Prior sensitization by transfusion or pregnancy to red blood cell antigens other than ABO may result in a transient rise in antibodies directed against those antigens. The antibody titer may wane to undetectable levels in as little as a few weeks. A second exposure prompts an anamnestic rise in antibody titer to a level sufficient to cause hemolysis.

The clinical manifestations of delayed hemolytic transfusion reactions are generally mild, with a fall in hematocrit accompanied by a slight increase in indirect bilirubin and lactic dehydrogenase levels about 1 week after transfusion. A repeat cross-match will demonstrate a "new" antibody. With some exceptions, hemolysis is extravascular and mild, without the serious sequelae that may follow acute hemolytic reactions. No specific therapy is necessary, but if clinically indicated, further transfusion should be given with red blood cells negative for the antigen. The blood bank should maintain a permanent record of the antibody, and all future red cell transfusions should be with antigen-negative blood. The patient should be informed of the antibody and of the need for screening of all future transfused red cells to avoid another such reaction. The patient should also be monitored for the development of other antibodies following subsequent transfusions.

Alloimmunization

Alloantibodies to red blood cell antigens other than ABO may occur in some recipients of red blood cell transfusions. Since there are over 300 red blood cell antigens, virtually all red blood cell transfusions expose the recipient to foreign antigens. Most antigens are not immunogenic, however, and rarely result in development of alloantibodies. Factors that influence the development of alloantibodies include the immunogenicity of the antigen, the frequency of the antigen in the population, the number of transfusions given, and the tendency of the recipient to form antibodies.

Because of the time required for the primary antibody response, alloantibodies do not complicate the sensitizing transfusion. Subsequent cross-match procedures will detect most clinically significant alloantibodies, but the development of multiple alloantibodies may make it difficult to find compatible units for transfusion-dependent recipients. Delayed hemolytic transfusion reactions may occur if the antibody is not detectable at the time of subsequent cross-match procedures. Red blood cell phenotyping may be useful for transfusion-dependent patients who demonstrate a tendency for antibody formation. When significant differences in the frequency of antigens exist between donor and recipient populations, empiric transfusion of red cells negative for certain antigens may be useful (eg, Duffy antigen-negative red cells for sickle cell patients) to prevent alloimmunization.

INFECTIOUS COMPLICATIONS OF TRANSFUSIONS

Current transfusion techniques minimize the risk of transmission of many potential pathogens (Table 3–4). The major factors that decrease the risk of transmission of disease include a closed, sterile system of collection of blood, proper storage and preservation of blood products, and screening. Screening includes obtaining historical information from potential donors to identify risk factors for infectious diseases and performing tests to identify carriers of known transmissible agents and those at high risk of being carriers. Current screening tests include VDRL, hepatitis B surface antigen and core antibody, hepatitis C antibody, HIV-1 and HIV-2 antibodies, HIV-1 p24 antigen, and antibodies to HTLV-1 and -2 and sometimes cytomegalovirus. Current screening practices reduce the incidence of but do not eliminate entirely the transmission of infectious disease by blood transfusion. Characteristics of agents transmissible by blood include the ability to persist in blood for a prolonged period in an asymptomatic potential donor and stability in blood stored under refrigeration. Table 3–4 sets forth the major clinical features of transfusion-transmitted infectious diseases.

NONHEMOLYTIC, NONINFECTIOUS COMPLICATIONS

Nonhemolytic, noninfectious transfusion reactions account for more than 90% of adverse effects of transfusions and occur in approximately 7% of recipients of

Table 3–4. Infectious complications of transfusion therapy.

Infection	Clinical Significance/Incidence
Viruses	
Hepatitis A	Rarely transmitted because of short period of viremia and lack of carrier state (1 in 1,000,000 units transfused).
Parvovirus B19	Estimated risk is 1 in 10,000 units transfused. Infection clinically insignificant except in pregnant women, patients with hemolytic anemia or who are immunocompromised.
Esptein-Barr virus	Rarely transmitted because of immunity acquired early in life.
Cytomegalovirus	Clinically significant transfusions complication in low-birth-weight neonates or immunocompromised hosts. Preventable by use of CMV-seronegative donors for all blood component therapy or by leukodepletion.
HTLV-1, HTLV-2	Estimated risk is 1 in 250,000 to 1 in 2,000,000 units transfused. Blood stored for more than 14 days and noncellular components are not infectious. Twenty to forty percent of recipients receiving infected blood become infected with virus; infection may lead to T cell lymphoproliferative disorder or myelopathy after long latency period. Donors are screened for both viruses.
Hepatitis B	Estimated risk is 1 in 30,000 to 1/150,000 units transfused. Usually causes anicteric and asymptomatic hepatitis 6 weeks to 6 months after transfusion. Ten percent become chronic carriers at risk for cirrhosis. All donors screened with surface antigen and core antibody.
Delta agent	Cotransmitted with hepatitis B, found primarily in drug abusers or patients who have received multiple transfusions. Superinfection of hepatitis B surface antigen carriers may result in fulminant hepatitis or chronic infectious state. Screening for hepatitis B eliminates the majority of infectious donors.
Hepatitis C	Previously the leading cause of posttransfusion hepatitis; donors are now screened, with estimated risk 1 in 30,000 to 1 in 250,000. Infection may be asymptomatic but 85% become chronic, 20% develop cirrhosis, and 1–5% develop hepatocellular carcinoma.
Hepatitis G (GB virus C)	Viremia may be present in 1–2% of donors, but no clear evidence that virus causes disease. Coinfection with HIV associated with prolonged survival. No approved screening test.
HIV	Screening program has been highly successful in eliminating transfusion-associated HIV disease; high risk donors excluded from donation; all donors tested for HIV antibody and p24 antigen. Estimated risk is 1 in 200,000 to 1 in 2,000,000 units transfused. Most recipients of infected blood develop HIV infection.
Bacteria	
Environmental contaminants	Closed, sterile collection techniques, use of preservatives and refrigeration, and natural bactericidal action of blood ensures extremely low risk, but improper storage or contamination with pathogens that survive refrigeration may result in serious bacterial infection.
Donor-transmitted	Asymptomatic carriers of certain bacteria may transmit infection; *Yersinia enterocolitica* is most common (1 in 65,000 units of red blood cells) and is highly fatal. Other organisms (salmonella, brucella) associated with chronic carrier state are transmitted less often. Platelet concentrates carry higher risk (1 in 12,000) due to high storage temperature (most common organisms are staphylococcus, klebsiella, serratia); pooled platelets have greater risk than single-donor apheresis units.
Spirochetes	
Syphilis	Short viability period (96 hours) in storage and donor screening with VDRL/RPR virtually eliminates possibility of transmission.
Lyme disease	*Borrelia burgdorferi* viable much longer than *Treponema pallidum,* but the period of blood culture positivity is associated with symptoms that preclude donation. No reported cases from transfusion.

(*continued*)

Table 3–4. Infectious complications of transfusion therapy. (*continued*)

Infection	Clinical Significance/Incidence
Parasites	
Malaria	Rare complication in USA because of exclusion from donation of asymptomatic individuals who have traveled to endemic areas within 1 year, or who have history of malaria or use of antimalarial prophylaxis, or who are former residents of endemic areas for 3 years. Unexplained fever 7–50 days after transfusion should prompt consideration of post-transfusion malaria.
Chagas' disease	*Trypanosoma cruiz* mainly a transfusion hazard in Central and South America, but immigration to the USA may result in increased incidence. No screening test currently available.
Babesiosis	Endemic to northeastern USA. Causes mild malaria-like illness. Major risk to asplenic or immunocompromised recipients.
Toxoplasmosis	Infrequent hazard of granulocyte transfusion in immunosuppressed hosts.
Prions	
Variant-Creutzfeldt-Jakob disease (v-CJD, mad cow disease)	No reported cases from transfusions thus far, but the FDA has recommended excluding from donation individuals who spent a significant amount of time or received blood transfusions in endemic areas (United Kingdom, France, certain other parts of Northern Europe) between 1980 and 1986; or those who used bovine insulin during this time period.

blood components. Major features of these unwanted complications are listed in Table 3–5.

CURRENT CONTROVERSIES & UNRESOLVED ISSUES

PERIOPERATIVE TRANSFUSION

The need for transfusion in the perioperative period should be determined by individual patient characteristics and by the type of surgical procedure rather than by hemoglobin level alone. Chronic mild to moderate anemia does not increase perioperative morbidity and by itself is not an indication for preoperative red blood cell transfusion. Intraoperative and postoperative blood loss should be managed first with crystalloids to maintain hemodynamic stability. Red blood cells should not be administered unless there is hemodynamic instability or the patient is at high risk for complications of acute blood loss (eg, coronary or cerebral vascular disease, congestive heart failure, or significant valvular heart disease). Patients who are at high risk or are unstable should be transfused on a unit-by-unit basis to maintain adequate perfusion of vital organs and to stabilize vital signs. It is reasonable to transfuse stable perioperative patients who have hemoglobin values around 7–8 g/dL if there are no significant risk factors for ischemia; in patients who are elderly, unstable, or at higher risk for ischemia, a higher threshold (eg, 10 g/dL) is probably safer.

Alternatives to homologous red blood cell transfusions in the perioperative period include autologous red blood cells donated in advance of elective surgery, acute normovolemic hemodilution, and intraoperative blood salvage. Preoperative autologous red blood cell donations are desirable whenever elective surgery likely to require red blood cell transfusion is planned and the patient is medically suitable for donation. Epoetin alfa (erythropoietin) use may enhance collection in patients with anemia or those likely to require large amounts of red blood cell transfusions. However, autologous donation is not without problems. Although autologous donation may decrease the use of allogeneic blood from an ever-decreasing donor pool, thus reserving it for emergencies, about half of the autologous blood collected is discarded, which is both wasteful and costly. Preoperative autologous donation may increase the risk of ischemic events, thereby outweighing the potential decrease in infectious risks, particularly in patients undergoing cardiovascular bypass surgery. In addition, collection of autologous blood preoperatively increases the risk of postoperative anemia and may actually in-

Table 3–5. Noninfectious complications of transfusion.

Complication	Clinical Manifestations., Pathogenesis, Prevention, and Treatment Strategies
Fever	Occurs in 0.5–3% of transfusion. Rigors or chills followed by fever during or shortly after transfusion due to prior sensitization to WBC or platelet antigens, or to pyrogenic cytokines released during storage. Prevent with antipyretics or leukocyte depletion of blood components.
Transfusion-related acute lung injury (TRALI)	Noncardiogenic pulmonary edema with fevers, chills, tachycardia, and diffuse pulmonary infiltrates shortly after transfusion, due to leukocyte incompatibility. Resolved in 1–4 days; rarely results in respiratory failure. Occurs in 1:5000 transfusions.
Allergic reactions	Occurs in 1-3% of transfusions. Urticaria, pruritus, bronchospasm, or frank anaphylaxis due to recipient sensitization to a cellular or plasma element. Rarely, due to allergy to medication donor is taking. If severe, evaluate recipient for IgA deficiency (2% of population). Leukocyte depletion or washed red cells may be necessary for subsequent transfusions.
Circulatory overload	Common following transfusion for chronic anemia or when patient has impaired cardiovascular reserve. Prevent by transfusing only when clearly indicated, using the minimum amount of blood required to reverse symptoms, and carefully reassessing patient after each unit. Treat with oxygen, diuretics, and, rarely, phlebotomy (save units for reinfusion if necessary).
Dilutional effects	Transfusing with more than one blood volume or red blood cells with dilute platelets and coagulation factors. Replacement indicated only for clinical bleeding.
Hypocalcemia	Due to citrate intoxication following massive transfusion. Treat only if symptomatic.
Hyperkalemia	May occur in patients with preexisting renal insufficiency and hyperkalemia or in neonates. Use of fresh blood or washed red cells decreases potassium load for these patients.
Hypothermia	After massive transfusion of refrigerated blood, hypothermia may cause cardiac arrhythmias. Refrigerated blood may accelerate hemolysis in patients with cold agglutinin disease. Prevent by warming blood.
Immune modulation	Mechanisms and clinical significance unclear for immunosuppression that follows transfusion; enhances results following renal transplantation; possible deleterious effect on outcome after colorectal cancer surgery; possible increased susceptibility to bacterial infections.
Graft-versus-host-disease	Immunocompetent donor T lymphocytes may engraft if the recipient is markedly immunosuppressed or if closely HLA-related. Symptoms and signs include high fever, maculopapular erythematous rash, hepatocellular damage, and pancytopenia 2–30 days after transfusion. Usually fatal despite treatment with immunosuppressives. Prevent by irradiating all blood components with 2500 cGy for immunocompromised recipients or when donor is first-degree relative.
Iron overload	Multiple transfusions in the absence of blood loss lead to excess accumulation of body iron with cirrhosis, heart failure, and endocrine organ failure. Prevent by decreasing total amount of red cells given, using alternatives to red cells whenever possible, using neocytes, and modifying diet to decrease iron absorption. Iron chelation indicated for patients with chronic transfusion dependence if prognosis is otherwise good.
Posttransfusion purpura	Acute severe thrombocytopenia about 1 week after transfusion due to alloantibodies to donor platelet antigen (usually P1A1). Self-limited, but treatment with steroids, high-dose IgG, plasmapheresis, or exchange transfusion recommended to prevent central nervous system hemorrhage. Platelet transfusions are ineffective even with compatible platelet. Pathogenesis poorly understood.
Miscellaneous	Increased supply of complement may accelerate hemolysis in paroxysmal nocturnal hemoglobinuria or make angioedema worse in patient with C_1 esterase inhibitor deficiency. Increased blood viscosity may occur in patients with Waldenström's macroglobulinemia, polycythemia, or leukemia with high white blood cell count. Sudden deterioration may follow platelet transfusion in patients with TTP/HUS or heparin-induced thrombocytopenia.

crease the need for perioperative transfusion. Transfusion of autologous blood is also associated with some of the same risks as allogeneic blood (administrative errors leading to ABO mismatch and hemolysis, bacterial contamination, volume overload, and reactions to preservatives). Therefore, criteria for transfusion of autologous units should be the same as those for transfusion of homologous red cells to avoid these unnecessary potential complications.

Acute normovolemic hemodilution may be suitable for patients undergoing surgical procedures with a significant risk of intraoperative bleeding (more than 20% of blood volume) who have baseline hemoglobin levels greater than 10 g/dL and who do not have severe ischemic heart disease or critical aortic stenosis. Phlebotomy with volume replacement by crystalloid is performed immediately after anesthetic induction. Blood lost intraoperatively results in loss of fewer red cells because of the lowered hematocrit, and subsequent reinfusion of the phlebotomized blood can restore oxygen-carrying capacity if necessary. Perioperative allogeneic transfusion requirements following acute normovolemic hemodilution or preoperative autologous donation appear to be about the same when compared directly in certain types of surgery, but there are some advantages favoring hemodilution. It is less costly because no testing is performed on the blood; the risks of bacterial contamination related to storage or ABO mismatch due to administrative error are reduced because the blood never leaves the operating room; and surgery does not have to be delayed to allow time for autologous donation.

Intraoperative blood salvage may be indicated for patients undergoing procedures with substantial blood loss or when transfusion is impossible (eg, patients who refuse blood transfusions and patients with rare blood groups or multiple red blood cell alloantibodies). Reinfusion of blood salvaged from the surgical field can reduce the requirement for standard homologous and autologous blood transfusions. Relative contraindications include the presence of infection, amniotic fluid or ascites in the operative field, malignancy, or the use of topical hemostatic agents in the field from which blood is salvaged. It has not been demonstrated, however, that use of salvaged blood decreases the need for allogeneic transfusion, and it may be expensive if automated cell-washing devices are used. The main value of intraoperative salvage is that blood is immediately available if rapid blood loss occurs.

Postoperative salvage from chest or pericardial tubes or from drains may also provide blood for autologous transfusion if persistent bleeding occurs. However, because the fluid collected is dilute (therefore providing a small volume of red cells for reinfusion), depleted of coagulation factors, and may contain cytokines, it is not clear how effective or safe reinfusion of recovered fluid is. Clinical trials have yielded conflicting results about the benefits of this procedure.

DIRECTED DONATIONS

Transfusions from ABO- and Rh-compatible family members or friends are frequently requested because of concerns about the safety of homologous transfusion. There is no evidence that directed donations are safer than volunteer donations, however, and some evidence exists that they may be less safe because blood from directed donors has a higher prevalence of serologic markers of infections than blood from volunteer donors. The patient and potential directed donors should be informed of the increased risk of transmission of infectious disease when directed donations are used. If the patient accepts this risk, potential donors should be given every opportunity to inform the blood bank of any conditions that would preclude use of their blood. Directed donations are not available immediately for transfusion because laboratory screening procedures are the same as for volunteer donor blood and require about 72 hours to complete. Blood donated from first-degree relatives should be irradiated prior to transfusion to prevent graft-versus-host disease, which can occur when the donor and recipient are closely HLA-matched.

INCREASING BLOOD PRODUCT SAFETY

Several strategies have been proposed and implemented in order to decrease further the risk of transfusion-related infections. Solvent/detergent-treated pooled plasma is now commercially available for treatment of coagulopathies and thrombotic thrombocytopenic purpura. Viruses with lipid envelopes are inactivated; however, there is concern that use of these products will result in transmission of viruses that do not have lipid envelopes. Plasma can be frozen and stored for a year, allowing for retesting beyond the window period between infection and serologic conversion of plasma donors prior to releasing the units for transfusion. Inactivation of viruses by exposure to psoralen and ultraviolet A irradiation (PUVA) can reduce the levels of HIV and hepatitis viruses, inactivate bacteria, and eliminate the problem of immunomodulation due to transfused lymphocytes. However, any toxicity from exposure of blood products to psoralen derivatives must be determined before this approach can be recommended. In addition, viability of platelets may be affected by PUVA.

Exposure of blood products to gamma irradiation (2500 cGy) results in inactivation of donor leukocytes, rendering them incapable of participation in the immune response. Graft-versus-host disease, a rare complication of blood transfusion that can occur in immunocompromised hosts or when the donor and recipient are closely related, can be prevented by irradiation of cellular blood components prior to transfusion. Alloimmunization, which can lead to poor response to subsequent platelet transfusions, can also be prevented with irradiation.

PATIENTS WHO REFUSE BLOOD TRANSFUSION

Even after extensive counseling regarding the risks and benefits of transfusion, some patients refuse some or all blood products even under life-threatening circumstances. Courts have affirmed the right of individuals to refuse medical care in part (eg, transfusions) without relinquishing the right to receive other care. This is true also for surrogate decision makers for adults who are not competent to make their own medical decisions. In such situations, it is important to determine how adamant the patient is in refusing to accept blood products and to have the patient affirm that refusal in writing if possible, even if death is imminent. Patients who have previously refused blood products should not be transfused if subsequently unable to give consent (eg, under general anesthesia). In an emergency, courts have generally granted permission to physicians to transfuse a patient over a family member's objections if no prior refusal by the patient has been documented and the patient is incompetent to give consent. It is preferable to avoid transfusions, however, rather than to obtain court permission to transfuse against a patient's or the family's wishes. Every effort should be made to treat existing anemia or acute blood loss with alternative therapy—volume expansion, erythropoietin (epoetin alfa), and (hematinics iron, vitamins)—whenever possible. Careful surgical technique, meticulous hemostasis, and reliance on aggressive volume support have eliminated the need for transfusion during many major surgical procedures in patients who refuse blood transfusion therapy.

EPOETIN ALFA (Erythropoietin)

Recombinant human erythropoietin is available (as epoetin alfa) for the treatment of anemia due to renal disease, for AIDS patients on zidovudine therapy with transfusion-dependent anemia, and for anemia associated with cancer or cancer chemotherapy. It may also be useful in the treatment of the anemia of chronic disease. Erythropoietin may be useful to augment autologous donations of red blood cells preoperatively even in the absence of anemia and may decrease the need for transfusion perioperatively when autologous blood is not collected. Because the cost of the drug is substantial, patient selection and modification of dosage will improve cost-effectiveness of this therapy. Those who will benefit most from preoperative erythropoietin treatment have baseline hematocrits between 33% and 39%, with expected blood loss of 1000–3000 mL. If more blood loss is anticipated, autologous donation in addition to erythropoietin may be needed to prevent preoperative polycythemia. Erythropoietin therapy may also improve the efficacy of acute normovolemic hemodilution. Its use reduces the need for red cell transfusion and significantly decreases the total amount of blood transfused in critically ill patients with anemia. It does not appear to influence other outcomes, including mortality or other serious events.

MASSIVE TRANSFUSION

Administration of a volume of blood and blood components equal to or exceeding the patient's estimated blood volume within a 24-hour period is accompanied by complications not often seen during transfusion of smaller volumes.

Deficiencies of platelets and clotting factors may occur, especially if extensive tissue injury or disseminated intravascular coagulation is present. However, prophylactic replacement with platelets or fresh frozen plasma results in unnecessary transfusions for many patients. It is preferable to base the decision to replace platelets and clotting factors on clinical criteria such as a generalized bleeding diathesis and laboratory abnormalities (platelet count and clotting times).

Clinically significant citrate (anticoagulant) intoxication is rare even with massive transfusions. Prophylactic calcium administration is not indicated, with the possible exception of patients with severe hepatic or heart failure in whom citrate metabolism may be impaired. Hyperkalemia occurs rarely following even massive blood transfusion. In fact, hypokalemia occurs more frequently as a result of metabolic alkalosis, which occurs as citrate is metabolized to bicarbonate. Interventions should be based on serum potassium levels. Although banked blood is acidic, massive transfusion does not complicate the lactic acidosis present in a patient with severe blood loss because improved tissue oxygenation results in metabolism of lactate and citrate to bicarbonate. Therefore, prophylactic administration of sodium bicarbonate is inadvisable in the massively transfused patient. The clinical significance of the low 2, 3-DPG found in stored red blood cells appears to be minor, since many other factors determine tissue oxygenation, including pH, tissue perfusion, hemoglobin concentration, and temperature. There appears to be no advantage in transfusing fresh red blood cells over stored cells.

Hypothermia may result from massive transfusion of refrigerated blood and may impair cardiac function.

Warming of blood prior to transfusion is recommended to prevent this complication. Microembolization of particulate debris in stored blood probably does not have any clinical significance. The use of microaggregate filters rather than standard blood filters has not been proved to be beneficial.

A significant potential hazard of massive transfusion is unrecognized acute hemolytic transfusion reaction. Many of the clinical signs and symptoms observed in the acutely bleeding patient are identical to those of an acute hemolytic event. Most fatal hemolytic transfusion reactions occur in emergency settings, both because of the difficulty in recognizing such reactions and because of the higher potential for human error in emergency situations. Strict attention to details of specimen labeling and patient identification and recognition of signs such as hemoglobinuria, fever, and generalized oozing from DIC can minimize the risks and complications of such reactions.

BLOOD SUBSTITUTES

Two main types of synthetic red-cell substitutes are under development—cell-free hemoglobin solutions and perfluorocarbon emulsions (synthetic oxygen carriers)—primarily for use in trauma or in patients undergoing surgery with or without acute normovolemic hemodilution. These compounds can be stored at room temperature for prolonged periods of time; they do not depend upon blood group compatibility for their therapeutic utility; and they can be treated so as to eliminate viruses without compromising function. The usefulness of these products in clinical practice remains to be demonstrated, and considerations of cost and blood supply will be important determinants of the role of artificial blood in the management of bleeding and anemia.

Recently, embryonic stem cells have produced human blood cells (hematopoietic stem cells), which could eventually lead to a new source of cells for blood transfusion. These cells were produced from one of the stem cell lines currently available for federally funded research under the current administration. It will be many years before it will be known if this development will be of any practical value in transfusion medicine.

PRETRANSPLANT TRANSFUSION THERAPY

Pretransplant blood transfusion may improve allograft survival in patients undergoing organ transplantation. Use of HLA-related blood donors in particular may induce immune tolerance to donor antigens that may decrease transplant rejection. However, better methods of immunosuppression of transplant recipients have decreased the clinical importance of pretransplant blood transfusion. In contrast, blood transfusion prior to bone marrow transplantation—particularly in patients with aplastic anemia—appears to decrease its success, especially if HLA-related donors are the source of blood.

USE OF NON-CROSS-MATCHED BLOOD IN EMERGENCY SITUATIONS

In the absence of unusual antibodies, complete cross-matching takes approximately 30–60 minutes. In most cases of acute hemorrhage, initial management with crystalloid is sufficient to maintain perfusion and hemodynamic stability. Occasionally, a delay in red blood cell transfusion poses a substantial risk to the patient, as in sudden massive blood loss or less massive blood loss occurring in a patient with myocardial or cerebral ischemia. In these circumstances, transfusion with non-cross-matched type O, Rh-negative blood or ABO-compatible blood tested with an abbreviated cross-match (5–20 minutes) may be necessary. Since Rh-negative blood is often in short supply, Rh-positive blood may be given to women beyond childbearing years or to males if emergent transfusion is required. If the recipient's blood type is known, unmatched blood of the same group may be used. Patients with group AB blood may receive either group A or group B cells. Type-specific plasma is preferred when plasma transfusion is necessary since naturally occurring anti-A or anti-B antibodies (or both) are present in plasma from all donors except those with type AB red cells, independent of prior sensitization. When type-specific plasma is not available, patients with type O blood can receive plasma of any type, but patients with types A and B can only receive plasma from AB donors. Patients with type AB blood can only receive type-specific plasma.

The disadvantages of using non-cross-matched blood include the possible transfusion of incompatible blood due to clinically significant antibodies to blood groups other than ABO, transfusion of anti-A and anti-B antibodies from plasma accompanying type O, Rh-negative red blood cells, and depletion of the supply of group O blood. Whenever possible, transfusion of cross-matched, type-specific blood should be used. ABO group-specific partially cross-matched blood is preferred over type O blood to avoid transfusion of ABO-incompatible plasma. Non-cross-matched type O blood should be reserved for truly extreme emergencies. A blood sample from the patient should always be obtained prior to any transfusion for complete cross-matching for subsequent transfusions and to aid in the evaluation of transfusion reactions.

CONSERVATION OF BLOOD RESOURCES

Conserving blood resources is one of the goals of the National Blood Resource Education Program of the National Institutes of Health. Recently, several controlled clinical trials examining the impact of transfusion on outcomes in a wide variety of clinical settings have been performed. These trials serve to promote rational use of blood products for the benefit of patients as well as protecting the limited supply of blood from waste. These trials have clearly influenced transfusion practices in well-defined clinical situations. There are many situations, however, where no empiric data exist and the clinician must determine the benefits of transfusion on an individualized basis. Massive repeated transfusion in patients with uncorrectable vascular defects or who are terminally ill—and platelet and plasma transfusions for patients without demonstrated response to such transfusions—may deplete the blood supply without substantially improving the outcome for those patients.

The medical team caring for a patient with massive uncontrollable bleeding or a terminal illness should make every effort to discuss the limits of care with the patient and family members, to establish long-term treatment goals and expectations, and to decide when continued blood transfusion is no longer of benefit to the patient. In addition, family members should be strongly encouraged to donate blood to help replace some of the units used. Ineffective therapy should not be given prophylactically (eg, daily platelet transfusions in patients with consumptive thrombocytopenia without bleeding, or plasma therapy for patients with multiple severe coagulation deficiencies not corrected with large doses of plasma).

REFERENCES

Consensus conference. Fresh-frozen plasma. Indications and risks. JAMA 1985;253:551–3.

Corwin HL et al: Efficacy of recombinant human erythropoietin in the critically ill patient: a randomized, double-blind, placebo-controlled trial. Crit Care Med 1999;27:2346–50.

Ely EW, Bernard GR: Transfusions in critically ill patients. (Editorial.) N Engl J Med 2000;340:467–8.

Goodnough LT et al: Erythropoietin therapy. N Engl J Med 1997;336:933–8.

Goodnough LT et al: Transfusion medicine—blood transfusion. (Two parts.) N Engl J Med 1999;340:438–47, 525–33.

Greenbaum BH: Transfusion-associated graft-versus-host disease: Historical perspectives, incidence, and current use of irradiated blood products. J Clin Oncol 1991;9:1889–1902.

Greenwalt TJ: Pathogenesis and management of hemolytic transfusion reactions. Semin Hematol 1981;18:84–94.

Hebert PC et al: A multicenter, randomized, controlled clinical trial of transfusion requirements in critical care. N Engl J Med 1999;340:409–17.

Hebert PC et al: Is a low transfusion threshold safe in critically ill patients with cardiovascular diseases? Crit Care Med 29:227–34.

Leukocyte reduction and ultraviolet B irradiation of platelets to prevent alloimmunizations and refractoriness to platelet transfusions. The Trial to Reduce Alloimmunization to Platelets Study Group. N Engl J Med 1997;337:1861–1870.

The National Blood Resource Education Program's Transfusion Alert: Indications for the use of red blood cells, platelets, and fresh frozen plasma. U.S. Department of Health and Human Services. NIH Publication No. 91-2974a, Revised September 1991.

Schiffer CA et al: Platelet transfusion for patients with cancer: clinical practice guidelines of the Society of Clinical Oncology. J Clin Oncol 2001;19:1519—38.

Starkey JM et al: Markers for transfusion-transmitted disease in different groups of blood donors. JAMA 1989;262:3452–4.

The use of autologous blood. The National Blood Resource Education Program Expert Panel. JAMA 1990;263: 414–7.

Valeri CR, Crowley JP, Loscalzo J: The red cell transfusion trigger: has a sin of commission now become a sin of omission? Transfusion 1998;38:602–10.

Wayne AS, Kevy SV, Nathan DG: Transfusion management of sickle cell disease. Blood 1993;81:1102–23.

Pharmacotherapy

4

Jennifer H. Cupo Abbott, PharmD, & Maria I. Rudis, PharmD

Design of optimal pharmacotherapeutic regimens for the critically ill patient is a significant challenge for the clinician. The frequent occurrence of renal failure and hepatic failure complicates drug dosing. The complexity of the drug regimen in critically ill patients makes them more susceptible to adverse drug events and interactions.

A basic knowledge of pharmacokinetics and pharmacodynamics is essential for monitoring a drug's therapeutic and toxic effects. **Pharmacokinetics** is the movement of a drug through the body over time and is defined by the following: absorption, distribution, metabolism, and elimination. **Pharmacodynamics** is the relationship between drug concentration and drug effect. Both pharmacokinetic and pharmacodynamic changes occur in critical illness. This chapter will review the principles of pharmacokinetics and pharmacodynamics as well as the mechanisms of the different types of drug interactions.

PHARMACOKINETIC PARAMETERS

In clinical practice, the most important pharmacokinetic parameters are half-life, clearance, and volume of distribution. The disposition of a parenterally administered drug is dependent upon both clearance (CL) and the volume of distribution (V_d). Clearance is the rate at which a drug is eliminated from the body. Volume of distribution is a proportionality constant, a theoretical volume that relates the concentration in the plasma to the amount of drug in the body. The elimination half-life ($t_{1/2}$) depends on the above independent variables and is described by the following mathematical relationship:

$$t_{1/2} = (0.693 \times V_d / CL)$$

Hence, either decreased clearance or an expanded volume of distribution will result in an increased pharmacologic half-life. A practical understanding of this mathematical relationship is essential for developing optimal dosing regimens.

PHARMACOKINETIC CONSIDERATIONS

ABSORPTION

Drug absorption is influenced by a variety of factors, including the site of absorption, the amount metabolized before reaching the systemic circulation ("first-pass effect"), and drug interactions. In critical illness, the site of absorption is of utmost importance. The extent of oral absorption—bioavailability—may be diminished as a result of low cardiac output or shunting of blood from the mesentery or peripheral circulation. Therapeutic "failures" may be due to inadequate bioavailability rather than absence of effect at the intended receptor site. One example is lack of anticipated antihypertensive effect after administration of an oral calcium channel blocker. This often necessitates conversion to a continuous infusion with either diltiazem or nicardipine for more predictable and controlled blood pressure response.

In general, the intravenous route is preferred and subcutaneous or intramuscular administration should be avoided. In patients with peripheral edema or hypoperfusion states (eg, septic shock), either intramuscular or subcutaneous administration is unsatisfactory because of the potential for erratic or decreased absorption. Subcutaneous administration of insulin may yield inadequate or variable insulin delivery and result in uncontrolled hyperglycemia. Conversely, hypoglycemia may occur with improvement of perfusion and subcutaneous absorption. Similarly, subcutaneous administration of low-molecular-weight heparins often results in inadequate absorption and anticoagulation, with potential failure of prevention or treatment of deep venous thrombosis or pulmonary embolism in the critically ill.

Intravenous administration circumvents these problems in the critically ill patient.

DISTRIBUTION

The distribution of drugs in the body depends on factors such as blood flow, body composition, and plasma protein binding (Table 4–1). In critical illness, fluid over-

Table 4–1. Protein binding.

Drug	Protein-Bound
Amphotericin B	90–95%
Ceftriaxone	93–96%
Chlordiazepoxide	94–97%
Clindamycin	93%
Diazepam	84–98%
Erythromycin	96%
Ethacrynic acid	95%
Furosemide	91–99%
Haloperidol	90–92%
Heparin	> 90%
Hydralazine	90%
Lorazepam	90%
Midazolam	94–97%
Nafcillin	70–90%
Nifedipine	89–92%
Oxacillin	89–94%
Phenytoin	90%
Prochlorperazine	90%
Rifampin	84–91%
Vecuronium	60–90%
Verapamil	90%

load can significantly increase a patient's volume of distribution, and insufficiently effective drug concentrations may result. For drugs with extensive tissue distribution, eg, digoxin, the volume of distribution is approximately 500 L. Thus, it is unlikely that changes in fluid status can significantly affect the distribution of digoxin. Conversely, tobramycin has a volume of distribution of about 0.3 L/kg of ideal body weight. An 80 kg patient would have a volume of distribution for tobramycin of 24 L. When that patient is given a 240 mg dose of tobramycin, the serum level would be 240 mg/24 mL (10 mg/mL). However, if this patient gains 15 L of fluid, the new volume of distribution would be 39 L. The same dose would then yield a serum level of about 6–7 mg/mL (240 mg/39 L), which is inadequate for treating serious infections such as nosocomially acquired pneumonia.

Body composition and the lipophilicity of a given drug are also important factors to consider. In general, lipophilic agents such as diazepam readily distribute into fat. For these agents, dosing should be based on total body weight. Since most agents used in the ICU setting are not lipophilic, such as pressors and most antimicrobials, it may be more accurate to use ideal body weight in dosing calculations.

Protein binding is another important determinant of distribution. Only the unbound fraction of a drug can diffuse or be transported into tissues. Thus, the influence of protein binding is a limiting factor in drug distribution for highly bound drugs (Table 4–1). Phenytoin, for example, is a highly protein-bound drug (about 90%) that is used in the critical care setting. The remaining 10% circulates as unbound or "free" drug and is the fraction responsible for the pharmacologic effect. If a patient with normal albumin has a phenytoin level of 12 mg/L, the free fraction would be 1.2 mg/L. However, with decreased serum albumin, as is found in patients with central nervous system trauma or those with end-stage liver disease, less serum protein is available to bind phenytoin. The laboratory reports total phenytoin concentrations, which includes bound and unbound drug. In a patient with hypoalbuminemia, the total phenytoin level will be unchanged, but the percentage of "free" drug (ie, pharmacologically available) will increase. For example, a patient with a serum albumin of 2 mg/dL and a measured phenytoin plasma concentration (Cmeas) of 12 mg/L has more free drug, resulting in an adjusted phenytoin plasma concentration (Cadj) of 24 μg/mL.

$$
\begin{aligned}
\text{Cadj} &= \frac{\text{Cmeas}}{(0.2)\,(\text{Alb}) + 0.1} \\
&= \frac{12\,\mu\text{g}/\text{mL}}{(0.2)\,(2.0\ \text{mg}/\text{dL}) + 0.1} \\
&= 24\,\mu\text{g}/\text{mL}
\end{aligned}
$$

The uremia accompanying renal failure also displaces phenytoin from its binding sites since endogenous competitors for binding accumulate. It is important to recognize that malnourished patients and those with renal failure will have a lower than normal "therapeutic range" for phenytoin. (Similarly, the adjusted total plasma phenytoin concentration may be calculated using the following equation: Cadj = Cmeas/[(0.1)(Alb) + 0.1]). For this reason, it is clinically more relevant to monitor free phenytoin concentrations or to use these values in calculation of dosage adjustments.

DRUG CLEARANCE (ELIMINATION)

With limited exceptions, most pharmacologic agents are eliminated either renally or hepatically. Since multiorgan dysfunction and fluid overload are commonly encountered in critically ill patients, drug accumulation and toxicity are of concern. Specific dosage adjustment is often required in the setting of renal or hepatic impairment. Some of the most frequently used agents with predominantly renal elimination are listed in Table 4–2. Most antimicrobials—including the aminoglycosides, vancomycin, and several beta-lactams and fluoroquinolones—are eliminated primarily via the kidney. Although some dosage adjustment is needed when these antimicrobials are used in critically ill patients with acute renal failure, one should have a high threshold for dosage adjustment given the low risk:benefit ratio. Since these patients are often infected with organisms that have marginal drug susceptibilities, ongoing assessments of renal function and clinical status are necessary to make certain that underdosing does not occur. Another drug with primarily renal elimination used in the critical care setting is enoxaparin, a low-molecular-weight heparin. Although there are no clear dosage adjustment recommendations at this time, recent evidence suggests that it is prudent to decrease the dose of enoxaparin by up to 50% in patients with renal impairment. Others have advocated avoiding use of enoxaparin in patients with an estimated creatinine clearance of less than 30 mL/min to reduce the likelihood of drug accumulation and subsequent bleeding events. Some drugs have mixed routes of elimination and require both renal and hepatic function for proper clearance. Vecuronium is an example of a drug with mixed renal and hepatic elimination of the parent drug and its active metabolite. In ICU patients with renal or hepatic insufficiency, monitoring of the depth of neuromuscular blockade and adjustment of vecuronium dosing with a peripheral nerve stimulator helps to individualize therapy and minimize accumulation of both the parent drug and its active metabolite, 3-hydroxydesacetylvecuronium—which has 30–50% of the pharmacologic activity of the parent drug—and to prevent adverse drug events such as prolonged neuromuscular blockade.

Renal Dysfunction

When the serum creatinine level is known, an estimate of creatinine clearance can be obtained to assist with dosage adjustment using the following equation:

$$\frac{(140-\text{Age}) \times \text{Weight (in kg)}}{72 \times \text{Serum creatinine}}$$

(For females, multiply numerator by factor of 0.85.)

Although this equation is frequently used in ICU patients, it has not been validated in that patient population. In situations where a more accurate determination of renal function is necessary, a 6-hour urine collection for measured creatinine clearance is advised.

Table 4–2. Drugs with primarily renal elimination.

Antimicrobials		
Acyclovir	Ciprofloxacin	Meropenem
Amikacin	Fluconazole	Penicillin G
Ampicillin	Flucytosine	Piperacillin
Cefazolin	Ganciclovir	Ticarcillin-clavulanate
Cefepime	Gatifloxacin	Tobramycin
Cefotetan	Gentamicin	Trimethoprim-sulfamethoxazole
Cefoxitin	Imipenem-cilastatin	Vancomycin
Ceftazidime	Levofloxacin	
Ceftizoxime		
Antihypertensives		
Diazoxide		
Methyldopa		
Nitroprusside		
Antiarrhythmic agents		
Bretylium		
Digoxin		
Procainamide		
Miscellaneous drugs		
Ranitidine		
Pancuronium		

Table 4–3. Drugs significantly removed by hemodialysis.

Antimicrobials		
Aminoglycosides	Ceftizoxime	Meropenem
Ampicillin	Chloramphenicol	Metronidazole
Cefazolin	Ciprofloxacin	Penicillin G
Cefepime	Gatifloxacin	Piperacillin
Cefotaxime	Imipenem-cilastatin	Quinupristin-dalfopristin
Cefotetan	Levofloxacin	Trimethoprim-sulfamethoxazole
Cefoxitin	Linezolid	
Ceftazidime		
Antihypertensives		
Diazoxide		
Methyldopa		
Nitroprusside		
Antiarrhythmic agents		
Bretylium		
Digoxin		
Procainamide		
Miscellaneous drugs		
Ranitidine		
Pancuronium		

For patients requiring hemodialysis, it is essential to know the extent to which drugs can be removed by dialysis. Knowledge of pharmaceutical properties such as hydrophilicity, low molecular weight, low plasma protein binding, and small volume of distribution (Table 4–3) can help distinguish those agents that are dialyzable. Aminoglycosides are a class of drug that fits the above criteria. Tobramycin concentrations decline by 30–50% following a 3-hour dialysis session. Conversely, drugs with extensive tissue distribution such as digoxin or the calcium channel blockers are not affected by dialysis. Other important considerations for drug clearance include the duration and type of dialysis. Short dialysis sessions are less likely to remove significant amounts of drug. New forms of dialysis are more efficient and remove drugs previously thought to be minimally dialyzable. Hemodialysis with high-flux filters removes significant amounts of vancomycin. Continuous renal replacement therapy is a much more efficient process than conventional hemodialysis and equates to a creatinine clearance of approximately 30 mL/min. It is essential to review the medication regimen closely when patients are dialyzed with high-flux filters or are switched from hemodialysis to continuous renal replacement, since the dosage of many drugs will have to be increased.

Hepatic Dysfunction

Some drugs require dosage adjustment in hepatic insufficiency (Table 4–4). Determining the degree of hepatic dysfunction is difficult, since no quantitative equations exist. In general, laboratory tests of hepatic synthetic function (prothrombin time, serum albumin, conjugated bilirubin) are the ones most predictive of drug elimination. For drugs metabolized by the liver, route of metabolism is important in determining the effects of liver disease on drug clearance. Some enzyme systems are remarkably well preserved even in end-stage liver disease. Drugs such as lorazepam that are metabolized primarily by conjugation with glucuronic acid are minimally affected in cirrhosis, so little dosage adjustment is required. For drugs whose clearance depends on oxidative metabolism (metronidazole, theophylline, opioids, sedative-hypnotics), cirrhosis reduces their elimination. Generally speaking, acute liver disease (eg, hepatitis) does not significantly alter drug clearance.

Table 4–4. Drugs requiring dosage adjustment in severe hepatic insufficiency.

Analgesics	**Antimicrobials**
Acetaminophen	Cefoperazone
Opioids	Ceftriaxone
Salicylates	Chloramphenicol
Antiarrhythmics	Clindamycin
Lidocaine	Erythromycin
Quinidine	Isoniazid
Verapamil	Metronidazole
Anticonvulsants	Nafcillin
Phenobarbital	Rifampin
Phenytoin	**Sedative-hypnotics**
Antihypertensives	Chlordiazepoxide
Hydralazine	Diazepam
Labetalol	Midazolam
Nitroprusside	**Miscellaneous**
	Haloperidol
	Theophylline

Table 4–5. Therapeutic ranges for drugs commonly used in critical care.

Drug	Therapeutic Range
Amikacin	Peak: 25–35 mg/L Trough: < 10 mg/L
Amiodarone	0.8–2.8 mg/L
Gentamicin, tobramycin	Peak: 8–12 mg/L Trough: < 1 mg/L
Digoxin	1–2 μg/L
Lidocaine	1–5 mg/L
Phenobarbital	10–30 mg/L
Phenytoin	10–20 mg/L
Procainamide *N*-Acetylprocainamide	4–8 mg/L < 30 mg/L
Salicylates	100–300 mg/L
Theophylline (in COPD)	8–10 mg/L
Vancomycin	Trough: 5–15 mg/L

THERAPEUTIC DRUG MONITORING

Agents with a narrow therapeutic index have small differences between therapeutic and toxic effects, and monitoring of serum drug concentrations is recommended (Table 4–5). Examples of agents with low therapeutic indices are the aminoglycosides, digoxin, theophylline, and phenytoin. Although the reported dosage ranges for these agents are considered to be therapeutic, they are intended to serve merely as a guide. Some patients may experience toxicity with levels at mid range, and some may require levels above the therapeutic range to achieve a therapeutic effect. One example of a drug with a revised therapeutic range is theophylline.

Given that toxicity was readily seen at the upper end of the previously recommended therapeutic range (10–20 mg/L), the more appropriate goal is 8–10 mg/L.

It is imperative to know when the sample was drawn relative to the timing of the previous dose to accurately assess and interpret serum drug concentration values. The clinician can then decide if sufficient time has elapsed to allow for the distribution phase of the drug, to decide if the sampling time is valid, and to assess whether the drug is at steady state concentration (not often achieved in ICU patients). Digoxin is an example of a drug that needs sufficient time for distribution from the blood to the tissue compartments. If a serum digoxin level is obtained within 2 hours after an intravenous dose, the level will be predictably elevated, and any clinical decision based on this level would be inappropriate. In the case of digoxin, it is best to take samples 4 hours after an intravenous dose or 6 hours after an oral dose to obtain an accurate assessment of levels once distribution is complete. Vancomycin is an example of a drug for which peak and trough levels were formerly advocated. However, given that the peak level is not associated with any measure of efficacy and that a peak level may appear falsely elevated if obtained during the distribution phase, only vancomycin trough levels are currently recommended. Drug distribution is also of concern following dialysis. It is important to allow at least 3 hours to elapse after dialysis to obtain drug levels to allow for redistribution of drug from other tissues into the main compartment (eg, intravascular space). This is illustrated also in the case of hemodialysis for a toxic ingestion of lithium. A lithium level of 10 meq/mL (therapeutic level is 0.5–2 meq/L) obtained before dialysis may decrease to 1 meq/L immediately after hemodialysis. However, a third level obtained 3–4 hours after dialysis may rebound to a toxic level of 5 meq/L, showing evidence of redistribution from the central nervous system back into the main compartment. This indicates the need for a longer or more frequent hemodialysis.

Aminoglycosides are another class of drugs for which recommendations for obtaining levels have recently been revised. With the advent of once-daily dosing strategies, there is little utility for measuring a peak aminoglycoside level that will appear transiently elevated. It is more relevant clinically to obtain a level 10–14 hours after administration as a surrogate marker for drug accumulation. Thus, although this level may be slightly higher than the previously acceptable trough range for aminoglycosides (< 2 mg/L), it is still therapeutic given the extended dosing interval. Finally, for many drugs, daily levels are inappropriate and may lead to improper dosage adjustments. Since digoxin and phenytoin possess half-lives in the range of 40 hours, levels should be ordered twice weekly as opposed to once daily.

DRUG INTERACTIONS

Given the number of drugs prescribed for critically ill patients, the potential for drug interactions is high. Drug interactions may occur as a result of pharmacodynamic, pharmaceutical, or pharmacokinetic effects. Pharmacodynamic interactions may enhance or antagonize a drug's effects depending on the pharmacology of the drugs involved. Pharmaceutical interactions can result from a number of causes, one of which is the relationship between two drugs. Pharmacokinetic interactions may occur because of a decrease in absorption, changes in distribution, or altered drug clearance.

Pharmacodynamic Interactions (Table 4–6)

Pharmacodynamic drug interactions can result in synergistic, additive, or antagonistic pharmacologic effects. A beneficial additive effect would be observed in a patient with poorly controlled hypertension who receives a second antihypertensive agent from a different class and then achieves optimal blood pressure control. Another example of an additive or synergistic pharmacologic effect is the concomitant use of opioid analgesics with benzodiazepines. This combination is useful to optimize sedation and analgesia in the ICU. It may also be associated with an increased risk of respiratory depression (of limited importance in mechanically venti-

Table 4–6. Pharmacodynamic interactions.

Drug	Effect
Additive	
Gentamicin and neuromuscular blocking agents	Additive blockade
Midazolam and morphine	Additive CNS depression
Synergistic	
Gentamicin and ampicillin	Increased activity vs enterococcus
Tobramycin and piperacillin	Increased activity vs pseudomonas
Antagonistic	
Propranolol and (or beta-agonist)	Decreased theophylline (beta-agonist) effect
Extended-spectrum penicilin and imipenem (vs *E cloacae, P aeruginosa*, citrobacter species)	Decreased antimicrobial killing or increased development of resistance

lated patients) or hypotension, particularly in hypovolemic patients. Synergistic combinations are noted when the resultant pharmacologic effect with combination therapy is greater than the expected sum of drug effects. This phenomenon occurs infrequently and is best described for antimicrobial combinations. A beta-lactam antimicrobial (eg, piperacillin or ceftazidime) in combination with an aminoglycoside is more effective than a beta-lactam plus a fluoroquinolone and results in a lower incidence of acquired bacterial resistance in the treatment of infections with aerobic gram-negative organisms. On the other hand, antagonism may be encountered when beta-blockers reverse the pharmacologic benefit of beta-agonists in patients with chronic obstructive pulmonary disease. While some beta-blockers such as atenolol are more cardioselective at lower doses, they still have the potential to antagonize bronchodilators such as albuterol and salmeterol. The concomitant use of antimicrobials from the same class also carries the potential for antagonism. For example, some beta-lactams induce production of chromosomal beta-lactamase. The combination of a strong inducing beta-lactam such as imipenem with a labile compound (eg, piperacillin) for the treatment of infections due to enterobacter species has been shown to produce antagonism in vitro and in animal models of infection. Hence, double beta-lactam combinations that include a weak and a strong inducer should be avoided.

Pharmaceutical Interactions

Pharmaceutical interactions may be caused by drug incompatibilities or drug adsorption to catheters and to intravenous administration materials. For example, intravenous administration of nitroglycerin requires special equipment to decrease the likelihood of adsorption. The complexity of drug regimens in the critically ill patient coupled with limited intravenous access makes intravenous drug compatibility a significant issue. Although a great deal is known about the compatibility of drug combinations, there are still many potential combinations for which no such information is available.

Pharmacokinetic Interactions

Although pharmacokinetic interactions occur as a result of alterations in drug absorption, distribution, metabolism, or elimination, the effects on drug metabolism are the most clinically significant. A commonly seen absorption interaction occurs when fluoroquinolones are administered concomitantly with multivalent cations (eg, antacids), causing decreased quinolone bioavailability. Similarly, enteral feeding should be withheld 2 hours before and after the administration of oral phenytoin formulations because of the decreased and delayed absorption of phenytoin that occurs.

Drug interactions due to altered distribution may also occur. When two drugs compete for binding sites on plasma proteins or tissues, the unbound or free serum concentration of one or both drugs may increase. Although this theoretically may increase a drug's effect, the enhanced pharmacologic effect is usually transient as more unbound drug is now available for elimination by the liver and kidney. Thus, the clinical significance of protein-binding displacement interactions is minimal.

Pharmacokinetic drug interactions due to altered metabolism involve the cytochrome P450 enzyme system that is responsible for oxidative metabolism. More than 30 isoenzymes have been identified, but the primary ones responsible for drug metabolism are CYP3A4, CYP2D6, CYP1A2, and the CYP2C subfamily. While a comprehensive list of drugs that are metabolized by these pathways is beyond the scope of this chapter, some practical examples can be presented. A drug may be a substrate for, an inducer to, or an inhibitor of these enzymes. Inhibition is a result of competitive binding between a substrate and an inhibitor at the enzyme's binding site. This interaction is dependent on several factors, including the substrate's affinity for the enzyme, the concentration of the enzyme required for inhibition, and the half-life of the inhibitor drug. The end result of this interaction is an increased concentration of the substrate drug. Conversely, enzyme induction occurs when the synthesis of cytochrome P450 enzymes is stimulated. Few drugs are known to be enzyme inducers, and carbamazepine, phenobarbital, phenytoin, and rifampin are the most common inducer agents. Chronic ethanol abuse typically induces hepatic cytochrome enzymes, and this is why frequent administration of larger doses of anxiolytics such as diazepam and midazolam and analgesics such as morphine are required for this group of critically ill patients. The immunosuppressants cyclosporine and tacrolimus are both eliminated via the cytochrome P4503A4 system. Their metabolism can either be inhibited (eg, erythromycin or some azole antifungals) or induced (eg, phenobarbital or phenytoin). In either situation, therefore, frequent monitoring of cyclosporine or tacrolimus blood concentrations is necessary to ensure that increased side effects or organ rejection does not occur. It may be more prudent to choose an alternative agent and avoid the interacting combination.

ADVERSE EFFECTS & DRUG TOXICITIES

Drugs may adversely affect all organ systems, but the kidney, liver, central nervous system, and vascular system are most frequently affected. In critically ill patients with multiple medical problems, it can be quite difficult to isolate drug toxicity as the sole cause of organ failure.

Nephrotoxicity

The most common causes of drug-induced nephrotoxicity are listed in Table 4–7. Nephrotoxicity in critically ill patients may be due to drug-induced causes or to hypoperfusion. Because the mortality rate for intensive care patients with acute renal failure approaches 80%, efforts should be directed at removing all potential causes of nephrotoxicity. Adequate fluid resuscitation and maintenance of renal perfusion is of paramount importance for preventing prerenal acute renal failure. Although low doses of dopamine have been used empirically for this purpose, recent controlled trials have demonstrated the failure of low-dose dopamine to improve renal perfusion, prevent acute renal failure, or avoid the need for hemodialysis in all critically ill patients, including those with septic shock (regardless of vasopressor use). Thus, the use of low-dose dopamine should be abandoned.

Despite adequate preventive measures, up to 20% of all cases of acute renal failure may be associated with drug toxicity. Drug-induced toxicity may take the form of acute tubular necrosis, interstitial nephritis, or glomerulonephritis. Of those drugs associated with acute tubular necrosis, the most notable are the aminoglycosides and amphotericin B. With once-daily dosing of aminoglycosides (5–7 mg/kg/d) and proper therapeutic drug monitoring, the incidence of acute tubular necrosis is significantly reduced. However, if renal insufficiency does develop, it is important to adjust the aminoglycoside dosing regimen to conventional dosing with lower daily doses at extended intervals to prevent drug accumulation. The novel amphotericin B formulations as well as the newly developed antifungals (eg, echinocandins) to be used in combination with amphotericin B may provide some alternatives to conventional amphotericin B dosing and its predictable nephrotoxicity. Interstitial nephritis and glomerulonephritis are due to hypersensitivity reactions or immune complex formation. The most common cause of drug-induced interstitial nephritis is methicillin, and for this reason it is replaced with either oxacillin or nafcillin at most institutions.

Table 4–7. Nephrotoxic drugs.

Acute tubular necrosis
Acyclovir
Aminoglycosides
Amphotercin B
Iodinated contrast dyes
Foscarnet
Pentamidine
Interstitial nephritis
Allopurinol
Cimetidine
Furosemide
Methicillin
Phenytoin
Rifampin
Thiazides
Trimethoprim-sulfamethoxazole
Vancomycin
Glomerulonephritis
ACE inhibitors
Gold salts
Hydralazine
Penicillamine
Rifampin
Renal hemodynamics
ACE inhibitors
Cyclosporine
NSAIDs
Tacrolimus

Table 4–8. Hepatotoxic drugs.

Hepatocellular
Acetaminophen
Allopurinol
Amiodarone
Azole antifungals
Ciprofloxacin
Dantrolene
Halothane
Isoniazid
Phenytoin
Pyrazinamide
Quinine
Rifampin
Salicylates
Tetracycline
Valproic acid
Cholestatic
Benzodiazepines
Chlorpromazine
Clindamycin
Erythromycin
Flucytosine
Haloperidol
HMG-CoA reductase inhibitors ("statins")
Nafcillin
Nitrofurantoin
NSAIDs
Oxacillin
Prochlorperazine
Trimethoprim-sulfamethoxazole

Hepatotoxicity

While a variety of drugs have been associated with altered liver function tests, these changes are usually reversible upon discontinuation of the offending agent. Since acute hepatic injury is classified according to morphology, drug-induced hepatic injury may cause either direct hepatocellular necrosis, cholestasis, or a mixed presentation of both (Table 4–8). Some drug combinations such as rifampin and isoniazid, amoxicillin and clavulanic acid, as well as trimethoprim and sulfamethoxazole may also increase the possibility of hepatotoxic reactions. This may occur because one agent alters the metabolism of the other, leading to the production of toxic metabolites. Phenytoin induces both hepatic necrosis and cholestasis in association, producing an immune response manifested by a rash, eosinophilia, atypical lymphocytosis, and serum IgG antibodies against phenytoin.

REFERENCES

Joy MS et al: A primer on continuous renal replacement therapy for critically ill patients. Ann Pharmacother 1998;32:362–75.

Michalets EL: Update: Clinically significant cytochrome P-450 drug interactions. Pharmacother 1998;18:84–112.

Mlynarek ME, Peterson EL, Zarowitz BJ: Predicting unbound phenytoin concentrations in the critically ill neurosurgical patient. Ann Pharmacother 1996;30:219–23.

Nicolau DP et al: Experience with a once-daily aminoglycoside program administered to 2,184 adult patients. Antimicrob Ag Chemother 1995;39:650–5.

Riker RR, Picard JT, Fraser GL: Prospective evaluation of the Sedation-Agitation Scale for adult critically ill patients. Crit Care Med 1999;27:1325–9.

Rudis MI et al: A prospective, randomized, controlled evaluation of peripheral nerve stimulation versus standard clinical dosing of neuromuscular blocking agents in critically ill patients. Crit Care Med 1997;25:575–83.

Trissel LA: *Handbook on Injectable Drugs,* 11th ed. American Socety of Health-System Pharmacists, 2001.

Van den Berghe G et al: Intensive insulin therapy in critically ill patients. N Engl J Med 2001;345:1359–67.

Intensive Care Anesthesia & Analgesia

5

Tai-Shion Lee, MD

PHYSIOLOGIC EFFECTS OF ANESTHESIA IN THE CRITICALLY ILL

Many critically ill patients undergo surgery and anesthesia before or after admission to the ICU. To take care of these patients perioperatively, an understanding of the physiologic effects of anesthesia is essential.

Anesthetics produce their primary effects by acting on the central nervous system. They also elicit a variety of physiologic changes throughout the body. The physiologic reserve of critically ill patients is limited because of concurrent or preexisting pathophysiologic disorders. Such individuals are thus more susceptible to physiologic derangements than normal and more apt to develop complications during the recovery period.

Recovery from the influences of anesthesia requires careful observation and specialized management. Since patients may be labile and vulnerable during this stage, they may stay in the postanesthetic care unit (PACU) until they have regained consciousness. The function of the PACU is to provide close monitoring of vital functions and to ensure prompt recognition of problems due to anesthesia and surgery. The same functions can be served in the ICU as well.

Benumof JL: Respiratory physiology and respiratory function during anesthesia. In: *Anesthesia,* 3rd ed. Miller RD (editor). Churchill Livingstone, 1990.

Gal TJ: Respiratory physiology during anesthesia. In: *Thoracic Anesthesia,* 2nd ed. Kaplan JA (editor). Churchill Livingstone, 1991.

Knight AA et al: Perioperative myocardial ischemia: Importance of the preoperative ischemia pattern. Anesthesiology 1988;68: 681–88.

Nunn JF: *Applied Respiratory Physiology,* 3rd ed. Butterworths, 1987.

Stoelting RK: *Pharmacology and Physiology in Anesthesia Practice,* 2nd ed. Lippincott, 1991.

Warner DO et al: Pulmonary resistance during halothane anesthesia is not determined only by airway caliber. Anesthesiology 1989;70:453–60.

ANESTHESIA & THE AIRWAY

Soft Tissue Obstruction

Under the influence of residual anesthesia and muscle relaxant effects, airway obstruction is a common and potentially catastrophic complication in the immediate postanesthesia period. It usually results from soft tissue obstruction by the tongue and laryngopharyngeal structures when recovery from neuromuscular function is incomplete. It can be detected by physical signs and symptoms with or without abnormal blood gas measurements. Management includes hyperextension of the head, chin lift-jaw thrust maneuvers, insertion of an oropharyngeal or nasopharyngeal airway, or positive-pressure ventilation.

Laryngospasm

As the patient is emerging from anesthesia, the vocal cords are sensitive and prone to develop spasms if blood or secretions accumulate in the area of the larynx. This may result in hypoxia, hypercapnia, and respiratory arrest if not corrected promptly. Suctioning corrects the problem in most cases. If spasms persist, positive-pressure ventilation by mask with or without small doses (10–20 mg) of succinylcholine may be necessary. Endotracheal reintubation is seldom required.

LARYNGOEDEMA

Edema of the laryngeal structures may occur following extubation after anesthesia. It is usually due to use of an oversized endotracheal tube or traumatic intubation, fluid overload, or allergic reaction. In women, it may be caused by preeclampsia. It usually responds best to high humidity and nebulized racemic epinephrine. Corticosteroids may be beneficial.

Aspiration

Recovery of laryngopharyngeal function may be incomplete after anesthesia with muscle relaxant drugs. Prolonged placement of the endotracheal tube may further aggravate the situation. With an incompetent larynx, aspiration may occur following vomiting or regurgitation.

CARDIOVASCULAR EFFECTS OF ANESTHESIA

Anesthesia may disrupt homeostatic regulation of the cardiovascular system by a variety of mechanisms.

Inhalation Anesthesia

A. Blood Pressure Response

All currently used inhalation anesthetics (halothane, enflurane, isoflurane, desflurane, and sevoflurane) cause dose-dependent reduction in mean arterial blood pressure. The decrease in blood pressure is primarily due to a decrease in cardiac output by myocardial depression with halothane and enflurane and a decrease in peripheral vascular resistance with isoflurane, desflurane, and sevoflurane.

B. Cardiac Effects

All inhalation anesthetics shift the left ventricular function curve downward and to the right, indicating depression of myocardial contractility. This may be due to a direct action of anesthetics on cardiac cells or on postganglionic receptors on the myocytes. The drugs may inhibit the slow Na^+-Ca^{2+} channels and reduce Ca^{2+} influx. The degree of depression varies with different agents and concentrations. There is a consistent decrease in stroke volume as well as cardiac output, while the heart rate response may vary. All agents decrease the slope of phase 4 and phase 0 depolarizations and increase the action potential duration at minimum alveolar concentrations.

C. Peripheral Resistance Effects

All inhalation agents cause vasodilation and decrease peripheral resistance, but to different degrees. This effect may be due to the direct vasodilating effects on vascular smooth muscle as well as the result of decrease in sympathetic vasoconstrictor tone. Anesthetics may interfere with the movement of Ca^{2+} across the vascular endothelial membranes and within the smooth muscle cells.

D. Cardiovascular Reflexes

Inhalation anesthetic agents depress homeostatic reflex regulation of the cardiovascular system. The baroreceptor reflex is attenuated or blocked via either a central or a peripheral effect. The cardiac chronotropic response is also blunted by higher anesthetic doses.

Narcotic Anesthesia

A. Cardiac Effects

Depression in myocardial contractility has been demonstrated in a variety of isolated heart muscle preparations using different opioids in concentrations much higher than those attained clinically. Opioid receptors may not be involved in this effect. It is not preventable with naloxone pretreatment.

With the exception of meperidine, opioids cause bradycardia by stimulation of vagal preganglionic neurons in the medulla oblongata. They may also cause direct depression of the sinoatrial node at very high doses. Bradycardia can be reversed by naloxone or atropine.

B. Peripheral Resistance Effects

Aside from histamine release, morphine may cause vasodilation of both resistance and capacitance vessels through direct local effects on vascular smooth muscle or the central vasomotor center. The degree of this effect is determined by the specific opioid, the rate of injection, the baseline status of the patient, and compensatory responses. The vascular effects of morphine may not involve opioid receptors or narcotic action. Clinically, opioid-induced vasodilation occurs predominantly in patients who are critically ill or in those with underlying cardiac disease with elevated sympathetic tone.

Anesthesia with opioids in high doses (morphine, 1–3 mg/kg; fentanyl, 50–150 μg/kg) normally causes little hemodynamic change and is well tolerated by patients with poor cardiovascular function. However, the potential risk of myocardial depression and peripheral vasodilation by opioids should not be underestimated. Adding nitrous oxide or benzodiazepines to high doses of fentanyl may produce hypotension due to myocardial depression or peripheral vasodilation.

Regional Anesthesia

Local anesthetic agents inhibit the excitation-conduction process in peripheral nerves. In sufficient tissue concentration, they may affect the heart and smooth muscles of blood vessels, resulting in hemodynamic depression.

A. Direct Effects

All local anesthetics produce a dose-related decrease in velocity of atrial conduction, atrioventricular conduction, and ventricular conduction. Lidocaine decreases the maximum rate of depolarization, action potential duration, and effective refractory period. Bupivacaine, etidocaine, and tetracaine, which are highly potent local anesthetics, tend to decrease conduction velocity through various parts of the heart at relatively low concentrations. Extremely high concentration of local anesthetics will depress spontaneous pacemaker activity in the sinus node, resulting in sinus bradycardia and sinus arrest.

All local anesthetics essentially exert a dose-dependent negative inotropic action. High doses of bupivacaine are cardiotoxic. A biphasic peripheral vascular effect of local anesthetic agents may be observed, with vasoconstriction followed by vasodilation in high concentration.

B. Indirect Effects

Spinal or epidural anesthesia is associated with sympathetic blockade that may result in profound hypotension due to peripheral vasodilation. The higher the spinal level of the blockade, the lower the blood pressure.

Below the T5 dermatomal level, epidural anesthesia is not usually associated with significant cardiovascular changes. From T5 to T1, it produces about a 20% decrease in blood pressure. At T1 or above, bradycardia and a fall in cardiac output may develop as a result of blockade of cardiac sympathetic accelerator nerves. In addition to peripheral vasodilation, myocardial contractility is depressed. Hypovolemic patients are more susceptible to sympathetic blockade; profound hypotension may occur when the preload is too low. High epidural anesthesia may decrease coronary and hepatic blood flow and may alter normal autoregulation of cerebral and renal blood flow as well.

ANESTHESIA & THE RESPIRATORY SYSTEM

Inhalation Anesthesia

A. Control of Ventilation

In general, all volatile anesthetics decrease ventilation in a dose-related manner. When the patient is allowed to breathe spontaneously, the decrease in tidal volume reflects the depth of anesthesia. Although anesthesia reduces metabolism and thus CO_2 production, it also increases dead space. Postoperative hypoventilation may occur under the residual effect of anesthesia on the respiratory center with resultant hypercapnia and hypoxemia.

With the exception of ether, all inhalation anesthetics cause not only a rise in resting $Paco_2$ but also a diminished responsiveness of ventilation to added CO_2. This shifts the CO_2 response curve downward and to the right, causing hypoventilation in the immediate postanesthesia period. Doxapram, which produces respiratory stimulation via peripheral carotid chemoreceptors, may be useful, but mechanical ventilation until the residual anesthesia effect completely wears off is the best treatment.

In general, inhalation anesthetics depress the hyperventilation response to hypoxemia by acting directly on the carotid body. This hypoxic ventilatory response is impaired in a dose-related manner; however, the dose required is much smaller than that required for depressing the hypercapnic ventilatory response. In the immediate postoperative period, the patient may fail to respond to hypoxemia by increasing ventilation because of impairment of this defense mechanism by residual anesthetic agent.

1. Response to loading and stimulations—In a conscious person, inspiratory effort increases when external resistance is imposed. This response is markedly depressed by anesthesia. Under the influence of anesthetics, patients with chronic obstructive pulmonary disease, in particular, may fail to increase ventilation when airway resistance is increased.

Ventilation increases with surgical stimulation during anesthesia. When all stimulation ceases at the conclusion of the procedure, spontaneous breathing may diminish or stop.

2. Apnea threshold—The apnea threshold is the $Paco_2$ level at which spontaneous ventilatory effort ceases. The difference between the $Paco_2$ during spontaneous breathing and during apnea is generally a constant value of 5–9 mm Hg, independent of anesthetic depth. When $Paco_2$ is too low as a result of prolonged hyperventilation during anesthesia, postoperative hypoventilation or apnea can occur and lead to hypoxemia.

3. Posthyperventilation hypoxemia—Following prolonged anesthesia with hyperventilation, the body stores of CO_2 are depleted. Refilling CO_2 stores leads to low $Paco_2$ and hypoventilation. Hypoxemia may occur if supplemental oxygen is not provided.

B. Mechanics of Respiration

General anesthesia and muscle paralysis have a significant impact on respiratory mechanics that may lead to impaired gas exchange.

1. Functional residual capacity—With induction of general anesthesia, functional residual capacity is reduced by about 500 mL within 30 seconds. The mechanisms of this effect remain unclear. Increased elastic recoil of the lung, decreased outward recoil of the chest wall, and peripheral alveolar atelectasis due to absorption or hypoventilation in the dependent portions of the lung are the most likely underlying mechanisms. Other possibilities include trapping of gas distal to the closed airways, increased activity of expiratory or decreased activity of inspiratory muscles, and increased thoracic or abdominal blood volume, alone or in combination.

Twenty-four hours after recovery from anesthesia—particularly following upper abdominal surgery—functional residual capacity continues to fall to the lowest value (70–80% of the preoperative level). It takes about 7–10 days to return to the preoperative volume. When closing capacity exceeds functional residual capacity, regions with a low ventilation-perfusion ($\dot{V}/\dot{Q}$) ratio develop, leading to atelectasis, shunting, and impaired gas exchange. Widening of the alveolar-arterial Po_2 gradient and some degree of hypoxemia are not uncommon in the immediate postoperative period.

2. Compliance of the lung and chest wall—The compliance of the total respiratory system and lungs is reduced. The pressure-volume curve shifts rightward, following induction of general anesthesia. This may be due to decrease in functional residual capacity, increase in recoil of the lung, and paralysis of the diaphragm. The reduction in total compliance results in a necessity for greater airway pressures to inflate the lungs to a given volume under anesthetic influence. A restrictive ventilatory pattern with impaired gas exchange may occur during the recovery period.

3. Airway resistance—Following induction of general anesthesia and endotracheal intubation, pulmonary resistance may be doubled. The size of the airway may be altered by the decrease of lung recoil, and bronchial smooth muscle tone may be diminished by some anesthetics. The pressure-flow relationship is affected, and dynamic compliance is also decreased.

4. Intrapulmonary gas distribution—Changes in the vertical pleural pressure gradient secondary to alterations in the shape or pattern of chest wall motion during anesthesia may influence the intrapulmonary distribution of inspired gas. In contrast to the awake state, preferential ventilation of the nondependent lung occurs in patients under general anesthesia. This redistribution does not depend on the use of muscle paralytic agents. Abnormal gas distribution and $\dot{V}/\dot{Q}$ mismatching may exist when there is a residual effect of anesthetics or muscle relaxant.

5. Postoperative vital capacity—The characteristic pulmonary function profile following abdominal or thoracic surgery is a restrictive pattern with markedly reduced inspiratory capacity and vital capacity. Patients usually breathe with a shallow volume at a higher rate and cough ineffectively. The vital capacity is reduced by 50–70% of preoperative values immediately after upper abdominal surgery and remains depressed for 7–10 days. Only moderate or minimal reduction in vital capacity is observed following extremity surgery. If not improved, this defect of pulmonary mechanics may lead to atelectasis and pneumonia during the postoperative period. Although residual effects of anesthetics and muscle relaxants may have some contribution during the immediate postoperative period, the reduction of vital capacity appears to be more related to surgical pain and the noxious reflex, which limit excursion of the diaphragm more than the anesthesia itself.

6. Diaphragmatic function—Normally, the muscles of the chest wall, the diaphragm, and the abdominal muscles have important roles in the regional distribution of inhaled gases. Anesthesia and muscle paralysis have a significant impact on the mechanics of the chest wall, particularly the diaphragm, causing irregularities of gas distribution and exchange. Both anesthesia and muscle paralysis move the diaphragm cephalad in the recumbent and decubitus positions at the end of expiration. This is of greatest significance for the dependent parts of the diaphragm, for which abdominal pressure has the greatest influence. While displacement of the diaphragm during spontaneous inspiration is maximal in dependent regions and minimal in nondependent regions, the relationship is reversed during paralysis with mechanical ventilation. Regional gas volume and distribution are in proportion to diaphragmatic movement. In states of anesthesia and paralysis, the anteroposterior diameters of both the rib cage and the abdomen decrease while the transverse diameters increase. Compliance of the rigid thoracic compartment increases and that of the abdomen and diaphragm decrease. The persistent tonic activity of the diaphragm throughout expiration is also abolished, and the motion of the diaphragm becomes passive. In contrast to active breathing, displacement of the diaphragm and the associated gas distribution will be different. Mismatch of ventilation and perfusion may be exaggerated.

C. Pulmonary Gas Exchange

Under general anesthesia, oxygen consumption normally decreases by approximately 10%. This may decline to 25% of normal depending on the fall in body temperature. It is raised substantially if shivering occurs. The production of CO_2 fluctuates with oxygen consumption. While it is not uncommon to mechanically hyperventilate a paralyzed patient, hypoventilation usually occurs during anesthesia with spontaneous breathing. Diffusing capacity for carbon monoxide remains unaltered, indicating that transfer across the alveolar-capillary membrane is not affected. Studies on gas exchange indicate the occurrence of ventilation-perfusion mismatching during anesthesia. The increase in $P(A\text{–}a)O_2$ gradient may be due to increased perfusion of regions with low $\dot{V}/\dot{Q}$ ratio or increased shunt (or both). The increase in alveolar dead space appears to be a result of the relative maldistribution of ventilation.

D. Pulmonary Circulation

Normally, hypoxic pulmonary vasoconstriction is a powerful physiologic response. The mechanism is triggered by regional alveolar hypoxia (low P_{AO_2} or low $P\bar{v}O_2$), which causes precapillary pulmonary arterial constriction. The increase of vascular tone in the hypoxic area diverts blood flow to areas of higher oxygen tension. This optimizes ventilation-perfusion matching in the lung and thus reduces venous admixture and maintains better gas exchange. All three currently used inhalation anesthetics inhibit hypoxic pulmonary vasoconstriction in a dose-dependent manner. This special effect of volatile agents may contribute to the inefficiency of oxygen exchange during anesthesia.

E. Diffusion Hypoxemia and Absorption Atelectasis

At the conclusion of inhalation anesthesia, when the patient starts to breathe spontaneously, diffusion hypoxemia may occur. Since nitrous oxide is 30 times more soluble than nitrogen, it will rapidly diffuse from the pulmonary capillary blood and dilute the inspired alveolar air. This causes a reduction in PaO_2 that can be corrected with supplemental oxygen.

When high concentrations of oxygen are used during anesthesia, the lung units with low ventilation/perfusion ratios may become unstable and collapse. This absorption atelectasis may widen the P_{AO_2}–PaO_2 gradient, particularly when ventilation is shallow and inadequate.

Narcotic Anesthesia

All opioid agonists produce a dose-dependent depression of ventilation by acting on the central respiratory center. The ventilatory effects of opioids include a decreased respiratory rate, decreased minute ventilation, increased arterial CO_2 tension, and decreased ventilatory response to CO_2. Although equianalgesic doses of opioids are likely to produce equivalent depression of ventilation, the peak effects and durations are determined by the pharmacokinetics of each drug. Depression of ventilation is augmented and prolonged in elderly and debilitated patients and in the presence of other central nervous system depressants. Airway reflexes are blunted, as is the hypoxic ventilatory response. Additionally, fentanyl may cause chest wall rigidity and compromise ventilatory function.

Regional Anesthesia

Diaphragmatic function is usually preserved even with high spinal anesthesia as long as the cervical portion of the spinal cord is not involved. With paralysis of the thoracic cage, the patient may appear to experience an incoordinate breathing pattern with paradoxic abdominal respiration even though ventilatory function is well maintained at the 75–85% level. The blockade of intercostal nerves leads to abdominal muscle paralysis that may limit the ability to cough and clear secretions. When anesthetics reach the cervical region or fourth ventricle, total apnea develops.

ANESTHESIA & BODY TEMPERATURE

Hypothermia may occur with general anesthesia. Not only are the thermoregulatory centers depressed by anesthetic agents, but the interior and exterior of the body are also exposed to a cool environment for hours. In addition, the peripheral vasodilatory effect associated with most types of anesthesia can aggravate heat loss and further decrease body temperature. Although hypothermia lowers total body oxygen consumption, severe depression may be fatal. Other complications of hypothermia include myocardial dysfunction, cardiac dysrhythmia, coagulopathy, and acidosis. Shivering during recovery may increase oxygen consumption as much as fourfold. During rewarming, circulatory collapse can occur if adequate fluid replacement is not provided to offset increased vascular capacitance.

EFFECTS OF NEUROMUSCULAR BLOCKADE

Neuromuscular blocking agents are commonly used in anesthesia to facilitate surgical procedures. Because of paralysis or weakness of skeletal muscles, such blockade has a significant influence on ventilation and airway maintenance if a residual effect persists during the recovery period. Neuromuscular blocking agents are classified as depolarizing or nondepolarizing depending on their effects at the neuromuscular junction. Depolarizing agents form strong attachments to the postsynaptic cholinergic receptor and result in persistent depolarization and paralysis. Nondepolarizing drugs bind competitively to postsynaptic cholinergic receptors and prevent acetylcholine from activating sodium channels. Residual neuromuscular blockade must be antagonized before extubation—otherwise, airway patency as well as respiratory function may be compromised postoperatively. If not completely reversed, residual neuromuscular blockade may persist into the recovery period. Recovery is monitored by peripheral nerve stimulators utilizing a train-of-four test. There are essentially two patterns of blockade: (1) Phase 1 (depolarizing) block is produced by succinylcholine and is associated with sustained tetanus, equal train-of-four responses (muscle responses to four consecutive 2-Hz electrical nerve stimuli), and absence of posttetanic potentiation, which refers to enhanced twitch responses after tetanic stimulation. (2) Phase 2 block is caused by nondepolarizing agents or the prolonged use of succinylcholine and is characterized by tetanic fade, fade of the train-of-four responses and posttetanic potentiation. Both can recover spontaneously. Nondepolarizing agents may be reversed with anticholinesterases such as edrophonium, neostigmine, or pyridostigmine. Persistent phase 1 block requires continuos ventilatory support.

AIRWAY MANAGEMENT

In the ICU, airway management is a common challenge in daily practice. For critical care physicians, its importance cannot be overemphasized. A variety of techniques must be mastered, ranging from merely lifting the chin to emergency tracheostomy. Physicians confronted with airway problems must decide whether to intervene. This requires rapid assessment of several factors such as the duration of hypoxia, the current status of the airway and ventilation, the presence of jaw-clenching, cervical spine stability, prior difficulties with intubation, and available equipment and skills. Contingency plans for various potential airway emergencies must be in place and familiar to all ICU personnel. The risk of irreversible hypoxic damage should always dictate priorities in the decision algorithm. Gloves and goggles are indicated for personal protection during manipulations of the airway.

SECURE A PATENT AIRWAY

Partial or complete obstruction of the airway results in ventilatory failure, hypoxemia, hypercapnia, and death. The first priority in management of any critically ill patient is establishment of airway patency. In the ICU, this may be accomplished urgently for cardiopulmonary resuscitation or electively for mechanical ventilation.

Mechanical Maneuvers

Whenever the airway is compromised at the pharyngolaryngeal area due to tongue or soft tissue occlusion, the chin lift-jaw thrust maneuver is useful initially to maintain patency, particularly in conjunction with insertion of oral or nasal airways. These techniques for temporary opening of the airway can be performed easily in any unconscious patient. They are commonly followed by mask ventilation and endotracheal intubation.

It is essential to exclude cervical spine injury by appropriate x-rays at the time of a patient's arrival in the unit so that further neurologic damage can be avoided in case emergent intubation is required. Neck lift and head tilt maneuvers are contraindicated in patients with cervical spine injury. Chin lifting or jaw thrusting may be performed while the neck is maintained in the neutral position.

Clearing of vomitus, secretions, blood, and foreign bodies should be done immediately when necessary to ensure an open airway. If the risk of aspiration is high and the spine is stable, the patient should be placed in the lateral position. Adequate suction devices, including large-bore rigid and flexible cannulas, should always be available.

Artificial Airways

Artificial airways are useful when the obstruction is above the laryngopharynx. They keep the tongue from falling back and aid in removal of secretions from the posterior pharynx. Oropharyngeal and nasopharyngeal airways are commonly used. Selection of an airway of appropriate size is required to achieve optimal effect. Oral airways may prevent undesirable clenching of the teeth. Nasal airways are usually better tolerated by agitated and semiconscious patients. Lubrication with local anesthetics prior to airway insertion can be helpful. Nasal airways are contraindicated in patients with suspected basilar skull fractures or coagulopathies because they may cause severe bleeding from the nasal mucosa.

Intermediate Airways

Intermediate airways include the esophageal obturator airway, the esophageal gastric tube airway, the pharyngeal-tracheal lumen airway, and the esophageal-tracheal combitube. The first two are designed to occlude only the esophagus, whereas the latter two can be inserted into either the trachea or the esophagus. These devices are designed to establish an airway rapidly, but they fail to control the airway completely. Because of the latter shortcoming, they are not often used in the ICU.

ENDOTRACHEAL INTUBATION

Endotracheal intubation is indicated if the chin lift-jaw thrust maneuver fails to establish or secure a patent airway; if the patient is obtunded and aspiration is a concern; if positive-pressure mechanical ventilation is required; if tracheobronchial secretions cannot be cleared; or if complete control of the airway is desirable. In critically ill patients, use of the esophageal obturator airway and its variants should be limited to situations in which endotracheal intubation has been unsuccessful and no other methods are available.

Any maneuver involving movement of the neck should be avoided in cases of confirmed or suspected cervical spine injury. However, if the patient sustains apnea or severe hypoxemia in spite of conservative management, immediate endotracheal intubation may become necessary. Oral endotracheal intubation may be attempted if stability of the neck can be maintained. The risk of further damage must be balanced by the overall risk to the patient's life due to failure to secure an airway. If time permits, fiberoptic nasotracheal intubation should be the first choice in such situations. Blind nasotracheal intubation is the alternative when a skilled operator with the necessary equipment for fiberoptic intubation is not available or when the oral approach is contraindicated, impossible, or difficult. Nevertheless, a careful orotracheal approach is common practice.

SPECIAL CONSIDERATIONS IN AIRWAY MANAGEMENT

Neuromuscular Blocking Agents

At the time of intubation, jaw clenching induced by neurologic dysfunction in various disease states can obstruct the oral passage and prevent not only access to the larynx but also clearing of secretions, vomitus, blood, and foreign bodies. Even though jaw clenching will usually subside when severe hypoxia develops, the risk of irreversible cerebral damage is very high if a patent airway cannot be established immediately. Rather than attempting intubation with force, neuromuscular blocking agents are indicated to overcome jaw clenching and facilitate intubation.

Time Factors

Irreversible brain damage can result within minutes if apnea is not corrected. The period of apnea that can be sustained without brain damage depends on the degree of preoxygenation and the patient's oxygen consumption, hemoglobin concentration, cardiac output, and functional residual capacity. Patients with low reserves can tolerate only brief periods of apnea. Without preoxygenation, the customary maximum interval of allowable apnea during intubation is 30 seconds. The interval can be extended to minutes in a healthy young person who has been preoxygenated. Ventilation with a mask that provides 100% oxygen is strongly recommended before attempts at reintubation are repeated. Prolonged and multiple attempts at intubation can injure the airway and cause decompensation of the cardiorespiratory system, including hypoxemia, arrhythmia, bradycardia, asystole, laryngospasm, bronchospasm, and apnea. An oxygen saturation monitor (pulse oximeter) and atropine should be available.

Endotracheal Tube Size

In adults, cuffed endotracheal tubes of different internal diameters (6.5–9 mm) should be available. Tubes with diameters of 7–8 mm are usually appropriate for females, whereas slightly larger tubes (7.5–8.5 mm) are appropriate for males. A slightly smaller tube (by 0.5 mm in each case) is usually adequate for nasal intubation. Tubes that are too large will cause laryngeal injury, particularly after prolonged intubation; tubes that are too small will increase airway resistance and the work of breathing. An endotracheal tube with a minimum internal diameter of 8 mm is advisable if bronchoscopy is anticipated. The cuff should be checked for any leak beforehand. After tube placement, the cuff should be inflated with the minimum volume necessary to prevent air leak around the tube. Breath sounds should be checked bilaterally immediately after tube placement, and the position of the tube should be checked by x-ray. When the tube is correctly placed, it is secured with tape and a bite block or oral airway to protect it from damage or crimping.

Improper Positioning

Esophageal placement of the endotracheal tube, if unrecognized, is a lethal complication. Unfortunately, esophageal intubation may not be detected immediately. Auscultation of breath sounds bilaterally is useful but not always reliable. Absence of breath sounds, increasing abdominal girth, or gurgling during ventilation in conjunction with desaturation and cyanosis should alert one to the possibility of esophageal intubation. End-tidal CO_2 measurement has become the best means of confirming proper placement of the endotracheal tube in most instances. A flexible fiberoptic bronchoscope, if available, is also helpful to ensure proper positioning under direct vision.

If a tube that is too long is inserted, main stem bronchus intubation results. This occurs most commonly on the right side. If unrecognized, one-sided intubations can cause atelectasis of the opposite lung, hypoxemia due to shunting, and an increased risk of barotrauma of the ipsilateral lung. Asymmetric breath sounds and chest movements are common findings. The tube should be withdrawn about 2–3 cm beyond the point where equal breath sounds are first heard. Chest radiographs are useful to confirm tube placement but do not always exclude main stem intubations.

Other than esophageal and main stem bronchus intubations, complications following nasal endotracheal intubation include epistaxis, nasal necrosis, retropharyngeal laceration, mediastinal emphysema, and intracranial placement of the tube. Nasal sinusitis is common and may be a cause of sepsis.

PERSISTENT AIR LEAK

Persistent air leak around an endotracheal tube may result in hypercapnia and hypoxemia secondary to inadequate ventilation. The leak may be due to damage to the balloon itself or to the pilot balloon. Other causes include tracheomalacia or malposition of the cuff at or above the vocal cords. Repositioning the tube or replacement with a tube of appropriate size is required.

Surgical Airway

When endotracheal intubation is impossible or has failed after several attempts, operative creation of an airway becomes imperative. Options include needle cricothyrotomy, surgical cricothyrotomy, and tracheostomy. Jet ventilation may be used initially with needle cricothyrotomy; however, adequate alveolar ventilation is not ensured, and a formal airway is usually required in less than 45 minutes. Surgical cricothyrotomy will rapidly stabilize and secure the airway, but pressure effects will lead to necrosis if the endotracheal tube is not removed within several days.

Airway Management in Patients Requiring Prolonged Ventilation

The use of high-volume, low-pressure cuffs has greatly reduced the incidence of tracheal injury from intubation. However, damage to the laryngeal area has been a continuing problem. Tubes with high-pressure, low-compliance cuffs should be avoided or replaced. Monitoring of the cuff pressure is useful but not reliable, since it does not reflect the lateral tracheal wall pressure and may fluctuate when high pressures are used to overcome poor lung compliance. Conversion to a tracheostomy is indicated when endotracheal intubation is prolonged and laryngeal damage is a concern. Other relative indications include patient comfort, easier nursing care, and facilitation of suction.

The time limit for change is debated. Three weeks is the empiric limit.

Benumof JL: Management of the difficult adult airway with special emphasis on awake tracheal intubation. Anesthesiology 1991; 75:1087–110.

Benumof JL, Scheller MS: The importance of transtracheal jet ventilation in the management of the difficult airway. Anesthesiology 1989;71:769–78.

Clinton JE, Ruiz E: Emergency airway management procedures. In: *Clinical Procedures in Emergency Medicine,* 2nd ed. Hedges R (editor). Saunders, 1991.

King TA, Adams AP: Failed tracheal intubation. Br J Anaesth 1990;65:400–14.

Norton ML, Brown ACD: Evaluating the patient with a difficult airway for anesthesia. Otolaryngol Clin North Am 1990; 23:771–85.

PAIN MANAGEMENT IN THE ICU

Pain control in the ICU has improved significantly over the last decade with greater understanding of neurophysiologic mechanisms, anatomic pathways, causes of pain perception, and clinical pharmacology. In a sense, pain serves as a means for detection of tissue damage, for prevention of further harm, and for promotion of healing through rest. Postoperative or posttraumatic pain, however, may have no such useful purpose and may in fact be detrimental and cause complications in many organ systems. The goal of pain management in the ICU is to minimize discomfort and promote faster recovery of normal function.

ANATOMIC PATHWAYS & PHYSIOLOGY OF PAIN

Pain is perceived through the nociceptors at nerve endings throughout the body. The impulses in response to mechanical, thermal, and certain chemical stimuli are transmitted through A δ and C fibers to the neuraxis at the dorsal horn of the spinal cord. The marginal layer cells in lamina I and the wide-dynamic-range neurons in lamina V are activated and send projections to the nociceptive areas of the thalamus. The spinothalamic tract is the predominant but not the only pathway. Others project to the reticular formation, midbrain, hypothalamus, and limbic forebrain structures. Impulses finally reach the cortex, where perception of pain is completed. Cells in the substantia gelatinosa modulate both segmental and descending input and exert an inhibitory effect on thalamic projection cells in the dorsal horn. Some visceral pain may pass through visceral afferents.

PATHOPHYSIOLOGY OF PAIN

Perception of pain at the neuraxis provokes both segmental reflexes and central responses. Segmentally, it causes a marked increase in local skeletal muscle tension, which not only impairs normal function but also intensifies pain. Centrally, the sympathetic nervous system is activated, and this leads to an increase in overall sympathetic tone, thereby increasing cardiac output, blood pressure, and cardiac work load. Cardiac metabolism—as well as whole body metabolism—and oxygen consumption are augmented. Tachypnea, ileus, nausea, bladder hypotonicity, and urinary retention are not uncommon.

Pain itself—as well as the associated anxiety and apprehension—also aggravates the hypothalamic neuroendocrine response. There are increased secretions of catabolic hormones such as catecholamines, ACTH, cortisol, ADH, aldosterone, and glucagon. Secretion of anabolic hormones such as insulin and testosterone is decreased. Persistent pain, if uncorrected, will result in a catabolic state and negative nitrogen balance.

PAIN & RESPIRATORY DYSFUNCTION

The incidence of postoperative pulmonary complications varies from 5% to 28%. Most of these complications are related to inappropriate control of postoperative pain. Pulmonary function can be significantly affected depending on the site and extent of surgery or trauma. Derangement of ventilation-perfusion relationships occurs, followed by abnormal gas exchange and hypoxemia. Surgery and postoperative pain cause involuntary splinting and reflex muscle spasm of the abdominal and thoracic muscles. Excursions of the diaphragm are markedly limited, particularly when ileus develops. Furthermore, in an attempt to minimize pain, the patient refrains from deep breathing and coughing. Pulmonary status deteriorates, and some patients progress to atelectasis and pneumonia. When narcotics are given in sufficient quantity, respiratory depression results. Apnea can occur in severe cases. Adequate monitoring and therapeutic facilities should always be available.

ANALGESIA WITH OPIOIDS

Intravenous Opioid Analgesia

Opioid analgesics alone or in combination with adjuvant agents such as nonsteroidal anti-inflammatory drugs have been conventionally used for pain relief. They are effective if properly prescribed. However, patients are frequently undertreated. The minimum effective analgesic dosage varies widely in different patients. Therefore, the dose of opioid should be individualized and titrated as needed.

The absorption of opioids following intramuscular or oral administration is variable. The intravenous route is usually appropriate for patients in the ICU because an effective plasma concentration level can be achieved promptly. Not uncommonly, small doses (3–5 mg) of morphine or other equally potent opioids are given for pain relief. Continuous infusion of small doses of morphine (0.1 mg/min) avoids peaks and valleys in plasma concentration and provides effective relief of pain in most instances.

Patient-controlled analgesia (PCA) allows the patient to self-administer a preset amount of opioid intravenously as needed. A lock-out interval can be set to prevent overdosage. PCA permits the patient to titrate his or her own analgesic requirements and maintains a relatively steady level of minimum effective analgesic concentration. PCA is generally well accepted by patients. Overall, it provides smoother and more adequate analgesia accompanied by relief of fear and anxiety. It improves pulmonary function in postoperative patients, reduces nocturnal sleep disturbances, and decreases the overall drug requirement. The patient must be thoroughly instructed about the device in order to maximize its advantages.

The ideal agent for PCA in the ICU should have a rapid onset, a predictable efficacy, a relatively short duration of action with minimal side effects (particularly on cardiopulmonary function), and no tendency to cause tolerance or dependency. A typical prescription of PCA with morphine is a loading dose of 2–10 mg over 15–30 minutes, followed by a patient-triggered bolus (1–2 mg) via the PCA pump programmed with a lock-out interval of 5–15 minutes. This regimen may be changed according to the patient's responses. Total doses and effective therapeutic concentrations cannot be predicted. Individualization is necessary.

The combination of PCA with continuous infusion has the advantage of providing a baseline plasma level of analgesic while allowing titration of boluses to overcome varying acute changes in the threshold of pain perception.

Epidural & Intrathecal Opioids

The use of epidural and intrathecal opioids for pain relief in the ICU has increased recently. Epidural and intrathecal narcotics act mainly on spinal receptors and produce long-lasting pain relief with relatively small amounts of drug. The major advantage of this modality over local anesthesia is that sympathetic and motor nerves are not blocked.

Morphine, a highly hydrophilic drug, has been shown to spread rostrally to reach the fourth ventricle and brain stem in about 6 hours following epidural administration. There are two phases of respiratory depression. The earlier phase reflects the rise of serum levels through absorption from epidural veins. It commonly occurs 20–45 minutes after an injection. The second phase coincides with rostral spread and appears approximately 6–10 hours after injection. It causes a decrease in respiratory rate. The risk of delayed respiratory depression rises greatly if opioid is given systemically at the same time.

Fentanyl, a lipophilic agent, also travels cephalad through the cerebrospinal fluid, but extends less than morphine. When given by lumbar epidural catheter, it may not be equianalgesic with morphine for thoracic pain. It tends to have fewer side effects than morphine, and most can be reversed with naloxone. These include nausea and vomiting (17–34%), pruritus (11–24%), and urinary retention (22–50%).

Epidural morphine has a relatively slow onset, prolonged action, and delayed occurrence of respiratory depression. Fentanyl has a rapid onset and short duration of action and is not uncommonly used for continuous epidural infusion. The addition of epinephrine to epidural narcotics is not recommended because of the increased incidence of side effects.

Intermittent epidural administration of opioids has the drawback of peak and trough concentrations, so that patients may suffer unacceptable pain before adequate analgesia is restored. Continuous infusion, PCA, or a combination of both may provide better pain control in certain situations.

The epidural route has been used more commonly than the intrathecal route for postoperative pain control. Potential risks, complications, and monitoring requirements are similar for the two techniques. Because of spinal cord toxicity, not all drugs used epidurally are safe for intrathecal use. Compared with regional anesthesia, epidural or intrathecal narcotics provide highly effective pain relief with no direct effects on hemodynamics and motor function. However, they may be less effective than regional anesthesia in blocking nociceptive perception and the associated metabolic and neuroendocrine reactions.

LOCAL ANESTHETIC ANALGESIA

Postoperative or posttraumatic pain control can also be managed with long-acting local anesthetics. Brachial plexus block, intercostal block, intrapleural block, and local infiltration of the wound area are available. When feasible, continuous infusion may be more effective and reliable.

Regional Analgesia

Regional analgesia with local anesthetic agents generally provides better pain relief than opioids because anesthetic agents block both the afferent and the efferent pathways of the reflex arc. This minimizes neuroendocrine and metabolic responses to noxious stimuli. Nevertheless, when local anesthetics are administered epidurally or intrathecally, care must be exercised to minimize side effects such as hypotension and limb paralysis or weakness secondary to sympathetic and somatic nerve blockade. A proper combination of opioids and local anesthetics may achieve the ideal goal of adequate analgesia with minimum metabolic and physiologic changes.

Local Anesthetic Agents

Local anesthetics produce both sensory and motor block when a sufficient quantity is deposited near neural tissue. They are used in the ICU to provide anesthesia and analgesia through regional, field, nerve block, or intravenous techniques.

Local anesthetics are classified as esters or amides depending on the chemical bond of their alkyl chain. The actions of local anesthetics are affected by multiple factors, including lipid solubility, pK_a, protein binding, metabolism, and local vasoactivity. Onset of block depends on availability of the nonionized form of the drug, which is determined by its pK_a and the tissue pH. The extent of binding to membrane protein and the time of direct contact with the nerve fiber affect its duration of action. Epinephrine (1:200,000) is frequently added to local anesthetic solutions to reduce their absorption and prolong the duration of action through local vasoconstriction.

Allergic reactions to local anesthetics are rare and more likely to occur with esters than with amides. High plasma concentrations of local anesthetics from either excessive absorption or inadvertent overdose lead to severe side effects. Hypotension, direct myocardial depression, arrhythmias, and cardiac arrest are potentially lethal complications. Perioral numbness, restlessness, vertigo, tinnitus, twitching, and seizures are common manifestations that involve the nervous system.

A. Lidocaine

Lidocaine is currently the most widely used local anesthetic in the ICU because it has a low incidence of side effects, a rapid onset of action, and an intermediate duration of action. It has a volume of distribution of 90 L, a clearance rate of 60 L/h, a distribution half-life of 57 seconds, and an elimination half-life of 1.6 hours. It is metabolized in the liver by oxidative dealkylation.

Lidocaine is used to provide pain control in spinal, epidural, caudal, nerve, and field blocks and in Bier block anesthesia (intravenous regional block). Lidocaine in concentrations of 2–4% has been used topically in the nose, mouth, laryngotracheobronchial tree, esophagus, and urethra. Lidocaine concentrations of 0.5–1.5% are used for local infiltration. An intravenous bolus of lidocaine (1.5 mg/kg) is useful to attenuate the increase of intracranial pressure and blood pressure during laryngoscopy and endotracheal intubation.

Systemic toxicity occurs when plasma concentrations of lidocaine are above 5–10 μg/mL. Doses of 6.5 mg/kg can cause central nervous system toxicity.

B. Bupivacaine

Bupivacaine, commonly used in obstetric anesthesia, is highly protein-bound and produces intense analgesia of prolonged duration but is relatively slow in onset. It has a volume of distribution of 72 L, a clearance rate of 28 L/h, a distribution half-life of 162 seconds, and an elimination half-life of 3.5 hours. It is primarily metabolized in the liver.

Bupivacaine is commonly used in epidural anesthesia and for intercostal nerve blocks. Central nervous system toxicity occurs with plasma concentrations of 1.5 μg/mL. Clinically, doses exceeding 2 mg/kg may cause systemic toxicity. Cardiac toxicity due to severe myocardial depression may be fatal. Other less commonly used agents include etidocaine, mepivacaine, chloroprocaine, and procaine (Table 5–1).

C. Ropivacaine

Ropivacaine, newly introduced, is one of the amide group of local anesthetics. It is 94% protein bound with a steady state volume of distribution of 41 ± 7 L and is extensively metabolized in the liver. Approximately 37% of the total dose is excreted in the urine. Unlike most other local anesthetics, the presence of epinephrine has no major effect on either the time of onset

Table 5–1. Commonly used anesthetics.

Agent	Half-Life (hours)	Use	Maximum Single Dose
Amides			
Bupivacaine	3.5	Epidural, spinal infiltration	3 mg/kg
Etidocaine	2.6	Epidural, caudal, infiltration, nerve block	3 (4)[1] mg/kg
Lidocaine	1.6	Epidural, caudal, infiltration, nerve block	4.5 (7)[1] mg/kg
Mepivacaine	1.9	Epidural, caudal, infiltration, nerve block	4.5 (7)[1] mg/kg
Esters			
Procaine	0.14	Spinal, infiltration, nerve block	12 mg/kg

[1]Maximum dose with epinephrine.

or the duration of action. At blood concentrations achieved with therapeutic doses, changes in cardiac conduction, excitability, refractoriness, contractility, and peripheral vascular resistance are minimal. Ropivacaine may cause depression of cardiac contractility. Although both are considerably more toxic than lidocaine, the cardiac toxicity of ropivacaine is less than that of bupivacaine.

NONSTEROIDAL ANTI-INFLAMMATORY DRUGS

Nonsteroidal anti-inflammatory drugs (NSAIDs) are a group of compounds with heterogeneous structures that relieve pain, lower fever, and decrease inflammatory reactions. The mechanism of their actions remains unclear but may involve an inhibitory effect on prostaglandin synthesis. They are useful for management of mild to moderate pain. Compared with opioids, they have both the advantages and the disadvantages of analgesia but without producing changes in sensorium or ventilatory depression without the possibility of dependency. NSAIDs cause platelet dysfunction and prolong bleeding time. They may produce gastric erosions and hemorrhage. Other adverse effects include interstitial nephritis, renal hypoperfusion, somnolence, nausea and vomiting, and palpitations.

Until recently, because of a lack of parenteral formulations, the use of NSAIDs in the ICU was limited. The advent of ketorolac tromethamine, which can be given parenterally, has made this class of agents more conveniently available for critically ill patients.

Ketorolac tromethamine has no direct effect on opiate receptors. It is a potent analgesic with a ceiling effect. Intramuscular doses of 30–90 mg have analgesic efficacy comparable to that of 10 mg of morphine. After intramuscular injection, maximum plasma concentrations are achieved within 45–60 minutes.

Ketorolac tromethamine is highly protein-bound and metabolized primarily by hepatic conjugation. Excretion is through the kidney. It is nonaddicting and has no effect on ventilation. Its side effects are similar to those of other NSAIDs. It should be avoided in patients with renal dysfunction and bleeding tendencies.

Barson WG, Jastremski MS, Syuerud SA: *Emergency Drug Therapy.* Saunders, 1991.

Bonica JJ: Management of postoperative pain. In: *The Management of Pain,* 2nd ed. Bonica JJ (editor). Lea & Febiger, 1990.

Crews JC: Epidural opioid analgesia. Crit Care Clin 1990; 6:315–42.

Eisenach JC, Grice SC, Dewan DM: Patient-controlled analgesia following Cesarean section: A comparison with epidural and intramuscular narcotics. Anesthesiology 1988;68:444–48.

King MJ, Bowden MI, Cooper GM: Epidural fentanyl and 0.5% bupivacaine for elective caeserean section. Anaesthesia 1990;45:285–88.

Ornato JP, Gonzalez ER: *Drug Therapy in Emergency Medicine.* Churchill Livingstone, 1990.

Stenseth R, Sellevold O, Breivik H: Epidural morphine for postoperative pain: Experience with 1085 patients. Acta Anaesthesiol Scand 1985;29:148–56.

Stoelting RK: *Pharmacology and Physiology in Anesthesia Practice,* 2nd ed. Lippincott, 1991.

Veselis RA: Sedation and pain management for the critically ill. Crit Care Clin 1988;4:167–81.

Vestergaard-Madsen J et al: Respiratory depression following postoperative analgesia with epidural morphine. Acta Anesthesiol Scand 1986;30:417–20.

ANALGESIA & ANESTHESIA FOR BEDSIDE PROCEDURES

Excision of Eschar in Burn Patients; Wound Debridement & Dressing Changes

The first excision may be performed without anesthesia on the fifth or sixth day following the burn. This is carried to the point of pain or bleeding and identifies the areas of second- and third-degree burn. Anesthesia with intramuscular ketamine in a dose of 3–4 mg/kg provides a satisfactory condition for subsequent excisions. The patient is usually semiresponsive, while respiratory function and the gag and cough reflexes are preserved. Emergence nightmares may occur and can be reduced by giving diazepam or midazolam (intramuscularly or intravenously) during induction of and emergence from ketamine anesthesia. Increased sympathetic activity following ketamine administration may be beneficial in critically ill patients with circulatory depression.

Cardioversion

In cases of elective conversion such as atrial flutter or atrial fibrillation, there is usually sufficient time to premedicate the patient to provide a period of amnesia or hypnosis. Intravenous diazepam, 5–10 mg, or midazolam, 2–3 mg, is effective and safe. Methohexital, a short-acting barbiturate, 1 mg/kg intravenously, is also useful. Thiopental (50–100 mg) and propofol (0.5–1 mg/kg) have also been used. Narcotics alone are not sufficient. Supplemental oxygen and equipment for intubation and ventilation should be available.

MUSCLE RELAXANTS IN INTENSIVE CARE

Neuromuscular blocking agents (Table 5–2) are used frequently in the intensive care unit. Their major drawbacks are the lack of titratable agents and the difficulty with bolus techniques. This, coupled with inadequate monitoring, may result in inappropriate blockade and markedly delayed recovery. Newly introduced bedside intravenous pumps and intermediate-acting nondepolarizing agents have redefined their role in intensive care management. Recent reports of prolonged paralysis, muscle weakness from neuromuscular junction dysfunction, and muscle atrophy following long-term treatment with neuromuscular blocking agents should alert the clinician to serious potential consequences. Whenever prolonged use of neuromuscular blocking agents is planned, the balance of benefits and complications should be carefully assessed.

There are some circumstances in critical care in which neuromuscular blocking agents are indicated but not indispensable. These include endotracheal intubation, postoperative rewarming with shivering, the presence of delicate vascular anastomoses, the need for protection of wounds with tension, tracheal anastomosis, increased intracranial pressure, insertion of invasive vascular catheters in agitated patients, and the facilitation of mechanical ventilation. In other specific areas (neurosurgical intensive therapy, management of tetanus, and severe status epilepticus), neuromuscular agents can either provide protection of the patient or facilitate procedures and management. Neuromuscular blocking agents in these situations are beneficial but not essential. If adequate sedation and analgesia are provided, the need for relaxants is frequently diminished. In most instances, muscle relaxation is required only when sedation and analgesia fail to achieve adequate ventilation or other therapeutic goals. Anxiety, apprehension, and confusion, together with pain and discomfort, often make patients agitated, combative, and more apt to fight against the ventilator. It is essential to provide appropriate levels of sedation and pain relief before and after a trial of neuromuscular blocking agents. Adequate intravenous administration of narcotics, either by bolus or by continuous infusion, accompanied by benzodiazepines, usually obviates the need for neuromuscular blocking agents.

Once paralysis is induced, the feeling of total dependency and helplessness can lead to extreme anxiety and fear. This psychosomatic impact must not be ignored. Sedation with narcotics or benzodiazepines is mandatory.

Table 5–2. Commonly used muscle relaxants.

Drug	Loading Dose	Maintenance Dose	Time of Onset	Duration of Action	Complications
Succinylcholine	1–2 mg/kg	Not recommended	0.5–1 min	5–10 min	Vagolytic, prolonged
Pancuronium	0.1 mg/kg	0.3–0.5 μg/kg/min	3 min	45–60 min	Minimal histamine release
Atracurium	0.5 mg/kg	3–10 μg/kg/min	1.5–2 min	20–60 min	Weak histamine release
Vecuronium	0.1 mg/kg	1–2 μg/kg/min	2–3 min	25–30 min	None
Doxacurium	0.05 mg/kg	Supplemental dose guided by twitch monitor	4 min	30–160 min	None
Pipecuronium	0.15 mg/kg		3 min	45–120 min	None
Mivacurium	0.15 mg/kg		2 min	15–20 min	Weak histamine release

MUSCLE RELAXANTS IN MECHANICAL VENTILATION

Only rarely does a mechanically ventilated patient require neuromuscular blockade. Therapy should be instituted to make certain the patient is properly sedated and free from pain before blockade is considered. The use of muscle relaxants is indicated for patients who have very poor thoracic or lung compliance, those who are fighting the ventilator, and those at increased risk of barotrauma from high airway pressures. If total control of ventilation is required with modalities such as inverted I:E ratio or high minute volume ventilation, muscle relaxants may be required.

Before initiating neuromuscular blockade, the patient-ventilator system should be thoroughly reviewed and evaluated. Any sudden development such as pulmonary edema, pneumothorax, or an obstructed endotracheal tube can cause contraction of the respiratory muscles, resulting in uncoordinated asynchronous breathing. On the other hand, the ventilator settings may no longer be appropriate. Adjustments in tidal volume, inspiratory flow rate, ventilator triggering sensitivity, or mode of ventilation often can avoid the need for neuromuscular blockade.

If there is no apparent change in the patient's clinical status and if adjustments in the mechanical ventilator fail to improve the situation, attention should be directed to the need for adequate sedation and analgesia.

DEPOLARIZING AGENTS

Succinylcholine

Succinylcholine is the only clinically available depolarizing neuromuscular blocking agent in the United States. It has a uniquely rapid onset (30–60 seconds) and a short duration of action (5–10 minutes). It acts as a false transmitter of acetylcholine by avidly binding to postsynaptic cholinergic receptors, resulting in persistent depolarization and muscle paralysis. Succinylcholine also stimulates all cholinergic receptors, including autonomic ganglia, postganglionic cholinergic nerve endings, and the acetylcholine receptors of the vascular system, which causes changes in blood pressure and heart rate. A peculiar bradycardia may occur after repeated bolus doses of succinylcholine, especially in children, when the interval of injections is shorter than 4–5 minutes. Use of succinylcholine in a hypoxic patient may cause irreversible sinus arrest. Muscle fasciculations from sustained depolarization following succinylcholine can increase serum K^+ by 0.5–1 meq/L and produce arrhythmias. This induced hyperkalemia is enhanced after burns, with paraplegia or hemiplegia, following skeletal muscle trauma, and with upper motor neuron injury following trauma or cerebrovascular accidents. Succinylcholine should be avoided under these situations and between 1 week and 6–12 months after injury. Severe fasciculations may also increase intragastric pressure, resulting in regurgitation and aspiration. Succinylcholine may also trigger malignant hyperthermia.

Succinylcholine is rapidly hydrolyzed by pseudocholinesterase in the plasma to succinylmonocholine, a relatively inactive metabolite. In patients with low levels of pseudocholinesterase or atypical cholinesterase enzyme, prolonged relaxation can occur. Furthermore, when very large doses of succinylcholine are used, a type II competitive block may develop.

Succinylcholine is used in the ICU mainly for endotracheal intubation, especially when jaw clenching or muscle tone make laryngoscopy difficult or impossible. The usual dose of succinylcholine is 1–2 mg/kg intravenously. This drug is particularly useful in critically ill patients with a full stomach, for whom a rapid-sequence intubation technique is needed.

NONDEPOLARIZING NEUROMUSCULAR BLOCKING AGENTS

Nondepolarizing neuromuscular blocking agents bind in a competitive manner principally to postsynaptic cholinergic receptors at the neuromuscular junctions, where they prevent depolarization by acetylcholine.

Pancuronium

Until recently, pancuronium bromide, a bisquaternary aminosteroid, has been the principal muscle relaxant used in critical care. It is a long-acting nondepolarizing agent, water-soluble, highly ionized, and excreted mainly through the kidney. Its clearance depends upon the glomerular filtration rate. It is also metabolized and broken down into less active hydroxyl metabolites in the liver. The elimination half-life of pancuronium is 90–160 minutes, which is greatly prolonged by hepatic or renal failure.

Pancuronium is administered intravenously as a bolus of 0.1 mg/kg. Onset of complete relaxation is 3–5 minutes, and the duration of action is 45–60 minutes. Unlike monoquaternary relaxants, pancuronium causes histamine release. In large doses, because of vagolytic and sympathomimetic effects, it may cause increases in heart rate and blood pressure. Prolonged paralysis can occur after relatively large doses of pancuronium, particularly in patients with renal or hepatic dysfunction.

Atracurium

Atracurium is a nondepolarizing muscle relaxant with an intermediate duration of action. It has the unique property of being hydrolyzed through the Hoffman degradation mechanism. Renal or hepatic disease does not prolong its short elimination half-life (19 minutes). Laudanosine, its metabolite, causes cerebral irritation in high doses in several animal species. This has not been noted clinically, however, even after prolonged use of atracurium. The route of laudanosine elimination is not certainly known, but it seems that renal failure itself will not affect metabolic accumulation significantly.

For intravenous administration, 0.5 mg/kg is given in adults. The onset of action is 1.5–2 minutes, with peak relaxation in 3–5 minutes. The duration of action is 20–60 minutes. There are no cumulative effects.

Administration of atracurium should be slow and adequate in amount, because rapid intravenous injection with a large bolus may result in histamine release and hypotension. Clinically, in most instances, recovery is rapid and complete once the infusion is stopped. Because of its relatively mild cardiovascular and cumulative effects, atracurium by continuous infusion appears to be useful when prolonged neuromuscular blockade is required.

Vecuronium

Vecuronium is a shorter-acting monoquaternary steroidal analog of pancuronium. It is classified as an intermediate-duration nondepolarizing muscle relaxant. Because it causes no vagolytic effects and does not provoke histamine release, its use is associated with marked cardiovascular stability. The metabolism and excretion of vecuronium are mainly through the liver, though about 15–25% is excreted by the kidneys. The elimination half-life is 70 minutes. The metabolite 3-desacetyl vecuronium has about half the potency of the parent compound.

The intravenous dose of vecuronium for adults is 0.1 mg/kg. Onset of action is 2–3 minutes; peak relaxation occurs within 3–5 minutes; and the duration of action is 25–30 minutes. Continuous infusion of vecuronium is recommended for prolonged paralysis in patients with cardiovascular instability. A lower dose should be used in patients with hepatic or renal failure. In patients with cardiac failure, modification of the dose is not required.

In patients with normal renal and liver function, recovery of neuromuscular function occurs rapidly when the infusion is stopped even after large doses. However, in patients with renal and hepatic failure, the effect may be more variable and the duration of action unpredictable.

Rocuronium

Depending on the dose, rocuronium is a nondepolarizing neuromuscular blocking agent with a rapid to intermediate onset. With rocuronium 0.6 mg/kg, good to excellent intubating conditions can be achieved within 2 minutes in most patients. The duration of action of rocuronium at this dose is approximately equivalent to the duration of other intermediate-acting neuromuscular blocking drugs. Generally there are no dose-related changes in mean arterial pressure or heart rate associated with injection. The rapid distribution half-life is 1–2 minutes, and the slower distribution half-life is 14–18 minutes. Rocuronium is eliminated primarily by the liver. Patients with liver cirrhosis have a marked increase in volume of distribution, resulting in a plasma half-life approximately twice that of patients with normal liver function. Currently, rocuronium is commonly used to replace succinylcholine when rapid-sequence intubation is needed and succinylcholine is contraindicated.

Other Nondepolarizing Neuromuscular Blocking Agents

Doxacurium, pipecuronium, and mivacurium are nondepolarizing neuromuscular blocking agents. Mivacurium is unique because of its short duration of action (15–20 minutes). Doxacurium and pipecuronium are as long-acting as pancuronium but are associated with better cardiovascular stability. Clinical experience with their use in the ICU is limited.

COMPLICATIONS OF USE OF MUSCLE RELAXANTS

Psychosomatic Effects

When paralysis is imposed without adequate explanation and sedation, severe psychosomatic stress and crisis may result. If both muscle relaxants and sedatives are appropriately titrated, the goal of management can be maintained in a cooperative and well-sedated but easily arousable patient.

Suppression of Cough Reflex

When all the respiratory muscles are paralyzed, the cough reflex is suppressed. Endotracheal suctioning may provoke no response or only an ineffective cough. Retention of secretions can precipitate atelectasis and lead to pneumonia.

NEUROMUSCULAR DYSFUNCTION & PROLONGED PARALYSIS

When controlled ventilation is indicated, prolonged use (more than 48 hours) of neuromuscular blocking agents is often necessary. Aside from delayed recovery from paralysis, there is evidence that some degree of neuromuscular dysfunction can occur. Clinically, these types of neuromuscular dysfunction range from generalized weakness, paresis, and areflexia to persistent flaccid paralysis for days or months. There are generally no sensory disturbances after discontinuation of relaxants.

Long periods of iatrogenic immobilization lead to disuse atrophy. Pathologic changes of motor endplates and muscle fibers have been demonstrated. Electrodiagnostic studies show evidence of neurogenic and myopathic abnormalities as well as transmission disturbances at the neuromuscular junction. Unless strongly indicated, the duration of relaxation should be as short as possible. Range of motion exercises may help to prevent atrophy and contracture.

MONITORING WITH A PERIPHERAL NERVE STIMULATOR

Without objective monitoring of responses, overdosing of muscle relaxant is not uncommon. During surgical anesthesia, train-of-four stimuli are used to detect the degree of muscle relaxation. In the ICU, paralysis with total ablation of twitches of a train-of-four is usually not necessary. The use of peripheral nerve stimulators is helpful to titrate the requirement of neuromuscular blocking agents.

REVERSAL OF NEUROMUSCULAR BLOCKADE

While there is no specific antagonist for depolarizing agents, nondepolarizing neuromuscular blockade can be reversed with intravenously administered anticholinesterase drugs. The commonly used anticholinesterases include edrophonium (0.5 mg/kg), neostigmine (0.05 mg/kg), and pyridostigmine (0.2 mg/kg). Anticholinergic agents such as atropine (0.01 mg/kg) or glycopyrrolate (0.008 mg/kg) are usually given simultaneously to offset the stimulation of muscarinic receptors.

Durbin CG Jr: Neuromuscular blocking agents and sedative drugs: Clinical uses and toxic effects in critical care units. Crit Care Clin 1991;7:489–505.

Griffiths RB, Hunter JM, Jones RS: Atracurium infusion in patients with renal failure on an ITU. Anaesthesia 1986;41:375–81.

Ornato JP Gonzalez ER: *Drug Therapy in Emergency Medicine.* Churchill Livingstone, 1990.

Segredo V et al: Prolonged neuromuscular blockade after long-term administration of vecuronium in two critically ill patients. Anesthesiology 1990;72:566–70.

Stoelting RK: *Pharmacology and Physiology in Anesthesia Practice,* 2nd ed. Lippincott, 1991.

SEDATIVE-HYPNOTICS FOR THE CRITICALLY ILL

Critically ill patients are constantly exposed to an unusual and frequently noxious environment that includes pain, noise, tracheal suctioning, sensory overload or deprivation, isolation, immobilization, physical restraints, lack of communication, and sleep deprivation. These unpleasant experiences can lead to anger, frustration, anxiety, and mental stress. This may result in a diagnosis of ICU psychosis unless organic and pharmacologic causes are excluded.

Sedative-hypnotic medications are frequently used to calm the patient or induce sleep for therapeutic or diagnostic purposes. Because of associated side effects, stable cardiopulmonary function must be assured prior to administration. Furthermore, because individual responses may vary greatly among patients—and even in the same patient at different stages of illness—dosage should be carefully adjusted. The conventional categories of sedative-hypnotic agents are the benzodiazepines, barbiturates, and narcotics. The ideal agent for use in the ICU should have a rapid onset of action, a predictable duration of action, no adverse effects on cardiovascular stability or respiratory function, a favorable therapeutic index, no tendency toward accumulation in the body, ease of administration, and available antagonists.

BENZODIAZEPINES

Benzodiazepines (Table 5–3) produce sedation, anxiolysis, and muscle relaxation. They also have anticonvulsant activity. Flumazenil is the specific antagonist for benzodiazepines in a dosage of 1 mg slowly intravenously up to a total dose of 3 mg.

Table 5–3. Commonly used benzodiazepines.

Agent	Intravenous Dose	Duration of Action
Diazepam	2–10 mg	4–6 hours
Lorazepam	0.04 mg/kg	6–10 hours
Midazolam	0.1 mg/kg	0.5–2 hours

Diazepam

Diazepam binds to specific benzodiazepine receptors in cortical limbic, thalamic, and hypothalamic areas of the central nervous system, where it enhances the inhibitory effects of γ-aminobutyric acid (GABA) and other neurotransmitters. Following an intravenous dose, its onset of action is within 1–2 minutes. Maximum effect is achieved in 2–5 minutes, and the duration of action is 4–6 hours. Diazepam is initially redistributed into adipose tissue and is metabolized in the liver by microsomal oxidation and demethylation. Its active metabolites are excreted by the kidney with a half-life of 45 hours. The intramuscular route should not be used because of poor bioavailability from unpredictable absorption. Abscesses may form at the injection site.

Diazepam is used to produce sedation and amnesia for reduction of anxiety and unpleasant stress. It is also useful for anticonvulsion, muscle relaxation, cardioversion, endoscopy, and management of drug or alcohol withdrawal.

For relief of anxiety in adults, a bolus injection of 2–10 mg is given slowly intravenously. This can be repeated every 3–4 hours if necessary. When used for cardioversion, 5–15 mg is administered intravenously 5–10 minutes before the procedure. For status epilepticus, 5–10 mg is administered intravenously and repeated every 10–15 minutes up to a maximum dose of 30 mg. For acute alcohol withdrawal, 5–10 mg is given intravenously every 3–4 hours as necessary.

Diazepam can cause prolonged dose-related drowsiness, confusion, and impairment of psychomotor and intellectual functions. Paradoxic excitement can occur. Hypotension, bradycardia, cardiac arrest, respiratory depression, and apnea have been associated with rapid parenteral injection, particularly in elderly and debilitated patients. Allergic reactions have been reported. Irritation at the infusion site and thrombophlebitis may occur.

Lorazepam

Lorazepam acts on benzodiazepine receptors in the central nervous system and enhances the chloride channel gating function of GABA by promoting binding to its receptors. The resulting increase in resistance to neuronal excitation leads to anxiolytic, hypnotic, and anticonvulsant effects. Lorazepam is highly lipid-soluble and protein-bound. It can be administered both intravenously and intramuscularly. The onset of action following intravenous injection is within 1–5 minutes, with a peak at 60–90 minutes. The duration of action is 6–10 hours. Seventy-five percent of the dose is conjugated in the liver and excreted in the urine. The elimination half-life is 12–20 hours.

Lorazepam is useful for the management of anxiety with or without depression, stress, and insomnia. It can be used for preoperative sedation as well as status epilepticus.

The common dosage for intravenous or intramuscular administration is 0.04 mg/kg. Normal maximum doses are 2 mg intravenously and 4 mg intramuscularly. The dose needs to be individualized to minimize adverse effects. For status epilepticus, 0.5–2 mg may be given intravenously every 10 minutes until seizures stop.

Side effects of drowsiness, ataxia, confusion, and hypotonia are extensions of the drug's pharmacologic effects. Cardiovascular depression, hypotension, bradycardia, cardiac arrest, and respiratory depression have been associated with parenteral use of lorazepam, especially in elderly and debilitated patients. Caution and adjustment of doses are required when administering this drug to patients with liver or kidney dysfunction.

Midazolam

Midazolam, an imidazole benzodiazepine derivative, exerts its sedative and amnestic effect through binding of benzodiazepine receptors. It is two to three times as potent as diazepam. Its onset of action begins within 1–2 minutes after an intravenous or intramuscular dose. Its duration of action is 0.5–2 hours. Midazolam reaches its peak of action rapidly (3–5 minutes) and has a plasma half-life of 1.5–3 hours. Its high lipid solubility results in rapid redistribution from the brain to inactive tissue sites, yielding a short duration of action. Metabolism is by hepatic microsomal oxidation with renal excretion of glucuronide conjugates. The drug's half-life can be extended up to 22 hours in patients with liver failure. It is water soluble and can be administered intravenously or intramuscularly. Pain and phlebitis at injection sites are less frequently seen than with other benzodiazepines.

Midazolam is indicated for sedation, creation of an amnesia state, anesthesia induction, and anticonvulsant treatment. It has become the benzodiazepine of choice for sedation in the ICU. Midazolam can be administered intravenously or intramuscularly at a rate of 0.1 mg/kg to a maximum dose of 2.5 mg/kg. Alternatively, intermittent doses of 2.5–5 mg may be given every 2–3 hours. A rate of 1–20 mg/h or 0.5–10 μg/kg/min can be used for continuous intravenous infusion.

Midazolam may cause unexpected respiratory depression or apnea, particularly in elderly and debilitated patients. In combination with some narcotics, midazolam may cause myocardial depression and hypotension in relatively hypovolemic patients. Monitoring of cardiopulmonary function is required.

BARBITURATES

The barbiturates possess sedative-hypnotic activities without analgesia.

Thiopental

This ultra-short-acting barbiturate is a potent coma-inducing agent. It blocks the reticular activating system and depresses the central nervous system to produce anesthesia without analgesia. It quickly crosses the blood-brain barrier and has an onset of action within 10–15 seconds after an intravenous bolus, a peak effect within 30–40 seconds, and a duration of action of only 5–10 minutes. This initial effect on the central nervous system disappears rapidly as a result of drug redistribution. Thiopental is metabolized by hepatic degradation, and the inactive metabolites are excreted by the kidney. The elimination half-life is 5–12 hours but can be as long as 24–36 hours after prolonged continuous infusion. In sufficient doses, thiopental can cause deep coma and apnea but poor analgesia. It also produces a dose-related depression of myocardial contractility, venous pooling, and an increase in peripheral vascular resistance. Thiopental reduces cerebral metabolism and oxygen consumption.

Thiopental is used for induction of general anesthesia but is also useful for sedation, particularly in patients with high intracranial pressures or seizures. It is also useful for short procedures such as cardioversion and endotracheal intubation.

For induction of anesthesia, an intravenous bolus of 3–5 mg/kg is given over 1–2 minutes. Individual responses are sufficiently variable so that the dose should be titrated to patient requirements as guided by age, sex, and body weight. In cases with cardiac, hepatic, or renal dysfunction, dose reduction is required. Slow injection is recommended to minimize respiratory depression. Convulsions can usually be controlled with a dose of 75–150 mg. When continuous infusion is required, the maintenance dose is 1–5 mg/kg/h in 0.2% or 0.4% concentration. After prolonged continuous use, thiopental will become a long-acting drug.

Side effects of thiopental include respiratory depression, apnea, myocardial depression with hypotension, laryngospasm, bronchospasm, arrhythmias, and tissue necrosis with extravasation. Thiopental is contraindicated in patients with porphyria or status asthmaticus and in those with known hypersensitivity to barbiturates.

OPIOIDS (NARCOTICS)

Opioids (Table 5–4) have the advantage of possessing both analgesic and sedative effects.

Table 5–4. Commonly used intravenous opioids.

Agent	Usual Initial Intravenous Dose	Duration of Action
Morphine	3–5 mg	2–3 hours
Meperidine	25–50 mg/kg	2–4 hours
Fentanyl	2–3 μg/kg	0.5–1 hours
Sufentanil	0.1–0.4 μg/kg	20–45 minutes
Alfentanil	10–15 μg/kg	30 minutes

Opioid Agonists

Opioid agonists acting at stereospecific opioid receptors at the level of the central nervous system are associated with dose-related sedation in addition to their pain-relieving effects. Titration to patient response is advisable. Alterations in sensorium such as nervousness, disorientation, delirium, and hallucinations can occur. It is essential to maintain a balance between the patient's comfort and level of awareness. Opioids can cause peripheral vasodilation, but their use has rarely been associated with clinically significant cardiovascular effects. Unlike local anesthetics, opioids do not block noxious stimuli via the afferent nerve endings or nerve conduction along peripheral nerves.

Opioid agonists include morphine, fentanyl, sufentanil, alfentanil, and meperidine as well as other drugs. Each produces particular pharmacologic effects depending on the types of receptors stimulated.

A. Morphine

Morphine, a pure agonist of opioid receptors, produces analgesia through its action on the central nervous system. It can also induce a sense of sedation and euphoria. Its volume of distribution is 3.2–3.4 L/kg; its distribution half-life is 1.5 minutes; and its elimination half-life is 1.5 hours in young adults. Elimination is prolonged up to 4–5 hours in the elderly. It has an onset of action within 1–2 minutes, a peak action at 30 minutes, and a duration of action of 2–3 hours. Morphine is metabolized primarily in the liver by conjugation with glucuronic acid. It is excreted principally through glomerular filtration. Only 10–50% is excreted unchanged in the urine or in conjugated form in the feces.

Morphine is widely used for management of moderate to severe pain. A variety of administration routes are available. These include the epidural, intrathecal, intramuscular, and intravenous routes (by bolus injection such as PCA). Morphine is also very useful for sedation, particularly in patients with some pain. Other indications are myocardial infarction and pulmonary edema.

Since absorption following intramuscular or subcutaneous administration is unpredictable, the intravenous route is preferable in critically ill patients. The initial intravenous dose is 3–5 mg. This may be repeated every 2–3 hours as necessary to titrate effect. For maintenance, it can be given by continuous infusion at a rate of 1–10 mg/h.

Morphine causes respiratory depression through direct action on the pontine and medullary respiratory centers. It decreases the response to CO_2 stimulation. Respiratory depression, which is dose-dependent, occurs shortly after intravenous injection but may be delayed following intramuscular or subcutaneous administration. In therapeutic doses, morphine produces little change in the cardiovascular system other than occasional bradycardia and mild venodilation. It also causes nausea and vomiting, bronchial constriction, spasm at the sphincter of Oddi, constipation, and urinary urgency and retention. In patients with renal, hepatic, or cardiac failure, smaller doses at less frequent intervals may be necessary. Respiratory depression can be treated with naloxone, 0.4–2 mg intramuscularly or intravenously.

B. Meperidine

Meperidine, a phenylpiperidine derivative opioid agonist, is one-tenth as potent as morphine and has a slightly faster onset and shorter duration of action. Meperidine is metabolized in the liver by demethylation to normeperidine, which is an active metabolite. It has a distribution half-life of 5–15 minutes, an elimination half-life of 3–4 hours, and a duration of action of 2–4 hours. Meperidine can cause direct myocardial depression and histamine release. It may increase the heart rate via a vagolytic effect. Overdosage of meperidine may depress ventilation. Compared with morphine, meperidine produces less biliary tract spasm, less urinary retention, and less constipation. It is useful as an analgesic for short procedures that produce moderate to severe pain. It is also used to induce sedation.

For intravenous administration, the initial dose is 25–50 mg every 2–3 hours as necessary. For intramuscular injection, 50–200 mg is given initially and repeated every 2–3 hours if required. Ventilatory depression can be reversed with naloxone. Other side effects include histamine release, hypotension, nausea and vomiting, hallucinations, psychosis, and seizures.

C. Fentanyl

Fentanyl, a highly lipid-soluble synthetic opioid agonist, crosses the blood-brain barrier easily. It is 75–125 times more potent than morphine as an analgesic. It has a rapid onset of action (< 30 seconds), a short duration of effect, a plasma half-life of 90 minutes, and an elimination half-time of 180–220 minutes. Initially, fentanyl is redistributed to inactive tissue sites such as fat and muscle. It is eventually metabolized extensively in the liver and excreted by the kidneys.

When fentanyl is administered in repeated doses or by continuous infusion, progressive saturation occurs. As a result, the duration of analgesia—as well as ventilatory depression—may be prolonged. Fentanyl does not cause histamine release and is associated with a relatively low incidence of hypotension and myocardial depression. It has been widely used in balanced anesthesia for cardiac patients.

Fentanyl is indicated for short painful procedures such as orthopedic reductions and laceration repair. The initial intravenous dose is 2–3 μg/kg over 3–5 minutes for analgesia. The dosing interval is 1–2 hours. A reduced dose and an increase in dosing interval may be necessary in hepatic or renal diseases.

Ventilatory depression is a potential complication following fentanyl. Muscle rigidity, difficult ventilation, and respiratory failure can develop and call for administration of naloxone.

D. Sufentanil

Sufentanil, a thienyl analog of fentanyl, has high affinity for opioid receptors and an analgesic potency five to ten times that of fentanyl. Its lipophilic nature permits rapid diffusion across the blood-brain barrier followed by quick onset of analgesic effect. The effect is terminated by rapid redistribution to inactive tissue sites. Repeated doses of sufentanil can cause a cumulative effect. Sufentanil has an intermediate elimination half-time of 150 minutes and a smaller volume of distribution. It is rapidly metabolized by dealkylation in the liver. Metabolites are excreted in urine and feces.

Sufentanil is given intravenously in doses of 0.1–0.4 μg/kg to produce a longer period of analgesia and less depression of ventilation than a comparable dose of fentanyl. Sufentanil may cause bradycardia, decreased cardiac output, and delayed depression of ventilation.

E. Alfentanil

Alfentanil, a highly lipophilic narcotic, has a more rapid onset and a shorter duration of action than fentanyl. The onset of action after intravenous administration is 1–2 minutes. Because of the agent's low pH, more of the nonionized fraction is available to cross the blood-brain barrier. The serum elimination half-life of alfentanil is about 30 minutes because of redistribution to inactive tissue sites and metabolism. The drug is metabolized in the liver and excreted by the kidney.

Continuous intravenous infusion of alfentanil does not lead to a significant cumulative effect. Alfentanil does not cause histamine release and thus tends not to cause hypotension and myocardial depression. It can be used in patients with chronic obstructive pulmonary disease or asthma. Respiratory depression can occur with large doses.

The initial dose for intravenous injection is 10–15 μg/kg over 3–5 minutes, repeated every 30 minutes as needed. For maintenance, continuous infusion is given at a rate of 25–150 μg/kg/h. Reduction of dosage and increase in dosing interval are required in hepatic and renal dysfunction. Muscle rigidity and respiratory depression may develop following administration of alfentanil.

Opioid Agonist-Antagonists

Opioid agonist-antagonists bind to opioid receptors and produce limited pharmacologic responses to opioids. They are effective analgesics but lack the efficacy of subsequently administered opioid agonists. The advantage of this group of drugs is the ability to provide analgesia with limited side effects, including ventilatory depression and physical dependence.

A. Butorphanol

Butorphanol, acting on different opioid receptors, has agonist and antagonist effects. It may be used for control of acute pain. However, in comparison with equianalgesic doses of morphine, it may cause similar ventilatory depression. It is metabolized in the liver to an inactive form that is largely eliminated in the bile. The onset of analgesia is within 10 minutes following intramuscular injection; peak activity is within 30–60 minutes; and the elimination half-life is 2.5–3.5 hours. Following intravenous doses, butorphanol may increase mean arterial pressure, pulmonary wedge pressure, and pulmonary vascular resistance. It is useful for postoperative or traumatic pain of moderate or severe degree.

For the average adult, the usual intravenous dose is 0.5–2 mg every 3–4 hours as required. Butorphanol may also be given by intramuscular injection in a dosage of 1–4 mg every 3–4 hours as indicated. Side effects include dizziness, lethargy, confusion, and hallucinations. Butorphanol may increase the cardiac workload, which limits its usefulness in acute myocardial infarction or coronary insufficiency and congestive heart failure.

B. Buprenorphine

Buprenorphine, is derived from the opium alkaloid thebaine. It has 50 times the affinity of morphine for the mu receptors and is a powerful analgesic drug. It is highly lipid-soluble and dissociates slowly from its receptors. After intramuscular administration, analgesia occurs within 15–30 minutes and persists for 6–8 hours, with a plasma half-life of 2–3 hours. Two-thirds of the drug is excreted unchanged in the bile and one-third in the urine as inactive metabolites. A buprenorphine dose of 0.3–0.4 mg is equivalent to 10 mg of morphine.

Buprenorphine is indicated for the control of moderate to severe pain such as that of myocardial infarction, cancer, renal colic, and postoperative or posttraumatic discomfort. For intramuscular or intravenous administration, 0.3–0.4 mg of buprenorphine is given every 6–8 hours as needed. Drowsiness, nausea, vomiting, and depression of ventilation are common side effects. The duration of ventilatory depression may be prolonged and resistant to antagonism with naloxone.

OPIOID ANTAGONISTS

Pure opioid antagonists act by a competitive mechanism in which they bind to receptors, making them unavailable to the agonist. Naloxone is the single agent used clinically.

Naloxone

Naloxone, a synthetic congener of oxymorphone, competitively displaces opioid agonists from the mu receptors and thus reverses opioid-induced analgesia and ventilatory depression. Following intravenous administration, naloxone has a rapid onset of effect (within 2 minutes) and a relatively short duration of action (30–45 minutes). For this reason, repeated doses or continuous infusions are usually required for sustained antagonist effects. Naloxone is metabolized in the liver by conjugation, with an elimination half-life of 60–90 minutes. Naloxone is most commonly used for the treatment of opioid-induced ventilatory depression and opioid overdosage.

Intravenous doses of 1–4 μg/kg are given to reverse opioid-induced ventilatory depression. Boluses of 0.4–2 mg (intravenously, intramuscularly, or subcutaneously) may be repeated every 2–3 minutes up to a total dose of 10 mg. Continuous infusion of 5 μg/kg/h may reverse ventilatory depression without affecting analgesia.

Reversal of analgesia, nausea, and vomiting can occur following naloxone administration when given to antagonize ventilatory depression. Larger doses of naloxone have been associated with increased sympathetic activity manifested by tachycardia, hypertension, pulmonary edema, and cardiac arrhythmias.

HALOPERIDOL

Haloperidol, a butyrophenone antipsychotic agent, produces rapid tranquilization and sedation of agitated or violent patients. The mechanism of action is unclear, though it may be related to antidopaminergic activity. Onset of action is 5–20 minutes when haloperidol is given intravenously or intramuscularly. Peak action is at 15–45 minutes, though the duration of effect is highly variable (4–12 hours). Haloperidol is metabolized in the liver and excreted through the kidneys. The plasma half-life is 20 hours. Haloperidol causes few hemodynamic or respiratory changes.

For control of agitated patients, administration begins with intravenous or intramuscular doses of 1–2 mg. This dosage can be increased to 2–5 mg every 8 hours. The dose may be doubled every 30 minutes until the patient is calmed. Maintenance dosage depends on individual response. As much as 50 mg over 1–2 hours has been used.

Haloperidol can cause extrapyramidal reactions and is absolutely contraindicated in patients with Parkinson's disease. Other complications include neuroleptic malignant syndrome, hypotension, seizures, and cardiac arrhythmias. Haloperidol may also antagonize the renal diuretic effect of dopamine.

INTRAVENOUS ANESTHETICS

Propofol

Propofol, an isopropylphenol, is increasingly used for sedation and induction of general anesthesia. Following intravenous administration, it produces unconsciousness within 30 seconds. In most cases, recovery is more prompt and complete than recovery from thiopental and without residual effect. Redistribution and liver metabolism are responsible for rapid clearance of propofol from the plasma. Elimination seems not to be affected by renal or hepatic dysfunction. The plasma half-life is 0.5–1.5 hours. Propofol has been used by continuous infusion without excessive cumulative effect. Hemodynamically, it may cause hypotension, especially in hypovolemic or elderly patients or those with heart failure. Propofol can produce transient ventilatory depression or apnea following rapid intravenous boluses.

In the ICU, propofol may be used for brief procedures such as cardioversion, endoscopy, and endotracheal intubation and for sedation of agitated, anxious patients. The dosage for sedation is 1–3 mg/kg/h; for anesthesia, the dosage is 5–15 mg/kg/h.

Propofol may cause ventilatory and cardiovascular depression, particularly if given rapidly or in large amounts. It has been noted to increase the prothrombin time.

Ketamine

Ketamine, a phencyclidine derivative, produces dissociative anesthesia with profound analgesia and hypnosis. In contrast to inhalation anesthetics, ketamine is characterized by slightly increased skeletal muscle tone, normal pharyngeal and laryngeal reflexes with a patent airway, and cardiovascular stimulation secondary to sympathetic discharge. It has a rapid onset of action (intravenously, < 1 minute; intramuscularly, 15–30 minutes). Its volume of distribution is 3 L/kg and its distribution half-life is 15–45 minutes. Ketamine is eliminated by hepatic biotransformation, with a plasma half-life of 2–3 hours. With doses lower than those needed for dissociative anesthesia, ketamine induces analgesia comparable to that achieved with the opioids. It also produces bronchodilation.

In the ICU, ketamine is useful as a sole anesthetic or analgesic agent for relatively short diagnostic and surgical procedures that do not require muscle relaxation. It has been used for treatment of persistent status asthmaticus. It is one of the agents of choice for the care of burn patients. An intravenous dose of 2 mg/kg or an intramuscular dose of 10 mg/kg may be used to produce surgical anesthesia. For maintenance, 10–30 μg/kg/min is given by continuous infusion. Ketamine at a dosage of 0.2–0.3 mg/kg produces analgesia with little change in the level of consciousness. It is particularly useful in patients who have cardiovascular depression and are in constant pain.

Transient emergence hallucinations, excitement, and delirium have been associated with ketamine administration in 5–30% of patients. Stimulation of the cardiovascular system may cause tachycardia, hypertension, and increased myocardial oxygen consumption. Other side effects include nystagmus, nausea, paralytic ileus, increased skeletal muscle tone, and slight elevation in intraocular pressure. Severe respiratory depression or apnea may occur following rapid intravenous administration of high doses. Ketamine is contraindicated in patients with increased intracranial pressure because it augments cerebral blood flow and oxygen consumption.

Barson WG, Jastremski MS, Syuerud SA: *Emergency Drug Therapy.* Saunders, 1991.

Durbin CG Jr: Neuromuscular blocking agents and sedative drugs: Clinical uses and toxic effects in critical care units. Crit Care Clin 1991;7:489–505.

Oldenhot H et al: Clinical pharmacokinetics of midazolam in intensive care patients: A wide interpatient variability. Clin Pharmacol Ther 1988;43:263–69.

Stone DJ: Sedation in the intensive care unit. Semin Anesth 1990; 9:162–68.

Veselis RA: Sedation and pain management for the critically ill. Crit Care Clin North Am 1988;4:167–81.

MALIGNANT HYPERTHERMIA

ESSENTIALS OF DIAGNOSIS

- *History of exposure to agents known to trigger malignant hyperthermia.*

- *Development of muscle rigidity.*
- *Signs of hypermetabolic activity with hyperthermia.*
- *Confirmation by muscle biopsy with caffeine-halothane contracture test.*

General Considerations

Malignant hyperthermia is a syndrome characterized by a paroxysmal fulminant hypermetabolic crisis in both skeletal and heart muscle. Massive heat is generated and overwhelms the body's normal dissipation mechanisms. It is a complication uniquely associated with anesthesia. Almost any anesthetic agent or muscle relaxant may trigger malignant hyperthermia. Halothane and succinylcholine are the most common offenders. Malignant hyperthermia can occur at any time perioperatively—before, during, or after the induction of anesthesia.

The incidence of malignant hyperthermia is difficult to assess because of various regional distributions. It is estimated to occur in 1:50,000 adults and 1:15,000 children undergoing general anesthesia.

Pathophysiology

Malignant hyperthermia is a genetically predisposed syndrome transmitted as an autosomal dominant with reduced penetrance and variable expressivity. The precise cause has not been fully elucidated. The central pathophysiologic event is a sudden increase in intracellular Ca^{2+} concentration in skeletal and perhaps also cardiac muscles triggered by causative agents. This may be due to any of the following mechanisms, singly or in combination: increased release of Ca^{2+} from the sarcoplasmic reticulum, inhibition of calcium uptake in the sarcoplasmic reticulum, defective accumulation of calcium in mitochondria, excessive calcium influx via a fragile sarcolemma, and exaggeration of adrenergic activity.

The excessive myoplasmic calcium activates ATPase and phosphorylase, thus causing muscle contracture and a massive increase in oxygen consumption, CO_2 production, and heat generation. The toxic concentrations of calcium within mitochondria uncouple oxidative phosphorylation that leads to increased anaerobic metabolism. The production of lactate, CO_2, and heat is accelerated. Membrane permeability increases when the ATP level eventually falls. This allows K^+, Mg^{2+}, and PO_4^{2-} to leak from and calcium to flow into myoplasm. As a result, severe respiratory and metabolic acidosis develops followed by dysrhythmias and cardiac arrest. Rhabdomyolysis, hyperkalemia, and myoglobinuria are common consequences of muscle damage.

Clinical Features

A. Symptoms and Signs

Unexplained tachycardia (96%) and tachypnea (85%) are usually the earliest and most consistent—but nonspecific—signs of malignant hyperthermia. The patient may also present with profuse sweating, hot and flushed skin, mottling and cyanosis, arrhythmias, and hypertension or hypotension. During anesthesia, the canister of CO_2 absorbent is overheated. Evidence of increased muscle tone may appear in the form of marked fasciculations or sustained muscle rigidity.

A rapid rise of body temperature (1 °C per 5 minutes) is a classic but relatively late sign. The magnitude and duration of fever directly affect the mortality rate. Conventionally, the diagnosis of malignant hyperthermia is based on the clinical triad of (1) a history of exposure to an agent or stress known to trigger the episode, (2) development of muscle rigidity, and (3) signs of hypermetabolic activity with hyperthermia. However, 20% of patients may never manifest any perceptible hyperthermia or muscle rigidity. Signs of pulmonary edema, acute renal failure, myoglobinuria, disseminated intravascular coagulation, and cardiovascular collapse may occur subsequently.

B. Laboratory Findings

Respiratory and metabolic acidosis with hypercapnia is the characteristic finding on arterial blood gas analysis. Clinically, a sudden marked increase in end-tidal CO_2 is the best early clue to the diagnosis. Hypoxemia, hyperkalemia, hypermagnesemia, myoglobinemia, hemoglobinemia, and increases in lactate, pyruvate, and creatine kinase may be seen.

C. Special Tests

The diagnosis can be confirmed by muscle biopsy with the caffeine-halothane contracture test. Clinically, rapid resolution after treatment with dantrolene is highly suggestive.

Complications

Late complications of malignant hyperthermia involve multiple organ systems (see Table 5–5).

Treatment

Early diagnosis and prompt drug treatment cannot be overemphasized. To be effective, dantrolene must be given before tissue ischemia occurs. Hyperthermia must be controlled as quickly as possible. Standard support-

Table 5–5. Late complications of malignant hyperthermia.

Site	Complication
Heart	Increase in myocardial oxygen consumption, decrease in myocardial contractility, decrease in cardiac output, hypotension, dysrhythmia, and cardiac arrest.
Lungs	Pulmonary edema.
Central nervous system	Cerebral edema and hypoxia, convulsion , of, coma, brain death, and increased sympathetic activity.
Kidneys	Acute renal failure, myoglobinuria, and hemoglobinuria.
Hematologic system	Disseminated intravascular coagulopathy, hemolysis.
Liver	Increased hepatic enzyme activity.
Musculoskeletal system	Muscle edema and necrosis.

ive and cooling measures should be started immediately and simultaneously with administration of dantrolene.

The treatment of malignant hyperthermia should proceed as follows:

(1) Immediately discontinue all possible triggering agents if any are still in use.

(2) Perform intubation and start hyperventilation with 100% oxygen.

(3) Initiate active cooling by internal and external measures; use intravenous refrigerated saline, iced saline lavage of the stomach or rectum, surface cooling with a thermal blanket, ice or alcohol, and fans.

(4) Dantrolene sodium is the only specific drug for treatment of malignant hyperthermia. A hydantoin derivative, it acts by inhibiting the release of calcium from sarcoplasmic reticulum. Intravenous dantrolene should be started at a rate of 1–2 mg/kg. Repeat the same dose every 15–30 minutes up to 10–20 mg/kg, if necessary, until signs of improvement become evident. Response is indicated by slowing of the heart rate, resolution of arrhythmia, relaxation of muscle tone, and decline in body temperature. Because retriggering may occur, dantrolene should be continued for 24–48 hours.

(5) Fluid resuscitation, diuretics, procainamide, and bicarbonate should be used as indicated.

(6) Continue to monitor the patient closely.

Prognosis

The mortality and morbidity rate, high 2 decades ago (70%), is now much lower (10%) because of earlier diagnosis and effective treatment.

Ellis FR, Smith G (editors): Symposium on malignant hyperthermia. Br J Anaesth 1988;60:251–319.

Larach MG et al: Standardization of caffeine halothane muscle contracture test. Anesth Analg 1989;69:511–5.

Kolb ME, Horne ML, Martz R: Dantrolene in human malignant hyperthermia: A multicenter study. Anesthesiology 1982; 56:254–62.

Rosenberg H, Fletcher JE: Masseter muscle rigidity and malignant hyperthermia susceptibility. Anesth Analg 1986;65:161–4.

Tomarken JL, Britt BA: Malignant hyperthermia. Ann Emerg Med 1987;16:1253–65.

Nutrition 6

John A. Tayek, MD

NUTRITION & MALNUTRITION IN THE CRITICALLY ILL PATIENT

In the critically ill patient, nutritional status plays a key role in recovery. The extent of muscle wasting and weight loss in the ICU is inversely correlated with long-term survival. However, because conventional parenteral nutritional therapy of malnourished critically ill patients has not been demonstrated to produce anabolism, blunting of the catabolic state may be the more effective strategy. The use of conventional nutritional support and the role of newer nutritional adjunctive techniques utilized in the critical care setting will be discussed in this chapter.

METABOLIC & NUTRITIONAL CHANGES DURING CRITICAL ILLNESS

Acute Phase Response

The acute phase response to sudden illness or trauma is one of the most basic features of the body's defenses against injury. Phylogenetically, this response could be considered the most primitive one that occurs, and it is similar for insults due to trauma, burns, or infections. It includes alterations in amino acid distribution and metabolism, an increase in acute phase globulin synthesis, increased gluconeogenesis, reductions in serum iron and zinc levels, and increased serum copper and ceruloplasmin levels. Fever and negative nitrogen balance follow as a consequence of these changes.

Changes in levels of cytokines and hormones occur as part of the acute response. For example, an infectious process in the lung will attract monocytes that will be transformed into macrophages at the site of infection. These macrophages will secrete proteins known as cytokines and other peptides that attract other white blood cells and initiate the inflammatory response common to many types of injury. These cytokines include tumor necrosis factor-α (TNFα) and interleukins 1–16. TNFα and other cytokines circulate to the liver, where they inhibit albumin synthesis and stimulate the synthesis of acute phase proteins, including (1) C-reactive protein, which promotes phagocytosis and modulates the cellular immune response; (2) α_1-antichymotrypsin, which minimizes tissue damage from phagocytosis and reduces intravascular coagulation; and (3) α_2-macroglobulin, which forms complexes with proteases and removes them from circulation, maintains antibody production, and promotes granulopoiesis. TNFα and some of the interleukins also circulate to the brain, where they are responsible for induction of fever and initial stimulation of adrenocorticotropic hormone release with a subsequent rise in serum cortisol. Recent data from studies of cultured fetal adrenal cells suggest that TNFα can inhibit the P450 enzymes responsible for cortisol synthesis, thereby inhibiting the overall cortisol response in acute injury or severe sepsis.

Hormonal Changes

A. Insulin Resistance

As a result of severe injury, many patients develop the syndrome of insulin resistance with hyperglycemia even though they had no history of diabetes prior to the injury. Both the injury response and the septic state are associated with a decrease in whole body glucose oxidation and an increase in the fasting hepatic glucose production rate. Conversely, both the injury response and the septic state are associated with an increase in fatty acid oxidation and plasma fatty acid appearance rates. Triglyceride hydrolysis is much greater than fat oxidation, so that albumin-bound fatty acids are used partially for energy production but most are utilized for reesterification of substrate back to triglyceride.

The rise in serum cortisol is one of the many factors responsible for the development of insulin resistance. Insulin resistance is easy to diagnose because the injured patient will develop an elevated blood glucose level (> 160 mg/dL) while being provided with a modest amount of glucose solution or during usual alimentation, either enterally or parenterally. In addition to cortisol, elevations in catecholamines, glucagon, and growth hormone in the injured patient also contribute to the development of insulin resistance. Increased catecholamine levels are a direct response to the injury via secretion of these hormones by the adrenal gland and sympathetic ganglia throughout the body. Glucagon levels increase in response to the injury. Like the glucagon response, the increase in growth hormone secretion is not well understood, but it occurs in most types of injury. Growth hormone is known to be a potent inhibitor of glucose uptake in skeletal muscle and may be one of the major contributors to the insulin resistance that occurs as part of the injury response. Growth hormone may also increase hepatic glucose production. One possible cause of the increase in growth hormone is a reduction in insulin-like growth factor-1 (IGF-1) levels in the critically ill patient. Reduced levels of IGF-1 would, via the feedback loop to the pituitary, increase growth hormone secretion and, together with exogenous glucose administration, cause hyperglycemia. A decrease in IGF-1 is not always noted in severe injury, so that abnormalities in IGF-binding proteins or other factors may be responsible for the elevated growth hormone levels noted in injury.

B. Thyroid Hormones

As a normal response to injury, the body's ability to convert the stored form of thyroid hormone, thyroxine (T_4), into the active form, triiodothyronine (T_3), becomes impaired. There is increased conversion of T_4 to an inactive thyroid hormone known as reverse T_3 (rT_3) rather than T_3. This may have evolved as an energy-saving response during severe injury or illness to reduce the known contribution of T_3 to increased resting energy expenditure. Thus, the syndrome of low T_3 ("sick euthyroid syndrome") seen in acute illness is an adaptive strategy that reduces the normal effects of T_3 on resting energy expenditure.

In clinical trials, normalization of T_3 values by replacement of thyroid hormone in critically ill patients has had no beneficial effect on clinical outcome.

Catabolism & Urine Urea Nitrogen

As part of the injury response resulting in protein breakdown, critically ill adult patients may lose about 16–20 g of nitrogen (in the form of urea) in the urine per day—compared with about 10–12 g/d in normals. In some septic patients, losses have been noted to be as high as 24 g of urinary urea nitrogen per day. The loss of 1 g of urinary urea nitrogen is equal to the nitrogen contained in 6.25 g of protein. This amount of protein is equal to approximately 1 oz of lean body mass. As one can calculate, the loss of 16 g of nitrogen as urinary urea is therefore equal to the loss of about 1 lb of skeletal muscle or lean body mass per day.

Specific areas of lean body mass loss may result in functional impairment of the respiratory muscles (including the diaphragm), heart muscle, and gastrointestinal mucosa, thus contributing to the development of respiratory failure, heart failure, and diarrhea. Rapid development of malnutrition can occur in the critically ill patient as a result of these large daily losses of lean body mass. The patient who enters the ICU at 100% of ideal body weight (IBW) will usually not survive a weight loss greater than 30%. However, because large changes in intravascular and extravascular fluid may occur in critically ill patients, body weight needs to be correlated with loss in lean body mass (estimated from urinary creatinine) to confirm that any weight changes are not just due to changes in fluid volume.

The injury response is associated with an increase in both protein synthesis and protein degradation as determined by either stable or radioactive amino acid tracer infusion studies. In contrast to increased whole body protein synthesis, skeletal muscle protein synthesis is usually reduced, so that the increased whole body protein synthesis may be due to production of acute phase proteins, leukocytes, complement, and immunoglobulins. Leukocytes have a 4- to 6-hour half-life during infection, so that adequate nutritional support is important for their replacement and function. It has been estimated that the average adult can break down and resynthesize up to 400 g of protein per day.

Conventional Total Parenteral Nutrition & Loss of Lean Body Mass

It has been demonstrated that conventional total parenteral nutrition (TPN) given at a rate of 39 kcal/kg/d and 1.8 g/kg/d of protein did not stop the loss of lean body mass in acute illness. Despite this aggressive feeding regimen, critically ill patients lost an average of 24 g of nitrogen (1.5 lb of lean body mass) per day over a 10-day period, resulting in a 15-lb loss of lean body mass. These patients were able to increase the fat content of their bodies by about 5 lb over this same period, but they were unable to increase lean body mass. It was concluded that conventional TPN in this study was able to ameliorate the overall nitrogen and lean body mass loss but was not able to produce a net protein anabolism. Because of the inability of conventional TPN to stop progressive loss of lean body mass in acute illness, several anabolic agents (insulin, anabolic steroids, and growth hormone) are currently being studied to see if they can prevent the loss of lean body mass and its functional consequences.

NUTRITIONAL ASSESSMENT & PREDICTION OF OUTCOME

Nutritional Markers

Conventional nutritional assessment in the critically ill patient is of limited value. Daily weights in critically ill patients are helpful more for the determination of fluid changes and less for the determination of actual loss of lean body mass. The 24-hour urine urea nitrogen measurement is the single best determination of the severity of the injury response, but it cannot be used in those who have oliguric renal failure. Daily measurement of urine urea nitrogen is inexpensive and provides a good marker of catabolism that may not be detected from systemic signs such as tachycardia, tachypnea, or fever. Unfortunately, the severity of the catabolic response to injury is the same in malnourished and nonmalnourished patients. Therefore, the absolute urine urea nitrogen content does not indicate who is initially more malnourished.

Serum Albumin

The serum albumin level is one of the best predictors of malnutrition because it provides the clinician with an index of visceral and somatic protein stores in most medical illnesses. Exceptions include anorexia nervosa, severe edema, and congenital analbuminemia (rare). However, the serum albumin level rarely increases during most hospital stays because of albumin's 21-day half-life. Thus, while serum albumin is a marker of initial nutritional status, serum transferrin (7-day half-life) responds more rapidly to nutritional support, and serum transferrin is preferred for sequential measurements.

Albumin is a 584-amino-acid protein with a net negative charge of 19, permitting transport of many compounds. A large portion of the plasma's calcium, magnesium, zinc, bilirubin, many drugs (anticoagulants, antibiotics, etc.), and free fatty acids are transported bound to albumin. Approximately 40% of whole body albumin reserves (4–5 g/kg) are intravascular, and albumin is responsible for about 76% of the colloid oncotic pressure of the plasma. Patients with normal serum albumin levels have less wound edema, and the inflammatory phase of wound healing is shortened.

A. Causes of Hypoalbuminemia

Except for the rare patient with analbuminemia, hypoalbuminemia results from an increase in plasma volume; an increase in skin, urine, or stool losses of albumin; an increase in albumin degradation, or a reduction in albumin synthesis. Bed rest is associated with an approximately 7% increase in plasma volume and an equal reduction in serum albumin. In patients who are hypoalbuminemic, plasma volume can increase by 18% with bed rest. Because the skin stores approximately 20% of the total albumin mass, excessive losses of albumin occur with burns and subsequent exudative losses. Massive losses of protein can occur in the nephrotic syndrome, in which 60% to as much as 90% of the protein lost in the urine is albumin. Gastrointestinal losses of protein can vary markedly, and the amount of albumin normally degraded and lost in the stool is not known. A third factor contributing to the development of hypoalbuminemia is impaired albumin synthesis in the liver. Albumin is synthesized in the hepatocyte as a larger precursor, preproalbumin, containing 24 additional amino-terminal amino acids referred to as the "signal peptide." The preproalbumin undergoes two sequential cleavages within the rough endoplasmic reticulum within 3–6 minutes after initial formation and is transported to the Golgi apparatus within 15–20 minutes for subsequent vesicular release. Albumin synthesis is inhibited by severe protein and calorie deprivation, ethanol, severe liver disease, malabsorption, early forms of injury, burns, infections, cancer cachexia, and aging.

B. Albumin Synthesis

The rate of albumin synthesis (normally 150 mg/kg/d) is stimulated by (1) reduction in colloid oncotic pressure; (2) antibiotic treatment; (3) glucocorticoid therapy in cirrhosis; and (4) amino acid administration. Albumin synthesis was increased to 350 mg/kg/d in a small group of patients with idiopathic tropical diarrhea following 2 weeks of tetracycline therapy. In a small group of patients with cirrhosis, prednisolone, 60 mg daily for 2 weeks, was associated with an increase of albumin synthesis from 130 mg/kg/d to 260 mg/kg/d.

In one study, albumin synthesis is more stimulated (240 mg/kg/d) after 300 kcal of amino acid administration than after 400 kcal of glucose administration (160 mg/kg/d). Furthermore, albumin synthesis is higher (360 mg/kg/d) when providing a total of 700 kcal/d rather than only 300 kcal/d (albumin synthesis rate 240 mg/kg/d) for the same protein intake (1 g/kg/d).

There is a positive correlation between albumin synthesis rate and serum concentrations of leucine, isoleucine, valine, and tryptophan. It appears that the albumin synthesis rate in cancer cachexia is also responsive to isonitrogenous amounts of a branched chain-enriched amino acid solution. In one study, cancer patients increased albumin synthesis from 100 mg/kg/d to 190 mg/kg/d as a result of increased administration of leucine, isoleucine, and valine (branched chain amino acids). These observations imply that providing a diet rich in tryptophan, leucine, isoleucine, and valine may stimulate albumin synthesis.

Nutritional Predictors of Outcome

Serum albumin is an excellent predictor of survival (Table 6–1). At least 21 studies to date have shown that a below-normal serum albumin level can be used to predict disease outcome in many groups of patients. Thirty-day mortality rates for a total of 2060 consecutive medical and surgical admissions were reported at a Veterans Affairs hospital. The investigators found that 24.7% of the patient population had a low albumin, defined as ≤ 3.4 g/dL. The 30-day mortality rate for hypoalbuminemic

Table 6–1. Serum albumin and increased mortality risk in various published studies.

Diagnosis or Study Group	n	Normal Serum Albumin (g/dL)[1]	Mortality,Normal Serum Albumin	Mortality Low Serum Albumin	Relative Mortality Risk of Low Serum Albumin
Medical and surgical patients	500	3.5	1.3%	7.9%	6.1
Critically ill	55	3.0	10.0%	76.0%	7.6
Surgical patients	243	3.5	4.7%	23.0%	4.9
Hodgkin's disease	586	3.5	1.0%	10.0%	10.0
Malnutrition	92	3.5	8.0%	40.0%	5.0
Colorectal surgery	83	3.5	3.0%	28.0%	9.3
Alcoholic hepatitis	352	3.5	2.0%	19.8%	9.9
Cirrhosis	139	2.9	32.0%	52.0%	1.6
Lung cancer	59	3.4	49.0%	85.0%	1.7
Heart disease	7,735	4.0	0.4%	2.3%	6.1
Multiple myeloma	23	3.0	25.0%	50.0%	2.0
Trauma	34	3.5	15.4%	28.6%	1.9
Sepsis	199	2.9	0.7%	15.9%	22.7
Pneumonia	456	3.5	2.1%	8.3%	4.0
Pneumonia	38	3.0	0.0%	10.0%	—
VA Hospital	152	3.5	3.3%	7.8%	7.8
VA Hospital	2,060	3.5	1.7%	14.5%	14.5
CABG/Cardiac valve surgery	5,156	2.5	0.2%	0.9%	5.7
Preoperative (VA hospital)	54,215	3.5	2.0%	10.3%	5.1
Beth Israel Hospital	15,511	3.4	4.0%	14.0%	3.5
Hemodialysis	13,473	4.0	8.0%	16.6%	2.1
Stroke	225	3.5	20.0%	55.0%	2.7

[1]Serum albumin, g/dL, separating normal and low albumin groups for each study.

patients was 24.6%, as opposed to 1.7% in patients with normal serum albumin levels. The investigators also demonstrated an excellent correlation between serum albumin levels and 30-day mortality rates. A 1 g/dL drop in serum albumin levels (eg, from 3.5 g/dL to 2.5 g/dL) translated into a 33% increase in mortality risk. Patients with an average albumin level of 1.8 g/dL had a mortality rate of 65%. It is interesting to note that 15 hypoalbuminemic patients in this study were provided with TPN, and only one of these patients died (7% mortality rate).

The relationship between albumin concentration and mortality is not linear. In 13,473 patients on hemodialysis, for example, mortality increased in an exponential fashion as serum albumin decreased. If one set the risk for death equal to 1 at an albumin of 4.25 g/dL, then the risk for death (odds ratio) increases 12.8-fold for patients with an albumin < 2.5 g/dL. In contrast, the odds ratio for death falls to 0.47 if serum albumin concentration > 4.4 g/dL. A simplified formula for estimating risk of death is: $128/(\text{albumin}^3)$, where albumin is in grams per deciliter. An albumin of 4 g/dL has a twofold risk of death and an albumin of 2 g/dL has a 16-fold risk of death (Figure 6–1). In a large group (54,215) of preoperative patients, there was also an exponential increase in 30-day mortality as albumin decreased. For example, 30-day mortality was 1% in patients with normal concentration (albumin > 4.6 g/dL), and mortality increased to 29% with an albumin of < 2.1 g/dL.

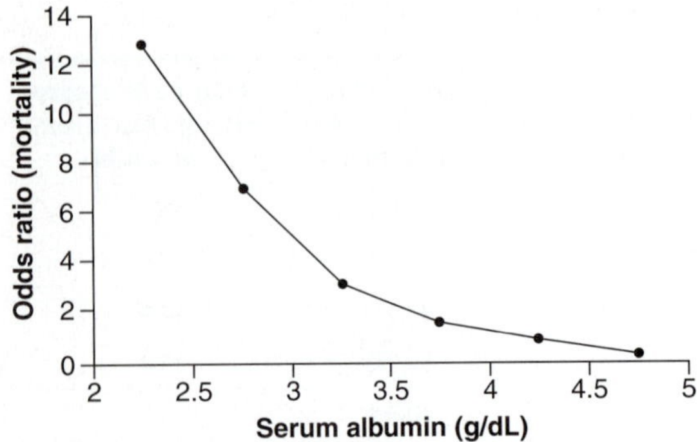

Figure 6–1. In patients undergoing hemodialysis, lower serum albumin is a predictor of increased mortality. The risk of death (odds ratio) is approximately $\frac{128}{\text{Albumin}^3}$.

An APACHE II score of 20 at the author's institution is associated with an approximately 50% mortality rate. However, APACHE II is poor at predicting outcomes in malnourished patients who are receiving parenteral nutritional support. APACHE III, a later version of this ICU prognostic scoring system, includes serum albumin as a variable, thereby factoring in the presence or absence of malnutrition.

In addition to the use of serum albumin, the patient's caloric intake predicts survival. Patients provided with an adequate caloric intake (1632 kcal/d versus 671 kcal/d) have an eightfold reduction in mortality (11.8% versus 1.5%). At the same albumin concentration (< 3 g/dL), survival is longer in those who have a normal caloric intake. This is also true for patients with advanced liver cirrhosis.

In summary, APACHE III score, serum albumin concentration, and caloric intake in critically ill patients provide the clinician with tools to help predict recovery or demise. Albumin levels should be monitored at regular intervals (weekly), and caloric intake should be determined daily in patients who are ill and at risk for malnutrition. Once hypoalbuminemia is documented, it is not an ideal indicator of nutritional repletion, since it returns to normal slowly (half-life 21 days) and lags behind other laboratory indices of nutritional status such as transferrin (half-life 7 days), prealbumin (half-life 1 day), IGF-1 (half-life 20 hours), and retinol-binding protein (half-life 4 hours). Albumin replacement itself does not reverse the metabolic process that the hypoalbuminemic state represents. The reduced level of protein reserves in the patient and the severity of the metabolic injury are the two most important determinants of serum albumin level.

FEATURES OF MALNUTRITION IN CRITICAL ILLNESS

Symptoms & Signs

It is important to ask patients if they have been able to maintain appetite and body weight over the last several months. A history of recent hospitalization is important because of the common development of protein malnutrition during a hospital stay. Physical examination should include an estimate of muscle mass, noting especially a loss of temporalis muscle mass, "squaring off" of the deltoid muscle, and loss of thigh muscle mass. Measurement of body weight should be standard on all ICU admissions, and weight should be followed on a daily basis. Daily weights are facilitated in the ICU by use of beds with built-in scales. Although it can be argued that body weight is not a good marker of nutritional status in the ICU—and this may be true for many patients—body weight is also useful as a marker of changes in fluid status.

Laboratory Findings

Up to 50% of hospitalized surgical and medical patients have either hypoalbuminemic malnutrition or marasmic-type malnutrition. Hypoalbuminemic (protein) malnutrition is diagnosed by finding reduced serum albumin, transferrin, prealbumin, or retinol-binding protein levels. Serum albumin is most commonly used. Marasmic malnutrition is identified in anyone who has lost 20% or more of usual body weight over the preceding 3–6 months or who is at less than 90% of ideal body weight. Of these two types of malnutrition, hypoalbuminemic malnutrition is the most common, and its presence in one study was associated with a fourfold increase in dying and a 2.5-fold increased risk of developing a nosocomial infection and sepsis. Table 6–1 shows that a low serum albumin level predicts a significant increase in mortality rate in a variety of types of patients and diseases.

Delayed Hypersensitivity

Delayed hypersensitivity as measured by skin testing is frequently abnormal or absent (anergic) in patients with hypoalbuminemic malnutrition. When five appropriate antigens are used for testing delayed hypersensitivity in such patients, failure to respond to more than one antigen was associated with an 80% 2-year mortality rate compared with an overall 35% mortality rate. In another study of over 500 patients, anergy was associated with a fivefold increase in numbers of deaths in trauma patients and a sixfold increase in those numbers in septic patients.

Lean Body Mass

The use of body weight as an index of muscle mass in ICU patients is very difficult because of fluid shifts that occur in the extracellular compartment. Body weight can be divided into three compartments: extracellular mass, lean body mass, and fat mass. Extracellular fluid is known to increase as a result of critical illness even in well nourished individuals, but the degree of increase in extracellular fluid is greater in the malnourished. Much of this is accounted for by fluid shifts into the extracellular space because of reduced plasma colloid oncotic pressure.

Lean body mass is the sum of skeletal muscle, plasma proteins, skin, skeleton, and visceral organs, with the skin and skeleton accounting for 50% of the total. There are no convenient markers to determine loss of nitrogen from skin or skeleton. The plasma proteins account for only 2% of the lean body mass, but measurement of plasma proteins can reflect the overall status of the lean body mass compartment. The viscera account for about 12% of the lean body mass, and decreases in size of some organs (gut atrophy, cardiac atrophy) are noted in critically ill patients. Unfortunately, there is no convenient marker of loss of lean body mass from the visceral organs.

The skeletal muscles account for 35% of lean body mass and provide the major storage area for amino acids needed during illness. Urinary creatinine is related to the size of the skeletal muscle mass. A standard way to assess the size of the skeletal muscle mass is to determine the creatinine-height index by collecting a 24-hour urine and comparing the value to normal tables of creatinine excretion for age, sex, and height. A simpler way is to divide the 24-hour creatinine excretion by the patient's usual body weight obtained from the history. The normal value for an adult man is 23 mg/kg of ideal body weight; the normal value for a woman is 18 mg/kg. A creatinine-weight index 10% less than normal would be consistent with a 10% loss in muscle mass. For example, if the usual weight for a woman was 50 kg, her 24-hour urine collection should contain 900 mg of creatinine. A value of 810 mg/24 h would reflect minimal loss of muscle mass. A value of 20% less than normal would classify patients as having mild muscle loss; a 20–30% loss would classify them as having a moderate loss; and a 30% or greater reduction in the 24-hour urinary creatinine would document severe muscle loss. The most accurate estimates result from measuring urinary creatinine over a 3-day period and repeating the measurements at intervals to document the loss of muscle mass over an extended period of time. Dietary creatine and creatinine intake has only a minor influence (< 20%) on urinary creatinine in the normally fed individual, and dietary influences will be very small in most critically ill patients. However, impairment of renal function reduces normal creatinine excretion and excludes the creatinine-height or creatinine-weight index as a marker of muscle mass.

Vitamins & Minerals

Many of the vitamins and minerals act as cofactors for essential processes in health and illness. The requirements for health have been well established and are published as the recommended daily requirements (Tables 6–2 and 6–3). The exact needs for the critically ill patient are not well documented.

Reduced levels of vitamin C, vitamin A, copper, manganese, and zinc are associated with poor wound healing. Abnormally low levels of minerals are known to occur as part of the cytokine-mediated inflammatory response and may also occur secondary to poor oral intake, increased requirements, and excessive urinary and stool losses in the critically ill patient.

Table 6–2. Adult daily nutritional requirements (RDA, 1989).

Nutrient	Oral	Intravenous	Special Requirements
Vitamin A	3300 IU	3300 IU (1 mg)	5000 + IU (serious infections)
Vitamin D	400 IU	200 IU (5 μg)	
Vitamin E	10 mg	10 mg	
Biotin	100 μg	60 μg	
Pantothenic acid	7 mg	15 mg	
Folic acid	0.2 mg	0.4 mg	5 mg (ICU patient; thrombocytopenia)
Thiamin	1.5 mg	3 mg	50 mg (alcoholics, Wernicke-Korsakoff)
Riboflavin	1.8 mg	3.6 mg	
Niacin	20 mg	40 mg	
Pyridoxine	2 mg	4 mg	
Vitamin C	60 mg	100 mg	
Vitamin B_{12}	2 μg	5 μg	
Vitamin K	80 μg	See note 1.	

[1]Vitamin K is routinely given as 10 mg subcutaneously on admission and then weekly.

Table 6–3. Adult daily nutritional requirement.

Nutrient	Oral	Intravenous	Special Requirements
Macronutrients			
Protein	1.5 g/kg	1.5 g/kg	2–3 g/kg (thermal injury)
Glucose	20–25 kcal/kg	20–25 kcal/kg	
Lipid	4% of kcal	4% of kcal	
Micronutrients			
Sodium	60–150 meq	60–150 meq	
Potassium	40–80 meq	40–80 meq	
Chloride	40–100 meq	40–100 meq	
Acetate	10–40 meq	10–40 meq	
Phosphorus	10–60 mmol	10–60 mmol	
Calcium	5–20 meq	5–20 meq	
Magnesium	10–20 meq	10–20 meq	50–100 meq (cardiac arrhythmias, diarrhea)
Zinc	3 mg	2.5–4 mg	10–50 mg (diarrhea, fistula, wounds)
Copper	1.5–3 mg	1–1.5 mg	
Chromium	50–200 μg	10–15 μg	40 μg (diarrhea, GI losses)
Molybdenum	75–250 μg	100–200 μg	
Manganese	2–5 mg	150–800 μg	
Selenium	40–120 μg	40–120 μg	120–200 μg (thermal injury, wounds)

A. Folate

In large studies of critically ill patients, 12–52% have been noted to have reduce folate levels. Not all of these will have folate deficiency because serum levels fall rapidly, despite normal tissue stores, when folate intake is restricted. Alcohol intake has a similar effect of falsely lowering folate levels. A prospective randomized clinical trial demonstrated that critically ill patients given only replacement doses of approximately 0.3 mg/d of folate continued to demonstrate decreased serum and red cell folate levels. A few of these patients developed severe hematologic disturbances that were reversed with administration of larger amounts of folate. Most of the patients who were given 50 mg of folate per week and all of the patients given 5 mg of folate per day demonstrated an increase in serum and red cell folate, and all patients who were initially deficient in folate were restored to normal serum folate status.

B. Vitamin A and Vitamin C

Critically ill patients, especially those with sepsis, can have significant reductions in plasma levels of vitamin A and vitamin C. A recent study in healthy elderly patients demonstrated that approximately 20% have reduced vitamin C levels (< 0.5 mg/dL) and 10% have a reduced serum vitamin A level (< 33 μg/dL). The administration of multiple vitamins and minerals containing 80 mg of vitamin C and 15,000 IU of vitamin A daily for 1 year resulted in a significant reduction in the number of days of infection-related illnesses (48 ± 7 to 23 ± 5 days per year; mean ± SEM). The multiple vitamin and mineral supplement improved the lymphocyte response to phytohemagglutinin and the natural killer cell activity. Vitamin A treatment in premature infants reduces the development of chronic lung disease or death (from 62% to 55%).

While plasma levels of vitamin C do reflect whole body stores, plasma levels of vitamin A may not be the best marker of actual deficiency states. Liver vitamin A measurements may be a better marker. Patients who die of infectious diseases have an 18–35% incidence of severe reduction of liver vitamin A. In other studies, serum vitamin A (retinol) levels are low in 30–92% of patients with serious infections. The mechanism for this loss may be via excessive urinary losses of vitamin A. Patients with pneumonia, sepsis, and severe injury can lose vitamin A (retinol) in the urine on a daily basis in an amount greater than the recommended dietary intake of vitamin A (5000 IU vitamin A). In contrast to what is noted in serious infections, trauma patients who die within 7 days after hospitalization have only a 2% incidence of severe liver vitamin A deficiency.

Several prospective randomized clinical trials have demonstrated that the administration of vitamin A to children who have measles or other infectious illnesses can reduce the mortality rate by up to 50%. Similar data are not available for adults. Nevertheless, because serum vitamin A levels are frequently reduced in critically ill patients who have serious infections, critically ill patients should start receiving the RDA of vitamin A upon admission.

In addition to the changes in folate, vitamin A, and vitamin C, excessive losses of several other vitamins have been observed in patients receiving medications that interfere with normal utilization or elimination (Table 6–4).

C. Magnesium

Normal levels for magnesium were determined by measuring serum magnesium in hospitalized patients, some of whom were probably alcoholics. Hypomagnesemia occurs in 34–44% of patients receiving TPN. Severe depletion is associated with cardiac arrhythmias and sudden death. Alcoholics are commonly found to have poor magnesium intake and also to have excessive urinary magnesium losses. For this reason and because of recent data on the antiarrhythmic effects of magnesium, the commonly used normal values for serum magnesium levels should probably be increased from 1.7–2.3 mg/dL to 2–2.6 mg/dL. Isolated bacteremia in otherwise healthy men is associated with a 60 mg (5 meq) magnesium loss in the urine per day. Large losses can occur in conditions such as ulcerative colitis, where the stool can contain up to 12 meq/L and urinary losses can be as much as 25 meq/d. Large urinary losses can also be seen in patients receiving aminoglycosides, diuretics, and amphotericin B, to mention a few medications commonly used in the ICU. Furthermore, large quantities of magnesium can be found in some of the intestinal fluids (Table 6–5). The effects of magnesium depletion and hypomagnesemia are discussed in the section on hypomagnesemia in Chapter 2.

Table 6–4. Drug-induced nutrient deficiencies.

Drug	Nutrients Affected
Aminoglycosides	Magnesium, zinc
Ammonium chloride	Vitamin C
Antacids	Phosphorus, phosphates
Aspirin	Vitamin C
Cholestyramine	Triglycerides, fat-soluble vitamins
Cisplatin	Magnesium, zinc
Corticosteroids	Vitamin A, potassium
Diuretics	Sodium, potassium, magnesium, zinc
Estrogen and progesterone compounds	Folic acid, vitamin B_6
Hydralazine	Vitamin B_6
Isoniazid	Vitamin B_6, niacin
Laxatives	Sodium, potassium, magnesium
Penicillamine	Vitamin B_6
Phenobarbital	Vitamin C, vitamin D,
Phenothiazines	Vitamin B_2
Phenytoin	Vitamin C, vitamin D, niacin
Tetracycline	Vitamin C
Tricyclic antidepressants	Vitamin B_2
Warfarin	Vitamin K

D. Phosphate

Hypophosphatemia occurs in 35–45% of patients receiving TPN. Severe hypophosphatemia results in cardiac standstill and sudden death. Recent data have demonstrated rapid and life-threatening reductions in serum phosphate associated with live-donor liver transplantation. Phosphate is an intracellular anion that must be administered in very large quantities to both the donor and the recipient. The profound hypophosphatemia is probably due to the rapid regeneration of the liver that is known to occur over the first few weeks after transplantation.

E. Zinc

Serum zinc levels drop as an early response to infection and injury. There are minor tissue stores of zinc in skin, bone, and intestine, but zinc is redistributed to liver, bone marrow, thymus, and the site of injury or inflammation in the critically ill patient. This redistribution is mediated by IL-1 and other cytokines secreted from macrophages. In one study of sepsis, low serum zinc (< 70 μg/dL) was found in 100% of patients. In burn injury, approximately 60–70% of patients have a reduced serum zinc level. The administration of approximately 50 mg of zinc a day to these patients was associated with normalization of the zinc level after 3 weeks of feeding. A study in healthy elderly patients demonstrated that approximately 15% have a reduced serum zinc level (< 67 μg/dL). The administration of 14 mg of zinc per day for 1 year resulted in a significant reduction in the number of days of infection-related illnesses (48 ± 7 to 23 ± 5 days per year; mean ± SEM).

Zinc supplementation in the critically ill patient is needed for cell mitosis and cell proliferation in wound repair. It has also been demonstrated that 600 mg of zinc sulfate (136 mg of elemental zinc) orally daily will improve wound healing in patients who had a serum zinc level upon admission of < 100 μg/dL. In this double-blind study, the healing rate increased more than twofold in those randomized to receive zinc supplementation. In addition, large losses of zinc can occur via intestinal losses (Table 6–5). It is important to note that intestinal fluids may contain up to 17 mg of zinc per liter, so that the replacement rate of zinc should

Table 6–5. Electrolyte and mineral content (meq/L) of body fluids.

Body Fluid	Na^+	K^+	Cl^-	HCO_3^-	Mg^{2+}	Zn^{2+} (mg/L)
Saliva	10	20–30	15	50	0.6	...
Stomach fluids	100	10	120	0	0.9	...
Duodenal fluid	130	5–10	90	10	1–2	12
Ileal fluids	140	10–20	100	20–30	6–12	17
Colonic fluids	50	30–70	15–40	30	6–12	17
Diarrheal fluids	50	35	40	45	1–13	17
Pancreatic juice	140	5	75	70–115	0.5	...
Bile	145	5	100	15–60	1–2	...
Urine	60–120	30–70	60–120	...	5	0.1–0.5
Urine (post furosemide)	1½–2 times normal	2 times normal	...	...	20 times normal	...

take into account the abnormal sources of zinc loss as well as the routine nutritional requirements.

F. Copper

Serum copper and ceruloplasmin increase with severe injury or sepsis. Cytokines are believed to be responsible for these changes. The reasons for these increases are not known.

G. Iron

Serum iron levels fall as a result of the cytokine-mediated response to infection or injury. The iron is stored in the Kupffer cells of the liver until the inflammation wanes. This is probably a beneficial effect, since many microbes use iron as a source of energy. Therefore, iron administration should be restricted in patients with serious infections, as iron therapy in one double-blind study demonstrated an increase in infectious episodes. In liver transplantation, patients who receive a liver high in iron concentration have an increased incidence of fatal infections (24% versus 7%) and reduced 5-year survival rates (48% versus 77%).

Engelman DT et al: Impact of body mass index and albumin on morbidity and mortality after cardiac surgery. J Thorac Cardiovasc Surg 1999;118:866–73.

Gibbs J et al: Preoperative serum albumin level as a predictor of operative mortality and morbidity: results from a National VA Surgical Risk Study. Arch Surg 1999;134:36–42.

Tayek JA et al: Improved protein kinetics and albumin synthesis by branched chain amino acid-enriched total parenteral nutrition in cancer cachexia, a prospective randomized crossover trial. Cancer 1986;58:147–57.

NUTRITIONAL THERAPY

ASSESSMENT OF NUTRITIONAL NEEDS

Catabolism in Critical Illness

The best marker of catabolism is the determination of urine urea nitrogen loss that occurs in the critically ill patient. Approximately 80% of the total urine nitrogen appears as urinary urea nitrogen, and this test can be performed at the cost of a single urea determination. A classification of catabolism is based upon the urine urea nitrogen loss over a 24-hour period plus approximately 2 g of nitrogen lost as creatinine, creatine, ammonia, and amino acids and approximately 2 g in skin, stool, and respiratory losses (though losses > 2 g can occur in thermal injury and severe diarrhea). Urinary loss of less than 6 g of urea nitrogen is normal; loss of 6–12 g/d is mild, 12–18 g/d moderate, and more than 18 g/d is severe catabolism. As mentioned above, 1 g of urea nitrogen in the urine is equal to 6.25 g of nonhydrated protein or 1 oz of lean body mass. Therefore, the loss of 16 g of urea nitrogen in the urine per day is roughly equal to the loss of 1 lb of skeletal muscle per day. Although the mobilized amino acids that are broken down into urea do not all come from the skeletal muscles, those muscles are the major source of the amino acids utilized during the catabolic process that occurs in all critically ill patients because they represent 50% of the fat-free body weight. In a patient with mild to moderate catabolism, 12 g of urinary urea nitrogen loss plus

4 g of nitrogen loss from other sources calls for replacement of about 100 g of nitrogen daily to maintain nitrogen balance. For a 70-kg adult, this is approximately 1.5 g of protein (or amino acid)/kg/d. In severely catabolic patients, protein requirements may be higher.

Energy Expenditure in the Critically Ill Patient

Resting energy expenditure (REE) is directly linked to lean body mass. REE is difficult to determine precisely in the ICU without measuring oxygen consumption and carbon dioxide production rates and without performing appropriate calculations for estimation of energy expenditure. Various equations used to estimate REE without actual measurements are not very accurate in critically ill patients. These equations, based on REEs in healthy individuals, do, however, provide an approximation of the energy requirements. Using these estimates, several authors have suggested that energy expenditure is increased by 30–100% above REE in critically ill patients. However, recent data based upon direct measurements of energy expenditure in critically ill patients do not support the need for higher estimates of energy requirements. Thus, more appropriate estimates would be between 20% and 50% above predicted needs. A convenient estimate that takes REE and added energy expenditure into account is to provide 30–35 kcal/kg/d (based on ideal body weight) to patients with mild to moderately severe critical illness. In those with severe pancreatitis, closed head injury, or thermal injury, caloric requirements may be close to 40 kcal/kg/d.

Vitamins & Minerals

The recommended oral and intravenous vitamin intakes are listed in Table 6–2. The mineral and trace element requirements are listed in Table 6–3. Also included are the few exceptions to the routine intravenous amounts for both tables. These vitamin, mineral, and trace mineral recommendations are for critically ill patients who do not have oliguric renal failure or cholestatic liver disease. In acute oliguric renal failure, vitamins A and D should be reduced or eliminated from the enteral or parenteral solutions. Potassium, phosphorus, magnesium, zinc, and selenium should be reduced or eliminated. Iron and chromium are known to accumulate in renal failure and should be removed from the parenteral or enteral formulations.

Copper and manganese are excreted via the biliary tree, and intake should be reduced or eliminated in patients with cholestatic liver disease to prevent toxicity. In comparison, large amounts of electrolytes and minerals can be lost in gastrointestinal fluids and in urine (Table 6–5). It is essential to replace the estimated amounts lost on a daily basis by appropriate supplementation of the parenteral nutrition fluid.

ENTERAL & PARENTERAL NUTRITION

Choice of Enteral or Parenteral Feeding

In all clinical situations, if the gut is functional then the gut should be used as the route of feeding. Gut atrophy predisposes to bacterial and fungal colonization and subsequent invasion associated with bacteremia. Sepsis due to microbial translocation or endotoxin translocation from the gut into the portal system is a frequent source of fever in those who do not have an obvious source of infection. Utilization of the gastrointestinal tract for feeding can reduce the incidence of bacterial translocation.

A recently published prospective randomized clinical trial of abdominal trauma patients has demonstrated that the use of enteral nutrition is associated with maintenance of serum albumin and a reduction in major infections from 20% to 3%. A study of over 200 abdominal trauma patients compared mortality rates of parenterally and enterally fed ICU patients who had similar illness severity at admission. The group that could not tolerate enteral feeding received total parenteral nutrition that averaged 35 kcal/kg/d and 1.2 g/kg/d of protein. The other group tolerated enteral feedings and received 30 kcal/kg/d and 1.1 g/kg/d of protein. The overall mortality rate was significantly lower (51% versus 25%) in patients who tolerated enteral nutritional support. It appears that patients with gastrointestinal intolerance may have a poorer clinical outcome even though they were given appropriate parenteral nutritional support.

The indications for TPN are listed in Table 6–6. Preoperative TPN should not be routinely used since the majority of prospective studies have shown no benefit and one has shown harm. However, recent evidence in malnourished cancer patients demonstrated that preoperative TPN reduces complications and may reduce mortality. Likewise, postoperative TPN should not be

Table 6–6. Indications for total parenteral nutrition (TPN).

Short bowel syndrome
High output gastrointestinal fistula
Hyperemesis gravidarum
Bone marrow transplantation
Nonfunctional gut with hypoalbuminemia (serum albumin < 2.8 g/dL)

Note: If the gastrointestinal tract is functional, *do not use TPN.*

routinely used since the majority of prospective trials showed no benefit and some showed an increased rate of complications. This lack of benefit and increased harm may be due to failure to maintain tight glucose control (< 110 mg/dL) in critically ill patients receiving TPN.

Enteral Nutrition

The feeding tube should be positioned in the small bowel up to the ligament of Treitz. This is best achieved with the aid of fluoroscopy but can also be achieved by passage of the feeding tube into the small bowel by a "corkscrew" technique after bending the distal tip of the feeding tube to about 30 degrees with the wire stylet in place. Upon placement in the stomach, the tube is rotated so that the tip can pass via the pylorus into the duodenum. The infusion of enteral products into the small bowel will reduce the incidence of aspiration because the infusion is below the pylorus. Patients with a cuffed endotracheal tube have a smaller risk of aspiration, so that placement of a feeding tube into the small bowel is less essential.

Supine patients had a 34% incidence of aspiration pneumonia, but the risk was only 8% when patients were kept semirecumbent. The CDC recommends that ICU patients be managed in this position to reduce the risk for nosocomial infections.

A. Protein

Protein is better absorbed in the peptide form than as free amino acids because of specific transporters in the small intestines for amino acids, dipeptides, and tripeptides. Supplementation of standard enteral feeding products with increased amounts of arginine has been shown to enhance immune function, though published data in humans are very limited. It is also important to point out that arginine is a precursor of nitric oxide, a vasodilator substance that may be involved in mediating some of the effects of sepsis. Branched chain-enriched amino acid enteral products have been shown to improve mental function and reduce mortality rates in patients with hepatic encephalopathy. Albumin synthesis is also stimulated by branched chain-enriched amino acids. However, data to date do not demonstrate decreased morbidity or mortality rates in trauma or sepsis patients randomized to receive branched chain-enriched amino acids as opposed to conventional feeding.

B. Lipid

The lipid composition of enteral feeding products is becoming an important consideration depending upon the type of disease. The use of omega-3 (fish oil) enriched fatty acids in the enteral product has been associated with modification of the inflammatory response. This effect may be related to increased arachidonic acid metabolism and decreased omega-6 pathway fatty acid metabolism. Because most commercially available enteral products that contain omega-3 fatty acids also have other additives such as arginine, glutamine, and nucleotides, the benefits attributed to the use of an omega-3 enriched fatty acid enteral diet await confirmation.

C. Enteral Feeding Products

A large variety of enteral feeding products are manufactured for use in the ICU and acute medical care settings, including elemental formulas (amino acids, mono- and oligosaccharides, and lipids), specialized products for certain critical care situations (renal failure, liver failure), products containing fiber, and lactose-free nonelemental products containing 1–2 kcal/mL. These formulations vary in terms of ratio of nitrogen to nonnitrogen calories, protein source, and concentration. They also vary in the amount and source of fat, electrolyte concentration, and other constituents. Most hospitals select a limited number of enteral feeding products for their formularies and have recommended products for each clinical situation.

D. Recommended Enteral Feeding Formulas

Lactose-free formulas should be used for ICU patients. The infusion rate should not exceed 30 kcal/h for the first 6–12 hours, and the rate should then be advanced as tolerated. If the patient has a serum albumin < 2.5 g/dL, the enteral infusion rate should be increased slowly (ie, every 24 hours).

The source of carbohydrate or protein appears not to be important except in patients with hepatic encephalopathy, in whom a formula high in the branched chain amino acids would be indicated. The addition of moderate amounts of glutamine may be helpful because only a few formulas have added glutamine. Until additional data become available, there are no specific recommendations for the source of fat calories in the enteral feeding formula, such as omega-3 fatty acids, omega-6 fatty acids, or medium-chain triglycerides.

Parenteral Nutrition

A. Central Versus Peripheral Parenteral Nutrition

The route of parenteral nutrition should be secondary to the principle of meeting the individual patient's calorie and protein goals. Peripheral parenteral nutrition (ie, given through a peripheral vein) can be used in patients who can tolerate the daily 3-L fluid requirement necessary to obtain adequate calorie administration or in patients in the early phase of enteral alimentation as a supplement. Currently, the permissible concentrations of glucose, amino acids, and other nutrients delivered via peripheral vein alimentation are limited by phlebitis caused by the high osmolality of the alimentation solution. Advances in catheter technology may allow for peripheral administration of solutions of > 600 mosm/L without damage to the vein. A solution of 900 mosm/L may be well tolerated and could reduce the volume of peripheral alimentation fluid to 2 L/d. Even with this new technology, patients requiring severe fluid restriction should receive central parenteral nutrition (via a central venous catheter) using one of several fluid-restricted formulas (Table 6–7).

B. Placement of Catheters for Total Parenteral Nutrition

Central and peripheral venous catheters are composed of scarified polyvinylchloride, standard polyvinylchloride, polyethylene, silicone, hydromer-coated polyurethane, standard polyurethane, fluoroethylene, propylene, or Teflon. The lowest rate of thrombogenicity is seen with the hydromer-coated polyurethane. The rate of thrombophlebitis is relatively low when catheters are used in a central vein owing to the rapid rate of dilution of the hyperosmolal solution. Peripheral venous access is associated with a higher rate of thrombophlebitis, which is secondary to the high-osmolality solution infused into a small vein. The size of the peripheral catheter is important, with the larger catheters having a more frequent rate of thrombophlebitis. Recent data would suggest that the use of a small silicone-coated catheter may increase the life span from 2 days to 5 days when infusing a fluid of very high osmolality through a peripheral vein. Osmolality above 900 mosm/kg is not recommended for peripheral infusion.

Traditional aseptic technique is required for placement of central venous catheters. The subclavian vein is the most commonly used site, followed by the internal jugular vein. Central venous access can also be obtained by the use of a long venous catheter placed in the upper arm vein and passed up near but not into the right atrium. Central catheters can also lead to thrombosis as a result of improper placement in the subclavian vein. The tip of the catheter should be positioned at the entry of the right atrium.

Heparin (1000 units/L) or hydrocortisone (5 mg/L) added to the TPN solution can reduce the occurrence of thrombophlebitis resulting from peripheral administration of hyperosmolar solutions. A nitroglycerin patch on the skin (5 mg) acts as a local vasodilator and has also been associated with a reduction in thrombophlebitis. Subcutaneous tunneling may help reduce the rate of catheter infection, but the best precaution is optimal nursing care and the use of chlorhexidine as an antiseptic for skin preparation.

Catheter-related infection is a major concern. The two most likely causes for catheter-related infections are

Table 6–7. Some selected typical parenteral nutrition formulas.

Name[1]	Amino Acids (g/L)	Dextrose (g/L)	Calories (kcal/L)	Osmolarity (mosm/L)	BCAA[2] (%)
Central A5% D15%	50	150	710	1250	19
Peripheral A3.5% D5%	35	50	310	760	19
Fluid-restricted (central) A7% D21%	70	210	994	1808	19
Severe fluid restriction (central) A10% D15%[3]	100	150	910	1750	19
High branched-chain amino acids (central) A3.5% D25%	35	250	990	1762	46
Renal failure (central) A2.7% D35%	27	350	1292	2426	39
Glycerin A3% G3%	30	0	222	735	23

Key: Dextrose (D) = 3.4 kcal/g, Amino acids (A) = 4.0 kcal/g, Glycerin (G) = 3.4 kcal/g
Each 1 g amino acids = 10 mosm; each 1 g dextrose = 5 mosm
Each 1% amino acids = 100 mosm; each 1% dextrose = 50 mosm
[1]Lipids are included in many of these formulas at 10–60% of total calories; these formulations are called "3 in1."
[2]Branched chain amino acids
[3]Contraindicated in renal failure and hepatic encephalopathy

migration of bacteria down the catheter sheath and trapping and growth of bacteria on the fibrin tip that accumulates at the distal end of the catheter. Replacement of the catheter involves either exchange over a guidewire or selection of a new site. If obvious infection is present at the original site, a new site must be selected. If there is no obvious infection at the catheter site, the catheter may be aseptically exchanged over a guidewire. The removed catheter tip should be sent for culture, and, if bacteria grow over the next 24–72 hours, the exchanged catheter should be discontinued and a new site selected. Central line placement has a 3–5% likelihood of causing pneumothorax or some other serious complication. Changes of catheter sites reserved solely for TPN usage are not needed on a regular basis but only when there is evidence of local or systemic infection or other complication of the catheter.

The most common complication of TPN is catheter-related infection. In a pediatric setting, 15% of patients may develop bacteremia or candidemia. Patients at highest risk are those with diabetes mellitus. It has been estimated that catheter-related infections occur in 3% of nondiabetic adults and in 17% of diabetic adults. The most serious infections are due to candida species, with mortality rates as high as 34% despite antifungal treatment.

C. Carbohydrate and Protein

Since the intravenous route is not the natural route for nutritional substrate administration, it is important to provide adequate but not excessive amounts of protein, carbohydrate, and fat on a daily basis. Most critically ill patients need 1.5 g/kg/d of protein. The ideal body weight value should be used in calculating the daily protein requirements. Dextrose administration to most critically ill patients should not exceed 3.5 mg/kg/min (5 g/kg/d). This generally translates into about 350 g of dextrose, or 2 L of 15% dextrose in a 70-kg adult. Administration of greater amounts of dextrose can result in glucose intolerance, abnormal liver function tests, and fatty infiltration of the liver.

D. Lipid

Currently available intravenous fat emulsion products are derived from soybean or a mixture of soybean and safflower oil. The products vary slightly in the amount of linoleic, linolenic, and oleic acids. Each product is available in 10% and 20% concentrations, but the 20% product is the best choice because of its caloric density and the lack of imbalance in the phospholipid-to-lipid ratio. Intravenous lipid can be administered as a separate 20% concentration over 20–24 hours or—more commonly—as part of the TPN called "3 in 1" with dextrose and amino acids. Maximum fat administration can be estimated at 2 g/kg/d or 140 g/d (1260 kcal).

The use of intravenous fat administration in critically ill patients was initially very controversial. Some of the early studies did not demonstrate any improvement in nitrogen retention when glucose calories were exchanged for fat calories. Intravenous lipid administration may still not be well utilized in the severely traumatized patient. On the other hand, fat is well utilized in the noncatabolic patient, who can routinely receive and utilize up to 50% of calories as fat.

The septic patient has a reduced ability to utilize calories provided as dextrose, so that any amount of dextrose in excess of 350 g/d (1190 kcal) may not be utilized as energy and could contribute to the development of fatty liver infiltration and mild elevation in liver function tests. Because septic patients have an approximately threefold increase in fat oxidation rate, fat calories may be readily utilized in these patients. As a precaution, however, and because excessive amounts of intravenous lipids in animals contribute to an increased incidence of sepsis and associated morbidity, a maximum of 60% of total calories as intravenous fat is acceptable in most critically ill patients.

There is some interest in the use of peripheral administration of lipid, amino acids, and dextrose in a single 3-L bag via a very small catheter. In theory, the catheter floats in the vein, causing less luminal damage. An option used by some is to administer the peripheral infusion of lipid emulsion for 18 of the 24 hours and to run in 5% dextrose over the 6-hour resting period. This makes physiologic sense, since fasting will permit clearance of lipid VLDL particles and allow for adaptation to the nonfed state.

Essential fatty acid requirements are estimated to be approximately 1–4% of total energy requirements and should be in the form of linoleic acid. An elevation of the eicosatrienoic acid (triene) to arachidonic acid (tetrane) ratio to ≥ 0.4 is indicative of essential fatty acid deficiency. Treatment of essential fatty acid deficiency requires approximately 10–20% of total energy to be in the form of linoleic acid.

E. Parenteral Nutrition Solutions

Some standard parenteral nutritional formulas and those containing higher amounts of branched chain-enriched amino acid formulas are listed in Table 6–7. Standard parenteral nutrition solutions do not contain glutamine owing to the instability of this amino acid in solution. Standard parenteral formulas also do not contain large amounts of arginine. Both glutamine and arginine can be added to the parenteral formulas before administration, but there is no convincing evidence that added arginine is helpful. Recent data would suggest that glutamine may be a preferred fuel for enterocytes and lymphocytes. The use of glutamine-enriched formulas can prevent postinjury expansion of the extracellular water compartment in bone marrow transplant patients. There may also be a slight reduction in the incidence of infection.

F. Recommendations for Ordering Central Parenteral Nutrition

Each hospital should have standard formulas for parenteral nutrition. Consider using central parenteral nutrition formula with 15% dextrose, 5% amino acids, and 5% lipid containing 1160 kcal/L and osmolarity of 1250 mosm/L (Table 6–7). Fluid-restricted formulas are often required for use in critically ill patients. These solutions contain more concentrated mixtures of amino acids. Special formulas may be useful in hepatic and renal failure.

G. Recommendations for Peripheral Parenteral Nutrition

A standard solution is 3–5% amino acid and 5–10% dextrose for peripheral vein administration, eg, 3.5% amino acid and 5% dextrose. Three liters of this solution provide 105 g protein (amino acids) and about 930 kcal.

Using a microcatheter that allows for a higher-osmolarity solution to be infused safely, more calories can be given via a peripheral vein by adding 20% lipid. For ICU patients, a solution of 5% amino acid, 5% dextrose, and 5% lipid contains 900 mosm/L. Two liters of this formula provides 100 g of protein and 1640 kcal (55% of calories from lipid).

NUTRITIONAL SUPPORT IN SPECIFIC DISEASES

MALNUTRITION

Patients with a serum albumin < 2.8 g/dL, a 20% weight loss over the preceding 3 months, or an ideal body weight less than 90% for height should be provided nutritional support upon entry to the ICU. Other patients should be evaluated for the likelihood of being able to ingest a minimum of 1500 kcal by the fifth day in the ICU. If this seems unlikely, it would be appropriate to provide nutritional support early in the ICU stay.

CARDIOPULMONARY DISORDERS

Hypo-oncotic Pulmonary Edema

Albumin provides about 78% of the total oncotic pressure in the plasma compartment, and hypo-oncotic edema can be misdiagnosed as ARDS. In conformity with Starling's law, pulmonary edema may evolve as (1) hydrostatic edema (fluid overload), (2) increased permeability of the epithelium, (3) hypo-oncotic edema (low plasma oncotic pressure from decreased plasma protein), and (4) lymphedema. Capillary fluid exchange is based upon the balance of forces moving fluid outward (hydrostatic pressure, negative interstitial pressure, and interstitial colloid pressure) and the only force moving fluid inward (plasma oncotic pressure). Therefore, the plasma proteins are the only force holding fluid inside the capillaries. If a patient has isolated hypo-oncotic edema, with serum albumin < 2.5 g/dL, then a 25–50 g infusion of albumin over 24 hours may resolve the edema.

Pneumonia

Both lymphopenia (< 1000/μL) and hypoalbuminemia (serum albumin < 2.5 g/dL) are predictors of poor prognosis in patients with pneumonia.

In hospitalized patients, the use of antacids or H_2 blockers is associated with an increased incidence of nosocomial pneumonia, and use of sucralfate in place of antacids or H_2 blockers has been associated with a significantly lower rate of nosocomial infection. The reduced incidence of nosocomial infections was also associated with a significant reduction in mortality rate (from 46%–24%). The decrease has been thought to be due to maintenance of gastric acidity to support the stomach's overall bactericidal activity. Although there is some controversy about increased risks of infection in patients receiving H_2 blockers in the ICU, current data also suggest that the rate of spontaneous gastritis or gastrointestinal ulceration in the ICU patient was actually falling prior to the increased use of these drugs for prophylaxis against upper gastrointestinal bleeding.

Emphysema

In malnourished patients with emphysema, energy expenditure is increased by as much as 23–26% above weight-matched controls. Unlike the preferred fat oxidation seen in sepsis, patients with emphysema have an increase in protein and carbohydrate oxidation in the fasting and fed states. Forced vital capacity and diaphragmatic mass and strength are reduced in malnourished patients. Even though there are no prospective studies demonstrating improved survival in patients with emphysema given aggressive nutritional support, the ability to maintain respiratory muscle strength and mass during acute illness should be beneficial.

Enteral nutrition should be used with caution, however, in patients with COPD due to increased mortality. This may be due in part to the common practice of nursing patients in the supine position (increased risk of aspiration pneumonia) instead of the safer 45-degree upright position. Another risk may be due to the elevated blood glucose and associated morbidity and mortality associated with patients on mechanical ventilators. If nutritional support is provided, it must be done safely. Recent evidence suggests that weight loss during hospitalization and a low body mass index increase the risk for unplanned readmission to hospital.

Congestive Heart Failure

Many patients awaiting heart valve replacement have a combination of marasmic and hypoalbuminemic malnutrition, placing them at a higher postoperative risk for subsequent morbidity and mortality. Feeding these patients can improve cardiac function, but certain precautions are necessary. A low-sodium intake is essential owing to the association of sodium administration and fluid retention, resulting in cardiac failure. Because fatty acids are used as cardiac muscle fuel, mixed-fuel nutritional support (lipid, carbohydrate, and protein) may be preferable. Cardiac muscle that is ischemic derives all of its energy from anaerobic metabolism, so that TPN with adequate glucose, potassium, and insulin may optimize substrate delivery to areas limited to anaerobic glycolysis. Patients with severe calorie or protein malnutrition (albumin < 2.5 g/dL) should be given adequate calories and protein for about 1 week before cardiac surgery to optimize the recovery period. Patients treated with diuretics (eg, furosemide) are at an increased risk for thiamin deficiency. The loss of thiamin in the urine can increase the risk for high-output congestive heart failure (wet cardiac beriberi).

GASTROINTESTINAL DISORDERS

Pancreatitis

Earlier work suggested that the benefits of parenteral nutrition were especially important in patients with acute pancreatitis who were malnourished upon entry into the ICU. However, nutritional status may be difficult to determine, since weight history and actual weights are frequently not accurate owing to fluid accumulation in this disorder. Several studies have evaluated the benefits of parenteral nutritional support in patients with acute pancreatitis. In one study, the overall mortality rate was decreased from 21% to 3% in patients who were able to receive an average of 37 ± 1 (mean ± SEM) versus 26 ± 4 kcal/kg/d over a 29-day period. In a recently published report, the mortality rate in 67 patients was reduced from 38% to 13% if patients with acute pancreatitis received parenteral nutritional support within 72 hours after admission. Other studies have not demonstrated decreased mortality rates with administration of parenteral nutrition. Septic complications are reduced in patients with acute necrotizing pancreatitis provided enteral nutritional support as compared with those given TPN (28% versus 50%). Mortality in this study was similar with TPN and enteral nutrition.

Hepatic Encephalopathy

A branched-chain-enriched amino acid formula has been shown to improve mental recovery in almost all studies to date. A meta-analysis of six large studies demonstrated that there was an improvement in overall survival if patients with liver disease are fed a parenteral formula containing increased amounts of branched-chain amino acids. The mortality rate in the branched-chain-enriched amino acid treatment group averaged 24%, and in the control group it was 43%. In contrast to the beneficial effects noted in hepatic encephalopathy, there is no evidence that high branched-chain-enriched nutritional regimens reduce the mortality rate in trauma or in sepsis.

Alcoholic Hepatitis

One of the earliest studies of protein administration to patients with alcoholic hepatitis was performed in 1948, and this study demonstrated an improved survival rate in patients given protein and calories. One study has evaluated patients with alcoholic hepatitis who were prospectively randomized to receive parenteral nutritional support with amino acid solutions or the regular hospital diet. This small study demonstrated that morbidity and mortality rates were reduced in patients given parenteral nutrition support. A more recent study between enteral feeding and steroid therapy demonstrated a reduced 1-year mortality in the enteral-treated group (37% versus 53%, $P < .05$). Survival in alcoholic hepatitis was linked to the level of protein malnutrition. Thirty-day mortality rates ranged from 2% in mild malnutrition to 15% in moderate malnutrition, and up to 52% in severe malnutrition. Contrary to what is still written in most textbooks, the administration of 1 g/kg of protein is not associated with deterioration in mental status in patients with alcoholic hepatitis. Increased nutritional intake has been associated with prolonged survival.

Gastrointestinal Dysfunction

Absolute indications for parenteral nutrition include pseudo-obstruction, radiation enteritis, massive small bowel obstruction, prolonged ileus, prolonged diarrhea, short bowel syndrome, and hyperemesis gravidarum. Parenteral or enteral nutritional support may be indicated for Crohn's disease, Whipple's disease, abetalipoproteinemia, and diarrhea associated with scleroderma. The benefits of parenteral nutrition in ulcerative colitis are no greater than the use of bowel rest and hydrocortisone. However, the potential benefit of parenteral nutrition is that the patient may be better nourished and thus better able to tolerate colectomy if needed. Dysfunctional bowel, as mentioned earlier, is predictive of a poor outcome. Methods to improve gastrointestinal function should be utilized when absolute contraindications to bowel utilization are not present. Osmotic diarrhea can sometimes be improved with the use of intravenous albumin supplementation when serum albumin levels are < 2.5 g/dL.

Gastrointestinal Fistulas

Fistulas with a fluid output of at least 500 mL/d have been routinely treated with parenteral nutrition and bowel rest. A recent study suggests that enteral nutrition can be successful in patients with high-output fistulas but that these patients should be cared for in a specialized unit where optimal conditions for artificial nutrition and local management are in place.

RENAL DISORDERS

Acute Renal Failure

Although early studies of parenteral nutrition (amino acids and vitamins) compared with dextrose infusion alone (no vitamins or amino acids) demonstrated better recovery in patients with acute renal failure, subsequent studies have not consistently demonstrated a clear benefit. The patient who develops acute renal failure with malnutrition should receive enteral nutrition if the gut is functional and parenteral nutrition if it is not. The combination of acute renal failure and severe malnutrition is associated with a 7.2-fold increase in mortality.

Chronic Renal Failure

In chronic renal failure the relative risk for mortality increases logarithmically as albumin decreases (Figure 6–1). The risk increases to 12.8-fold for serum albumin < 2.5 mg/dL. In contrast, the relative risk decreases to 0.47 when the serum albumin is > 4.4 g/dL. In addition to serum albumin, serum ferritin is a marker of increase morbidity. Chronic renal failure patients with serum ferritin levels > 500 g/mL have a 19-fold increase in sepsis episodes compared with chronic renal failure patients who do not have as high an iron load. Treatment with deferoxamine mesylate, an iron-chelating agent, reduces the sepsis rate 24-fold. Selected renal failure patients and those with iron overload should be carefully watched for a higher than expected incidence of infection. The increased use of epoetin alfa (erythropoietin) has virtually eliminated the iron overload problem seen in patients with chronic renal failure. However, methods to remove the excess iron storage may be indicated to reduce the incidence of serious infections.

HEMATOLOGIC DISORDERS & CANCER

Bone Marrow Transplantation

Conventional nutritional therapy in bone marrow transplant patients in some studies can increase the engraftment rate of the donor's cell in the recipient's bone marrow, but in some studies has shown no benefit. Early parenteral nutritional support rather than a hospital diet in well-nourished bone marrow recipients can increase overall survival. Recent evidence suggests that the use of glutamine-enriched parenteral nutritional support after bone marrow transplantation improves nitrogen balance, reduces the incidence of infection, and shortens the hospital stay by about 7 days.

Cancer Cachexia

A meta-analysis concluded that parenteral nutritional support does not improve survival and may in fact increase the risk for infection in nonmalnourished cancer patients. A possible source of error in interpretation of these results is that many of the studies did not control for the severity of the malnutrition. In a few studies, the more severely ill and malnourished patients were selected to receive parenteral nutritional support. Those who were less ill or who could tolerate a hospital diet were given enteral support. Aggressive nutritional support should be provided as routine care to the cancer cachexia patient, using the gastrointestinal route if available.

Iron Deficiency Anemia

Critically ill patients are often found to be anemic. This is most often found to be anemia of chronic infection (or illness). If iron deficiency anemia is diagnosed, the standard of care has been to provide the patient with iron replacement after causes of iron deficiency anemia are evaluated. Data from a prospective clinical trial have demonstrated, however, that iron replacement is associated with a significant increase in rates of infection or reactivation of malaria, brucellosis, schistosomiasis, and tuberculosis. Iron replacement should therefore be confined to those who do not have a high risk for subsequent infection and who do not have a current serious infection.

Thrombocytopenia

Sepsis and disseminated intravascular coagulation are the most common causes of thrombocytopenia in ICU patients. Folate deficiency is relatively common in acute illness and can be seen in approximately 19–52% of the ICU population. A small proportion of cases of thrombocytopenia may actually be due to isolated deficiency of folate. Critically ill patients who are not eating should be given 5 mg/d of folate to prevent thrombocytopenia.

TRAUMA & POSTSURGERY

Severe Head Injury & Spinal Trauma

Closed head injury is one of the most highly catabolic illnesses in ICU patients. Urinary urea nitrogen excretion can approach that seen in thermal injury. Several prospective trials have evaluated the risks and benefits of parenteral and enteral nutritional support in these patients. One early study demonstrated improved survival in parenterally fed patients compared with nonfed controls. A second trial failed to demonstrate improvement in survival over that of enterally fed patients. A clinical trial demonstrated that TPN could improve morbidity but that the improvement in mortality was not significant. Data to date support in general the notion that adequate nutritional support (enteral or parenteral) will reduce morbidity in head injury patients. Recently, patients given enteral feeding for non-traumatic coma were shown to have improved survival. Enteral diets containing glutamine reduced the incidence of pneumonia (17% versus 45%), bacteremia (7% versus 42%), and sepsis (3% versus 26%). The addition of arginine, omega-3 fatty acids, and nucleotides reduced infectious complications (6% versus 41%).

Abdominal Trauma

Enteral nutritional support compared with parenteral nutritional support is associated with maintenance of serum albumin levels and a significant reduction in major infections from 20% to 3%. Patients who tolerate enteral feedings have better survival rates than those who cannot tolerate enteral feeding and therefore must receive parenteral feeding.

Abdominal Wound Dehiscence & Wound Healing

Appropriate nutrient administration is important for rapid and safe wound closure. Parenteral nutrition increases hydroxyproline levels and tensile strength in wounds. Wound dehiscence is eight times more common with decreased vitamin C levels. This is probably because vitamin C enhances capillary formation and decreases capillary fragility and is essential for hydroxylation of proline and lysine in collagen synthesis. Vitamin A enhances collagen synthesis and cross-linking of new collagen, enhances epithelialization, and antagonizes the inhibitory effects of glucocorticoids on cell membranes. Manganese is a cofactor in the glycosylation of hydroxylysine in procollagen. Copper acts as a cofactor in the polymerization of the collagen molecule and in the formation of collagen cross-links. Zinc supplementation also speeds up the wound healing rate. Vitamin, mineral, and nutritional support are essential for prompt wound repair.

Burns

Parenteral nutrition may be indicated in the early management of burn patients who develop burn-related ileus. After that time, the gut is the preferred route of feeding. In a small study of 18 burned children, providing 4.9 g/kg/d of protein versus 3.9 g/kg/d reduced the mortality rate from 44% to nil.

SEPSIS & MULTIPLE ORGAN FAILURE SYNDROME

Preoperative nutritional support of malnourished and nonmalnourished patients reduces the rate of septic complications (wound infections, pneumonia, intra-abdominal abscess, and sepsis), but the overall mortality rate has not been consistently affected. A study of blunt abdominal trauma patients who were prospectively randomized to receive either enteral or parenteral nutritional support has demonstrated a significant reduction in the incidence of pneumonia (from 31% to 12%), intra-abdominal abscesses (from 13% to 2%), and catheter sepsis (from 13% to 2%) in the group receiving enteral nutritional support.

The ability to provide adequate protein and calories to septic ICU patients has been associated with adequate IL-1 production and a significant improvement in hospital survival rates. Early enteral nutrition during sepsis does not prevent the development of multiple organ failure. Treatment for this disorder remains supportive.

ENDOCRINE & METABOLIC DISORDERS

Diabetes Mellitus

Metabolic stress syndrome is a condition of elevated blood glucose (> 109 mg/dL) in the ICU setting. The incidence of MSS ranges from 45–50% in patients receiving TPN to 99% of patients on mechanical ventilation. Severe elevation in blood glucose (> 199 mg/dL) occurs in 21–31% of patients on TPN. Nondiabetic ICU patients with a blood glucose > 109 mg/dL have a 3.9-fold increase risk of death, and a blood glucose > 144 mg/dL in non-diabetics was associated with an increased risk for congestive heart failure or cardiogenic shock. Diabetic patients with a glucose concentration > 179 mg/dL have a 1.7-fold increase in mortality. Survival in diabetic patients with acute myocardial infarctions is improved with aggressive blood glucose control.

Metabolic stress syndrome is probably not due to caloric intake alone but to elevated counterregulatory hormones and insulin resistance. Reducing caloric intake from 1400 kcal to 1000 kcal per day does not reduce the incidence of the syndrome. Aggressive regular insulin administration to maintain blood glucose under 110 mg/dL in 765 mechanically ventilated patients reduced mortality by 43%. In this prospective randomized trial, patients were randomized to either intensive insulin therapy or standard therapy. The goal in the intensive therapy group was to maintain blood glucose concentrations under 110 mg/dL. This was obtained with the intravenous administration of insulin. Ninety-nine percent of patients required insulin at an average dose of 71 units of regular insulin per day. Both groups were equally randomized according to age, gender, body mass index, injury score, incidence of type 2 diabetes (13%), and incidence of cancer. The intensive treatment group had a significant reduction in mean early morning blood glucose (103 ± 18 mg/dL versus 173 ± 32 mg/dL; $P < .001$). Improved blood glucose control reduced the incidence of bacteremia by 50%, the need for hemodialysis by 42%, and the need for prolonged mechanical ventilation by 37% ($P < .01$). ICU mortality was reduced by 43% (from 8.1% to 4.6%) and hospital mortality was reduced by 34% (from 10.9% to 7.2%; $P < .01$).

Both type 1 and type 2 diabetic patients frequently have low levels of vitamin C. Type 1 diabetics also have a lower serum retinol (vitamin A) level than normal volunteers. The exact mechanisms responsible for reduced serum vitamin C and vitamin A levels in these patients are not known. In diabetic animals treated with vitamin A, abnormally low hydroxyproline levels and decreased wound breaking strength return to normal. Type 1 diabetics also have reduced serum and white blood cell zinc levels and excessive losses of zinc in the urine. Both type 1 and type 2 diabetics can have increased magnesium losses in the urine and reduced serum magnesium levels.

Diabetics also have alterations in neutrophil function, putting them at an increased risk of infection, including decreased adhesiveness, poor chemotaxis, decreased opsonization, decreased phagocytosis, and decreased intracellular killing. The lymphocyte also behaves differently in diabetics, especially if the patient is malnourished, and the lymphocyte count is decreased in proportion to the degree of malnutrition. Diabetics have decreased cell-mediated immunity with decreased lymphocyte transformation, reduced macrophage-lymphocyte interaction, and an impaired delayed-type hypersensitivity. One may be able to improve leukocyte dysfunction by maintaining excellent glucose control in the diabetic with blood glucose < 200 mg/dL at all times. A blood glucose level below 250 mg/dL improves but does not correct white blood cell phagocytic function; improves but does not correct granulocyte adherence; and improves but does not correct leukocyte bacterial killing.

Diabetic patients receiving TPN frequently have serum electrolyte and glucose levels that are difficult to control. Hyperglycemia is associated with an osmotic diuresis and loss of sodium, potassium, and minerals (including trace minerals). Effective insulin administration is important to optimize the administration of TPN to the diabetic patient. TPN should be initiated in the diabetic patient with only 150 g of dextrose over the first 24 hours (eg, as 1 L of 15% dextrose at 40 mL/h or 1 L 25% dextrose with 5% amino acid at 24 mL/h). Approximately one-third to one-half of the patient's usual total daily subcutaneous insulin dose should be added to the TPN solution. Additional subcutaneous insulin should be administered using a "sliding scale" regimen written as a standing order, with the dose of insulin based on bedside glucose measurements and serum glucose from venous blood measured every 3–4 hours. After the first 24 hours, approximately half of the additional regular subcutaneous insulin administered over the 24-hour period is then added to the TPN solution prior to increasing the rate of TPN administration or the concentration of dextrose.

The optimal intravenous insulin infusion rate may take 2–3 days to determine because of the variable loss of insulin to different types of plastic and glass bottles used in hospitals. However, once serum glucose is less than 140 mg/dL over a 24-hour period, the overall rate of the TPN infusion or the dextrose concentration can be increased. If the rate of the infusion is increased, there should be no need to alter the dextrose:insulin ratio in the TPN solution. If the concentration of the dextrose is increased, the original ratio of dextrose to insulin should be maintained in the TPN solution by adding insulin to the bottle. To prevent hypoglycemia, it is advisable not to add excessive amounts of insulin to the TPN solution. Insulin *must* be added to the TPN solution for any patient who has a blood glucose > 140 mg/dL. The use of separate intravenous infusions of insulin and TPN solution has been associated with severe hypoglycemia and death.

Immune-Enhancing Diet

The use of an immune-enhancing diet in severe trauma can reduce major infectious complications (6% versus 41%) and hospital stay (18 days versus 33 days). A recent review of these diets demonstrates that most of the benefit is in surgical patients, with a reduction in infections of 33%, a reduction of time on the ventilator of 2.6 days, and a reduction in the length of the hospital stay of 2.9 days.

Acute Hepatic Porphyria

This rare cause of abdominal pain is treated with dextrose, 500 g/d (2 L of 25% dextrose at a rate of 80 mL/h).

NEW TREATMENT STRATEGIES FOR THE MALNOURISHED CRITICALLY ILL PATIENT

Insulin

Prior to the development of severe malnutrition, critically ill patients without diabetes frequently have elevated blood glucose due to metabolic stress syndrome. The syndrome is due to insulin resistance and elevations in counterregulatory hormones. This response may interfere with nutritional therapy. The metabolic abnormalities of insulin resistance include glucose intolerance, increased hepatic glucose production, increased whole body amino acid flux, and decreased whole body glucose utilization. Insulin resistance resulting in the metabolic stress syndrome is type 2 diabetic in character, since the patients are not insulinopenic but are insulin-resistant. The more severe the malnutrition or illness, the greater the hepatic glucose production. Amino acid flux is also greater the more severe the malnutrition or illness. Recognizing the presence of metabolic stress syndrome in patients is important since insulin administration appears to be protein-sparing in catabolic postinjury patients and reduces mortality in ICU patients when blood glucose is maintained under 110 mg/dL. The use of insulin or other agents that reduce hepatic glucose production in critical illness may be helpful in reducing protein breakdown from the lean body mass for amino acid gluconeogenic precursors.

A randomized study of tight glycemic control with intravenous insulin intended to keep blood glucose between 80 and 100 mg/dL (compared with conventional therapy with a target blood glucose of 180–215 mg/dL) in postoperative cardiac surgery patients resulted in lower mortality (4.6% compared with 8%), fewer bloodstream infections, less need for hemodialysis, and shorter duration of mechanical ventilation. Of note is that only a small proportion of patients had a history of diabetes. Hypoglycemia (blood glucose < 40 mg/dL) occurred in 5% of the intensively treated group and < 1% of the conventionally treated patients. The median daily amount of insulin needed for tight control was 71 units per day compared with 33 units per day for the others. While this study was on surgical patients, these data support the beneficial effect of insulin and a considerably lower target blood glucose for ICU patients than previously recognized.

Growth Hormone

Exogenous growth hormone in postoperative patients can significantly reduce and almost abolish the loss of lean body mass over the postinjury period. In a prospective blinded study, administration of growth hormone to burned children has been associated with an improved healing time. In a retrospective state, growth hormone treatment increased survival in adults with severe burns. However, the use of growth hormone was also associated with an increase in insulin resistance and the need to administer an increased insulin dose. Growth hormone probably improves wound healing by increasing protein synthesis without increasing protein oxidation, so that there is a net protein deposition in the body. However, small changes in nitrogen balance may represent a change in a labile nitrogen pool that may be as large as 30–50 g. Studies documenting marked changes in liver size during alimentation suggest that the liver accounts for much of the positive nitrogen balance.

At present, use of growth hormone is restricted to those children who are growth hormone-deficient. Growth hormone should not be used in critically ill patients because mortality can increase 1.9-fold to 2.4-fold. Prospective double-blind trials are needed prior to use of growth hormone in patients who are seriously ill.

Anabolic Steroids

Anabolic steroids have been used in several clinical trials of malnourished patients with mixed results. Nitrogen balance has been shown to be improved in some but not all of the clinical trials. The improved nitrogen balance was generally seen in patients with benign diseases (hip replacement surgery, vagotomy, or pyloroplasty). In a prospective study of burns, oxandrolone 20 mg/d reduced weight loss (3 kg versus 8 kg), nitrogen loss (4 g/d versus 13 g/d), and healing time (9 days versus 13 days). On the other hand, oxandrolone treatment in trauma patients failed to reduce nitrogen loss (17 g/d versus 19 g/d), length of hospital stay (31 days versus 27 days), or length of ICU stay (17 days versus 15 days). The mixed success of anabolic steroids in critically ill patients may be due to the antianabolic effects of elevated counterregulatory hormones and insulin resistance, reduced enteral food intake, or limited total dose of anabolic steroids.

Albumin

Normal serum albumin is associated with a shorter inflammatory phase of wound healing and normal angiogenesis, collagen synthesis, and wound remodeling. Albumin levels < 2.5 g/dL represent a 50% loss in the normal plasma colloid oncotic pressure and may contribute to gastrointestinal mucosal edema and diarrhea. A serum albumin level of 2.5 g/dL can be used to predict those patients who will develop diarrhea when fed by mouth. In fact, several authors have found that up to 100% of patients with a serum albumin below 1.5 g/dL have diarrhea with enteral feeding.

Limited clinical trials have demonstrated some benefit from albumin administration and nutritional support in critically ill patients with noninfectious causes of diarrhea and in nontraumatic hypovolemic shock such as septic shock. Less convincing evidence exists for a beneficial effect of albumin administration in primary lung injury such as acute respiratory distress syndrome (ARDS). This is probably because the permeability defect in ARDS is due to an abnormal pore size and not a simple loss of normal plasma oncotic pressure. A few cases of what appeared to be ARDS with low serum albumin levels have resolved following restoration of a normal colloid oncotic pressure by continuous administration of albumin until a normal level is reached. However, the use of albumin should be restricted to specific indications until the clinician is able to measure oncotic pressure and make certain that a very low level is responsible for the hemodynamic changes seen in the lung.

Arguments against the use of intravenous albumin include its shorter half-life in the critically ill patient than in normal individuals and the fact that it is rapidly lost into the extracellular space. It is important to note that only 40% of the albumin pool is in the plasma compartment, so that approximately 60% of the albumin administered is distributed to the extracellular space (skin, gastrointestinal tract, etc.). If intravenous albumin is administered, it is advisable to administer it with the TPN fluid or over a prolonged period of time. Even though the 50 mL vial of 25% human albumin can be given as a rapid intravenous infusion, one 50 mL vial of 25% albumin can rapidly expand the plasma compartment by as much as 300 mL, which may be enough to cause a sudden onset of pulmonary edema in susceptible patients.

Beta-Adrenergic Blockade

A small study showed that 2 weeks of propranolol given to children with 40% or more third-degree burns resulted in lower heart rate, oxygen consumption, and energy expenditure by about 20%. Propranolol increased protein synthesis and prevented net whole body protein loss by approximately 10% over a 1-month period. Beta-adrenergic blockade may be useful in decreasing metabolic demands, but this possibility awaits confirmation in larger trials.

REFERENCES

Abou-Assi S, O'Keefe SJ: Nutrition in acute pancreatitis. J Clin Endocrinol 2001;32:203–9.

Boelens PG et al: Glutamine alimentation in catabolic state. J Nutr 2001;131(9 Suppl):2569S–77S.

Capes SE et al: Stress hyperglycaemia and increased risk of death after myocardial infarction in patients with and without diabetes: a systemic review. Lancet 2000;355:773–78.

Consensus Recommendations from the U.S. summit on immune-enhancing enteral therapy. JPEN J Parenteral Enteral Nutr 2001;25(2 Suppl):S61–3.

McCowen KC, Malhotra A, Bistrian BR: Stress-induced hyperglycemia. Crit Care Clin 2001;17:107–24.

Marchesini G et al: Nutritional treatment with branched-chain amino acids in advanced liver cirrhosis. J Gastroenterol 2000;35(Suppl 12):7–12.

Murray MJ et al. The adverse effect of iron repletion on the course of certain infections. BMJ 1978;2:1113–5.

Stratov I et al: Candidaemia in an Australian teaching hospital: relationship to central line and TPN use. J Infect 1998;36:203–7.

Takala J et al: Increased mortality associated with GH treatment in critically ill adults. N Engl J Med 1999;341:785–92.

Torosian MH: Perioperative nutritional support for patients undergoing gastrointestinal surgery: critical analysis and recommendations. World J Surg 1999;23:565–9.

van den Berghe G et al: Intensive insulin therapy in critically ill patients. N Engl J Med 2001;345:1359–67.

Yanagawa T et al: Nutritional support for head-injured patients (Cochrane Review). In: The Cochrane Database Library, Issue 4, 2001. Oxford: Update Software.

Imaging Procedures

7

Kathleen Brown, MD, Steven S. Raman, MD, & Cindy Kallman, MD

An unprecedented array of imaging options is now available to the physician in the ICU. The choice of a particular imaging modality is occasionally difficult, based on recommendations in the literature, local expertise, type of equipment available, and the experience of the radiologists. Given the increasing emphasis on cost-effective practice, clinicians and radiologists must maximize the diagnostic and therapeutic yield of procedures while minimizing costs.

Optimal management of critically ill patients also requires close communication between the critical care team and the diagnostic and interventional radiologist. An established practice of daily ICU radiology rounds with the participation of the radiologist facilitates this level of communication.

In a traditional model, all ICU films would be placed on a designated mechanical film alternator within either the ICU or the radiology department. With rapid advances in imaging options and telecommunications feasibility, new models for ICU imaging are being developed. In one model, films are acquired electronically and displayed in a patient archival and communications system (PACS) or on web-based servers. The PACS unit is able to display plain radiographs, ultrasound studies, computed tomography (CT), and magnetic resonance images (MRI). Suboptimal exposures may be corrected in part by adjusting contrast and window levels. High-resolution monitors may be placed at designated sites in the ICU and throughout the hospital. An ideal system would integrate PACS with the hospital information system (HIS) and the radiology information system (RIS) to display efficiently clinical and radiologic information. These systems could greatly improve the efficiency of clinicians, nurses, and support staff.

TECHNIQUES FOR IMAGING OF THE CHEST

Most radiographic examinations in the ICU are obtained at the bedside utilizing conventional analog or digital equipment. Other imaging methods, including ultrasound, CT, nuclear medicine techniques, and MRI, are used to supplement plain film radiography. Interventional procedures, either at the bedside or in the radiology suite, are also frequently performed under imaging guidance.

Chest Radiographs

Chest radiographs are the most common imaging examination, accounting for approximately 40% of the volume in a radiology department. As many as one-third of these chest radiographs may be obtained at the bedside (portable radiographs), and in the ICU almost all chest radiographs are taken using the portable technique. The utility and effectiveness of routine daily portable chest radiographs has been studied, and—despite limitations of the technique—these films play an important role in identifying and following pulmonary and cardiac disorders in ICU patients. In addition, digital radiographic systems are increasingly being used in the ICU for portable chest imaging. With these systems, images are obtained using a stimulable phosphor imaging plate instead of film. The exposed imaging plate is scanned, read, and processed by computer, and the image can be transmitted to an ICU console or viewed as hard copy on a conventional view box. Conventional radiographs may also be converted into digital format for transmission to PACS or storage.

Ultrasound

Ultrasound examination at the bedside in the ICU is relatively inexpensive and does not utilize ionizing radiation. In the thorax, ultrasound is most often used to evaluate and localize pleural fluid collections, to determine whether such collections are free or loculated, and as a guide to thoracentesis. Ultrasound is also helpful in clarifying peridiaphragmatic processes, since the diaphragm is easily visualized, allowing differentiation of supradiaphragmatic and infradiaphragmatic fluid collections. The greatest utility of ultrasound, however, is in the evaluation of abdominal disease. Ultrasound provides rapid assessment of hepatobiliary and genitourinary disease and may be used to guide percutaneous drainage of intra-abdominal abscesses.

Computed Tomography

By virtue of transaxial imaging capabilities and improved contrast resolution, CT has been shown to be very valuable in increasing diagnostic accuracy and guiding therapeutic procedures for critically ill patients. Multidetector CT and spiral CT allow for more rapid scanning of patients and have facilitated the use of CT for evaluation of vascular disorders such as aortic dissection and pulmonary embolism. In one study evaluating the utility of thoracic CT in critically ill patients, thoracic CT added clinically useful information not available from plain radiographs in 70% of examinations. Similar findings have been reported in the evaluation of abdominal disease. Transportation of the ICU patient to the CT scanner requires coordinated effort from hospital personnel, including ICU physicians and nurses, respiratory therapists, radiology technologists, and radiologists. Careful monitoring during transport and during the procedure is essential and must include arrhythmia monitoring and pulse oximetry.

Nuclear Scintigraphy

Nuclear scintigraphy has a number of applications in the critically ill patient. Myocardial perfusion and infarct scanning in cardiac disease, ventilation-perfusion scanning in patients with suspected pulmonary embolism, evaluation of gastrointestinal hemorrhage and acute cholecystitis, and localization of occult infection are among the most common indications for radionuclide imaging in the ICU patient.

Magnetic Resonance Imaging

MRI has supplanted CT in the evaluation of many disorders because it does not employ ionizing radiation, because it provides excellent differentiation of vascular and nonvascular structures without the use of intravenous contrast, and because it provides cross-sectional images in multiple planes. However, in many cases, MRI is not feasible in the evaluation of the critically ill patient because of interference caused by ferromagnetic monitoring devices, the difficulty of adequately ventilating and monitoring patients within the narrow MRI gantry, and long scan times.

MacMahon H, Grigor M: Portable chest radiography techniques and teleradiology. Radiol Clin North Am 1996;34:1–20.

Maffessanti M, Berlot G, Bortolotto P: Chest roentgenology in the intensive care unit: an overview. Eur Radiol 1998;8:69–78.

Miller WT Jr, Tino G, Friedburg JS: Thoracic CT in the intensive care unit: assessment of clinical usefulness. Radiology 1998; 209:491–8.

Schilling R: infoRAD: Computers for clinical practice and education in radiology. Teleradiology, information transfer, and PACS: implications for diagnostic imaging in the 1990s. Radiographics 1993;13:683–6.

IMAGING OF SUPPORT & MONITORING DEVICES IN THE ICU

ENDOTRACHEAL & TRACHEOSTOMY TUBES

Both endotracheal intubation and tracheostomy may cause potentially serious complications. Malpositioning of the endotracheal tube into the right main stem bronchus occurs in approximately 9% of endotracheal intubations. Such malpositioning may lead to atelectasis of the left lung, hyperinflation of the right lung, and possible pneumothorax. The clinical assessment of tube location is frequently inaccurate, and a chest radiograph should be obtained immediately following intubation. Tubes currently in use are usually radiographically visible by virtue of a metallic wire or barium marker in the wall of the tube. Periodic radiographs are required to exclude inadvertent displacement of the tube by cough, suctioning, or the weight of respiratory apparatus.

Since endotracheal tubes are typically fixed in position at the nose or mouth, flexion and extension of the neck may result in motion of the tube relative to the carina, with the tube descending during flexion and ascending during extension. With the neck in neutral position, the ideal position of the tube tip is 5–7 cm above the carina, which allows for a tolerable change in tube position during flexion and extension. In 90% of patients, the carina projects between the fifth and seventh thoracic vertebrae on the portable radiograph; when the carina cannot be clearly seen, the ideal positioning of the endotracheal tube is at the T2–T4 level. The balloon cuff should not be greater in diameter than the trachea, since cuff overinflation can cause pressure necrosis of the tracheal wall.

Inadvertent placement of the endotracheal tube into the esophagus is uncommon but may be catastrophic when it does occur. Esophageal intubation may be difficult to diagnose on the portable chest film because the esophagus frequently projects over the tracheal air column. Gastric or distal esophageal distention, location of the tube lateral to the tracheal air column, and deviation of the trachea secondary to an overinflated intraesophageal balloon cuff are radiographic signs of esophageal intubation. The right posterior oblique view with the patient's head turned to the right allows ease of separation of the esophagus and trachea and should be obtained in equivocal cases.

Intubation may result in injury to the trachea, with tracheal stenosis developing in approximately 19% of patients following endotracheal intubation and approximately 65% of patients with tracheostomy. In patients with translaryngeal intubation, the most frequent sites of stenosis are the cuff site and the subglottic region.

Tracheostomy is typically performed in the patient who requires relatively long-term ventilatory support. Although the surgical mortality rate is less than 2%, the long-term complication rate may be as high as 60%. Pneumothorax, pneumomediastinum, subcutaneous emphysema, hemorrhage, and tube malposition may occur as early complications, whereas late complications include tracheal stenosis, tracheo-innominate artery fistula, tracheoesophageal fistula, stomal infection, aspiration, and tube occlusion. In addition, the incidence of nosocomial pneumonia is increased secondary to airway bacterial colonization.

Brunel W et al: Assessment of routine chest roentgenograms and the physical examination to confirm endotracheal tube position. Chest 1989;96:1043–5.

Heffner JE, Miller S, Sahn SA: Tracheostomy in the intensive care unit: 2. Complications. Chest 1986;90:430–6.

Salem MR: Verification of endotracheal tube position. Anesthesiol Clin North Am 2001;19:813–39.

Smith GM, Reed JC, Choplin RH: Radiographic detection of esophageal malpositioning of endotracheal tubes. AJR Am J Roentgenol 1990;154:23–6.

CENTRAL VENOUS PRESSURE CATHETERS

Central venous pressure catheters are used frequently in the ICU patient for venous access, especially for purposes of parenteral alimentation, monitoring central venous pressure, and hemodialysis. Such catheters are visible on the chest radiograph, and knowledge of normal thoracic venous anatomy is required to assess catheter location. The subclavian vein, the internal jugular vein, and the femoral veins are the sites of venous access used most often. Central venous lines inserted via a thoracic vein are optimally positioned when the tip is past the valves in the subclavian or brachiocephalic veins or within the superior vena cava. Union of the subclavian and internal jugular veins to form the brachiocephalic vein usually occurs behind the sternal end of the corresponding clavicle. Whereas the right brachiocephalic vein has a vertical course as it forms the superior vena cava, the left brachiocephalic vein crosses the mediastinum from left to right in a retrosternal position to enter the superior vena cava. Although seldom obtained in ICU patients, the cross-table lateral view may be helpful to localize catheters malpositioned in the internal mammary or azygos vein or in extravascular positions.

In a study of 300 central venous lines, approximately one-third of catheters were incorrectly positioned at the time of the initial chest radiograph. The malpositioned catheter tip may result in venous thrombosis or perforation as well as inaccurate venous pressure readings. Positioning of the catheter tip within the right atrium may result in cardiac perforation and tamponade, while a right ventricular location may result in arrhythmias secondary to irritation of the endocardium or interventricular septum.

Complications of central venous catheterization include pneumothorax, hemothorax, and perforation, which may result in pericardial effusion, hydrothorax, mediastinal hemorrhage, or ectopic infusion of intravenous solutions (Figure 7–1). Less common complications include air embolism and catheter fracture or embolism. The incidence of pneumothorax ranges between 1% and 12% and is higher with a subclavian approach than with an internal jugular approach. Pneumothorax may be clinically occult, and a chest radiograph should be obtained to exclude a pneumothorax following line placement. A radiograph should be obtained even following an unsuccessful attempted line placement and is more critical when contralateral venous cannulation is anticipated to avoid the development of bilateral pneumothoraces.

Venous air embolism is an uncommon complication of central venous catheterization. Radiographically, air in the main pulmonary artery is diagnostic, but other features include focal oligemia, pulmonary edema, and atelectasis. Intracardiac air or air within the pulmonary artery is easily seen on CT. Long-term complications of venous access devices include delayed perforation, pinch-off syndrome, thrombosis, catheter knotting, and catheter fragmentation. A gentle curve at the tip of the catheter may be a forewarning of perforation. In one study, this was seen 4 hours to 7 days prior to clinical or radiographic recognition of perforation, and the authors recommended prompt catheter repositioning when this curved-tip sign was identified. In pinch-off syndrome, the catheter lumen is compromised by compression between the clavicle and the first rib, leading to catheter malfunction and possible catheter fracture. This is frequently first observed as subtle focal narrowing of the catheter as it crosses the intersection of clavicle and rib. As increasing numbers of chronically ill patients with long-term venous catheters—including liver and bone marrow transplant recipients—are transferred to the ICU during their hospital course, more such complications may be seen.

Chang TC, Funaki B, Szymski GX: Are routine chest radiographs necessary after image-guided placement of internal jugular central venous access devices? AJR Am J Roentgenol 1998;170:335–7.

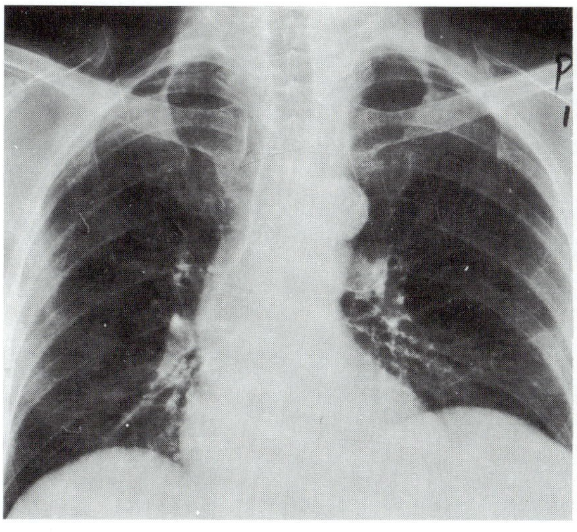

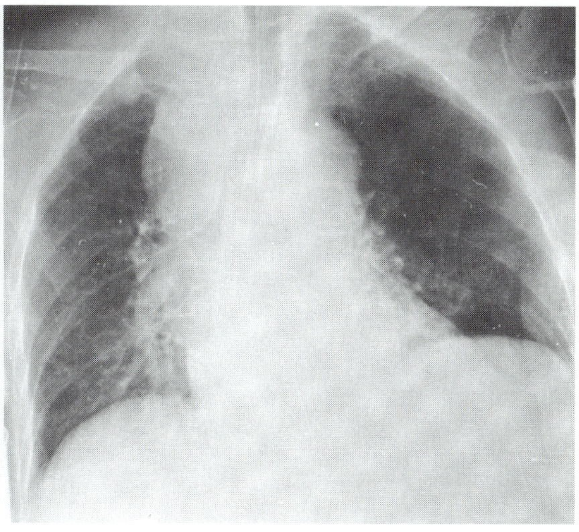

A B

Figure 7–1. Mediastinal hematoma following attempted central venous catheterization. ***A:*** Mediastinum appears unremarkable prior to catheter placement. ***B:*** Following attempted central line placement, there is widening of the superior mediastinum secondary to mediastinal hemorrhage due to a lacerated subclavian artery.

Hinke DH et al: Pinch-off syndrome: A complication of implantable subclavian venous access devices. Radiology 1990; 177:353–6.

Tocino IM, Watanabe A: Impending catheter perforation of the superior vena cava: Radiographic recognition. AJR Am J Roentgenol 1986;146:487–90.

Wechsler RJ, Steiner RM, Kinori I: Monitoring the monitors: The radiology of thoracic catheters, wires, and tubes. Semin Roentgenol 1988;23:61–84.

PULMONARY ARTERY CATHETERS

The pulmonary artery catheter has enhanced the management of the ICU patient, allowing monitoring of left atrial and left ventricular end-diastolic pressures and calculation of vital data such as cardiac output and vascular resistance. Complications associated with their use include arrhythmias, pneumothorax, vascular perforation, venous air embolism, and catheter-related sepsis. Knotting, kinking, and coiling of the catheter also occur. In a prospective study of pulmonary artery catheterization in 500 patients, a 24% overall complication rate was noted, with serious complications (including sepsis, pulmonary infarction, and cardiac arrhythmias) occurring in 4.4%.

Pulmonary infarction, thrombosis, pulmonary artery rupture, and infection represent other major complications associated with indwelling pulmonary artery catheters. There is a 7% incidence of pulmonary ischemic lesions due to direct injury from the use of pulmonary artery catheters. The majority of these lesions are thought to be due to vascular occlusion by the catheter itself. Continuous wedging of the catheter tip in a peripheral pulmonary artery and central pulmonary artery obstruction by the inflated balloon were cited as precipitating causes. In a smaller number of cases, emboli arose from peripheral thrombosis around the catheter.

Pulmonary infarction secondary to a pulmonary artery catheter has a radiographic appearance like that of infarction from other causes. Typically, a wedge-shaped parenchymal opacity is seen in the distribution of the vessel distal to the catheter (Figure 7–2). Pleural effusion is variable. Management consists of removal of the catheter; anticoagulation is not required. Resolution of consolidation usually occurs in 2–4 weeks.

Pulmonary artery rupture is a catastrophic complication of pulmonary artery catheterization, with a reported mortality rate of 46%. The incidence is low—no more than 0.2% of catheter placements. Risk factors include pulmonary hypertension, advanced age, and improper balloon location or inflation. The mortality rate increases in anticoagulated patients. Pseudoaneurysm formation has been reported secondary to rupture or dissection by the balloon catheter tip. This appears radiographically as a well-defined nodule at the site of the aneurysm, but it may initially be obscured by extravasation of blood into the adjacent air spaces. Chest radiographic findings often precede clinical manifestations, and death due to rupture of pseudoaneurysm may occur weeks following catheterization. The CT appearance of pulmonary artery pseudoaneurysm has been described as

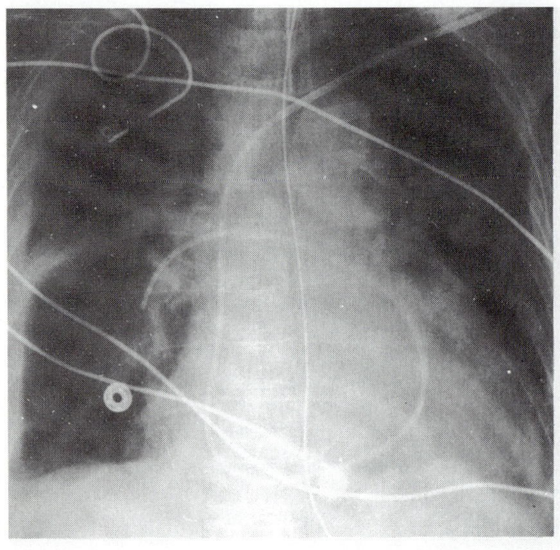

A

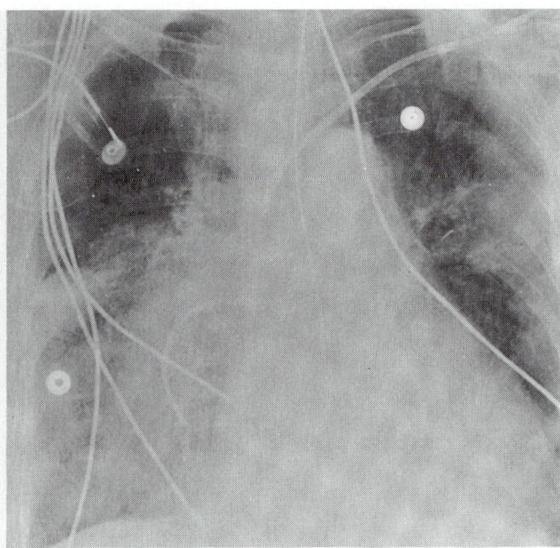

B

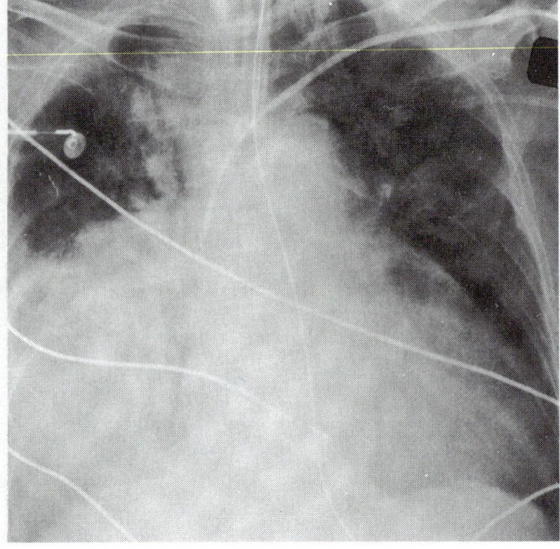

C

Figure 7–2. Lung infarction secondary to pulmonary artery catheterization. ***A:*** Initial radiograph after catheterization shows the tip of the catheter at the level of the right interlobar pulmonary artery. Mild redundancy of the catheter is present within the dilated heart. ***B:*** At 24 hours, the patient developed hemoptysis. Radiograph now shows migration of the catheter into a segmental arterial branch with increased density in the right lower lobe. ***C:*** Follow-up film demonstrates dense consolidation of the right middle and lower lobes secondary to infarction. (Reproduced, with permission, from Aberle DA, Brown K: Radiologic considerations in the adult respiratory distress syndrome. Clin Chest Med 1990;2:737–54.)

a sharply defined nodule with a surrounding halo of faint parenchymal density. Pulmonary artery pseudoaneurysm may now be treated in some patients with transcatheter embolization rather than surgical resection.

Location of the catheter tip should be monitored with serial radiographs. Softening of the catheter over time may result in migration of the catheter tip peripherally. Redundancy of the catheter within the right heart favors peripheral migration, and the intracardiac loop gradually becomes smaller (Figure 7–2). The ideal position for the pulmonary artery catheter is within the right or left main pulmonary artery, below the level of the left atrium. This generally corresponds to the lower lobes in supine patients.

Dieden JD, Friloux L, Renner JW: Pulmonary artery false aneurysms secondary to Swan-Ganz pulmonary artery catheters. AJR Am J Roentgenol 1987;149:901–6.

Foote GA, Schabel SI, Hodges M: Pulmonary complications of the flow-directed balloon-tipped catheter. N Engl J Med 1974;290:927–31.

Guttentag AR, Shepard JO, McLoud TC: Catheter-induced pulmonary pseudoaneurysm: The halo sign on CT. AJR Am J Roentgenol 1992;158:637–79.

Hannan AT, Brown M, Bigman O: Pulmonary artery catheter-induced hemorrhage. Chest 1984;85:128–31.

INTRA-AORTIC BALLOON COUNTERPULSATION

Intra-aortic balloon counterpulsation is used to improve cardiac function in patients with cardiogenic shock and in the perioperative period in cardiac surgery patients. The device consists of a fusiform inflatable balloon surrounding the distal portion of a catheter that is placed percutaneously from a femoral artery into the proximal descending thoracic aorta. The balloon is inflated during diastole, thereby increasing diastolic pressure in the proximal aorta and increasing coronary artery perfusion. During systole, the balloon is forcibly deflated, allowing aortic blood to move distally and decreasing the afterload against which the left ventricle must contract, thus decreasing left ventricular workload. The timing of inflation and deflation is controlled by the ECG.

The tip of the balloon should ideally be positioned just distal to the origin of the left subclavian artery at the level of the aortic knob, maximizing the effect on the coronary arteries while reducing the possibility of occlusion of the left subclavian artery, embolization to cerebral vessels, or occlusion of the abdominal vessels by the balloon. Complications associated with the device are most often secondary to malpositioning of the catheter and include obstruction of the subclavian artery and cerebral embolism. Aortic dissection has been described, and an indistinct aorta on chest radiographs has been suggested as an early clue to intramural location, requiring confirmation by angiography. Balloon leak or rupture has also been described.

CARDIAC PACEMAKERS

Cardiac pacemakers can be inserted by three approaches: transvenous, epicardial, and subxiphoid. Most often the transvenous approach is used, whereby wires are introduced via the subclavian or jugular vein and fluoroscopically guided into the right atrium and ventricle.

When viewed on a chest radiograph, the pacemaker lead should curve gently throughout its course; regions of sharp angulation will have increased mechanical stress and enhance the likelihood of lead fracture. Excessive lead length may predispose to fracture secondary to sharp angulation or may perforate the myocardium, and a short lead can become dislodged and enter the right atrium. Leads may also become displaced and enter the pulmonary artery, coronary sinus, or inferior vena cava. When possible, a lateral chest radiograph is recommended to confirm pacemaker lead location, with the electrodes located at least 3 mm deep to the epicardial fat stripe. Other complications include venous thrombosis or infection, either at the pulse generator pocket or within the vein. Myocardium perforation may result in hemopericardium and cardiac tamponade.

AUTOMATIC IMPLANTABLE CARDIOVERTER DEFIBRILLATOR

The automatic implantable cardioverter defibrillator (AICD) is used for treatment of ventricular tachyarrhythmias unresponsive to conventional antiarrhythmic drugs. The device consists of a fine titanium mesh placed on the cardiac surface and attached to a generator source that provides an electrical output in the event of ventricular arrhythmia. Opaque marker wires delineate the margins of the mesh pad, and sensing electrodes are also visible. Radiographs may be helpful in assessing the location of wires.

NASOGASTRIC TUBES

Nasogastric tubes are frequently used to provide nutrition and administer oral medications as well as for suctioning gastric contents. Ideally, the tip of the tube should be positioned at least 10 cm beyond the gastroesophageal junction. This ensures that all sideholes are located within the stomach and decreases the risk of aspiration. Complications of nasogastric intubation include esophagitis, stricture, and perforation.

Small-bore flexible feeding tubes have been developed to facilitate insertion and improve patient comfort. However, inadvertent passage of the nasogastric tube into the tracheobronchial tree is not uncommon, most often occurring in the sedated or neurologically impaired patient. In patients with endotracheal tubes in place, low-pressure high-volume balloon cuffs do not prevent passage of a feeding tube into the lower airway. If sufficient feeding tube length is inserted, the tube may actually traverse the lung and penetrate the visceral pleura (Figure 7–3). Removal of the tube from an intrapleural location may result in tension pneumothorax, and preparations should be made for potential emergent thoracostomy tube placement at the time of

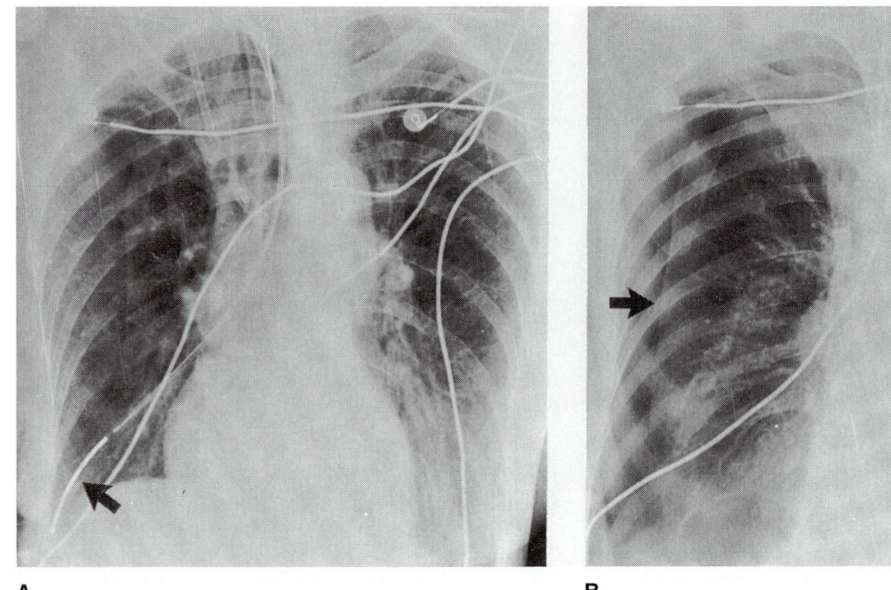

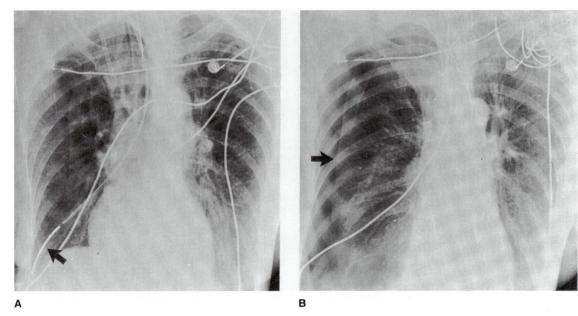

Figure 7–3. Malpositioned feeding tube. ***A:*** Feeding tube courses via the right main stem bronchus with the tip (arrow) overlying the right costophrenic angle. An endotracheal tube is present. ***B:*** Following removal of the feeding tube, a pneumothorax is seen (arrow).

removal. Although fluoroscopic placement is advocated by some authors, at many institutions small feeding tubes are used so frequently that fluoroscopic guidance is not feasible. Placement of the tube in two stages may prevent malpositioning. In the two-stage procedure, the tube is inserted initially to a predetermined length equaling the distance from the earlobe to the xiphoid process. This distance is too short to penetrate the pleura if the tube has inadvertently been placed in the airway. A radiograph of the chest is then obtained to confirm the tube location, and if the tube is within the esophagus, it can be advanced into the stomach. If the tube is situated endobronchially, it is immediately withdrawn and repositioned. The stylet is withdrawn after a second film confirms the final location of the tube in the stomach. The additional expense of two radiographs during tube placement is more than justified by the reduced incidence of complications such as pneumothorax, intrapulmonary feeding, and infection.

In addition to feeding tubes, balloon tamponade tubes occasionally are used for nasogastric intubation in the treatment of bleeding esophageal and gastric varices. The balloon can be easily recognized when distended, and correct positioning can be evaluated radiographically. Esophageal rupture complicates approximately 5% of cases in which balloon tamponade tubes are used.

Ghahrenami GC: Complications due to the inadvertent tracheobronchial placement of feeding tubes. (Letter.) Radiology 1988;167:875.

Roubenhoff R, Ravich WJ: Pneumothorax due to nasogastric tubes: report of four cases, review of the literature, and recommendations for prevention. Arch Intern Med 1989;149:184–8.

Smith GM, Reed JC, Choplin RH: Radiographic detection of esophageal malpositioning of endotracheal tubes. AJR Am J Roentgenol 1990;154:23–6.

Woodall BH, Winfield DF, Bissett GS III: Inadvertent tracheobronchial placement of feeding tubes. Radiology 1987;165:727–9.

CHEST TUBES

Thoracostomy tubes ("chest tubes") are used for the evacuation of air or fluid from the pleural space. When chest tubes are used for relief of pneumothorax, apical location of the tip of the tube is most effective, whereas a tube inserted to drain free-flowing effusions should be placed in the dependent portion of the thorax. Chest radiographs, ultrasound, or CT should be used to guide correct placement of the tube for adequate drainage of a loculated effusion. Failure of the chest tube to decrease the pneumothorax or the effusion within several hours should arouse suspicion of a malpositioned tube. Tubes located within the pleural fissures are usually less effective in evacuating air or fluid collections. An interfissural location is suggested by orientation of the tube along the plane of the fissure on frontal radiographs and by lack of a gentle curvature near the site of penetration of the pleura, indicating failure of the tube to be deflected anteriorly or posteriorly in the pleural space. The lateral view may be confirmatory. Uncommonly, thoracostomy tubes may penetrate the lung, resulting in pulmonary laceration and bronchopleural fistula. Unilateral pulmonary edema may occur following rapid evacuation of a pneumothorax or pleural effusion that is of long standing or has produced significant compression atelectasis of lung.

Gayer G et al: CT diagnosis of malpositioned chest tubes. Br J Radiol 2000;73:786–90.

Webb WR, LaBerge JM: Radiographic recognition of chest tube malposition in the major fissure. Chest 1984;85:81–3.

IMAGING IN PULMONARY DISEASES

ROUTINE DAILY CHEST RADIOGRAPHS: UTILITY & EFFICACY

Portable chest radiographs are frequently obtained on a daily basis on ICU patients and as indicated by changes in the clinical situation. Several factors related to portable radiography may lead to difficulty in evaluation of radiographs in a critically ill patient. The equipment used for portable radiographs requires longer exposure time than standard radiographs obtained in the radiology department, sometimes resulting in artifacts due to respiratory, cardiac, and gross patient motion. Inadequate exposure may result from the limited power output of portable equipment. Special attention must be paid to the multiple monitoring devices required by the ICU patient, and considerable physical effort by the technologists is required to transport portable equipment.

Limitations imposed by the portable technique often complicate image interpretation. Almost all portable chest radiographs are taken with the patient supine and with the film placed behind the back of the patient (anteroposterior) rather than in the conventional upright, posteroanterior position used in the radiology department. Supine chest radiographs result in decreases in lung volume and can alter the size and appearance of the lungs, the pulmonary vasculature, and the mediastinum. Anteroposterior chest radiographs cause cardiac magnification, making evaluation of true cardiac size more difficult. Inspiratory films may be difficult to obtain because of respiratory distress, pain, sedation, or alterations of mental status. These technical limitations complicate diagnostic interpretation. Nonetheless, portable radiography continues to be a primary method of imaging critically ill patients.

Several studies have examined the efficacy of chest radiography in the ICU setting. When applied to imaging procedures, efficacy can be defined in three ways: (1) diagnostic efficacy, or the influence of a test on diagnosis; (2) therapeutic efficacy, or the influence of a test on management; and (3) outcome efficacy, or the influence of a test on eventual patient outcome. Since patient outcome depends primarily on the underlying disease process, few studies have been performed assessing the influence of chest radiography on the outcomes of patients receiving care in the ICU. In one prospective study, the diagnostic and therapeutic efficacy of chest radiography in a respiratory ICU was evaluated. Overall, 35% of chest radiographic examinations demonstrated either new or increased abnormalities or abnormalities of tube or catheter placement. Approximately 39% of routine and 50% of nonroutine films led to further diagnostic procedures, a change in therapy, or adjustment of a tube or catheter (therapeutic efficacy). When catheter position adjustments were excluded, a change in the diagnostic approach or therapy occurred after 24% of routine examinations. Not surprisingly, films obtained following a change in clinical condition had greater diagnostic efficacy than routine morning films, with an impact on patient management in 43% of cases. In another prospective study, the efficacy of bedside chest radiographs was investigated. Sixty-five percent of all radiographs showed moderate or marked cardiopulmonary abnormalities or tube or line malpositioning that affected clinical management. In a separate study, 45% of portable chest examinations showed new radiographic findings.

The utility of daily radiographs may depend on the underlying disease process. In a prospective study in ICU patients, clinically unsuspected abnormalities were observed on 17% of routine radiographs obtained on critically ill patients with pulmonary or complicated cardiac disease but in only 3% of patients without pulmonary or complicated cardiac disease. From these studies it would appear that chest radiographs obtained following an interventional procedure or change in clinical status of the patient are the most useful diagnostically. Routine daily radiographs are of greatest utility in patients with pulmonary or complicated cardiac disease. The American College of Radiology Thoracic Expert Panel concluded that daily chest radiographs are indicated on patients with acute cardiopulmonary problems and those receiving mechanical ventilation. In patients requiring cardiac monitoring or stable patients admitted for extrathoracic disease, an initial admission film is recommended. Additional radiographs are indicated when new support devices are placed or a specific question arises regarding cardiopulmonary status.

Bekemeyer WB et al: Efficacy of chest radiography in a respiratory intensive care unit. Chest 1985;88:691–6.

Henschke CI et al: Accuracy and efficacy of chest radiography in the intensive care unit. Radiol Clin North Am 1996;34:21–31.

Strain DS et al: Value of routine daily chest x-rays in the medical intensive care unit. Crit Care Med 1985;13:534.

Tocino I et al: Routine daily portable x-ray. American College of Radiology. ACR Appropriateness Criteria. Radiology 2000;215(Suppl):621–6.

ATELECTASIS

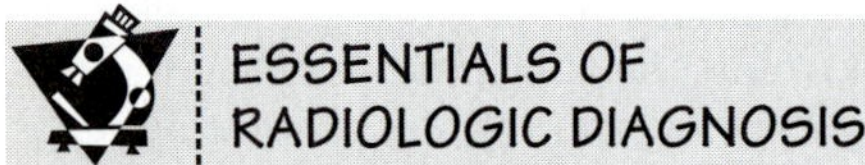

ESSENTIALS OF RADIOLOGIC DIAGNOSIS

- *Shift in position of a fissure or change in position of hila or mediastinum.*
- *Elevation of hemidiaphragm.*
- *Compensatory hyperexpansion of uninvolved lobes.*
- *Increased opacity of the atelectatic lung.*
- *Air bronchograms.*
- *Narrowing of rib interspaces.*

General Considerations

Atelectasis is the most common pulmonary parenchymal abnormality seen in ICU patients. Multiple factors contribute to the development of atelectasis. In the bedridden patient, hypoventilation results in atelectasis of the dependent lung. Central neurogenic depression, anesthesia, or splinting may decrease alveolar volume, reducing surfactant and promoting diffuse microatelectasis. Bronchial obstruction from retained secretions and mucous plugging may lead to postobstructive collapse of the distal lung, particularly in patients with pulmonary infection or chronic airway disorders. In the intubated or postoperative patient, other factors are contributory. A malpositioned endotracheal tube with right main stem bronchial intubation can cause atelectasis of the nonventilated left lung. Following cardiac surgery, left lower lobe collapse occurs frequently, owing in part to the weight of the heart unsupported by pericardium, which compresses the left lower lobe bronchus. Phrenic nerve paresis secondary to intraoperative cold cardioplegia results in diaphragmatic elevation and is also thought to contribute to lower lobe atelectasis.

Radiographic Features

The radiographic appearance of atelectasis depends largely on the degree and cause of lung collapse. Findings noted on the chest radiograph in atelectasis range from subtle diminution in lung volume without visible opacification to complete opacification of a segment, lobe, or lung. Dependent atelectasis occurring in supine patients may be demonstrated on thoracic CT even in healthy individuals but is usually not appreciated on plain chest radiography. Linear bands of opacity may be seen in "discoid" or "plate-like" atelectasis, whereas patchy opacity is seen with atelectasis of lung subtended by a segmental or subsegmental bronchus. With more extensive volume loss such as collapse of an entire lobe or lung, radiographic signs include an increase in opacity of the atelectatic lung; shift in the position of a fissure; change in the position of the mediastinum, hila, or diaphragm; and hyperexpansion of the uninvolved lung (Figure 7–4). In some cases, signs of volume loss may be absent because of exudation of fluid into the atelectatic lung.

Air bronchograms are linear lucencies coursing through opacified lung and represent patent bronchi and bronchioles surrounded by opacified air spaces. Air bronchograms are radiographically nonspecific and occur in any disorder in which patent air-containing bronchi are situated within consolidated lung, including atelectasis, pulmonary edema, pneumonia, and hemorrhage. The presence of air bronchograms is also variable in atelectasis and depends on the patency of the major airways and the cause of atelectasis. Air bronchograms may be useful predictors of the effectiveness of bronchoscopy in patients with lobar collapse. Patients without air bronchograms are more likely to demonstrate improvement following fiberoptic bronchoscopy than those with air bronchograms. The absence of air bronchograms in lobar collapse suggests that central airways may be plugged by secretions which by virtue of their proximal location are amenable to bronchoscopic removal. In contrast, the presence of air bronchograms suggests that the collapse is more apt to be due to small airway collapse or peripheral mucous plugs that are not effectively treated by therapeutic fiberoptic bronchoscopy.

The left lower lobe is the most frequent location of lobar atelectasis, with collapse occurring two to three times more often in the left lower than in the right lower lobe. The cause is uncertain, though many of the factors cited above are contributory. The radiographic

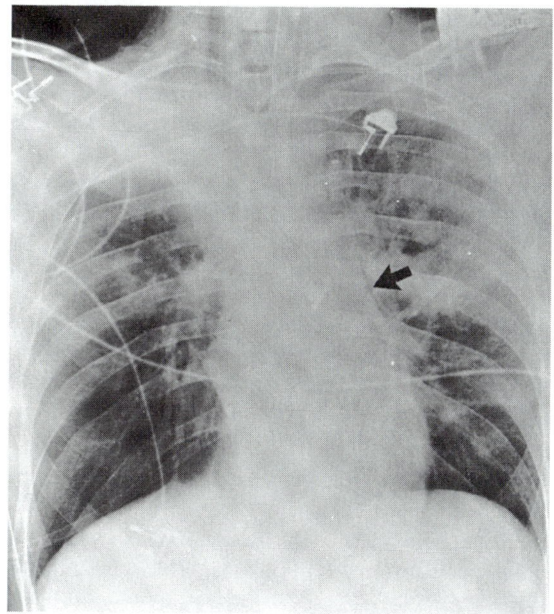

Figure 7–4. Atelectasis in a 22-year-old man with status asthmaticus. The right upper lobe is opaque, and there is elevation of the minor fissure consistent with right upper lobe collapse. Areas of increased density in the left lung are also due to atelectasis. Lucency adjacent to the left heart border secondary to pneumomediastinum is present (arrow), and there is subcutaneous emphysema in the right supraclavicular region.

features of left lower lobe collapse include a triangular opacity in the retrocardiac region and loss of definition of the descending aorta and left hemidiaphragm—as well as other signs of volume loss outlined above (Figure 7–5). Adequate penetration and patient positioning are important in assessing left lower lobe disease. Left lower lobe collapse may be falsely diagnosed secondary to faulty radiologic technique. Cephalic angulation of the radiographic beam by 10–15 degrees (lordotic positioning) may cause projection of extrapleural fat onto the base of the left lung and result in loss of tangential imaging of the apex of the hemidiaphragm and subsequent loss of definition of the diaphragm in the absence of left lower lobe disease. In instances in which patients are examined radiographically with even a small degree of lordosis, loss of definition of the diaphragm therefore cannot be assumed to be secondary to left lower lobe collapse. Ancillary findings, including depression of the hilum, crowding of vessels, and air bronchograms, must be used to diagnose true left lower lobe disease.

Many other causes of parenchymal opacification may be confused with atelectasis, including pneumonia and pulmonary infarction. In addition to other features previously discussed, temporal sequence may be helpful in distinguishing atelectasis from other causes of focal parenchymal opacification. Whereas atelectasis may appear within minutes to hours and may also clear rapidly, pneumonia and infarction typically resolve over days to weeks.

Woodring JH, Reed JC: Types and mechanisms of pulmonary atelectasis. J Thorac Imaging 1996;11:92–108.

Zylak CJ, Littleton JT, Durizch ML: Illusory consolidation of the left lower lobe: A pitfall of portable radiography. Radiology 1988;167:653–5.

PNEUMONIA

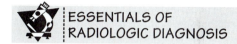

- *May present as lobar pneumonia, bronchopneumonia, or interstitial pneumonia.*
- *Parapneumonic effusions and cavitation may be present.*
- *Hilar or mediastinal densities may lead to suspicion of obstruction due to cancer.*

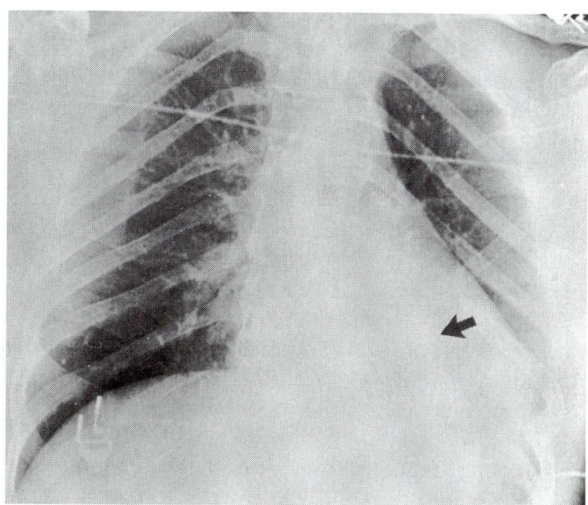

Figure 7–5. Left lower lobe collapse in a 20-year-old man with head trauma sustained in a motor vehicle accident. A triangular region of increased opacity is present in the retrocardiac region secondary to left lower lobe collapse. The major fissure is displaced inferiorly (arrow).

- *In ICU patients, development of new or worsening parenchymal pulmonary infiltrates may indicate nosocomial pneumonia, especially if accompanied by cavitation.*

General Considerations

Patients with severe pneumonia complicated by sepsis, respiratory failure, hypotension, or shock are frequently seen in the ICU. Some patients will have acquired pneumonia outside of the hospital (community-acquired), but an important problem is that of nosocomial pneumonia, defined as lower respiratory tract infection occurring more than 72 hours after admission. Nosocomial pneumonia is the most common infection leading to death among hospitalized patients. Factors contributing to the high incidence of hospital-acquired pneumonias include endotracheal intubation or tracheostomy, aspiration, and impaired host defenses. Prior antibiotic therapy promotes colonization of the tracheobronchial tree.

Most radiologists sort the radiographic appearance of pneumonias into three categories that may aid in differentiation: lobar (alveolar or air space) pneumonia, lobular pneumonia (bronchopneumonia), and interstitial pneumonia. Lobar pneumonia is characterized on x-ray by relatively homogeneous regions of increased lung opacity and air bronchograms. The entire lobe need not be involved, and in fact, with early therapy, consolidation does not usually affect the entire lobe. Pathologically, the infecting organism reaches the distal air spaces, resulting in edema filling the alveoli. The infected edema fluid spreads centripetally throughout the lobe via communicating channels to adjacent segments. Air bronchograms are common. *Streptococcus pneumoniae* (pneumococcal) pneumonia is the classic lobar pneumonia, though other organisms, including *Klebsiella pneumoniae* and *Legionella pneumophila,* may produce an identical pattern. Since the airways are not primarily involved, volume loss is not conspicuous. Indeed, expansion of the lobe may occur in klebsiella or pneumococcal pneumonia.

Bronchopneumonia (lobular pneumonia) results from inflammation involving the terminal and respiratory bronchioles rather than the distal air spaces. Since the process focuses in the airways, the distribution is more segmental and patchy, affecting some lobules and sparing others. Pathologically, there is less edema fluid and more inflammation of the mucosa of bronchi and bronchioles. In bronchopneumonia, the consolidation is patchy, sparing some segments while involving others. Mild associated volume loss may be present. Air bronchograms are not as common a feature in bronchopneumonia as in lobar pneumonia. The most common organisms producing classic bronchopneumonia are *Staphylococcus aureus* and pseudomonas species.

Interstitial pneumonia is typically caused by viruses or *Mycoplasma pneumoniae.* In the immunocompromised patient, *Pneumocystis carinii* is an important cause of interstitial pneumonia. The pathologic process is primarily located in the interstitium, and the classic radiograph reflects the interstitial process and demonstrates an increase in linear or reticular markings in the lung parenchyma with peribronchial thickening and occasionally septal lines (Kerley A and B lines). Although the pathologic process is primarily located in the interstitium, proteinaceous fluid is exuded into the air spaces and consequently may progress to a pneumonia that radiographically appears alveolar.

Radiographic Features

A. Plain Films

Although plain films cannot provide a specific microbial diagnosis in a patient with pneumonia, radiology has a central role in both initial evaluation and treatment. The chest radiograph documents the presence and extent of disease. Associated parapneumonic effusions, mediastinal or hilar adenopathy, cavitation, and abscess formation—as well as predisposing conditions such as central bronchogenic carcinoma—may be identified. Such information can guide the clinician to a high-yield diagnostic procedure such as thoracentesis or bronchoscopy, which may be necessary in a patient who cannot produce adequate sputum for bacteriologic culture. The chest radiograph is also critical in evaluating the patient's response to therapy. Antibiotic therapy is frequently empiric, and the chest radiograph may be the first indicator of failure of antibiotics and a need for change in management. A pneumonia that does not clear despite antibiotic therapy should raise the suspicion of central airway obstruction by a mass or foreign body or may represent a bronchoalveolar cell carcinoma mimicking pneumonia.

Localization of the consolidation to a specific lobe is important not only to correlate with the physical examination but also to guide the bronchoscopist when necessary. In addition, different types of pneumonia may be more likely to occur in specific regions, eg, reactivation tuberculosis in the apical and posterior segments of the upper lobes and the superior segment of the lower lobes. The silhouette sign is useful in determining the site of pneumonia. When consolidation is adjacent to a structure of soft tissue density (eg, the heart or the diaphragm), the margin of the soft tissue structure will be obliterated by the opaque lung. For example, right middle lobe consolidation may cause loss of the margin of the right heart border, lingular consolidation may cause loss of the left heart border, and lower lobe pneumonia may obliterate the diaphragmatic contour.

Intrathoracic nodal enlargement may be a useful diagnostic feature. Enlargement of the hilar or mediastinal lymph nodes is uncommon in bacterial pneumonia and most viral pneumonias. Tuberculosis, atypical mycobacterial infections, fungal infections such as coccidioidomycosis and histoplasmosis, and viral infections such as measles and infectious mononucleosis may be associated with adenopathy.

Pleural effusion occurs in up to 40% of patients with bacterial pneumonia. A parapneumonic effusion consists of intrapleural fluid in association with pneumonia or lung abscess. Empyema is defined as pus in the pleural space. Thoracentesis is required for differentiation of a simple parapneumonic effusion from empyema, and the decision to place a chest tube is dependent on the characteristics and the quantity of the effusion. Pleural effusion is usually identified radiographically on a plain film, though ultrasound or CT may be necessary in some cases.

1. Lung abscess and cavitation—Cavitation of pneumonia results from destruction of lung tissue by the inflammatory process, leading to lung abscess formation (Figure 7–6). Although often seen in pneumonias due to gram-negative organisms such a pseudomonas and klebsiella, cavitation is rare in pneumococcal pneumonia. Pneumonias due to *Mycobacterium tuberculosis,* atypical mycobacteria, and fungi and those due to anaerobes and staphylococci also frequently cavitate. Cavitary lung abscesses must be distinguished from bullae, pneumatoceles, cavitary lung cancers, and other lucent lesions. Most abscesses have a wall thickness between 5 mm and 15 mm, allowing differentiation from bullae and pneumatoceles, which usually have thin, smooth walls. Lung abscess is usually surrounded by adjacent parenchymal consolidation, which may serve to differentiate abscess from cavitary bronchogenic carcinoma. Complications of lung abscess include sepsis, cerebral abscess, hemorrhage, and spillage of contents of the cavity into uninfected lung.

In one review, 18% of lung abscesses were radiographically occult, with only nonspecific lung opacities or nodules identified. In these patients, the diagnosis was made at surgery or at postmortem examination. One reason lung abscesses were not identified was probably failure to use a horizontal beam in obtaining the chest radiographs. With semierect or supine positioning, air-fluid levels within the cavity were obscured. In cases where erect chest films are unobtainable, decubitus or cross-table lateral views can be obtained with a horizontal beam and may be diagnostic.

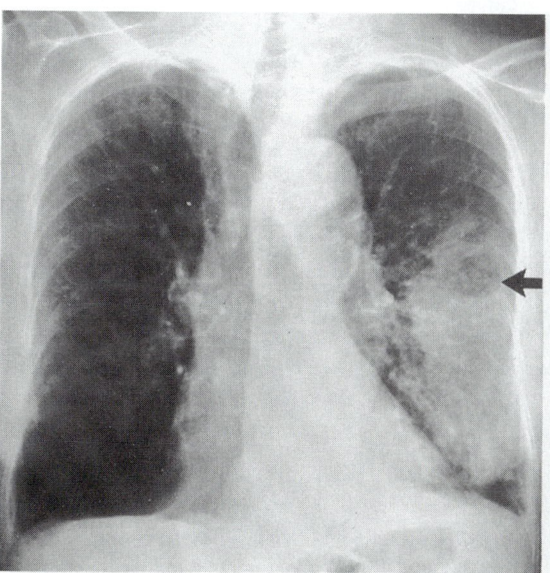
A

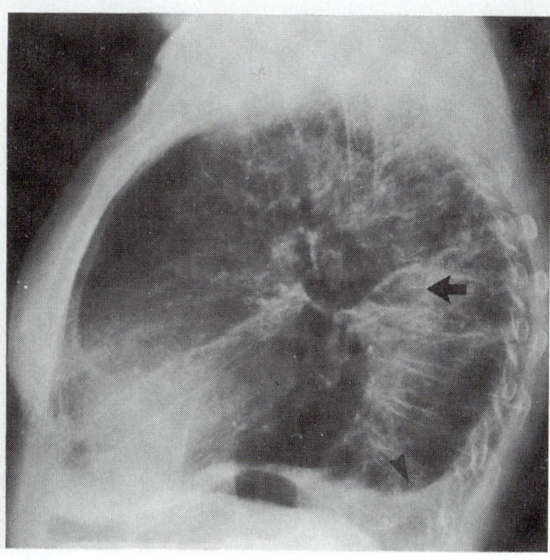
B

Figure 7–6. Cavitary pneumonia. Posteroanterior ***(A)*** and lateral ***(B)*** chest radiographs demonstrate consolidation with cavitation (arrows) in the superior segment of the left lower lobe secondary to pseudomonas pneumonia. A small left pleural effusion is present, best seen on the lateral view (arrowhead). Changes of chronic obstructive pulmonary disease are present.

2. Nosocomial pneumonia—Definitive diagnosis of nosocomial pneumonia is difficult because both the clinical features and the chest radiographic findings may be present in other disease processes and because abnormalities on chest radiographs are often present prior to development of nosocomial pneumonia. Clinical suspicion in patients with underlying heart and lung disease is important. For example, the incidence of nosocomial pneumonia is increased in patients with ARDS as well as in other patients with respiratory failure. In a multi-institutional study of pneumonias in patients admitted to the ICU, a 31% risk of developing pneumonia followed intubation. Since virtually all intubated patients develop colonization of the tracheobronchial tree by approximately 48 hours after intubation, sputum cultures may be unreliable. Fever and leukocytosis are nonspecific. The overall mortality rate in this study was 40%; the mortality rate was 47% in nosocomial pneumonia versus 17% in community-acquired pneumonia. A bacteriologic diagnosis was

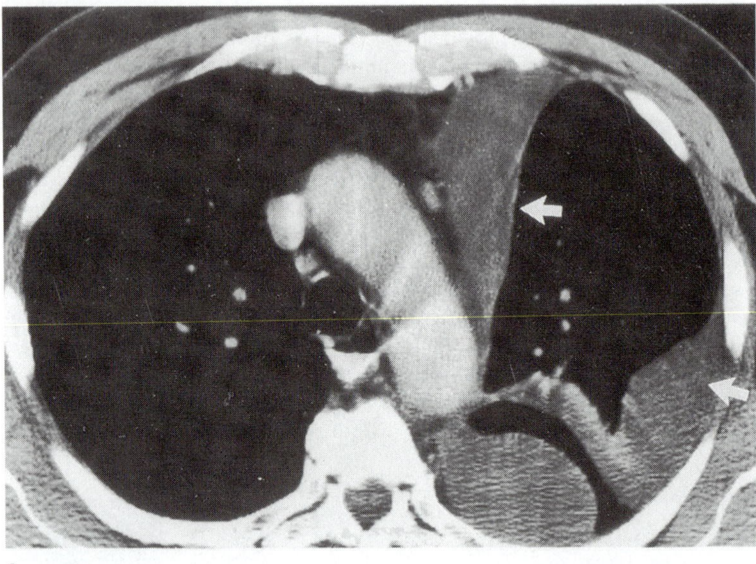

A

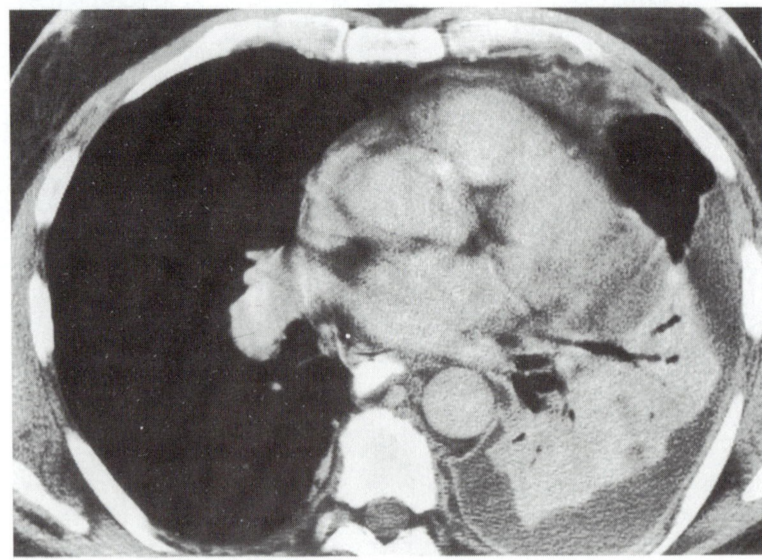

B

Figure 7–7. Pneumonia with loculated empyema. ***A:*** CT shows a loculated pleural effusion in the left hemithorax (arrows). ***B:*** More caudally, dense consolidation with air bronchograms secondary to pneumonia is present in the left lower lobe. The consolidated lung enhances with contrast and is easily distinguished from the surrounding pleural effusion.

made in only 38% of nosocomial pneumonias, with the majority caused by gram-negative aerobic bacteria. *S aureus* is also an important pathogen in nosocomial pneumonias in tertiary care centers.

Radiographically, nosocomial pneumonia is heralded by the development of new or worsening parenchymal opacities, usually multifocal. Since nosocomial pneumonias are most often due to aerobic gram-negative organisms or staphylococci, abscesses and pleural effusions may develop. Development of cavitation helps to distinguish nosocomial pneumonia from other causes of parenchymal opacification such as atelectasis, lung contusion, or pulmonary edema.

B. Computed Tomography

The cross-sectional imaging plane and superior contrast resolution make CT useful in the evaluation of complicated inflammatory disease. Cavitation, which may be obscured on plain films, is easily identified on CT. Localization of parenchymal disease facilitates the direction of invasive studies such as bronchoscopy or open lung biopsy. Superimposed pleural and parenchymal processes are more easily differentiated on CT than on plain films (Figure 7–7). Loculated pleural effusion or empyema associated with pneumonia may be difficult to evacuate, and CT may serve to guide thoracentesis, chest tube placement, or percutaneous drainage of large lung abscesses.

Empyema and lung abscess are more easily distinguished on CT than on conventional radiographs. In one study, CT was able to correctly localize 100% of inflammatory thoracic lesions of the lung or the pleura. Separation of thickened visceral and parietal pleural surfaces ("split pleura sign") and compression of lung were specific for empyema and were not identified in any cases of lung abscess. Other useful findings included wall characteristics, with smooth uniform walls seen in empyema and thick irregular walls more commonly seen in lung abscess. The size and shape of the lesion were less helpful; though lung abscesses generally tended to be round—as opposed to lenticular in empyemas—this finding was not absolute. The administration of intravenous contrast facilitates differentiation of pleural and parenchymal disease, since the lung parenchyma will enhance with contrast whereas the pleural effusion will retain its low attenuation.

Armstrong P, Wilson AG, Dee P (editors): *Imaging of Diseases of the Chest.* Year Book, 1990.

Bowton DL, Bass DA: Community-acquired pneumonia: The clinical dilemma. J Thorac Imaging 1991;6:1–5.

Ely EW, Maponik EF: Pneumonia in the elderly patient. J Thorac Imaging 1991;6:45–61.

Groskin SA et al: Bacterial lung abscess: A review of the radiographic and clinical features of 50 cases. J Thorac Imaging 1991;6:62–7.

Light RW (editor): *Pleural Diseases,* 2nd ed. Lea & Febiger, 1990.

Lipchik RJ, Kuzo RS: Nosocomial pneumonia. Radiol Clin North Am 1996;34:47–58.

Norwood SH, Civetta JM: Evaluating sepsis in the critically ill patient. Chest 1987;92:137–44.

Ruiz-Santana S et al: ICU pneumonias: A multi-institutional study. Crit Care Med 1987;15:930–2.

ASPIRATION PNEUMONIA

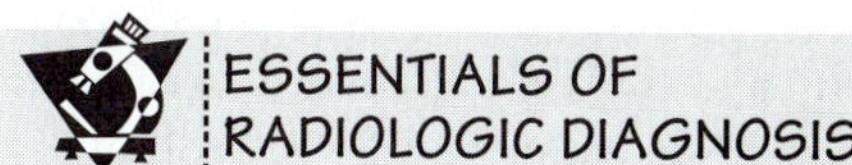
ESSENTIALS OF
RADIOLOGIC DIAGNOSIS

- *Consolidation in dependent regions of the lung, varying with position of patient at time of aspiration, but may be multilobar and bilateral.*
- *Cavitation and abscess formation may be seen, but pleural effusions are infrequent.*
- *May lead to necrotizing pneumonia and lung abscess.*
- *Aspiration of gastric contents may result in noncardiogenic pulmonary edema, cavitation, and atelectasis.*

General Considerations

Aspiration pneumonia results from endotracheal aspiration of oropharyngeal or gastric secretions. Aspiration is thought to be a common occurrence in the healthy adult, with the incidence during sleep estimated to be as high as 45%. Small-volume aspirates are cleared by physical entrapment and coughing along with the mucociliary elevator action of the respiratory epithelium. Inactivation by IgA antibodies and opsonization and ingestion of bacteria by phagocytic cells play a role as well. Although organisms are present in pathogenic numbers even in small-volume aspirates, normal individuals are able to clear these organisms without sequelae.

Several clinical conditions predispose patients to aspiration. Depressed levels of consciousness secondary to medications, alcoholic excess, seizures, anesthesia, or neurologic disease result in impaired upper airway reflexes. Endotracheal intubation increases the rate of aspiration, with both high-volume, low-pressure cuffs and uncuffed or low-volume, high-pressure tubes implicated. The incidence of aspiration is even higher in patients with tracheostomies as compared with endotracheal tubes. Nasogastric and feeding tubes, gastric distention, gastroesophageal reflux, hiatal hernia, decreased esophageal mobility, and vomiting have all been cited as predisposing factors for aspiration. Bacterial colonization of gastric secretions also plays a role in the development of aspiration pneumonia. Although gastric acidity prevents significant bacterial colonization, antacid therapy for prophylaxis for stress ulcers may change gastric pH, resulting in increased bacterial colonization of gastric secretions.

Aspiration pneumonia occurs when a normal host aspirates a large amount of contaminated matter, overwhelming host defenses, or when smaller amounts are aspirated in a patient with impaired defenses. Aspiration pneumonia is caused by mixed anaerobic and aerobic infection, with up to 80% of cases caused by multiple organisms. The organisms responsible for the pneumonia vary with the clinical setting—community-acquired, nursing home, or hospitalized patients—and reflect colonization of the upper airway. Aerobic bacteria associated with community-acquired aspiration pneumonia are mostly streptococci, whereas gram-negative organisms, particularly klebsiella and *Escherichia coli,* are seen more often in nosocomial infection. The major anaerobic organisms include *Fusobacterium nucleatum,* peptostreptococcus, *Bacteroides melaninogenicus,* and *Bacteroides intermedius.*

There are three general clinical patterns that may be seen following aspiration: (1) respiratory compromise followed by rapid clinical and radiographic improvement; (2) rapid clinical and radiographic progression; and (3) transient stabilization followed by protracted worsening of clinical and radiographic status, with bacterial superinfection or ARDS.

Aspiration of acidic gastric contents resulting in an acute pulmonary reaction with pulmonary edema is sometimes called Mendelson's syndrome. Manifestations depend on the volume, pH, and distribution of the aspirate. The absorption of acid by the pulmonary vasculature and subsequent pulmonary injury are almost immediate and lead to consolidation, alveolar hemorrhage, and collapse with transudation of fibrin and plasma into the alveoli. Aspiration of a combination of acid and gastric particulate material produces a more severe injury pattern than either acid or gastric particulate matter alone.

Radiographic Features

Aspiration pneumonia results in consolidation in dependent regions of the lung. The location of the pneumonia will vary according to the patient's position at the time of aspiration. In the supine patient, the superior segments of the lower lobes, the posterior segment of the right upper lobe, and the posterior subsegment of the left upper lobe are involved—whereas in the upright patient, the basal segments of the lower lobes are more often affected, particularly on the right. The more obtuse angle between the trachea and the right main stem bronchus compared with the angle of the trachea and the left main stem bronchus results in a higher percentage of right-sided abnormalities in the supine patient. Consolidation is usually multilobar and bilateral (Figure 7–8). Because of frequent infection with anaerobes, cavitation and abscess formation may be seen. Effusions are infrequent.

Complications of simple aspiration pneumonia include necrotizing pneumonitis and lung abscess. Necrotizing pneumonia results in multiple small cavities within the involved lung and may extend into the pleural space, leading to empyema. Lung abscess radiographically appears as a cavitary lesion within a focus of consolidation, usually solitary. Empyema is less likely in lung abscess since extension of infection into the pleural space is usually impeded by the barrier effect of the fibrous wall of the abscess cavity.

Patients who aspirate gastric contents may develop a chemical pneumonitis that shows characteristics consistent with noncardiogenic pulmonary edema. ARDS and features of secondary bacterial infection may follow, including lung necrosis and cavitation. Atelectasis may be a feature of airway obstruction with food particles.

Elpern EH, Jacobs ER, Bone RC: Incidence of aspiration in tracheally intubated adults. Heart Lung 1987;16:527–31.

Pennza PT: Aspiration pneumonia, necrotizing pneumonia, and lung abscess. Emerg Med Clin North Am 1989;7:279–307.

Shifrin RY, Choplin RH: Aspiration in patients in critical care units. Radiol Clin North Am 1996;34:83–96.

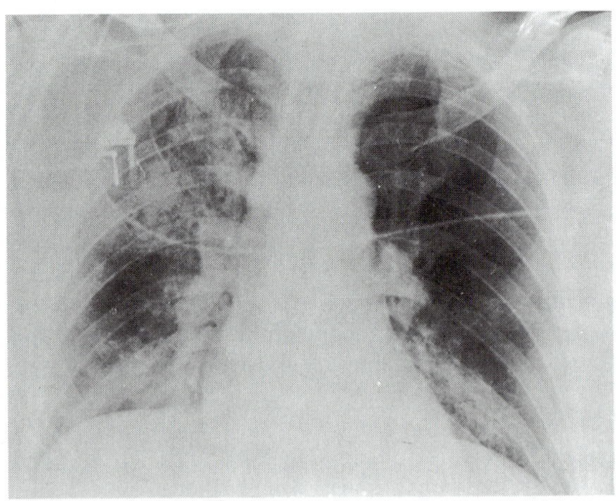

Figure 7–8. Aspiration pneumonia. Multiple areas of pulmonary opacification are present bilaterally—secondary to aspiration pneumonia following drug overdose.

CHRONIC OBSTRUCTIVE PULMONARY DISEASE

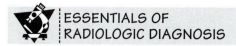

- *Hyperinflation.*
- *Bullae or blebs.*
- *Pulmonary arterial deficiency pattern (areas of decreased pulmonary vasculature).*
- *Features of pulmonary hypertension.*

General Considerations

Chronic obstructive pulmonary disease (COPD) is any pulmonary disorder characterized by airflow obstruction. Emphysema and chronic bronchitis are the most common examples. Emphysema is defined as a lung condition characterized by enlargement of the air spaces distal to the terminal bronchiole, accompanied by destruction of the walls and without obvious fibrosis. Four principal types of emphysema are described: centrilobular, panlobular, paraseptal, and paracicatricial. Chronic bronchitis is usually defined in clinical terms, manifested by chronic productive cough for at least 3 months for a minimum of 2 consecutive years and characterized by excessive secretion of mucus in the bronchi. Emphysema and chronic bronchitis frequently coexist.

Radiographic Features

There is considerable controversy regarding the utility of the chest radiograph in the evaluation of emphysema. Although moderate to severe emphysema is usually apparent on the chest radiograph, mild disease is difficult to appreciate. Hyperinflation results from obstruction of small airways, resulting in air trapping. Radiographic features include an increase in size of the retrosternal clear space, flattening of the hemidiaphragms, increased height of the lung, and increased radiolucency (Figure 7–9). Measurements obtained from chest x-rays have shown that the height of the lung and the height of the arc of the right hemidiaphragm correlate best with spirometric measures such as the forced expiratory volume in 1 second (FEV_1) and forced vital capacity (FVC). A lung height of 29.9 cm or greater, as measured from the tubercle of the first rib to the dome of the right hemidiaphragm, will identify 70% of patients with abnormal pulmonary function tests. A height of the right hemidiaphragm of less than 2.6 cm on the lateral projection identifies 68% of patients with abnormal pulmonary function tests.

Bullae and blebs appear as focal regions of hyperlucency. Although good indicators of emphysema, they may also be seen in patients without COPD. Bullae are recognized as hyperlucent or avascular regions and are occasionally demarcated peripherally by a fine curvilinear wall. The lung adjacent to large bullae may be compressed, and redistribution of pulmonary blood flow away from areas of extensive bullous disease may occur. The arterial deficiency pattern refers to regions of radiolucent, hypovascular pulmonary parenchyma characterized by a decrease in the size and number of vessels. This appearance may be due to multiple bullae. Emphysema can eventually lead to pulmonary arterial hypertension, manifested radiographically by disproportionate enlargement of the central pulmonary arteries and right heart chambers.

The radiographic appearance of the lungs in chronic bronchitis is even less specific. Unlike that of emphysema, the diagnosis of chronic bronchitis is based on clinical symptoms and not morphologic appearance. In addition, chronic bronchitis and emphysema frequently coexist, making pure chronic bronchitis difficult to characterize. Radiographic findings suggesting chronic bronchitis include thickening of bronchial walls and increased linear markings ("dirty lungs"). Hyperinflation and hypovascularity have been described but are probably due to concomitant emphysema.

High-resolution CT (HRCT) is more sensitive than plain radiographs in the detection of emphysema. On HRCT, emphysema appears as regions of low attenuation, lung destruction, or simplification of the pulmonary vasculature. The type of emphysema can often be defined by its pattern and distribution on CT, with centrilobular CT predominantly upper zone in distribution and panlobular emphysema more diffuse or more severe within the lower lobes. The CT appearance of chronic bronchitis may be overshadowed by coexisting emphysema. Bronchial wall thickening and centrilobular abnormalities have been described.

Cleverley JR, Muller NL: Advances in radiologic assessment of chronic obstructive pulmonary disease. Clin Chest Med 2000;21:653–63.

Johnson MM et al: Radiographic assessment of hyperinflation: correlation with objective chest radiographic measurements and mechanical ventilator parameters. Chest 1998;113:1698–704.

Lillington GA, Müller NL: Radiological imaging in the detection and differentiation of diffuse obstructive airway diseases. Clin Rev Allergy 1990;8:277–90.

Reich SB, Weinshelbaum A, Yee J: Correlation of radiographic measurements and pulmonary function tests in chronic obstructive pulmonary disease. AJR Am J Roentgenol 1985;144:695–9.

Thurlbeck WM, Müller NL: Emphysema: Definition, imaging and quantification. AJR Am J Roentgenol 1994; 163:1017–25.

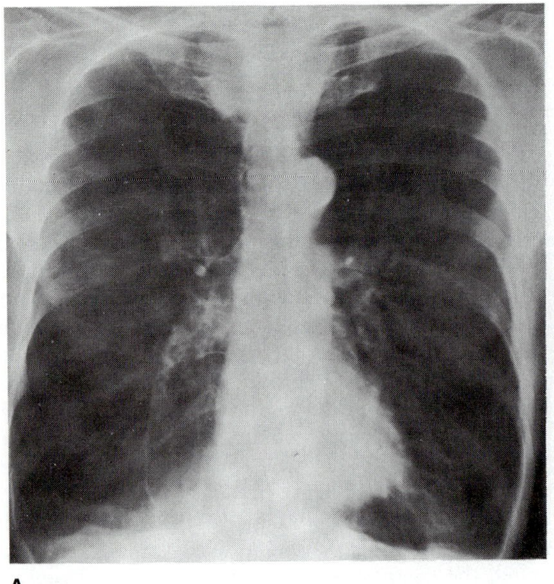
A

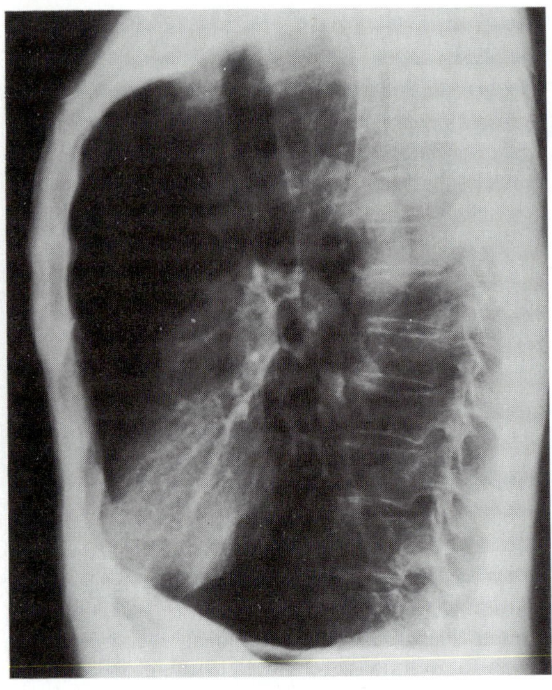
B

Figure 7–9. Chronic obstructive pulmonary disease. Posteroanterior ***(A)*** and lateral ***(B)*** chest radiographs show hyperinflated lungs with increased anteroposterior diameters, flattening of the diaphragm, and increased retrosternal clear space.

Webb WR: Radiology of obstructive pulmonary disease. AJR Am J Roentgenol 1997;169:637–47.

ASTHMA

ESSENTIALS OF RADIOLOGIC DIAGNOSIS

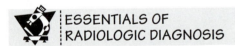

- *Hyperinflation.*
- *Peribronchial thickening.*
- *Increased lung markings centrally.*
- *Subsegmental atelectasis.*

General Considerations

Asthma is a disease characterized by widespread narrowing of the airways that fluctuates in severity over short periods of time either spontaneously or following therapy. Hyperactivity of airways may be induced by a variety of stimuli, and asthma is usually divided into two types: intrinsic and extrinsic. Pathologic changes include smooth muscle hypertrophy, mucosal edema, mucous hypersecretion, and plugging of airways by thick, viscid mucus. The result is narrowing of the airway diameter.

Radiographic Features

The radiographic manifestations of asthma vary from a normal radiograph to hyperinflation, atelectasis, or barotrauma. Radiographic findings may be categorized as (1) those common features of asthma that do not affect management and are therefore not unanimously considered abnormalities, and (2) findings that influence patient management. The incidence of radiographic abnormalities is dependent upon the age of the patient and the definition of "abnormal" by the investigator.

A. Uncomplicated Asthma

Hyperinflation, bronchial wall thickening, and prominent perihilar vascular markings are all features commonly seen in uncomplicated asthma that do not alter patient management. Hyperinflation, characterized by flattening of the hemidiaphragms and an increase in the retrosternal clear space, results from air trapping. Bowing of the sternum, another sign of hyperinflation, is more frequently seen in the pediatric population, probably secondary to more pliable osseous structures. Hyperinflation is not specific for asthma and occurs in other pulmonary diseases associated with air trapping, including emphysema and cystic fibrosis.

Bronchial wall thickening results from edema of the bronchial wall and can be diagnosed when the walls of secondary bronchi peripheral to the central bronchi appear abnormally thickened. Identification of bronchial wall thickening may be difficult and is best made when serial films are compared. Mucous plugs may be identified as tubular or branching soft tissue densities; plugging of large airways may result in atelectasis. Prominent perihilar vascular shadows and prominence of the main pulmonary artery segment are probably due to transient pulmonary arterial hypertension and are more often seen in children.

B. Complications of Asthma

Radiographic findings that alter medical management and are therefore considered as manifestations of complicated asthma consist of pneumonia, segmental or lobar atelectasis, and barotrauma, including pneumomediastinum and pneumothorax. Exacerbation of asthma secondary to pneumonia is usually secondary to viral infection. Although subsegmental atelectasis from mucous plugging is common in uncomplicated asthma, plugging of large airways may result in lobar collapse (Figure 7–4). Lobar atelectasis occurs more often in children, with an incidence between 5% and 10%.

Pneumomediastinum complicating asthma is uncommon but has been reported in 1–5% of cases of acute asthma. This complication occurs primarily in children; the presumed mechanism is an increase in intra-alveolar pressure and subsequent alveolar rupture secondary to mucous plugging, giving rise to pulmonary interstitial emphysema. Central dissection of air along the perivascular sheaths results in pneumomediastinum and may eventuate in subcutaneous emphysema and pneumothorax. In aerated lung, pulmonary interstitial emphysema is usually not identifiable, but the sequelae of pneumomediastinum and pneumothorax may be recognized.

C. Assessment of Asthma Severity

Several studies have addressed the usefulness of chest radiography in acute asthma. Although the findings of hyperinflation, increased perihilar markings, bronchial wall thickening, and subsegmental atelectasis are frequently seen, identification of these abnormalities does not change medical management. For example, in 95% of pediatric patients evaluated for asthma, vital signs and pretreatment auscultation identified those children with complicated asthma. A respiratory rate of 60/min or higher, a heart rate of 160/min or higher, a body temperature of 38.3 °C or higher, localized rales, or localized decreased breath sounds prior to therapy allowed identification of 20 of 21 children with complicated asthma. In another study, only 2.2% of adult asthmatics had radiographic abnormalities, compared with 13% of children. The authors concluded that a chest radiograph in an adult asthmatic is unnecessary unless the patient is unresponsive to therapy and requires hospitalization. Most investigators agree that a chest radiograph should be obtained when asthma is initially diagnosed to rule out other causes of wheezing such as airway obstruction by tumor or foreign body, congestive heart failure, bronchiectasis, or pulmonary embolism.

D. High-Resolution CT

HRCT is rarely used to evaluate patients with asthma. Bronchial wall thickening with mild bronchiectasis may be seen with mucous plugging of small centrilobular bronchioles, resulting in a tree-in-bud appearance. Air trapping may be identified with focal or diffuse hyperlucency, accentuated on expiratory images.

Blair DN, Coppage L, Shaw C: Medical imaging in asthma. J Thorac Imaging 1986;1:23–35.

Friedman PJ: Radiology of the airways with emphasis on the small airways. J Thorac Imaging 1986;1:7–22.

Lynch DA: Imaging of asthma and allergic bronchopulmonary mycoses. Radiol Clin North Am 1998;36:129–142.

EPIGLOTTITIS

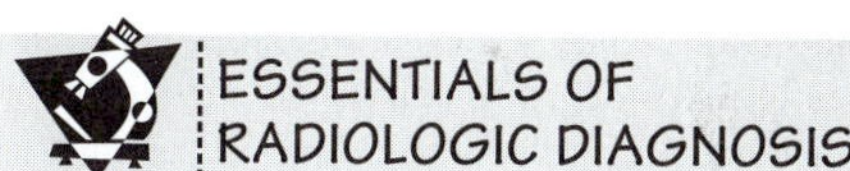
ESSENTIALS OF
RADIOLOGIC DIAGNOSIS

- *Enlargement of the epiglottis and thickening of the aryepiglottic folds on lateral radiographs of the neck.*
- *Ballooned hypopharynx, narrowed tracheal air column, prevertebral soft tissue swelling, and obliteration of the vallecula and piriform sinuses.*

General Considerations

Epiglottitis is a potentially lethal infection of the epiglottis and larynx resulting in supraglottic airway obstruction. Although usually a disorder of children aged 3–6 years, epiglottitis can occur in adults as well. In the pediatric patient, the causative organism is usually *Haemophilus influenzae,* whereas in adults the etiologic agents also include *Haemophilus parainfluenzae,* pneumococci, group A streptococci, and *S aureus.* Epiglottitis results in edema of the epiglottis, aryepiglottic folds, false cords, and subglottic region and may involve the entire pharyngeal wall. The clinical presentation differs somewhat in children and adults, with fever more common in the pediatric patient.

Radiographic Features

The radiologic examination may be diagnostic. However, sudden death from airway obstruction is known to occur, and patients should be accompanied by a physician during the examination in the event that emergency endotracheal intubation or tracheostomy is necessary. Films should be obtained in the erect position to minimize respiratory distress; manipulation of the neck should be avoided. A single lateral radiograph of the neck should be confirmatory. In the patient with obvious (classic) epiglottitis, roentgenographic diagnosis is not necessary, and airway management is started immediately.

In acute epiglottitis, enlargement of the epiglottis and thickening of the aryepiglottic folds are noted in 80–100% of patients. The normal epiglottis has a shape like a little finger, whereas the enlarged epiglottis has been likened to a thumb ("thumb sign"). Other radiographic features of acute epiglottitis include a ballooned hypopharynx, narrowed tracheal air column, prevertebral soft tissue swelling, and obliteration of the vallecula and the piriform sinuses. In one report of an affected adult, CT examination demonstrated enlargement of the epiglottis and aryepiglottic folds as well as induration of preepiglottic fat. CT is not appropriate in children with suspected epiglottitis and is rarely required in an adult.

Radiography may be useful in distinguishing epiglottitis from other causes of upper airway obstruction in the pediatric patient such as croup, retropharyngeal abscess, or foreign body aspiration.

Flom LL: Upper airway obstruction in the pediatric patient. Emerg Med Clin North Am 1991;9:757–66.

Hodge KM, Ganzel TM: Diagnostic and therapeutic efficiency in croup and epiglottitis. Laryngoscope 1987;97:621–5.

Waeden CA, Rogers LF: CT evaluation of adult epiglottitis. J Comput Assist Tomogr 1989;13:883–5.

PULMONARY EMBOLISM

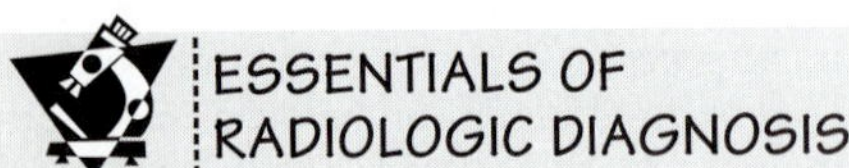
ESSENTIALS OF
RADIOLOGIC DIAGNOSIS

- *Chest radiograph usually abnormal but nonspecific, showing atelectasis. Useful to exclude pneumonia, pneumothorax, and pulmonary edema.*
- *In pulmonary embolism, chest radiograph may show focal oligemia and radiolucency. In pulmonary infarction, may show peripheral parenchymal opacities.*
- *Pleural effusions frequently occur.*
- *Ventilation-perfusion lung scan used to assess probability of pulmonary embolism in a given patient.*
- *Spiral or electron beam CT allows for direct visualization of thrombus and parenchymal and pleural changes secondary to pulmonary embolism.*
- *If clinical suspicion of pulmonary embolism is strong but the patient has an indeterminate, intermediate, or low-probability ventilation-perfusion scan, pulmonary angiography is necessary for diagnosis.*

General Considerations

Pulmonary embolism is a common life-threatening disorder that results from venous thrombosis, usually arising in the deep veins of the lower extremities. In situ pulmonary arterial thrombosis is exceedingly rare. The signs and symptoms of pulmonary embolism are nonspecific, seen in a variety of pulmonary and cardiovascular diseases. The clinician must stay alert to the possibility of pulmonary embolism in any patient at risk for Virchow's triad of venous stasis, intimal injury, and hypercoagulable state. The high morbidity and mortality rates of pulmonary embolism and the not inconsequential risk of anticoagulant therapy make accurate diagnosis of thromboembolism crucial. A variety of imaging resources, including chest radiography, ventilation-perfusion scans, pulmonary angiography, and spiral or helical CT, play a role in the diagnosis of pulmonary embolism.

Radiographic Features

A. Chest Radiograph

Although the chest x-ray is abnormal in 80–90% of cases, findings are nonspecific. In one study, the average sensitivity, specificity, and predictive value of chest radiography were 33%, 59%, and 40%, respectively. Despite its low sensitivity and specificity, the chest radiograph may exclude other diseases that can mimic pulmonary embolism, such as pneumonia, pneumothorax, or pulmonary edema. In addition, the chest radiograph is necessary for proper interpretation of the ventilation-perfusion radionuclide scan.

Radiographic findings include atelectasis, pleural effusion, alterations in the pulmonary vasculature, or consolidation. Linear opacities (discoid or plate atelectasis) occur commonly in pulmonary embolism as well as in several other disorders in which ventilation is impaired. These line shadows are most prevalent in the lung bases and are presumed to be secondary to regions of peripheral atelectasis from small mucous plugs. Some investigators have suggested that these linear opacities are caused by infolding of subpleural lung in low-volume states with hypoventilation, distal airway closure, and decreased surfactant production. Linear shadows may also occur secondary to regions of fibrosis due to pulmonary infarction or prior inflammatory disease. Pleural effusions are a frequent finding, occurring in up to 50% of patients. The effusions are usually small and unilateral. Effusions may be present with or without pulmonary infarction, though patients with lung infarction tend to have larger, more slowly resolving effusions that are often hemorrhagic. Alterations in the pulmonary vasculature are manifested radiographically by focal oligemia and radiolucency (Westermark's sign). These findings result from obstruction of pulmonary vessels either by thrombus or by reflex vasoconstriction. Focal oligemia usually requires occlusion of a large portion of the vascular bed and is uncommonly observed. Associated enlargement of the central pulmonary artery may be seen secondary to a large central embolus or acute pulmonary hypertension.

It is estimated that approximately 10–15% of pulmonary thromboemboli cause pulmonary infarction. By virtue of dual blood supply via the pulmonary and bronchial arterial circulations, infarcts are relatively uncommon, occurring more often peripherally, where collateral flow via bronchial arteries is reduced. The incidence of pulmonary infarction is also greater in patients with left ventricular failure, in whom there is compromise of the bronchial circulation. Infarcts are more common in the lower lobes and vary in size from less than 1 cm to an entire lobe. Radiographically, they appear as regions of parenchymal opacity adjacent to the pleura, typically developing 12–24 hours following the onset of symptoms. Initially ill-defined, the lesion becomes more discrete and well-demarcated over several days. Air bronchograms are uncommon, presumably because the bronchi are filled with blood. Hampton and Castleman described the classic appearance of a pulmonary infarct as a wedge-shaped, well-defined opacity abutting the pleura (Hampton's hump), but this is observed in a minority of cases.

Infarcts may resolve entirely or may clear with residual linear scars or pleural thickening. The appearance of a resolving infarct has been likened to a melting ice cube in that the infarct shrinks in size while maintaining its basic configuration. This is in contrast to infectious processes, which show gradual resolution or fading of the entire involved area.

B. Ventilation-Perfusion Lung Scan

The ventilation-perfusion ($\dot{V}/\dot{Q}$) scintigraphic lung scan is usually the next imaging procedure performed in the patient with suspected pulmonary embolism. A normal perfusion scan virtually excludes pulmonary embolism. The interpretation of $\dot{V}/\dot{Q}$ scans is complex, and an abnormal $\dot{V}/\dot{Q}$ scan does not make a definitive diagnosis of pulmonary embolism. Instead, the $\dot{V}/\dot{Q}$ scan in conjunction with the chest radiograph may be used to determine the probability of pulmonary embolism in a given patient. The results of a $\dot{V}/\dot{Q}$ scan in an individual patient must then be evaluated in conjunction with the clinical data to determine the course of action for that specific patient. Based on these combined data, the decision to treat the patient or not or to perform additional diagnostic procedures is made.

Ventilation-perfusion scans are based on the premise that pulmonary thromboembolism results in a region of lung that is ventilated but not perfused. The study consists of two scans—the perfusion scan and the ventilation scan—that are compared for interpretation. The perfusion scan involves injection of an agent such as macroaggregated albumin labeled with technetium Tc 99m (^{99m}Tc). This agent is trapped via the precapillary arterioles and identifies areas of normal lung perfusion. Following injection, the patient is immediately scanned in multiple projections. Regions of the lung with absent perfusion will appear photon-deficient. The ventilation scan is performed by having the patient inhale a radionuclide, usually xenon (^{133}Xe), krypton (^{81m}Kr), or ^{99m}Tc. Images are obtained during an initial breath-hold of approximately 15 seconds, while breathing in a closed system (equilibrium), and during a "washout" phase. Most images are obtained in a posterior projection, allowing for evaluation of the largest lung volume. Ventilation scans can also be performed using a radionuclide aerosol. This has the advantage of allowing multiple images to be made with the patient in the same positions as during the perfusion scan.

Although the concept behind $\dot{V}/\dot{Q}$ scanning is simple, image interpretation is quite complex. Perfusion scans are quite sensitive in the detection of perfusion abnormalities. However, several disorders other than pulmonary thromboembolism may cause perfusion defects, including chronic obstructive pulmonary disease, pulmonary edema, lung cancer, pneumonia, atelectasis, and vasculitis. In an attempt to increase the specificity of radionuclide lung scans, ventilation scans were added to perfusion scans. Whereas pulmonary embolism results in a region of nonperfused lung, ventilation to this region is maintained, resulting in a perfusion defect without an associated ventilation defect (mismatch). In obstructive pulmonary disease, both perfusion and ventilation are impaired, resulting in a matched perfusion and ventilation defect.

There has been considerable controversy regarding the efficacy, reliability, and interpretation of $\dot{V}/\dot{Q}$ scans. The majority of these studies were retrospective, resulting in bias secondary to patient selection. Standardized criteria have been established that are most often used in the interpretation of the $\dot{V}/\dot{Q}$ scan. The chest radiograph, the size and number of perfusion defects, and the match or mismatch of ventilation defects are all taken into consideration in assigning probability categories for pulmonary embolism. There are four probability categories: normal, low, indeterminate or intermediate, and high. Fewer than 8% of patients in the low-probability category had pulmonary embolism documented by angiography, whereas those in the high-probability category had pulmonary embolism documented in approximately 90% of cases. Of the intermediate-probability group, 20–33% had pulmonary embolism documented angiographically. In a multicenter prospective study (PIOPED) of the value of the ventilation-perfusion study in acute pulmonary embolism, 88% of patients with high-probability scans had pulmonary embolism, whereas 33% of those with intermediate-probability scans and 12% of those with low-probability scans had pulmonary embolism. However, only a minority of patients with pulmonary embolism had high-probability scans. Angiography was required for a substantial number of patients in order to make a definitive diagnosis of pulmonary embolism.

C. CT Pulmonary Angiography

The search for a noninvasive study that can detect thrombus rather than the secondary effects of thrombi has lead to the use of CT scanning for the evaluation of pulmonary embolism. Contrast-enhanced helical (spiral) or electron beam CT has sensitivities and specificities of approximately 90% in the diagnosis of pulmonary embolism involving segmental or larger pulmonary arteries. Although subsegmental thrombi may be missed, the clinical significance of isolated subsegmental clot is uncertain, as is the incidence of isolated subsegmental clot. Given the relatively noninvasive nature of the technique and its high sensitivity and specificity for central clot, many institutions have chosen to perform CT pulmonary angiography as the initial study in the investigation of suspected pulmonary embolism, bypassing the ventilation-perfusion scan.

CT findings of pulmonary embolism include partial or complete filling defects within the pulmonary artery due to nonocclusive or occlusive thrombi, contrast streaming around a central thrombus, or mural defects (Figure 7–10). Oligemia of lung parenchyma distal to the occluded vessel may be present. Parenchymal and pleural changes that occur with pulmonary emboli are also easily detected on CT. Pulmonary embolism may result in hemorrhage that is visible as ground-glass opacification or consolidation on CT. An infarct may appear as a peripheral region of consolidation, typically wedge-shaped with a central region of lower attenuation due to uninfarcted lobules. Pleural effusions are commonly seen. CT may also provide an alternative diagnosis in patients with suspected pulmonary embolism.

Pitfalls in the interpretation of CT pulmonary angiography include breathing artifacts in patients unable to breath-hold, inadequate contrast opacification of the pulmonary arteries, and suboptimal visualization of vessels that are obliquely oriented relative to the transverse imaging plane (eg, the segmental branches of the right middle lobe and lingula). Partially opacified veins may

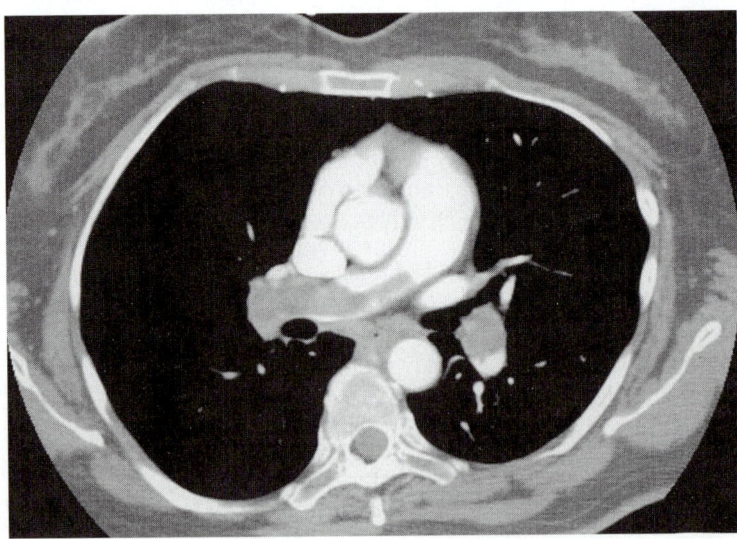

Figure 7–10. Acute pulmonary embolism. CT pulmonary angiogram demonstrates low attenuation filling defects within the right pulmonary artery and within the left lower lobe pulmonary artery. There is distention of the left lower lobe pulmonary artery.

be confused with thrombosed arteries, and hilar lymph nodes may be misinterpreted as thrombi.

D. Pulmonary Angiography

Pulmonary angiography is generally considered the most sensitive and specific imaging method for the diagnosis of pulmonary embolism. Angiography is indicated when there is disagreement between the results of the $\dot{V}/\dot{Q}$ scan and the clinical suspicion of pulmonary embolism; when the $\dot{V}/\dot{Q}$ scan is indeterminate or is of intermediate probability; when there is a contraindication to anticoagulant therapy; or when therapy involves more complicated treatment such as an inferior vena cava filter, surgical embolectomy, or thrombolytic therapy. Complications of pulmonary angiography are related to the catheter and its manipulation through the heart and to reactions to intravenous contrast material. Dysrhythmias, heart block, cardiac perforation, cor pulmonale, and cardiac arrest may occur. Relative contraindications to pulmonary angiography include elevated right ventricular and pulmonary arterial pressures, bleeding diathesis, renal insufficiency or failure, left heart block, and a history of contrast allergy. Pulmonary angiography can be performed in all of these settings if appropriate measures are taken to reduce the risk of the procedure.

At angiography, the diagnosis of pulmonary embolus is made when an intraluminal filling defect or an occluded pulmonary artery is identified. Secondary findings include decreased perfusion, delayed venous return, abnormal parenchymal stain, and crowded vessels, which, though suggestive, may be seen in other pulmonary disorders.

E. MRI

The role of MRI and MR angiography (MRA) in the diagnosis of pulmonary embolism remains unclear. Although central and peripheral emboli have also been detected on MRA, computed tomography is more readily accessible and suitable for imaging of the critically ill patient.

F. Imaging Techniques in Chronic Pulmonary Embolism

Chronic pulmonary embolism may lead to right ventricular failure and pulmonary arterial hypertension. Radiographic findings include enlargement of the right heart and of the main and proximal pulmonary arteries and decreased peripheral vascularity. Bronchial arteries distal to the occluded pulmonary artery may become dilated. As in patients with acute pulmonary embolism, evaluation of the patient with suspected chronic pulmonary embolism includes $\dot{V}/\dot{Q}$ scanning, CT pulmonary angiography, and pulmonary angiography. In addition to direct visualization of clot, other signs of chronic pulmonary embolism include abrupt narrowing of the vessel diameter, cut-off of distal lobar or segmental arterial branches and an irregular or nodular arterial wall. Recanalization and eccentric location of thrombi also suggest chronicity.

Buckner CB, Walker CW, Purnell GL: Pulmonary embolism: Chest radiographic abnormalities. J Thorac Imaging 1989;4:23–7.

Gottsater A et al: Clinically suspected pulmonary embolism: is it safe to withhold anticoagulation after a negative spiral CT? Eur Radiol 2001;11:65–72.

Kim K, Müller, Mayo JR: Clinically suspected pulmonary embolism: utility for spiral CT. Radiology 1999;210:693–7.

Lorut C et al: A noninvasive diagnostic strategy including spiral computed tomography in patients with suspected pulmonary embolism. Am J Respir Crit Care Med 2000;162:1413–8.

Ost D et al: The negative predictive value of spiral computed tomography for the diagnosis of pulmonary embolism in patients with nondiagnostic ventilation-perfusion scans. Am J Med 2001;110:16–21.

Perrier A et al: Performance of helical computed tomography in unselected outpatients with suspected pulmonary embolism. Ann Intern Med 2001;135:88–97.

PIOPED Investigators: Value of the ventilation-perfusion scan in acute pulmonary embolism. JAMA 1990;263:2753–9.

Remy-Jardin M et al. Diagnosis of pulmonary embolism with spiral CT: comparison with pulmonary angiography and scintigraphy. Radiology 1996;200:699–706.

Remy-Jardin M et al. Spiral CT of pulmonary embolism: technical considerations and interpretive pitfalls. Journal Thorac Imaging 1997;12:103–17.

Swensen SJ et al: Outcomes after withholding anticoagulation from patients with suspected acute pulmonary embolism and negative computed tomographic findings: a cohort study. Mayo Clin Proc 2002;77:130–8.

Teigen CL et al: Pulmonary embolism: diagnosis with contrast-enhanced electron-beam CT and comparison with pulmonary angiography. Radiology 1995;194:313–9.

SEPTIC PULMONARY EMBOLI

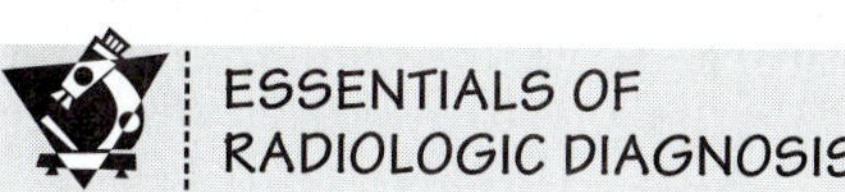
ESSENTIALS OF
RADIOLOGIC DIAGNOSIS

- *Wedge-shaped or rounded peripheral opacities of varying size, usually multiple and more numerous in the lower lobes.*
- *Thin-walled cavities, sometimes with necrotic debris, are common.*
- *On CT scan, peripheral nodules, wedge-shaped peripheral opacities, and cavitation.*

General Considerations

Infections of the right side of the heart or of the peripheral veins may give rise to septic pulmonary emboli. Risk factors include intravenous drug use, indwelling catheters, pelvic inflammatory disease, organ transplantation, and immunologic deficiencies such as lymphoma or AIDS. Infectious thrombophlebitis may also result from infection of the pharynx extending to the parapharyngeal space and internal jugular venous system (Lemierre's syndrome, or post-anginal sepsis). Tricuspid valve endocarditis is the most common source of septic emboli in the intravenous drug user. *S aureus* is the most commonly isolated organism, followed by streptococci.

Radiographic Features

Septic pulmonary emboli appear radiographically as wedge-shaped or rounded peripheral opacities. Septic emboli are usually multiple and are more numerous in the lower lobes, reflecting increased blood flow to the dependent lung. The lesions may vary in size by virtue of variations in timing of embolization. Cavitation, typically thin-walled, is common, and necrotic debris may be identified within the cavity. Hilar and mediastinal adenopathy can occur.

The CT features of septic emboli have been described. Peripheral nodules with identifiable feeding vessels, wedge-shaped peripheral opacities, and cavitation are the most diagnostic features. Peripheral enhancement along the margins of the wedge-shaped densities has been reported following administration of intravenous contrast material (Figure 7–11). It has been suggested that CT can detect disease earlier than the plain radiograph and that it better characterizes the extent of disease. Moreover, the cross-sectional perspective of CT affords better identification of embolic lesions that may be obscured on chest radiographs by edema or other diffuse consolidations.

Huang RM et al: Septic pulmonary emboli: CT-radiographic correlation. AJR Am J Roentgenol 1989;153:41–5.

Kuhlman JE, Fishman EK, Teigen C: Pulmonary septic emboli: Diagnosis with CT. Radiology 1990;174:211–3.

PULMONARY EDEMA

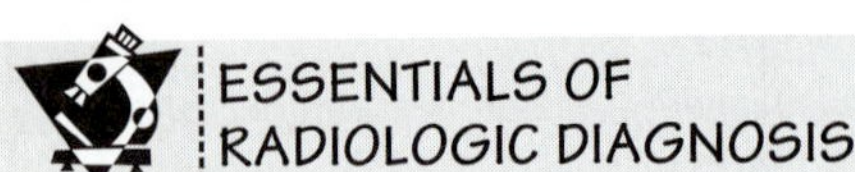
ESSENTIALS OF
RADIOLOGIC DIAGNOSIS

Interstitial edema:

- *Kerley B (most common), A, and C lines.*
- *Peribronchial cuffing.*
- *Indistinct pulmonary vessels.*
- *Hilar haze.*

Alveolar edema:

- *Poorly marginated, coalescent opacities.*
- *Air bronchograms.*
- *"Butterfly" pattern.*

General Considerations

Pulmonary edema—an excess of water in the extravascular space of the lung—is a frequent cause of respiratory distress in the critically ill patient. The three main categories of pulmonary edema are cardiac edema secondary to myocardial or endocardial disease; overhydration due to renal failure or excess administration of fluid; and increased capillary permeability, which may result from a variety of insults to the microvasculature of the lung. In the ICU patient, more than one mechanism may contribute to the formation of edema, increasing the difficulty of diagnostic interpretation on radiographs.

There are four principal mechanisms that result in the development of edema: elevated capillary hydrostatic pressure, decreased plasma oncotic pressure, increased capillary permeability, and obstruction of lymphatic drainage. Decreased plasma oncotic pressure and obstruction to lymphatic drainage only rarely lead to pulmonary edema but may be contributing factors in the setting of increased hydrostatic pressure. The most common cause of edema is hydrostatic pressure elevation due to cardiac disease. Acute myocardial infarction, acute volume overload of the left ventricle, and mitral stenosis are common causes of cardiogenic edema.

Radiographic Features

The chest radiograph is the most commonly used noninvasive test in the evaluation of the patient with pulmonary edema. Interstitial edema may be present radiographically in the absence of clinical signs and symptoms, and the chest radiograph may be the first indication of edema.

A. Cardiogenic Pulmonary Edema

In the patient with heart failure, pulmonary edema is preceded by pulmonary venous hypertension. In patients with left ventricular failure, elevated left ventricular end-diastolic pressure (pulmonary venous hypertension) is reflected in the pulmonary vasculature by dilation and redistribution of pulmonary blood flow to the upper lobes. In the normal erect patient, the upper zone vessels are smaller than the lower zone vessels, and a significant fraction of the pulmonary circulation, particularly to the

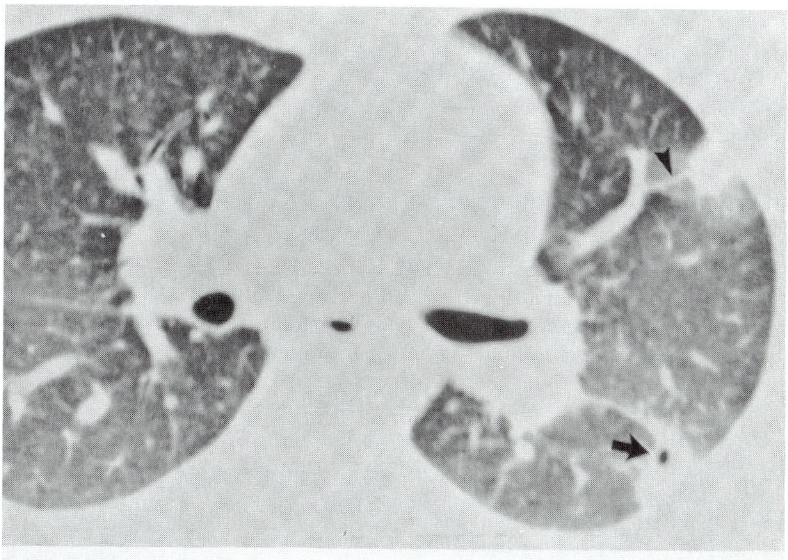

A

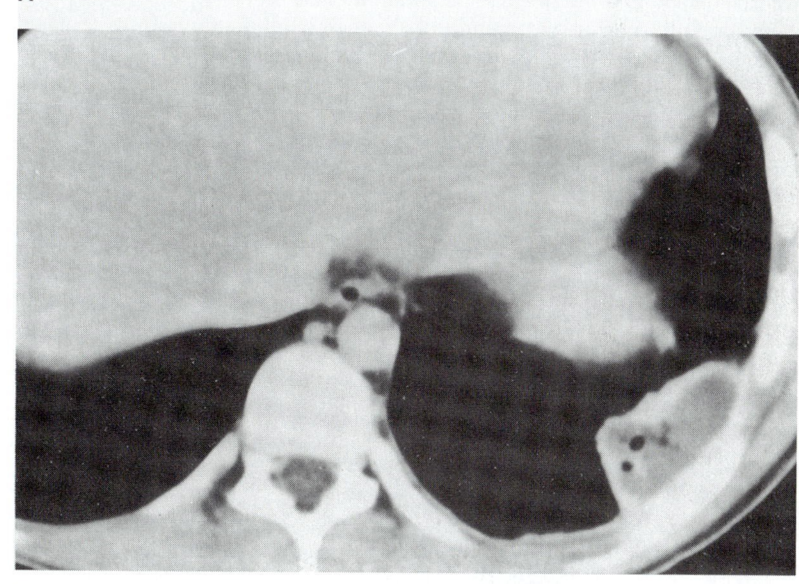

B

Figure 7–11. Young woman with septic emboli secondary to intravenous drug abuse. Blood cultures were positive for *Staphylococcus aureus*. ***A:*** Peripheral nodular opacities are present with evidence of cavitation (arrow). A feeding vessel is identified leading to a pulmonary nodule, consistent with hematogenous dissemination (arrowhead). ***B:*** Wedge-shaped subpleural lesion is noted with peripheral enhancement after administration of intravenous contrast.

upper lobes, is not perfused. In conditions of increased pulmonary blood volume or left ventricular failure, there is recruitment of these nonperfused reserve vessels in the upper lobes, and reflex hypoxic vasoconstriction of lower lobe vessels occurs. These and other pathophysiologic factors contribute to the phenomenon of upper lobe arterial and venous redistribution. Vascular redistribution is often difficult to observe on radiographs, particularly in critically ill patients imaged in the semierect or supine position. As the pulmonary venous pressure continues to increase, pulmonary edema develops.

Pulmonary edema may be present within the pulmonary interstitium, the alveoli, or both. Radiographic evidence of interstitial edema includes Kerley A, B, and C lines; peribronchial cuffing; hilar haze; indistinct vascular markings; and subpleural edema. Kerley lines represent thickened interlobular septa, with Kerley B lines the most easily and most frequently seen. These lines are horizontal linear densities measuring 1–2 cm in length and 1–2 mm in width. They are located peripherally, extend to the pleural surface, and are best seen at the lung bases on the frontal film (Figure 7–12). Kerley A lines are longer and more randomly oriented and are best seen in the upper lobes, directed toward the hila. Kerley C lines are presumably a superimposition of many thickened interlobular septa and appear as a fine reticular pattern. Other signs of interstitial edema, including peribronchial cuffing, hilar haze, and indistinct vascular markings, result from accumulation of fluid in the perivascular and peribronchial interstitium. Accumulation of fluid in the subpleural interstitium is best demonstrated along the pleural fissures.

Alveolar edema occurs as fluid fills the air spaces of the lungs (Figure 7–13). Although interstitial edema precedes alveolar edema and continues to be present in the alveolar filling stage, the interstitial component is frequently obscured by concomitant air space edema. With filling of the air spaces, the lung becomes opaque, with poorly defined confluent opacity. Air bronchograms are identified as tubular lucencies representing normal patent bronchi surrounded by fluid-filled air spaces. The butterfly pattern, appearing as a dense perihilar opacification, has been described in overhydration and cardiac edema.

In general, cardiogenic pulmonary edema is bilateral and symmetric. Atypical edema patterns may be seen in patients with underlying acute or chronic lung disease or as a consequence of gravitational forces related to patient positioning. Destruction of the lung due to emphysema may cause a patchy, asymmetric distribution of edema that spares regions of bullous disease. Gravitational forces also affect the distribution of edema, with increased edema in the dependent lung, and shifting the patient's position can change the appearance of edema. Such maneuvers may help distinguish atypical edema from other air space processes such as pneumonia. The temporal sequence of parenchymal opacification is also crucial because the onset and resolution of hydrostatic edema may be rapid, whereas in other conditions such as pneumonia and ARDS, changes are more gradual.

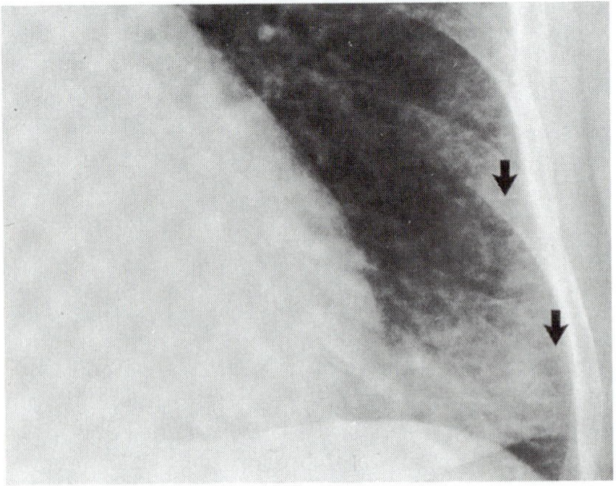

Figure 7–12. Interstitial edema. Kerley B lines are identified at the lung bases (arrows).

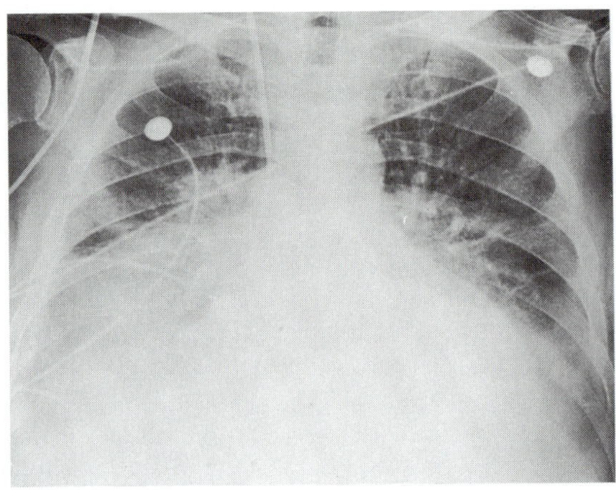

Figure 7–13. Alveolar edema. Air space opacities with vascular redistribution, perihilar haze, cardiomegaly, and bilateral pleural effusions are secondary to cardiogenic edema. A pulmonary artery catheter and nasogastric tube are present.

B. Distinguishing Cardiogenic From Noncardiogenic Pulmonary Edema

Three principal features have been proposed to distinguish cardiogenic and noncardiogenic pulmonary edema radiographically: distribution of pulmonary flow, distribution of pulmonary edema, and width of the vascular pedicle. Ancillary features include pulmonary blood volume, peribronchial cuffing, septal lines, pleural effusions, air bronchograms, lung volume, and cardiac size. The vascular pedicle width his defined as the width of the mediastinum just above the aortic arch, with normal ranging from 43 mm to 53 mm in an erect patient. The vascular pedicle is enlarged in 60% of patients with cardiac failure and in 85% of patients with renal failure or overhydration. This is in contrast to patients with capillary permeability edema, who had a normal or narrowed vascular pedicle in 70%

of cases. The distribution of flow is also a discriminating feature in that patients with hydrostatic edema more typically have balanced flow or vascular redistribution. In contrast, patients with capillary permeability edema usually demonstrate a normal or balanced distribution of flow. Finally, the distribution of edema is symmetric and perihilar or basilar in patients with cardiac or overhydration edemas, whereas capillary permeability edema appears patchy and peripheral.

Heart size and the presence or absence of septal lines may also be useful criteria for differentiating cardiogenic from permeability edema, with an accuracy of 83%. Thus, if the heart is enlarged or of normal size and septal lines are present, cardiogenic edema is likely, but if the heart size is normal and septal lines are absent, permeability edema is more likely. There may be considerable overlap. In one study, a classic hydrostatic pattern occurred in 90% of patients with hydrostatic edema, but 40% of patients with increased permeability edema had radiographic features consistent with hydrostatic edema. A peripheral or patchy air space pattern was relatively specific for capillary permeability edema. Overlapping features may arise from differences in patient populations, including differences in severity of edema, underlying heart or lung disease, and radiologic technique and patient positioning.

Thus, the radiographic diagnosis of edema may be complicated by several factors. However, general guidelines can be suggested. In general, noncardiogenic edema typically demonstrates normal cardiac size with air space opacities (Figure 7–14) and infrequent Kerley lines, peribronchial cuffing, or pleural effusions. In contrast, hydrostatic edema is associated with cardiac enlargement, septal lines, and frequent pleural effusions. The accuracy of chest radiographic diagnosis is dependent upon the integration of all available clinical and physiologic data.

Aberle DR et al: Hydrostatic versus increased permeability pulmonary edema: Diagnosis based on radiographic criteria in critically ill patients. Radiology 1988;168:73–9.

Gluecker T et al: Clinical and radiologic features of pulmonary edema. Radiographics. 1999;19:1507–31.

Milne EN et al: The radiologic distinction of cardiogenic and noncardiogenic edema. AJR Am J Roentgenol 1985; 144:879–94.

Ravin CE: Pulmonary vascularity: Radiographic considerations. J Thorac Imaging 1988;3:1–13.

Smith RC et al: Radiographic differentiation between different etiologies of pulmonary edema. Invest Radiol 1987;22:859–63.

Thomason JW et al: Appraising pulmonary edema using supine chest roentgenograms in ventilated patients. Am J Respir Crit Care Med 1998;157:1600–8.

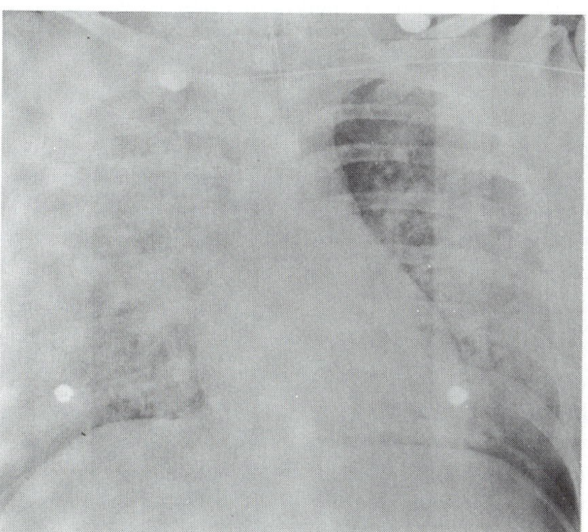

A

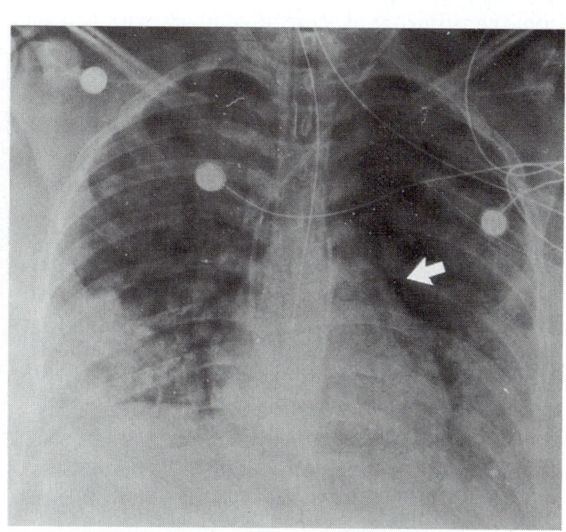

B

Figure 7–14. Noncardiac edema secondary to near drowning. ***A:*** Anteroposterior chest radiograph demonstrates asymmetric air space opacities bilaterally. Heart size is normal, and there are no pleural effusions. Endotracheal tube is high in position, and a nasogastric tube is present. ***B:*** Radiograph 48 hours after admission shows heterogeneous parenchymal opacification, with worsening at the lung bases. A left thoracostomy tube and pulmonary artery catheter are now present, and the endotracheal tube is in satisfactory position. There is evidence of barotrauma with pneumomediastinum (arrow).

ACUTE RESPIRATORY DISTRESS SYNDROME

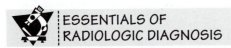

- *Early ARDS: Decrease in lung volumes, but lungs are generally clear. If ARDS is caused by aspiration or pneumonia, parenchymal opacifications may be present.*
- *Later: Air space opacification is usually bilateral but may be asymmetric and patchy and may progress later to more uniform consolidation. Air bronchograms are usually present.*
- *Late ARDS associated with collagen deposition shows less dense parenchymal consolidations with interstitial or "ground glass" opacities.*
- *Complications include pulmonary interstitial emphysema, pneumomediastinum, and pneumothorax.*

General Considerations

Acute respiratory distress syndrome (ARDS) is a catastrophic consequence of acute lung injury, with damage to the alveolar epithelium and pulmonary vasculature resulting in increased capillary permeability edema. Despite numerous attempts at clarification in the literature, there is still disagreement about the best way to describe this disorder. It is usually characterized clinically by refractory hypoxemia, decreased lung compliance, severe acute respiratory distress, and pulmonary parenchymal consolidations on chest radiographs. A variety of disorders are associated with ARDS, including both direct insults to the lungs and nonpulmonary systemic conditions.

Radiographic Features

A. Chest Radiographs

The radiographic manifestations correlate with the pathologic changes seen in the lungs and vary with the stage of lung injury. Three stages have been described in ARDS. Stage I is the earliest and most transient stage of lung injury and occurs during the first hours after the insult. Pathologically, this stage is characterized by pulmonary capillary congestion, endothelial cell swelling, and extensive microatelectasis. Fluid leakage is confined to the interstitium and is limited. Clinically, respiratory distress with tachypnea and hypoxemia is present. In patients with ARDS secondary to systemic insults, diffuse microatelectasis and diminished lung compliance may result in a decrease in lung volumes, but the lungs are generally clear. Interstitial fluid is usually too mild to be radiographically apparent (Figure 7–15). In primary pulmonary insults causing ARDS, such as aspiration or pneumonia, parenchymal opacifications may be present (Figure 7–16). Physiologic changes due to therapy are also reflected on the radiograph, including overhydration and barotrauma. The

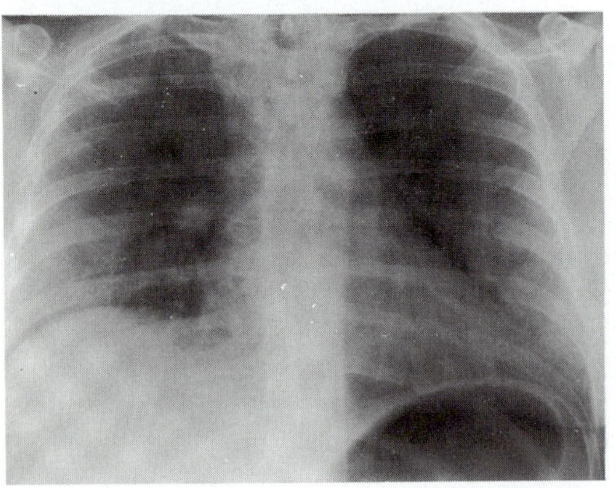

A

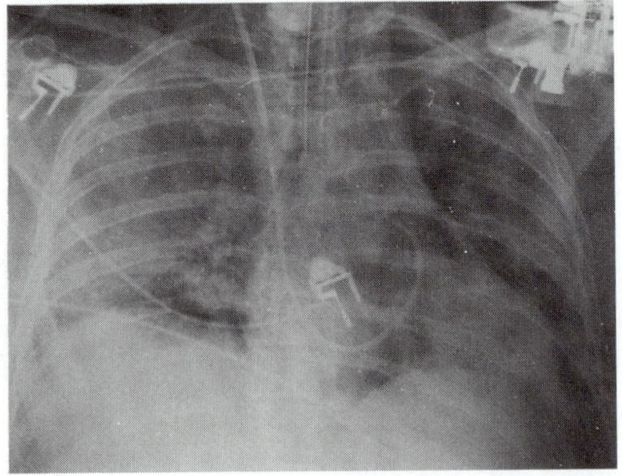

B

Figure 7–15. ARDS secondary to sepsis in an immunocompromised patient following bone marrow transplantation. ***A:*** Stage I ARDS. The lungs are clear, despite marked dyspnea and hypoxemia. Lung volumes are slightly decreased. ***B:*** Stage II ARDS. Within 24 hours, the chest radiograph shows diffuse parenchymal opacification consistent with ARDS.

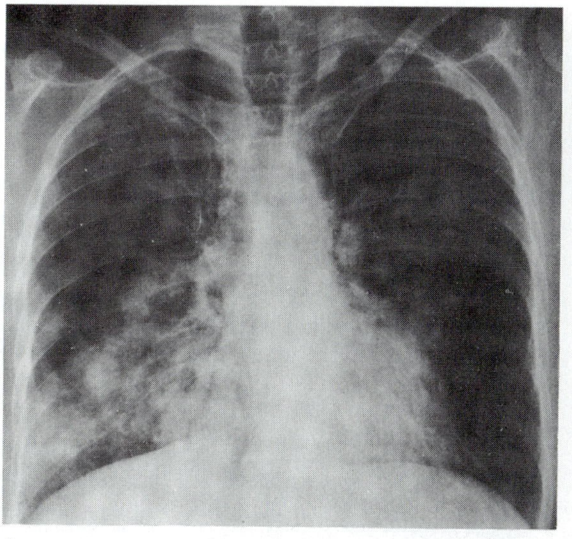

A

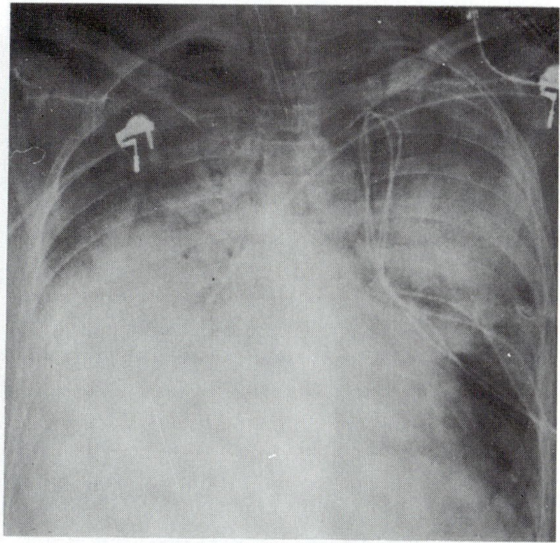

B

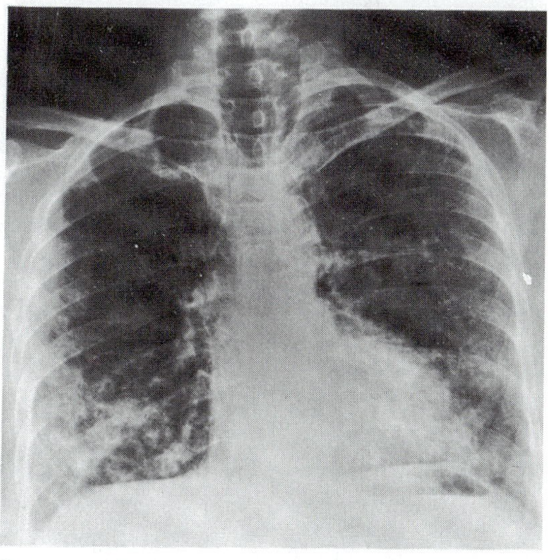

C

Figure 7–16. ARDS secondary to pneumococcal pneumonia in a patient with a history of Hodgkin's disease and splenectomy several years earlier. ***A:*** Initial chest radiograph demonstrates patchy bilateral consolidation. ***B:*** Within 12 hours after admission, dense air space consolidation is present, necessitating intubation. Clinical course was consistent with ARDS. ***C:*** Follow-up radiograph 5 weeks after admission to the intensive care unit shows a coarse reticular pattern bilaterally. Lung volumes are slightly decreased in comparison with the admission radiograph.

use of positive end-expiratory pressure (PEEP) may cause improvement in aeration on the chest radiograph without physiologic or clinical improvement. In fact, occasionally there is paradoxic worsening of oxygenation from alveolar overdistention with subsequent diversion of pulmonary flow to poorly ventilated regions. In stage II, the pathologic features of hemorrhagic fluid leakage, fibrin deposition, and hyaline membrane formation result in radiographic consolidation. Air space opacification is usually bilateral but may be asymmetric and patchy and may progress later to more uniform consolidation. Air bronchograms are usually present and become more conspicuous with severe consolidation. The transition to stage II may occur 1–5 days following the pulmonary insult, depending on its type and severity. More severe injuries result in a more rapid transition. Pleural effusions are uncommon and, when present, are small.

Stage III is characterized by hyperplasia of type II alveolar cells and collagen deposition. Decreased lung compliance, ventilation-perfusion imbalance, diffusion impairment, and destruction of the microvascular bed result in abnormal gas exchange and lung mechanics.

Radiographically, parenchymal consolidations become less dense and confluent. Interstitial or ground-glass opacities develop as fluid is replaced by the deposition of collagen. Subpleural lucencies may develop in regions of peripheral ischemia and ischemic necrosis. The treatment of ARDS, including positive-pressure ventilation, sometimes results in barotrauma that is manifested as pulmonary interstitial emphysema, pneumomediastinum, and pneumothorax (Figure 7–17).

Long-term sequelae of ARDS are variable. The overall mortality rate is approximately 50%. Although long-term survivors may have complete recovery of pulmonary function, respiratory impairment may result from pulmonary fibrosis and microvascular damage. Improvement in lung function is relatively rapid during the first 3–6 months, reaching maximum recovery within 6–12 months following onset of ARDS. The chest radiograph may continue to show hyperinflation and some residual lung opacities, but most often it returns to normal.

B. CT Scans

The CT appearance of ARDS has been described by numerous investigators. In general, CT demonstrates a variable and patchy distribution, with most marked involvement in the dependent lung regions. These opacities probably represent severe diffuse microatelectasis as

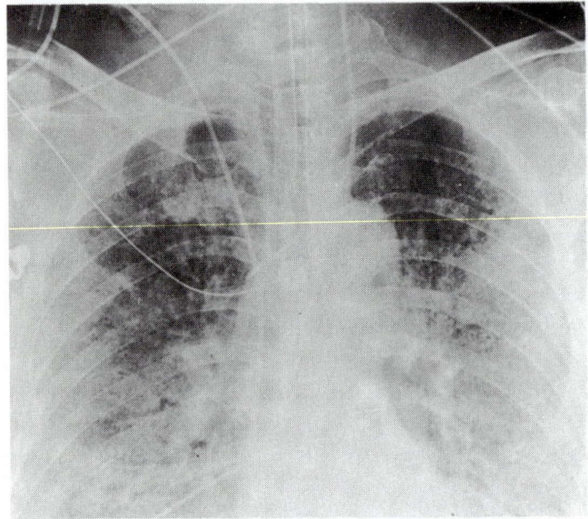

A

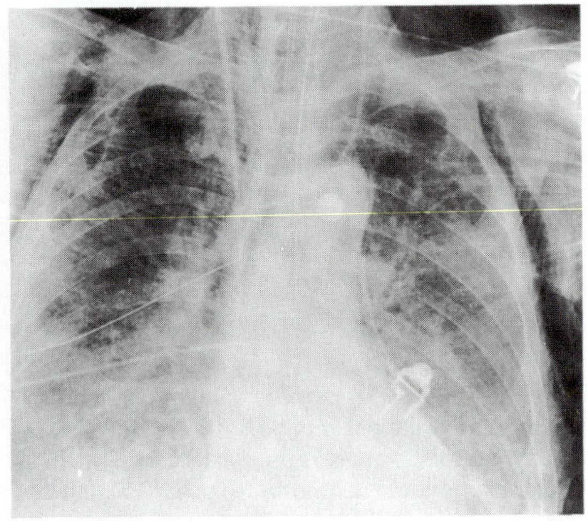

B

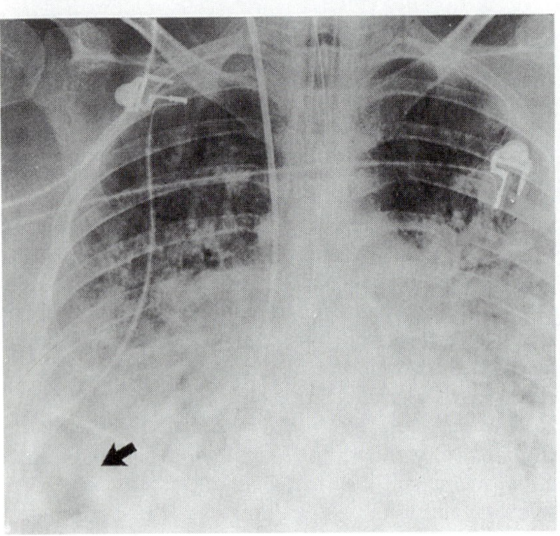

C

Figure 7–17. Barotrauma in ARDS. ***A:*** Chest radiograph demonstrates diffuse lung consolidation secondary to ARDS. Parenchymal stippling is present, with lucent perivascular halos secondary to pulmonary interstitial emphysema. ***B:*** On chest radiograph 4 days later, pneumomediastinum is now identified with extensive subcutaneous emphysema. ***C:*** In another patient with ARDS, subpleural cysts (arrow) and parenchymal stippling due to pulmonary interstitial emphysema are present.

well as edema fluid and have been observed to migrate under the influence of gravity. Air bronchograms are frequent, and pleural effusions, typically small, occur in approximately one-half of patients. The distribution of consolidation may be dependent on the stage of ARDS. Early changes may show patchy areas of ground-glass opacity or consolidation diffusely but not uniformly, without central or gravity dependence. Later changes show more homogeneity as the lung becomes more edematous, and gravity-dependent atelectasis increases. On CT, barotraumatic lung cysts and infectious complications such as cavitation or empyema are better identified than on projectional radiographs (Figure 7–18).

Aberle DR, Brown K: Radiological considerations in the adult respiratory distress syndrome. Clin Chest Med 1990;11:737–54.

Gattinoni L et al: Adult respiratory distress syndrome profiles by computed tomography. J Thorac Imaging 1986;1:25–30.

Gattinoni L et al: What has computed tomography taught us about the acute respiratory distress syndrome? Am J Respir Crit Care Med 2001;164:1701–11.

Goodman LR: Congestive heart failure and adult respiratory distress syndrome: new insights using computed tomography. Radiol Clin North Am 1996;34:33–46.

Goodman LR et al: Adult respiratory distress syndrome due to pulmonary and extrapulmonary causes: CT, clinical, and functional correlations. Radiology 1999;213:545–52.

Maunder RJ et al: Preservation of normal lung regions in the adult respiratory distress syndrome: Analysis by computed tomography. JAMA 1986;255:2463–5.

Stark P et al: CT-findings in ARDS. Radiology 1987;27:367–9.

Ware LB, Matthay MA: The acute respiratory distress syndrome. N Engl J Med 2000;342:1334–49

IMAGING IN PLEURAL DISORDERS

PLEURAL EFFUSIONS

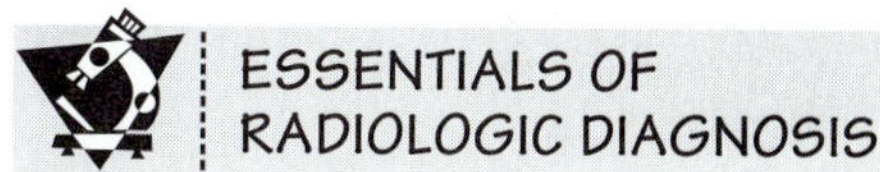

ESSENTIALS OF RADIOLOGIC DIAGNOSIS

- *Blunting of the lateral costophrenic angle (meniscus sign).*
- *Elevation of the apparent level of the diaphragm. Increased separation between the lung and the stomach bubble.*
- *Homogeneous increased density of the involved hemithorax.*
- *Fluid capping the lung apex.*
- *Decreased visibility of pulmonary vessels below the diaphragm.*
- *Increased density within the pleural fissures ("pseudotumor").*

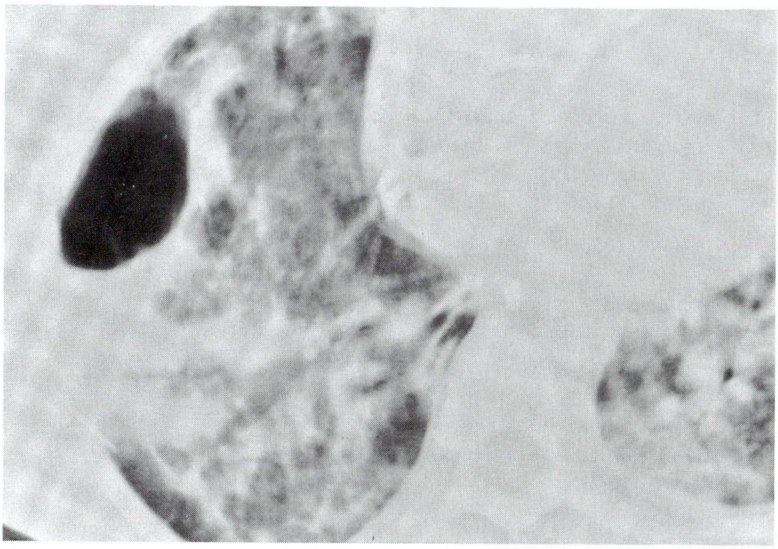

Figure 7–18. Adult respiratory distress syndrome. CT shows heterogeneous consolidation with subpleural air cyst secondary to barotrauma.

General Considerations

Pleural fluid is primarily formed on the parietal pleural surface and absorbed on the visceral pleural surface, with approximately 25 mL of fluid present normally in the pleural space. Pleural effusion is an excess accumulation of intrapleural fluid. A wide variety of disorders result in excess pleural fluid. Although the chest radiograph is useful for detecting and estimating the amount of pleural effusion, the differentiation between transudate, exudate, empyema, and hemorrhagic pleural effusion requires thoracentesis. In the ICU population, congestive heart failure is the most common cause of pleural effusion.

Radiographic Features

The distribution of fluid within the pleural space is greatly affected by lung elastic recoil and gravity. On erect frontal and lateral radiographs, free pleural effusions typically have a concave, upward-sloping contour (the meniscus appearance). Since the posterior costophrenic angles are usually deeper than the lateral costophrenic angles, small pleural effusions are typically best seen on the lateral view. Blunting of the lateral costophrenic angle—detectable on an erect posteroanterior chest radiograph—may occur with as little as 175 mL of fluid, though in some cases as much as 525 mL will be present before blunting is noted. Pleural effusion may also accumulate in a subpulmonary location between the lung base and diaphragm without causing blunting of the lateral costophrenic sulcus. These subpulmonary collections simulate elevation of the diaphragm; on the left, the distance between the gastric air bubble and the "pseudodiaphragm" will be increased. The pulmonary vessels are not seen through the basilar pulmonary parenchyma. The pseudodiaphragm is elevated and flattened, with the dome appearing more lateral than normal.

Pleural effusions may extend into the fissures, with the radiographic appearance depending on the shape and orientation of the fissure, the location of the fluid, and the direction of the radiographic beam. Collections of fluid in the fissures may mimic a mass, resulting in a "pseudotumor" appearance.

Although the above radiographic appearances of pleural effusion are well known and easily recognized on posteroanterior and lateral chest radiographs, these projections are infrequently obtained in the ICU patient, and recognition of pleural effusion in the supine patient may be difficult. In supine patients, the most dependent regions of the pleural space are the posterior aspects of the bases and the lung apex. Free pleural effusions layer posteriorly, resulting in a homogeneous increased density of the lower involved hemithorax. Fluid may also accumulate at the apex of the thorax, resulting in apical capping. These findings, however, are frequently seen only in moderate or large pleural effusions, and small effusions may not be detected on supine radiographs. Although very small accumulations of pleural effusion can be detected on lateral decubitus views, this projection is logistically difficult to obtain in the ICU patient.

Atelectasis and other lung consolidations may be difficult to distinguish from pleural effusion because they too may result in elevation of the hemidiaphragm and decreased visibility of lower lobe vessels. Cross-sectional imaging using ultrasound or CT is very helpful in detecting small amounts of pleural effusion and in distinguishing complicated pleural and parenchymal processes. These imaging methods are also frequently used to guide interventional procedures, including diagnostic thoracentesis, drainage of empyema or malignant pleural effusions, and sclerotherapy. Ultrasound can be performed at the bedside and can easily detect both free pleural effusions and loculated collections (Figure 7–19). In most situations, ultrasound is the imaging method of choice for guiding thoracentesis and may decrease the incidence of iatrogenic pneumothorax. The percutaneous drainage of pleural fluid collections with small catheters instead of large-bore thoracostomy tubes has been shown to be effective in treating both sterile and infected effusions.

Computed tomography is extremely sensitive in detecting even small amounts of free pleural effusion, demonstrating loculations, and evaluating the underlying lung parenchyma. The excellent contrast resolution of CT allows demonstrations of regions of high attenuation secondary to blood or proteinaceous collections and shows calcifications that are not apparent on chest radiographs. By virtue of the cross-sectional perspective, air-fluid levels are easily identified. In complicated cases, intravenous contrast administration will help to differentiate pulmonary and pleural processes in that perfused, consolidated lung will be enhanced whereas pleural processes will not (Figure 7–7). The disadvantages of CT are its relatively high cost and the necessity for transporting the critically ill patient to the radiology department.

Ruskin JA et al: Detection of pleural effusions on supine chest radiographs. AJR Am J Roentgenol 1987;148:681–3.

Stavas J et al: Percutaneous drainage of infected and noninfected thoracic fluid collections. J Thorac Imaging 1987;2:80–7.

PNEUMOTHORAX

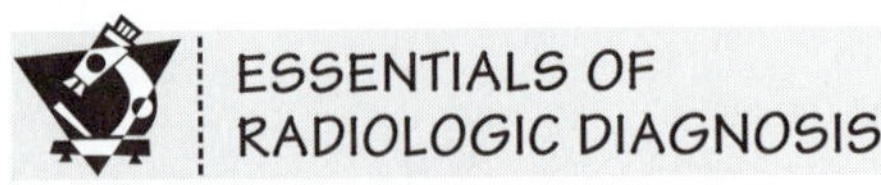
ESSENTIALS OF
RADIOLOGIC DIAGNOSIS

- *Identification of a visceral pleural line.*
- *Absence of pulmonary vessels peripheral to visceral pleural line.*

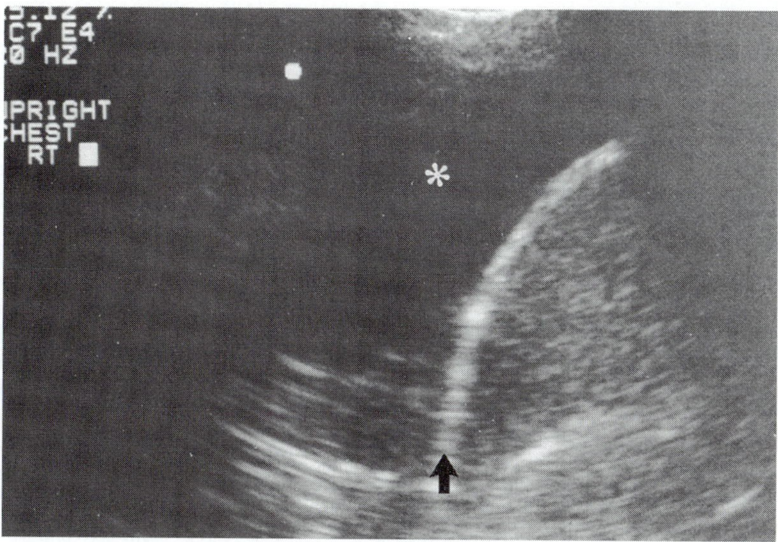

Figure 7–19. Pleural effusion on ultrasound. Right pleural effusion is seen as a region of low echogenicity (asterisk) above the hyperechoic diaphragm (arrow).

- *Basilar hyperlucency in the supine patient.*
- *Deep sulcus sign (supine patient).*

General Considerations

Pneumothorax is a frequent complication in the ICU. Iatrogenic pneumothorax may develop as a sequela of invasive diagnostic or therapeutic procedures, including central venous catheterization, endotracheal intubation, tracheostomy, thoracentesis, pleural biopsy, percutaneous lung biopsy, bronchoscopy, cardiothoracic or abdominal surgery, and interventional abdominal procedures to the liver and upper abdominal viscera. Pneumothorax may also result from blunt chest trauma or underlying lung diseases such as COPD, asthma, cystic fibrosis, and interstitial lung disease. Pneumothorax can complicate the course of cavitary pneumonias due to infections with *M tuberculosis,* staphylococci, klebsiella and other gram-negative organisms, or fungi; similarly, there is an increased incidence of pneumothorax in patients with AIDS who develop pneumocystis pneumonia. Finally, in patients receiving positive-pressure mechanical ventilation, pneumothorax may result from pulmonary interstitial emphysema due to barotrauma.

Radiographic Features

A. Simple Pneumothorax

As with fluid in the pleural space, the distribution of pneumothorax is influenced by gravity, lung elastic recoil, potential adhesions in the pleural space, and the anatomy of the pleural recesses. In the upright patient, air accumulates in the nondependent region of the pleural space, the apex. Radiographically, pneumothorax is identified by separation of the visceral pleural surface from the chest wall and the absence of pulmonary vessels peripheral to the pleural line. Pneumothorax is typically better seen on expiratory images because of a relative decrease in lung volumes compared with the air in the pleural space.

Imaging in the supine position alters the radiographic appearance of pneumothorax. In this position, the least dependent regions of the pleural space are the anteromedial and subpulmonary regions. Pleural air in the anteromedial space results in sharp delineation of mediastinal contours, including the superior vena cava, the azygos vein, the heart border, the inferior vena cava, and the left subclavian artery. The accumulation of air in the subpulmonary region is seen as a hyperlucent upper quadrant of the abdomen; a deep, hyperlucent lateral costophrenic sulcus ("deep sulcus sign"); sharp delineation of the ipsilateral diaphragm; and visualization of the inferior surface of the lung (Figure 7–20). Air can accumulate in the apicolateral pleural space in the supine patient just as in the erect patient, especially when a large pneumothorax is present. In the presence of lower lobe collapse, air can accumulate in the posteromedial pleural recess. This results in sharp delineation of the posterior mediastinal structures, including the descending aorta and the costovertebral sulcus.

Subtle pneumothoraces may require other projections for detection, such as decubitus or cross-table lateral views. Computed tomography is an excellent method for diagnosing a small pneumothorax not demonstrated on plain chest radiographs.

Several conditions may be confused with pneumothorax. Pneumoperitoneum may result in a hyperlucent upper abdomen, mimicking pneumothorax. Skin folds can be confused with apicolateral pneumothorax but should be recognized when they extend outside the bony thorax or are traced bilaterally. Pneumomediastinum may simulate medial pneumothorax, but pneumomediastinum may cross the midline and extend into the retroperitoneum.

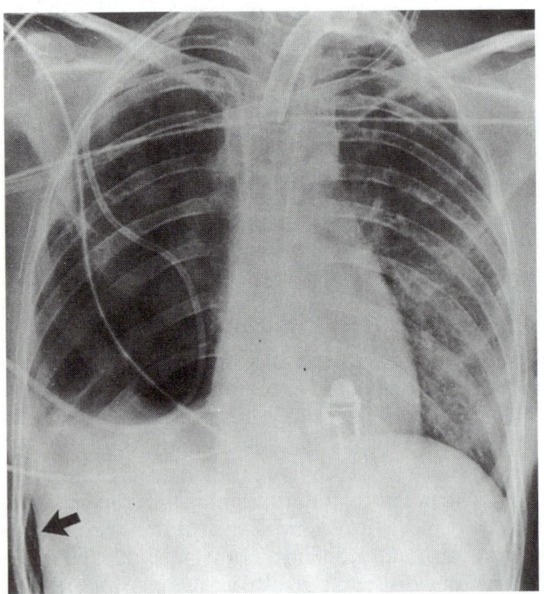

Figure 7–20. Pneumothorax in a supine patient with ARDS. Chest radiograph demonstrates a large right pneumothorax with intrapleural air adjacent to the diaphragm and evidence of a deep sulcus (arrow). The margin of the right hemidiaphragm is obliterated by adjacent adhesions.

B. Tension Pneumothorax

Recognition of even small pneumothoraces is crucial to prevention of progressive accumulation of pleural air collections, particularly in patients being maintained on mechanical ventilation. Tension pneumothorax occurs when the pressure of air in the pleural space exceeds ambient pressure during the respiratory cycle. With this pressure gradient, air enters the pleural space on inspiration but is prevented from exiting the pleural space during expiration owing to a check-valve mechanism. Tension pneumothorax may result in acute respiratory distress and, if untreated, cardiopulmonary arrest and death. The diagnosis of tension pneumothorax is made clinically, reflecting the hemodynamic sequelae of impaired venous return to the right heart. Radiographic signs include displacement of the mediastinum toward the contralateral thorax, inferior displacement or inversion of the diaphragm, and total lung collapse (Figure 7–21). However, significant hemodynamic compromise can exist in the absence of these findings. Adhesions may prevent mediastinal shift, and lung collapse may not occur in patients with stiff lungs such as those with ARDS. A small pneumothorax may convert to a tension pneumothorax, particularly in patients receiving mechanical ventilatory support.

Rankine JJ, Thomas AN, Fluechter D: Diagnosis of pneumothorax in critically ill adults. Postgrad Med J 2000;76:399–404.

Raptopoulos V et al: Factors affecting the development of pneumothorax associated with thoracentesis. AJR Am J Roentgenol 1991;156:917–20.

Tocino IM, Miller MH, Fairfax WR: Distribution of pneumothorax in the supine and semirecumbent critically ill adult. AJR Am J Roentgenol 1985;144:901–5.

PULMONARY INTERSTITIAL EMPHYSEMA & PNEUMOMEDIASTINUM

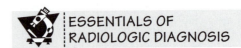

- *Pulmonary interstitial emphysema: Perivascular "halo" (air surrounding pulmonary vessels seen on end), linear radiolucencies radiating toward the hila, irregular radiolucent mottling, parenchymal cysts, or collections of air along visceral pleural surface.*
- *Pneumomediastinum: Linear lucencies adjacent to the heart and aortic arch, descending aorta, and great vessels. May have subcutaneous em-*

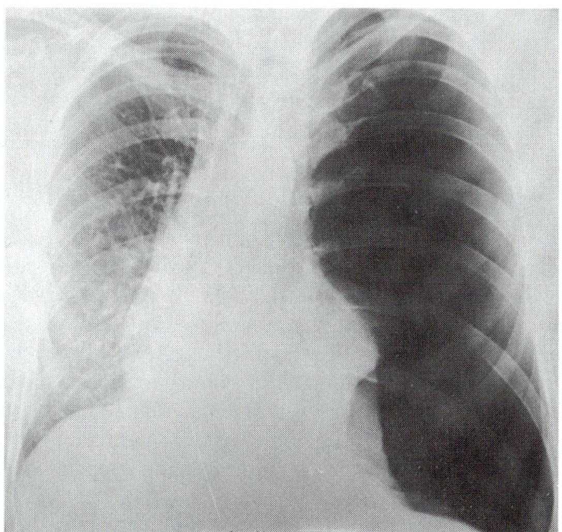

Figure 7–21. Spontaneous tension pneumothorax. The left lung is completely collapsed, with visualization of a visceral pleural line and hyperlucency of the thorax. The mediastinum is shifted to the right, and there is depression of the left hemidiaphragm consistent with tension pneumothorax.

physema with linear radiolucencies extending along tissue planes in the chest wall and neck.

General Considerations

Barotrauma is a serious and frequent complication in the ICU patient. Defined as damage secondary to the presence of extra-alveolar or extraluminal air, the incidence is highest in patients being supported by mechanical ventilation. Alveolar overdistention and an increased intra-alveolar pressure gradient from alveolus to vascular sheath allow rupture of air into the interstitial space along the perivascular sheaths, resulting in pulmonary interstitial emphysema. Reduction in the caliber of pulmonary vessels—as well as general and local alveolar overinflation—contributes to the pressure gradient, causing alveolar rupture. Although commonly associated with mechanical ventilation, barotrauma may also result from coughing, straining, trauma, pneumonia, a Valsalva maneuver, anesthesia or resuscitation, parturition, positive-pressure breathing, and asthma. Other manifestations of barotraumas develop because air from ruptured alveoli follows the path of least resistance. Air dissects centrally to cause pneumomediastinum and dissects via the cervical fascial planes, resulting in subcutaneous emphysema in the neck and chest wall. Air can also dissect from the mediastinum into the abdomen, leading to retroperitoneal air and pneumoperitoneum or into the pleural space resulting in a pneumothorax.

Barotrauma has a high incidence in patients with ARDS. In one study of 15 patients with ARDS—all requiring positive-pressure ventilation—radiographic evidence of pulmonary interstitial emphysema was found in 87%. Although there was no correlation with positive end-expiratory pressure or mean airway pressure, in all but one of the patients barotrauma was noted when peak airway pressure was > 40 cm H_2O. Other studies report an incidence of about 50% and suggest that PEEP does contribute to the development of barotrauma. Decreased compliance of the lungs in patients with ARDS necessitates higher ventilatory pressures to maintain adequate oxygenation, which results in an increased risk of barotrauma. Pulmonary diseases that increase lung compliance may also promote barotrauma since there is greater overdistention of the lung.

Radiographic Features

Radiographic findings of pulmonary interstitial emphysema include visualization of perivascular air along pulmonary vessels seen on end (producing a perivascular "halo"), linear radiolucencies radiating toward the hila, irregular radiolucent mottling, parenchymal cysts (pneumatoceles), and linear or rounded collections of air along the visceral pleural surface (subpleural air cysts). Pulmonary interstitial emphysema may be difficult to detect and to distinguish from air bronchograms. Moreover, pulmonary interstitial emphysema is usually not apparent radiographically unless present in conjunction with pulmonary opacification.

Pneumomediastinum may be recognized radiographically by linear lucencies adjacent to the heart and aortic arch, descending aorta, and great vessels. Visibility of the wall of a main bronchus, air outlining the thymus, and air between the parietal pleura and diaphragm have also been described. Pneumomediastinum is usually easier to identify than pulmonary interstitial emphysema and is often the first evidence of barotrauma. Subsequent dissection of air from the mediastinum along fascial planes may result in subcutaneous emphysema, with linear radiolucencies extending along tissue planes in the chest wall and neck (Figure 7–17). Less often, dissection of air along the descending aorta into the retroperitoneum will occur, with rare rupture into the abdomen giving rise to pneumoperitoneum. In such instances, clinical correlation is essential to exclude a perforated abdominal viscus. Early diagnosis of pulmonary interstitial emphysema may alert clinicians to pneumothorax, a potentially catastrophic consequence of barotrauma. Although other manifestations of barotrauma are usually self-limited, even a small pneumothorax may progress to tension pneumothorax in critically ill patients, particularly in patients being maintained with mechanical ventilators. As previously discussed, pneumothorax in the supine patient may be difficult to diagnose and must be considered or it will be missed. Occasionally, tension pneumomediastinum may occur, though this is usually of greater clinical likelihood in pediatric patients. Concomitant pulmonary interstitial emphysema will result in further respiratory embarrassment secondary to compression of lung parenchyma by interstitial air and decreases in both ventilation and perfusion. Pneumopericardium arises infrequently secondary to barotrauma but may progress to tension, in which there is increased intrapericardial pressure and impairment in venous return and cardiac function.

Beyers JA, Melonas CF: The visible wall of a main bronchus: A new radiological sign of pneumomediastinum. Br J Radiol 1987;60:877–9.

Haake R et al: Barotrauma pathophysiology, risk factors, and prevention. Chest 1987;91:608–13.

Unger JM, England DM, Bogust GA: Interstitial emphysema in adults: Recognition and prognostic implications. J Thorac Imaging 1989;4:86–94.

Woodring JH: Pulmonary interstitial emphysema in the adult respiratory distress syndrome. Crit Care Med 1985;13:786–91.

IMAGING OF THE ABDOMEN & PELVIS

General Principles

Imaging of the gastrointestinal tract should generally begin with plain radiographs since these are readily obtained and provide useful information regarding perforation, bowel obstruction, and ileus. However, because the overall sensitivity of plain radiographs remains low, further imaging with computed tomography may be necessary to confirm suspected pneumoperitoneum or intra-abdominal abscess and to inspect the features of the small and large bowel walls and surrounding fat. Imaging of abdominal and pelvic solid organs, including the gallbladder and urinary bladder, should begin with ultrasound, since it is nonionizing and portable at the bedside.

Plain Films

Plain abdominal radiographs are probably the most common radiographic test obtained to evaluate abdominal complaints or abnormal physical findings. Supine radiographs are most appropriate for verifying nasogastric or feeding tube placement and for investigation of renal stones and possible ileus or bowel obstruction. Additional views (semi-upright, left lateral decubitus, cross-table lateral) may be helpful in cases of bowel perforation, ileus, or obstruction.

Ultrasound

The versatility and portability of ultrasound aid in bedside diagnosis and guide therapeutic interventions in the ICU. Lack of ionizing radiation is another advantage. Ultrasound is very useful for evaluation of the hepatobiliary system, gallbladder, kidneys, pelvic organs, and scrotal disorders. Ultrasound provides a rapid assessment of vascular flow, parenchymal blood flow, and direction of flow, especially in transplanted organs. This technique also helps guide bedside biopsies and drainage of fluid collections.

Computed Tomography

Despite advances in other imaging procedures, computed tomography remains the single most useful imaging test for diagnosis of occult disease in the abdomen and pelvis. Multidetector row helical scanners can scan the chest, abdomen, and pelvis in less than a minute. A number of studies have consistently shown that significant additional information is obtained from CT when compared with plain radiography. However, transportation of critically ill ICU patients to and from the CT scanner must involve careful coordination between physicians, nurses, and respiratory therapists.

Nuclear Medicine

Nuclear medicine examinations are generally considered complementary functional imaging techniques for imaging organs and processes. Evaluation of the brain, lungs, heart, kidneys, lymphatics, and gastrointestinal tract is possible. Generalized searches for occult malignancies, infections, and active gastrointestinal bleeding may be conducted portably in the ICU. Portable organ-based examinations include study of biliary tract abnormalities with technetium Tc 99m imidodiacetic acid agents and of native and transplant renal function with technetium Tc 99m mercaptoacetyltriglycine (MAG-3) agents.

Magnetic Resonance Imaging

In most institutions, MR imaging is considered a problem-solving tool rather than a primary imaging modality. Routine MR imaging is generally more challenging in the ICU population. Most ICU equipment is ferromagnetically incompatible with MR imaging, and it is difficult to ventilate and monitor patients during MR imaging. However, with adequate investment in MR-compatible equipment and on-site equipment, MR imaging in the ICU may be feasible. Owing to its lack of ionizing radiation, multiplanar capability, and the low risk to renal function of gadolinium-DTPA contrast agents, MR imaging is generally considered the single best imaging method for evaluation of the central nervous system, head and neck, liver, and musculoskeletal system.

GASTROINTESTINAL PERFORATION

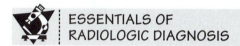

- *Lucency over the liver or abdomen.*
- *Lucency under a hemidiaphragm on upright views.*
- *"Double wall sign."*
- *Visualization of the falciform ligament.*
- *"Football sign."*
- *Inverted "V" sign.*
- *Triangle sign.*

General Considerations

In the ICU, bowel perforation usually results from an upper abdominal source, such as a penetrating gastric or duodenal ulcer, a lower GI tract source, such as diverticulitis or toxic megacolon, or from complications of upper and lower endoscopic procedures. Other causes of perforation include severe intestinal inflammation, bowel obstruction, bowel infarction, or neoplasm.

Radiographic Features

An experienced abdominal radiologist may identify even small amounts of free air on a supine abdominal radiograph, finding small bubbles or generalized increased lucency over the abdomen, right upper quadrant, or subhepatic space. Other signs include the "double wall sign" of Rigler, the "triangle sign," the "football sign," or the falciform ligament sign (Figure 7–22). For less experienced readers, a second view must be added to the supine radiograph to increase sensitivity. Most commonly, this is an upright abdominal film in which air rises to outline the thin curvilinear hemidiaphragm. However, to obtain this view properly is nearly impossible in the ICU. Useful alternatives include the left lateral decubitus view (where the patient maintained in the left side down position for at least 5–10 minutes), allowing free air to rise toward the right subphrenic space. A right lateral decubitus view is usually nondiagnostic because of confusion arising from the adjacent stomach bubble. In immobile patients, a cross-table lateral view may be obtained in which the patient remains supine but the x-ray beam is tangential to the anterior abdominal wall. However, small amounts of free air may be missed on this view. If plain films are equivocal and perforation is suspected, an abdominal CT (Figure 7–23) offers an excellent means of detecting even tiny amounts of free air and possibly localizing a source.

Differential Diagnosis

Pneumoperitoneum has a variety of causes and is not synonymous with bowel perforation, its most serious and surgically urgent cause. In the ICU, the most common reason for pneumoperitoneum is probably the postoperative state. Pneumoperitonem may persist for up to 14 days after surgery, the amount of air decreasing progressively and never increasing over time. Other forms of pneumoperitoneum requiring urgent attention include peritonitis caused by gas forming microorganisms. Benign causes include dissection of gas from the thoracic cavity in patients with COPD receiving mechanical ventilation.

Gore RM et al: Helical CT in the evaluation of the acute abdomen. AJR Am J Roentgenol 2000;174;901–13.

Mori PA, Mori KW: Abdomen. In: *Emergency Radiology*, 2nd ed. Keats TE (editor). Year Book, 1989.

Shaffer HA Jr: Perforation and obstruction of the gastrointestinal tract: Assessment by conventional radiology. Radiol Clin North Am 1992;30:405–26.

BOWEL OBSTRUCTION

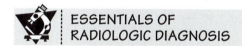

- *Asymmetric dilation of proximal bowel loops.*
- *Normal or collapsed distal bowel loops.*
- *Small bowel obstruction: dilated U-shaped loops with air-fluid levels (upright or decubitus films) or a single loop with air fluid at different heights.*
- *Large bowel obstruction: cecal distention, absence of rectal gas.*
- *CT scan: excellent for detecting bowel obstruction and confirming the cause.*

General Considerations

Mechanical obstruction of the bowel is a relatively common occurrence in hospitalized patients. In the general population, bowel obstructions account for approxi-

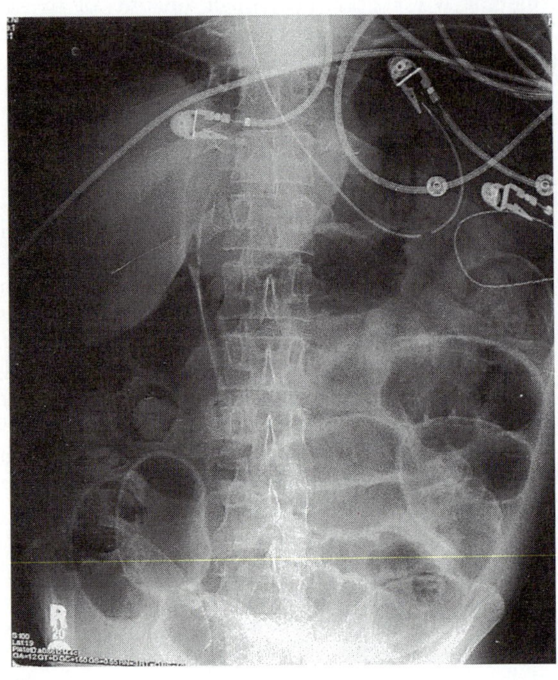

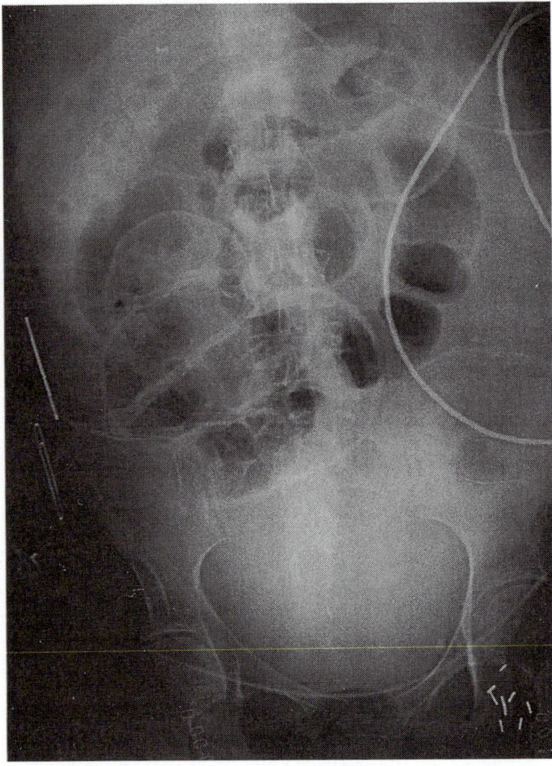

A B

Figure 7–22. ***A:*** Pneumoperitoneum in a 72-year-old man with perforated sigmoid diverticulitis. On a supine radiograph, there is lucency over the right upper quadrant, with visualization of falciform ligament. Both sides of small bowel wall are visualized (Rigler's sign) with characteristic triangles. ***B:*** Pneumoperitoneum in an 80-year-old man after recent abdominal surgery. Supine radiograph demonstrates a more subtle example of Rigler's sign.

mately 20% of acute abdominal conditions. Obstruction usually results from extrinsic compression but can occur from luminal obstruction. Without prompt attention, bowel obstruction may progress to bowel infarction because of disruption of venous outflow and subsequent arterial blood supply. Bowel infarction may progress to mucosal ulceration, necrosis, and perforation. Mortality rates for untreated obstruction have been as high as 60%.

Approximately three-fourths of bowel obstructions are related to the small bowel (enteric) and one-fourth to the colon. Small bowel obstructions are most commonly due to adhesions from prior abdominal surgery. Adhesions can form rapidly, sometimes within 4–10 days after surgery, or may develop manifestations many years later. Other causes of small bowel obstruction include hernias (external and internal), primary and metastatic tumor, intussusception, inflammatory bowel disease, abscesses, and trauma.

Large bowel obstructions are most often (60%) caused by primary carcinomas of the distal (left) colon. Metastatic tumor or invasion from cancers of surrounding organs, diverticulitis, volvulus, and fecal impaction may also cause colonic obstruction.

Radiographic Features

A. Plain Abdominal Radiographs

An abdominal series that includes supine plus upright or decubitus views of the abdomen is only 50–60% sensitive for small bowel obstruction. Objective evidence of small bowel obstruction includes asymmetric dilation (luminal diameter > 3 cm) of small bowel proximal to the site of obstruction, with normal or decompressed small bowel loops distally and normal to absent colonic gas. However, these findings may not be seen in an individual patient with small bowel obstruction. More valu-

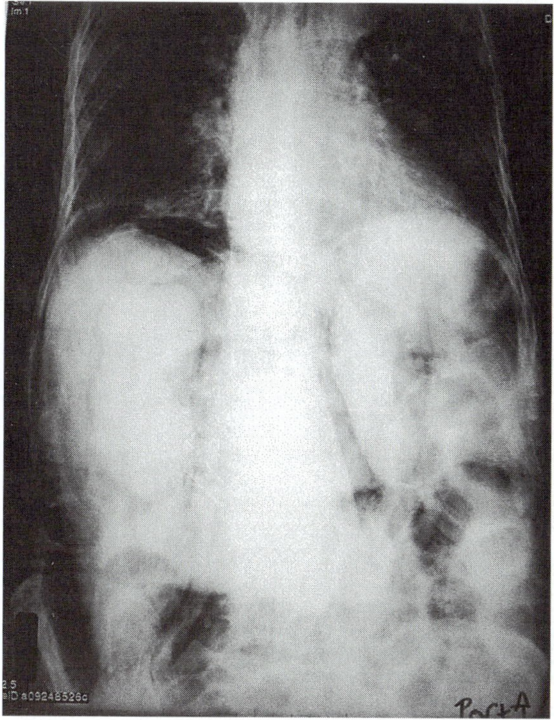

A

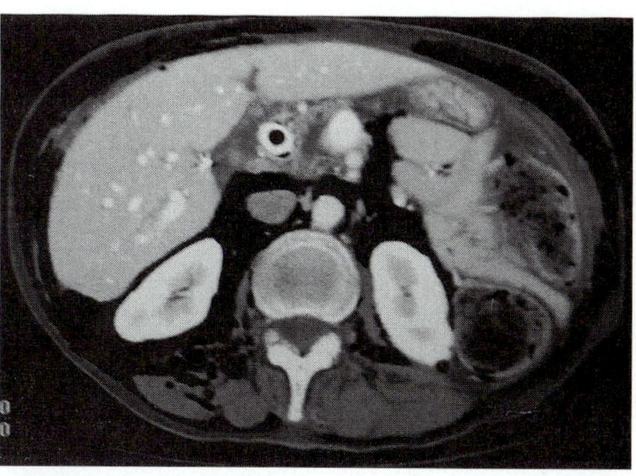

B

Figure 7–23. ***A:*** Pneumoperitoneum and pneumoretroperitoneum in a 76-year-old man after biliary stent placement because of obstruction from pancreatic cancer. A supine radiograph shows characteristic air under the diaphragm and surrounding liver. The psoas muscles and kidneys are also outlined by gas, confirming the presence of pneumoretroperitoneum. ***B:*** Abdominal CT demonstrates ectopic gas and confirms the diagnosis of pneumoperitoneum in the patient in Figure 7–21B.

able is the relative change in distention over time, and for this reason comparison of a series of studies is prudent. Other radiographic signs include an inverted U-shaped loop of dilated small bowel with air-fluid levels, multiple air-fluid levels, and dynamic loops (air-fluid levels at varying heights in different limbs of a loop) In some cases, a "string of pearls" sign will be seen (Figure 7–24).

On a single supine film of the abdomen, dilated small bowel loops may be mostly fluid-filled, with a minimal amount of gas, or may be completely devoid of gas. In this case, the film will be nonspecific, and additional views or CT may be required. Diagnosis of small bowel obstruction may be difficult because the presence of radiographic signs will depend on the site, duration, and degree of obstruction. Bowel distal to a complete obstruction takes 12–48 hours to evacuate all of its gas. Serial plain films are sometimes required to capture these changes, since films may be nonspecific if imaging is performed too early.

Because of the limited utility of plain radiographs, helical CT is now the preferred method for evaluating suspected bowel obstruction (Figure 7–25). In patients who cannot undergo CT or if CT is unavailable, serial radiographs may be taken after ingestion of enteric contrast material. Although water-soluble contrast agents are preferred, especially for patients who are surgical candidates, they are hypertonic and become progressively more dilute, limiting the ability of the study to accurately identify the site of obstruction. Barium is preferred in nonsurgical patients since progressive dilution does not occur and the site of obstruction is more easily identified. However, in high-grade obstructions, barium may thicken and become difficult to evacuate. The high density of retained barium also degrades CT images because of a beam hardening artifact that results in a nondiagnostic CT examination. Given these problems, CT is the initial imaging procedure of choice if small bowel obstruction is suspected.

In general, colonic obstruction (Figure 7–26) tends to occur distally since most obstructing colon cancers occur in the distal large bowel. A single supine radiograph often fails to identify the site of obstruction, and supplementary views—an upright view, a right lateral decubitus view, or a prone view—may be necessary to work up a possible obstruction and distinguish it from ileus. In large bowel obstruction, the cecum distends to a greater degree than does the remainder of the colon regardless of the site of obstruction. This follows from Laplace's law, which states that the pressure required to distend the walls of a hollow structure is inversely proportionate to its radius. The cecum has the largest radius

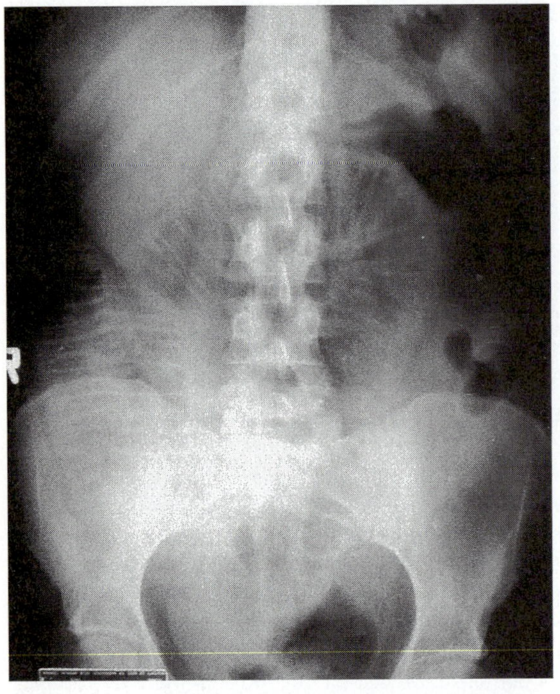

A

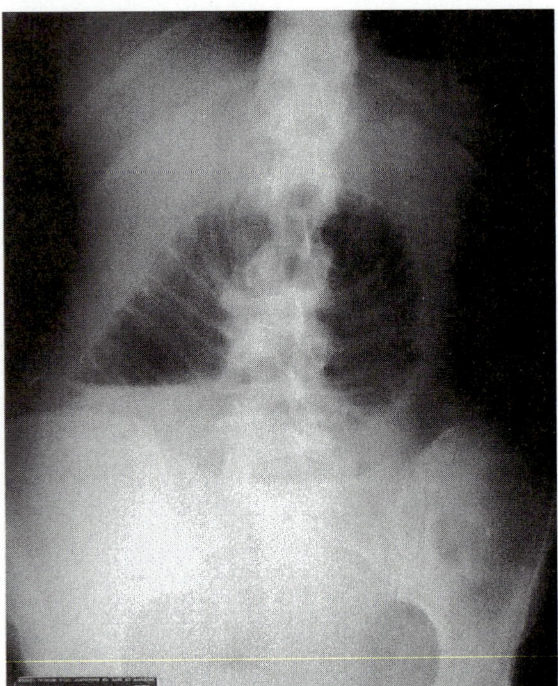

B

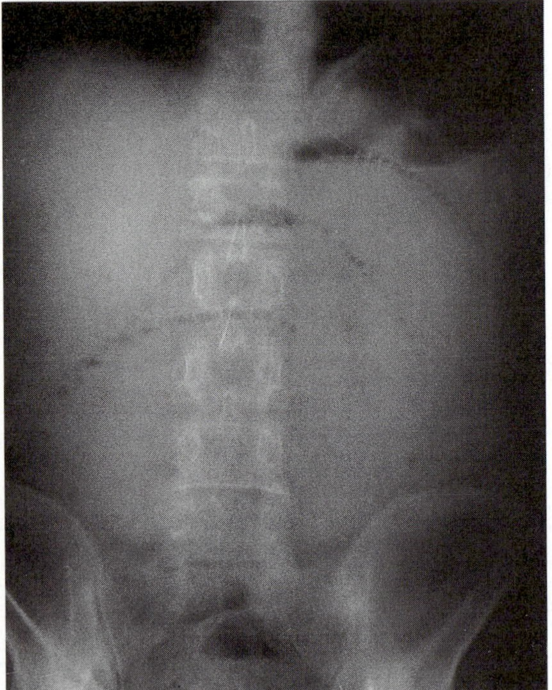

C

Figure 7–24. ***A:*** Small bowel obstruction. Because of their widespread availability, conventional upright and supine radiographs are a good first step in suspected small bowel obstruction, although sensitivity and specificity are low. A supine radiograph demonstrates asymmetric dilation of the proximal small bowel (note plicae circulares) without significant gas in the colon. ***B:*** In the same patient, an upright abdominal radiograph demonstrates a prominent air-fluid level from proximal small bowel obstruction. ***C:*** The "string of pearls" sign in small bowel obstruction; an upright radiograph demonstrates numerous air-fluid levels.

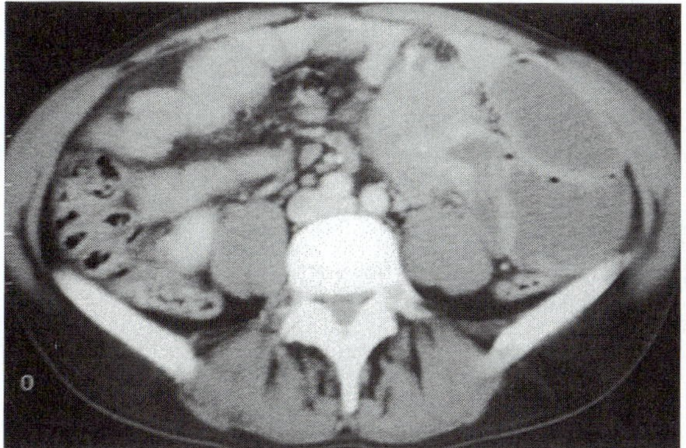
A

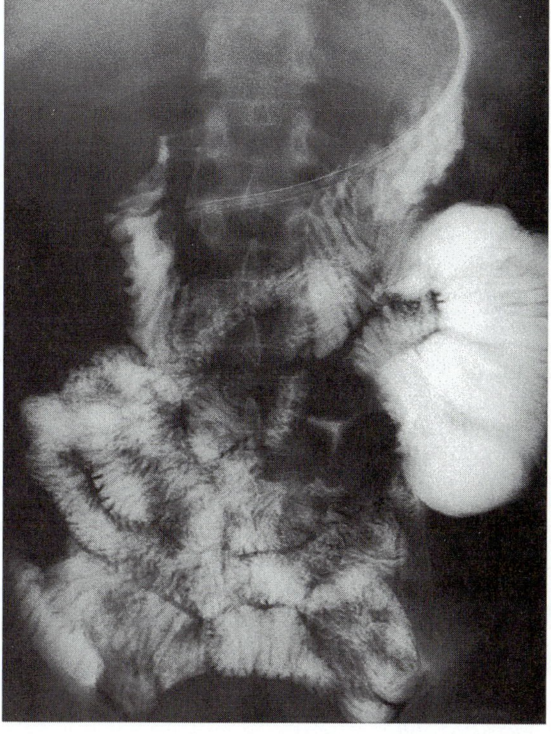
B

Figure 7–25. ***A:*** CT is excellent for diagnosing small bowel obstruction and detecting a cause (mass, intussusception, hernia). In this patient, a large leiomyosarcoma caused a high-grade small bowel obstruction. ***B:*** In certain situations, following luminal contrast through the small bowel ("small bowel follow-through") may be helpful for detecting small bowel obstruction. This study from the same patient demonstrates an abrupt tapering of the bowel lumen with dilated proximal bowel due to the mass.

of any part of the large bowel. Generally, the upper limits of normal for the transverse diameter of a large bowel loop is 6 cm; for the cecum it is 9 cm. However, these are rough estimates only and may not hold true for a given patient. Again, one must interpret, if possible, the relative change in distention over time with comparison studies over time. Perforation is a dread complication of obstruction. The overall risk of cecal perforation is low—approximately 1.5%—but may increase to 14% with delay in diagnosis. There is an increased risk of cecal perforation if the luminal diameter exceeds 9 cm and persists for more than 2–3 days.

B. Computed Tomography

Over the last 10 years, several investigators have emphasized the value of CT scanning in detecting bowel obstruction. Helical CT can help determine whether obstruction is present, the severity and level of obstruction, the cause of obstruction, and whether strangulation or ischemia is present. Current helical and multidetector row technology permits evaluation of the abdomen and pelvis in 20 seconds to 2 minutes. Oral and intravenous contrast may not be required if experienced radiologists interpret the scans. In most cases of small bowel obstruction, a transition point between dilated and nondilated bowel can be demonstrated. Although adhesions themselves are too thin to be imaged, most other common causes of small bowel obstruction—including hernia, tumor, intussusception, postradiation fibrosis, and gallstone ileus—may be identified. The accuracy of CT is 90–95% in high-grade bowel obstruction but somewhat less in low-grade obstruction.

Brolin RE, Krasna MJ, Mast BA: Use of tubes and radiographs in the management of small bowel obstruction. Ann Surg 1987;206:126–33.

Ericksen AS et al: Use of gastrointestinal contrast studies in obstruction of the small and large bowel. Dis Colon Rectum 1990;33:56–64.

Lappas JC, Reyes BL, Maglinte DD: Abdominal radiography findings in small-bowel obstruction: relevance to triage for additional diagnostic imaging. AJR Am J Roentgenol 2001;176:167–74.

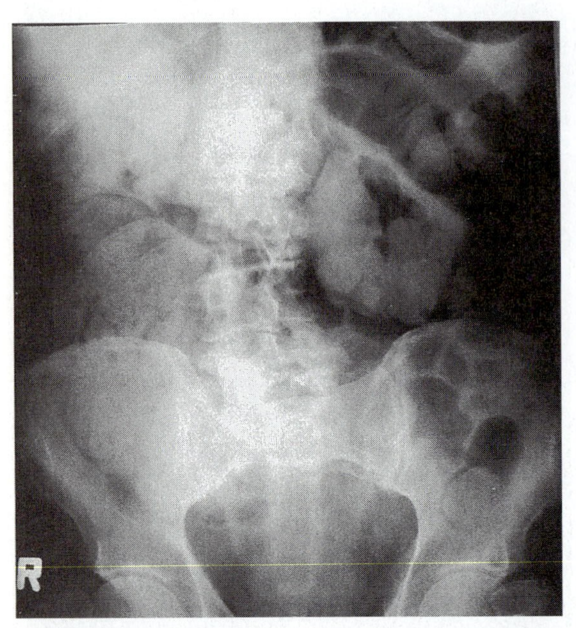

A

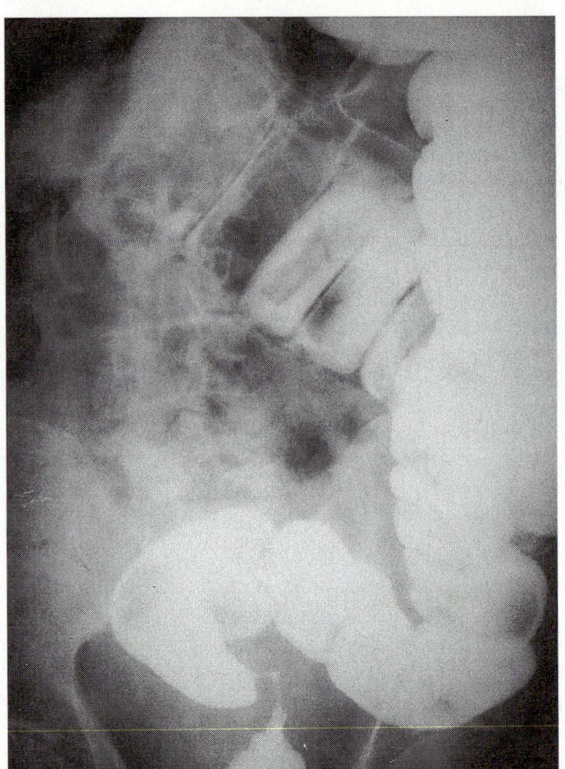

B

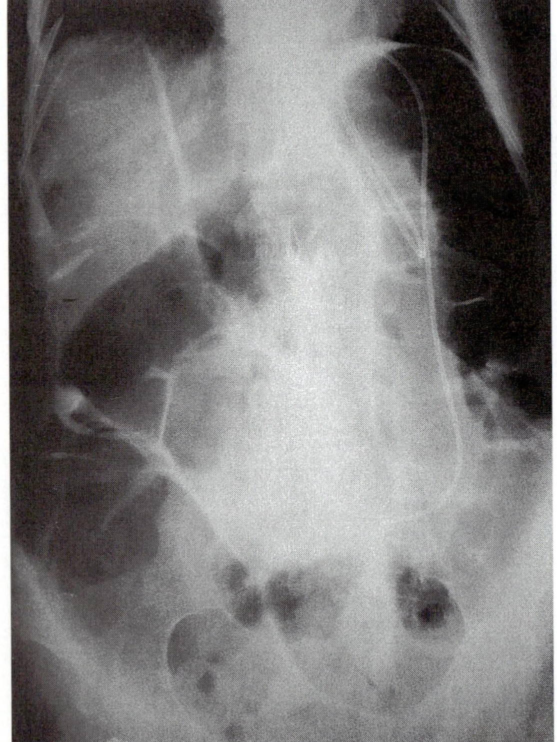

C

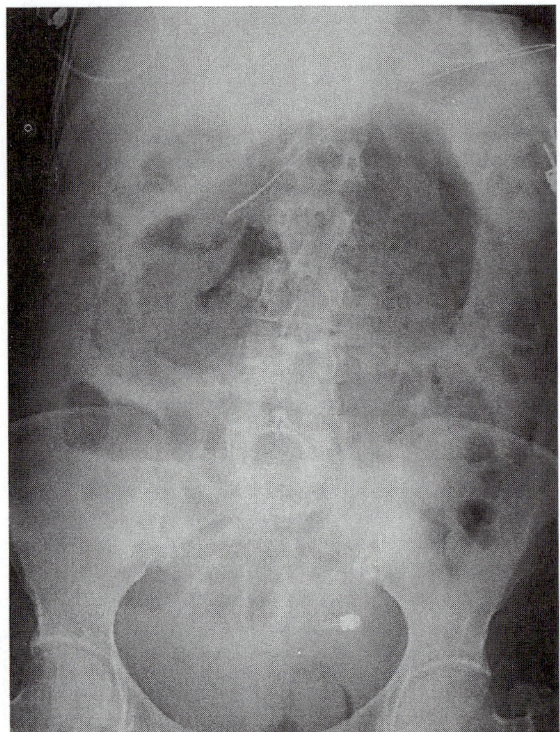

D

Maglinte DD et al: The role of radiology in the diagnosis of small-bowel obstruction. AJR Am J Roentgenol 1997;168:1171–80.

Maglinte DD et al: Small-bowel obstruction: optimizing radiologic investigation and nonsurgical management. Radiology 2001;218:39–46.

Megibow AJ et al: Bowel Obstruction: Evaluation with CT. Radiology 1991;180:313–8.

Shaffer HA Jr: Perforation and obstruction of the gastrointestinal tract: Assessment by conventional radiology. Radiol Clin North Am 1992;30:405–26.

ILEUS

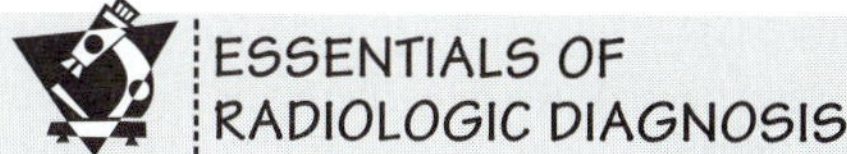

ESSENTIALS OF RADIOLOGIC DIAGNOSIS

- *Diffuse symmetric dilation of small and large bowel.*
- *May be focal when adjacent to an inflammatory source.*
- *Colonic ileus (Ogilvie's syndrome) may be seen alone or in conjunction with small bowel ileus.*

General Considerations

Ileus is generalized dysfunction of bowel related to an underlying disorder, usually most severe in the 2–4 days following abdominal surgery with extensive bowel manipulation. Dysfunction due to humoral, metabolic, and neural factors contributes to the overall process. Other common causes include abdominal infections, peritonitis, active inflammatory bowel disease, opioid or chemotherapy use, electrolyte imbalances, visceral pain syndrome (biliary or ureteral colic, ovarian torsion), and myocardial infarction.

Radiographic Features

In the generalized form of ileus, the small and large bowel are dilated but generally to a lesser degree than seen in moderate to severe bowel obstruction (Figure 7–27). In many cases, there is a significant overlap with clinical and radiologic features of small bowel obstruction, and differentiation on the basis of a single study may not be possible. Serial radiographs, contrast studies with water-soluble contrast agents or barium, or CT may be required.

An intra-abdominal inflammatory event (acute pancreatitis) or trauma may produce a focal form of ileus. The dysfunctional segment of bowel may lose peristaltic activity and enlarge. This is known as a sentinel loop.

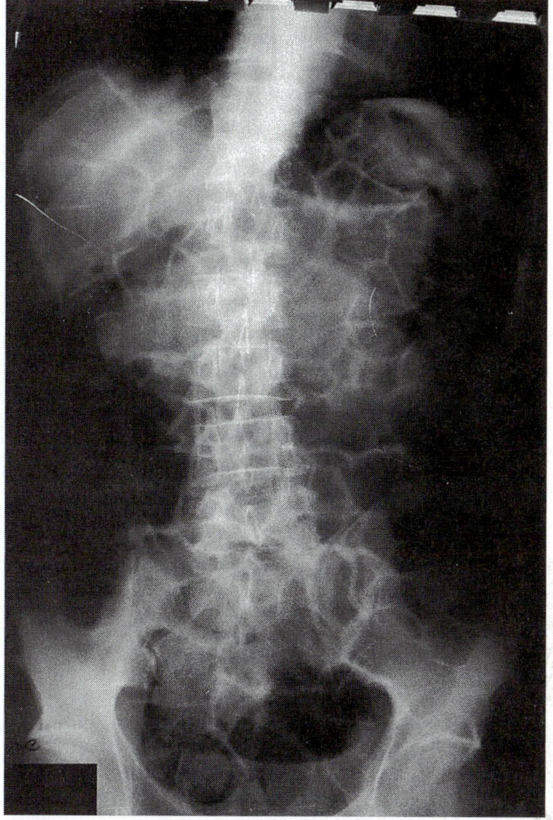

Figure 7–27. Ileus. Plain abdominal radiograph demonstrates mild diffuse gaseous dilation of both the small and the large bowel. No transition point is present.

Figure 7–26. Large bowel obstruction. ***A:*** Most large bowel obstructions occur distally and are due to tumors or diverticulitis. In this patient, the large bowel is diffusely dilated and filled with stool. ***B:*** A single-contrast barium enema depicts a short segment annular carcinoma causing sigmoid colon obstruction. ***C:*** Sigmoid volvulus. On plain radiograph, the dilated sigmoid colon may project over the right upper quadrant with a "coffee bean" appearance. The remainder of the colon is dilated. ***D:*** Cecal volvulus: On plain radiographs, the dilated cecum is filled with stool and projects over the mid abdomen or sometimes the left upper quadrant. The small bowel is diffusely dilated.

Colonic ileus—also known as intestinal pseudoobstruction, or Ogilvie's syndrome—usually presents in elderly debilitated or bedridden patients with major underlying systemic abnormalities, severe infection, cardiac disease, or recent surgery. Progressive large bowel distention is variably accompanied by small bowel distention. Massive cecal distention compromises blood flow and may be complicated by perforation, with a mortality rate of 30–45%. As in the small bowel, colonic ileus is not always diffuse and may be segmental, typically in the cecum. In cecal ileus, there is massive dilation of the cecum. If the cecum is mobile, this condition may be difficult to distinguish from cecal volvulus and a contrast examination may be necessary to make the differentiation.

Conservative treatment, consisting of nasogastric tube, rectal tube, or colonoscopic decompression, is successful in 78% of cases. Alternatively, surgical cecostomy may be necessary. Percutaneous cecostomy may be offered to high-risk patients.

Eisenberg RL: *Gastrointestinal Radiology*, 3rd ed. Lippincott Williams Wilkins, 1995.

Johnson CD et al: The radiologic evaluation of gross cecal distension: emphasis on cecal ileus. AJR Am J Roentgenol 1985;145:1211–7.

vanSonnenberg E et al: Percutaneous cecostomy for Ogilvie syndrome: laboratory observations and clinical experience. Radiology 1990;175:679–82.

INTESTINAL ISCHEMIA

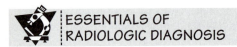

ESSENTIALS OF RADIOLOGIC DIAGNOSIS

- *Plain films: Early, nonspecific dilation of bowel; later: focal, edematous, thick-walled bowel loops, gas in the superior mesenteric and portal veins, pneumatosis intestinalis, ileus, and gasless abdomen.*
- *Abdominal CT: bowel wall thickening, pneumatosis, portal venous gas.*
- *CT or MR angiography provides excellent evaluation of the larger mesenteric arteries and veins.*
- *Conventional angiography is infrequently needed but may be confirmatory in some situations.*

General Considerations

Early diagnosis of bowel ischemia and infarction remains difficult because of limited clinical and radiologic sensitivity. Vascular insufficiency must be considered in elderly patients or for any patient with atherosclerotic vascular disease, hypotension, cardiac failure, or arteritis. In young patients, vasculitis, a hypercoagulable state, pregnancy, illicit use of cocaine, or embolic sources (eg, patent foramen ovale) must be suspected. Morbidity and mortality rates remain high (30–80%).

Ischemia has a variety of underlying causes, including mesenteric arterial occlusion (thrombus, embolus, dissection), venous occlusion (hypercoagulable states, malignancy), nonocclusive mesenteric ischemia (hypoperfusion, myocardial infarction, shock), and mechanical obstruction, including colonic pseudo-obstruction. Any portion of the small bowel may be affected; the cecum and distal left colon are the large bowel segments most commonly affected. Rectal ischemia is infrequent because of the rectum's dual blood supply, but it may be seen in patients who have had prior radiation therapy to that area.

Clinical symptoms are variable. Generally, abdominal pain out of proportion to physical findings and bloody diarrhea may be suggestive of ischemic colitis. Segmental ischemia often resolves spontaneously, but fibrotic strictures may develop. Infarcted bowel must be surgically resected. In selected cases, clots identified on intravenous contrast-enhanced CT may be treated with angiographic interventional techniques, including thrombolysis or stent placement.

Radiographic Features

A. Plain Radiographs

Edematous, thick-walled bowel, pneumatosis intestinalis, and portal venous gas are the most specific signs of ischemia and infarction but are insensitive. More commonly, plain films are normal, show lack of abdominal gas, or suggest focal ileus or small bowel obstruction (Figure 7–28).

B. Computed Tomography

Helical CT is important for detecting early changes of ischemia. A high-quality helical CT is usually performed with oral contrast to opacify and distend the small bowel along with rapid intravenous contrast injection (3 mL/s) to optimize opacification of the superior mesenteric artery and vein. The CT features of intestinal ischemia vary with its cause, chronicity, and severity. Bowel wall thickening is a sensitive but nonspecific early finding and may be accompanied by a "target sign" appearance of bowel caused by submucosal edema. Indirect signs of ischemia include focal ascites, bowel distention, and mesenteric edema. In more advanced stages of bowel ischemia, the presence of gas within the bowel wall or within the superior mesenteric or portal vein makes the prognosis more grave. Colonic ischemia generally results from hypoperfusion or hy-

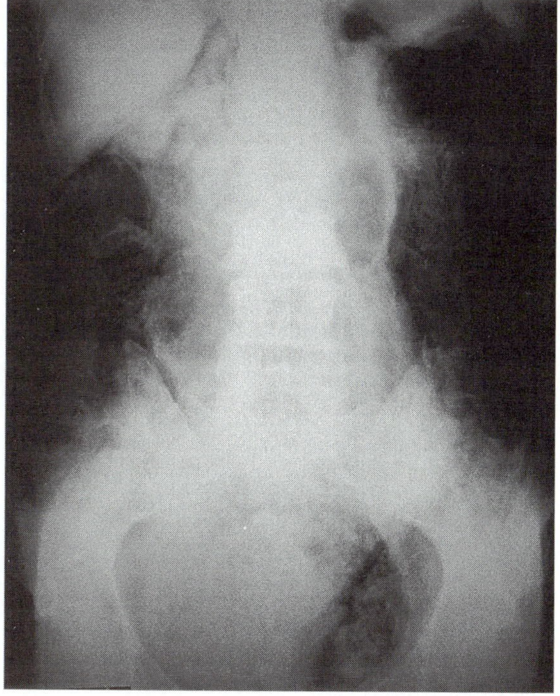

A

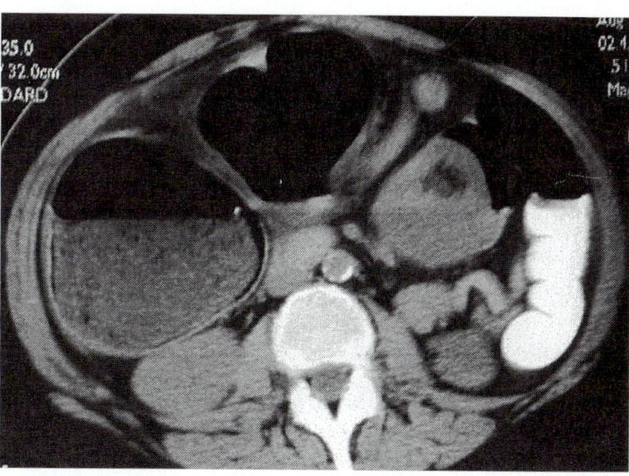

B

Figure 7–28. Colonic ischemia. ***A:*** Plain radiograph demonstrates mottled lucency of the wall of the ascending colon consistent with pneumatosis. ***B:*** Abdominal CT is excellent for confirmation of pneumatosis.

potension, and mesenteric thrombosis is rare. With the advent of multidetector row helical scanners, CT angiography may help to evaluate vascular patency. Thrombus in the major mesenteric vessels may be detected. However, a normal CT does not exclude ischemia, and if a strong clinical suspicion is present—especially in patients with vasculitis—angiography or surgery may be required.

C. Catheter Angiography

Angiography may be both diagnostic and therapeutic. Vasodilators may be used in conjunction with thrombolytic agents in certain patients. Due to its unparalleled spatial resolution, it is the diagnostic test of choice in patients with vasculitides. Angiography has a limited role in colonic ischemia since low blood flow states rather than occlusion of the vasculature are most often the cause.

Balthazar EJ, Yen BC, Gordon RB: Ischemic colitis: CT evaluation of 54 cases. Radiology 1999;211:381–8.

Levine JS, Jacobson ED: Intestinal ischemic disorders. Dig Dis 1995;13:3–24.

Smerud MJ, Johnson CD, Stephens DH: Diagnosis of bowel infarction: A comparison of plain films and CT scans in 23 cases. AJR Am J Roentgenol 1990;154:99–103.

COLITIS

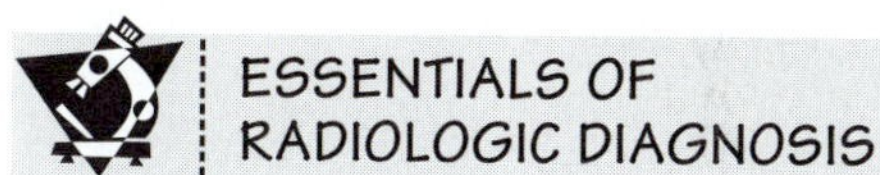
ESSENTIALS OF
RADIOLOGIC DIAGNOSIS

- *Colonic wall thickening and nodularity associated with paralytic ileus.*
- *Infiltration of pericolonic fat, often seen on CT.*
- *Plaque-like filling defects are suggestive of pseudomembranous colitis.*

General Considerations

Inflammatory bowel disease, ischemia, and infections are the most common causes of colitis. Patients present with pain, bloody diarrhea, cramping, fever, and leukocytosis. Infectious colitis may be bacterial, viral, fungal, or parasitic. Stool cultures, serologic tests, or colonic biopsy may be required.

Pseudomembranous colitis—the most common cause of colitis in hospitalized populations—is a complication of antibiotic therapy. *Clostridium difficile* produces an enterotoxin that causes mucosal ulceration and edema and the development of pseudomembranes. The process may be focal or diffuse.

Neutropenic colitis is typically seen in patients undergoing chemotherapy or bone marrow transplantation with myelosuppression. Although involvement can be diffuse, it typically affects the ascending colon, cecum, appendix, and terminal ileum. If cecal inflammation is present, then the term typhlitis is used.

Radiographic Features

Although usually normal or nonspecific, plain radiographs may reveal colonic fold thickening and nodularity. Features of paralytic ileus may be present. Contrast studies such as a barium enema should be avoided, but can be performed carefully with water-soluble agents only if absolutely necessary (Figure 7–29). Although abdominal CT is an excellent test, it may be normal in early infectious colitis. In more advanced cases of infectious colitis and in pseudomembranous colitis, mural thickening is more severe, averaging 15–20 mm, with a target or halo pattern. An accordion-like pattern reflecting haustral thickening may be produced in addition to pericolonic inflammatory changes and lymphadenopathy. In neutropenic colitis (typhlitis), similar features are present, but most commonly in the right colon. Occasionally in advanced cases, pneumatosis intestinalis and frank perforation may develop.

Johnson GL, Johnson PT, Fishman EK: CT evaluation of the acute abdomen: bowel pathology spectrum of disease. Crit Rev Diagn Imaging 1996;37:163–90.

Kawamoto S, Horton KM, Fishman EK: Pseudomembranous colitis: can CT predict which patients will need surgical intervention? J Comput Assist Tomogr 1999;23:79–85.

Ruiz-Healy F, Manzanilla-Sevilla M, Orozco-Vazquez J: Acute abdomen caused by inflammatory colonic non-parasitic pathology: staging by CT. Int Surg 1996;84:39–42.

TOXIC MEGACOLON

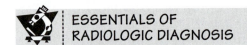

ESSENTIALS OF RADIOLOGIC DIAGNOSIS

- *Gaseous colonic distention, which may be diffuse or segmental.*

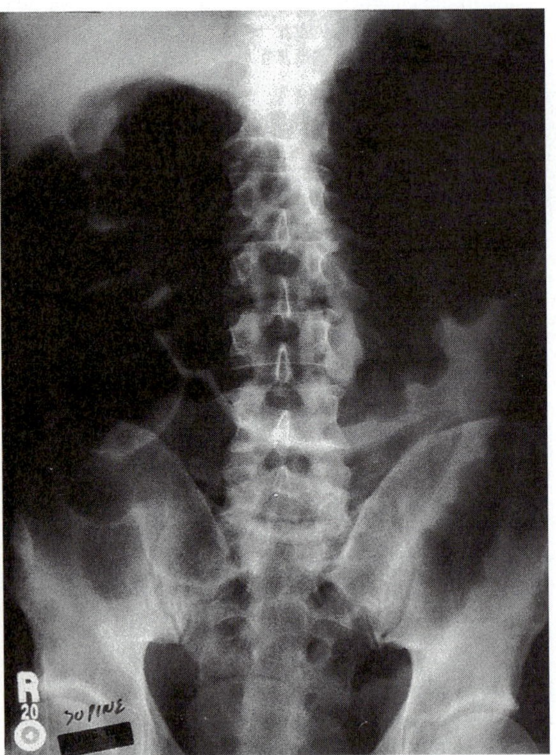

A

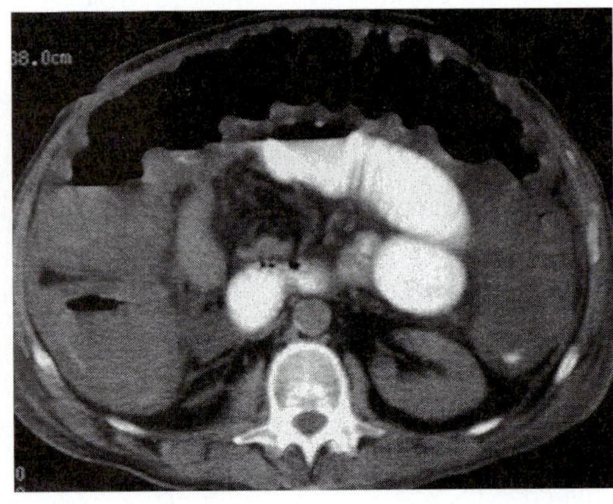

B

Figure 7–29. ***A:*** Colitis. Plain radiograph demonstrates mild dilation and severe fold thickening (thumbprinting) of transverse colon in this case of pseudomembranous colitis. ***B:*** Abdominal CT also demonstrates mural colonic thickening with associated infiltration of the pericolonic fat.

- *Effacement of haustra, edematous folds (thumbprinting), relative paucity of feces.*
- *Common complication of a number of inflammatory conditions, notably ulcerative colitis.*

General Considerations

Toxic megacolon is a complication of many different types of ischemic, inflammatory, or infectious conditions of the colon but is most closely associated with ulcerative colitis. Patients are usually in extremis, complaining of fever and bloody diarrhea. Tachycardia and abdominal pain may be present. Clinical features are accompanied by thickened colonic haustra on plain radiographs. Owing to the transmural nature of the inflammation, the neuromuscular and neurohumoral tone of the colon is disrupted. Without treatment, the mortality rate is nearly 20%.

Radiographic Features

Generally, plain radiographs will reveal varying degrees of colonic dilation (generally > 6.5 cm) with or without associated fold thickening. Thickened or effaced haustra are present, with edematous or inflamed folds, and there is a paucity of feces. An enema is contraindicated if toxic megacolon is suspected (Figure 7–30). These features are seen to better advantage on abdominal CT, and complications such as perforation and gas within the colonic wall are easier to detect. The pericolonic fat is usually infiltrated, and both colon and fat are sometimes hyperemic.

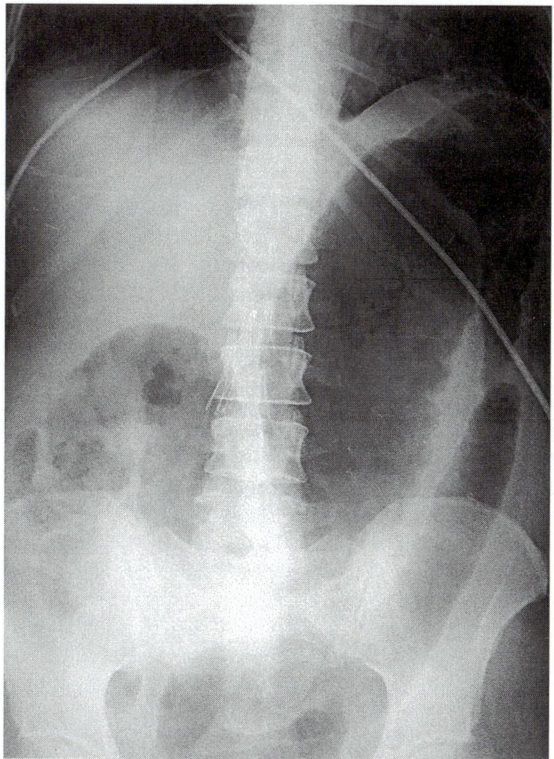

Figure 7–30. Toxic megacolon. Plain radiograph demonstrates diffuse dilation and severe thickening of mucosal folds (thumbprinting) of the colon. There is no stool. The patient was in extremis with a severe flare of ulcerative colitis.

INTRA-ABDOMINAL ABSCESS

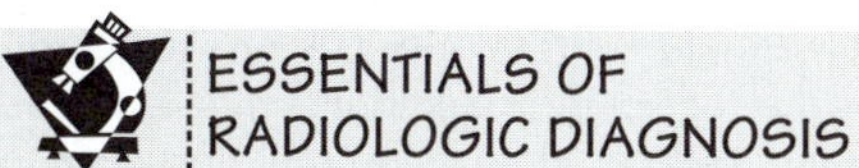

ESSENTIALS OF RADIOLOGIC DIAGNOSIS

- *Plain film: usually invisible except when abscess is gas-filled or produces a mass effect.*
- *Ultrasound: well circumscribed collection of variably echogenic fluid.*
- *Abdominal CT: Well-circumscribed fluid-filled mass, which may contain gas. Wall is of variable thickness and enhancement.*
- *Radionuclide scintigraphy: Radionuclide-tagged white blood cell scan may be useful in search for occult abscess or other sources of infection.*

General Considerations

Over the past 25 years, imaging has revolutionized the diagnosis and management of abdominal and pelvic abscesses, often precluding the need for laparotomy and for incision and drainage in the vast majority of patients.

Intra-abdominal abscesses are typically caused by perforated appendicitis in the young and diverticulitis in the elderly. Overall, most cases are iatrogenic, occurring after intra-abdominal surgery. The mortality remains high, ranging from 80% to 100% without treatment and 30% in patients receiving appropriate treatment.

Radiographic Features

A. Plain Radiographs

These may be helpful in evaluating the gastrointestinal tract but are not generally able to localize an abscess.

On occasion, the abscess will appear as a gasless fluid collection mimicking a mass with defined radiodense contours that displaces bowel or bladder.

B. Ultrasound

Ultrasound is an excellent means for bedside evaluation of defined areas such as the upper quadrants, the paracolic gutters, and the pelvis. Features that suggest an infected fluid accumulation on sonography include rounded or ovoid collections with thick walls, with variable internal echoes, and without evidence of central vascularity as demonstrated by color, power, or spectral Doppler signals. Focal bright echoes with variable shadowing within collections may suggest the presence of gas. However, these signs are not specific for infected fluid; a hematoma or seroma may appear identical. On the other hand, noninfected collections generally have angular margins, conform to anatomic spaces, and tend to lack significant internal echogenicity.

Ultrasound is especially valuable for evaluating the subdiaphragmatic regions or the low pelvis. However, one should bear in mind its limitations. Ultrasound will not reliably evaluate the retroperitoneum and retroperitoneal organs such as the pancreatic body and tail. Evaluation of complex collections in postoperative patients or in patients with open abdominal incisions or surgical dressings is likely to be suboptimal. Imaging of abscesses within organs may be difficult.

C. Computed Tomography

Computed tomography is the method of choice for evaluation of an intra-abdominal abscess (Figure 7–31). Although preparation with oral and intravenous contrast agents is preferred for optimal diagnosis in most patients, contrast is not always required when using the latest-generation equipment. This is especially true in obese patients because of inherent contrast provided by intra-abdominal fat. Actual scanning time with a multidetector row helical scanner is typically on the order of 20–40 seconds.

Abscesses generally appear as round or ovoid collections with thick surrounding rims. Intraluminal gas due to anaerobic bacterial infection may be present in up to 50% of collections. If intravenous contrast is given, enhancement of the surrounding rim may be noted in up to 50% of abscesses. Abscesses under the diaphragm and surrounding the liver or kidney may have crescentic margins. However, in many cases, the CT signs of an abscess are nonspecific. Necrotic tumor may have an identical appearance, and percutaneous aspiration may be required to distinguish between them.

D. Radionuclide Scintigraphy

Although unnecessary in the vast majority of patients, nuclear medicine studies with indium (^{111}In)-labeled or gallium citrate (^{67}Ga)-labeled white blood cells are useful for the detection of occult abscesses, especially in patients with fever of unknown origin. Both indium-oxine-labeled and gallium citrate-labeled cells are injected intravenously, and scans are typically obtained 48–72 hours later. Although gallium is highly sensitive for detection of intra-abdominal abscess (80–90%), specificity is limited by intestinal secretion at 48–72 hours. Overall, indium-labeled white blood cell scans are more accurate for abdominal applications.

E. Algorithm for Imaging the Patient With Suspected Abdominal Abscess

In patients without localizing signs or symptoms and varying degrees of suspicion of abdominal abscess, the test of choice is helical or multidetector row CT with intravenous and oral contrast. This study helps exclude potential peritoneal and retroperitoneal sources of infection. CT is necessary for adequate visualization of the pancreas, psoas muscles, other retroperitoneal structures, and complex collections. CT is superior to other imaging methods in patients with ileus, open incisions, dressings, indwelling catheters, and drains. If symptoms are localized to the upper abdominal quadrants or to the pelvis, ultrasound is an excellent choice for diagnosis and can be quickly performed at the bedside. Furthermore, bedside percutaneous incision and drainage may be performed with sonographic guidance. Scintigraphy has a limited role in diagnosing abscess in an acutely ill patient.

F. Percutaneous Image-Guided Drainage

Percutaneous drainage has revolutionized the management of infected fluid collections. Expanded criteria render only a small minority of collections unsuitable for such drainage. General criteria include a fluid collection at least 2–3 cm in diameter and safe access to the collection without intervening blood vessels, pleura, bladder, or bowel. One should confirm with CT or sonographic Doppler that the collection in question is not a pseudoaneurysm. Fluid collections may be multiloculated or communicate with the gastrointestinal, biliary, or genitourinary tracts. Solid organ and tubo-ovarian abscesses may be safely drained, though the latter frequently respond to antibiotics and needle aspiration alone.

A variety of catheter types and sizes are available. Noninfected serous collections can usually be drained with 6–8F catheters, while infected, thick purulent collections may be drained with 10–14F catheters. Multiple catheters or larger catheters (16–18F) may occasionally be needed for multiloculated noncommunicating thick-walled collections. Guidance for drainage procedures includes ultrasound, fluoroscopy, or CT. Ultrasound is especially versatile since cavitary probes (endovaginal or endorectal) can help diagnose deep pelvic

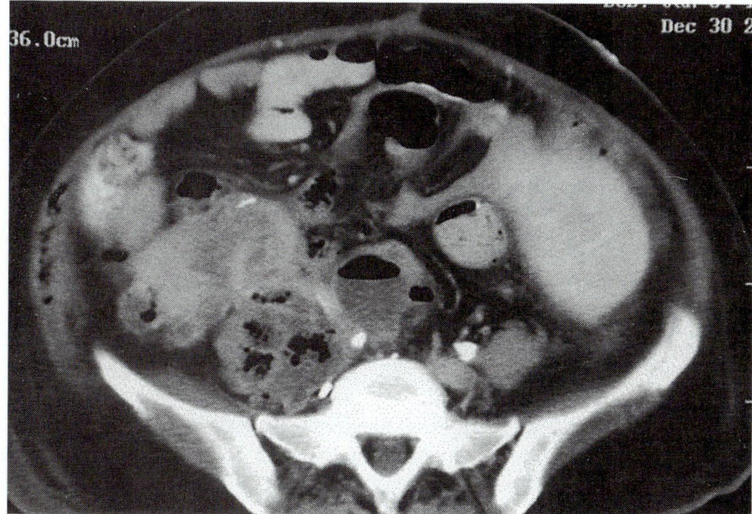

A

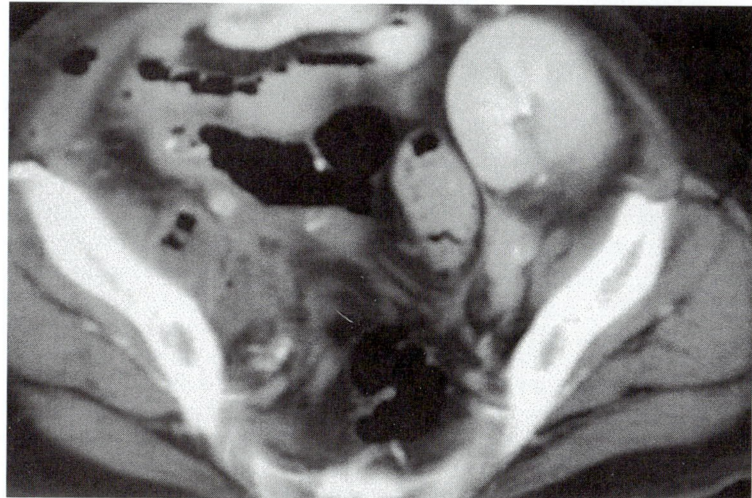

B

Figure 7–31. Psoas abscess. Young woman with pain and fever 1 month after renal and pancreas transplantation. ***A:*** CT demonstrates a multiloculated right psoas abscess with air and gas tracking into the right psoas sheath. ***B:*** Air in the right abdominal wall is from a recent biopsy.

abscesses and guide transrectal or transvaginal drainage. Catheters should be left to gravity drainage and flushed gently with 5 mL of normal saline at 8-hour intervals to ensure patency. Drainage output should be recorded on the nursing flow sheet.

Catheter position may be confirmed by fluoroscopic injection of contrast or by ultrasound or CT. General criteria for catheter removal include resolution of symptoms and signs, decrease in net catheter output to under 10 mL/d, and closure of the cavity as determined by follow-up imaging studies.

Gerzof SG et al: Percutaneous catheter drainage of abdominal abscesses: a five year experience. N Engl J Med 1981; 305:653–7.

Gerzof SG et al: Expanded criteria for percutaneous abscess drainage. Arch Surg 1985;120:227–32.

Lambiase RE et al: Percutaneous drainage of 335 consecutive abscesses: results of primary drainage with 1-year followup. Radiology 1992;184:167–79.

vanSonnenberg E et al: Percutaneous abscess drainage: current concepts. Radiology 1991;181:617–26.

ACUTE PANCREATITIS

ESSENTIALS OF RADIOLOGIC DIAGNOSIS

- *Plain radiographs: Gallstones, ileus of regional bowel (sentinel loop), transverse colon ileus (colon cut-off), pancreatic calcifications (chronic pancreatitis), and pleural effusion.*
- *Ultrasound: Peripancreatic fluid, enlarged pancreas with variable echogenicity, localized fluid collections, cholelithiasis, choledocholithiasis, biliary tract obstruction.*
- *Helical CT: pancreatic enlargement, necrosis, or hemorrhage; thoracic and intra-abdominal fluid or fluid collections; cholelithiasis, choledocholithiasis.*

General Considerations

Imaging studies in acute pancreatitis help to confirm the diagnosis, suggest possible causes (eg, choledocholithiasis, pancreas divisum), detect features suggesting chronicity, and demonstrate the extent of complications, such as abscess, pseudocyst, hemorrhage, and necrosis. Imaging findings may add to prognostic information derived from clinical and serum laboratory parameters.

Acute pancreatitis is mainly caused by alcohol abuse or choledocholithiasis. In the ICU, iatrogenic causes such as postoperative state, medications (antiretrovirals, chemotherapeutics), or endoscopic retrograde cholangiopancreatography may cause acute pancreatitis. Other causes include trauma, peptic ulcer disease, and structural congenital anomalies.

By imaging criteria, acute pancreatitis may be subdivided broadly into acute interstitial (edematous) pancreatitis and acute necrotizing or hemorrhagic pancreatitis. While acute interstitial pancreatitis is usually self-limited and requires supportive care, acute necrotizing pancreatitis is difficult to manage and carries a significant risk of high morbidity and mortality. In up to 60% of cases, peripancreatic and pancreatic fluid collections are present. Pseudocysts, which are collections of pancreatic juice and debris, are lined by a fibrous capsule and by definition are at least 5 weeks old. In the acute phase, the behavior of a phlegmon or nonliquified inflammatory pancreatic tissue is difficult to predict, though most resolve. If a pancreatic abscess is detected, prompt percutaneous or surgical debridement must be performed since it is associated with a high mortality.

Radiographic Features

A. Plain Abdominal Radiographs

Several indirect signs in a patient with acute back or epigastric pain suggest acute pancreatitis (Figure 7–32). However, none of the following are specific for pancreatitis: (1) duodenal ileus—gas in the second portion of the duodenum, reported in up to 50% of patients; (2) jejunal ileus—focal gaseous distention of a jejunal loop ("sentinel loop sign"); (3) transverse colon ileus—gaseous distention of the transverse colon with a paucity of gas in the descending colon, compatible with the "colon cutoff sign"; and (4) left-sided pleural effusion, reported in 10–15% of patients.

B. Fluoroscopic Contrast Studies

Upper gastrointestinal studies may be indicated to look for peptic ulcer disease. Although they are not indicated for the diagnosis of acute pancreatitis, one may sometimes observe a widening of the C loop with thickening of the duodenal folds due to edema.

C. Ultrasound

An ultrasound examination may be necessary to confirm or exclude the presence of gallstones within the gallbladder or common duct. Sonographic imaging of the pancreas may reveal diffuse edema.

D. Abdominal CT

Current CT techniques allow detailed pancreatic imaging tailored to the particular clinical situation. In the setting of acute pancreatitis, a single or multidetector row helical CT may be performed, imaging the pancreas with a minimum of 3-mm collimation with intravenous contrast enhancement in the "pancreatic phase," approximately 40 seconds after bolus contrast injection in patients with normal cardiac output. In addition to highly detailed pancreatic images, the remainder of the abdomen and pelvis should be imaged to exclude distant complications, including fluid collections and phlebitis. CT is the single best imaging method for pancreatic evaluation since it provides excellent evaluation and the ability to treat complications percutaneously.

Uncomplicated acute pancreatitis has an extremely variable presentation. The pancreas may be normal or edematous, increasing the attenuation of the intrapancreatic fat. The peripancreatic fat planes may become infiltrated by edema and products of the nonspecific inflammatory response. In patients with severe pancreatitis, sections of the gland undergo necrosis and may become hemorrhagic or infected. On CT, lack of diffuse and homogenous pancreatic enhancement with intravenous contrast reflects poor parenchymal perfusion and is typical of necrotizing pancreatitis. In areas of necrosis, the pancreas becomes ill-defined, with a severe peripancreatic inflammatory re-

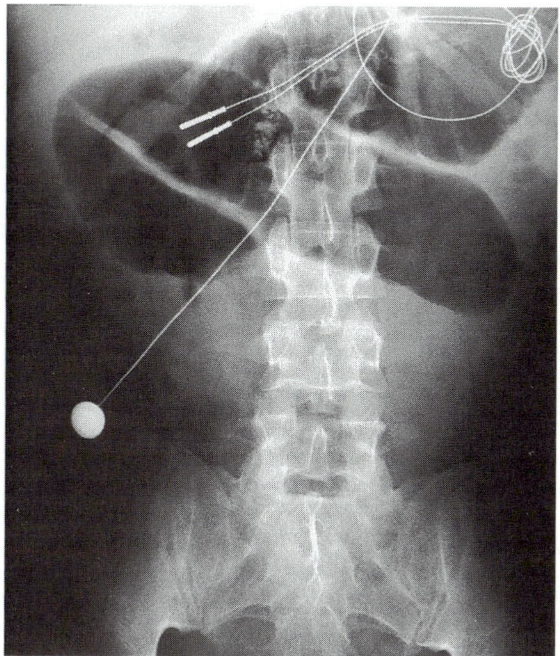

A

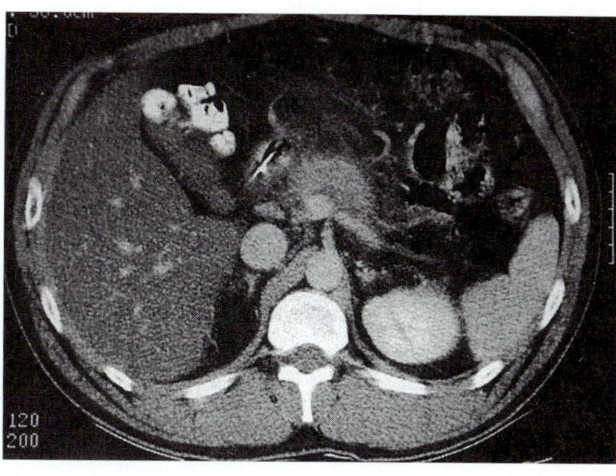

B

Figure 7–32. Acute pancreatitis. ***A:*** Plain film demonstrates focal dilated "sentinel loops" resulting from localized ileus. ***B:*** Abdominal CT in the same patient shows peripancreatic stranding and a fatty liver from recent ethanol abuse.

sponse and local and distant free and contained fluid. Splenic vein thrombosis may be present, and other complications such as pseudoaneurysm formation and pseudocyst formation may be seen at local and distant sites (Figure 7–33). A proposed CT grading system is used in some centers to estimate the amount of pancreatic injury and to predict outcome. Hemorrhagic complications are well seen because recent hemorrhage (< 1 week) is usually of high attenuation compared with surrounding tissue. Over time as the hematoma ages, its attenuation gradually decreases.

A pancreatic abscess, which may complicate acute pancreatitis in up to 9% of patients, implies a poor prognosis, with reported mortality rates of 40–70% in the pre-CT era. Prompt CT diagnosis and treatment have reduced the mortality rate to 20%. CT appearance of a pancreatic abscess can be variable and can range from a contained fluid collection to a more typical rim-enhancing lesion with central low attenuation and gas collection. The latter findings are present in only 20–30% of all pancreatic abscesses, and percutaneous aspiration is usually necessary for confirmation. The presence of gas bubbles may also suggest a fistulous communication with bowel.

Treatment

Acute pancreatitis complicated by necrosis or infection can often be treated successfully by aggressive percutaneous catheter drainage with large bore catheters. In more complex or severe cases, percutaneous management may help temporize a critically ill patient until surgical debridement is possible.

The management of pseudocysts is complex. Generally, pseudocysts may be managed expectantly since most will regress over time. By definition, a true pseudocyst has a mature fibrous wall developed over at least 5 weeks. Indications for percutaneous drainage or internal drainage into the stomach are the following: infection, enlargement, pain, bowel, bile or urinary obstruction, and diameter > 5 cm. For noninfected pseudocysts, success rates for internal or external drainage are high. For the 20–30% of pseudocysts communicating with the pancreatic duct, external drainage will be difficult and a cyst gastrostomy performed percutaneously, surgically or laparoscopically may be better.

Superinfection of a previously sterile pseudocyst occurs in < 5% of cases. As with most fluid collections, identification of infection within a pseudocyst requires clinical suspicion and confirmation by percutaneous aspiration. Successful drainage of an infected pseudocyst uses the same principles of drain placement and management as for most intra-abdominal abscesses.

Balthazar EJ et al: Acute pancreatitis: Value of CT in establishing prognosis. Radiology 1990;174:331–6.

Baron TH, Morgan DE: Acute necrotizing pancreatitis. N Engl J Med 1999;340:1412–7.

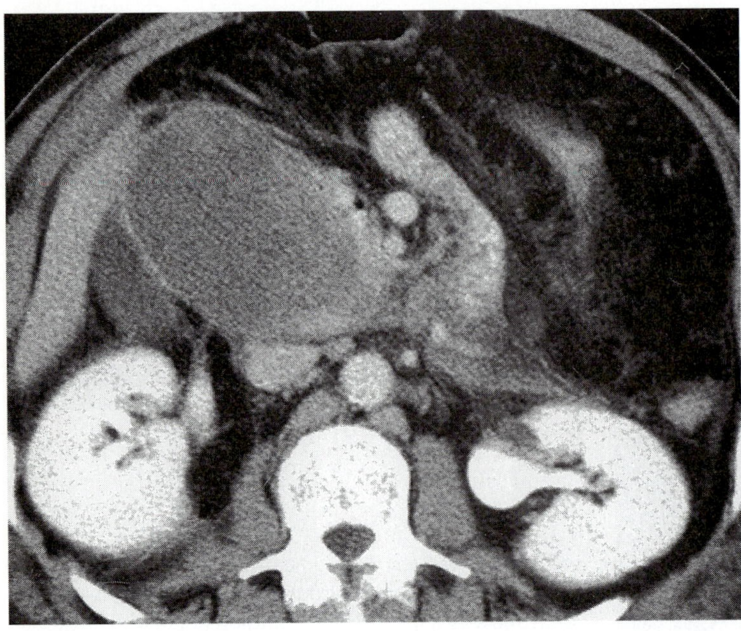

Figure 7–33. Complicated pancreatitis. CT demonstrates a large pseudocyst in the head of the pancreas.

De Sanctis JT et al: Prognostic indicators in acute pancreatitis: CT vs APACHE II. Clin Radiol 1997;52:842–8.

Freeny PC et al: Infected pancreatic fluid collections: percutaneous catheter drainage. Radiology 1988;167:435–41.

Paulson EK et al: Acute pancreatitis complicated by gland necrosis: spectrum of findings on contrast-enhanced CT. AJR Am J Roentgenol 1999;172:609–13.

vanSonnenberg E et al: Percutaneous drainage of infected and noninfected pancreatic pseudocysts: experience in 101 cases. Radiology 1989;170:757–61.

vanSonnenberg E et al: Percutaneous radiologic drainage of pancreatic abscesses. AJR Am J Roentgenol 1997;168:979–84.

Yassa NA, Agostini JT, Ralls PW: Accuracy of CT in estimating the extent of pancreatic necrosis. Clin Imaging 1997;21:407–10.

IMAGING OF ACUTE GALLBLADDER & BILIARY TRACT DISORDERS

ACUTE CALCULOUS CHOLECYSTITIS

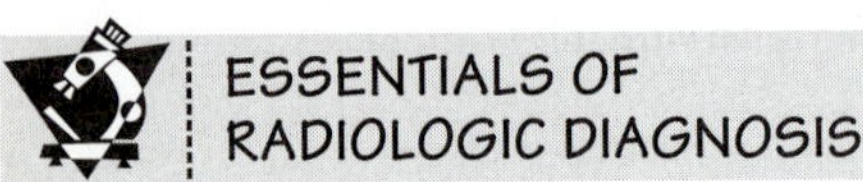

ESSENTIALS OF RADIOLOGIC DIAGNOSIS

- *Plain films: 15–20% of gallstones are radiopaque; distended gallbladder may be present in the right abdomen and produce a rounded radiodensity; gas may be present in the lumen or wall in emphysematous cholecystitis.*
- *Ultrasound: Thickening of gallbladder wall (> 3 mm); intraluminal gallstones and sludge; pericholecystic fluid and focal tenderness over gallbladder (sonographic Murphy sign).*
- *CT: Nearly 100% of gallstones visualized. Distended gallbladder with thickened wall; rim enhancement; pericholecystic fat stranding; gas in lumen or wall in emphysematous cholecystitis.*
- *Hepatobiliary scintigraphy: Uptake of iminodiacetic acid analogs into liver but nonvisualization of gallbladder within 60 minutes of injection.*

General Considerations

In acute calculous cholecystitis, cystic duct obstruction results from a lodged gallstone in almost 95% of cases. The gallbladder distends, with resulting mucosal inflammation and edema from bile stasis. Both distention and mural edema may lead to venous obstruction and subsequent mural ischemia and possible perforation.

Clinical parameters are of limited utility in the critical care setting. There is a significant clinical overlap among a variety of conditions such as acute pancreatitis, perforated peptic ulcer, pyelonephritis, and thoracic abnormalities such as pneumonia and myocardial infarction.

Radiographic Features

A. Plain Abdominal Radiographs

Plain radiographs can detect the 15% of gallstones that are radiopaque. In emphysematous cholecystitis, typically seen in diabetics, gas within the gallbladder wall and lumen may be seen. Plain films may also be useful to distinguish other causes of right upper quadrant pain, such as perforated viscus or pneumonia.

B. Ultrasound

Ultrasound should be the test of choice for rapid diagnosis of acute cholecystitis at the bedside. Features highly suggestive of acute calculous cholecystitis include a thick walled distended gallbladder with gallstones, pericholecystic fluid, and focal tenderness overlying the gallbladder (sonographic Murphy sign) (Figure 7–34). However, in patients who have been in the ICU for a few days or longer, the gallbladder tends to look abnormal on sonography, usually having a thickened wall and internal echoes. In these patients, a reliable sonographic Murphy sign should be absent.

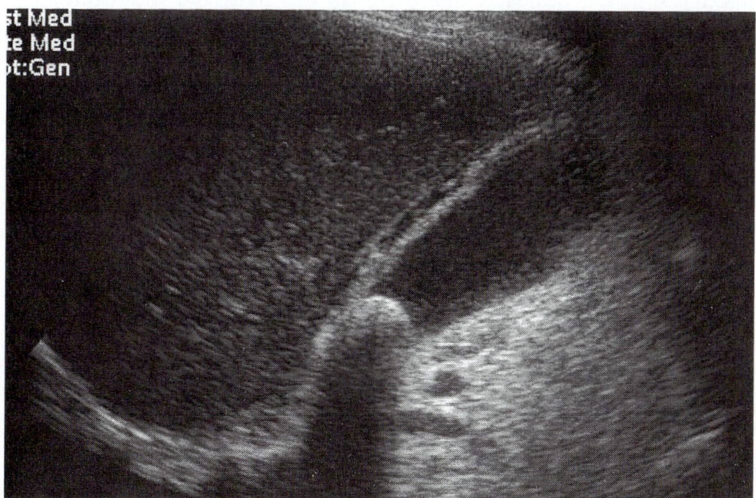

A

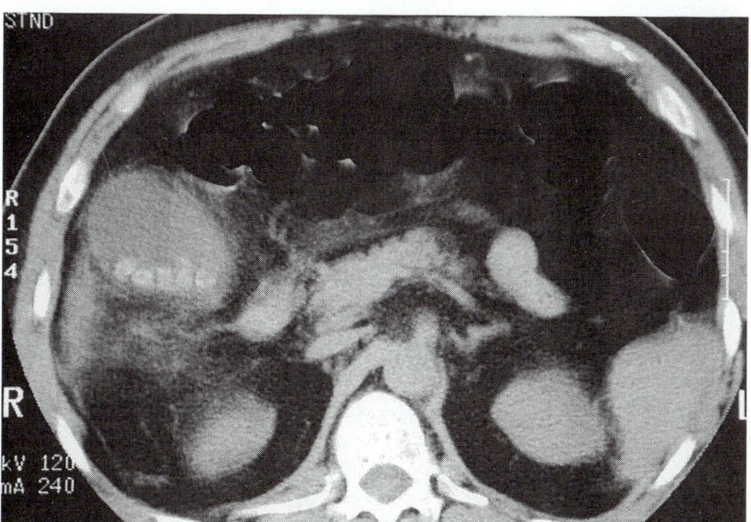

B

Figure 7–34. Acute cholecystitis. ***A:*** Ultrasound demonstrates a stone at the gallbladder neck with thickening of the gallbladder wall, pericholecystic fluid, and tenderness on compression (sonographic Murphy sign). In combination, these features are highly specific for acute cholecystitis. ***B:*** In another patient, abdominal CT shows distended gallbladder with gallstones and surrounding infiltration of the fat.

Sonography may also be limited by body habitus, overlying bowel gas, gangrenous cholecystitis, or overlying dressings. Pericholecystic fluid is an unreliable sign in patients with ascites. Gallbladder wall thickening alone in the absence of other findings may have many causes, including acute hepatitis, HIV cholangiopathy, interleukin-2 therapy, and anasarca.

C. Scintigraphy

In patients with equivocal signs and sonography, scintigraphy may provide complementary information in acute calculous cholecystitis. Technetium (Tc 99m-) iminodiacetic acid-derived agents have been shown to have high sensitivity and specificity for the diagnosis of acute cholecystitis. These agents are injected intravenously, and sequential imaging is performed over the liver with a SPECT camera. Sequential liver uptake and excretion into the biliary tree and intestine are imaged for up to 1 hour after injection. Normally, the gallbladder should fill with the radiotracer within 1 hour. Lack of filling confirms the diagnosis of acute calculous cholecystitis. However, lack of filling is also seen with intrinsic gallbladder dysfunction.

Although scintigraphy is an excellent test, it is cumbersome to perform at the bedside in the ICU compared with sonography. An accurate test requires that the patient fast for at least 2–4 hours prior to the procedure, and delayed images up to 4 hours may be needed. Scintigraphy has high negative predictive value; filling of the gallbladder within 1 hour excludes the diagnosis of acute calculous cholecystitis. However, there are many causes that prevent radiotracer flow into the cystic duct, and false-positive examinations have been reported in up to 40% of severely ill or debilitated patients. The most common causes of false-positive tests are bile stasis, bile hyperviscosity, and gallbladder distention. Specific causes include chronic cholecystitis, hyperalimentation, severe jaundice, hepatic dysfunction, pancreatitis, prolonged fasting, and recent nonfasting state. Causes of false-negative tests include pancreatitis and poor hepatic function. Hepatobiliary scintigraphic agents may also be used to confirm complications such as total common duct obstruction or bile leak.

ACALCULOUS CHOLECYSTITIS

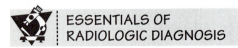

- *Ultrasound: gallbladder wall is thickened; no intraluminal stones; sonographic Murphy sign usually present.*
- *CT: mural thickening and inflammatory infiltration of the pericholecystic fat.*

General Considerations

Acalculous cholecystitis is associated with a variety of clinical conditions, including chronic debilitation, prolonged intubation, nasogastric suction and hyperalimentation, burns, and pancreatitis. Although comprising 10–15% of all cases of cholecystitis, acalculous cholecystitis predominates in the postoperative and posttraumatic patient population, accounting for up to 90% of all cholecystitis cases in that group. Mechanisms are poorly understood and probably multifactorial. Bile stasis, bile hyperconcentration, and edema with pressure in the gallbladder wall leading to progressive ischemia have been linked to pathogenesis. In addition, reflux of pancreatic juices through biliary enteric anastomoses and pancreatitis has been suggested. The clinical presentation of acalculous cholecystitis is similar to that of calculous cholecystitis. However, typical symptoms may be masked by concomitant problems.

Radiographic Features

Like the clinical diagnosis, radiologic diagnosis is also difficult. In the patient population most prone to acalculous cholecystitis, intrinsic functional and morphologic abnormalities of the gallbladder limit the specificity of both scintigraphy and sonography (Figure 7–35). Scintigraphy relies on technetium (Tc 99m-) iminodiacetic acid to fill the gallbladder, and scans are often done with pharmacologic intervention to improve accuracy. Morphine may causes contraction of the sphincter of Oddi, resulting in increased back pressure; cholecystokinin can be used to first empty the gallbladder. Although the sensitivity of scintigraphy has been reported to be as high as 95%, specificity is significantly lower than in calculous cholecystitis. This is because of the high number of false negatives resulting from coexisting conditions such as prolonged intubation, nasogastric suction, and hyperalimentation.

Sonographic features suggesting cholecystitis are similarly compromised in these patients. They may have mild wall thickening from edema and mild contraction. Often, right upper quadrant tenderness mimicking a sonographic Murphy sign is present in these patients in the absence of acalculous cholecystitis. Although the sensitivity of sonography is high, specificity is poor.

If results are equivocal, both scintigraphy and ultrasound may be necessary, or a CT scan may be performed. Using intravenous contrast-enhanced CT, mural thickening, mucosal enhancement, and subtle pericholecystic inflammatory changes may improve specificity.

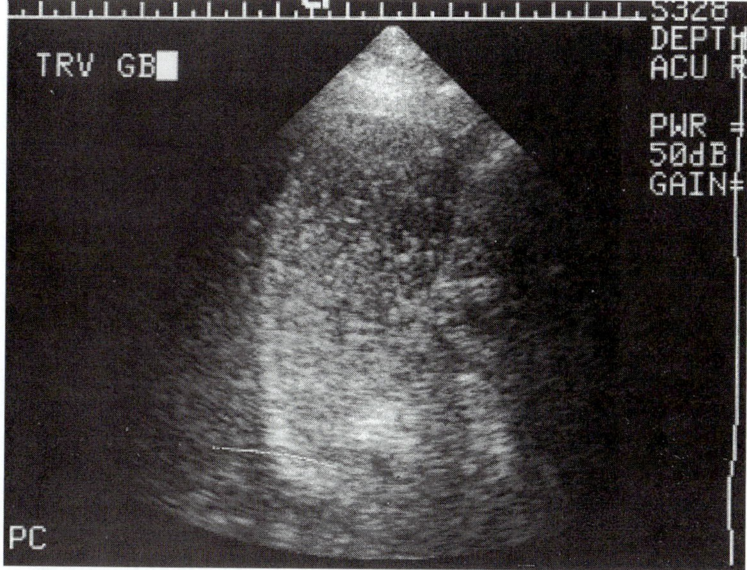

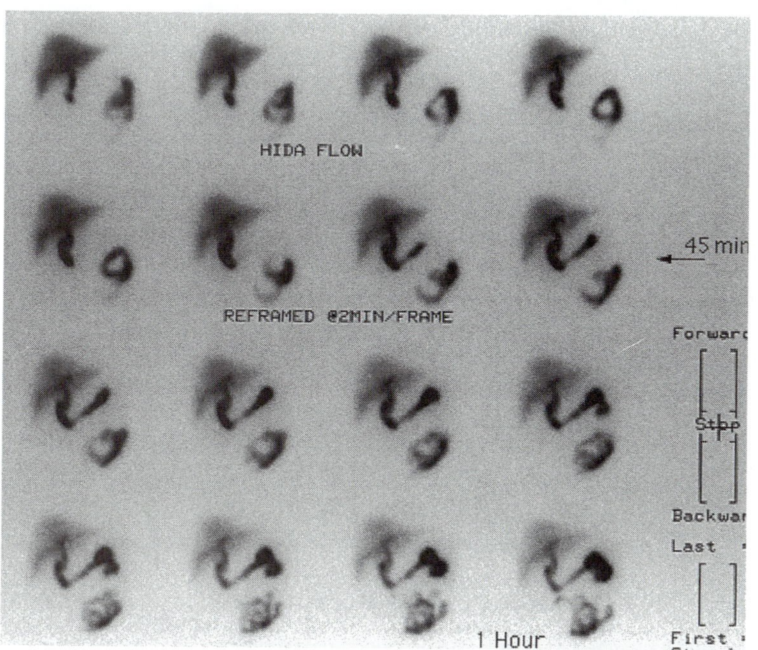

Figure 7–35. Acalculous cholecystitis. ***A:*** Ultrasound demonstrates diffuse echoes throughout the gallbladder, a marginally thickened wall, and positive sonographic Murphy sign. ***B:*** HIDA scan. The gallbladder does not fill with tracer by 60 minutes despite provocative maneuvers.

Treatment

In patients with uncomplicated acute cholecystitis, intravenous antibiotics contain the inflammatory response and suppress further inflammation, allowing patients to undergo less invasive surgery with fewer complications.

Although percutaneous aspiration can usually be performed in patients with acute cholecystitis, its role is debated because there is a high incidence of false-negative sterile aspirates resulting from effective antibiotic treatment.

Temporary gallbladder decompression by percutaneous cholecystostomy is beneficial in patients with acute cholecystitis who are high surgical risks. The procedure is performed with sonographic and fluoroscopic guidance in most institutions, but it may be performed with CT guidance. It can also be performed with sonographic guidance alone at the bedside. Complications, including bile leak, hemobilia, and vagal reaction, have been reported in 5–10% of cases—less than the complication rate associated with surgery (24% of cases). Other indications for percutaneous drainage include decompression of the biliary tract in cases of distal common duct obstruction with only mild dilation of the intrahepatic ducts. Some have advocated performing percutaneous cholecystostomy in critically ill patients as a means of diagnosing and treating acute cholecystitis. With this approach, in one study, 58% of critically ill patients improved.

Fidler J, Paulson EK, Layfield: CT evaluation of acute cholecystitis: findings and usefulness in diagnosis. AJR Am J Roentgenol 1996;166:1085–8.

Jeffrey RB Jr, Sommer FG: Follow-up sonography in suspected acalculous cholecystitis: preliminary clinical experience. J Ultrasound Med 1993;12:183–7.

Mariat G et al: Contribution of ultrasonography and cholescintigraphy to the diagnosis of acute acalculous cholecystitis in intensive care unit patients. Intensive Care Med 2000;26:1658–63.

Mirvis SE et al: The diagnosis of acute acalculous cholecystitis: a comparison of sonography, scintigraphy, and CT. AJR Am J Roentgenol 1986;147:1171–5.

Laing FC et al: Ultrasonic evaluation of patients with acute right upper quadrant pain. Radiology 1981;140:449–55.

Laing FC: The gallbladder and bile ducts. In: Rumack CM, Charboneau JW, Wilson SR (editors): *Diagnostic Ultrasound,* 2nd ed. Mosby, 1998.

Ralls PW et al. Prospective evaluation of the sonographic Murphy sign in suspected acute cholecystitis. J Clin Ultrasound 1982;10:113–5.

Ralls PW et al: Real time sonography in suspected acute cholecystitis. Radiology 1985;155:767–71.

Teefey SA et al: Gallbladder wall thickening: an in vitro sonographic study with histologic correlation. Acad Radiol 1994;1:121–7.

vanSonnenberg E et al: Percutaneous gallbladder puncture and cholecystostomy: results, complications, and caveats for safety. Radiology 1992;183:167–70.

IMAGING IN EMERGENT & URGENT GENITOURINARY CONDITIONS

ACUTE RENAL FAILURE

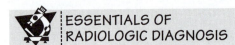

- *Ultrasound: In obstructive uropathy, dilation of the calices and renal pelvis with visualization of echogenic calculi; in intrinsic renal disease, increased cortical echogenicity correlates with chronic medical renal disease.*
- *CT: In obstructive uropathy, signs of acute obstruction on CT include dilation of the collecting system, a source of obstruction such as stone, swollen kidney with increased stranding in the perinephric space; CT urography (noncontrast helical CT) provides a rapid method of detecting renal calculi and obstructive nephropathy from a passing stone.*
- *MR urography: Rapid assessment of cause and level of obstruction; with gadolinium enhancement, differential rates of enhancement permit assessment of renal perfusion.*
- *Renal scintigraphy: Technetium Tc 99m-MAG 3 scan permits rapid assessment of differential renal function, including flow, uptake, and excretion. Especially valuable in transplanted kidneys to assess a vascular occlusion from intrinsic renal abnormality.*

General Considerations

The workup of acute renal failure has been traditionally focused on identifying prerenal, intrinsic renal, and postrenal causes. Prerenal causes (eg, cardiac or liver failure) and systemic hypotension account for 75% of all causes of renal failure. Intrinsic causes such as acute tubular necrosis and glomerulonephritis account for 20%, and postrenal causes such as obstructive nephropathy account for less than 5% of cases. Imaging is used mainly to exclude an obstructive cause of acute renal failure. These causes include obstruction from a lower urinary tract source such as bladder tumor, prostatic enlargement, or urethral stricture. Concomitant reflux may also decrease renal function. Ureteral causes of obstruction include luminal stones, tumors, blood clots, fungus balls, and sloughed papillae as well as extraluminal causes such as mural strictures or extramural causes such as retroperitoneal fibrosis, lymphadenopathy, or inadvertent ureteral ligation.

Radiographic Features

Azotemia due to obstruction is usually easily and rapidly treatable. Cross-sectional imaging allows rapid identification of hydronephrosis and its causes as well as clues to evaluate pyonephrosis, pyelonephritis, or abscess.

Sonography is the imaging method of choice to evaluate hydronephrosis in the critically ill patient. It may be performed at the bedside. Since it detects the presence of a dilated collecting system, pitfalls in interpretation may be present. In acute hydronephrosis, sonography may be normal in 50% of cases since dilation is suboptimal, especially in the first 72 hours. In subacute situations, a ruptured calix may decompress the collecting system, leading to a false-negative diagnosis if perinephric fluid is minimal or absent. A volume-depleted patient may also have poor distention of the collecting system due to low urine output. Patients with retroperitoneal fibrosis or neoplastic encasement of the ureters may have only minimally distended collecting systems. Conversely, patients with vesicoureteral reflux, parapelvic cysts, or prior episodes of inflammation may receive a false-positive diagnosis of hydronephrosis. Sonography may suggest the diagnosis of pyonephrosis or renal bleeding by the presence of echoes in the collecting system.

In a large series of patients with azotemia undergoing renal sonography, hydronephrosis was detected in 29% of those known to be at high risk (pelvic malignancy, palpable abdominal or pelvic mass, renal colic, known nephrolithiasis, bladder outlet obstruction, recent pelvic surgery or sepsis). However, in patients without these risk factors, hydronephrosis was detected in only 1%. Sixty-five percent of patients in the low-risk group had medical renal disease compared with 36% of high-risk patients. The simplicity and relatively low cost of a sonogram must be weighed against a typically negative result in the vast majority of patients and the risk of missing an obstructive cause of renal failure.

Helical noncontrast CT has emerged over the past few years as the imaging procedure of choice for the evaluation of renal colic (Figure 7–36). Helical CT detects over 99% of all types of calculi—with the exception of the stones caused by crystallization of the antiretroviral protease inhibitor indinavir. Helical CT images not only stones in the renal collecting system but also the ureters, bladder, and posterior urethra. CT also images the retroperitoneum and pelvis, allowing detection of processes such as retroperitoneal fibrosis and lymphadenopathy. CT is excellent for the detection of perirenal abscesses and abscesses in other areas of the abdomen and pelvis.

When a potentially obstructing stone is found in the urinary tract, the specific signs of obstruction include hydronephrosis and hydroureter to the level of obstruction, unilateral infiltration of perirenal and periureteral fat, and a swollen kidney. Hydronephrosis may not be distinguishable from pyonephrosis. However, high-density debris or, especially, gas within the collecting system suggests pyonephrosis.

MR imaging is emerging as a tool for evaluating urinary tract disease. However, it is currently impractical in critically ill patients.

URINARY TRACT INFECTION

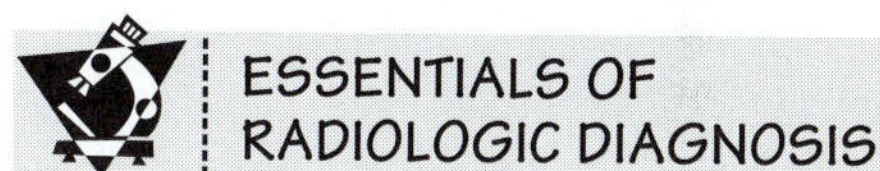
ESSENTIALS OF
RADIOLOGIC DIAGNOSIS

- *Ultrasound: Usually normal in uncomplicated pyelonephritis. However, the kidneys may be enlarged, with variable echogenicity. Focal nephritis may appear as a solid renal mass. A renal abscess appears as a complex cystic or hypoechoic mass.*
- *CT: Pyelonephritis is typically associated with nonspecific findings. Kidneys may be enlarged, with perinephric stranding. With intravenous contrast, a striated nephrogram may be seen with delayed function in infected areas. Focal nephritis appears as an ill-defined region of low attenuation in a lobar distribution. Renal abscesses are well-defined masses, often with an enhancing rim, increased attenuation of the adjacent perirenal fat, and thickening of the renal fascia.*

General Considerations

Pyelonephritis is typically a clinical diagnosis. Imaging is helpful to detect complications of pyelonephritis or urosepsis or in patients who have failed to respond to standard medical therapy. Complications of pyelonephritis include pyonephrosis, renal or perirenal abscess, or other conditions requiring surgical or percutaneous intervention.

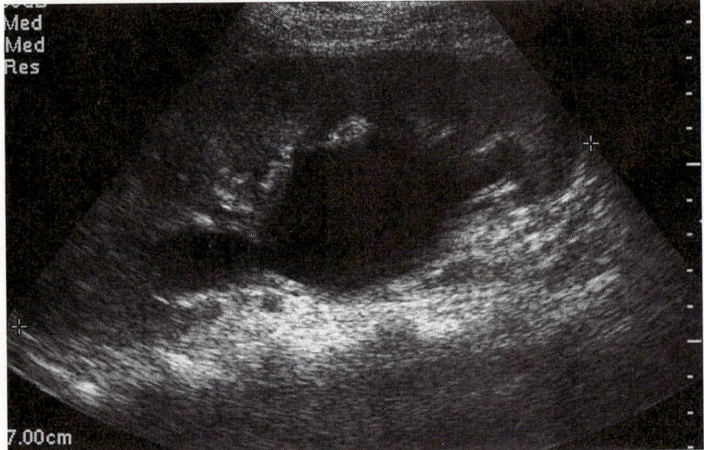

A

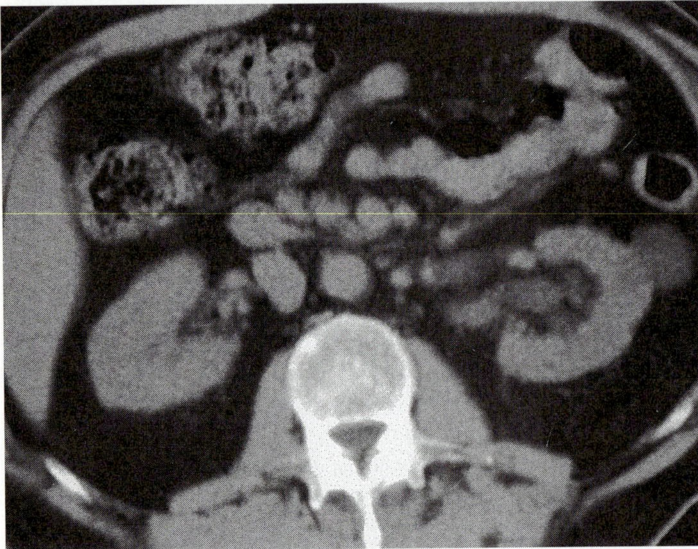

B

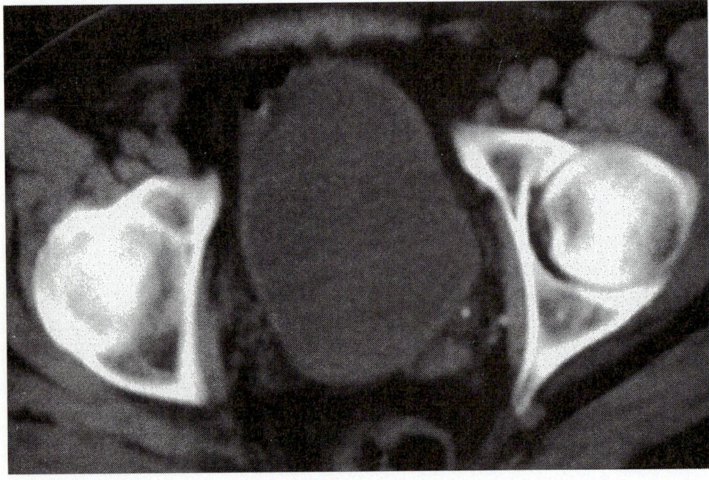

C

Figure 7–36. Obstructive uropathy. ***A:*** Ultrasound shows moderate hydronephrosis in the left kidney. ***B:*** CT scan demonstrates moderate left hydronephrosis with hydroureter. ***C:*** There is a tiny calculus obstructing the left ureterovesical junction.

Radiographic Features

Sonography is relatively insensitive and nonspecific in diagnosing acute pyelonephritis. It is useful to exclude hydronephrosis and possibly pyonephrosis as well as renal or perirenal abscess. However, sonography cannot diagnose changes in the perinephric fat or inflammatory thickening of the perirenal fascia.

Barbaric ZL: *Principles of Genitourinary Radiology,* 2nd ed. Thieme, 1994.

Erwin B et al: Renal infarction appearing as an echogenic mass. AJR Am J Roentgenol 1982;138:759–61.

Hoddick W et al: CT and sonography of severe renal and perirenal infections. AJR Am J Roentgenol 1983;140:517–20.

Lowe LH et al: Role of imaging and intervention in complex infections of the urinary tract. AJR Am J Roentgenol 1994;163:363–7.

Sacks D et al: Renal and related retroperitoneal abscesses: percutaneous drainage. Radiology 1988;167:447–51.

Smith RC et al: Diagnosis of acute flank pain: value of unenhanced helical CT. AJR Am J Roentgenol 1996;166:97–101.

Smith RC, Levine J, Rosenfeld AT: Helical CT of urinary tract stones. Epidemiology, origin, pathophysiology, diagnosis, and management. Radiol Clin North Am 1999;37:911–52.

Intensive Care Monitoring

8

Kenneth Waxman, MD, Frederic S. Bongard, MD, & Darryl Y. Sue, MD

A major function of the intensive care unit is to provide a setting where advanced physiologic monitoring is available for appropriate indications. Monitoring should be selected and applied to detect pathophysiologic abnormalities in patients at high risk of developing them and to aid in the titration of therapy to appropriate physiologic end points.

ELECTROCARDIOGRAPHY

Continuous electrocardiography permits monitoring of heart rate and rhythm, ie, detection of arrhythmias and evaluation of pacemaker function. It may also help detect myocardial ischemia or electrolyte abnormalities. Continuous electrocardiographic monitoring is indicated for patients with potential for developing arrhythmias—particularly those with acute myocardial infarction, traumatic cardiac contusion, following cardiac surgical procedures, and for patients with a prior history of arrhythmia. It is also useful for those in whom heart rate monitoring is indicated, such as patients at risk of hemorrhage or those undergoing fluid resuscitation. Monitoring of the ST segments is indicated for patients at risk of myocardial ischemia, such as those with coronary artery disease who have an injury, illness, or operation. Monitoring of the ECG may also be useful to detect certain electrolyte abnormalities such as hypokalemia during treatment of diabetic ketoacidosis.

The cardiac electrical potential available for skin surface monitoring is between 0.5 mV and 2.0 mV. Because of this low signal level, electrocardiographic systems must have good sensing, amplifying, and display capabilities. The electrodes used for electrocardiographic monitoring are usually composed of silver/silver chloride gel (Ag/AgCl) inside an adhesive pad. Prior to placement, the skin should be clean and dry. The stratum granulosum has an electrical resistance of 50,000 ohms/cm^3, which can be reduced to 10,000 ohms/cm^3 simply by cleansing, which removes oils and dead cells. Difficulties with a low signal are often remedied by reapplying the electrode after cleaning the skin.

Optimum electrode placement (Figure 8–1) allows proper detection of the electrocardiographic signals with a minimum of extraneous noise. A "modified lead II" configuration is appropriate for routine diagnostic monitoring, with limb leads extended proximally to lie over the shoulders. Placing them over bony prominences reduces electrical noise from muscle contractions.

Connecting cables should be inspected routinely for breaks and frayed insulation. Cables should be shielded and spiraled around each other to reduce noise interference and to prevent them from acting as antennas for electromagnetic radiation produced by equipment such as intravenous pump motors and heating blankets.

Most electrocardiographic amplifiers and display modules can be used for both diagnostic and monitoring applications. The diagnostic setting permits greater amplifier bandwidth (0.05–100 Hz) when compared with the monitor setting (0.5–50 Hz). For routine rate and arrhythmia detection, the monitor setting is preferred because it decreases baseline wander, reduces unwanted interference, and improves overall trace quality. However, because it may falsely elevate or depress ST segments, the diagnostic mode should be selected when myocardial ischemia is the primary concern.

Clinical Applications

A. Electrocardiographic Monitoring

Lead placement at the shoulders and in the lead II position parallels the atria and results in the greatest P wave voltage of any surface lead configuration. This facilitates recognition of arrhythmias and inferior wall ischemia. When placed in the V_5 position along the anterior axillary line, both anterior and lateral wall ischemia can be detected. Because patient positioning may make a true lead V_5 position difficult, a modified arrangement (CS_5), in which the left arm lead is placed just lateral to the left nipple and the lower limb lead is placed over the iliac crest, is a good alternative. When possible, leads II and V_5 should be monitored simultaneously. Esophageal leads are better than lead II for the detection of arrhythmias, but their use is difficult in patients who are not paralyzed and sedated, and they are rarely utilized in the ICU setting.

B. Complications

Difficulties associated with electrocardiography are usually due to technical error or equipment malfunction. Electrodes may not function properly when they are old and dry or if they are not attached securely. Electrical noise accompanying the displayed ECG is usually due to loose electrodes, broken wires, or poorly fitting contacts,

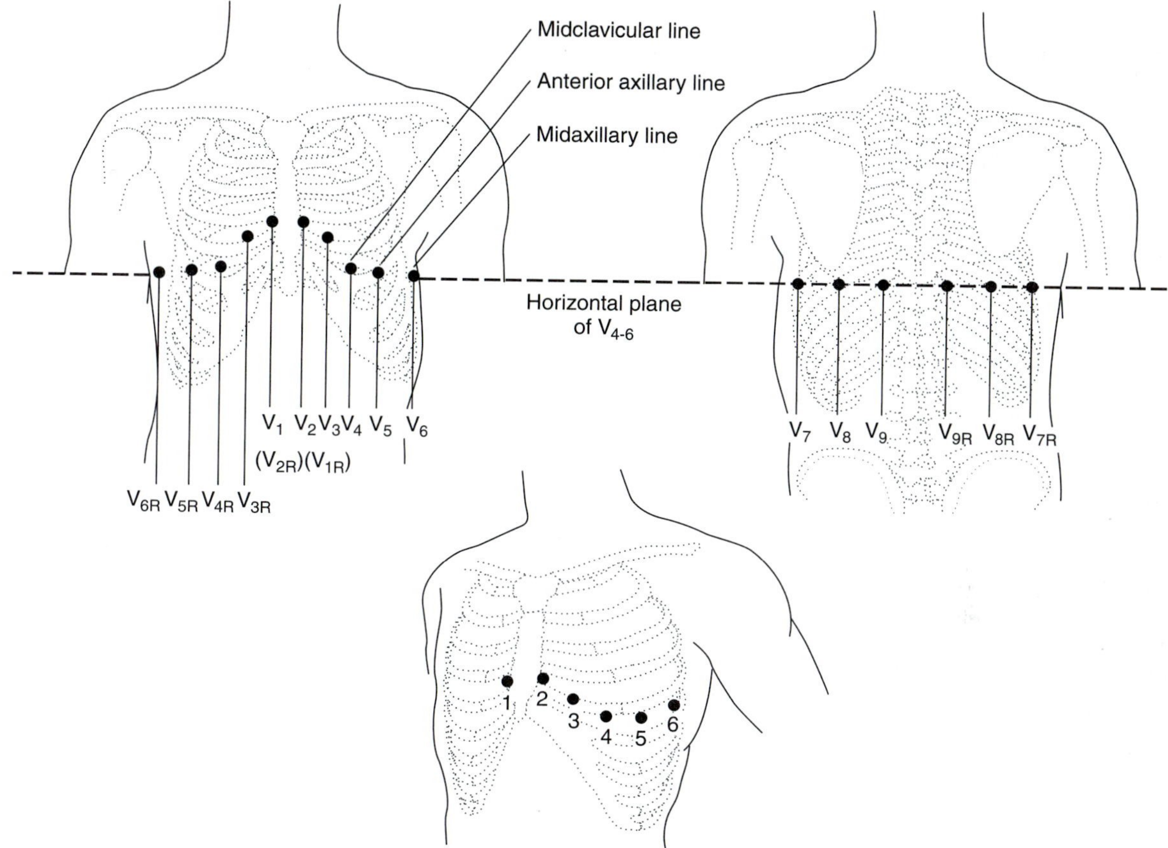

Figure 8–1. **Locations of the unipolar precordial leads on the body surface.** (Reproduced, with permission, from Goldschlager N, Goldman MJ: Principles of Clinical Electrocardiography, 13th ed. Originally published by Appleton & Lange. Copyright © 1989 by The McGraw-Hill Companies, Inc.)

or problems with associated electrical equipment. For any given patient, electrodes of the same type and from the same manufacturer should be used to prevent the creation of "half-cell" voltages, which arise because of different reduction-oxidation potentials between electrode gels. Proximity of the patient to electrical lines (power cords, etc) produces a potential difference through capacitive coupling known as common mode voltage. Typically as low as a few millivolts, coupling can cause voltages as high as 20 V. Common mode voltage interference usually presents as 60 Hz interference and can often be reduced by using properly placed shielded wires, good skin preparation, and use of an electrocardiographic amplifier that offers common mode rejection.

Proper sensitivity setting of the amplifier and recorder is essential to make certain that large T waves are not "double-counted" in the rate determination. Additional filtering is occasionally required for patients who have pacemakers—in whom the pacer spike is interpreted as a QRS complex.

Blitt CD: *Monitoring in Anesthesia and Critical Care Medicine,* 2nd ed. Churchill Livingstone, 1990.

Gardner RM, Hollingsworth KW: Optimizing the electrocardiogram and pressure monitoring. Crit Care Med 1986;14:651–8.

BLOOD PRESSURE MONITORING

A variety of techniques are available for blood pressure monitoring in the ICU. Because systemic blood pressure is related to both cardiac function and the peripheral circulation, blood pressure monitoring provides information related to the overall circulatory condition. While blood pressure monitoring is standard and universal for critically ill patients, the type of blood pressure monitoring and its frequency should be chosen based upon the individual patient's diagnosis and condition.

Blood pressure represents lateral force exerted on the vasculature by flowing blood. Pressure is maximal shortly after ventricular systole (SBP). The diastolic pressure (DBP) follows cardiac diastole and is the lowest pressure in the cycle. The mean arterial pressure (MAP) represents the standing pressure in the arterial circuit and is calculated as follows:

$$\mathrm{MAP}\frac{(\mathrm{SBP}+2\times\mathrm{DBP})}{3}$$

Pulse pressure is the arithmetic difference between the systolic and diastolic pressures. Pulse pressures vary with stroke volume or vascular compliance. Pulse pressures less than 30 mm Hg are common with hypovolemia, tachycardia, aortic stenosis, constrictive pericarditis, pleural effusions, and ascites. Widened pulse pressures may be due to aortic regurgitation, thyrotoxicosis, patent ductus arteriosus, arteriovenous fistula, and coarctation of the aorta.

The initial upstroke and peak of the arterial waveform is produced by left ventricular ejection. The end of systole is marked by a brief decline in pressure until the aortic valve closes and redirects backflowing blood into the aorta. The "dicrotic notch" so created may be detected on recordings obtained from aortic or proximal arterial sites. The waveform becomes more peaked and of higher amplitude as it progresses distally. The initial upstroke is prolonged, producing a higher systolic and a lower diastolic pressure (Figure 8–2).

The velocity of blood flow is slowest in the largest arteries because they are distensible and absorb energy from the pressure wave front. The pulse wave travels at a rate of 7–10 m/s in large arteries such as the subclavian artery and increases to 15–30 m/s in smaller distal arteries.

When a pressure wave front enters a small nondistensible artery, part of the wave may be reflected back proximally. If a reflected wave strikes an oncoming wave, the two summate, causing a higher pressure than would otherwise occur. This phenomenon produces pressures in the distal peripheral arteries that may be more than 20–30 mm Hg above those recorded in the aorta.

Arterial pressure is dependent upon cardiac output (CO) and systemic vascular resistance (SVR). The latter is calculated as follows:

$$\mathrm{SVR}=\frac{(\mathrm{MAP}-\mathrm{CVP})}{\mathrm{CO}}\times 80$$

When MAP and CVP (central venous pressure) are in millimeters of mercury and CO is in liters per minute, SVR is expressed in dynes×s×cm^{-5}. Evaluation of the equation indicates that an increase in either SVR or CO will increase mean arterial pressure.

Clinical Applications

Arterial blood pressure can be assessed either by direct instrumentation of the vascular tree or by indirect means. The indirect technique usually involves inflating a cuff to occlude an artery. As the cuff is deflated and inflow resumes, arterial pressure can be determined.

A. Noninvasive Arterial Pressure Monitoring:

1. Palpation—A blood pressure cuff is placed above an easily palpated artery and inflated until pulsation

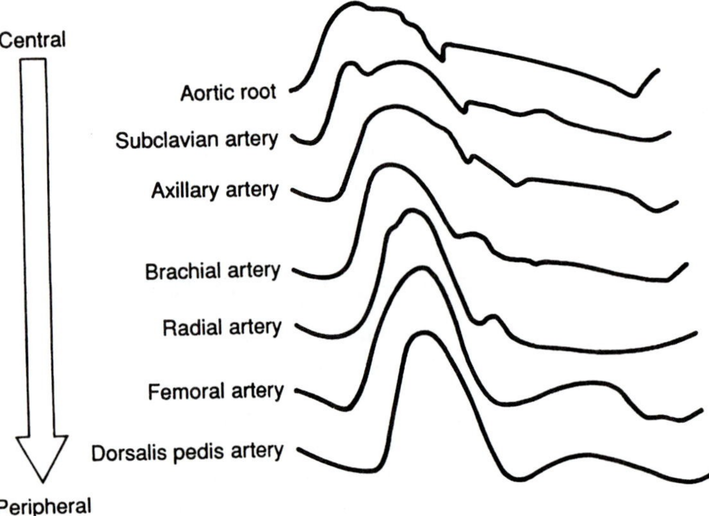

Figure 8–2. The shape of the arterial pressure wave front changes as it progresses distally. The systolic peak becomes more pronounced, as does the dicrotic notch. (Reproduced, with permission, from Morgan GE, Mikhail MS: *Clinical Anesthesiology*. Originally published by Appleton & Lange. Copyright © 1992 by The McGraw-Hill Companies, Inc.)

ceases. Upon cuff deflation, systolic pressure is estimated as that pressure at which pulsation resumes. This method is limited because it underestimates true arterial pressure and does not provide a diastolic pressure.

2. Auscultation (Riva-Rocci method)—When an occluding proximal cuff is deflated below systolic pressure, flow begins through the compressed artery. The turbulent flow thus created strikes the walls of the vessel, causing them to reverberate (Korotkoff sounds). As long as the cuff pressure is higher than diastolic pressure, no flow will occur during diastole. The sound thus produced is rhythmic in nature. Once the pressure in the cuff is below diastolic pressure, flow occurs throughout the cardiac cycle and the sounds disappear. A cuff 20% wider than the diameter of the limb must be used in order to obtain correct sphygmomanometric pressures. If the cuff is too narrow, the systolic and diastolic pressures will be artificially increased, and vice versa. Other sources of error include too tight or too loose cuff application and too rapid or too slow cuff deflation. Unduly slow deflation produces venous congestion, which decreases the amplitude of the Korotkoff sounds as the cuff pressure nears the diastolic pressure.

When compared with intra-arterial pressure measurements, those obtained by auscultation differ by 1–8 mm Hg systolic and 8–10 mm Hg diastolic. At intra-arterial pressures below 120 mm Hg systolic, auscultation tends to overestimate pressure, while above 120 mm Hg, auscultation underestimates arterial pressure.

3. Oscillometry—The oscillometer uses two cuffs in series; one occludes the artery proximally, while the other detects the onset of pulsations. Slow deflation of the proximal cuff produces aneroid needle oscillation or mercury column variation at systolic pressure. Oscillometry is the only noninvasive technique capable of indicating mean arterial pressure, which coincides with maximum deflection of the manometer. Although diastolic pressure is defined as that point at which oscillation ceases, measurement of diastolic pressure is in fact inaccurate. Oscillometry requires several cardiac cycles to measure blood pressure accurately.

Automated oscillometry devices generally use single bladder cuffs that are alternately inflated and deflated. On deflation, alterations in cuff pressure are sensed by a transducer inside the instrument. Pairs of oscillations and corresponding cuff pressures are stored electronically to permit measurement of the systolic and diastolic pressures. Use of these automated devices is limited in those with irregular rhythms or when motion cannot be minimized. In addition, measurements tend to be unreliable in low-flow states.

4. Plethysmography—Arterial pulsations produce minute changes in the volume of an extremity. Such alterations in finger volume can be detected photometrically with a plethysmograph. These devices tend to be less accurate than alternative pressure monitoring techniques, particularly during low flow and stress conditions.

5. Doppler—The Doppler principle states that any moving object in the path of a sound beam will alter the frequency of the transmitted signal. The sound beam used to "insonate" tissue is created by applying an electrical potential to a crystal that causes it to oscillate in the radio frequency spectrum. This sound is coupled to the tissue of interest through an acoustic gel.

When the beam strikes moving blood cells, the frequency of the reflected beam is altered in a manner proportionate to the velocity of the reflecting surface. Continuous and pulsed wave Doppler equipment is currently available. Continuous wave transducers have two crystals mounted together in a single probe. One is continuously transmitting, and the other is continuously receiving. Only the velocity of flow and its direction can be determined by a continuous wave device. Because a Doppler shift occurs only when blood moves relative to the transducer, an angle correction must be applied:

$$\Delta f = \frac{2\,feV\,(\cos\,\theta)}{C}$$

where Δf = frequency shift, fe = frequency of insonating beam, V = blood velocity, θ = incident angle of insonation, and C = velocity of sound in tissue.

The depth of tissue penetration by the sound beam is inversely proportionate to the frequency of insonation. Because arteries of interest are typically superficial, a 10-MHz probe can be used. As can be seen from the equation, the largest frequency shift is obtained when the probe is held parallel to the artery. Perpendicular positioning decreases the frequency shift ($\cos\,\theta \rightarrow 0$). Doppler blood pressure measurements are obtained by placing an ultrasonic probe on an artery distal to a compressing cuff.

Doppler sounds become apparent when cuff pressure falls below arterial pressure. Arterial pressures obtained using a Doppler probe are usually higher than those obtained by palpation and lower than those obtained by direct measurement, though the overall correlation is excellent. An automated device (Arteriosonde) is available for Doppler measurements. It uses a 2-MHz insonation frequency directed at the brachial artery. Overall accuracy is very good—especially at low pressures, when ultrasonic and palpatory techniques are more accurate than auscultation. Disadvantages include motion sensitivity, requirement for accurate placement, and the need to use a sonic transmission gel.

6. Tonometry—Arterial tonometry measures blood pressure by sensing the occlusive pressure required to stop flow through a superficial artery as it is compressed against a bony prominence. The device consists of several independent pressure transducers affixed to the skin over an artery. The stress applied between the transducer over the artery and the skin approximates intraluminal pressure. When monitored continuously, the waveform produced closely resembles that obtained from intraluminal recordings. Motion artifacts severely limit use of the technology.

B. Invasive Arterial Pressure Monitoring

Insertion of a catheter into an artery is the most accurate technique for pressure monitoring. Such catheters are connected by tubing to pressure transducers which convert pressure into electrical signals. Because arterial pressure waves are themselves too weak to generate electrical impulses, most transducers actually measure the displacement of an internal diaphragm. This diaphragm is connected to a resistance bridge (Whetstone bridge) such that motion of the diaphragm modulates an applied current. The transducer's sensitivity is the change in applied current for a given pressure change.

Because transducers are ultimately mechanical, they absorb energy from the systems they monitor. If absorbed energy in the transducer's diaphragm is suddenly released, it will begin to vibrate at its natural (resonant) frequency. The tendency for this oscillation to stop depends on the damping of the system. Oscillating frequency increases as damping decreases. The resonant frequency is a function of the natural frequency and the damping coefficient. Classically, a system's damping coefficient is determined by applying and releasing a square pressure wave (Figure 8–3).

Damping increases when compliance increases. Soft (compliant) connecting tubing absorbs transmitted pressure waves and damps the system. Other factors that increase damping include air in the transducer dome or tubing, excessively long or coiled tubing, connectors containing diaphragms, and the use of stopcocks. Because air is more compressible than water, even small bubbles increase the system damping. Excessive damping results in underestimation of systolic pressure and overestimation of diastolic pressure. There is little effect on mean pressure. Underdamped systems produce the opposite effects. Additionally, systems with insufficient compliance tend to "ring" when rapid pressure changes cause oscillations within the system. Conversely, overdamping decreases the frequency response to the point that rapid changes in pressure may not occur. The effect of damping on the natural frequency of the system is illustrated in Figure 8–4. The optimal damping coefficient is near 0.7 because there is essentially no effect on amplitude until the measured frequency approaches the natural frequency of the measuring system.

Clinical Applications

The arteries commonly used for invasive blood pressure monitoring, in order of usual preference, are the radial, ulnar, dorsalis pedis, posterior tibial, femoral, and axillary arteries. The radial artery is preferred because of its ease of cannulation and relatively low incidence of serious complications. The ulnar artery is the dominant artery to the hand in 90% of patients. It connects with the radial artery through the palmar arches in 95% of patients. Because vascular insufficiency may result from occlusion of the dominant artery, all patients should undergo an Allen test prior to catheter insertion and results entered into the medical record. However, one prospective study has demonstrated that vascular complications were not reliably related to the results of the Allen test. Overall, there is a 10% incidence of arterial occlusion in adults cannulated with 20-gauge Teflon catheters for a period of 1–3 days. The use of 22-gauge catheters seems to reduce this incidence.

For unknown reasons, women have a lower incidence of arterial thrombosis than men. When thromboses do occur in women, occlusions are usually temporary. Distal occlusion of the radial artery may cause overestimation of systolic pressure because of increased wave reflection, while proximal occlusion usually causes reduction in pressure due to overdamping. Another complication of arterial catheters is infection, most commonly limited to the skin but sometimes involving the artery as well; distal septic emboli rarely occur. The incidence and severity of such infections can be minimized by strict adherence to policies of daily catheter inspection, sterile dressing changes, and limiting catheterization to 5 days or less at any single site. Pseudoaneurysm formation may be a late complication of arterial catheters. The incidence of pseudoaneurysms may be minimized by utilizing smaller catheters, minimizing the duration of catheterization, and preventing catheter infections.

Physiologic pressures are measured with reference to the tricuspid valve, where intravascular pressure is defined as zero. This phlebostatic axis is independent of changes in body habitus. Postural changes affect the reference pressure by less than 1 mm Hg. The phlebostatic point is identified as (1) 61% of the way from the back to the front, (2) exactly in the midline, and (3) one-quarter of the distance above the inferior tip of the xiphoid process. A convenient method of system calibration is to move an open stopcock attached by fluid-

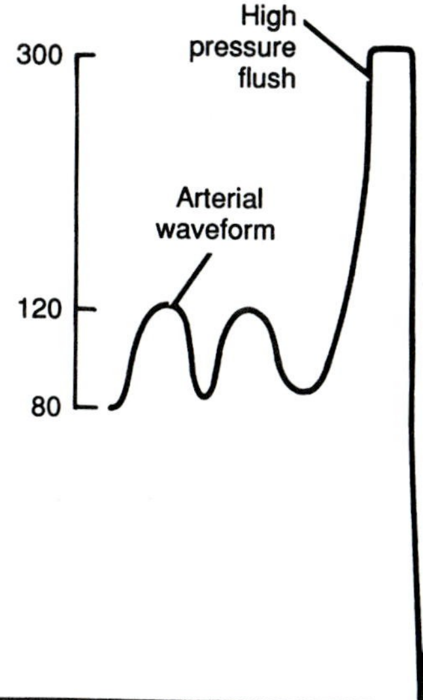

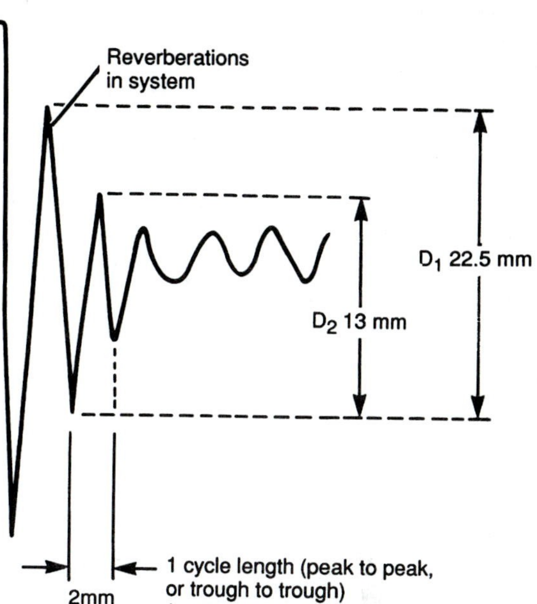

DAMPING:

$$\text{Amplitude ratio} = \frac{D_2\ (\text{mm})}{D_1\ (\text{mm})} = \frac{13}{22.5} = 0.58$$

$$\text{Damping coefficient} = \beta = \sqrt{\frac{\left(\ln \frac{D_2}{D_1}\right)^2}{\pi^2 + \left(\ln \frac{D_2}{D_1}\right)^2}} = 0.17$$

Amplitude ratio (D_2/D_1)	Damping coefficient
.9	.034
.8	.071
.7	.113
.6	.160
.5	.215
.4	.280
.3	.358
.2	.456
.1	.591

NATURAL FREQUENCY:

$$\text{Natural frequency} = f_n = \frac{1}{2\pi}\sqrt{\frac{\pi D^2\,\Delta P}{4\rho\, L \Delta V}} = \frac{\text{Paper speed (mm/sec)}}{\text{Length of 1 cycle (mm)}}$$

$$= \frac{25\ \text{mm/sec}}{2\ \text{mm}} = 12.5\ \text{HZ}$$

D = Internal diameter of tubing

ρ = Density of blood

L = Length of tubing

$\frac{\Delta P}{\Delta V}$ = Compliance ("stiffness") of system

Figure 8–3. **The amplitude ratio obtained by measuring the amplitude of oscillations after pressure release. Either the listed formula or the tables can then be used to calculate the damping coefficient.** (Reproduced, with permission, from Morgan GE, Mikhail MS: *Clinical Anesthesiology*. Originally published by Appleton & Lange. Copyright © 1992 by The McGraw-Hill Companies, Inc.)

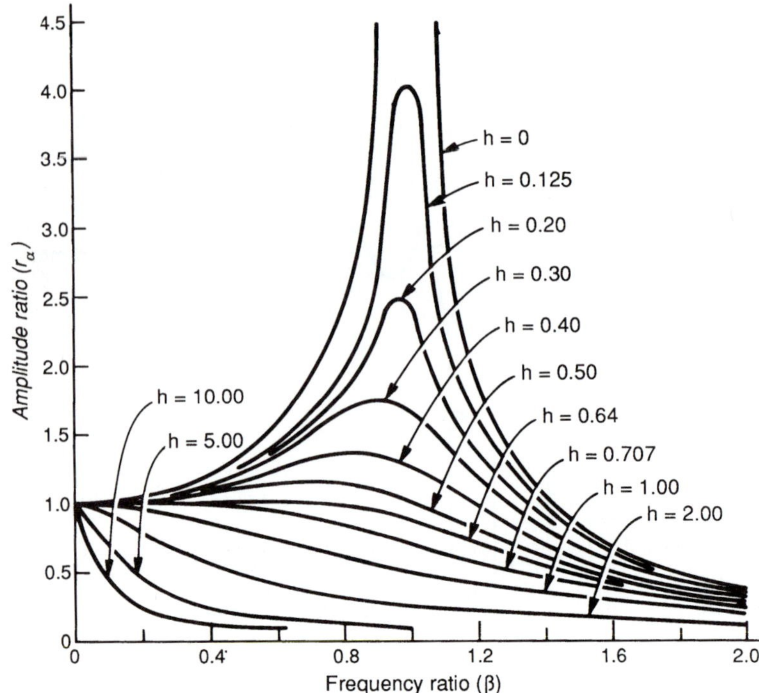

Figure 8–4. **The amplitude ratio depends upon the natural frequency of the system and the damping ratio (h). A system that operates below its natural frequency and with a damping ratio near 0.7 is desirable.** (Reproduced, with permission, from Fry DL: Physiologic recording by modern instruments with particular reference to pressure recording. Physiol Rev 1960;40.)

filled connecting tubing to the transducer up against the patient's midaxillary line. The digital display on the monitor indicates whether the midaxillary line is above (positive pressure) or below (negative pressure) the transducer. The bed is then moved up or down until the pressure reads zero (Figure 8–5).

Calibration of the monitor for nonzero pressure can be done internally or externally. External calibration can be done with a mercury manometer for systemic arterial pressures. A convenient method adequate for the lower pressure range required for a pulmonary artery catheter (up to 60 cm H_2O) takes advantage of the fluid-filled connecting tubing. After establishing the zero reference, move an open stopcock connected to the transducer above the transducer a measured amount. The height above the transducer in *centimeters* (cm H_2O pressure) should be read by the monitor system in *millimeters of mercury* as height in centimeters divided by 1.36. Therefore, if the system is accurately calibrated, the pressure reading should be about 14.8 mm Hg when the stopcock is raised 20 cm above the transducer.

An additional use of arterial catheterization is to provide access for arterial blood sampling. This is often indicated in patients who require frequent sampling of blood for arterial blood gases or other blood tests. Monitors are now available which also allow continuous monitoring of arterial blood gases, but the reliability and cost-effectiveness of such monitors is controversial at this time.

Abrams JH et al: Use of a needle valve variable resistor to improve invasive blood pressure monitoring. Crit Care Med 1984;12:978–82.

Cameron JN: *Principles of Physiologic Measurement.* Academic Press, 1986.

Fry DL: Physiologic recording by modern instruments with particular reference to pressure recording. Physiol Rev 1960;40:753–88.

Gardner RM, Hollingsworth KW: Optimizing the electrocardiogram and pressure monitoring. Crit Care Med 1986;14:651–8.

Gardner RM: Direct blood pressure measurements: Dynamic response requirements. Anesthesiology 1981;54:227–36.

Gibbs NC, Gardner RM: Dynamics of invasive pressure monitoring systems: Clinical and laboratory evaluation. Heart Lung 1988;17:43–51.

Harrington GR, Hratiuk OW: Noninvasive monitoring. Am J Med 1993;95:221–8.

Rubin SA: *The Principles of Biomedical Instrumentation: A Beginner's Guide.* Year Book, 1987.

Shapiro GG, Krovetz JL: Damped and underdamped frequency responses of underdamped catheter manometer systems. Am Heart J 1970;80:226–36.

Slogoff S, Keats AS, Arlund C: On the safety of radial artery cannulation. Anesthesiology 1983;59:42–7.

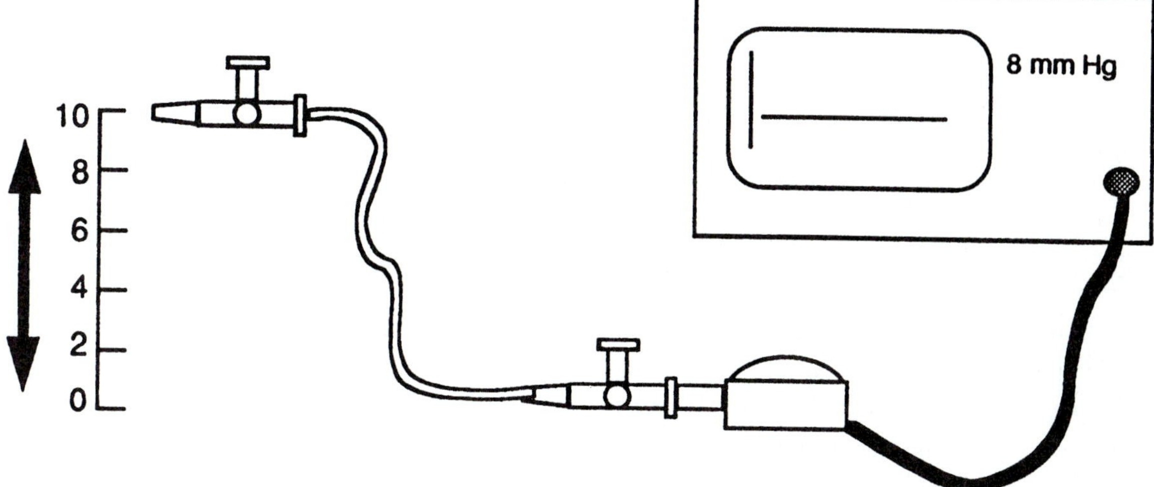

Figure 8–5. The height of the transducer must be adjusted to the phlebostatic axis to ensure accuracy of the pressure measurements.

CENTRAL VENOUS PRESSURE

Central venous pressure (CVP) reflects the balance between systemic venous return and cardiac output. Although classically defined in terms of myocardial end-diastolic fiber length (correlating with end-diastolic volume), the relationship between preload and cardiac contractility (law of Frank-Starling) is often applied clinically by correlating right atrial pressure (preload) and cardiac output. However, this substitution of central venous pressure for right ventricular end-diastolic volume is not always reliable, as ventricular contractility and afterload may alter end-diastolic volume at the same right atrial pressure. Nonetheless, CVP monitoring may provide useful information in selected settings, which may aid in clinical decision making.

In the normal heart, the right ventricle is more compliant than the left. This difference in compliance accounts for the slope of their corresponding Frank-Starling curves. The use of central venous pressure to assess left-sided preload causes difficulty because CVP primarily reflects changes in right ventricular end-diastolic pressure and only secondarily reflects changes in pulmonary venous and left-sided pressures. The relationship between CVP and venous return is shown in Figure 8–6A. Decreasing right atrial pressure below zero does not significantly increase CVP because of collapse of the vasculature leading to the chest. The figure also demonstrates that changes in mean systemic pressure cause a parallel change in venous return. Alterations in vascular resistance (decreased by anemia, arteriovenous fistulas, pregnancy, thyrotoxicosis) change the slope of the respective curves (Figure 8–6B).

A water or mercury manometer may be used to measure central venous pressure. Because mercury is more dense than water, pressures obtained with a water manometer must be divided by 1.36 to account for the difference. The normal range of CVP is between –4 and +15 mm Hg.

An electronic strain-gauge transducer has the advantage not only of providing pressure information but also of displaying the corresponding waveform. The bandwidth of a catheter-transducer system used to monitor CVP can be significantly narrower than that used for arterial pressure.

A typical CVP waveform consists of three positive deflections *(a, c,* and *v)* and two descents *(x* and *y)* (Figure 8–7). The increase in venous pressure caused by atrial contraction produces the *a* wave. The *c* wave is created when the tricuspid valve is displaced into the right atrium during initial ventricular contraction. The *x* descent corresponds to the period of ventricular ejection, when blood empties from the heart; it is inscribed when the ventricle draws down on the floor of the atrium and decreases the central venous pressure. The *v* wave is produced by the increase in atrial pressure that takes place as venous return continues while the tricuspid valve is closed. The *y* descent occurs when the tricuspid valve opens at the conclusion of ventricular contraction and blood enters the right ventricle. The *a* wave is absent during atrial fibrillation and is magnified by tricuspid stenosis (cannon wave). The *x* descent may

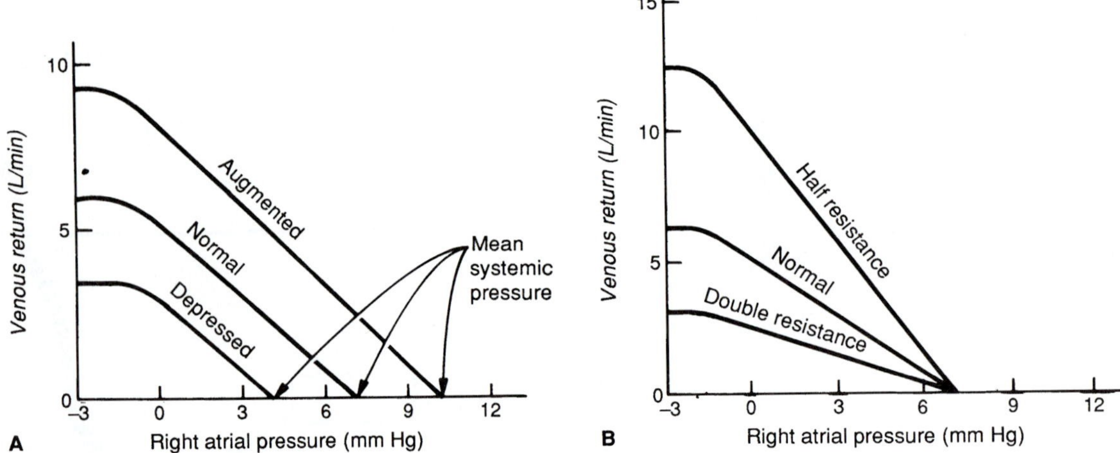

Figure 8–6. ***A:*** **Effect of mean systemic pressure on venous return.** ***B:*** **Effect of systemic vascular resistance on venous return.** (Reproduced, with permission, from Otto CW: Central venous pressure monitoring. In: *Monitoring in Anesthesia and Critical Care.* Blitt CD [editor]. Churchill Livingstone, 1985.)

also be absent with atrial fibrillation. The *x* and *y* descents are both exaggerated by constrictive pericarditis. Cardiac tamponade magnifies the *x* descent while abolishing the *y* descent. When tricuspid regurgitation occurs, the *c* wave and the *x* descent are replaced by a large single regurgitant wave. Pulmonary hypertension decreases right ventricular compliance and accentuates the *v* wave.

Clinical Applications

A. Application of CVP Monitoring

Central venous pressure monitoring is best used for patients without preexisting cardiac disease as one indicator of the adequacy of venous return and cardiac filling. A rapid intravenous fluid challenge is employed to aid in determining whether decreased blood pressure is due to hypovolemia or to cardiogenic failure (Table 8–1). Measurements of CVP are affected by ventilation because transthoracic pressure is transmitted through the pericardium and the thin-walled venae cavae. During spontaneous ventilation, inspiration lowers CVP while exhalation increases it. The situation is reversed in patients being mechanically ventilated, in whom inspiration increases intrathoracic pressure and elevates CVP.

The degree of this elevation depends on the compliance of the lungs and intravascular volume and will vary between patients. For this reason, CVP measurements are best made and compared at the same point in the ventilatory cycle—usually end-expiration. When positive end-expiratory pressure (PEEP) is applied, the positive pressure is transmitted through to the right atrium, causing a decrease in venous return and a rise in CVP. Again, the magnitude of this effect of PEEP on CVP varies with pulmonary compliance and blood volume. Some argue that the patient should be temporarily removed from PEEP while the measurement is taken. This is both impractical and potentially dangerous. In critical

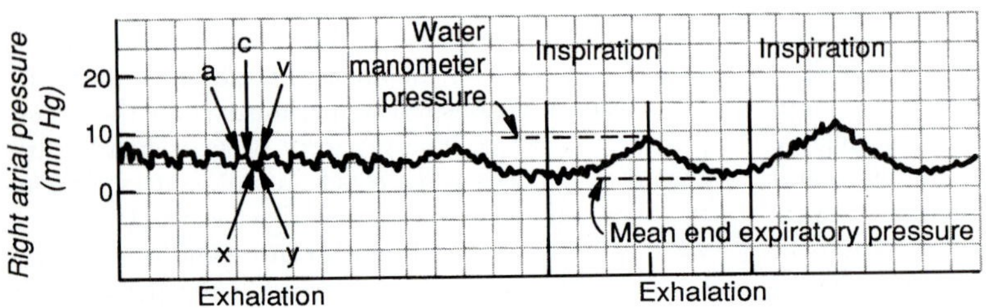

Figure 8–7. **Effect of mechanical ventilation on central venous pressure. The *a, c,* and *v* waves along with the *x* and *y* descents are shown.** (Reproduced, with permission, from Otto CW: Central venous pressure monitoring. In: *Monitoring in Anesthesia and Critical Care.* Blitt CD [editor]. Churchill Livingstone, 1985.)

Table 8–1. Response of CVP to volume infusion.[1]

CVP	Initial Increase	Return to Baseline	Cardiac Status	Vascular Volume	Cardiac Output
Below Normal	+	Rapid	Normal	Reduced	Low
			Hyperdynamic	Reduced	Low to normal
	+ to ++	Moderate	Depressed	Reduced	Very low
			Hyperdynamic	Normal	High
Normal	+ to ++	Rapid	Normal	Reduced	Low to normal
	++	Moderate	Normal	Normal	Normal
			Hyperdynamic	Normal	High
	++	Slow	Normal	Elevated	High
			Hyperdynamic	Elevated	Very high
	+++	Rapid	Depressed	Reduced	Very Low
	+++	Moderate	Depressed	Normal	Low
	+++	Slow	Depressed	Elevated	Low to normal
Above normal	++	Moderate	Normal	Elevated	High
			Hyperdynamic	Elevated	Very high
	+++	Moderate	Depressed	Reduced	Very low
	+++	Slow	Depressed	Normal	Low
			Depressed	Elevated	Low to normal

[1]From Otto CW: Central venous pressure monitoring. In: Blitt CD: *Monitoring in Anesthesia and Critical Care.* Churchill Livingstone, 1985.
Key: + = minimal; ++ = moderate; +++ = large

situations, an esophageal probe can be inserted to estimate transthoracic pressure. Subtracting the transthoracic pressure from the CVP provides transmural pressure, which is a better estimate of right atrial pressure in the presence of elevated transthoracic pressure.

B. Complications

Inadvertent arterial insertion occurs about 2% of the time; such insertion is particularly dangerous if large rigid "introducer" catheters are inserted. Perforation of the superior vena cava is associated with a 67% mortality rate, while the rate associated with laceration of the right ventricle approaches 100%. Such perforations may occur either from guidewires or from catheter erosion—again, particularly with introducer catheters. Other structures that may be injured on insertion include the brachial plexus, the stellate ganglion, and the phrenic nerve. Air emboli occur but are uncommon. Late complications are due to catheter migration, embolization, and infection. The incidence of cannula-related thrombosis of the axillary and subclavian veins varies between 16.5% and 46%. A recent report that used angiography to study patients receiving parenteral nutrition revealed an 80–90% incidence of some degree of venous thrombosis. However, less than one-fourth of these patients were clinically symptomatic. Central venous catheter infections occur in approximately 5% of insertions. The organisms most commonly involved are *Staphylococcus epidermidis,* 30%; *Staphylococcus aureus,* 8%; streptococci, 3%; gram-negative rods, 18%; diphtheroids, 2%; candida species, 24%; and other pathogens, 15%. Both colonization of central venous catheters and systemic sepsis are reduced by routine catheter care and periodic removal and reinsertion. A study that examined catheters changed over a "J wire" every 48 hours with alternation of the insertion site every 4 days reported no cases of suppurative thrombophlebitis among burn patients during a 3-year period.

Aldridge HE, Jay AWL: Central venous catheters and heart perforation. Can Med Assoc J 1986;135:1082–4.

Bozzetti F: Central venous catheter sepsis. Surg Gynecol Obstet 1985;161:293–301.

Cobbs CG, Carr MB: Endocarditis and other intravascular infections in the critically ill. In: *Principles of Critical Care.* Hall JB, Schmidt GA, Wood LDH (editors). McGraw-Hill, 1992.

Karnauchow PN: Cardiac tamponade from central venous catheterization. Can Med Assoc J 1986;135:1145–7.

Longerbeam JK: Central venous pressure monitoring: A useful guide to fluid therapy during shock and other forms of cardiovascular stress. Am J Surg 1965;110:220–30.

Mark JB: Central venous pressure monitoring: clinical insights beyond the numbers. J Cardiothorac Vasc Anesth 1991; 5:163–73.

Otto CW: Central venous pressure monitoring. In: *Monitoring in Anesthesia and Critical Care Medicine.* Blitt CD (editor). Churchill Livingstone, 1985.

Purdue GF, Hunt JL: Placement and complications of monitoring catheters. Surg Clin North Am 1991;71:723–31.

Scott WL: Complications associated with central venous catheters. Chest 1988;94:1221–4.

Sise MJ, Pistone FJ: The swollen arm. In: *Decision Making in Vascular Surgery.* Scribner RG, Brown WH, Tawes RL (editors). BC Decker, 1987.

PULMONARY ARTERY CATHETERIZATION

Catheterization of the pulmonary artery is a useful addition to central venous pressure monitoring. It provides information related to left heart filling pressures and allows sampling of pulmonary artery blood for determination of mixed venous oxygen saturation. When combined with a thermistor, it allows measurement of cardiac output.

As the balloon flotation catheter is advanced through the heart, characteristic pressure waveforms are obtained that indicate the position of the catheter's distal port (Figure 8–8). Simultaneous electrocardiographic monitoring is essential to ensure that ventricular tachyarrhythmias will be detected as the catheter traverses the right ventricle. After a pulmonary capillary wedge tracing is obtained, the catheter should be deflated and withdrawn until only 1–1.5 mL of balloon inflation is required to advance from a pulmonary artery to a capillary wedge tracing. Insertion of excessive catheter length contributes to intracardiac knotting. If subsequent pressure tracings are not obtained within 15 cm of additional insertion, looping should be suspected. When the catheter is placed through either the subclavian or the jugular vein, the typical distances required are as follows: right atrium, 10–15 cm; right ventricle, 20–30 cm; pulmonary artery, 45–50 cm; and pulmonary capillary wedge, 50–55 cm. As the catheter passes through the right ventricle, a wedge-like pressure tracing may be obtained. This "pseudo-wedge" is due to engagement of the catheter tip beneath the pulmonary valve or within trabeculations. Withdrawal of 10 cm of the catheter will solve the problem. Overinflation of the balloon, causing it to herniate over the tip of the catheter, results in a pressure tracing that continues to rise to high levels. The balloon should be deflated and a short length of catheter withdrawn before further advancement is attempted.

The final position of the catheter tip within the pulmonary artery is critical. This may be described with reference to three lung zones that depend upon the relationship of airway and vascular pressures (Figure 8–9). In zones I and II, mean airway pressure is intermittently greater than pulmonary venous pressure, which results in collapse of the vasculature between the catheter tip and the left atrium. In this position, observed pressures will be more indicative of airway pressure than of left atrial pressure. Only in zone III is there an uninterrupted column of blood between the catheter

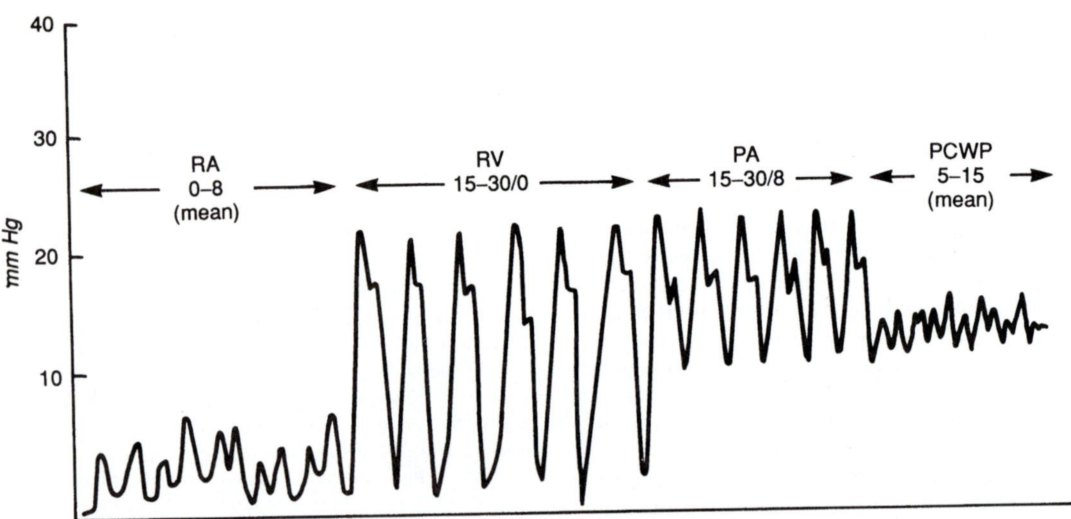

Figure 8–8. Normal pressures and waveforms obtained as a pulmonary artery flotation catheter is advanced from the right atrium to a pulmonary artery wedge position. (Reproduced, with permission, from Morgan GE, Mikhail MS: *Clinical Anesthesiology.* Originally published by Appleton & Lange. Copyright © 1992 by The McGraw-Hill Companies, Inc.)

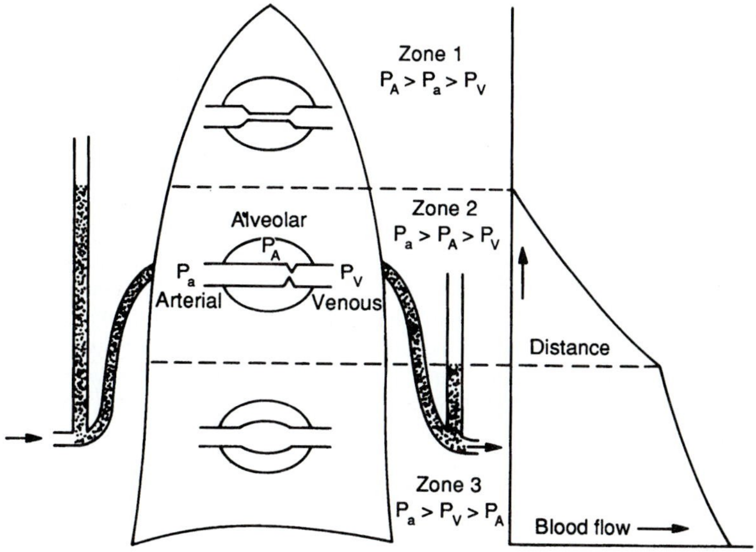

Figure 8–9. The effect of airway pressure on the pulmonary vasculature is divided into three zones. A pulmonary artery flotation catheter should wedge in zone III, where there is a continuous column of blood between the pulmonary capillary and the left atrium. (From West JB, Dollery CT, Naimark A: Distribution of blood flow in isolated lung: relation to vascular and alveolar pressures. J Appl Physiol 1964;19:713.)

and the left atrium. In the supine position, zone III assumes a more dependent position, caudal to the atrium. Decreased airway pressures change the ventilation-perfusion relationship, producing a relative increase in zone III. Hypovolemia decreases vascular pressures and decreases zone III.

Correct catheter position should be ensured by chest x-ray. Although most catheters migrate caudally and to the right, an occasional catheter will become wedged anterior to the vena cava. In this position, true pulmonary capillary pressures may be less than alveolar pressures, resulting in spuriously elevated measurements. A lateral chest x-ray will demonstrate when the catheter has assumed this position. Indicators of proper tip placement include (1) a decline in pressure as the catheter moves from the pulmonary artery into the "wedged" position, (2) ability to aspirate blood from the distal port (eliminating the possibility of overwedging), and (3) a decline in end-tidal CO_2 concentration with inflation of the balloon (produced by a rise in alveolar dead space).

The pulmonary capillary wedge (pulmonary capillary occlusion) pressure estimates left ventricular end-diastolic pressure and thus serves as an estimate of left ventricular preload. Because the pulmonary vasculature forms a low-resistance circuit, the pulmonary artery end-diastolic pressure is usually only 1–3 mm Hg higher than the mean pulmonary capillary wedge pressure and can be used to estimate left ventricular pressure when the PCWP is not available—in the absence of severe lung disease. Normal values for pulmonary artery catheter pressures are shown in Figure 8–8.

Pulmonary capillary filtration pressure (P_{cap}) is a measure of the potential difference that drives fluid from the pulmonary vasculature into the perivascular interstitial and alveolar spaces. The contribution of hydrostatic and osmotic pressure differences to fluid filtration is described by Starling's law. The equation relating mean PA pressure, PCWP, and P_{cap} is as shown below:

$$P_{cap} = PWCP + 0.4 \times (PA - PCWP)$$

Adult respiratory distress syndrome widens the PA to PCWP gradient and increases P_{cap}, contributing to pulmonary edema.

Clinical Applications

A. Pressure Measurements

In most instances, PCWP is an accurate indicator of left ventricular end-diastolic pressure and of left ventricular preload. Correlation between CVP and PCWP may be poor in critically ill patients with cardiopulmonary disease because of differences between right and left ventricular function. In this group, both absolute values and relative changes in CVP are unreliable because alterations in the pulmonary vascular bed affecting the right heart do not equally affect the left ventricle. This is of particular importance following pulmonary embolization, which increases right ventricular afterload without affecting left ventricular end-diastolic pressure. Central venous pressure and pulmonary systolic and diastolic pressures are all elevated, while pulmonary capillary wedge pressure is decreased because of the decline in forward flow.

Pulmonary capillary wedge pressure correlates best with left atrial pressure (LAP) when the latter is less than 25 mm Hg. However, PCWP will be lower than LAP in hypovolemic patients, whose pulmonary vasculature collapses during peak inspiration. When LAP increases to more than 25 mm Hg—which may occur after acute myocardial infarction with decreased left ventricular compliance—PCWP tends to underestimate LVEDP. As left ventricular function deteriorates, the contribution that atrial contraction makes to left ventricular filling is increased, and LVEDP can be significantly higher than PCWP. Several conditions affect the accuracy of PCWP as an indicator of LVEDP. Mitral stenosis results in an elevated PCWP because left atrial pressure at end-diastole may be significantly higher than left ventricular pressure. This is diagnosed by the presence of large *v* waves on a PCWP tracing. Large left atrial myxomas also elevate PCWP. Aortic regurgitation produces an underestimation of LVEDP by PCWP because the mitral valve closes early in spite of increasing left ventricular pressure. Mitral regurgitation results in accentuation of LVEDP because of backward flow during systole. Pericardial tamponade restricts filling of all four cardiac chambers and results in an equalization of CVP, MPAP, and PCWP. This occurs because all such pressures are under the restrictive influence of the tamponade. Positive end-expiratory pressure (PEEP) adversely affects the ability of PCWP to monitor left ventricular preload. High positive airway pressures (PEEP > 15 mm Hg) result in pulmonary vascular collapse, causing PCWP to reflect airway pressure instead of left atrial pressure. As with CVP, an esophageal pressure transducer permits calculation of transmural rather than transthoracic pressures. However, because pulmonary compliance is not disturbed uniformly, the pressure obtained through the esophageal probe may not correctly reflect the pressure that surrounds the pericardium.

B. Mixed Venous Oxygen Saturation

The distal port of the pulmonary artery catheter can be used to withdraw blood samples for measurement of mixed venous oxygen saturation ($S\bar{v}O_2$). Oxyhemoglobin saturation of peripheral and central venous samples is usually higher than that of mixed venous blood, because they do not contain the highly desaturated blood that drains from the coronary sinus into the right atrium. Blood from the superior vena cava normally has a lower $S\bar{v}O_2$ than blood from the inferior vena cava.

Mixed venous oxygen saturation is an indicator of *systemic* oxygen utilization. Normally, peripheral oxygen consumption ($\dot{V}O_2$) is independent of oxygen delivery (DO_2). Therefore, as cardiac output and oxygen delivery decline, peripheral oxygen extraction increases to keep consumption constant. This results in decreased mixed venous oxygen saturation. Conversely, sepsis causes a reduction in peripheral oxygen consumption, thereby increasing mixed venous oxygen saturation.

The partial pressure of oxygen in mixed venous blood is normally 40 mm Hg, resulting in a hemoglobin saturation of 75%. Oxygen content can be calculated for both arterial and venous hemoglobin saturations (% Sat Hb) using the following formula:

$$CXO_2 = 1.34 \times Hb \times \%Sat + (.0031 \times PXO_2)$$

If hemoglobin concentration is in grams per deciliter, oxygen content is expressed in milliliters per deciliter. Dissolved oxygen ($0.0031 \times PO_2$) contributes minimally to oxygen content but may become significant in patients who are profoundly anemic. The normal arteriovenous oxygen content difference—$(a\text{–}v)DO_2$—is 5 mL/dL. Hypovolemia and cardiogenic shock both increase the gradient (> 7 mL/dL), while sepsis decreases it (< 3 mL/dL). Left-to-right intracardiac shunts produce a significant step-up in hemoglobin saturation in the right ventricle and therefore decrease the $(a\text{–}v)DO_2$ gradient.

Mixed venous saturation can be obtained continuously from pulmonary artery catheters with integral fiberoptic oximetry capabilities. Two or three infrared wavelengths are used to detect the amount of oxygenated and deoxygenated hemoglobin flowing past the catheter tip in a branch of the pulmonary artery. A dedicated bedside module attached to the catheter continuously displays the results. Dual oximetry combines mixed venous and arterial pulse oximetry ($SpaO_2$) to provide continuous estimates of oxygen extraction and intrapulmonary shunting. From continuous oximetry data, the ventilation-perfusion index ($\dot{V}/\dot{Q}I$) can be calculated by the following equation:

$$VQI = \frac{1.32 \times Hb \times (1 - Sp_aO_2) + (0.0031 \times PAO_2}{1.32 \times Hb \times (1 - S\bar{v}O_2) + (0.0031 \times PAO_2}$$

where PAO_2 is alveolar oxygen tension, calculated from the alveolar gas equation.

$\dot{V}\dot{Q}I$ correlates well with shunt ($\dot{Q}s/\dot{Q}t$) over a wide range of parameters and clinical conditions.

C. Complications

Complications of pulmonary arterial catheterization may occur both on insertion and subsequently. Problems at the time of insertion are usually related to technical factors. The incidence of a pneumothorax with either the subclavian or internal jugular approach is 2–3%. Catheter knotting is related to the size of the catheter and the insertion length. Smaller catheters knot more frequently, as do those with excessive redundancy in the ventricle. If a pulmonary artery pressure tracing is not obtained within 15 cm after entering the right ventricle, the catheter should be withdrawn and reinserted. The incidence of catheter-induced transient right bundle branch block is between 0.1% and 0.6% and is thought to be caused by direct trauma to the bundle of His. The incidence increases to as high as 23% in patients with preexisting left bundle branch block. Ventricular arrhythmias may also occur, though they are usually transient and do not require treatment. Other complications that may occur during insertion include tracheal laceration, innominate artery injury, and bleeding.

Pulmonary artery rupture may occur at the time of placement, as a result of laceration by the catheter tip; or subsequently, from overinflation of the balloon in the distal pulmonary artery. The overall incidence of rupture is substantially less than 1%. Contributory factors include distal position of the catheter, decreased vessel diameter (primary pulmonary hypertension), systemic anticoagulation, and prolonged balloon inflation. Hemoptysis is usually the presenting sign. Chest radiography may show pulmonary infarction with a watershed distribution. The need for complete removal of the catheter is debatable because the requirements for monitoring are compounded by the complication. The catheter should be withdrawn to a more proximal site and the patient positioned with the affected side down to optimize ventilation-perfusion relationships. Some have argued that the balloon should be reinflated in a more proximal pulmonary artery to restrict blood flow to the site of injury. Emergency thoracotomy is required in rare cases when uncontrolled bleeding occurs.

Air embolism occurs most commonly with tubing changes and transducer calibrations. Approximately 20 mL/s of air is required in adults before symptoms appear, with 75 mL/s required to produce hemodynamic collapse and death. These volumes are substantially lower in children. The precipitating cause is mechanical obstruction of right ventricular outflow by the air embolus. Patients should be placed in the left decubitus and steep Trendelenburg position. This puts the outflow tract in a dependent location and allows the air to rise in the ventricle. Aspiration of air through the pulmonary artery catheter has been reported with varying results. Obstruction of the pulmonary vasculature by the embolus results in hypoxemia, increased pulmonary artery pressure, and right ventricular dysfunction. Passage of air through a patent foramen ovale may cause cerebral embolization and stroke.

Thromboemboli may originate from the tip or body of the catheter and can result in pulmonary emboli. Catheters left in place for long periods may lead to subclavian or jugular venous thrombosis. Other complications include infective endocarditis, sepsis, aseptic thrombotic endocarditis, and rupture of the chordae tendineae.

The avoidance of sepsis with pulmonary arterial catheters is identical to the protocols for central venous catheters. Daily sterile catheter care, dressing changes, and regular rotation of insertion sites are critical to minimize catheter-related infections.

Benumof JL et al: Where pulmonary artery catheters go: Intrathoracic distribution. Anesthesiology 1977;47: 455–65.

Bongard FS, Leighton TA: Continuous dual oximetry in surgical critical care: Indications and limitations. Ann Surg 1992;216:60–8.

Chandrakant P et al: Acute complications of pulmonary artery catheter insertion in critically ill patients. Crit Care Med 1986;14:195–7.

Ellis JE: Con: Pulmonary artery catheters are not routinely indicated in patients undergoing elective abdominal aortic reconstruction. J Cardiothorac Vasc Anesth 1993;7:753–7.

Filbuch EE, Tuohy GF: Intracardiac knotting of a flow-directed balloon tipped catheter. Anesth Analg 1980;59:217–8.

Garnett RL: Pro: A pulmonary artery catheter should be used in all patients undergoing abdominal aortic surgery. J Cardiothorac Vasc Anesth 1993;7:750–2.

Hannan AT, Brown M, Bigman O: Pulmonary artery catheter-induced hemorrhage. Chest 1984;85:128–1.

Iberti TJ et al: Ventricular arrhythmias during pulmonary artery catheterization in the intensive care unit. Am J Med 1985;78:451–4.

Raper RL, Sibbald WJ: Misled by the wedge? Swan-Ganz catheter and left ventricular preload. Chest 1986;89:427–34.

Sise MJ et al: Complications of the flow-directed pulmonary artery catheter. A prospective analysis of 219 patients. Crit Care Med 1981;9:315–20.

Swan HCJ et al: Catheterization of the heart in man with use of a flow-directed balloon-tipped catheter. N Engl J Med 1970;283:447–51.

Walston A, Kendall ME: Comparison of pulmonary wedge and left atrial pressure in man. Am Heart J 1973;86:159–64.

West IB: Ventilation-perfusion relationships. Am Rev Resp Dis 1977;116:919.

CARDIAC OUTPUT

The bedside technique of measuring cardiac output by thermodilution added a new dimension to intensive care monitoring. When a known quantity of hot (or cold) solution (indicator) is injected into the circulation, a time-temperature curve may be produced that allows calculation of flow. The area under the time-temperature curve is inversely proportionate to cardiac output. This is calculated using the Stewart-Hamilton indicator dilution equation:

$$\text{Cardiac output} = \frac{V_I \times (T_B - T_I) \times S_I \times C_I \times 60}{S_B \times C_B}$$

where V_I = volume of injectate (mL) and T_B, T_I, S_I, S_B, C_B, and C_I = temperature, specific gravity, and specific heat of blood (B) and indicator (I), respectively.

$$\frac{S_I \times C_I}{S_B \times C_B} = 1.08 \text{ for } D_5W$$

Either iced or room temperature thermal boluses can be used, though the use of iced fluid improves the signal-to-noise ratio. For best results, the difference between the blood's temperature and that of the injectate should be at least 12 °C. Bolus injection speed and warming of the indicator as it passes through the catheter have only minimal effects (± 3%). When technique is optimal, measurement repeatability is within 10%. Severe cardiac arrhythmias may reduce repeatability and yield results that may not accurately reflect average cardiac output. Timing of injection with a particular phase of respiration (end-expiration) improves consistency of measurements. Excessive patient movement may also produce erratic results.

Other Methods to Measure Cardiac Output

A. Indicator Dilution Cardiac Output

This technique relies on principles similar to those governing thermodilution but uses color instead of heat as an indicator. A bolus of dye is injected intravenously (usually through a central venous catheter) at the same time that peripheral arterial blood is withdrawn. The arterial sample is continuously passed through a densitometer that calculates dye concentration based on light absorption. The area under the dye curve is calculated, and a modification of the Stewart-Hamilton equation is applied:

$$\text{Cardiac output} = \frac{60 \times \text{Indicator dose (mg)}}{\text{Average concentration} \times \text{Time}}$$

Indicator dilution is complicated because of the need to simultaneously infuse dye and withdraw blood. Indocyanine green is the dye most commonly used. It is protein-bound, rapidly metabolized, and nondiffusible in the lungs. Results may be inaccurate due to right-to-left shunts, in which indicator reaches the circulation prematurely; and to left-to-right shunts, in which peak concentration of the dye is decreased. Common to both dye and indicator dilution techniques are the requirements for stable blood flow, constant blood volume, absence of recirculation, and constant indicator distribution times.

B. Doppler Ultrasound

Doppler devices measure ascending aortic flow and calculate cardiac output. A continuous wave Doppler probe is placed in the sternal notch to measure the velocity of aortic blood flow. A separate A-mode pulsed Doppler probe is centered in the third or fourth anterior intercostal space to measure the cross-sectional diameter of the aortic root. The stroke volume is the product of the cross-sectional area and the average blood velocity. Cardiac output is calculated by multiplying the heart rate and the stroke volume. Potential sources of error include (1) misalignment of the Doppler beam, which produces errors in measurement of blood velocity; (2) the assumption that the aorta is circular; and (3) the assumption that aortic blood flow is laminar. Each of these factors accounts for a cardiac output error that approaches 15% when compared with determinations obtained by other means. The difference between suprasternal Doppler ultrasound cardiac output and standard thermodilution has been reported to range from −4.9 L/min to +5.8 L/min. An esophageal probe is now available that measures descending aortic flow. An insertion depth of about 30 cm is required to reach the esophageal "window." The aortic root is sized using an A-mode pulsed Doppler, and a single measurement of ascending aortic flow is performed with a continuous mode suprasternal probe. The esophageal probe is then calibrated against the cardiac output obtained by the suprasternal technique. This method yields results as good as those obtained with the suprasternal technique and offers the added advantage of providing data continuously. A recently developed transtracheal probe uses a pulsed Doppler probe attached to the distal end of an endotracheal tube. Controlled studies have shown good accuracy, but extensive clinical experience is wanting.

C. Thoracic Bioimpedance

This noninvasive technique measures stroke volume by passing a small alternating current (2.5–4.0 mA) through the chest at radio frequency 70–100 kHz. Four pairs of electrodes (one transmitter and one sensor) are required. Two pairs are placed at the base of the neck and two at the level of the xiphoid process in the midcoronal plane. The change in thoracic impedance is due to blood flow, ventilation, and body movement. Respiratory variations occur much more slowly than those associated with blood flow and can be eliminated by the computer algorithm. Similarly, motion artifacts can be rejected by special circuitry. The majority of systolic blood flow is due to pulsatile blood flow in the descending thoracic aorta. Stroke volume is obtained by analyzing the impedance change over a cardiac cycle. Heart rate is determined at the same time and multiplied by stroke volume to yield cardiac output. Other parameters obtained include ejection velocity index, thoracic fluid index, and ventricular ejection time. The thoracic fluid index is thought to correlate with extravascular lung water, while ejection time has been used as a parameter of cardiac function.

Because bioimpedance cardiac output measurements are noninvasive, they can be repeated frequently. The volume of electrically participating tissue (VEPT) is critical in determination of the stroke volume. Although changes in body habitus are included in the nomogram used to calculate VEPT, small changes can produce significant error. Similarly, electrode placement is important. A 2 cm change in the distance between the sensing electrodes will produce a 20% variation in recorded cardiac output. Overall correlation with thermodilution in adults has been only fair. The method is further limited by inaccuracies caused by dysrhythmias. Furthermore, readings are difficult during patient movement, including shivering. Cardiac output is overestimated when preload is reduced; in low-flow states, when inotropes are required; and with aortic insufficiency. Underestimation is produced by hyperdynamic sepsis, hypertension, and intracardiac shunts.

D. Fick's Method

Cardiac output may be calculated by relating oxygen consumption to arterial and mixed venous oxygen saturation using Fick's equation:

$$\text{Cardiac output} = \frac{\dot{V}O_2}{(a-v)\,DO_2 \times 10}$$

Calculation of cardiac output using Fick's equation is the reference with which all other techniques are compared. The arteriovenous oxygen content difference requires that a pulmonary artery catheter be placed to obtain mixed venous blood. Oxygen consumption is calculated by measuring the oxygen content difference between inspired and exhaled gas.

E. Continuous Cardiac Output

The usefulness of cardiac output monitoring has now been further enhanced by the recent development of reliable continuous cardiac output monitoring devices. The devices now available utilize electrical impulses to generate heat in coils mounted on the right atrial portion of the pulmonary arterial catheter. Multiple small heat signals are generated that result in a corresponding pattern of changes in pulmonary arterial blood temperature, measured by the pulmonary arterial thermistor. Utilizing recently developed computer algorithms, the monitoring devices are programmed to analyze these patterns of heat and temperature to calculate a cardiac output value which reflects the average cardiac output for the previous 3–5 minutes. This period of time is necessary to minimize errors produced by the signal-to-noise ratio problem caused by the small increases in temperature inherent in this technique. Hence, this technique generates cardiac output data that do not change instantaneously and may not reflect transient changes in cardiac output, as do techniques such as bolus thermodilution. When instantaneous cardiac output is needed, bolus thermodilution injections may be useful to complement the continuous data.

This continuous thermodilution technique requires pulmonary arterial catheter placement and is thus subject to all of its previously discussed complications. A potential complication of damage to the endocardium by the heat coil is avoided by limiting the amount of energy applied and heat generated to safe levels.

A major advantage of continuous cardiac output techniques is that cardiac output data are continuously available and may thus help detect important physiologic alterations that may not be evident between intermittent measurements. The continuous data may also be coupled with other data such as arterial and mixed venous oximetry to provide continuous data reflecting oxygen delivery and oxygen consumption.

Alternative methods of continuous cardiac output measurement are also in development but as yet have not been widely utilized. These include ultrasonic techniques, automated bolus thermodilution techniques, and continuous indirect calorimetry and dual oximetry with a resulting continuous calculated cardiac output by the Fick principle.

Sources of Error

Use of correct temperatures and volumes is the most important factor contributing to accurate thermodilution cardiac output results. If the amount of indicator injected is less than the amount used in calculation, the fall in indicator temperature will be less than anticipated and the cardiac output will be falsely elevated. Cardiac output will also be falsely elevated if the injectate is warmer than that used in the calculation. The latter problem has been largely overcome with the introduction of new cardiac output computers that measure the injectate's temperature and automatically enter the value into the calculation.

Right-to-left intracardiac shunt will result in loss of the indicator, resulting in a falsely elevated cardiac output. Left-to-right shunts permit recirculation of indicator that has already passed through the lungs. This produces multiple peaks in the time-temperature curve that cannot be interpreted by the cardiac output computer, resulting in a bad curve alert. When tricuspid regurgitation occurs, blood and indicator mix, resulting in prolongation of transit time. The curve produced has a slow upstroke and decay, thereby increasing the area underneath it. This causes sporadic readings and underestimation of the true cardiac output.

Derived Parameters

Cardiac output measurements may be combined with systemic arterial, venous, and pulmonary artery pressure determinations to calculate a number of hemodynamic variables useful in assessing the overall hemodynamic status of the patient (Table 8–2). Oxygen transport parameters may also be calculated (see below).

Bernstein DR: Continuous noninvasive real-time monitoring of stroke volume and cardiac output by thoracic electrical bioimpedance. Crit Care Med 1986;14:898–903.

Davies GD, Jebson PJ, Glasgow BM: Continuous Fick cardiac output compared to thermodilution cardiac output. Crit Care Med 1986;14:881–5.

Donovan KD et al: Comparison of pulsed Doppler and thermodilution methods for measuring cardiac output in critically ill patients. Crit Care Med 1987;15:853–7.

Elkazan V et al: Cardiac output by the thermodilution technique: Effect of injectate's volume and temperature on accuracy and reproducibility in the critically ill patient. Chest 1983;84:418–22.

Hillis LD, Firth BG, Winniford MD: Analysis of factors affecting the variability of Fick versus indicator dilution measurements of cardiac output. Am J Cardiol 1985;56:764–8.

Marini JJ: Obtaining meaningful data from the Swan-Ganz catheter. Respir Care 1985;30:572–85.

Mihaljevic T et al: Continuous thermodilution measurement of cardiac output: in-vitro and in-vivo evaluation. Thorac Cardiovasc Surg 1994,42:32–5.

Moore FA, Haenel JB, Moore EE: Alternatives to Swan-Ganz cardiac output monitoring. Surg Clin North Am 1991;71:699–721.

Salandin V et al: Comparison of cardiac output estimation by thoracic electrical impedance, thermodilution, and Fick methods. Crit Care Med 1988;16:1157–8.

Swan HJC, Ganz W: Hemodynamic measurements in clinical practice: A decade in review. J Am Coll Cardiol 1983;1:103–13.

PULSE OXIMETRY

Pulse oximetry affords a noninvasive estimate of arterial oxygen saturation using the change in light absorption across a vascular bed during the arterial pulse. In the intensive care unit, pulse oximetry has important uses and has become a standard of care in many institutions. There are, however, a number of issues that should be understood and considered with this monitoring technique. In particular, the reliability of this method may be limited in patients with severe hypoxemia, abnormal arterial pulsations, and hypoperfusion of the site of measurement.

Table 8–2. Hemodynamic formulas and normal ranges.[1]

Variable	Formula	Normal	Units
Cardiac index	$\frac{\text{Cardiac output (L/min)}}{\text{Body surface area (m}^2\text{)}}$	2.8–4.2	L/min/m^2
Total systemic vascular resistance	$\frac{\text{MAP (mm Hg)} - \text{CVP (mm Hg)} \times 80}{\text{Cardiac output (L/min)}}$	1200–1500	dynes•s•cm^{-5}
Pulmonary vascular restistance	$\frac{\text{PA (mm Hg)} - \text{PCWP (mm Hg)} \times 80}{\text{Cardiac output (L/min)}}$	100–300	dynes•s•cm^{-5}
Stroke volume	$\frac{\text{Cardiac output (L/min)} \times 1000}{\text{Heart rate (beat/min)}}$	60–90	mL/beat
Stroke index (SI)	$\frac{\text{Stroke volume (mL/beat)}}{\text{Body surface area}}$	30–65	mL/beat/m^2
Right ventricular stroke-work index	$0.0136\ (\overline{PA} - CVP) \times SI$	5–10	g-m/beat/m^2
Left ventricular stroke-work index	$0.0136\ (MAP - PCWP) \times SI$	45–60	g-m/beat/m^2

[1]From Morgan GE, Mikhail MS: *Clinical Anesthesiology.* Appleton & Lange, 1992.

When light of a particular wavelength is transmitted through a clear solvent containing solute that absorbs light at that wavelength, the amount of light absorbed is the product of solute concentration, path length, and the extinction coefficient (determined by the solute and the wavelength). For a hemoglobin solution, the relative concentrations of oxy- and deoxyhemoglobin can be determined in a spectrophotometer because the extinction coefficients are different for these two hemoglobin species at certain wavelengths.

Pulse oximetry uses the beat-to-beat changes in light absorption through a vascular bed to estimate arterial O_2 saturation, discarding any nonvariable light absorption by considering only the difference between peak and nadir light intensities. The method determines O_2 saturation by a complex calculation that includes several important assumptions. With the use of two light-emitting diodes (LEDs) producing light in the red and infrared ranges, pulse oximetry is able to estimate oxyhemoglobin as a proportion of the sum of oxyhemoglobin plus deoxyhemoglobin—the so-called **functional oxyhemoglobin saturation.** Pulse oximeters are "calibrated" by comparison of arterial blood oxygen saturation in volunteers to calculated values; the devices utilize a "look-up table" to translate the measured proportion to the displayed saturation. Pulse oximetry is subject to artifact-caused errors. Movement of the oximeter probe, extraneous incident light (especially if pulsatile), variations in arterial pulsation, dependent position, venous pulsations, and other factors may result in incorrect O_2 saturation readings.

Validity

The accuracy of pulse oximetry is generally considered good in the range of normoxia to mild hypoxemia. However, accuracy may be suspect during more severe hypoxemia, such as when arterial O_2 saturation is below 75%. In this range, differences between measured O_2 saturation and pulse oximetry saturation range from 5–12%.

A. Patient Factors

Patients in the ICU frequently have hypotension, poor distal extremity perfusion, and impaired oxygen delivery—or are being given pharmacologic vasopressors or vasodilators. These factors affect blood flow to the site of pulse oximetry and vary the contour and intensity of the beat-to-beat pulse used to calculate O_2 saturation. Most devices are programmed to avoid reporting O_2 saturation when low perfusion or a poor pulse signal is being measured. In some of the few studies considering these issues in the ICU, failure of the pulse oximeter to measure O_2 saturation was not infrequent in patients with hemodynamic instability (12–15%). However, other studies have demonstrated that some pulse oximeters continue to measure and report O_2 saturation despite very poor blood flow and severe hypotension. These results may not be reliable, and there is concern that pulse oximeter O_2 saturation under these conditions may be misleadingly high.

B. Abnormal Hemoglobins

The pulse oximeter cannot measure carboxyhemoglobin nor accurately measure oxyhemoglobin in the presence of carboxyhemoglobin. The oxygen saturation displayed is essentially equal to the difference between total hemoglobin and deoxygenated hemoglobin (100% minus the percentage of deoxyhemoglobin), but the relative concentrations of oxy- and carboxyhemoglobin are unknown. Other substances in the blood may or may not affect pulse oximetry. Bilirubin has little effect on pulse oximetry; methemoglobin, generated in the presence of oxidizing agents such as nitrites and sulfonamides, usually increases the difference between functional O_2 saturation and oxyhemoglobin, but methemoglobin may also have the peculiar effect of causing the pulse oximeter always to read 85%. A variety of dyes such as indocyanine green and methylene blue also have effects on the accuracy of measurement.

Clinical Applications

Pulse oximetry has widespread usefulness in the ICU, especially in adjusting inspired oxygen, during weaning from mechanical ventilation, and in testing different levels of PEEP, inverse I:E ratio, or other mechanical ventilator adjustments. Other uses include monitoring during procedures such as bronchoscopy, gastrointestinal endoscopy, cardioversion, hemodialysis, and radiography. Pulse oximetry is particularly accurate in following O_2 saturation in patients who have mild to moderate hypoxemia (O_2 saturation > 75%) but without severe hypoperfusion or hypotension. It cannot be regarded as a complete substitute for arterial blood gases, partly because of the lack of P_{O_2} and pH determinations but also because of the relationship between P_{O_2} and O_2 saturation when the latter is above 90–95%. Results of pulse oximetry should be interpreted cautiously in patients with carboxyhemoglobinemia or methemoglobinemia.

Barker SJ, Tremper KK: The effect of carbon monoxide inhalation on pulse oximeter signal detection. Anesthesiology 1987; 67:599–603.

Bongard F, Sue D: Pulse oximetry and capnography in intensive and transitional care units. West J Med 1992;156:57–64.

Clark JS et al: Noninvasive assessment of blood gases. Am Rev Respir Dis 1992;145:220–32.

Haessler R et al: Continuous intra-arterial oximetry, pulse oximetry, and co-oximetry during cardiac surgery. J Cardiothorac Vasc Anesth 1992;6:668–73.

Schnapp LM, Cohen NH: Pulse oximetry. Chest 1990;98:1244–50.

Severinghaus JW, Naifeh KH: Accuracy of response of six pulse oximeters to profound hypoxia. Anesthesiology 1987; 67:551–8.

Severinghaus JW, Spellman MJ: Pulse oximeter failure thresholds in hypotension and vasoconstriction. Anesthesiology 1990;73:532–7.

Tremper KK, Barker SJ: Pulse oximetry. Anesthesiology 1989;70:98–108.

AIRWAY CO_2 MONITORING

Airway CO_2 monitoring is achieved with a rapidly responding infrared CO_2 analyzer or mass spectrometer using a sidestream sample of gas or an infrared analyzer that measures CO_2 directly at the end of the endotracheal tube. **Capnography** is a continuous display or recording of CO_2 concentration during each breath.

Other devices display the end-tidal CO_2 fraction or partial pressure (P_{ETCO_2}).

The infrared analyzer uses an appropriate wavelength of infrared light for which the CO_2 concentration is proportionate to the absorption of the light. It has the advantage of relatively low cost, real-time sampling, reliability, ease of calibration, and acceptable response time. Small alterations in CO_2 measurement at high O_2 concentrations can be accounted for by changes in the calculation algorithm. The mass spectrometer is a highly accurate device that separates respiratory gases by molecular weight and charge. The CO_2 (or other gas) concentration is expressed as the quotient of CO_2 molecules counted divided by the total number of measured molecules counted. Mass spectrometry is considerably more expensive than infrared CO_2 measurements. However, most mass spectrometers used in the ICU have an elaborate series of sampling tubing, allowing several patients to share the device, and has a very rapid response time.

With either device—infrared analyzer or mass spectrometer—capnography shows a continuous display of expired and, if desired, inspired CO_2 concentration or partial pressure. The expired CO_2 waveform can give a qualitative assessment of the degree of ventilation-perfusion mismatching. For example, the steepness of the slope of the "alveolar plateau" indicates more severe $\dot{V}/\dot{Q}$ mismatching because it demonstrates emptying of progressively less well ventilated lung units compared with a waveform showing a flatter alveolar plateau in a patient with less severe $\dot{V}/\dot{Q}$ mismatching. The inspiratory segment should also be inspected to confirm that the inspired gas is free of CO_2 as a result of malfunction of the ventilator's expiratory valve or some other component.

A newer technique utilizes a disposable colorimetric device to detect the presence of CO_2. This is a qualitative technique which is designed only to confirm endotracheal tube placement and position. When the device tests positively for CO_2, this confirms that the endotracheal tube is in the trachea. However, a negative result is not as reliable, and alternative means for checking tube placement must be utilized.

End-Tidal & Mixed Expired P_{CO_2}

In normal subjects at rest breathing at a normal tidal volume and respiratory rate, P_{ETCO_2} is close numerically to arterial P_{CO_2}, with the usual difference between Pa_{CO_2} and P_{ETCO_2} 0–4 mm Hg ($P[a–ET]_{CO_2}$). In patients with respiratory failure, contribution to expired gas from dead space and high $\dot{V}/\dot{Q}$ lung units decreases CO_2 concentration during expiration and at end-expiration. The $P(a–ET)_{CO_2}$ becomes increasingly large, with a strong correlation between $P(a–ET)_{CO_2}$ and the dead space/tidal volume ratio. The P_{ETCO_2} should not be used as a substitute for Pa_{CO_2} in patients with lung disease. Furthermore, $P(a–ET)_{CO_2}$ cannot be assumed to remain constant in the face of lung disease and mechanical ventilation. Therefore, the difference between the two values may not be fixed, and the practice of obtaining a single simultaneous pair of Pa_{CO_2} and P_{ETCO_2} readings at one time and subsequently estimating Pa_{CO_2} from P_{ETCO_2} plus the difference should be discouraged.

The mixed expired CO_2 fraction or partial pressure (P_{ECO_2}) is usually determined from collection of expired gas for several minutes. This should be distinguished from P_{ETCO_2} sampled at the end of a single breath. The mixed expired CO_2 fraction can be used with Pa_{CO_2} to calculate the dead space/tidal volume ratio (V_D/V_T) using the modified Bohr equation:

$$\frac{V_D}{V_T} = \frac{Pa_{CO_2} - P_{ECO_2}}{Pa_{CO_2}}$$

In addition, if minute ventilation is measured,

$$\dot{V}CO_2\ (\text{L/min, STPD}) = 0.826 \times \dot{V}_E\ (\text{L/min, BTPS}) \times \frac{P_{ECO_2}}{P_B}$$

where P_B is barometric pressure.

Validity

As described above, end-tidal P_{CO_2} should not be used as an accurate estimate of Pa_{CO_2}. Patients with either worsening of gas exchange function (increased Pa_{CO_2}) or improvement in function (decreased Pa_{CO_2}) can have a fall in P_{ETCO_2}. The former occurs because of an increase in $P(a–ET)_{CO_2}$; the latter represents a parallel fall in both P_{ETCO_2} and Pa_{CO_2}.

However, among the relatively few reports involving ICU patients—most of whom were receiving mechanical ventilation—some indicate that $PaCO_2$ and $PETCO_2$ track together relatively well, with mean differences less than 5 mm Hg and no change in difference during weaning or extubation. In COPD patients, the difference was considerably higher (as much as 9 mm Hg), but again relatively constant. In contrast, other studies have found that $P(a\text{–}ET)CO_2$ varies considerably, and, while there was correlation with VD/VT, there was a lack of a constant value for $P(a\text{–}ET)CO_2$ that would allow "tracking" of $PaCO_2$ from $PETCO_2$ alone. In particular, one study demonstrated that both increases and decreases in $P(a\text{–}ET)CO_2$ may result from mechanical ventilator adjustments.

Clinical Applications

Airway CO_2 monitoring has the advantage of being noninvasive, and studies are available that indicate a decrease in the number of arterial blood gases obtained when this modality is used. However, it is clear that the critically ill patient with respiratory failure will have the largest and most unpredictable difference between $PaCO_2$ and $PETCO_2$; in these patients, $PETCO_2$ is an unreliable estimate of $PaCO_2$. On the other hand, the difference between $PaCO_2$ and $PETCO_2$ can be used as a measure of dead space/tidal volume ratio and therefore as a measure of the severity of gas exchange derangement.

Although studies are lacking on the benefit of routine monitoring of airway CO_2, capnography and $PETCO_2$ monitoring have been used in several clinical situations. First, airway CO_2 monitoring can provide rapid noninvasive assurance of correct endotracheal tube placement. The capnogram should show increasing CO_2 concentration during expiration, and $PETCO_2$ should be a plausible value. Second, $PETCO_2$ has been used during cardiopulmonary resuscitation as a measure of the effectiveness of artificial circulatory assistance; a very low $PETCO_2$ suggests that venous blood is not adequately returning to the central circulation. Third, the combination of arterial and end-tidal PCO_2 provides an estimate of the inefficiency of ventilation (VD/VT). Some researchers have suggested that $P(a\text{–}ET)CO_2$ can be used to titrate the optimal amount of PEEP. While the smallest difference in $P(a\text{–}ET)CO_2$ has correlated with the highest degree of tissue oxygen delivery, this measurement has not proved ideal in all studies. Finally, it has been suggested that capnography can help in weaning patients from mechanical ventilation, but the predictive value of airway CO_2 monitoring in this clinical situation is unclear.

Bhende MS et al: Validity of a disposable end-tidal CO_2 detector in verifying endotracheal tube placement in infants and children. Ann Emerg Med 1992 21:142–5.

Bongard F, Sue D: Pulse oximetry and capnography in intensive and transitional care units. West J Med 1992;156:57–64.

Clark JS et al: Noninvasive assessment of blood gases. Am Rev Respir Dis 1992;145:220–32.

Hoffman RA et al: End-tidal carbon dioxide in critically ill patients during changes in mechanical ventilation. Am Rev Respir Dis 1989;140:1265–8.

Murray IP et al: Titration of PEEP by arterial minus end-tidal carbon dioxide gradient. Chest 1984;85:100–4.

Murray IP, Modell JH: Early detection of endotracheal tube accidents by monitoring carbon dioxide concentration in respiratory gas. Anesthesiology 1983;59:344–6.

Trillo G, von Planta M, Kette F: $ETCO_2$ monitoring during low flow states: clinical aims and limits. Resuscitation 1994 27:1–8.

Yamanaka MK, Sue DY: Comparison of arterial-end tidal PCO_2 difference and dead space/tidal volume ratio in respiratory failure. Chest 1987;92:832-35.

TRANSCUTANEOUS BLOOD GASES

Utilizing transcutaneous blood gas monitors, partial pressures of oxygen and carbon dioxide may be measured in the tissue beneath heated skin electrodes. This monitoring technique has value because it reflects tissue levels, but it should not be employed as a substitute for blood gas monitoring.

Principle

The Clark electrode, similar to that used in blood gas analyzers, has been modified to be used on the skin surface. The skin in the area of the electrode is heated to 43–45 °C. This heating is necessary to make the skin permeable to oxygen, but it has the additional effect of increasing perfusion in the tissues beneath the probe. As transcutaneous PO_2 ($PtcO_2$) reflects the oxygen tension level of the tissue beneath the probe, values may be affected either by arterial oxygenation or by systemic and regional perfusion. At relatively normal cardiac output and with normal regional blood flow, $PtcO_2$ values reflect arterial PO_2 values. In adults, the ratio of transcutaneous to arterial PO_2 is normally about 0.8, while in children it tends to be higher. (Values in neonates may be very close to equal.) However, when either cardiac output or regional perfusion is decreased, the ratio of transcutaneous to arterial PO_2 is decreased in proportion to the level of decreased perfusion. Hence, transcutaneous oxygen monitoring may be utilized as a monitor of both oxygenation and perfusion. A low $PtcO_2$ value is an indicator that the patient is either hypoxemic or in a low-flow state (or has reduced regional perfusion).

Transcutaneous PCO_2 ($PtcCO_2$) has been measured using a modified PCO_2 electrode or by a small-sample infrared analyzer, both attached to the skin surface. In contrast to $Ptco_2$, however, CO_2 is more soluble than O_2, so that tissue stores of CO_2 act as a buffer, reducing the dependence of $Ptcco_2$ on blood flow and metabolism. In theory, $Ptcco_2$ should mirror $Paco_2$ more closely than $Ptco_2$ reflects Pao_2, and there is no need to heat the skin at the monitoring site.

Both $Ptco_2$ and $Ptcco_2$ devices should be calibrated against known Po_2 and Pco_2. Because of the heating of the $Ptco_2$ electrode site, the location must be changed every 4–6 hours to minimize the risk of thermal injury.

Clinical Applications

Many neonatal intensive care units routinely employ $Ptco_2$ monitoring and have found good correlation with arterial blood gases except in patients with severe cardiac compromise. In adults, $Ptco_2$ measurement is best utilized as a measure of tissue *hypoperfusion.* A reduction of $Ptco_2$ may be an early indicator of low flow, particularly if pulse oximetry does not indicate severe hypoxemia.

Transcutaneous Pco_2 has been shown to correlate with $Paco_2$ in several clinical trials, but the average $Ptcco_2$–$Paco_2$ difference is generally in the range of 20 mm Hg in ICU patients. The difference may be considerably smaller in hemodynamically stable individuals.

Clark JS et al: Noninvasive assessment of blood gases. Am Rev Respir Dis 1992;145:220–32.

Hasibeder W et al: Factors influencing transcutaneous oxygen and carbon dioxide measurements in adult intensive care patients. Intensive Care Med 1991;17:272–5.

Tobin MJ: Respiratory monitoring in the intensive care unit. Am Rev Respir Dis 1988;138:1625–42.

Tremper KK: Interpretation of non-invasive oxygen and carbon dioxide data. Can J Anaesth 1990;37:627–38.

RESPIRATORY MECHANICS

Monitoring of respiratory system mechanics in the ICU includes both measured and derived parameters. Measured parameters commonly monitored are tidal volume, vital capacity, airway pressure, and intrathoracic pressure. Commonly monitored derived parameters include lung compliance, airway resistance, and work of breathing. A discussion of compliance and resistance is found in Chapter 12.

Tidal Volume

In the ICU, tidal volume is most commonly measured in patients who have endotracheal tubes and require mechanical ventilation. Ventilators measure expired tidal volume using bellows, ultrasonic flowmeters, or pneumotachographs. For the latter two, tidal volume is calculated by summing expired flow. Respiratory inductive plethysmography can provide a noninvasive estimate of tidal volume. Tidal volume measurements should be frequently monitored in patients receiving mechanical ventilation. When volume-preset modes are used, a difference in expired volume compared with preset volume indicates that there is a leak in the ventilator circuit, that inspiratory flow demand is extremely high, or that inspiratory peak pressure exceeds the preset limit. In pressure-controlled ventilation, tidal volume is used to adjust the level of set airway pressure, and any change in expired tidal volume indicates a change in lung or chest wall compliance or airway resistance. During spontaneous respiration, tidal volume monitoring using noninvasive measurement can be used to help identify patients with obstructive sleep apnea or abnormal breathing patterns (Cheyne-Stokes respiration). Tidal volume monitoring is also an important part of the care of patients with neuromuscular disorders or spinal cord injury and during weaning from the ventilator.

Maximum Inspiratory & Expiratory Airway Pressure

Inspiratory and expiratory maximum pressures are determined by a manometer connected either to a mouthpiece or to tubing adapted to fit onto the endotracheal tube. These pressures are correctly measured starting at functional residual volume, so that lung and chest wall elastic recoil are neutralized and the pressures reflect only respiratory muscle strength. In practice, this detail is often omitted. Normal maximum inspiratory pressure is more than −80 to −100 cm H_2O; maximum expiratory pressure in normal individuals exceeds 120–150 cm H_2O. Maximum negative inspiratory and positive expiratory pressures are useful in assessment of respiratory failure in patients with neuromuscular disorders. Studies support the use either of the average of maximum inspiratory and expiratory pressures or of vital capacity in roughly predicting the onset of hypercapnia in these patients when pressures fall by about 70% or when vital capacity is less than about 55% of predicted. These direct measures are notably better than extrapolations of respiratory muscle strength from measurements of the strength of the extremities. These measurements are also useful in determining whether a patient may be weaned from ventilatory support.

Intrathoracic (Intraesophageal) Pressure

Intrathoracic pressure requires a pressure sensor within the chest—almost always a balloon placed in the lower third of the esophagus, connected to a suitable pressure manometer. The balloon must be carefully filled with a small amount of air so that the changes in intrathoracic pressure are faithfully recorded without the confounding effects of the balloon's compliance. Care must be taken to position the balloon within the chest and not in the stomach. Systems for measuring esophageal pressure are commercially available. Esophageal pressure is most often used to determine lung or chest wall compliance or work of breathing, but it can also be helpful in identifying auto-PEEP. A potential use is to "correct" pulmonary artery or pulmonary artery wedge pressures for large swings in intrathoracic pressure during the respiratory cycle.

Lung & Chest Wall Compliance

Calculation of compliance of the respiratory system (chest wall and lungs together) is reviewed in Chapter 3. The components of respiratory system compliance can be subdivided into chest wall and lung compliances. Lung compliance (CL) is calculated as the ratio of change in volume (ΔV) to change in pressure (ΔP), where ΔV is usually the tidal volume and ΔP is the difference between end-inspiratory and end-expiratory transpulmonary pressure. Transpulmonary pressure is the pressure difference between the pressure in the airway and the esophageal pressure. Normal lung compliance is about 200 mL/cm H_2O. If determination of chest wall compliance (CCW) is desired, the formula $1/C_{RS} = 1/C_L + 1/C_{CW}$ can be used where RS = respiratory system). Decreased lung compliance has been used as a criterion of ARDS in some clinical studies but is not usually required for its clinical diagnosis. Low lung compliance does suggest increased work of breathing (if tidal volume remains unchanged) and could suggest that weaning would be difficult or inappropriate. Patients being given PEEP can be followed by changes in lung compliance; ideally, lung compliance increases with PEEP as unventilated lung units are recruited, but this measurement is not often applied outside of research settings. Because lung compliance and respiratory system compliance are usually measured together, chest wall compliance assessment is also available. On occasion, abnormal chest wall compliance as a cause of respiratory failure is not identified until this measurement is made. If chest wall noncompliance is found to be contributing to respiratory failure, a very different approach to treatment may be warranted. For example, in patients with chest wall burns, worsening compliance may be an indication for escharotomy.

Work of Breathing

A measurement of the work required for breathing is derived from the formula for mechanical work: W = force × distance. For breathing in which the force is applied over a predetermined volume, substitute pressure for work, and for distance substitute change in volume. Thus, work of breathing is the product of $\Delta P \times \Delta V$. Work of breathing can be calculated for the patient-ventilator system, with the result indicating the work being done *by the mechanical ventilator* for a particular tidal volume. The same work, of course, would be done by the patient breathing spontaneously, but this is usually not relevant because the patient is unlikely to breathe at the same rate, tidal volume, and I:E ratio. For spontaneous breathing, tidal volume should be measured nonintrusively, and the pressure difference between end-expiration and end-inspiration is measured inside the thorax (esophageal pressure). Thus, a setup for measuring mechanical work of breathing generally measures tidal volume (noninvasive or through the endotracheal tube) and esophageal pressure. A different and more elaborate approach is to determine metabolic rate by indirect calorimetry (oxygen consumption) and to subtract an estimate of the nonrespiratory energy requirement. The remainder is then considered to represent the energy requirement or work rate of the respiratory muscles. This method depends in part on accurate indirect calorimetry but more importantly on an estimate of the O_2 consumption of the rest of the body.

Work of breathing calculated from tidal volume and esophageal pressure may underestimate actual work being performed by a significant amount. Some of the difference arises from nonuniform expansion of the lung or chest wall or compression of intrathoracic gas, and the calculation does not consider the expiratory work of breathing. In practice, work of breathing is rarely measured for clinical purposes. Theoretically, increased work of breathing should be a good predictor of the success of weaning from mechanical ventilation and could provide a guide to maximizing respiratory muscle strength, maximizing lung and chest wall compliance, and minimizing airway resistance. In the area of research in critically ill patients, work of breathing has been used to characterize an excessive burden on the respiratory muscles from high resistance in the ventilator circuit, poorly functioning expiratory and inspiratory valves, development of auto-PEEP, and other factors.

Black LF, Hyatt RE: Maximal respiratory pressures: normal values and relationship to age and sex. Am Rev Respir Dis 1968;99:696–702.

Braun NMT, Arora NS, Rochester DF: Respiratory muscle and pulmonary function in polymyositis and other proximal myopathies. Thorax 1983;38:616–23.

Marini JJ: Monitoring during mechanical ventilation. Clin Chest Med 1988;9:73–100.

Tobin MJ: Respiratory monitoring in the intensive care unit. Am Rev Respir Dis 1988;138:1625–42.

Valta P et al: Evaluation of respiratory inductive plethysmography in the measurement of breathing pattern and PEEP-induced changes in lung volume. Chest 1992;102: 234–8.

MONITORING OF OXYGEN TRANSPORT

There is increasing evidence that the best currently available physiologic endpoints by which to titrate therapy in critically ill patients are oxygen delivery and oxygen consumption. Oxygen delivery is defined as cardiac output × arterial oxygen content.

It is most commonly measured intermittently but may now be estimated continuously, utilizing pulse oximetry and continuous cardiac output methodology. Oxygen consumption may be monitored by measurement of respired gases or may be calculated by the Fick equation.

Measurement of respired gases includes determination of CO_2 output ($\dot{V}CO_2$) and O_2 uptake ($\dot{V}CO_2$). In the steady state, these are considered equivalent to CO_2 production and O_2 consumption. The ratio $\dot{V}CO_2/\dot{V}O_2$ is the respiratory gas exchange ratio, which is equal to the respiratory quotient (RQ) in the steady state.

$\dot{V}CO_2$ and $\dot{V}O_2$ are measured by comparing inspired and expired gas concentrations of O_2 and CO_2 and knowing the inspired or expired minute ventilation. Gas concentrations are measured using discrete O_2 and CO_2 analyzers or a respiratory mass spectrometer. Oxygen analyzers most often measure PO_2 using an electrochemical method to generate current proportionate to PO_2. Infrared CO_2 analyzers are most common and are highly reliable and accurate. Both inspired and expired gas concentrations are needed.

The traditional method is to collect a timed sample of expired gas either from a spontaneously breathing patient or from the expiratory side of the mechanical ventilator circuit into a nonporous balloon or bag. The volume is determined using large calibrated syringes (3–4 L) or a suitable spirometer. The product of mixed expired CO_2 fraction ($FECO_2$) and expired minute ventilation is $\dot{V}CO_2$ (L/min) expressed at standard temperature and pressure, dry (STPD). For $\dot{V}O_2$ (L/min), the calculation is more complex, having to take into account the inspired oxygen fraction and the small but significant difference between inspired and expired minute ventilation due to the gas exchange ratio.

Automated instruments for measuring $\dot{V}CO_2$ and $\dot{V}O_2$ have been developed for use in the ICU. These measure ventilation by pneumotachographs or other flow or volume sensors and have built-in O_2 and CO_2 analyzers. These devices allow for continuous measurement of $\dot{V}CO_2$ and $\dot{V}O_2$ and often report these results in tables or graphs. Results can also be transferred directly to computers for storage and later analysis. Indirect calorimetry uses $\dot{V}O_2$ and an estimate of the substrate mix being used for energy production (RQ) to estimate the energy expenditure or caloric requirement of the patient:

$$\text{kcal/d} = \dot{V}O_2\ (\text{L/min}) \times 1440\ \text{min/d} \times (3.82 + 1.23 \times \text{RQ})\ \text{kcal/L}VO_2$$

$\dot{V}O_2$ and $\dot{V}CO_2$ can also be measured using the Fick equation with knowledge of arterial and mixed venous O_2 and CO_2 contents (mL/dL or mL/L of blood) and cardiac output (thermodilution or other technique). For critically ill patients, this requires a pulmonary artery catheter, and it has most commonly been an intermittent calculation. However, with continuous cardiac output technology, continuous mixed venous oximetry, and arterial pulse oximetry, a continuous calculated oxygen consumption is now possible.

Validity

Carbon dioxide output ($\dot{V}CO_2$) determination is generally accepted as satisfactory in the ICU, including its use with patients receiving mechanical ventilation. During high inspired O_2 breathing, CO_2 analyzers may require adjustment according to the manufacturer's instructions, but when the need for adjustment is anticipated this does not detract from the accuracy of the test.

On the other hand, $\dot{V}O_2$ is most often calculated using the difference between inspired and expired fraction of O_2 and an adjustment that accounts for the small difference between inspired and expired minute ventilation. This formula is notoriously sensitive to inaccuracy in inspired O_2 concentration, especially when $FIO_2 > 0.50$. In fact, some investigators are suspicious of $\dot{V}O_2$ determinations from expired gas when FIO_2 exceeds 0.21, and many commercial systems are not reliable when FIO_2 is > 0.30–0.40. Water vapor has an effect on PO_2 and PCO_2 measurement except when a mass spectrometer is used; water vapor pressure must be considered in the calculation of $\dot{V}O_2$, or the measured gas should be dried or otherwise treated so that the PH_{2O} is known.

Calculation of oxygen consumption by the Fick equation also has significant inherent inexactness. Intermittent bolus thermodilution measurements of cardiac output have significant variance, as do measurements of arterial and venous saturation as well as hemoglobin. Any errors in these measurements are increased geometrically during calculation of oxygen consumption—so-called mathematical coupling. However, the importance of this limitation to the accuracy of this methodology in clinical practice is a matter of controversy. It is possible that continuous cardiac output monitoring techniques may have less variance and thus allow more accurate calculation of oxygen consumption.

Clinical Applications

Monitoring of oxygen delivery and oxygen consumption allow titration of intensive care interventions to the best physiologic end point for individual patients. In many conditions, such as following sepsis, hemorrhage, shock, operations, trauma, or burns, it is known that patient survival is more likely if oxygen delivery and oxygen consumption are supernormal. Specific supernormal values of oxygen delivery and oxygen consumption have been suggested as goals of therapy. Alternatively, for an individual patient, the optimal cardiac output and oxygen delivery may be discovered operationally by determining at what point flow-limited oxygen consumption is no longer present.

Oxygen uptake by indirect calorimetry in the ICU may also be utilized to determine metabolic requirements, so that appropriate caloric requirements as well as substrate utilization may be monitored.

Becker CS, Feurer ID: Individualization of nutrient prescriptions with indirect calorimetry. In: *Nutritional Medicine: A Case Management Approach.* Blackburn GL, Bell SJ, Mullen JL (editors). Saunders, 1989.

Bongard FS, Leighton TA. Continuous dual oximetry in surgical critical care. Indications and limitations. Ann Surg 1992, 216:60–8.

Browning JA et al: The effects of a fluctuating $F_{I}O_2$ on metabolic measurements in mechanically ventilated patients. Crit Care Med 1982;10:82–5.

Campbell SM, Kudsk KA: "High tech" metabolic measurements: useful in daily clinical practice? JPEN J Parenter Enteral Nutr 1988;12:610–2.

Cortes V, Nelson LD: Errors in estimating energy expenditure in critically ill surgical patients. Arch Surg 1989;124:287–90.

Hanique G et al: Significance of pathologic oxygen supply dependency in critically ill patients: comparison between measured and calculated methods. Intensive Care Med 1994,20:12–8.

Hankeln KB et al: Use of continuous noninvasive measurement of oxygen consumption in patients with adult respiratory distress syndrome following shock of various etiologies. Crit Care Med 1991;19:642–9.

Russell JA; Phang PT: The oxygen delivery/consumption controversy. Approaches to management of the critically ill. Am J Respir Crit Care Med 1994:533–7.

Shoemaker WC, Appel PL, Kram HB: Role of oxygen debt in the development of organ failure, sepsis and death in high risk surgical patients. Chest 1992:102:208-214.

Sue DY, Wolff C: A method for increasing confidence in respiratory gas exchange measurements in mechanically ventilated patients. JPEN J Parenter Enteral Nutr 1991;15:625–9.

Weissman C et al: Resting metabolic rate of the critically ill patient. Measured vs. predicted. Anesthesiology 1986;64:673–9.

Transport

9

Samuel J. Stratton, MD, MPH

This chapter will describe and discuss **interfacility transport** of the critically ill. As technology advances (with its associated costs) and as fiscal realities increase the incentive to control health care spending, increased regionalization will result in transport of the critically ill to the hospital that can best manage the patient. Lessening the need for duplicate resources by regionalization of specialized healthcare services may achieve optimal patient outcomes at minimal costs. With the shift in delivery of health care to the managed care model, repatriation of health plan participants with their primary care providers has led to a dramatic increase in interfacility transport of persons requiring hospitalization or extended emergency evaluation.

Current literature supports the development and maintenance of specialized centers where higher levels of care can be provided. Management of resource-intensive critical illness in these centers has been shown to improve medical outcomes and cost effectiveness. Most studies support the concept that patient volume in tertiary care centers (Table 9–1) leads to better patient outcomes because staffs of these centers maintain high experience and proficiency levels. With medical evidence strongly supporting regionalized medical specialty centers, methods for transport of patients to these centers must be developed using practices based on the best scientific and management evidence.

Alter DA et al: Long-term MI outcomes at hospitals with or without on-site revascularization. JAMA 2001;285:2101–8.

Dardik A et al: Surgical repair of ruptured abdominal aortic aneurysms in the state of Maryland: factors influencing outcome among 527 recent cases. J Vasc Surg 1998;28:413–20.

Konvolinka CW, Copes WS, Sacco WJ: Institution and per-surgeon volume versus survival outcome in Pennsylvania's trauma centers. Am J Surg 1995;170:333–40.

Thiemann DR et al: The association between hospital volume and survival after acute myocardial infarction in elderly patients. N Engl J Med 1999;340:1640–8.

INTERHOSPITAL TRANSPORT

Composition of the Transport Team

Once the referring physician decides that a patient needs a higher level of care, the mode of transport must be chosen as well as the composition of the transporting crew. For interfacility transfers, there are no standard guidelines regarding which patients may be transferred solely with paramedics, which require a nurse in attendance, and which patients require a physician in attendance. Local regulations may restrict the role of paramedics, who should not, for example, give medications or manipulate unfamiliar equipment such as ventilators unless they have documented evidence of training and competence. The scope of such training may be limited by the paramedic licensing or certification board.

There are no national data on overall transport volumes or team composition within transport systems. Two medical attendant teams are most common, consisting of combinations of ambulance attendants, emergency medical technicians (EMTs) who receive 100–150 hours of initial education, paramedics who receive 1000–3000 hours of initial education, and licensed registered nurses as the team members. In urban areas, ground transport is most common; in rural areas, air transport is more often required because of the distances and the difficulties of road travel. In most settings, the EMT is the highest-level care provider on the interfacility transport team, but for critical care transports a physician, nurse, or paramedic may be the highest-level provider. EMTs, paramedics, and nurses usually have defined scopes of practice in the jurisdiction where they are licensed. This scope of practice limits what the individual may or may not do during the transport process. A survey of hospital-based air medical programs disclosed that 97% utilize two medical attendants. Of the small number of programs that use only one medical attendant, 75% use registered nurses and 25% use paramedics. The most common crew mix was a flight nurse and flight paramedic (53%), followed by nurse and other (usually respiratory therapist), 20%; nurse and physician, 11%; nurse and nurse, 11%; and other combinations, 5%. Many of the programs stating that they have physicians on board the aircraft are utilizing resident physicians–there is little information about whether the level of training of the physicians is a factor in outcome. Lastly, all of the studies looking at outcome use mortality as an end measure rather than length of hospital stay, cost, or morbidity. It is possible that short-term mortality may not be the best outcome on which to base a judgment about transport effectiveness. Many programs ascribe considerable value to the presence of physicians; this despite the fact that only 11% of programs fly

Table 9–1. Medical services most effectively delivered in specialized referral centers.

Burn injuries
Trauma
High-risk blunt and penetrating injuries
Neurologic injuries
Vascular injuries
Complex orthopedic injuries
Pediatric-age trauma
Oro-maxillary-facial injuries
Obstetric, high-risk
Neonatal care
Pediatric critical care
Cardiac
Invasive coronary revascularization
High-risk cardiac care
Cerebrovascular ("stroke") management
Rehabilitation, intensive

with physicians on board. Nonphysicians can safely use paralytic pharmacologic agents and perform intubation, cricothyrotomy, and tube thoracostomy; nurses or respiratory therapists may be more familiar with ventilators than a resident physician.

Studies are needed to discern whether those transfers that require a physician can be ascertained beforehand. It would be of value also to specify what pertinent skills the physicians should have, since some might be acquired by alternative flight personnel.

Mode of Transport

Current options for mode of transport are the ground ambulance, either a helicopter or a fixed-wing aircraft, and watercraft. In many urban centers, all options are available, and in rural areas—Alaska is an example—the airplane is essential. Decisions that will influence the mode of transport (if all options are available) include the distance and thus the duration of transport; the diagnosis and thus the complications that may arise during transport; the level of training and the techniques the transporting personnel can provide; the urgency of access to tertiary care; and the local weather conditions and geography. In general terms, ground ambulances are more available than air vehicles; ground ambulances may be dispatched from a local facility, though an outreach team from the tertiary care center may be requested; mobilization time of such a team and their arrival will have to be taken into consideration.

A. Ground Ambulance

Ground ambulance vehicles are usually the most readily available and may be categorized as vehicles for basic life support (BLS) or advanced life support (ALS). BLS ambulances are most often staffed with two EMTs and can provide basic first aid, automatic external defibrillation, and oxygen without cardiac monitoring. ALS ambulances are staffed with a paramedic, nurse, or physician as the highest-level provider. ALS ambulance personnel can provide cardiac monitoring and advanced airway management and can deliver the drugs and intravenous fluids commonly used for resuscitation of medical and trauma patients. ALS ambulances may have the necessary outlets for managing ventilators or balloon pumps for interfacility critical transfers. However, if the ambulance belongs to the local Emergency Medical Services (EMS) jurisdiction, the administrators may not allow the vehicle to be out of service for a long trip to a tertiary center. In many urban areas, ambulance companies maintain some ALS ambulances for interfacility transports so that the primary EMS system is not affected. Ground ambulances are limited by surface conditions or traffic congestion. Equipment utilized to support patients during transport should have a backup supply (batteries, extra oxygen tanks) in case of need. The United States Department of Transportation (DOT) has published standards that have been adopted by most states which relate to minimum ambulance configuration and equipment requirements. Communication between the ground ambulance and the receiving facility or designated medical control center can be a consideration during long transport. The ground ambulance is the most widely utilized and the least expensive mode of interfacility transfer. This method should be considered for transport distances of 30 miles or less.

B. Helicopter

Helicopters should be considered for transports over distances of 30–150 miles. They travel at ground speeds of 120–180 miles per hour and often are dispatched from the receiving tertiary facility or urban area. Helicopters usually require a warm-up time of 2–3 minutes before liftoff and–allowing for communication time–can be launched within 5-6 minutes after the flight request is received. Under normal weather conditions, helicopters can fly point-to-point and land at accident scenes or sending facilities; the liftoff capability depends on the type of helicopter utilized. Helicopter transports are limited by available landing sites (often a problem in densely populated areas) and weather. Helicopters are expensive—the capital cost is between $1.5 million and $6 million depending on whether a single- or dual-engine model is selected; likewise, the number of patients that can be transported is determined by aircraft selection and configuration.

Helicopters can fly from point to point under visual flight rules (VFR). In inclement weather, several helicopter programs can fly under instrument flight rules

(IFR). This, however, requires that they take off and land at an airport with appropriate instrumentation. Helicopters cannot fly in freezing rain or dense fog.

C. Fixed-Wing Aircraft

Fixed-wing aircraft should be considered for transport over distances exceeding 150 miles. Fixed-wing aircraft will have IFR capability and can fly from airport to airport, with ground transportation required at both ends. Aircraft cabins are normally pressurized between 6000 and 8000 feet, and this may have effects not only on the patient's clinical condition but also on apparatus such as endotracheal tubes or Swan-Ganz catheters; in addition, ventilators may need to be recalibrated. Some patients—eg, those being transferred to hyperbaric facilities for treatment of decompression sickness—may require pressurization at ground level.

Liability & Legal Issues

Interfacility transport of patients received increased legal visibility by the passage in 1986 of COBRA 1985, Section 9121, Amendments to the Social Security Law; and Section 1867, Special Responsibilities for Hospitals in Emergency Cases. These rules have undergone repeated emendation and the regulations have been renamed the Emergency Treatment and Active Labor Act (EMTALA), further amending Section 1867. Briefly, these laws refer to emergency transfers of unstable patients and were drafted to address the problem of transfers of uninsured patients. Indeed, the EMTALA regulations are often referred to as "anti-dumping legislation." EMTLLA provides a framework of legal liability under which the sending facility is responsible for initiating the transfer and selecting the mode of transportation (including the level of expertise of transferring personnel) and thus indirectly the equipment on the transporting vehicle. The sending facility is responsible for ensuring that the receiving facility has space and personnel available for care of the patient, and the sending physician is responsible for the risks of transfer and for deciding that the benefits to the patient following successful transfer outweigh the risks. A receiving facility that has specialized units (specified in the regulations as burn units, shock trauma units, and neonatal intensive care units) shall not refuse to accept an appropriate transfer if that hospital has the capability to treat the individual. This is a nondiscrimination clause and is an attempt to prevent receiving facilities from accepting only funded patients. All emergency critical care and transferring personnel should understand the implications of these statutes.

As of April 2003, all ambulance and transport providers who engage in transactions that transmit protected health information in electronic form will be required to comply with the United States Federal Health Insurance Portability and Accountability Act (HIPAA). Protected health information includes any information identifiable to a specific person which relates to that individual's past, present, or future physical or mental health. HIPAA provides criminal and civil penalties for the improper use of protected health information, requiring that consent be given to obtain health information and that safeguards be in place to protect such information. Records pertaining to the use and disclosure of protected health information must be maintained for inspection by appropriate parties.

In addition to the legal requirements of transfer, the transferring personnel have certain liability concerns–particularly if they perform air medical transport.

The high degree of acuteness of these patients and the potential for adverse outcomes mandate medical malpractice coverage for the transferring personnel; the premiums will vary according to the staffing pattern selected. Medical directors also may need to make certain that they are appropriately covered for giving off-line medical direction and may find that although some of their responsibilities are covered by medical malpractice insurance, directors' and officers' insurance may be needed to cover their management decisions.

Outcome

The data that support the validity of transfer of the critically ill emphasize five recurring themes:

(1) Outcomes of the critically ill in tertiary centers are better than outcomes in community hospitals (matched for severity).

(2) Transport of the critically ill does not adversely affect the patient during transport–and therefore, by implication, the patient receives the benefit of (1).

(3) Transport of critically ill patients improves outcome when compared with national norms.

(4) Established systems of care (encompassing critical transport as a component) have societal outcomes better than those of comparable communities without such a system and better than those in the same community before the system was in place.

(5) Regionalization of specialized care is cost-effective and improves utilization of community resources.

An outcome study of all critically injured children with respiratory failure and head trauma in Oregon for 6 months compared mortality in 71 nontertiary and three tertiary facilities. Using the pediatric risk of mortality score, they demonstrated that outcomes in the nontertiary facilities were lower than those in tertiary facilities–and, further, that the difference in outcome was more pronounced the higher the expected mortality. For the most critical group (mortality risk > 30%), the odds ratio of dying in a nontertiary versus a tertiary facility was 8:1. The study concluded that "pediatric survival from a broad range of disorders might be improved by regional organization of pediatric care."

Improved outcome of the critically ill has been related to the volume of patients. This has been shown for coronary artery bypass surgery, trauma management, acute cardiac disease, abdominal aortic aneurysm, and stroke. For example, using Trauma and Injury Severity Score (TRISS) methodology, it has been shown that rapid transport or transfer by helicopter of trauma patients to a specialized trauma center resulted in a 13% reduction in mortality when compared with the outcome expected from the benchmark Multiple Trauma Outcome Study database. Studies demonstrating improved outcomes of the critically ill in regionalized specialty centers are in strong support of critical patient transport systems that facilitate movement of patients to these centers.

Transfer of the critically ill has been shown to be safe in cardiac cases, patients with respiratory distress, and pediatric patients. Transfer of patients sustaining acute myocardial infarction by air does not appear to be detrimental to patient outcome. In one study, 104 patients with infarctions were transferred, and no deaths occurred during transport.

Systems of care involving not only identification of the critically ill but also appropriate triage, transport, and definitive care have been shown to benefit the multiple trauma patient and the head-injured patient. All of these studies provide support for critical care regionalization, of which transport is an essential component.

Asaeda G et al: Utilization of air medical transport in a large urban environment: a retrospective analysis. Prehosp Emerg Care 2001;5:36.

Boyd CR, Tolson MA, Copes WS: Evaluating trauma care: The TRISS method. J Trauma 1987;27:370–8.

Boyle M, Sheets C: Surgical cricothyrotomy performed by air ambulance flight nurses: A five year experience. J Air Med Transp 1989;8:60.

De Wing MD et al: Cost-effective use of helicopters for the transportation of patients with burn injuries. J Burn Care Rehabil 2000;21:535.

Domeier RM, Hill JD, Simpson RD: The development and evaluation of a paramedic-staffed mobile intensive care unit for inter-facility patient transport. Prehosp Disaster Med 1996;11:37.

Dunn JD: Legal aspects of transfers. Probl Crit Care 1990: 4:447–8.

Gervin AS: Cricothyrotomy by flight paramedics. Aeromed J 1988;3:22.

Gorman SP: CRAMS scale: Field range of trauma victims. Ann Emerg Med 1982;11:132–35.

Jacobs LM et al: Helicopter air medical transport: ten-year outcomes for trauma patients in a New England program. Conn Med 1999;63:677.

Kaplan L, Walsh D, Burney RE: Emergency aeromedical transport in patients with acute myocardial infarction. Ann Emerg Med 1987;16:55–57.

Pollack NM et al: Improved outcomes from tertiary center pediatric intensive care: A statewide comparison of tertiary and non-tertiary care facilities. Crit Care Med 1991; 19:50.

Selevan JS et al: Critical care transport:outcome evaluation after interfacility transfer and hospitalization. Ann Emerg Med 1999;33:33.

Smith RF et al: The impact of volume on outcome of seriously injured trauma patients: Two years' experience in the Chicago trauma system. J Trauma 1990;30:1066–76.

EQUIPMENT & MONITORING

Interfacility critical care transport requires continuous monitoring and clinical management of the patient throughout the transport environment. The transporting vehicle should have the necessary power converters for all equipment that could be needed during a transfer; in addition, much of the equipment needs battery backup in case of electrical failure and backup oxygen supply in case of vehicle breakdown. In cold climates, provision must be made for maintenance of a warm environment in case of vehicle failure.

Airway Management

Critical care transport often involves patients who require advanced airway management. Often patients have had an endotracheal tube placed prior to transport, but transport team members must always be prepared to reintubate or establish an advanced airway should the need arise. In addition to standard endotracheal intubation equipment, a backup system such as the laryngeal mask or pharyngotracheal lumen tube should be available for those in whom intubation cannot be accomplished. Emergency cricothyrotomy has been successful in establishing a temporary airway during transport when performed by properly trained personnel. In addition to advanced airway management, ALS transport crews should have equipment available for decompression of tension pneumothorax (either needle or chest tube thoracostomy).

Medications

Medication lists have been published for the management of the obstetric patient, the neonatal patient, the pediatric patient, and the adult patient during transport. Additional medications may be required that are dependent upon patient profiles, and protocols should be prepared for the use of these medications. Care must be taken to ensure that expiration dates on medications are recognized, and guidelines should be in place beforehand for authorization to use them. Utilization of critical care transport under these circumstances allows a higher level of pharmacologic intervention—eg, many flight programs routinely use paralytic agents to facilitate endotracheal intubation.

Blood Utilization

Blood product transfusion during interfacility transport is controversial. It has been shown that in rotor-wing programs utilizing flight nurses, the transfusion of blood can be safely performed and is feasible during transport. Use of blood product transfusions is limited to lengthy transports during which crystalloid infusion alone will not stabilize a patient. Use of blood products during transport requires adherence to strict standard blood transfusion protocols, with blood administered by properly trained transport personnel.

Ventilators

Several types of ventilators are available for the transport environment. The choice of ventilator will depend upon the mission profile, compatibility with sponsoring ICUs, and the preferences of the medical director. Mechanical ventilation of intubated patients during transport has been shown to be optimal in comparison with manual ventilation. FDA-approved transport ventilators have performance indexes comparable to those of ICU area ventilators. Transport ventilators must be continually monitored during transport and, because of the unique transport environment, are subject to problems such as power failure and disconnection. Pressure-controlled ventilators are most commonly used during transport and in aircraft must be adjusted to correct for altitude changes. Most programs now continually monitor their patients by oximetry; in one study, continuous oximetry monitoring identified clinically unrecognized hypoxia. Different types of pulse oximeters have been evaluated, and some models had a greater number of failures than others.

Monitoring

The ECG, blood pressure, and, if necessary pulmonary artery pressure, intra-arterial pressure, and intracranial pressure should be monitored during transport. Successful defibrillation has been performed during flight, and use of this equipment does not interfere with other systems on helicopters and fixed-wing aircraft. If the patient does not have an intra-arterial line, occlusion oscillometry or Doppler measurement will give a satisfactory indication of blood pressure; normal auscultation of the blood pressure using a sphygmomanometer cuff is difficult in the transport environment, as ambient noise may exceed 110 db.

Medications should be administered by infusion pump throughout transport to ensure smooth and accurate dosing. Many small rugged infusion pumps are available and can be rapidly reprogrammed to manage unstable patients. In addition, portable intra-aortic balloon pumps and left ventricular assist devices are now commercially available that weigh less than 150 lb and can be transported on most helicopters.

Barillo DJ et al: Pressure-controlled ventilation for the long-range aeromedical transport of patients with burns. J Burn Care Rehabil 1997;18:200.

Berns KS, Zietlow SP: blood usage in rotor-wing transport. Air Med J 1998;17:105.

Davey AL, Macnab AJ, Green G: Changes in pCO_2 during air medical transport of children with closed head injuries. Air Med J 2001;20:27.

Day S et al: Pediatric interhospital critical care transport: Consensus of national leadership conference. Pediatrics 1991; 88:696-704.

Evans A, Winslow EH: Oxygen saturation and hemodynamic response in critically ill, mechanically ventilated adults during interhospital transport. Am J Crit Care 1995;4:106.

Gudgell S, Vukov LF, Farrell MB: Pulse oximetry in rotor wing transport. Aeromed J 1987;2:81–84.

Martin SE et al: Use of the laryngeal mask airway in air transport when intubation fails. J Trauma 1999;47:352.

Miyoshi E et al: Performance of transport ventilator with patient-triggered ventilation. Chest 2000;118:1109.

Short L et al: A comparison of pulse oximeters during helicopter flight. J Emerg Med 1989;7:639–43.

Sing RF et al: Rapid sequence induction for intubation by an aeromedical transport team: a critical analysis. Am J Emerg Med 1998;16:598.

Sumida MP et al: Prehospital blood transfusion versus crystalloid alone in the air medical transport of trauma patients. Air Med J 2000;19:104.

EDUCATION & TRAINING

Crew Composition Decisions

Once the mission profile of the transport program has been specified, decisions must be made concerning the qualifications of the personnel. The mission profile may also dictate the qualifications of the medical director.

Physicians: On- & Off-Line

In addition to their duties in off-line medical control (supervising training, development of medical protocols and standing orders, quality assurance), physicians must be available on-line 24 hours a day (by cellular phone or radio) to help manage critical situations. Most on-line medical control is provided by emergency physicians. These individuals have experience conveying instruction by radio to paramedics, are immediately available 24 hours a day, and are familiar with radio equipment and the rules and regulations covering their use. Occasionally, on-line medical direction may be obtained through an ICU or from a neonatologist at a tertiary care facility.

Crew Qualifications

Training modules for all transporting personnel should be developed in such a way that their training is consistent with the policies and practices of the receiving facility. The facilities and the crew should be subjected to ongoing curriculum development and quality assurance by the medical director.

A. The Emergency Medical Technician

Emergency medical technicians (EMTs) have completed a course of training outlined by the DOT and are usually required to recertify every 2–4 years. EMTs are taught first aid and basic rescue skills in programs composed of 100–150 contact hours. EMTs receive training in the basic management of trauma, medical, pediatric, obstetric, and psychiatric emergencies. Many EMTs are proficient in the use of automatic external defibrillators. EMTs know basic noninvasive airway techniques. Generally, EMTs do not have training in cardiac rhythm recognition, intravenous access, drug administration, or invasive procedures.

B. The Paramedic

Paramedics have completed a course curriculum outlined by the DOT and are usually required to pass a state licensing examination and to seek recertification every 2 or 4 years. Most United States paramedics obtain initial certification by taking a nationally recognized testing program. In the United States, paramedic training programs vary from 1000 to 3000 contact hours. Paramedics have knowledge of all emergency situations, including the acute management of trauma and of cardiac arrhythmias. Under state or regional guidelines, they can usually perform defibrillation and are able to recognize and treat lethal dysrhythmias. They are trained in endotracheal intubation and cricothyrotomy, interosseous lines, needle thoracostomy, and transthoracic cardiac pacing, though not all of these skills are sanctioned for performance by paramedics in all states. Paramedic training corresponds to what is required for Aeromedical Crew Level 2 personnel by the American College of Surgeons.

C. The Critical Care Transport RN

Some schools for flight nursing have been developed, along with a generally recognized curriculum. In addition to other nursing skills, transport nurses should be trained to perform endotracheal intubation, needle thoracostomy, and cricothyrotomy and to insert and maintain interosseous lines and central venous lines. They are also expected to be familiar with the operation of transport ventilators and, if the mission profile includes intra-aortic balloon pumping, the management of a balloon pump (though many programs utilize pump technicians for this function). They should have knowledge of the critical care management of obstetric, neonatal, pediatric, and burn patients as well as cardiac, central nervous system, and psychiatric patient management. Transport teams involved in aerospace medicine should have knowledge about altitude physiology, aircraft safety, aviation communications, and emergency aeromedical procedures such as crash response and survival. Training guidelines have been developed and are in concert with the suggestions outlined in the ACS publication cited below.

Adams K et al: Comparison of intubation skills between interfacility transport team members. Pediatr Emerg Care 2000;16:5.

Committee on Trauma: *Resources for Optimal Care Of The Injured Patient.* American College of Surgeons, 1990.

Jones AE et al: A national survey of the air medical transport of high-risk obstetric patients. Air Med J 2001;20:17.

Wright AE, Campos JA, Gorder T: The effect of an in-flight, emergency training program on crew confidence. Air Med J 1994;13:127.

REIMBURSEMENT STANDARDS & COSTS

Standards

Any medical interfacility aero-ground transport vehicle will have to be licensed by the designating agency as a transferring ambulance. Ambulance licensing varies considerably from state to state but may depend upon minimal equipment requirements, staffing availability, staff licensing, and record keeping. Non-public sector aeromedical programs are required also to comply with Federal Aviation Administration regulations with respect to equipment, qualification, and hours of pilot duty. If transport vehicles cross state lines, the program may require licensing of both staff and vehicle in neighboring states unless an interstate agreement has been reached covering medical practice and emergency response contingencies. Voluntary standards have been developed by the Society of Aeromedical Systems, and an accreditation track is available.

Reimbursement

For hospital-based transport teams involving ground ambulances, the sponsoring facilities often support the medical crew and contract with an ambulance company for the ambulances, drivers, and in some cases the services of paramedical personnel. Ground ambulance services may be covered by third-party insurers. A medical necessity form is usually required justifying the transfer before payment is made.

Helicopter programs usually lease the helicopter together with pilots, support mechanics, and a backup for service during scheduled or unscheduled maintenance procedures. Hospital support is provided by the medical crew. Most programs bill third-party payers for the transport service. Both fixed-wing and helicopter rates and reimbursement vary widely nationally, and most continue to require support by sponsoring institutions in order to maintain financial viability. Charges and reimbursements are variable–and, indeed, charge structure may vary from one program to another because the medical costs such as crew salaries and equipment may be part of the hospital's or the flight program's cost base. Third-party payer reimbursement also varies nationally and usually requires utilization review. Medicare traditionally reimburses for transport only to the closest medical facility capable of managing the patient, and this policy may not be congruent with the emergency medical services plan for the state or region. Medicare reimbursement is made by a prospective payment system similar to what is used for hospital ambulatory care billing.

Schneider C: Counting the cost. Emergency 1989 (Nov): 39–43.

CURRENT CONTROVERSIES & UNRESOLVED ISSUES

The beneficial and cost-effective use of air transport continues to be studied. With regard to intermediate transport distances of about 50 miles (80.5 km), data are conflicting with regard to the benefit of air transport versus ground transport. Generally, rural areas must rely on air transport systems because of travel distances. In urban areas, a large number of variables determine the risks and benefits of a particular mode of transport.

The use of opioid analgesia during transport of the critically ill has been reviewed in descriptive reports. The judicious use of opioid agents seems to be supported by current practice and literature. Recommendations are for use of short acting agents with close monitoring of hemodynamic parameters and respiratory status. When opioids are used during transport, naloxone or other appropriate reversal agents should be readily available.

Chemical restraint for combative or agitated patients has been reported to be appropriate, particularly during air transport. Benzodiazepines are most commonly used. As with opioid analgesic use, patients must be closely monitored when chemical restraint is used.

Whether parents should be accommodated as passengers during transport of pediatric patients is another area of controversy, with most reports supporting the practice when space is available. Potential parent anxiety or agitation can result in crew distraction and must be considered as a potential risk in individual cases.

Although critical care transport is a common practice, truly comparative studies that address controversial practices are not yet available. Because of the nature of transport and the large number of variables to consider in transport research, most of the literature published is qualitative and descriptive. Qualitative research methods are appropriate for addressing many of the issues of critical care transport and should be done in conformity with proper research design techniques.

DeVellis P et al: Prehospital fentanyl analgesia in air-transported pediatric trauma patients. Pediatr Emerg Care 1998;14:321.

DeVillis P, Thomas SH, Wedel SK: Prehospital and emergency department analgesia for air-transported patients with fractures. Prehosp Emerg Care 1998;2:293.

Lewis MM, Holditch-Davis D, Brunssen S: Parents as passengers during pediatric transport. Air Med J 1997;16:38.

McMullan P et al: The use of chemical restraint in helicopter transport. Air Med J 1999;18:136.

Ethical & Legal Considerations 10

Paul A. Selecky, MD

Advances in modern medicine have increased the ability of the physician and the health care team to prolong life by utilizing a wide variety of life support modalities, including medications, mechanical devices, and the transplantation of vital organs. Despite their scientific success, these treatments can prolong life of a quality that in many cases is not meaningful or rewarding to the patient. The result has been that the physician and the health care team must sometimes help their patients make decisions about whether to withhold or withdraw life support medications or mechanical devices—and sometimes whether even to withhold basic life support measures such as nutrition and hydration.

Life support decision making in the intensive care unit often presents ethical or legal dilemmas that must be resolved by staff and patients and the patients' families or surrogates. This chapter will attempt to review the basic principles that form the ethical framework of the modern practice of medicine. The purpose of this discussion will not be to erect standards of practice or give legal advice but to offer a system for applying ethical principles in the effort to avoid or resolve conflicts. These principles are also applied in the light of the health care worker's personal and professional values, institutional policies and statutory mandates, and the published statements of professional bodies.

ETHICAL PRINCIPLES

The principles of medical ethics are rooted in religious and philosophical traditions, which include the absolute values of good and evil, right and wrong, and that human life is of infinite worth and sanctity. Ethics is the system of principles by which these beliefs govern our behavior and our interaction with others. The application of these beliefs may therefore change over time to adapt to the needs of society, but the boundaries of the absolute values are maintained.

Four basic ethical principles flowing from these absolute values strongly influence the practice of medicine, particularly in critical care medicine. The first is **beneficence,** which directs the physician and health care worker to do good, specifically by restoring health and relieving suffering. This has been a fundamental goal of medical practice since the time of Hippocrates in the fourth century BC, but it is not the only goal.

The ethical companion of beneficence is **nonmaleficence,** compelling health care workers *first of all* to do no harm ("primum non nocere"). Nonmaleficence is not merely a corollary of beneficence, since these two principles must sometimes be in conflict. For example, it is considered ethically justified to administer morphine to relieve pain (beneficence) in the terminally ill patient even though the morphine might increase the risk of death, an act which may violate the principle of nonmaleficence.

The third ethical principle is **autonomy,** which dictates that any legally competent adult patient who has been appropriately informed has the right to accept or refuse medical treatment, including life support measures—ie, the right of self-determination. This does not include the right to commit suicide or to require a physician to assist in suicide or perform euthanasia. Although Oregon legalized physician-assisted suicide under limited circumstances in 1997, physicians' participation remains voluntary. The physician and the health care team have a mandate to preserve patient autonomy, however, by being honest and truthful in providing clinical information to the patient in order to obtain informed consent to treatment. Table 10–1 lists the patient's rights adopted by the American Hospital Association. The Joint Commission on Accreditation of Healthcare Organizations (JCAHO) has drawn up a similar list of patient rights.

The fourth ethical principle is **justice,** dictating that individuals be treated fairly in relation to other patients and the overall distribution of medical resources. When medical resources are limited, this principle states that treatment should be administered to patients who are most likely to benefit from them. The overriding consideration for the physician is an obligation to care for the individual patient at hand. Thus, ethicists have argued that physicians involve themselves in the process of providing medical care to society in general but not use arguments about limited resources in making decisions about an individual patient.

CONFLICTS BETWEEN ETHICAL PRINCIPLES

The practice of medicine often generates conflicts among these fundamental principles. Efforts have been made to prioritize them, often putting autonomy first as the most important ethical guideline, but the matter

Table 10–1. A Patient's Bill of Rights.[1]

The patient has a right to—
Considerate and respectful care
Information about diagnosis, treatment, and prognosis
Make decisions about treatment
Have an advance directive
Consideration of privacy
Expect confidentiality
Review medical records
Request medical services
Be informed about health care business practices
Consent or decline to participate in research
Expect reasonable continuity of care
Be informed of hospital policies on patient care, including resources for conflict resolution

[1]With permission from the American Hospital Association.

is controversial. Nonetheless, the physician and health care team are required to address any conflicts among these principles in the light of the circumstances presented in each individual case.

Patient autonomy must be preserved, but the physician may sometimes find that the patient's wishes are in conflict with the physician's own professional, personal, or religious values. In these situations, the patient's wishes take precedence, while the physician attempts to transfer the responsibility for the patient's care to another physician.

Medical Futility

A conflict also may arise if the physician feels that the therapy requested by the patient is medically futile—particularly if it is a life support measure. A method of treatment is judged to be futile if reason and experience indicate that it would be highly unlikely to result in meaningful survival. One need not conclude that success of the treatment is impossible—it is enough to decide that a good result would be highly unlikely, eg, one proposed working definition of futility is no successful outcomes in the last 100 reported or observed attempts of that treatment. The physician is best qualified to judge whether the treatment is medically futile, but only the patient can decide whether continued survival would be personally acceptable. An example might be the decision whether or not to initiate ventilatory support for a patient with severe progressive chronic lung disease. Ideally, the treatment goals of the physician and the patient should be identical and consensually derived.

The current consensus among ethicists holds that the physician has no ethical obligation to provide life-sustaining treatment he or she considers to be futile but does have the responsibility to inform the patient of the reasons for that opinion. If the patient requests the treatment nonetheless, the physician is required to take measures necessary to transfer the patient's care to another physician or institution that would follow the patient's wishes. At the same time, all other care that is both medically indicated and agreed to by the patient must be continued.

ETHICAL DECISION-MAKING

Assessing Decision-Making Capacity

Medical decisions made in the ICU are governed by the principle of patient autonomy, but the patient's illness may have significantly diminished his or her decision-making capacity. This capacity is generally defined as the patient's ability to (1) receive and understand pertinent information, (2) reflect on this information in an appropriate way, and (3) communicate decisions and desires to the caregivers.

Surrogate Decision-Makers

When this decision-making capacity is diminished or lost, a surrogate decision-maker can be sought. Ideally, this will be an individual previously so designated by the patient in a written advance directive. Alternatively, it may be an appropriate family member in an order of authority and responsibility identified by local institutional or legal guidelines. A common hierarchy progresses from the patient's spouse to an adult child, then to a parent, then to an adult sibling, and then to a grandparent. Rarely, a court-appointed individual (conservator) undertakes this role.

In the absence of specific decisions about health care previously made by the patient, the surrogate is obliged to act in the patient's best interests, weighing the potential benefits and burdens of treatment—ie, applying the concept of proportionality. The surrogate should ideally therefore be someone who (1) is willing to accept these duties; (2) understands and accepts the personal values of the patient; (3) has no major emotional opposition to fulfilling the role; and (4) has no conflict of interest.

For circumstances when an appropriate surrogate decision-maker cannot be identified (eg, "patient John Doe"), the health care institution should have a mechanism in place for naming someone to act in the patient's best interests. Such a mechanism should be governed by factors such as local medical practice, legal precedents, and institutional policies. Consultation might be sought from an appropriate resource, such as a bioethicist or a hospital health care ethics committee.

Although rarely necessary, a legal decision can be sought from the courts, such as in situations in which (1) the state of the patient's decision-making capacity is in doubt, or (2) the surrogate decision-maker cannot make or refuses to make the decision, or (3) the health care team feels that the surrogate's decision is not in the patient's best interests, or (4) the surrogate's decision is contrary to the patient's advance directive.

Shared Decision Making

Decision making in the ICU should be a shared responsibility between the physician and the patient or surrogate decision maker. The physician should avoid making independent paternalistic medical decisions for the patient involving life support measures even though doing so might seem to be in the patient's best interests. The physician is singularly qualified to determine the medical futility of a specific treatment, but only the patient or surrogate decision-maker can decide quality-of-life issues, ie, whether prolongation of life would be meaningful and valuable to the patient. The physician should seek input from other members of the patient's health care team, including nurses and other care providers.

ADVANCE DIRECTIVES

In an attempt to support the fundamental ethical principle of patient autonomy, legislation has been enacted to facilitate the process by which the patient's wishes may be carried out when he or she is no longer able to make decisions—ie, the patient gives the physician and health care team advance notice of what he or she wants to be done or not done. Federal legislation requires hospitals and skilled nursing facilities that receive Medicare or Medicaid funding to inform all patients of their right to complete such an advance directive. These documents exist in most states, but the legal requirements and implications vary in different jurisdictions.

The **living will** is the most common document by which the patient may request or refuse life-sustaining treatment if he or she becomes terminally ill and no longer able to make medical decisions or becomes permanently unconscious. These documents are not legally binding in all states but serve as guides for the physician and surrogate decision-maker. A legally binding natural death declaration can include the decision to forgo basic life support measures of artificially administered nutrition and hydration.

The **Advance Health Care Directive** appoints a health care agent ("attorney-in-fact") to act in the patient's best interests when the patient can no longer do so. Such an advance directive is most helpful when the patient has expressed his or her wishes in writing in some detail rather than merely using general terms such as "no heroic measures." Ideally, individuals executing these directives should discuss their intentions, beliefs, and value systems with their health care agent, family, and physician, in addition to completing the advance directive document. It is also important that these wishes and the directive be reviewed on a regular basis, particularly each time the patient is hospitalized.

MEDICOLEGAL ASPECTS OF DECISION-MAKING

Critical care practices have been influenced by court actions that were pursued to resolve ethical conflicts regarding individual patients. While the actions are not legally binding outside those jurisdictions, they are used as legal precedents to guide behavior and to aid in arriving at future court decisions.

A number of cases have strengthened the ethical principle of patient autonomy and have helped to clarify the role of the surrogate decision-maker in exercising the process of "substituted judgment" when acting for the patient. For example, in 1976 the New Jersey Supreme Court allowed the family of Karen Quinlan to withdraw her from mechanical ventilation because it agreed with her parents that this treatment would not allow her to return to a cognitive and sapient life but would merely keep her in a persistent vegetative state. Similarly, legal decisions surrounding the care of Nancy Cruzan in Missouri in 1990 ultimately acknowledged that her parents as surrogate decision-makers, based on past comments the patient had made, could refuse life-sustaining treatment, including nutrition and hydration.

Patient autonomy was further strengthened by the legal determination in 1991 concerning the care of Helga Wanglie, who was in a persistent vegetative state on a ventilator in Minneapolis. The hospital had requested permission from her husband to discontinue life support treatment based on the medical decision that Ms Wanglie had no chance for recovery, ie, that the treatment was futile. Her husband refused, deciding that based on her religious beliefs, Ms Wanglie would have wished to continue living. The court affirmed Mr Wanglie's decision and refused to appoint an independent conservator to replace him as decision-maker.

These precedents reaffirm the principle of patient autonomy, but ethical conflicts nonetheless remain, particularly for individuals who stress the principle of justice and the fair allocation of medical resources.

WITHHOLDING & WITHDRAWING LIFE SUPPORT

Based on the ethical principles discussed in the preceding paragraphs, the patient or the surrogate decision-maker can request that life support treatments be withheld or withdrawn. Current judgment does not distinguish an ethical or legal difference between the act of withholding and the act of withdrawing life support measures. Nevertheless, the patient, the family, and the health care team may find it more difficult to withdraw life support than to withhold it. In addition, Orthodox Jewish tradition does not permit the withdrawing of life support measures, including nutrition or hydration, feeling that this would be equivalent to suicide. There is usually less concern about the more passive act of withholding treatment.

Decisions to withhold or withdraw treatment are best made in advance of a life-threatening situation, allowing the patient and family to consider the potential outcome of life support measures. This is particularly important in patients who are terminally ill or who have an illness that is severe and irreversible.

"Do Not Resuscitate" (DNR) Orders

In the event of cardiac or respiratory arrest in a hospitalized patient, cardiopulmonary resuscitation (CPR) is initiated automatically. In some cases, it may be desired to forgo CPR, in which case a "do not resuscitate" order is written. This decision is made jointly by the patient (or surrogate) and the physician, but either party may initiate discussion about the decision. In general, physicians should initiate discussions about CPR and DNR—ideally, before the patient becomes critically ill and before the disease progresses to a life-threatening stage despite optimal therapy.

The physician should choose an appropriate setting for this discussion with the patient and family, allowing ample time for discussion. The DNR order should be presented in a positive light, emphasizing the continuation of supportive care, relief of physical suffering such as pain and dyspnea, and support for emotional suffering. It should be made clear that such a decision does not mean that the health care team is "giving up" but that the focus of therapy is altered, emphasizing comfort while avoiding futile or unnecessary treatment.

When the outcome is bleak, the discussion should focus not only on whether CPR should be initiated but also on whether life support measures should be withheld or withdrawn. The "do not resuscitate" decision does not, by itself, imply any decisions about other medical care, including ICU admission, surgery, or other treatment. Thus, if the patient's outcome is likely to be poor, offering CPR may give the patient and family false hope about the likelihood of a good outcome. A better approach is to discuss whether to withhold or withdraw life support measures when a crisis develops if such measures are judged to be futile. The treatment plan thus should be presented in an atmosphere that will allow the patient, family, and health care team to "hope for the best but prepare for the worst."

There may be situations in which a physician recommends that a DNR order be written but the patient or family disagrees and wishes CPR to be initiated at the time of cardiac or respiratory arrest. In this situation, several steps can be taken. First, the physician and patient (or surrogate) should continue the discussion, with clarification about the reasons for each person's decision, misconceptions about CPR, and the continuation or discontinuation of other medical care. Second, the AMA Council on Ethical and Judicial Affairs has decided that a physician who determines that CPR may be futile may initiate a DNR order against the patient's wishes. In this situation, the patient must be informed of the decision and its reasons. Third, in the event of disagreement, the patient should be transferred to the care of another physician able to reconcile the wishes of the patient with his or her own medical judgment.

Once the decision for a DNR order is made by the patient or physician, institutional policies and procedures should govern how such an order should be written in order to avoid miscommunication. Major points of the discussion with the patient and family should be documented in the medical record, including who participated, the decision-making capacity of the patient, the medical diagnosis and prognosis, and the reasons for the DNR decision.

Withholding or Withdrawing Treatment

A. A Stepwise Approach

Decisions to withhold or withdraw life support treatment must not be made hastily. Several steps are recommended: (1) The physician should have a clear understanding of the patient's diagnosis, physiologic and functional status, and any coexisting morbid states. (2) The physician should seek unanimity among the health care team for the decision to withhold or withdraw life support measures. (3) The next step is to seek informed consent from a legally competent patient. If the patient is not legally competent, the surrogate decision-maker must be contacted. It is wise to include the family and the patient's referring or primary care physician in the process, though the patient or the surrogate decision-maker holds responsibility for the ultimate decision. (4) If a decision cannot be made in a timely fashion and life support measures are imminently required, the physician might consider recommending a limited trial of the life support measure—eg, ventilatory support for the next 72 hours, with reassessment at that time. In the absence of a firm decision, life support measures should be initiated or continued.

Physicians and other health care workers may fear that their actions in withholding or withdrawing life support may subject them to litigation or even criminal prosecution. While no one is immune from criticism or challenge, health care workers who act thoughtfully and rationally, with concern for the patient and in the open company of their peers, should not fear legal retribution.

B. Establishing a Treatment Plan

Once a decision has been made to withhold life support measures, a specific treatment plan should be formulated with emphasis on providing comfort and support and continually adjusting the plan to meet the changing needs of the patient. A DNR order should not automatically preclude care for a patient in the intensive care unit. All efforts should be made to avoid giving the patient and family a feeling of abandonment. Forgoing treatment does not mean forgoing care. It may be helpful to involve the services of a medical social worker or chaplain to make certain that the patient and family receive appropriate emotional support and attention to their physical comfort.

C. Withdrawing Life Support

When a decision to withdraw life support measures has been made, the order should be executed in a timely manner, paying close attention to the emotional needs of the patient and family.

After the life support measure is discontinued—eg, disconnecting the patient from mechanical ventilation—the family should be allowed access to the patient to the extent possible, and attention should be given to their emotional and physical needs. If the dying process is prolonged, the patient may be transferred to a separate room for more privacy. Medications appropriate to control pain, dyspnea, and other symptoms should be administered liberally. Nursing care and physician attention should be as diligent as before the decision was made. The primary training and practice of critical care clinicians is to prevent and treat life-threatening medical crises, but they must also be prepared to administer to the dying patient and his or her family.

ORGAN DONATION

Organ transplantation has progressed rapidly in recent years and now offers hope to patients who would otherwise die because of failure of a vital organ. One of the limiting factors, however, is the short supply of donor organs from individuals who have suffered irreversible cessation of brain stem function.

In order to establish the diagnosis of brain death, a physician who has no conflict of interest must verify by appropriate clinical evaluation that the patient has suffered irreversible cessation of all brain function. Such a diagnosis must be made in the absence of hypothermia, drug effect, or metabolic intoxication that can temporarily suppress the central nervous system. It must also be made with caution in patients in shock, because reduced brain perfusion may make the examination unreliable.

Because of the possibility that some patients may become candidates for organ donation, physicians and health care professionals in the intensive care unit should be aware of the processes by which donations can be made. Some patients may have already disclosed in an advance directive that they wish to donate body organs or tissues under these circumstances. Otherwise, authorization for such organ donation must be obtained from the surrogate decision-maker or appropriate family member unless the religious beliefs of the patient preclude such donation (eg, Christian Science, Orthodox Judaism, Jehovah's Witnesses).

Organ donation is a sensitive issue that health care providers are often reluctant to raise, particularly at a time when the potential donor patient's family is suffering the impending loss of their loved one. It is therefore necessary to discuss these issues in a sensitive and timely manner once the family has accepted the irreversibility of the brain damage. Legislation in some states requires that such a discussion take place. In the absence of any known family members or other appropriate surrogate decision-maker, the institution may be permitted to arrange a donation in accordance with statutory guidelines. It is important that all health care personnel be familiar with the policies and procedures for organ donation in order to identify potential transplant donors.

ROLE OF THE HEALTH CARE PROFESSIONAL

Education

All health care professionals who work in the critical care setting should be intimately familiar with the ethical and legal principles that influence their medical decision-making. A number of professional bodies have published position statements on the ethical implications of critical care, and some of these resources are listed in the references at the end of this chapter. Copies of these statements should be readily available to critical care personnel. Skilled legal resources should also be available.

Discussions with patients concerning life support measures are potentially within the purview of all health care workers, so that this education should be offered to the entire medical staff and all hospital medical personnel. The patient's primary physician should ideally initiate discussion about advance directives and decisions concerning treatment long before a crisis occurs. Such discussions can be encouraged through public education and by taking advantage of opportunities to document decisions such as when preparing wills and other estate planning instruments.

Communication Skills

In addition to possessing knowledge about the ethics of critical care medicine, health care workers should be skilled in communicating these principles and their conflicts to patients and families as well as among the health care team. The physician traditionally assumes the role of the leader of that team, but critical care nurses and respiratory care practitioners often develop close relationships with patients and their families as well and can aid in the process.

Communication is aided by allowing ample time for discussing these issues in an appropriate setting—ideally, long before a critical decision must be made. This would allow general discussion of such sensitive issues as whether to initiate or withhold cardiopulmonary resuscitation or other life support measures and other decisions about which the patient may wish to express a preference.

Medical institutions should establish mechanisms by which ethical conflicts can be satisfactorily resolved. This might include the availability of ethics consultations, patient care conferences, and resources such as patient advocates, medical social workers, and the hospital's retained legal advisers or others who are knowledgeable about critical care and ethical issues.

Development of Institutional Policies

Institutional policies and procedures should be drafted to aid the health care worker in responding to ethical issues in the critical care arena and other areas of the hospital. A number of such policies are listed in Table 10–2. They are designed as much to prevent ethical conflicts as to aid in resolving them. Guidelines for formulating these policies may be found in the references listed below. Some state hospital associations are also a resource for such policies.

Table 10–2. Institutional policies to help prevent or resolve ethical conflicts in critical care.

Intensive Care Unit admission and discharge criteria
Methods for resolving ethical conflicts
Do Not Resuscitate orders
Guidelines for withholding and withdrawing life support
Care of the dying patient
Definition of and procedure for determining brain death
Requesting organ or tissue donation
Organizational ethics

REFERENCES

ACCP/SCCM Consensus Panel. Bone RC et al: Ethical and moral guidelines for the initiation, continuation, and withdrawal of intensive care. Chest 1990;97:949–58.

AMA Council on Ethical and Judicial Affairs: Guidelines for the appropriate use of do-not-resuscitate orders. JAMA 1991; 265:1868–71.

AMA Council on Scientific Affairs and Council on Ethical and Judicial Affairs: Persistent vegetative state and the decision to withdraw or withhold life support. JAMA 1990;263:426–30.

American Academy of Neurology: Guidelines on the vegetative state. Commentary on the American Academy of Neurology statement, and position of the American Academy of Neurology on certain aspects of the care and management of the persistent vegetative state. Neurology 1989;39:123–6.

American College of Physicians: Ethics Manual. Fourth Edition. Ann Intern Med 1998;128:576–94.

American Hospital Association: *A Patient's Bill of Rights.* American Hospital Association, 1992.

American Thoracic Society: Withholding and withdrawing life-sustaining therapy. Am Rev Respir Dis 1991;144:727–32.

American Thoracic Society Bioethics Task Force: Fair allocation of intensive care unit resources. Am J Respir Crit Care Med 1997;156:1282–1301.

Anderson GR, Glesnes-Anderson VA (editors): *Health Care Ethics: A Guide for Decision Makers.* Aspen Publishers, 1987.

Asch DA, Hansen-Flaschen J, Lanken PN: Decisions to limit or continue life-sustaining treatment by critical care physicians in the United States: conflicts between physicians' practices and patients' wishes. Am J Respir Crit Care Med 1995;151(2 Pt 1):288–92.

Brock DW, Wartman SA: When competent patients make irrational choices. N Engl J Med 1990;322:1595–9.

Brody H et al: Withdrawing intensive life-sustaining treatment—recommendations for compassionate clinical management. N Engl J Med 1997;336:652–7.

Dunn PM et al: Medical ethics: an annotated bibliography. Ann Intern Med 1994;121:627–32.

Etchells E et al: Bioethics for clinicians: 3. Capacity. CMAJ 1996;155:657–61.

Faber-Langendoen K, Lanken PN: Dying patients in the intensive care unit: forgoing treatment, maintaining care. Ann Intern Med 2000;133(11):886–93.

Ganzini L et al: Physicians' experiences with the Oregon Death with Dignity Act. N Engl J Med 2000;342:557–63.

Goold SD, William B, Arnold RM: Conflicts regarding decisions to limit treatment: A differential diagnosis. JAMA 2000; 283:909–14.

Hofmann JC et al: Patient preferences for communication with physicians about end-of-life decisions. Ann Intern Med 1997;127:1–12.

Holmquist M et al: A critical pathway: guiding care for organ donors. Crit Care Nurse 1999;19:84–98. (Many other articles on organ donation, pages 21–83.)

Joint Commission on Accreditation of Healthcare Organizations (JCAHO): Patient rights. In: *Comprehensive Accreditation Manual for Hospitals.* Vol 1: *Standards.* JCAHO, 2000.

Jonsen AR, Siegler M, Winslade WJ: *Clinical Ethics: A Practical Approach to Ethical Decisions in Clinical Medicine,* 2nd ed. Macmillan, 1986.

Leonard CT, Doyle RL, Raffin TA: Do-not-resuscitate orders in the face of patient and family opposition. Crit Care Med 1999;27:1045–7.

Levin PD, Sprung CL: Are ethics consultations worthwhile? Crit Care Med 2000;28:3942–4.

Levy MM, Carlet JM (editors): Compassionate end-of-life care in the intensive care unit. Crit Care Med 2001;29:N1–N61.

Luce JM, Alpers A: Legal aspects of withholding and withdrawing life support from critically ill patients in the United States and providing palliative care to them. Am J Respir Crit Care Med 2000;162:2020–32.

Meisel A, Kuszewski M: Legal and ethical myths about informed consent. Arch Intern Med 1996;156:2521–6.

Meisel A, Snyder L, Quill T and the ACP-ASIM End-of-life Care Consensus Panel: Seven legal barriers to end-of-life care. JAMA 2000;284:2495–2501.

NIH Workshop Summary: Withholding and withdrawing mechanical ventilation. Am Rev Respir Dis 1986;134:1327–30.

Prendergast TJ, Luce JM: Increasing incidence of withholding and withdrawal of life support from the critically ill. Am J Respir Crit Care Med 1997;155:15–20.

Quill TE, Byock IR: Responding to intractable terminal suffering: the role of terminal sedation and voluntary refusal of food and fluids. ACP-ASIM End-of-life Care Consensus Panel. Ann Intern Med 2000;132:408–14.

Quill TE, Dresser R, Brock DW: The rule of double effect—a critique of its role in end-of-life decision making. N Engl Med 1997;337:1768–71.

Raffin TA: Ethical issues in respiratory care. In: *Foundations of Respiratory Care.* Pierson DJ, Kacmarek RM (editors). Churchill Livingstone, 1992.

Razek T, Olthoff K, Reilly PM: Issues in potential organ donor management. Surg Clin North Am 2000;80:1021–32.

Rivin AU: Futile care policy: lessons learned from three years' experience in a community hospital. West J Med 1997;166:389–93.

Ruark JE, Raffin TA, and Stanford University Medical Center Committee on Ethics: Initiating and withdrawing life support: Principles and practice in adult medicine. N Engl J Med 1988;318:25–30.

Rubenfeld GD, Curtis JR: State-of-the-art conference on palliative respiratory care. Part 1. Respir Care 2000;45:1318–1410. Part 2: 1460–1540.

Schneiderman LJ, Gilmer T, Teetzel HD: Impact of ethics consultations in the intensive care setting: a randomized, controlled trial. Crit Care Med 2000;28:3920–4.

Schneiderman LJ, Jecker NS, Jonsen AR: Medical futility: Its meaning and ethical implications. Ann Intern Med 1990;112:949–54.

Silverman HJ, Vinicky JK, Gasner MR: Advance directives: Implications for critical care. Crit Care Med 1992;20:1027–31.

Smedira NG et al: Withholding and withdrawal of life support from the critically ill. N Engl J Med 1990;322:309–15.

Snider GL: The do-not-resuscitate order: Ethical and legal imperative or medical decision? Am Rev Respir Dis 1991;143:665–74.

Snyder L, Caplan AL: Assisted suicide: finding common ground. Ann Intern Med 2000;132:468–9.

Sullivan AD, Hedberg K, Fleming DW: Legalized physician-assisted suicide in Oregon—the second year. N Engl J Med 2000;342:598–604.

Sulmasy DP et al: The accuracy of substituted judgments in patients with terminal diagnoses. Ann Intern Med 1998;128:621–9.

Tulsky JA et al: Opening the black box: how do physicians communicate about advance directives? Ann Intern Med 1998;129:441–9.

Wilson WC et al: Ordering and administration of sedatives and analgesics during the withholding and withdrawal of life support from critically ill patients. JAMA 1992;267:949–53.

WEB SITES FOR HEALTH CARE ETHICS INFORMATION & POLICIES

American Medical Association: http://www.ama-assn.org

Canadian Medical Association Bioethics for the Clinician Online: http://www.cma.ca/cmaj/series/bioethic.htm

The Hastings Center for Bioethics: http://www.thehastingscenter.org

Institute of Medicine. Non-heart-beating organ transplantation: practice and protocols (2000): http://books.nap.edu/catalog/9700.html

Medical College of Wisconsin Center for the Study of Ethics: http://www.mcw.edu/bioethics

University of Pennsylvania Center for Bioethics. American Journal of Bioethics Online: http://ajobobline.com

University of Pittsburgh Consortium Ethics Program: http://www.pitt.edu/~cep

University of Toronto Joint Center for Bioethics: http://www.utoronto.ca/jcb

University of Washington School of Medicine Ethics in Medicine: http://eduserv.hscer.washington.edu/bioethics

University of Wisconsin Biomedical Ethics: http://www.uwc.edu/fonddulac/faculty/rrigteri/biomed.htm

Shock & Resuscitation

11

Frederic S. Bongard, MD

The diagnosis and management of shock are among the most common challenges the intensivist must deal with. Shock may be broadly grouped into three pathophysiologic categories: (1) hypovolemic, (2) distributive, and (3) cardiac. Failure of end-organ cellular metabolism is a feature of all three. Hemodynamic patterns vary greatly and constitute the diagnostic features of the three types of shock.

HYPOVOLEMIC SHOCK

ESSENTIALS OF DIAGNOSIS

- *Tachycardia and hypotension.*
- *Cool and frequently cyanotic extremities.*
- *Collapsed neck veins.*
- *Oliguria or anuria.*
- *Rapid correction of signs with volume infusion.*

General Considerations

Hypovolemic shock occurs as a result of decreased circulating blood volume. The most common cause is trauma resulting in either external hemorrhage or concealed hemorrhage from blunt or penetrating injury. Hypovolemic shock may occur also as a result of sequestration of fluid within the abdominal viscera or peritoneal cavity.

The severity of hypovolemic shock depends not only upon the volume deficit but also upon the age and premorbid status of the patient. The rate at which the volume was lost is a critical factor in the compensatory response. Volume loss over extended periods, even in older, more severely compromised patients, is better tolerated than rapid loss. Clinically, hypovolemic shock is classified as mild, moderate, or severe depending upon the blood volume lost (Table 11–1). While these classifications are useful generalizations, the severity of preexisting disease may create a critical situation in a patient with only minimal hypovolemia.

Hypovolemic shock produces compensatory responses in virtually all organ systems.

A. Cardiovascular Effects

The cardiovascular system responds to volume loss through homeostatic mechanisms for maintenance of cardiac output and blood pressure. The two primary responses are increased heart rate and peripheral vasoconstriction, both mediated by the sympathetic nervous system. The neuroendocrine response, which produces high levels of angiotensin and vasopressin, enhances the sympathetic effects. Adrenergic discharge results in constriction of large capacitance venules and small veins, which reduces the capacitance of the venous circuit. Because up to 60% of the circulating blood volume resides in the venous reservoir, this action displaces blood toward the heart to increase diastolic filling and stroke volume. It is probable that venular constriction is the single most important circulatory compensatory mechanism in hypovolemic shock.

Precapillary sphincter and arteriolar vasoconstriction results in redirection of blood flow. The greatest decrease occurs in the visceral and splanchnic circuits. Flow to bowel and liver decreases early in experimental shock. Intestinal perfusion is depressed out of proportion to reductions in cardiac output. Reduction in flow to the kidneys accounts for the decline in glomerular filtration and urine output, while decreased skin flow is responsible for the cutaneous coolness associated with hypovolemia. The cutaneous vasoconstrictive response diverts flow to critical organs and has the further effect of reducing heat loss through the skin. The reduced diameter of the small, high-resistance vessels increases the velocity of flow and decreases the viscosity of blood as it reaches the ischemic vascular beds, thus permitting more efficient microcirculatory flow.

Increased flow velocity in the microcirculation may have the additional benefit of improving oxygen delivery while reducing tissue acidosis. A countercurrent exchange mechanism has been postulated in which oxygen diffuses from arterioles into adjacent venules. Normally, the amount of arterial oxygen lost by this mechanism is small. However, as flow decreases through dilated arterioles, more oxygen can leave the slowly flowing arterial

Table 11–1. Pathophysiology and clinical features of hypovolemia.[1]

	Pathophysiology	Clinical Features
Mild (< 20% of blood volume)	Decreased perfusion of organs that are able to tolerate ischemia (skin, fat, skeletal muscle, bone). Redistribution of blood flow to critical organs.	Subjective complaints of feeling cold. Postural changes in blood pressure and pulse. Pale, cool, clammy skin. Flat neck veins. Concentrated urine.
Moderate (deficit = 20–40% of blood volume)	Decreased perfusion of organs that withstand ischemia poorly (pancreas, spleen, kidneys).	Subjective complaint of thirst. Blood pressure is lower than normal in the supine position. Oliguria.
Severe (deficit > 40% of blood volume)	Decreased perfusion of brain and heart.	Patient is restless, agitated, confused, and often obtunded. Low blood pressure with a weak and often thready pulse. Tachypnea may be present. If allowed to progress, cardiac arrest results.

[1]From Holcroft JW, Wisner DH: Shock and acute pulmonary failure in surgical patients. In: Current Surgical Diagnosis and Treatment, 9th ed. Way LW (editor). Originally published by Appleton & Lange. Copyright © 1991 by the McGraw-Hill Companies, Inc.

blood and diffuse to the venous circuit. Arteriolar constriction increases flow velocity and decreases blood residence time. This effectively reduces the peripheral oxygen shunt. In a similar fashion, CO_2 diffuses from the postcapillary venules into the arterioles. In the absence of arteriolar vasoconstriction, such diffusion could increase the volume of CO_2 reaching the tissues and result in worsening of tissue acidosis.

The balance of fluid shifts between the intravascular and extravascular spaces is governed by Starling's law, which relates net transvascular flux to differences in hydrostatic and osmotic pressure:

$$\dot{Q} = K[(P_c - P_i) - \sigma(\Pi_c - \Pi_i)]$$

where Q is fluid flux, $(P_c - P_i)$ is the hydrostatic pressure gradient, $(P_c - P_i)$ is the osmotic pressure gradient, K is the permeability coefficient, and σ is the reflection coefficient.

Under normal circumstances, intravascular hydrostatic pressure (P_c) is greater than interstitial hydrostatic pressure (P_i), and fluid tends to move from the capillaries into the interstitium. Interstitial osmotic pressure (P_i) is usually less than the intravascular osmotic pressure (P_c), favoring the movement of fluid back into the capillary. This results in a small net movement of water, Na^+, and K^+ out of the capillaries. When hypovolemia occurs, intravascular pressure falls, facilitating the movement of fluid and electrolytes from the interstitium back into the vascular space. The degree of this translocation is limited, because as fluid moves back into the capillaries, the albumin remaining in the interstitium exerts an increased extravascular osmotic pressure. Compensatory vasoconstriction facilitates this process because fluid can be recovered more easily if the vascular space is collapsed than if it is dilated. The degree of such translocation is probably limited to a total of 1–2 L. This vascular refill accounts not only for the decrease in intravascular osmotic pressure; it is also primarily responsible for the decline in hematocrit observed in hypovolemic patients before resuscitation is started.

Increased heart rate and contractility are important homeostatic responses to hypovolemia. Both the direct adrenergic response and the epinephrine secreted by the adrenal medulla are responsible for these reflexes. Cardiac output is the product of heart rate and stroke volume. It is supported both by tachycardia and by translocated fluid. Because blood pressure is the product of systemic vascular resistance and cardiac output, peripheral vasoconstriction is an essential factor in supporting blood pressure.

B. Metabolic Effects

Tissue metabolic pathways require ATP as an energy source. Normally, ATP is produced through the Krebs cycle via the aerobic metabolism of glucose. Six molecules of oxygen are consumed when six molecules of glucose are used to convert six molecules of ADP into six molecules of ATP, CO_2, and water. When oxygen is not available, ATP is generated through anaerobic glycolysis, which not only yields smaller quantities of ATP for the amount of glucose consumed but also produces lactic acid. This latter product is largely responsible for the acidosis of ischemia. The point at which tissues change from aerobic to anaerobic metabolism is defined as the anaerobic threshold. This theoretic point varies between tissues and clinical situations. Recent work indicates that lactic acidosis may be a useful marker to detect the anaerobic threshold. The most important factor influencing the conversion to anaerobic glycolysis is oxygen availability.

The delivery of oxygen is dependent upon the quantity of oxygen present in the blood and the cardiac output. The former, defined as the oxygen content, is calculated as follows:

$$Ca = 1.34 \times Hb \times Sao_2 + (0.0031 \times Pao_2)$$

where CaO_2 is arterial oxygen content (in mL/dL), Hb is hemoglobin concentration (in g/dL), SaO_2 is hemoglobin saturation of arterial blood (in percent), and PaO_2 is partial pressure of dissolved oxygen in arterial blood (in mm Hg).

The principal determinants of oxygen content are the concentration of hemoglobin and its saturation. Although PaO_2 is the most commonly used indicator of oxygenation, the dissolved oxygen component contributes only minimally to oxygen content in patients with normal hemoglobin concentration and saturation. When anemia is profound, the relative contribution of dissolved oxygen increases. Systemic oxygen delivery is defined as shown below:

$$Do_2 = Cao_2 \times CO \times 10$$

where DO_2 is systemic oxygen delivery (in mL/min), CaO_2 is arterial oxygen content (in mL/dL), and CO is cardiac output (in L/min).

Normally, DO_2 is in excess of 1000 mL/min. When cardiac output falls with hypovolemic shock, DO_2 declines as well. The extent depends not only upon the cardiac output but also upon the fall in hemoglobin concentration. As oxygen delivery declines, most organs increase their extraction of oxygen from the blood they receive and return relatively desaturated blood to the venous circuit. Systemic oxygen consumption is calculated by rearranging Fick's equation:

$$\dot{V}o_2 = (a-v)Do_2 \times CO \times 10$$

Systemic oxygen consumption is typically 200–260 mL O_2/min for a 70 kg patient under baseline conditions. The arteriovenous oxygen content difference—(a–v)DO_2—is approximately 5 ± 1 mL/dL under these conditions. With hypovolemia, increased peripheral oxygen extraction increases the (a–v)DO_2 to values typically greater than 7 mL/dL. The oxygen extraction ratio (O_2ER), which is defined as $\dot{V}O_2/DO_2$, is also augmented. Increased (a–v)DO_2 and O_2ER are metabolic hallmarks of hypovolemic shock.

Tissues vary greatly in their ability to increase oxygen extraction. The normal extraction ratio is near 0.3 and may increase to as much as 0.8 in conditioned athletes. The heart and brain maximally extract oxygen under normal circumstances, making them extremely flow-dependent. Peripheral oxygen consumption ($\dot{V}O_2$) remains essentially constant during hypovolemia until a critical threshold is reached, at which point increased extraction can no longer keep pace with delivery. There is conflicting evidence about whether oxygen consumption decreases in the face of reduced oxygen delivery in humans. This so-called pathologic supply dependence may, however, occur in patients with distributive shock and with ARDS.

C. Neuroendocrine Effects

Adrenergic discharge and the secretion of vasopressin and angiotensin are neuroendocrine compensatory mechanisms which together produce vasoconstriction, translocation of fluid from the interstitium into the vascular space, and maintenance of cardiac output. A number of other humoral responses have been described as well.

1. Secretion of aldosterone and vasopressin—Together, these hormones increase renal retention of salt and water to assist in maintaining circulating blood volume.

2. Secretion of epinephrine, cortisol, and glucagon—These hormones increase the extracellular concentration of glucose and make energy stores available for cellular metabolism. Fat mobilization is increased. Serum insulin levels are decreased.

3. Endorphins—Although their exact role is unclear, these endogenously occurring opioids are known to decrease pain. They promote deep breathing, which might increase venous return by decreasing intrathoracic vascular resistance. Endorphins have a vasodilatory effect and may actually counteract the sympathetic influence.

D. Immunologic Effects

Hypovolemic shock initiates a series of inflammatory responses that may have deleterious effects. Stimulation of circulating and fixed macrophages induces the production and release of tumor necrosis factor (TNF), which in turn leads to production of neutrophils, inflammation, and activation of the clotting cascade. Neutrophils are known to release free oxygen radicals, lysosomal enzymes, and leukotrienes C_4 and D_4. These mediators may disrupt the integrity of the vascular endothelium and result in vascular leaks into the interstitial space. Activated complement and products of the arachidonic acid pathway serve to augment these responses.

Adhesion molecules are glycoproteins that cause leukocyte recruitment and migration after hemorrhagic shock. The most frequently involved cell adhesion molecules are the selectins, integrins, and immunoglobulins. Although the roles of the adhesion molecules are still under investigation, some authorities have reported a correlation between the severity of injury and the release of soluble cell adhesion molecules (SCAMs). Others have also noted a relationship between the development of multiple organ failure and the expression of SCAMs.

The feasibility of using monoclonal antibodies to SCAMs—as well as pathway blockade—is under study.

Oxygen metabolites, including superoxide anions, hydrogen peroxide, and hydroxyl free radicals, are produced when oxygen is incompletely reduced to water. These radical intermediates are extremely toxic because of their effects on lipid bilayers, intracellular enzymes, structural proteins, nucleic acids, and carbohydrates. Phagocytes normally generate oxygen radicals to assist in killing ingested material. Antioxidants protect surrounding tissue if these compounds leak from the phagocytes. Ischemia, followed by reperfusion, has been shown to accelerate the production of toxic oxygen metabolites independently of the activity of inflammatory cells. This ischemia-reperfusion syndrome may lead to extensive destruction of surrounding tissue and may play a significant role in determining the ultimate outcome of an episode of hypovolemic shock.

Animal experiments have identified a number of other potentially important immunologic responses to hypovolemia, including failure of antigen presentation by Kupffer cells in the liver and translocation of bacteria from the gut into the systemic circulation. This latter mechanism may explain the occurrence of sepsis after hypotension without other sources of infection.

E. Renal Effects

Blood flow to the kidneys decreases quickly with hypovolemic shock. The decline in afferent flow causes glomerular filtration pressure to fall below the critical level required for filtration into Bowman's capsule. The kidney has a high metabolic rate and requires substantial blood flow to maintain its metabolism. Therefore, sustained hypotension may result in tubular necrosis.

F. Hematologic Effects

When hypovolemia is due to loss of fluid volume without loss of red blood cells, which occurs with emesis, diarrhea, or burns, the intravascular space becomes concentrated, with increased viscosity. This sludging may lead to microvascular thrombosis with ischemia of the distal bed.

G. Neurologic Effects

Sympathetic stimulation does not cause significant vasoconstriction of the cerebral vessels. Autoregulation of the brain's blood supply keeps flow constant as long as arterial pressure does not decrease to less than 70 mm Hg. Below this level, consciousness may be lost rapidly, followed by decline in autonomic function.

H. Gastrointestinal Effects

Hypotension causes a decrease in splanchnic blood flow. Animal models have shown a rapid decrease in gut tissue oxygen tension which may lead to the ischemia-reperfusion syndrome or to translocation of intestinal bacteria. Increased concentrations of xanthine oxidase occur within the mucosa and may also be responsible for bacterial translocation. Pentoxifylline has aroused recent interest as a potential agent for increasing intestinal microvascular blood flow after periods of ischemia.

Clinical Features

A. Symptoms and Signs

The findings associated with hypovolemic shock vary with the age of the patient, the premorbid condition, the extent of volume loss, and the time period over which such losses occur. The physical findings associated with different degrees of volume loss are summarized in Table 11–1. Heart rate and blood pressure measurements are not always reliable indicators of the extent of hypovolemia. Younger patients can easily compensate for moderate volume loss by vasoconstriction and only minimal increases in heart rate. Furthermore, severe hypovolemia can result in bradycardia as a preterminal event. Orthostatic blood pressure testing is often helpful. Normally, transition from the supine to the sitting position will decrease blood pressure by less than 10 mm Hg in a healthy person. When hypovolemia is present, the decline is greater than 10 mm Hg, and the pressure does not return to normal within several minutes. Older patients who present with apparently normal blood pressures while supine often become hypotensive when brought to an upright position. Such testing must be used with caution in patients who have sustained multiple injuries because potentially unstable vertebral injuries may be present.

Decreased capillary refilling, coolness of the skin, pallor, and collapse of cutaneous veins are all associated with decreased perfusion. The extent of each depends upon the severity of the underlying shock. These findings are not specific to hypovolemic shock and may occur with cardiac shock or shock from pericardial tamponade or tension pneumothorax. Collapsed jugular veins are commonly found in hypovolemic shock, though they may also occur with cardiac compression in a patient who is not adequately fluid-resuscitated. Examination of the jugular veins is best performed with the patient's head elevated to 30 degrees. A normal right atrial pressure will distend the neck veins approximately 4 cm above the manubrium.

Urine output is usually markedly decreased in patients with hypovolemic shock. **Oliguria** in adults is defined as urine output less than 0.5 mL/kg/h. If oliguria is not present in the face of clinical shock, the urine should be examined for the presence of osmotically active substances such as glucose and radiographic dyes.

B. Laboratory Findings

Laboratory studies may be useful in determining the cause of hypotension. However, resuscitation of a patient in shock should never be withheld pending the results of laboratory determinations.

The hematocrit of a patient in hypovolemic shock may be low, normal, or high depending on the cause and duration of shock. When blood loss has occurred, evaluation prior to capillary refill by interstitial fluid will yield a normal hematocrit. On the other hand, if the patient has bled slowly, if recognition is delayed, or if fluid resuscitation has been instituted, the hematocrit will be low. When hypovolemia results from loss of nonsanguineous fluid (emesis, diarrhea, fistulas), the hematocrit is usually high.

Lactic acid accumulates in patients with shock that is severe enough to cause anaerobic metabolism.

Other nonspecific findings include decreased serum bicarbonate and a minimally increased white blood cell count.

C. Hemodynamic Monitoring

Assessment of central venous pressure is seldom required to make the diagnosis of hypovolemic shock. Because the decreased volume allows venous collapse, insertion of central venous monitoring catheters can be particularly hazardous. If the patient's blood pressure and mental status do not respond to fluid administration, a continued source of bleeding should be suspected. Central venous pressure monitoring may be useful in older patients with a known or suspected history of congestive heart failure because excessive fluid administration may rapidly result in pulmonary edema. In extreme cases, a pulmonary artery flotation catheter may be required to optimize fluid status.

Capnographic monitoring will reflect a decrease in end-tidal CO_2. This is produced by a decrease in blood flow to the lungs. When compared with arterial blood gases, a widening of the arterial-end tidal CO_2 gradient is apparent. If pulmonary function is normal, only minimal changes in arterial hemoglobin saturation will be present. Hence, pulse oximetry indicates normal saturation.

Differential Diagnosis

Shock due to hypovolemia may be confused with shock due to other causes (Table 11–2). Cardiac shock produces signs similar to those found with hypovolemia with the exception that neck veins are usually distended. Absence of such distention may be due to inadequate fluid resuscitation. Central venous pressure monitoring will help make the differentiation. Following trauma, peripheral vasodilation due to spinal cord injury may produce shock that is relatively resistant to fluid administration. Hypovolemia is the primary cause of shock in trauma victims, and it should never be assumed that other causes are responsible until fluid in adequate amounts has been administered.

Alcoholic intoxication may make the diagnosis of hypovolemia difficult. Serum ethanol elevation causes the skin to be warm, flushed, and dry. The patient usually makes dilute urine. These patients may be hypotensive when supine, with exaggerated postural blood pres-

Table 11–2. Clinical findings associated with shock.[1]

	Cardiogenic Shock	Cardiac Compressive Shock	Hypovolemic or Traumatic Shock			Low-Output Septic Shock	High-Output Septic Shock	Neurogenic Shock
			Mild	Moderate	Severe			
Skin perfusion	Pale	Pale	Pale	Pale	Pale	Pale	Pink	Pink
Urine output	Low	Low	Normal	Low	Low	Low	Low	Low
Pulse rate	High	High	Normal	Normal	High	High	High	Low
Mental status	Anxious	Anxious	Normal	Thirsty	Anxious	Anxious	Anxious	Anxious
Neck veins	Distended	Distended	Flat	Flat	Flat	Flat	Flat	Flat
Oxygen consumption	Low	Low	Low	Low	Low	Low	Low	Low
Cardiac index	Low	Low	Low	Low	Low	Low	High	Low
Cardiac filling pressures	High	High	Low	Low	Low	Low	Low	Low
Systemic vascular resistance	High	High	High	High	High	High	Low	Low

[1]From Holcroft J, Robinson MK: Shock: Identification and management of shock states. In: *Care of the Surgical Patient.* Scientific American, 1992.

sure changes. Hypoglycemic shock due to excessive insulin administration is not uncommon in critical care units. The patients are cold, clammy, oliguric, and tachycardiac. A history of recent insulin administration should arouse suspicion of hypoglycemic shock. After samples have been taken for blood glucose determinations, intravenous administration of 50 mL of 50% glucose should improve the situation.

Treatment

A. General Principles

Unlike acute posttraumatic situations, resuscitation of patients with hypovolemic shock in the ICU typically proceeds from a more controlled baseline. As in any emergent situation, the priorities of airway, breathing, and circulation must be addressed sequentially. Although many ICU patients will already have an established airway, attention to this area of concern is always the first priority. Techniques to control the airway and reestablish adequate breathing are discussed in Chapter 11.

Intravenous access through at least two large-bore (16-gauge) intravenous catheters is mandatory. The relatively small ports on pulmonary artery and triple-lumen catheters are inadequate for rapid fluid resuscitation and should be used only until larger catheters can be put in place. Central venous catheters should never be placed in hypovolemic patients for emergent resuscitation.

A quick search should be made for sources of blood and fluid loss. Potential sources include gastrointestinal bleeding, accelerated fluid loss through fistulas, disconnection of intravenous access lines with retrograde bleeding, and disruption of vascular suture lines. When external bleeding is present, direct pressure over the site should be applied until definitive surgical control can be secured. Blind probing of a bleeding wound with clamps almost invariably fails to control the bleeding and may cause further injury.

B. Fluid Resuscitation

Rapid fluid resuscitation is the cornerstone of therapy for hypovolemic shock. Fluid should be infused at a rate sufficient to rapidly correct the deficit. In younger patients, infusion is typically at the maximum rate sustainable by the delivery equipment and the access vein. In older patients or those with prior cardiac disease, infusion should be slowed once a response is detected to prevent complications associated with hypervolemia.

Parenteral solutions for the intravenous resuscitation of hypovolemic shock are generally classified as crystalloids or colloids depending upon the highest molecular weight of the species they contain.

1. Crystalloids—Crystalloid solutions have no species with a molecular weight greater than 6000. Although a large number of crystalloids are available, only those isotonic with human plasma that have sodium as their principle osmotically active particle should be used for resuscitation. Commonly available solutions are listed in Table 11–3. Because they have low viscosity, crystalloids can be administered rapidly through peripheral veins.

Because isotonic fluids have the same osmolality as body fluids, there are no net osmotic forces tending to move water into or out of the intracellular compartment. Therefore, the electrolytes and water partition themselves in a manner similar to the body's extracellular water content: 75% extravascular and 25% intravascular. When isotonic crystalloids are used for resuscitation, administration of approximately three to four times the vascular deficit is required to account for the distribution between the intra- and extravascular spaces. This partitioning typically occurs within 30 minutes after the fluid is given. Within 2 hours, less than 20% of the infused fluid remains within the intravascular space.

Crystalloid solutions are safe and effective for resuscitation of patients in hypovolemic shock. The major complications associated with their use are undertreatment and overtreatment. Because defined endpoints for resuscitation are lacking, clinical parameters such as restoration of urine output, decreased heart rate, and increased blood pressure should be used to determine when a sufficient quantity of fluid has been given. Restoration of mental status, skin turgor, and capillary refill are also useful parameters. Central venous or pulmonary artery pressure monitoring is useful in patients with preexisting cardiopulmonary disease.

Excessive administration of crystalloids is associated with generalized edema. Unless quantities sufficient to increase the pulmonary hydrostatic pressure to very high levels are given (typically > 25–30 mm Hg), pulmonary edema does not occur. Subcutaneous edema may be a significant problem because it limits patient mobility, increases the potential for decubitus ulcers, and potentially restricts respiratory excursions.

The choice of the specific crystalloid for resuscitation is largely a matter of individual preference. Normal saline has the advantages of being universally available and being the only crystalloid that can be mixed with blood. Because its chloride concentration is significantly higher than that of plasma, patients resuscitated with normal saline often develop a fixed hyperchloremic metabolic acidosis, which requires renal chloride excretion for correction. Lactated Ringer's solution has the advantage of a more physiologic electrolyte composition. The added lactate is converted to bicarbonate in the liver. Such conversion occurs readily in all but the sickest of patients.

Hypertonic saline solutions are crystalloids that contain sodium in supraphysiologic concentrations. They

Table 11–3. Composition of balanced salt solutions.[1]

Solutions	Glucose (g/L)	Na^+	Cl^-	NCO_3^-	K^+	Ca^{2+}	Mg^{2+}	HPO_4^-	NH_4^+
		(meq/L)							
Extracellular fluid	1000	140	102	27	4.2	5	3	3	0.3
5% dextrose and water	50								
10% dextrose and water	100								
0.9% sodium chloride (normal saline)		154	154						
0.45% sodium chloride (0.5 normal saline)		77	77						
0.21% sodium chloride (0.25 normal saline)		34	34						
3% sodium chloride (hypertonic saline)		513	513						
Lactated Ringer's solution		130	109	28[2]	4	2.7			
0.9% ammonium chloride		168							168

[1]From Miller TA, Duke JH: Fluid and electrolyte management. In: *Manual of Preoperative and Postoperative Care.* Dudrick SJ et al (editors). Saunders, 1983.
[2]Present in solution as lactate but is metabolized to bicarbonate.

expand the extracellular space by exerting an osmotic effect that displaces water from the intracellular compartment. They may also exert a mild positive inotropic effect as well as producing systemic and pulmonary vasodilation. In comparison with isotonic crystalloids, hypertonic saline decreases wound and peripheral edema. Recent studies have indicated, however, that hypertonic saline resuscitation may increase the incidence of bleeding. Animal models indicate that this may be due to decreased ADP-mediated platelet aggregation.

2. Colloids—As a group, colloids are solutions that rely on high-molecular-weight species for their osmotic effect. Because the barrier between the intra- and extravascular spaces is only partially permeable to the passage of these molecules, colloids tend to remain in the intravascular space for longer periods than do crystalloids. Smaller quantities of colloids are required to restore circulating blood volume. Because of their oncotic pressure, colloids tend to draw fluid from the extravascular to the intravascular space. They are significantly more expensive to use than crystalloids even though smaller absolute volumes are required.

a. Albumin—Albumin (normal serum albumin) is the most commonly used colloid. It has a molecular weight of 66,000–69,000 and is available as a 5% or 25% solution. Normal serum albumin is approximately 96% albumin, while plasma protein fraction is 83% albumin. Each gram of albumin can hold 18 mL of fluid in the intravascular space. The serum half-life of exogenous albumin is less than 8 hours, though less than 10% leaves the vascular space within 2 hours after administration. When 25% albumin is administered, it results in increased intravascular volume approaching five times the administered quantity.

Like crystalloid infusion, the end points for the administration of colloid to patients in hypovolemic shock are largely subjective. Because albumin has been implicated as a cause of decreased pulmonary function, strict attention to resuscitation endpoints is required. Other reported complications include depressed myocardial function, decreased serum calcium concentration, and coagulation abnormalities. The latter two may be due simply to volume effects.

b. Hetastarch—Hetastarch (hydroxyethyl starch) is a synthetic product available as a 6% solution dissolved in normal saline. It has an average molecular weight of 69,000. Forty-six percent of an administered dose is excreted by the kidneys within 2 days, and 64% is eliminated within 8 days. Detectable starch concentrations may be found 42 days after infusion. Hetastarch is an effective volume expander, with effects that typically last between 3 and 24 hours. Intravascular volume increases by more than the volume infused. Most patients respond to between 500 and 1000 mL. Renal, hepatic, and pulmonary complications may occur when dosing exceeds 20 mL/kg/d.

Hetastarch may cause a decreased platelet count and prolongation of the partial thromboplastin time due to its anti-factor VIII effect. Anaphylaxis is rare. A combination product containing 6% hetastarch in a balanced salt solution is now available. Because it may cause inhibition of factor VIII, its use for large-volume resuscitation requires further review. When used, it is typically administered at doses of 500–1000 mL.

A similar five-carbon preparation (pentastarch) is currently available only for leukapheresis but is also a useful volume expander. It may have fewer effects on the coagulation cascade than does hetastarch.

c. **Dextrans**—Two forms of dextran are generally available: dextran 70 (90% of molecules have MW 25,000–125,000) and dextran 40 (90% have MW 10,000–80,000). Both may be used as volume expanders. The extent and duration of expansion are related to the type of dextran used, the quantity infused, the rate of administration, and the rate of clearance from the plasma. The lower-molecular-weight molecules are filtered by the kidney and produce diuresis; the heavier ones are metabolized to CO_2 and water. The higher-MW dextrans remain in the intravascular space longer than do the lighter compounds. Dextran 70 is preferred for volume expansion because it has a half-life of several days. A 10% solution of dextran 40 has a greater colloid oncotic pressure than the 70% solution but is cleared from the plasma rapidly.

Several complications are associated with dextran administration, including renal failure, anaphylaxis, and bleeding. Dextran 40 is filtered by the kidney and may result in an osmotic diuresis that actually decreases plasma volume. It should be avoided in patients with known renal dysfunction. Dextran 70 has infrequently been associated with renal failure. Anaphylactic reactions occur in patients with high anti-dextran antibody titers. The incidence of reactions is between 0.03% and 5%.

Both dextrans inhibit platelet adhesion and aggregation probably via factor VIIIR:ag activity. The clinical effect is similar to von Willebrand's disease. The effect is greater with dextran 70 than with dextran 40. Both preparations may interfere with serum glucose determinations and blood cross matching.

d. **Other colloids**—Modified fluid gelatin (MFG) and urea-bridged gelatins are prepared as 3.5% and 4% solutions in normal saline, respectively. Both are effective plasma volume expanders. Their low molecular weight leads to rapid renal excretion. Anaphylactoid reactions (0.15%) are the most common complication. Rapid infusion of the urea-bridged formulation causes histamine release from mast cells and basophils. The incidence of allergic reactions is less for modified fluid gelatin. Gelatins may cause depression of serum fibronectin. They are not associated with renal failure and do not interfere with blood banking techniques. These preparations are used widely in Europe and in the military for mass casualties. They are currently unavailable in the United States.

Oxygen-carrying solutions such as stroma-free hemoglobin and perfluorocarbons are the subjects of active research. At present, however, they are available only for limited use and in clinical trials.

Current Controversies & Unresolved Issues

A. Crystalloids Versus Colloids

The relative advantages of crystalloid and colloid solutions for fluid resuscitation have long been debated. The advantages of crystalloids are that they are readily available, inexpensive and do not cause allergic reactions. Proponents of colloids claim that more efficient resuscitation is possible with lower volumes and that decreased peripheral edema is advantageous. At present, however, there is no clear advantage to the use of colloid-containing solutions.

B. Ischemia-Reperfusion

Ischemia-reperfusion is an area of critical investigation. Clarification of the mechanism of oxygen radical tissue destruction with tissue reperfusion may help prevent some of the complications of ischemia. A number of compounds including diltiazem, amiloride, and pentoxifylline have been explored in an effort to improve cardiac, peripheral vascular, and renal function after reperfusion.

C. End Points

The end points of resuscitation are parameters such as blood pressure, heart rate, and urine output. Tissue-specific monitors such as tissue oxygen tension (TPo_2) and intramucosal pH (pH_i) have received recent attention as objective indices. Because of the time required for pH_i sample collection, it is unlikely to become a clinically useful tool for resuscitation. It may, however, be valuable for monitoring patients after they have stabilized. Tissue oxygen measurements use several modalities, including electrodes and fluorescence-quenching optodes. The latter has proved to be a reliable indicator of oxygen tension in the subcutaneous and visceral tissues during shock and resuscitation. Its clinical usefulness remains to be demonstrated.

D. Bacterial Translocation

The anomalous appearance of sepsis in patients who develop hypovolemic shock has raised the question of intestinal bacterial translocation. This theory proposes that ischemia of the intestinal mucosa allows luminal bacteria to pass through or between cells and into the portal venous system. The mechanism has been clearly demonstrated in animals, but definitive evidence in humans is lacking. Elucidation of this mechanism may provide information on the prevention of sepsis in this setting.

Cross JS et al: Hypertonic saline fluid therapy following surgery: A prospective study: J Trauma 1988;29:817–25.

Dawidson I: Fluid resuscitation of shock. Current controversies. Crit Care Med 1989;17:1078–80.

Emerson TE: Unique features of albumin - a brief review. Crit Care Med 1989;17:690–4.

Gastinne H et al: A controlled trial in intensive care units of selective decontamination of the digestive tract with nonabsorbable antibiotics. N Engl J Med 1992;326:594–9.

Griffel MI, Kaufman BS: Pharmacology of colloids and crystalloids. Crit Care Clin 1992;8:235–53.

Holcroft JW, Robinson MK: Shock: Identification and management of shock states. In: *Care of the Surgical Patient.* Scientific American, 1992.

Holcroft JW, Trunkey DD: Extravascular lung water following hemorrhagic shock in the baboon: Comparison between resuscitation with Ringer's lactate and Plasmanate. Ann Surg 1974;180:408–17.

Krausz MM et al: Hypertonic saline treatment of uncontrolled hemorrhagic shock at different periods from bleeding. Ann Surg 1992;127:93–6.

Lowell JA et al: Postoperative fluid overload: Not a benign problem. Crit Care Med 1990;18:728–33.

Martinez-Mier G, Toledo-Pereyra LH, Ward PA: Adhesion molecules and hemorrhagic shock. J Trauma 2001;51:408–15.

Mazzoni MC et al: Amiloride-sensitive Na^+ pathways in capillary endothelial cell swelling during hemorrhagic shock. J Appl Physiol 1992;73:1467–73.

Morales J et al: The effects of ischemia and ischemia-reperfusion on bacterial translocation, lipid peroxidation, and gut histology: studies on hemorrhagic shock in pigs. J Trauma 1992;33:221–6.

Wang P et al: Diltiazem restores cardiac output and improves renal function after hemorrhagic shock and crystalloid resuscitation. Am J Physiol 1992;262:435–40.

Zikria BA et al: A biophysical approach to capillary permeability. Surgery 1989;105:625–31.

DISTRIBUTIVE SHOCK

Distributive shock is so named because of the redistribution of blood flow to the viscera. The three types of distributive shock commonly treated in intensive care units are septic, anaphylactic, and neurogenic shock.

SEPTIC SHOCK

ESSENTIALS OF DIAGNOSIS

- *Increased cardiac output in the face of decreased blood pressure.*
- *Decreased peripheral oxygen consumption.*
- *Decreased systemic vascular resistance.*
- *Decreased ventricular ejection fraction.*
- *Associated multiple system organ failure.*

General Considerations

The incidence of septic shock has been increasing in the United States over the past several years. Approximately 100,000–300,000 people develop bacteremia each year, and one-half of these cases progress to septic shock. The overall mortality rate from septic shock is between 40% and 60%. Higher death rates occur in the aged and in those with compromised immune status as a result of trauma, diabetes, malignancy, burns, cirrhosis, or treatment with antitumor chemotherapeutic agents. Aerobic gram-negative bacillary infections are the most common cause. The predominant organisms are *Escherichia coli* and klebsiella. Gram-positive organisms such as staphylococci and fungi may also cause septic shock.

A. Pathogenesis

It is unlikely that bacteria per se are responsible for septic shock. Rather, interactions between their products and normal host defenses probably elicit the usual reactions. Gram-negative organisms have complex walls composed of lipopolysaccharides and proteins. Endotoxin is a lipopolysaccharide component of the outer membrane. It is composed of oligosaccharide side chains, a core polysaccharide, and lipid A. The chemical and physical structure of the latter is highly conserved between different bacterial species and is highly antigenic. In both animal and human studies it has been shown that infusion of lipid A causes many of the same effects observed in clinical sepsis. Endotoxin has effects on multiple regulatory systems, including complement, kinins, coagulation, plasma phospholipases, cytokines, β-endorphins, leukotrienes, platelet-activating factor, and prostaglandins.

Cytokines are a group of proteins produced by white blood cells in response to a number of stimulating factors. Although multiple cytokines have been identified, those known to be involved in the human septic response are TNF and interleukins-1, -2, and -6. These agents are likely to have both beneficial and deleterious effects. Increased levels of TNF, IL-1, and IL-6 have been correlated with a poor outcome. TNF produces hypotension and decreased ventricular function in animal studies. The cytokines are known to induce the release of counterregulatory hormones such as glucagon, epinephrine, and cortisol, which are necessary to support the response to sepsis. Cytokines responsible for modulation of the immune response include IL-4, IL-6,

IL-10, IL-11, IL-13, and IL-1 Ra (receptor antagonist). Compounds responsible for amplification of the immune response include IL-8, IL-12, IL-18, platelet activating factor, serotonin, and the eicosanoids.

Circulating endotoxin induces the production of a number of white blood cell products that arise from the release of arachidonic acid from leukocyte cell membranes mediated by phospholipase A_2. The mobilized arachidonic acid can then follow one of two pathways: conversion to leukotrienes via the lipoxygenase pathway or creation of prostaglandins and thromboxanes via the cyclooxygenase pathway (Figure 11–1). The lipoxygenase and cyclooxygenase compounds have distinct actions (Table 11–4). Phospholipase A_2 also releases membrane-bound alkyl phospholipids that may be converted into platelet-activating factor (PAF), the most potent lipid mediator known. The actions of PAF include activation of phagocytes as well as of platelets, production of oxygen-free radicals, increase of vascular permeability, and decrease of cardiac output and blood pressure. Cells known to produce PAF include neutrophils, basophils, endothelial cells, and platelets.

Several plasma proteases are activated in septic shock. These include the kinin system, the clotting cascade, and the complement system. Endotoxin and gram-positive bacteria both activate the complement cascade via the extrinsic pathway. The effects of complement activation include (1) increased vascular permeability, (2) release of toxic oxygen metabolites by activated phagocytes, and (3) increased opsonization and phagocytosis by neutrophils and macrophages. It is likely that the increased vascular permeability so produced plays an important role in the hemodynamic picture characteristic of septic shock. A correlation has been demonstrated between increased concentration of activated complement and mortality rates. Concomitant activation of Hageman factor (XIIa) may be responsible for the disseminated intravascular coagulopathy associated with sepsis. Factor XIIa may also lead to the conversion of prekallikrein to kallikrein and ultimately to the release of bradykinin, which causes severe hypotension.

Recent interest has focused on the roles of toxic oxygen metabolites and nitric oxide. Activated phagocytes

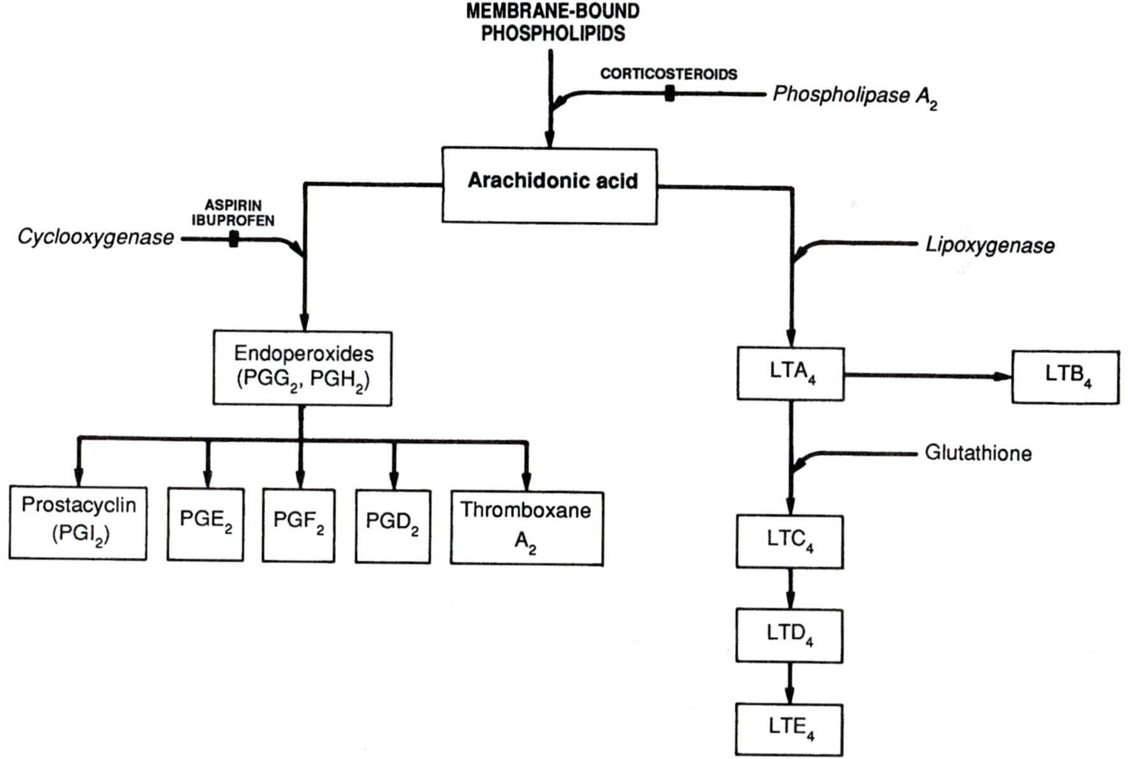

Figure 11–1. Pathways of arachidonic acid. (Adapted from Holcroft J, Robinson MK: Shock: Identification and management of shock states. In: *Care of the Surgical Patient.* Scientific American, 1992.)

Table 11–4. Actions of arachidoinic acid mediators.

Mediator	Actions
Prostacyclin (PGI_2)	Vasodilation Decreased platelet aggregation
PGE_2	Vasodilation Immunomodulation Platelet aggregation
PGF_2	Vasodilation
PGD_2	Vasodilation
Thromboxane A_2	Vasoconstriction Increased platelet aggregation
LTB_4	Chemotaxis Leukocyte-endothelial cell adhesion
LTC_4	Immunomodulation Vasoconstriction Bronchoconstriction Increased vascular permeability
LTD_4	Vasoconstriction Bronchoconstriction Increased vascular permeability
LTE_4	Vasoconstriction Bronchoconstriction Increased vascular permeability

produce oxygen radicals that kill ingested bacteria. When these products leak from the cell, they may cause severe tissue damage. Endothelium-derived relaxing factor (EDRF) is another toxic free radical species. Chemically, it is nitric oxide (NO). While small quantities of nitric oxide may improve blood flow in the microcirculation, higher concentrations produce vasodilation and hypotension. Nitric oxide may arise from several cell lines, including neutrophils, the vascular endothelium, and Kupffer cells. Nitric oxide synthetase is induced by both endotoxin and TNF. It produces nitric oxide from L-arginine.

B. Hemodynamic Effects

The distinguishing hemodynamic features of septic shock are elevated cardiac output, decreased systemic vascular resistance, and decreased blood pressure. Tachycardia is partially responsible for maintaining the blood pressure. Earlier investigators described hyperdynamic and hypodynamic phases of septic shock. More recent investigations have shown, however, that cardiac output remains elevated until decreased output develops as a preterminal event. It is likely that the earlier observations were made in patients who were inadequately fluid-resuscitated.

Right and left ventricular ejection fractions are decreased in septic shock, as is left ventricular stroke work. In contrast to hypovolemic shock, increasing preload by administering volume only minimally increases left ventricular stroke work. This may be due to altered compliance characteristics of the ventricles. Pulmonary artery hypertension, which frequently develops early, may also be partially responsible for right ventricular dysfunction. Cardiac adrenergic down-regulation also occurs. The number of receptors and their affinities are reduced. Patients who recover from septic shock increase their left ventricular stroke work index, whereas those who succumb do not. Radionuclide scans have shown that left ventricular dilation occurs within 1–2 days after the onset of shock. This increased end-diastolic volume permits a greater stroke volume in the face of decreased ejection fraction. Left ventricular dilation improves as patients recover. In spite of the ventricular abnormalities, the coronary circulation exhibits above-normal flow, normal myocardial oxygen consumption, and net myocardial lactate extraction.

The myocardial depressant factor (MDF) of sepsis has been characterized as a low-molecular-weight protein (< 1000). Patients with cardiac disease and sepsis without shock fail to exhibit such activity. MDF may originate from the intestinal tract in patients with hypovolemic shock. The cytokines and endotoxin have been suspected as the origin of MDF. However, TNF has a molecular weight of 17,000. Lipopolysaccharide, IL-1, and IL-2 in high concentrations fail to duplicate the effect of MDF. The decrease in circulating plasma volume due to increased capillary permeability is a major influence in the hemodynamic pathophysiology of sepsis. In addition to actual transudation of fluid from the intravascular into the interstitial space, peripheral pooling, hepatosplanchnic venous pooling, and gastrointestinal and wound losses–along with idiopathic polyuria–also reduce cardiac preload.

Changes in the pattern of blood flow distribution are characteristic of septic shock. It was once thought that shunting of blood through cutaneous arteriovenous pathways was responsible for decreased peripheral oxygen extraction, but the anatomic presence of such shunts has not been demonstrated. Rather, it is likely that a mismatching of blood flow and metabolic demand occurs. Thus, some organs receive supranormal oxygen delivery, whereas others are rendered ischemic. This is of particular importance in the splanchnic circulation, where hepatic venous desaturation has been reported in septic patients. Oxygen extraction is also affected, resulting in flow-dependent oxygen consumption. A normal or elevated mixed venous oxygen saturation and decreased arterial-venous oxygen content difference is present. Lactic acidosis may indicate the presence of pathologic oxygen delivery-dependent consumption. It is unlikely that oxygen utilization is limited by mitochondrial dysfunction.

C. Metabolic Abnormalities

The extent of the metabolic response to sepsis is dependent not only upon the duration and severity of the illness but also upon the premorbid nutritional and immunologic status. Even though systemic oxygen consumption is decreased, the metabolic rate in sepsis is markedly elevated. Mixed fuels serve as the energy source, with an increase in the respiratory quotient (RQ) to between 0.78 and 0.82. Hepatic glucose production is markedly increased, with lactate and alanine serving as the major gluconeogenic precursors. Hyperglycemia is common, as is insulin resistance. The elaboration of catechols in response to the cytokines induces lipolysis, although ketosis is reduced as a result of decreased hepatic production. Hypertriglyceridemia may occur as a result of increased hepatic synthesis and decreased lipoprotein lipase activity. Protein turnover is greatly increased as a result of the breakdown of skeletal muscle, connective tissue, and visceral proteins as acid sources. Branched-chain amino acids serve as the preferred fuel source for skeletal muscle. Production of acute phase reactants is increased, while the production of albumin and transferrin is decreased.

D. Multiple Organ Failure

Septic shock affects virtually all organ systems (Table 11–5). Although the exact mechanism responsible is not clear, this may result from microvascular injury and local inflammatory responses. Ischemia results from tissue hypoperfusion as blood flow is redistributed away from tissues with high metabolic demands.

The usual progression of organ system failures is pulmonary, hepatic, and renal. The mortality rate is proportionate to the number of organ systems that fail and reaches 80–100% when three or more systems are involved. Respiratory failure occurs in 30–80% of patients with septic shock and usually is in the form of ARDS. Hypoxemia refractory to increasing levels of support is characteristic. An elevated intrapulmonary shunt ($\dot{Q}s/\dot{Q}t$) makes the hypoxia resistant to increased concentrations of inspired oxygen. Pulmonary hypertension, increased extravascular lung water, and decreased pulmonary compliance accompany the syndrome. Respiratory muscle fatigue and depressed diaphragmatic contractility further complicate the situation.

Liver failure is manifested as hyperbilirubinemia and elevation of the aminotransferase and alkaline phosphatase concentrations. Decreased hepatic amino acid clearance with an elevation of serum amino acid concentrations are preterminal events. Histologic examination reveals intrahepatic cholestasis with minimal necrosis.

Renal failure may occur as a consequence of hypotension, from nephrotoxic drug administration (aminoglycosides, amphotericin B), or from intrarenal corticomedullary shunting.

Clinical Features

A. Symptoms and Signs

Before shock is overtly manifested, patients may show signs that shock is approaching. The septic syndrome is typically exhibited before hemodynamic compromise occurs (Table 11–6). Patients with the septic syndrome may be at high risk for the development of septic shock.

Septic shock is classically defined as a mean blood pressure of less than 60 mm Hg (systolic pressure < 90 mm Hg)—or a decrease in systolic blood pressure of more than 40 mm Hg from baseline—in a patient with clinical evidence of infection. Accompanying findings include fever or hypothermia, tachycardia, and tachypnea. Patients are frequently obtunded. The skin may be warm if hypovolemia is not present.

If a pulmonary artery catheter is placed for monitoring, an elevated cardiac output in the face of decreased systemic vascular resistance will be found. When decreased cardiac output is noted, hypovolemia should be suspected. Increased pulmonary artery pressures are common as a result of vascular reactivity and increased pulmonary vascular resistance. A pulmonary artery catheter capable of ejection fraction measurement will indicate a decrease in right ventricular ejection fraction and stroke volume. The left ventricular stroke work index is similarly depressed. Pulmonary capillary wedge pressure is usually low or normal. Volume infusion to increase the PCWP generally produces only minimal increases in cardiac output.

B. Laboratory Findings

Leukocytosis with an increased percentage of juvenile band forms is the usual finding. Neutropenia occurs in a small percentage of patients and portends a poor outcome. Disseminated intravascular coagulation (DIC) with increased prothrombin time, elevated fibrin split products, and decreased fibrinogen concentration are also common. Thrombocytopenia occurs in 50% of patients and may be due to endothelial adherence of platelets to reactive vascular endothelium. Overt bleeding is noted in less than 5% of patients.

Table 11–5. Recognition and assessment of organ system dysfunction.[1]

	Indicators of Dysfunction	Degree of Dysfunction		
		Mild	Moderate	Severe
Respiratory tract	PaO_2, FIO_2, PaO_2/FIO_2, PEEP number of days on ventilator; peak airway pressure; use of high-frequency ventilation or extra-corporeal membrane oxygenation	$PaO_2/FIO_2 > 250$	PaO_2/FIO_2 150–250	$PaO_2/FIO_2 < 150$
Kidneys	Creatinine level, creatinine clearance, BUN, need for dialysis to regulate serum potassium and bicarbonate	Creatinine < 150 μmo/L	Creatinine 150–300 μmo/L	Creatinine > 300 μmo/L; need for dialysis
Liver	Bilirubin, albumin, cholesterol, ALT, AST, γ-glutamyltransferase, alkaline phosphatase, ammonia	Bilirubin < 30 μmo/L	Bilirubin 30–80 μmo/L; elevation of transaminases or alkaline phosphatase to twice normal values	Bilirubin > 80 μmo/L; elevation of serum ammonia
Gastrointestinal tract	Stress-related mucosal ulceration and bleeding, mucosal acidosis, failure of pH regulation, volume of nasogastric drainage, ileus, diarrhea, intolerance of enteral feeding, acalculous cholecystitis, pancreatitis	Nasogastric drainage < 300 mL/ 24 h, diarrhea in response to enteral feeding	Nasogastric drainage 300–1000 mL/24 h, visible blood in drainage fluid	Nasogastric drainage > 1000 mL/ 24 h, upper GI bleeding necessitating transfusion, acalculous cholecystitis, pancreatitis
Heart	Supraventricular arrhythmias, elevated pulmonary artery wedge pressure and mean arterial pressure, reduced ventricular stroke-work index, requirement for inotropes or vasopressors to maintain adequate mean arterial pressure	Development of superventricular tachycardias with heart rate < 140 beats/min and no fall in mean arterial pressure	PAWP 16–30 mm Hg; requirement for dopamine or dobutamine at dosage of < 10 μg/kg/min to maintain satisfactory cardiac output and PAWP	Requirement for vasopressors (eg, dopamine, epinephrine, norepinephrine, phenylephrine) to maintain mean arterial pressure > 80 mm Hg
Central nervous system	Glasgow Coma Scale score, especially on components reflecting level of consciousness	Glasgow score 13–14	Glasgow score 10–12	Glasgow score ≤ 9
Hematologic system	Thrombocytopenia, elevated PT and PTT, elevated fibrin degradation products	Platelet count > 60,000/μL	Platelet count 20,000–60,000/μL; mild elevation of PT or PTT in absence of anticoagulation	Platelet count 20,000/μL; DIC
Metabolic and endocrine systems	Insulin requirements, levels of T_4 and reverse T_3	Insulin requirement ≤ 1 unit/h	Insulin requirement 2–4 units/h	Insulin requirement ≥ 5 units/h
Immunologic system	Impaired DTH responsiveness, reduced in vitro lymphocyte proliferation, infection with ICU pathogens (eg, *S epidermidis*, candida, pseudomonas, enterococcus)	Reduced delayed type hypersensitivity reactivity	Cutaneous anergy	Cutaneous anergy, recurrent infection with ICU pathogens
Wound healing	Wound infection, impaired formation of granulation tissue, would dehiscence	Wound infection	Impaired formation of granulation tissue	Decubitus ulcers wound dehiscence

[1]From Holcroft J, Robinson MK: Shock: Identification and management of shock states. In: *Care of the Surgical Patient.* Scientific American, 1992.

Table 11–6. Diagnostic criteria of the septic syndrome.

Clinical evidence of an infection site
Hypotermia (< 96 °F) or fever (> 101 °F)
Tachycardia (> 90 beats/min)
Tachypnea (> 20 beats/min)
Inadequate organ perfusion or dysfunction as evidenced by one of the following:
1. Poor or altered cerebral function
2. Hypoxemia ($PaO_2 < 75$ mm Hg)
3. Elevated plasma lactate
4. Oliguria (urine output < 30 mL/h or < 0.5 mL/kg body weight/h)

Hyperglycemia is common and probably reflects the action of counterregulatory hormones such as epinephrine, cortisol, and glucagon. Elevation of the serum glucose concentration in a patient receiving intravenous hyperalimentation may be the first indicator of impending sepsis. Hypoglycemia is frequently a preterminal event. Increased lactate concentration is common and reflects cellular hypoperfusion. Liver chemistries reveal an increase in bilirubin, aminotransferase, and alkaline phosphatase concentrations.

Mixed substrate fuel consumption increases the respiratory quotient to near 0.8. Hypermetabolic protein turnover is reflected by a negative nitrogen balance. Total serum amino acid levels are increased with the exception of branched-chain amino acids (leucine, isoleucine, and valine), which are decreased.

Arterial blood gas determinations typically indicate moderate hypoxemia and metabolic acidosis. Unless severe respiratory muscle weakness is present, Pa_{CO_2} is usually normal or only minimally elevated. The extent of arterial hypoxemia is related to the severity of the accompanying respiratory distress syndrome. The decrease in bicarbonate concentration may be greater than the increase in lactic acid level. Venous blood gases reveal an increased hemoglobin saturation. Although peripheral oxygen delivery is elevated, peripheral oxygen consumption and oxygen extraction are depressed. The arterial-venous oxygen content gradient is narrowed and may be less than 3 mL/dL. As volume is administered and oxygen delivery is increased, a corresponding increase in $\dot{V}O_2$ may also be noted. This supply dependency of oxygen consumption is characteristic of sepsis.

C. Microbiology

Positive blood cultures are present in about 45% of patients with the septic syndrome and septic shock. The frequency of organisms present varies in different studies, though gram-negative aerobic species usually predominate. A recent study found that 26% of patients with aerobic gram-negative bacteremia developed shock, while only 12% of those with gram-positive bacteremia went on to shock. There are no consistent differences in the laboratory findings of those with and without positive blood cultures. Furthermore, the mortality rates in the two groups are about the same (30% without versus 36% with). Other infecting organisms include *Candida albicans* and *Bacteroides fragilis.* Fungal infections are particularly common in patients with disorders associated with systemic immunocompromise such as diabetes. The prolonged use of antimicrobials and a history of polymicrobial bacterial infections also predispose to fungal sepsis.

Differential Diagnosis

The difference between true septic shock and the septic syndrome is a matter of degree. The major differential factor is that hypotension is not part of the septic syndrome. Other forms of distributive shock include anaphylaxis and neurogenic shock. A history of recent drug administration in the former and trauma in the latter should aid in diagnosis. Hemodynamic and cardiac shock rarely cause differential problems.

Treatment

A. Fluid Resuscitation

Restoration of adequate circulating blood volume is the first and most important therapy for septic shock. Loss of intravascular volume may be through capillary leaks, fistulas, diarrhea, or emesis. Patients may not have been receiving adequate oral intake or may have received insufficient maintenance intravenous fluid. Crystalloid is preferred by most physicians as the initial fluid for resuscitation. A pulmonary artery flotation catheter should be inserted to guide therapy. Administration of volume should be titrated against left ventricular filling pressures and cardiac output. Because of the relative myocardial depression that accompanies sepsis, PCWP frequently needs to be elevated to higher than normal levels before an adequate cardiac output and blood pressure are achieved. Typically, a PCWP between 10 mm Hg and 15 mm Hg will be required. This may call for the administration of several liters of balanced salt solution. Ongoing capillary leakage calls for continuing aggressive fluid replacement. Hemodilution may occur, calling for blood transfusion. The optimal level of hemoglobin is not known. If cardiac output remains depressed, increased peripheral oxygen delivery can be augmented by increasing the hematocrit. Similarly, patients who are hypoxemic with severe arterial hemoglobin desaturation should be transfused to increase their oxygen-carrying capacity and oxygen delivery.

B. Respiratory Support

Many patients with septic shock will have severe respiratory distress syndrome. They may also be unable to meet the increased demands of the work of breathing. Semi-elective endotracheal or orotracheal intubation is recommended prior to the development of respiratory arrest. After intubation, mechanical ventilation should always be instituted to decrease the work of breathing. Many will require high inspired oxygen concentrations and positive end-expiratory pressures (PEEP). Inverse I:E ratio and pressure-controlled ventilation may be required if pulmonary compliance is severely compromised. Treatment of respiratory failure is discussed in Chapter 3.

C. Pharmacologic Support

If intravascular volume resuscitation fails to restore blood pressure toward normal, pharmacologic support with pressor drugs is indicated. Both peripheral and cardiac adrenergic receptors appear to be down-regulated in sepsis, making the required dose of pressors higher than might otherwise be expected.

1. Dopamine—Dopamine is the most commonly used inotropic agent for blood pressure support in septic shock. It is the immediate precursor of endogenous norepinephrine. Dopamine's hemodynamic effects are due to the release of norepinephrine from sympathetic nerves and the direct stimulation of alpha, beta, and dopaminergic receptors. Approximately 50% of dopamine's effect is due to the release of norepinephrine. When compared with dobutamine, dopamine's effect is less pronounced after endogenous norepinephrine stores have been depleted. At lower doses (2–5 μg/kg/min), dopamine increases cardiac contractility and cardiac output without increasing heart rate, blood pressure, or systemic vascular resistance. Renal blood flow and urine output increase in response to doses of 0.5-2 μg/kg/min as a result of selective stimulation of dopaminergic receptors. When doses reach 10 μg/kg/min, dopamine has both a chronotropic as well as an inotropic effect. At infusion rates in excess of 10 μg/kg/min, alpha-adrenergic stimulation occurs along with an increase in systemic vascular resistance. The metabolic effects of dopamine administration include decreased aldosterone secretion, inhibition of thyroid-stimulating hormone and prolactin release, and inhibition of insulin secretion. Because it increases cardiac output, dopamine can increase pulmonary shunting by augmenting flow to poorly ventilated lung regions.

After ensuring adequate fluid resuscitation, dopamine infusion is usually started at a dose of 5 μg/kg/min and advanced until blood pressure increases. Used in low doses with norepinephrine, dopamine's selective effect on the renal vasculature may continue to allow adequate urine production, while norepinephrine supports the blood pressure by its vasoconstrictive effect.

2. Dobutamine—Dobutamine has predominantly β-adrenergic inotropic effects. It has a relatively minor chronotropic effect. Unlike dopamine, it does not cause the release of endogenous norepinephrine. It produces less increase in heart rate and peripheral vascular resistance than an equally inotropic dose of isoproterenol. It is the pressor of choice in patients with adequate blood pressure but depressed cardiac output. Onset of action is within 1–2 minutes, though the peak effect may not be reached until 10 minutes after administration. The plasma half-life is 2 minutes. The drug is methylated and excreted in the urine. Dobutamine tends to lose its hemodynamic effect after prolonged administration, probably because of down-regulation of receptors. However, dobutamine is a better choice for long-term infusion than dopamine, because the latter depletes myocardial norepinephrine stores. Dosage typically ranges from 5 to 15 μg/kg/min. Increased urine output may also be achieved after dobutamine administration because of increased renal perfusion from elevated cardiac output. Infusion is begun at a rate of 2-5 μg/kg/min and titrated to the desired effect. Maximal benefit is usually achieved at levels between 10 and 15 μg/kg/min.

Dopexamine is a newly developed inotropic agent not yet approved in the United States. It has strong β-adrenergic and dopaminergic effects but no α-adrenergic properties. It is both an inotrope and a vasodilator. While it appears that this agent might be most useful for the treatment of congestive heart failure, one study in septic patients reported an increase in cardiac index and heart rate and no increase in mean arterial pressure. Significantly, dopexamine appears to increase splanchnic blood flow. Animal studies indicate that dopexamine increases renal plasma flow and glomerular filtration rate more than dobutamine. Recommendations for this drug await further study and licensing.

3. Isoproterenol—Isoproterenol is a nonselective β-adrenergic agonist that is a positive inotrope and chronotrope. Venous return to the heart is increased because of decreased venous compliance. Pulmonary and systemic vascular resistance are decreased and may cause a fall in blood pressure. Isoproterenol increases both cardiac and renal blood flow. Duration of action is brief (half-life 2 minutes), with major metabolism by the catechol-*O*-methyltransferase pathway in the liver. The agent is occasionally useful in patients who fail to respond to dopamine or dobutamine and is usually used in the preterminal phase of cardiac decompensation. For routine elevation of blood pressure and cardiac output, dopamine or dobutamine are better choices. Treatment with isoproterenol is begun with an intravenous infusion at a rate of 0.01 μg/kg/min and increased to produce the desired effect.

4. Alpha-adrenergic agents—In spite of adequate volume resuscitation and improved cardiac output, blood pressure may remain depressed. Phenylephrine and norepinephrine are two agents commonly used to increase systemic vascular resistance.

Norepinephrine is the biosynthetic precursor of epinephrine, and as such posses both α- and β-adrenergic activity. In low doses, its major effect is β-adrenergic. It increases cardiac contractility, conduction velocity, and heart rate. At higher doses, both α- and β-adrenergic effects occur, which include peripheral vasoconstriction, increased cardiac contractility, cardiac work, and stroke volume. Norepinephrine causes splanchnic vasoconstriction, which may lead to end-organ ischemia. The drug is rapidly cleared from the plasma with a half-life of approximately 2 minutes. Initial infusion rates are 0.05–0.1 μg/kg/min. The usual maximum dose is 1 μg/kg/min.

5. Vasopressin—Vasopressin (antidiuretic hormone) is normally released by the hypothalamus and produces vasoconstriction of vascular smooth muscle in addition to its antidiuretic effect on the renal collecting system. At low plasma concentrations it causes vasodilation of the coronary, cerebral, and pulmonary vessels. Vasopressin levels increase in early septic shock and later fall as sepsis worsens. When given in doses of 0.01–0.04 units/min, vasopressin infusion increases serum vasopressin levels and decreases the need for other vasopressors. At this dose, urinary output may increase and pulmonary vascular resistance may decrease. Doses higher than 0.04 units/min can cause undesirable vasoconstrictive effects. Experience with this agent in sepsis is limited, and a controlled study is needed before it can be recommended routinely.

6. Vasodilators—Because decreased vascular resistance is the primary cause of hypotension in septic shock, further pharmacologic vasodilation is contraindicated. Occasionally, severe myocardial depression is accompanied by an increase in systemic vascular resistance. This preterminal event puts further strain on the left ventricle and may cause complete hemodynamic collapse. Judicious use of vasodilators such as nitroprusside may be tried. Nitroglycerin is probably an inferior choice because it also reduces preload.

D. Antimicrobial Agents

Identification of the source of sepsis is imperative. If the offending tissue bed is not drained or if bacteremia is not treated, outcome will be adversely affected. Evaluation of the patient's history is essential to determine likely sources. Once the probable origin has been identified, appropriate antimicrobial therapy can be instituted to provide coverage for organisms commonly encountered. The details of diagnosis and therapy of infections are presented in Chapters 15 and 16. When a likely source cannot be identified, empiric broad-spectrum therapy should be instituted with drugs known to be effective against gram-positive, gram-negative, and anaerobic organisms. In surgical patients who have had abdominal procedures, enteric gram-negative and anaerobic organisms are of particular concern. Attention must be given to dosing in these patients because alterations in renal function may affect degradation and because an expanded plasma volume affects the volume of distribution and therefore the size of the loading dose that must be given.

E. Supportive Care

Although not a part of the treatment of septic shock per se, attention must be given to nutritional support. These patients are in a severely catabolic state and continue to utilize structural protein as energy precursors. Hyperalimentation is frequently necessary to supply adequate protein and calories. The details of metabolic support are presented in Chapter 6.

F. Other Modalities

Corticosteroids have been studied both experimentally and clinically as adjuncts to the treatment of septic shock. They stabilize lysosomal membranes and may decrease the inflammatory response. Two recent large multicenter studies failed to demonstrate increased survival among patients who received steroids when compared with those who did not. Furthermore, the use of steroids afforded no protection against the development of ARDS. The only indication for the use of steroids in septic shock is for suspected adrenal insufficiency.

Naloxone is a competitive opioid inhibitor that also blocks the effect of endogenous endorphins. Because endorphins are vasodilators, they may be partially responsible for decreasing systemic vascular resistance. High doses of naloxone repeated over short periods have been shown to improve survival in some animal studies. Clinical studies, however, have failed to yield consistent results. Furthermore, the doses of naloxone used have been extremely high (0.4 mg/kg/h). Presently, naloxone cannot be recommended for routine use in the treatment of septic shock.

Nitric oxide synthase induction probably contributes to septic shock, and its inhibition by a number of agents, including methylene blue, may be useful, but this requires further study.

Current Controversies & Unresolved Issues

A. Fluid Resuscitation

The choice of fluid for the initial and continued resuscitation of septic patients is widely debated. Proponents of balanced salt solutions claim that pulmonary dysfunction is not worsened by judicious administration guided by endpoints such as ventricular filling pressure and cardiac output. Colloids increase the circulating plasma volume more effectively than do crystalloids, but they are expensive. When pulmonary microvascular permeability is increased, colloids may actually worsen respiratory function by increasing the osmotic gradient favoring translocation of fluid into the alveolar and pulmonary interstitial spaces.

B. Immunotherapy

Because of the apparently important role the cytokines, leukotrienes, and prostaglandins play in the pathogenesis of septic shock, inhibitors of many of these mediators have been developed. Specifically, inhibitors of prostaglandins, platelet-activating factor, leukotrienes, and thromboxanes have been found to decrease cardiac dysfunction and improve survival. The nonsteroidal anti-inflammatory drug ibuprofen is a potent inhibitor of the cyclooxygenase pathway. Animal studies have demonstrated that pretreatment with ibuprofen attenuates the cardiovascular response to IL-1 and TNF. Experimental evidence also indicates that pentoxifylline may inhibit the actions of TNF. Identification of lipid A from gram-negative bacteria has allowed the preparation of antibodies. The original polyclonal preparation, J5, was shown to improve the outcome of patients in septic shock, but because it was prepared from human volunteers it carried a high risk of disease transmission. Monoclonal antibodies have been prepared against lipid A and tested in clinical trials. Of the two agents tested, one was found to improve outcome in patients both with and without septic shock, while the second was shown to be effective only in patients not in shock. At this writing, clinical trials on one of the agents have been suspended. Efficacy of these products would be greatly improved if a simple laboratory test could be developed to detect the presence of circulating endotoxin.

Multiple clinical trials have been conducted with a number of novel immunotherapeutic agents. By and large, these trials have failed to provide usable agents. Recently, however, an agent directed at the coagulation cascade has been approved for use in the United States. Drotrecogin alfa is a glycoprotein analog of protein C that is activated by thrombin. Activated protein C inhibits coagulation, increases fibrin breakdown, and possibly inhibits the synthesis of tumor necrosis factor. A large clinical study of drotrecogin alfa found a reduction in mortality from 30.8% in patients treated with placebo to 24.7% in those treated with the drug. The most important adverse effect of the drug is bleeding, which occurred in 3.5% of those treated with the drug compared with 2% treated with placebo. Although the incidence of bleeding did not reach statistical significance, the drug is contraindicated in patients with active or recent bleeding or a high risk of bleeding, an epidural catheter, or intracranial hemorrhage. It should be used cautiously in those who are at risk for bleeding. Drotrecogin alfa is administered intravenously at a continuous dose of 24 μg/kg/h for 96 hours. No alteration in the dose is required for those with renal or hepatic compromise. The drug's cost is approximately $8000 for a 4-day regimen in a 70-kg patient.

Activated protein C (Xigris) for severe sepsis. Med Lett Drugs Ther 2002;44:17–18.

Bernard GR et al: Efficacy and safety of recombinant human activated protein C for severe sepsis. N Engl J Med 2001;344:699–709.

Beutler B, Cerami A: Cachectin: more than a tumor necrosis factor. N Engl J Med 1987;316:379–85.

Bone RC et al: Sepsis syndrome: a valid clinical entity. Crit Care Med 1989;17:389–93.

Bone RC: A critical evaluation of new agents for the treatment of sepsis. JAMA 1991;266:1686–91.

Bone RC: Sepsis, the sepsis syndrome, multiorgan failure: a plea for comparable definitions. Ann Intern Med 1991;114:332–3.

Brown G, Frankl D, Phang T: Continuous infusion of methylene blue for septic shock. Postgrad Med J 1996;72:612–4.

Cohen J, Glauser MP: Septic shock: treatment. Lancet 1991; 338:736–9.

Cunion RE, Parillo JE: Myocardial dysfunction in sepsis. Crit Care Clin 1989;5:99–118.

Dal Nogare AR: Southwestern internal medical conference: septic shock. Am J Med Sci 1991;302:50–65.

Holcroft JW, Robinson MK: Shock: identification and management of shock states. In: *Care of the Surgical Patient.* Scientific American, 1992.

Holmes CL et al: Physiology of vasopressin relevant to management of septic shock. Chest 2001;120:989–1002.

Lefer A: Significance of lipid mediators in shock states. Circ Shock 1989;27:3–12.

Luce J et al: Ineffectiveness of high dose methyl-prednisolone in preventing parenchymal lung injury and improving mortality in patients with septic shock. Am Rev Resp Dis 1988; 138:62–8.

Mecher CM et al: Unaccounted anion in metabolic acidosis during septic shock in humans. Crit Care Med 1991;19:705–11.

Parillo JE et al: Advances in the understanding of pathogenesis, cardiovascular dysfunction, and therapy. Ann Intern Med 1990;113:227–42.

Leighton TA, Klein SR, Bongard FS: Time course of cardiopulmonary effects of tumor necrosis factor and endotoxin are similar. Am Surg 1991;57:836–42:

Opal SM, Cross AS: Clinical trials for severe sepsis. Infect Dis Clin North Am 1999;13:285–97.

Petros A, Bennett D, Vallance P: Effect of nitric oxide synthase inhibitors on hypotension in patients with septic shock. Lancet 1991;338:1557–8.

Rackow EC, Astiz ME, Weil MH: Cellular oxygen metabolism during sepsis and shock: the relationship of oxygen consumption to oxygen delivery. JAMA 1988;259:1989–93.

Rackow EC, Astiz ME: Pathophysiology and treatment of septic shock. JAMA 1991;266:548–54.

Reuhaug A et al: Inhibition of cyclooxygenase attenuates the metabolic response to endotoxin in humans. Arch Surg 1988;123:162–70.

Smith AL: Treatment of septic shock with immunotherapy. Pharmacotherapy 1998;18:565–80.

Snell RJ, Parillo JE: Cardiovascular dysfunction in septic shock. Chest 1991;99:1000–9.

Suffredini A et al: The cardiovascular response of normal humans to the administration of endotoxin. N Engl J Med 1989;321:280–86.

Vincent JL, Preiser JC: Inotropic agents. New Horiz 1993; 1:137–44.

Ziegler E: Treatment of gram-negative bacteremia and septic shock with HA-1A human monoclonal antibody against endotoxin. N Engl J Med 1991;324;429–36.

ANAPHYLACTIC SHOCK & ANAPHYLACTOID REACTIONS

ESSENTIALS OF DIAGNOSIS

- *Cutaneous flushing, pruritus.*
- *Abdominal distention, nausea, vomiting, diarrhea.*
- *Airway obstruction due to laryngeal edema.*
- *Bronchospasm, bronchorrhea, pulmonary edema.*
- *Tachycardia, syncope, hypotension.*
- *Cardiovascular collapse.*

General Considerations

Anaphylactic shock and anaphylactoid reactions are due to the sudden release of preformed inflammatory mediators from mast cells and basophils. After exposure to the offending stimulus, initial symptoms may appear within seconds to minutes or may be delayed as long as 1 hour. **Anaphylactic shock** is differentiated from anaphylactoid reactions in that the former is a true anamnestic response in which a sensitized individual comes in contact with an antigenic substance. This reaction stimulates membrane-bound IgE, causing mast cells and basophils to release histamine and platelet-activating factor into the circulation. These mediators result in vasodilation, bronchoconstriction, pruritus, bronchorrhea, platelet aggregation, and increased vascular permeability. The latter may lead to laryngeal edema that culminates in airway obstruction. The frequency and outcome of anaphylactic reactions are summarized in Table 11–7. **Anaphylactoid reactions** occur when the offending agent causes the direct release of these substances without mediation by IgE. This may involve a number of pathways including complement-mediated reactions, nonimmunologic activation of mast cells, and production of arachidonic acid mediators. Reactions to NSAIDs are particularly dangerous because NSAID inhibition of the cyclooxygenase pathway favors the formation of lipoxygenase pathway mediators from arachidonic acid. Some of these include leukotrienes C_4, D_4, E_4 (slow-reacting substance of anaphylaxis), and LTB_4. These leukotrienes and their intermediate products (5-HETE and 5-HPETE) increase vascular permeability and produce bronchoconstriction. Leukotriene B_4 is an eosinophilic and neutrophilic chemoattractant. If the cyclooxygenase pathway is activated by the inciting agent, the production of prostaglandin D_2 furthers bronchoconstriction. The most common agents causing anaphylactic shock and anaphylactoid reactions are listed in Tables 11–8 and 11–9. Anaphylactoid reactions may

Table 11–7. Frequency of anaphylactic events and deaths.[1]

Agent	Frequency of Events: Mild	Frequency of Events: Severe	Deaths per Year (USA)
Penicillin	0.5–1%	0.04%	400–800
Hymenoptera stings	0.5%	0.05%	≥ 100
Contrast media	5%	0.10%	250–1000

[1]From Lavine SJ, Shelhamer JH: Anapyhlaxis. In: *Critical Care.* Civetta JM, Raylor RW, Kirby RR (editors). Lippincott, 1992.

Table 11–8. Etiologic agents responsible for anaphylactic shock.[1]

Haptens	Foods	Venoms
Beta-lactam antibiotics	Nuts	Stinging insects, especially Hymenoptera, fire ants
Sulfonamides	Shellfish	**Hormones**
Nitrofurantoin	Buckwheat	Insulin
Demeclocycline	Egg white	Adrenocorticotropic hormone
Streptomycin	Cottonseed	Thyroid-stimulating hormone
Vancomycin	Milk	**Enzymes**
Local anesthetics	Corn	Chymopapain
Others	Potato	L-Asparaginase
Serum products	Rice	**Miscellaneous**
Immune globulin	Legumes	Seminal fluid
Immunotherapy for allergic diseases	Citrus fruits	Others
Heterologous serum	Chocolate	
	Others	

[1]Modified from Austen KF: Systemic anaphylaxis in man. JAMA 1965;192:108; and from Kaliner M: Anaphylaxis. NER Allergy Proceedings 1984;5:324.

Table 11–9. Etiologic agents for anaphylactoid reactions.[1]

Complement-mediated reactions
Blood
Serum
Plasma
Plasmanate (not albumin)
Immunoglobulins
Nonimmunologic mast cell activators
Opioids
Radiocontrast media
Dextrans
Neuromuscular blocking agents
Others
Arachidonic acid modulators
Nonsteroidal anti-inflammatory drugs
Tartrazine (possibly)
Idiopathic
Most common conclusion after thorough evaluation

[1]Adapted from Kaliner M: Anaphylaxis. NER Allergy Proceedings 1984;5:324.

occur in up to 10% of patients. When an initial reaction occurs after the infusion of radiocontrast agents, the risk of a similar reaction upon reexposure approaches 35%.

Clinical Features

A. Symptoms and Signs

The initial symptoms are often complaints of pruritus and a sense of impending doom. These can progress to overt signs over several seconds or may be delayed for up to an hour. Respiratory symptoms may start with complaints of a lump in the throat, progressing to dyspnea, dysphonia, hoarseness, and cough. If pulmonary edema develops as a result of increased capillary permeability, dyspnea and cyanosis result. Cardiovascular findings begin with symptoms of weakness and faintness that may be accompanied by palpitations. As shock progresses, tachycardia appears along with arrhythmias, conduction disturbances, and myocardial ischemia. Cutaneous symptoms include flushing and pruritus that progress to urticaria, angioedema, and diaphoresis. Patients may complain of abdominal pain or bloating, cramps, and nausea. These progress to emesis, diarrhea, and occasionally hematemesis and hematochezia. Other signs include syncope, seizures, conjunctival injection, lacrimation, rhinorrhea, and nasal congestion.

B. Laboratory Findings

An increased hematocrit is found commonly as a result of hemoconcentration from vascular permeability. Serum mast cell tryptase is usually elevated.

Differential Diagnosis

Several common disorders seen in the ICU may be confused with anaphylactic shock and anaphylactoid reactions: myocardial ischemia and infarction, cardiac arrhythmias, hypovolemic shock, septic shock, pulmonary embolism, aspiration of feedings, bronchitis, acute exacerbation of COPD, seizure disorder, hypoglycemia, and cerebrovascular accidents. Relationship to administration of medications, blood, and new intravenous solutions should suggest the possibility of anaphylaxis.

Treatment

A. Airway

The first mandate is to ensure a secure airway. If the patient was intubated prior to the reaction, one should take care that the endotracheal or nasotracheal tube does not become dislodged during resuscitation. If the patient was not intubated, emergency airway control by bag and mask or intubation will probably be necessary. It is far better to intubate these patients before laryngeal edema develops, because subsequent intubation is extremely difficult. Some clinicians recommend the use of inhaled racemic epinephrine (0.3 mL in 3 mL of saline administered by nebulizer) if upper airway compromise occurs because of edema. It is far safer to intubate the patient.

B. Circulatory Support

Most patients who develop anaphylactic shock or an anaphylactoid reaction in the ICU will already have intravenous access. However, this catheter may be small and will not permit the administration of large volumes of fluid over a short period of time. Large-bore peripheral intravenous lines are mandatory for fluid and drug administration. Do not attempt central line placement in a hypotensive patient who is hypovolemic. Collapse of the large veins normally used for central catheter placement increases the risk of a life-threatening complication.

1. Epinephrine—Drug therapy should begin with epinephrine (1:1000), 0.3–0.5 mL subcutaneously. The dose of epinephrine may be repeated every 5–10 minutes as needed. If the patient does not respond to the initial dose–or if severe laryngospasm or frank cardiovascular collapse is present—5–10 mL of epinephrine (1:10,000) may be administered intravenously. If intravenous access is not available, either 0.5 mL of a 1:1000 dilution may be given intramuscularly or 10 mL of a 1:10,000 dilution may be instilled into the endotracheal tube. When epinephrine is given intravenously, severe tachycardia, myocardial ischemia, vasospasm, and hypertension may result. Epinephrine decreases mediator synthesis by increasing intracellular concentrations of cAMP. Furthermore, it counteracts many of the deleterious effects of the mediators of anaphylaxis.

2. Histamine antagonists—Histamine antagonists should be administered as early as possible. Diphenhydramine (1 mg/kg intravenously) and ranitidine (50 mg intravenously over 5 minutes) are the preferred drugs. Cimetidine must be used with extreme caution because rapid intravenous administration may result in hypotension or asystole.

3. Pressors—If hypotension persists after the repeated administration of epinephrine and histamine antagonists, aggressive fluid resuscitation is required. If this fails, dopamine may be started at an initial dose of 5 μg/kg/min and increased until the dose reaches 20 μg/kg/min. A plateau effect occurs above this dose, requiring that a second pressor be used if an adequate response has not yet been achieved. Because of the extreme vasodilation, norepinephrine should be started in the range of 3-4 μg/min and titrated until a mean arterial pressure between 60 and 80 mm Hg is reached. The patient should be weaned from pressors as quickly as possible.

C. Other Measures

Continued observation in the intensive care unit is indicated. An arterial catheter should be inserted for pressure monitoring and to aid in securing blood gas samples for ventilator management. In patients who remain unstable or who require continuing pressor infusion, a pulmonary artery catheter should be placed. Biphasic anaphylaxis may occur in up to 25% of patients. Life-threatening reactions reappear after an asymptomatic interval of up to 8 hours following resuscitation. Hydrocortisone, 100–250 mg intravenously every 6 hours, may help prevent the late manifestations of biphasic anaphylaxis. Steroids probably have no role in the immediate treatment of acute anaphylaxis.

Patients who are receiving beta-blockers at the time of an anaphylactic reaction may be resistant to the effects of administered epinephrine. Atropine and glucagon may be useful adjuncts to reverse the cardiac manifestations of anaphylaxis in such cases.

Prognosis

The patient's overall medical condition, the delay between exposure to the antigen and the onset of anaphylaxis, and the severity of symptoms all influence the outcome.

Anderson JA: Allergic reactions to drugs and biological agents. JAMA 1992;268:2844–57.

Atkinson TP, Kaliner MA: Anaphylaxis. Med Clin North Am 1992;76:841–55.

Goust JM: Immediate hypersensitivity. Immunol Ser 1993; 58:343–59.

Levine SJ, Shelhamer JH: Anaphylaxis. In: *Critical Care.* Civetta JM, Taylor RW, Kirby RR (editors). Lippincott, 1992.

Levy JH, Levi R: Diagnosis and treatment of anaphylactic/anaphylactoid reactions. Monogr Allergy 1992;30:145–55.

Marone G, Stellato C: Activation of human mast cells and basophils by general anesthetic agents. Monogr Allergy 1992;30:54–73.

Raper RF, Fisher MM: Profound reversible myocardial depression after anaphylaxis. Lancet 1988;1:386–9.

White MV: The role of histamine in allergic disease. J Allergy Clin Immunol 1990;86:599–605.

NEUROGENIC SHOCK

ESSENTIALS OF DIAGNOSIS

- *Preceded by trauma or spinal anesthesia.*
- *Hypotension with tachycardia.*
- *Cutaneous warmth and flushing in the denervated area.*
- *Venous pooling.*

General Considerations

Neurogenic shock is produced by loss of peripheral vasomotor tone as a result of spinal cord injury, regional anesthesia, or administration of autonomic blocking agents. Blood becomes pooled in the periphery, venous return is decreased, and cardiac output falls. If the level of interruption is below the mid thorax, the remaining adrenergic system above the level of injury is activated, resulting in increased heart rate and contractility. If the cardiac sympathetic outflow is affected, bradycardia results. Blood pressure can decrease to extremely low levels as blood pools peripherally in the venous reservoir. All patients who have sustained spinal trauma should be assumed to have hypovolemic shock from associated injuries until proved otherwise.

Clinical Features

A. Symptoms and Signs

Patients may be alert and responsive if head injuries are absent. Extremities are warm above the level of injury and cool below. Blood pressure may be extremely low, with a very rapid heart rate. Skeletal musculature is affected after trauma. Loss of the peripheral venous muscular pump may further decrease venous return. Signs and symptoms of spinal cord injury and spinal shock will be present.

B. Laboratory Findings

Laboratory studies are not helpful in diagnosis. Because capillary permeability is normal, plasma leaks do not occur. Prior to volume resuscitation, hematocrit is usually normal.

C. Imaging Studies

Radiographs of the cervical, thoracic, and lumbosacral spine are important to determine whether fractures are present that may be unstable. These will typically have been completed before the patient was admitted to the ICU, but the intensivist must review the films so that patient manipulations will not cause further spinal cord injury. CT and MRI may be useful to determine whether fragments within the spinal canal may be causing cord compression. When present, they may be amenable to neurosurgical decompression.

Differential Diagnosis

Trauma patients considered for admission to a critical care unit after spinal injury must have thorough surgical and neurosurgical evaluation before transfer. The presence of concomitant hypovolemic shock from unrecognized bleeding sites within the abdomen, chest, and extremities must be excluded. Isolated head injury does not cause shock. Rather, it may increase the blood pressure while slowing the heart rate (Cushing's reflex).

Treatment

A. Supportive Measures

A secure airway and adequate intravenous access are urgent priorities. If intubation is required and there is concern regarding the stability of the cervical spine, fiberoptic or nasotracheal intubation may be required. A diligent search must be made for other injuries in trauma patients. When neurogenic shock arises from a spinal anesthetic procedure in which the level of blockade has become too high, intubation may also be necessary because of compromise of the muscles of respiration.

Depending upon the level of the injury, patients may have loss of bladder function. A Foley catheter should be inserted to decompress the bladder and aid in monitoring urine output.

B. Fluid Resuscitation

Effective circulating blood volume decreases dramatically because of venous pooling. Fluid resuscitation is usually necessary and typically begins with several liters of balanced salt solution. In some patients, this may be all that is required to increase blood pressure.

C. Pharmacologic Support

If volume infusion fails to restore the blood pressure, infusion of an alpha-adrenergic agent is required to provide direct vasoconstriction. Either phenylephrine or norepinephrine may be used. These drugs are started in low doses and increased slowly until just sufficient to restore blood pressure to a mean between 60 and 80 mm Hg. Weaning can usually be achieved fairly quickly, so that central venous or pulmonary artery catheterization is not often required.

D. Surgery

If spinal cord transection is complete, the only role for surgery is stabilization of vertebral fractures to prevent further injury. If a foreign body is present, removal may promote return of function if the cord is intact.

E. Rehabilitation

After the acute stage has passed and the patient has been stabilized, planning should be undertaken to provide long-term care. This is the most difficult part of the management of these patients. Demands on nursing and support personnel are extreme in order to prevent pressure ulcers and urinary and respiratory tract infections and to provide nutritional support. Early consultation with a psychiatrist is recommended to help the patient adjust to complete and permanent loss of function.

CARDIAC SHOCK

Cardiac shock occurs when the heart fails to adequately pump the blood volume presented to it. There are two general categories: cardiogenic shock and cardiac compressive shock. Cardiogenic shock develops when the heart loses its ability to function as a pump. Cardiocompressive shock is due to compression of the great veins and cardiac chambers, restricting their normal filling and emptying.

CARDIOGENIC SHOCK

ESSENTIALS OF DIAGNOSIS

- *Decreased urine output.*
- *Impaired mental function.*
- *Cool extremities.*
- *Distended neck veins.*
- *Hypotension with evidence of peripheral and pulmonary venous congestion.*

General Considerations

Cardiogenic shock most commonly occurs either after relentless progression of cardiac disease or after an acute event such as myocardial infarction or rupture of a cardiac valve or septum. These causes are summarized in

Table 11–10. The absolute amount of myocardium involved is probably the most important prognostic factor. When more than 45% of the left ventricular myocardium is necrotic, cardiogenic shock becomes evident clinically.

Bradycardia and arrhythmias may underlie cardiogenic shock. Heart rates less than about 50 beats/min may be inadequate to support cardiac output. Similarly, arrhythmias may significantly alter cardiac filling patterns and prevent adequate pumping.

A staging system has been developed for the classification of cardiogenic shock that develops on a chronic basis.

A. Stage I (Compensated Hypotension)

The decreased cardiac output and resulting hypotension invoke compensatory mechanisms able to restore blood pressure and tissue blood flow to normal levels. These reflexes are mediated by the arterial baroreceptors, which increase the systemic vascular resistance.

B. Stage II (Decompensated Hypotension)

Cardiac output falls below that which enables the peripheral vasculature to maintain blood pressure by vasoconstriction. Blood pressure and tissue perfusion fall.

C. Stage III (Irreversible Shock)

Profound reduction in flow activates ischemic mediators such as the complement cascade. Membrane injury develops that further aggravates the ischemic insult. Irreversible myocardial and peripheral tissue damage occur.

Clinical Features

A. Symptoms and Signs

When cardiogenic shock occurs as a result of an acute event, pain may be a prominent finding. Details of diagnosis and management of acute myocardial infarction are presented in Chapter 22. When shock is an acute exacerbation of a relentless process or the result of another disease, symptoms may be less pronounced.

Table 11–10. Causes of cardiogenic shock.[1]

Nonmechanical Causes	Mechanical Causes
Acute myocardial infarction	Rupture of septum or free wall
Low cardiac output syndromes	Mitral or aortic insufficiency
Right ventricular infarction	Papillary muscle rupture or dysfunction
End-stage cardiomyopathy	Critical aortic stenosis
	Pericardial tamponade

[1]From Farmer JA: Cardiogenic Shock. In: *Critical Care.* Civetta JM, Taylor RW, Kirby RR (editors). Lippincott, 1992.

Physical examination will reveal signs consistent with the underlying pathophysiologic mechanism of decreased cardiac output and absolute hypervolemia. Blood pressure is less than 90 mm Hg. The heart rate may be extremely high and exceed the maximum aerobic limit (230 minus the patient's age in years). When decompensation occurs, bradycardia usually develops. Neck veins are distended, and pulsations can frequently be observed more than 4 cm above the clavicle with the patient in the semierect position. Peripherally, the extremities are cool, reflecting inadequate perfusion. Abdominal examination may reveal a congested and distended liver that is tender to palpation. Rales are detected on auscultation of the lungs in a patient who has a normal right ventricle. With biventricular failure or pulmonary hypertension, pulmonary auscultation may be normal. Cardiac examination typically reveals a third heart sound, and there may be a murmur characteristic of valvular disease.

B. Hemodynamic Effects

Virtually all patients with cardiogenic shock will require a pulmonary artery catheter for monitoring and evaluation of the response to therapy. The usual findings are elevation of central venous and pulmonary capillary wedge pressures and a cardiac index less than about 1.8 L/min/m^2.

C. Laboratory Findings

If acute myocardial infarction is the precipitating cause, elevated cardiac bands of creatine kinase will be observed. Plasma drug levels of medications the patient has been receiving should be measured to determine whether they are in the toxic or subtherapeutic ranges. A routine chemistry panel is required to evaluate K^+ and HCO_3^-. Serum lactate may be elevated when shock has been prolonged. Hematocrit and hemoglobin should be determined to evaluate the need for transfusion.

D. Imaging Studies

Chest radiography will often reveal a pattern of pulmonary edema. Radionuclide ventriculography may be helpful in evaluating ventricular ejection fraction. Echocardiography is also useful in the evaluation of valvular and ventricular function. If pericardial tamponade is suspected, echocardiography is the examination of choice to establish that diagnosis.

Differential Diagnosis

Cardiogenic shock should be suspected in patients with chronic myocardial disease who experience a sudden worsening of symptoms. Acute myocardial infarction may be complicated by ventricular septal rupture, papillary muscle rupture, and papillary muscle dysfunction, which can lead to cardiogenic shock. Constrictive pericarditis and rupture of a cardiac ventricular aneurysm may lead to cardiac compressive shock. Rupture of an abdominal aortic aneurysm in a patient with coronary artery disease may cause diagnostic confusion. Abdominal pain due to rupture of the aneurysm may simulate the pain of acute myocardial infarction. Electrocardiography typically reveals myocardial ischemia. The absence of distended neck veins is the critical distinguishing feature. Myocardial contusion after blunt trauma may cause severe cardiogenic shock.

Treatment

A. General Measures

Patient comfort and relief of anxiety should be addressed immediately. Opioids not only relieve pain and provide sedation—they also block adrenergic discharge and lessen cardiac stress. Intravenous morphine should be given starting with a bolus of 2–4 mg. Dosing should be titrated to both subjective response and effect on blood pressure. Because morphine is a vasodilator, it may decrease right ventricular filling and adversely affect blood pressure in a hypovolemic patient. An arterial catheter and a pulmonary artery flotation catheter are usually mandatory to manage these patients effectively.

When cardiogenic shock is the result of acute myocardial infarction, early efforts should be directed at controlling the infarct size. An imbalance between oxygen delivery and increased oxygen consumption prompted by changes in heart rate, blood pressure, and contractility may extend the size of the infarction. If therapy is begun within 3 hours after myocardial infarction, the incidence of cardiogenic shock is 4%. However, if therapy is delayed, cardiogenic shock occurs in up to 13% of patients. Intravenous nitroglycerin and beta-blockers are the main features of early treatment.

Nitroglycerin reduces right ventricular preload and decreases left ventricular afterload. The reduction in afterload decreases end-diastolic pressure and reduces wall stress and myocardial oxygen consumption. Furthermore, it dilates epicardial vessels and may improve oxygen delivery to ischemic areas. The early use of nitroglycerin both decreases infarct size and reduces early mortality. The possibility of right ventricular infarction and pericardial tamponade must be excluded before therapy with nitroglycerin is begun.

Beta-blockers decrease myocardial oxygen demand, antagonize circulating catechols, and have antiarrhythmic activity. A particular benefit may accrue when beta-blockers are combined with thrombolytic agents. Beta-blockers are best started within 2 hours after infarction. Calcium channel blockers have also been investigated for this purpose but have failed to demonstrate efficacy in acute situations. The mortality rate may be increased if calcium channel blockers are used in patients with pulmonary edema.

B. Resuscitation

Although cardiogenic shock may occur in patients with whole body fluid overload, they may be effectively hypovolemic. If PCWP is less than 10–12 mm Hg, balanced salt solution should be administered in an attempt to increase filling pressures. Cardiac output should be measured after each change of 2-3 mm Hg in PCWP. Filling pressures near 20 mm Hg may be required before cardiac output increases.

If laboratory studies reveal that the patient is hypoxemic, supplemental oxygen should be provided. Oxygen delivery should be maximized by ensuring complete arterial hemoglobin saturation. Intubation with positive end-expiratory pressure (PEEP) may be required to accomplish this when pulmonary edema is present. Judicious use of PEEP is required because it adversely affects ventricular preload and cardiac output.

C. Pharmacologic Support

Once volume status has been optimized, support of the failing myocardium is often necessary. Inotropes, vasodilators, and diuretics may all be used.

1. Inotropes—

Dobutamine—Dobutamine is the inotropic drug of choice for the management of congestive heart failure and cardiogenic shock. It is a β_1-adrenergic agonist that has minimum chronotropic and peripheral vasoconstrictive effects. It has a significant advantage over dopamine in that it does not cause the release of norepinephrine. Furthermore, it does not require the presence of norepinephrine at the nerve terminals for effect. Because of its minimum chronotropic effect, dobutamine can improve ventricular performance without significantly increasing myocardial oxygen demand. Dobutamine's greatest potential is realized in patients with reduced cardiac indices and increased filling pressures. Because it is a vasodilator, dobutamine reduces filling pressures and wall tensions in patients with dilated ventricles. This permits better myocardial nutrient flow during diastole. A recent study found a 33% improvement in cardiac index, a decrease in systemic vascular resistance, and no change in heart rate or systemic blood pressure when dobutamine was given in doses that averaged 8.5 μg/kg/min. The drug may be given in doses up to 40 μg/kg/min without significantly increasing heart rate. When three-vessel coronary artery disease is present, dobutamine may create a steal and direct blood away from ischemic areas.

b. Dopamine—The effects of dopamine are dependent on the dose administered. In lower doses (< 4 μg/kg/min), dopamine increases renal blood flow by stimulating dopaminergic (D_1) receptors in the kidney and causes peripheral vasodilation through D_2 receptors that inhibit the release of norepinephrine. At intermediate dosages (5–10 μg/kg/min), dopamine improves cardiac function and increases blood pressure without elevating myocardial oxygen consumption. Systemic vascular resistance is usually not increased. At higher doses (> 10 μg/kg/min), dopamine elevates systemic vascular resistance by stimulating alpha-adrenergic receptors and heart rate by stimulating beta-adrenergic receptors. A recent study found that an average dose of 17 μg/kg/min was needed to optimize coronary perfusion pressure in a group of patients that developed cardiogenic shock after myocardial infarction. Dopamine at such high levels increases myocardial oxygen demand, produces tachycardia, and may limit renal perfusion. It should be used with caution in patients with cardiogenic shock because it may adversely influence the balance of myocardial oxygen delivery and consumption.

c. **Digoxin**—Although digitalis preparations have modest inotropic effects, they are probably of little importance in the treatment of cardiogenic shock except for the treatment of atrial fibrillation with rapid ventricular response. Small intravenous doses of digoxin may improve diastolic filling time and increase cardiac output in these situations.

d. **Isoproterenol**—This agent causes tachycardia, increased myocardial contractility, and decreased peripheral vascular resistance through its stimulation of both β_1 and β_2 receptors. Myocardial oxygen consumption is dramatically increased. Although isoproterenol increases coronary blood flow, it may actually shunt blood away from ischemic areas and increase the infarct size. Highly restricted indications include the presence of bradycardia and severe aortic valvular insufficiency. Intravenous administration is started at a dose of 0.01 μg/kg/min and increased until the desired effect is obtained.

e. **Norepinephrine**—Norepinephrine has both alpha- and beta-adrenergic effects. At low doses, it causes beta stimulation of the heart and increases blood pressure and cardiac output. At higher doses, it primarily affects the alpha-adrenergic receptors and supports blood pressure by increasing systemic vascular resistance. At higher doses it also tends to produce tachycardia, arrhythmias, and peripheral visceral ischemia. Norepinephrine should be used with extreme caution because at higher doses it increases left ventricular afterload and may worsen myocardial ischemia. If cardiogenic shock proves resistant to both dobutamine and dopamine, norepinephrine may be started in doses of 1–2 μg/min and increased until blood pressure increases. Of particular concern are the visceral and renal vasoconstrictive effects that may produce end-organ ischemia in the face of apparently satisfactory blood pressure.

f. **Other agents**—**Amrinone** is a weak inotrope that increases contractility independently of the catechol pathways. Although its exact mechanism of action is not known, it increases intracellular cAMP and calcium concentrations. The increased cAMP concentration in smooth muscle decreases peripheral and pulmonary vascular resistance and dilates coronary arteries. Amrinone increases stroke volume without increasing heart rate. The usual loading dose is 0.75 mg/kg over 3–5 minutes, followed by a second bolus 30 minutes later. The boluses are followed by a continuous intravenous infusion of 5–10 μg/kg/min. The total daily dose should not exceed 10 mg/kg. After the bolus is given, effects are seen within several minutes.

Glucagon increases cardiac contractility and decreases peripheral vascular resistance. The onset of action is extremely rapid. A test dose of 4–6 mg should be given intravenously to determine whether any effect is produced. If successful, this is followed by a constant infusion of 4–12 mg/h. The agent appears to be useful for the treatment of cardiogenic shock and left ventricular failure. It probably merits consideration in patients who have failed to respond to other agents or when dysrhythmias develop. It may be helpful when left ventricular dysfunction is a result of treatment with beta-blockers. Hyperglycemia is a side-effect of the drug.

2. Vasodilators—Vasodilators are used to lower left ventricular afterload, which decreases myocardial oxygen consumption. Their use is limited by their hypotensive effect, which may compound the difficulties associated with peripheral oxygen delivery.

a. **Nitroprusside**—Nitroprusside decreases both afterload and preload. When nitroprusside is used optimally, the increase in left ventricular ejection fraction partially offsets the decrease in systemic vascular resistance. Therapy begins with a dose of 5– 10 μg/min and is advanced in increments of 2.5–5 μg/min every 10 minutes until an increase in cardiac output is noted. The dose should be reduced if systolic blood pressure falls below 90 mm Hg. Nitroprusside may produce an intracoronary steal that may aggravate areas of ischemia. The drug is metabolized to cyanide and subsequently to thiocyanate. Doses above 3 μg/min may lead to toxicity, especially when the drug is used for more than 3 days. Free cyanide ions combine with cytochromes, leading to anaerobic metabolism and increased lactate levels. This results in a metabolic acidosis that eventually culminates in confusion, hyperreflexia, and coma. Thiocyanate levels should be monitored and not permitted to rise above 10 mg/dL. Prophylactic infusion of hydroxocobalamin may avert toxicity by combining with cyanide to form cyanocobalamin.

b. **Nitroglycerin**—Nitroglycerin is a nitrate derivative whose greatest effect is preload reduction, which reflexly decreases left ventricular filling. It has the additional advantage of dilating the coronary vasculature and is the drug of choice when cardiogenic shock is due to ischemia. Nitroglycerin is also effective in the treatment of acute valvular incompetence. Care must be exercised to ensure that patients are not hypovolemic prior to its administration, because the increased venous capacity will decrease venous return and further lower the cardiac output. The normal starting dose is 10 μg/min, which can be increased by 10 μg/min every 5–10 minutes to a total dose of 50–100 μg/min. Doses as high as 400 μg/min can be tolerated for several days.

D. Other Modalities

The management of acute myocardial infarction is discussed in Chapter 22. Newer modalities available to improve cardiac function after infarction include thrombolytic therapy, percutaneous angioplasty, balloon pumping, and left ventricular assist devices. Emergency coronary artery bypass grafting is an option for patients who fail to respond to other forms of treatment.

Prognosis

Fulminant cardiogenic shock continues to carry a mortality rate of 90% when only pharmacologic therapy is used. Application of percutaneous transluminal coronary angioplasty, left ventricular assist devices, and early surgical revascularization may help improve this outcome.

Farmer JA: Cardiogenic shock. In: *Critical Care.* Civetta JM, Taylor RW, Kirby RR (editors). Lippincott, 1992.

Handler CE: Cardiogenic shock. Postgrad Med J 1985;61:705–12.

Holcroft JW, Wisner DH: Shock and acute pulmonary failure in surgical patients. In: *Current Surgical Diagnosis & Treatment,* 9th ed. Way LW (editor). Appleton & Lange, 1991.

Mueller HS: Inotropic agents in the treatment of cardiogenic shock. World J Surg 1985;9:3–10.

CARDIAC COMPRESSIVE SHOCK

ESSENTIALS OF DIAGNOSIS

- *Hypotension with tachycardia.*
- *Oliguria.*
- *Mental status changes.*
- *Distended neck veins.*

General Considerations

Cardiac compressive shock is a low-output state that occurs when the heart or great veins are compressed. Compression either impedes the return of blood to the heart or prevents effective pumping action of the heart itself. Pericardial tamponade is due to fluid within the pericardial sac that constricts the cardiac chambers and prevents them from filling properly. This may occur acutely after penetrating trauma with laceration of a coronary artery, or it may be progressive with chronic diseases such as uremia and connective tissue disorders. Distention of the abdomen with elevation of the diaphragm compresses the heart and may produce a form of shock. Positive end-expiratory pressure used with mechanical ventilation increases the intrathoracic pressure, which both collapses the superior and inferior vena cava and reduces the transmural pressure gradient, thereby decreasing cardiac filling. In similar fashion, tension pneumothorax increases the intrathoracic pressure and decreases venous return.

Clinical Features

A. Symptoms and Signs

Signs associated with poor peripheral perfusion such as hypotension, tachycardia, cool extremities, oliguria, and altered mental status are usually present. The presence of distended neck veins is central to the diagnosis, though they may be absent if the patient is hypovolemic. When tension pneumothorax is the cause, hyperresonance is noted on thoracic percussion, breath sounds are absent on the affected side, and the mediastinum is shifted away from the involved chest. Displacement of the trachea in association with distended neck veins is pathognomonic of tension pneumothorax. For patients who are breathing spontaneously, inspiration increases the degree of venous distention (Kussmaul's sign). Paradoxic pulse may also occur with spontaneous breathing and consists of a decrease in systolic pressure of more than 10 mm Hg with inspiration.

When cardiac compressive shock occurs after injury, penetrating trauma to the chest is usually present. Pericardial tamponade is uncommon after blunt injuries. Patients admitted for exacerbations of chronic disease often have a history of pericardial effusion. When mechanical ventilation is used, cardiac compressive shock occurs because (1) the inflated lungs compress the superior and inferior vena cava, (2) the right atrium and ventricle are compressed, and (3) expansion of the lungs compresses the pulmonary vasculature and increases the resistance to right ventricular ejection. Hypotension and tachycardia worsen in these patients as PEEP is increased. The correlation between the two may not be apparent at first, though careful examination of the patient's flowsheet will reveal changes in hemodynamics that correspond to ventilator manipulations.

B. Hemodynamic Monitoring

Central venous pressure is increased, as are pulmonary artery and pulmonary capillary wedge pressures. Equalization of central venous pressure, pulmonary artery, and pulmonary capillary wedge pressures strongly suggests pericardial tamponade.

C. Imaging Studies

Upright posteroanterior chest radiographs may show an enlarged cardiac shadow, but this is nonspecific. If tension pneumothorax is suspected, treatment must not be delayed while x-rays are obtained. If an incidental chest radiograph is available, it will reveal hyperlucency of one or both hemithoraces with displacement of the mediastinal structures to the contralateral side. Transesophageal two-dimensional echocardiography is very sensitive and can be used to establish the diagnosis in nonemergent situations. Treatment of suspected decompensated traumatic pericardial tamponade should never be postponed while awaiting imaging studies.

Differential Diagnosis

Primary cardiogenic shock without compression presents the major differential dilemma because both types present with low cardiac output and high venous pressure. An acute myocardial infarction or progressive deterioration in a critically ill patient suggests cardiogenic shock. Most patients who develop tension pneumothorax or pericardial tamponade after injury will have had the diagnosis established and therapy instituted before arrival in the critical care unit. Missed injuries occasionally occur and must be differentiated from traumatic air embolism to the coronary arteries. The latter usually causes severe dysrhythmias and a rapid downhill course.

Treatment

A. Fluid Resuscitation

Rapid fluid infusion may transiently compensate for the decrease in ventricular filling. Central venous pressure cannot be used to guide such infusion, because central venous pressure will always be elevated prior to the administration of fluid.

B. Operative Treatment

Surgical decompression of the offending site is indicated. For tension pneumothorax, immediate insertion of a large-bore intravenous catheter into the affected hemithorax will rapidly release the increased pressure. After pulse and blood pressure return to normal, this small catheter can be replaced with a larger tube thoracostomy connected to a chest evacuation device. Placement of the smaller catheter should never be delayed pending procurement and placement of a more definitive thoracostomy tube. If cardiac compression is due to gastric distention, placement of a nasogastric tube may be helpful. When distention is due to other causes, surgical exploration is usually warranted. Pericardial decompression should be performed for pericardial tamponade. Reduction of ventilatory pressures and augmentation of the circulating blood volume, if possible, usually correct compression resulting from the use of PEEP.

Respiratory Failure

12

Darryl Y. Sue, MD, & David A. Lewis, MD

PATHOPHYSIOLOGY OF RESPIRATORY FAILURE

Respiratory failure is inability of the respiratory system to maintain a normal state of gas exchange from the atmosphere to the cells as required by the body. Simply, the role of the respiratory system is to maintain normal arterial blood P_{O_2}, P_{CO_2}, and pH. Respiratory failure can result from disorders of the lungs, heart, chest wall, respiratory muscles, and central ventilatory control mechanisms. While not considered respiratory failure, dysfunctions of the heart, the pulmonary and systemic circulations, the oxygen-carrying capacity of the blood, and systemic capillaries have important implications for patients with respiratory failure.

Definition

Respiratory failure is present (1) if arterial P_{O_2} (Pa_{O_2}) is < 60 mm Hg, or (2) if arterial P_{CO_2} (Pa_{CO_2}) is > 45 mm Hg, except when the elevation in P_{CO_2} is compensation for metabolic alkalosis. A Pa_{O_2} < 60 mm Hg, indicating hypoxemic respiratory failure, is valid during room air breathing (inspired O_2 fraction [F_{IO_2}] = 0.21), but hypoxemia while breathing supplemental oxygen also indicates respiratory failure. An exception to the rule that Pa_{CO_2} > 45 mm Hg defines hypercapnic respiratory failure may occur during metabolic acidosis. Patients with metabolic acidosis normally decrease Pa_{CO_2} as compensation for low pH, but if Pa_{CO_2} is abnormally elevated even though below 45 mm Hg during metabolic acidosis, this may also be considered respiratory failure of the hypercapnic type.

Effectiveness & Efficiency of the Respiratory System

It is useful to distinguish between the *effectiveness* and the *efficiency* of the respiratory system in maintaining arterial blood gases. An arterial P_{O_2} of 100 mm Hg indicates effective oxygenation of the arterial blood. Effective elimination of CO_2 would be evidenced by an arterial P_{CO_2} of 40 mm Hg if this Pa_{CO_2} is consistent with an acceptable acid-base status. On the other hand, there is an obvious difference between two patients who each have an arterial P_{O_2} of 100 mm Hg if the first patient is breathing room air (F_{IO_2} = 0.21) and the other is breathing 100% O_2 (F_{IO_2} = 1.0). The first patient is exchanging oxygen more efficiently from the atmosphere to the arterial blood than the latter. Pa_{O_2} measures the effectiveness of oxygenation; the relationship between inspired oxygen concentration and Pa_{O_2} is a marker of the efficiency of oxygenation.

Arterial P_{CO_2} is a measure of the effectiveness of ventilation. Two patients who each have an arterial P_{CO_2} of 40 mm Hg have equally effective ventilation. But if one of them needs a higher minute ventilation (respired gas volume in 1 minute) than the other, the patient requiring the higher minute ventilation is less efficiently eliminating CO_2 than the one with the lower minute ventilation. Thus, Pa_{CO_2} is a measure of the effectiveness of ventilation; the relationship between Pa_{CO_2} and minute ventilation ($\dot{V}_E$) reflects the efficiency of ventilation. Measurement of the degree of inefficiency of oxygenation and ventilation is discussed below.

Classification of Respiratory Failure

One useful classification of respiratory failure separates disorders that affect the lungs (including airways, alveolar spaces, interstitium, and pulmonary circulation) from those that affect primarily the nonlung components of the respiratory system. Respiratory failure from diseases that directly affect the lungs almost always presents with hypoxemia, but these patients may or may not have hypercapnia depending on the specific type of disease and its severity. Examples include bacterial or viral pneumonia, aspiration of gastric contents, acute respiratory distress syndrome, pulmonary embolism, asthma, and interstitial lung diseases. Alteration of the anatomic and physiologic relationship between air in the alveoli and blood in the pulmonary capillaries is responsible for hypoxemia.

Respiratory failure resulting from disorders of the respiratory system other than the lungs usually causes hypercapnia. Examples include diseases that result in weakness of the respiratory muscles, central nervous system diseases that disrupt ventilatory control, and conditions that affect chest wall shape or size, such as kyphoscoliosis. In these kinds of hypercapnic respiratory failure, the lungs may be normal, and hypoxemia out of proportion to hypercapnia most likely is a marker of additional lung involvement. An example might be a patient with neuromuscular weakness from myasthenia gravis initially presenting with hypercapnic respiratory failure but who subsequently develops pneumonia from inability to clear tracheal secretions. At this point, the patient may add hypoxemic respiratory failure to the original hypercapnia.

HYPERCAPNIC RESPIRATORY FAILURE

By definition, patients with hypercapnic respiratory failure have abnormally high arterial PCO_2 levels ($PaCO_2$). Because CO_2 is elevated in the alveolar spaces, O_2 is displaced from the alveoli and arterial PO_2 decreases. Thus, these patients usually have both hypercapnia and hypoxemia unless the inspired gas is enriched with oxygen. The lungs themselves may or may not be abnormal in patients who have hypercapnic respiratory failure, especially if the primary disease affects nonlung parts of the respiratory system such as the chest wall, respiratory muscles, or brain stem. However, severe chronic obstructive lung disease not infrequently leads to hypercapnic respiratory failure, and some patients with severe asthma, end-stage pulmonary fibrosis, and severe ARDS can develop hypercapnia.

Physiologic Considerations

A. Alveolar Hypoventilation

In the steady state, a patient produces a quantity of CO_2 from metabolic processes each minute and must eliminate that amount of CO_2 from the lungs each minute. If the minute output of CO_2 ($\dot{V}CO_2$) exchanges into the gas-exchanging spaces of the lungs, the fractional concentration of CO_2 in the alveolar space is as shown below:

$$F_ACO_2 = \frac{\dot{V}CO_2\ (\text{L/min STPD})}{\dot{V}_A\ (\text{L/min BTPS}) \times 0.826}$$

where F_ACO_2 is the fractional concentration of CO_2 in the alveoli, $\dot{V}_A$ is the volume of air exchanging in the alveoli during that minute (alveolar ventilation), and 0.826 adjusts for temperature and water vapor. The sum of the partial pressures of individual gases is equal to the total pressure, so the fraction of alveolar gas that is CO_2 can also be written as follows:

$$F_ACO_2 = \frac{P_ACO_2\ (\text{mm Hg})}{P_B\ (\text{mm Hg})}$$

where P_ACO_2 is the alveolar partial pressure of CO_2 and P_B is barometric pressure. Because alveolar PCO_2 cannot be measured, arterial PCO_2 ($PaCO_2$) is usually substituted. Substituting and rearranging the equation above

$$\dot{V}CO_2\ (\text{L/min}) = PaCO_2\ (\text{mm Hg}) \times \dot{V}_A\ (\text{L/min}) \times \frac{1}{863}$$

where 863 includes factors that adjust for $\dot{V}CO_2$ at standard temperature and pressure, dry (STPD); for $\dot{V}_A$ at body temperature and pressure, saturated (BTPS); and for $PaCO_2$ in mm Hg. For constant CO_2 output, the relationship between $PaCO_2$ and $\dot{V}_A$ describes a "ventilatory hyperbola," in which $PaCO_2$ and $\dot{V}_A$ are inversely related. Thus, hypercapnia is always equivalent to alveolar hypoventilation, and hypocapnia is synonymous with alveolar hyperventilation. Because alveolar ventilation cannot be measured, estimation of alveolar ventilation can only be made by using arterial PCO_2 and this formula.

B. Minute Ventilation

In a patient with alveolar hypoventilation, $\dot{V}_A$ is reduced (and $PaCO_2$ is increased). Although $\dot{V}_A$ cannot be directly measured, the total amount of gas moving into and out of the lungs each minute can be easily measured. This is defined as the minute ventilation ($\dot{V}_E$, L/min). A useful physiologic concept is to assume that $\dot{V}_E$ is the sum of the $\dot{V}_A$ (the portion of $\dot{V}_E$ participating in gas exchange) and any wasted or dead-space ventilation ($\dot{V}_D$):

$$\dot{V}_E = \dot{V}_A + \dot{V}_D \text{ and } \dot{V}_A = \dot{V}_E - \dot{V}_D$$

Substituting, $\dot{V}_A = f \times V_A$; $\dot{V}_E = f \times V_T$; and $\dot{V}_D = f \times V_D$—where f is the respiratory frequency, V_T is tidal volume, and V_D is dead space volume:

$$V_A = V_E \times \left(1 - \frac{V_D}{V_T}\right),\ \text{where} \frac{V_D}{V_T} = \frac{\text{Dead space}}{\text{Tidal volume}} \text{ratio}$$

Substituting $\dot{V}_E \times (1 - V_D/V_T)$ for $\dot{V}_A$ above:

$$VCO_2 = PaCO_2 \times V_E \times \frac{(1 - V_D/V_T)}{863}$$

V_D/V_T reflects the degree of inefficiency of ventilation of the lungs. In a resting normal subject, V_D/V_T is about 0.30, meaning that about 30% of the minute ventilation is not participating in gas exchange. In most lung diseases, the wasted proportion of $\dot{V}_E$ increases, so V_D/V_T rises. From the above formula for a constant V_D/V_T and constant $\dot{V}CO_2$, the relationship of $PaCO_2$

and $\dot{V}_E$ is described by a hyperbola transposed upward from the hyperbola described by the relationship between Pa_{CO_2} and $\dot{V}_A$. For different values of V_D/V_T, these relationships are described by a family of hyperbolic curves (Figure 12–1). These curves are useful in estimating V_D/V_T from measurement of Pa_{CO_2} and $\dot{V}_E$, or they can be used to determine the appropriate change in $\dot{V}_E$ needed to cause a desired change in Pa_{CO_2}.

C. Mechanisms of Hypercapnia

Hypercapnia (alveolar hypoventilation) occurs when $\dot{V}_E$ is abnormally low, when $\dot{V}_E$ is normal or high but V_D/V_T is abnormally increased, or when both conditions are met. It is emphasized that the term "hypoventilation" refers to alveolar hypoventilation, and for that reason hypercapnia may be present even though the patient's minute ventilation is greater than normal if V_D/V_T is abnormally high or CO_2 output is increased (exercise or other increased metabolic rate).

Alveolar dead space and the dead space/tidal volume ratio are useful physiologic concepts that may or may not have anatomic counterparts. The trachea and airways serve as conduits for gas moving into and out of the lungs during the respiratory cycle but do not participate in gas exchange with the pulmonary capillary blood. These spaces make up the anatomic dead space. An artificial airway or part of a mechanical ventilator circuit that is common to both inspiratory and expiratory pathways also contributes to anatomic dead space. However, in patients with lung disease, most of the increase in total dead space consists of "physiologic dead space," in which regional ventilation exceeds the amount of regional blood flow (ventilation-perfusion [$\dot{V}/\dot{Q}$] mismatching). While $\dot{V}/\dot{Q}$ mismatching is usually considered as a mechanism of hypoxemia rather than hypercapnia, it theoretically should cause elevated Pa_{CO_2} as well. However, in all but severe instances of $\dot{V}/\dot{Q}$ mismatching, hypercapnia stimulates increased ventilation, returning Pa_{CO_2} to normal. Thus, $\dot{V}/\dot{Q}$ mismatching does not usually result in hypercapnia but in normocapnia with increased $\dot{V}_E$. As can be seen in Figure 12–1, increased $\dot{V}_E$ in the face of normal Pa_{CO_2} indicates increased V_D/V_T—in this case, an increase in physiologic dead space.

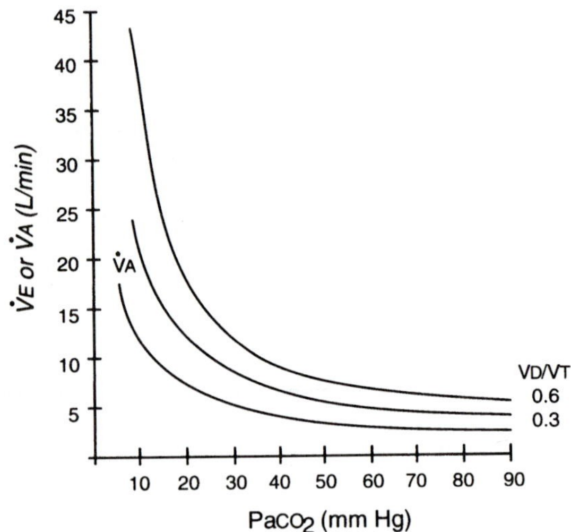

Figure 12–1. Alveolar ventilation ($\dot{V}_A$) or minute ventilation ($\dot{V}_E$) as a function of Pa_{CO_2} for a constant CO_2 output of 200 mL/min. Increased Pa_{CO_2} (hypercapnia) is due to alveolar hypoventilation; decreased Pa_{CO_2} (hypocapnia) is the same as alveolar hyperventilation. The other two curves show the relationship of $\dot{V}_E$ and Pa_{CO_2} for normal dead space/tidal volume ratio ($V_D/V_T = 0.3$) and abnormal dead space/tidal volume ratio ($V_D/V_T = 0.6$).

Clinical Features

Acute hypercapnia acts largely on the central nervous system (Table 12–1). Increased arterial Pa_{CO_2} is a central nervous system depressant, but the mechanism is primarily through a fall of pH in the cerebrospinal fluid resulting from acute elevation of Pa_{CO_2}. Because CO_2 freely and rapidly diffuses into the cerebrospinal fluid, pH falls rapidly and severely with acute hypercapnia. With chronic elevation of Pa_{CO_2}, however, the increase of Pa_{CO_2} has been present long enough to allow for serum and cerebrospinal fluid bicarbonate to increase in compensation for the chronic respiratory acidosis. This explains why the low pH rather than the absolute level of Pa_{CO_2} best correlates with altered mental status and other clinical changes.

Symptoms of hypercapnia may overlap those of hypoxemia. In addition, while hypercapnia stimulates

Table 12–1. Clinical manifestations of hypercapnia and hypoxemia.

Hypercapnia	Hypoxemia
Somnolence	Anxiety
Lethargy	Tachycardia
Coma	Tachypnea
Asterixis	Diaphoresis
Restlessness	Arrhythmias
Tremor	Altered mental status
Slurred speech	Confusion
Headache	Cyanosis
Papilledema	Hypertension
	Hypotension
	Seizures
	Lactic acidosis

ventilation in normal subjects, patients with hypercapnia may have either decreased or increased minute ventilation depending on the primary disorder leading to respiratory failure. Thus, dyspnea, tachypnea, and hyperpnea may be associated with hypercapnic respiratory failure just as often as bradypnea and hypopnea.

Patients with acute hypercapnic respiratory failure should be examined to determine the mechanism. The major differential diagnostic point is between hypercapnic respiratory failure due to lung disease versus nonlung disorders. Patients with lung disease will often have hypoxemia out of proportion to the degree of hypercapnia. This can be assessed using the alveolar-arterial P_{O_2} difference. However, patients with nonlung problems may have secondary hypoxemia as the effects of neuromuscular weakness (for example) result in atelectasis or aspiration pneumonia. Disorders of the lung—in contrast to disorders of other components of the respiratory system—are associated with increased V_D/V_T and, therefore, often with elevated $\dot{V}_E$ and respiratory frequency. However, patients with respiratory muscle weakness also may be tachypneic. The effects of hypercapnia and hypoxemia may mask neurologic disorders, overmedication with sedatives, myxedema, or head trauma. Alteration of mental status may make it difficult to assess muscle strength, and the strength of muscles in the extremities may not correlate with respiratory muscle strength.

HYPOXEMIC RESPIRATORY FAILURE

Hypoxemic respiratory failure is much more commonly encountered than hypercapnic respiratory failure. These patients have abnormally low arterial P_{O_2} but normal or low Pa_{CO_2}. The latter distinguishes them from hypercapnic respiratory failure, in which the primary problem is alveolar hypoventilation. Outside of unusual environments in which the atmosphere has a severely reduced amount of oxygen, such as high altitude or when oxygen has been replaced with other gases, hypoxemic respiratory failure indicates disease affecting the lung parenchyma or pulmonary circulation. Examples of common clinical situations in which hypoxemia without elevated Pa_{CO_2} are seen include pneumonia, aspiration of gastric contents, pulmonary embolism, asthma, and acute respiratory distress syndrome (ARDS).

Physiologic Considerations

A. Hypoxemia and Hypoxia

The term "hypoxemia" most often denotes low P_{O_2} in arterial blood (Pa_{O_2}), but it can be used in reference to capillary, venous, or pulmonary capillary P_{O_2} as well. It may also be used to signify low blood O_2 content or reduced saturation of hemoglobin with oxygen. Hypoxemia should be distinguished from hypoxia, which generally means decreased O_2 delivery to the tissues or the effects of decreased tissue O_2 delivery. While hypoxia will result from severe hypoxemia, hypoxia can also be a consequence of decreased O_2 delivery due to low cardiac output, anemia, septic shock, or carbon monoxide poisoning, in which the arterial P_{O_2} may be normal or even elevated.

B. Mechanisms of Hypoxemia

The physiologic mechanism of arterial hypoxemia has important implications for identifying the type of lung disease and the response to therapy with oxygen or other treatment. Five distinct mechanisms of hypoxemia can be identified, but these five can be divided conceptually into two major groups (Table 12–2): (1) decreased alveolar P_{O_2}; and (2) increased influence of venous admixture.

Table 12–2. Mechanisms of hypoxemia.

Mechanism	Pa_{CO_2} ($P_{A_{CO_2}}$)	$P_{A_{O_2}}$	$P(A-a)_{O_2}$[1]	P_{O_2} on 100% O_2 (mm Hg)[2]	Example
Alveolar P_{O_2}					
↓ Inspired P_{O_2}	↓	↓	Normal[3]	> 550	High altitude.
Hypoventilation	↑	↓	Normal	> 550	Neuromuscular disease, obesity-hypoventilation syndrome.
Venous admixture					
Right-to-left shunt	Normal or low	Normal	Increased	< 550	ARDS, septal defect.
V/Q mismatching	Normal or low	Normal	Increased	> 550	Pneumonia, asthma, COPD.
Diffusion limitation	Normal or low	Normal	Increased	> 550	Alveolar proteinosis.

[1] $P(A-a)_{O_2}$ on room air. Normal < 15–20 mm Hg.
[2] Pa_{O_2} while breathing 100% O_2 distinguishes right-to-left shunt from other mechanisms.
[3] $P(A-a)_{O_2}$ calculated using $P_{A_{O_2}}$ from alveolar gas equation.

Mechanisms of arterial hypoxemia can be demonstrated by analysis of the possible extremes of oxygenation of the arterial blood. If desaturated systemic venous blood returning to the lungs gained no oxygen during transit through the lungs, the arterial blood would have the same oxygen content and partial pressure as the systemic venous blood (obviously a situation incompatible with life). Systemic venous blood PO_2 ($P\bar{V}O_2$) determines the lower limit for arterial PO_2. On the other hand, if all of the desaturated venous blood passing through the lungs reaches equilibrium with gases in the alveolar space, then $PO_2 = PAO_2$. Thus, alveolar PO_2 (PAO_2) determines the hypothetical upper limit for arterial PO_2. If all of the desaturated venous blood passing through the lungs reaches equilibrium with gases in the alveolar space, then $PO_2 = PAO_2$. Therefore, all possible values of arterial PO_2 must be between $P\bar{V}O_2$ and PAO_2.

Arterial hypoxemia is always the result either of decreased alveolar PO_2 or of a greater quantity or an increased amount of desaturated venous blood (venous admixture) mixing with pulmonary capillary blood (Table 12–2). In many patients with hypoxemic respiratory failure, both of these mechanisms play a role.

C. Decreased Alveolar PO_2

The total pressure in the alveolar space is the sum of PO_2, PCO_2, PH_2O, and PN_2. If PH_2O and PN_2 do not change appreciably, any increase in $PACO_2$ must cause a fall in PAO_2. Thus, alveolar hypoventilation causes decreased PAO_2, which must result in decreased PaO_2, assuming that the arterial blood is in equilibrium with the gases in the alveolar space. The alveolar gas equation, in simplified form, shows the relationship between alveolar PO_2 and PCO_2:

$$PAO_2 = FIO_2 \times PB - \frac{PACO_2}{R}$$

where FIO_2 is the oxygen fraction of the inspired gas, PB is the barometric pressure, and R is the respiratory gas exchange ratio, indicating the steady-state ratio of CO_2 entering and O_2 leaving the alveolar space. In practice, arterial PCO_2 is used as an approximate value of alveolar PCO_2 ($PACO_2$). PAO_2 decreases in the presence of increased $PACO_2$. Thus, alveolar hypoventilation is a cause of hypoxemia (reduced PaO_2).

The alveolar gas equation also indicates that hypoxemia must occur if total barometric pressure is reduced, such as at high altitude, or if FIO_2 is low (such as when a person is breathing a gas mixture in which some of the oxygen has been replaced by another gas). This is again because PAO_2 falls. In hypoxemia due to reduced PAO_2 alone, the decrease in PaO_2 approximately equals the fall in PAO_2, and the difference between PAO_2 and PaO_2 does not appreciably change. The alveolar-arterial PO_2 difference is normal in hypoxemia due to hypoventilation alone.

D. Venous Admixture

The other causes of hypoxemia result from increased amounts of deoxygenated venous blood reaching the arterial blood without becoming fully oxygenated by exposure to the alveolar gas. The alveolar-arterial PO_2 difference ($P[A–a]O_2$) is increased in the presence of hypoxemia because of increased venous admixture. During room air breathing, $P(A–a)O_2$ is normally between 10 mm and 20 mm Hg, increasing with age and when the subject is in the upright position.

During room air breathing, $FIO_2 = 0.21$; if $R = 0.8$, $PaCO_2 = 40$ mm Hg, and $PaO_2 = 55$ mm Hg, then

$$PAO_2 = (0.21 \times 713) - \frac{40}{0.8} = 150 - 50 = 100 \text{ mm Hg}$$

and

$$P(A-a)O_2 = 100 - 55 = 45 \text{ mm Hg}$$

In this example, arterial hypoxemia is present ($PaO_2 < 60$ mm Hg) and $P(A–a)O_2$ is increased (> 20 mm Hg). It should be concluded that hypoxemia is due to one of the causes of increased venous admixture.

1. Right-to-left shunt—If some systemic venous blood bypasses the alveoli and then mixes with blood that did go through the lungs, the resultant arterial mixture of systemic venous and pulmonary capillary blood must have a PO_2 between PAO_2 and $P\bar{V}O_2$. The exact PO_2 depends on the proportion of blood that bypassed the lungs and the values of PAO_2 and $P\bar{V}O_2$. This mechanism of hypoxemia is known as right-to-left shunt, one of the mechanisms of hypoxemia due to increased venous admixture. Right-to-left shunt may occur because of complete collapse or atelectasis of a lung or lobe in which blood flow is maintained or may be seen in patients with congenital heart disease in which there is a right-to-left shunt through a cardiac septal defect. Patients with ARDS may have such severe pulmonary edema, localized atelectasis, or alveolar collapse that severe right-to-left shunt occurs. Clues to the presence of right-to-left shunt include severe hypoxemia while breathing room air, only very small increases in PaO_2 when supplemental oxygen is administered, a need to give $FIO_2 > 0.6$ to achieve an acceptable PaO_2, and $PaO_2 < 550$ mm Hg while breathing 100% O_2. By convention, when $PaO_2 < 550$ mm Hg while breathing 100% O_2, right-to-left shunt is confirmed.

2. Ventilation-perfusion mismatching—A second cause of hypoxemia due to venous admixture is ventilation-perfusion ($\dot{V}/\dot{Q}$) mismatching. This mechanism, sometimes termed $\dot{V}/\dot{Q}$ inequality, is the most frequent cause of hypoxemia. In contrast to right-to-left shunt, hypoxemia in $\dot{V}/\dot{Q}$ mismatching does not result from venous blood completely bypassing ventilated areas of lung. Rather, some regions of the lungs have insufficient ventilation for the amount of blood flow, whereas others have excessive ventilation for the amount of regional blood flow. Pulmonary capillary blood draining those parts of the lungs that have relative "hypoventilation" is less well oxygenated than normal and contributes to hypoxemia of the arterial blood. The effects of $\dot{V}/\dot{Q}$ mismatching on gas exchange are often quite complicated, but for practical purposes any lung disease that alters the distribution of ventilation or blood flow can result in $\dot{V}/\dot{Q}$ mismatching. Thus, hypoxemia due to $\dot{V}/\dot{Q}$ mismatching is seen in asthma and other chronic obstructive lung diseases in which variations in airway resistance tend to distribute ventilation unevenly. $\dot{V}/\dot{Q}$ mismatching also contributes to hypoxemia in pulmonary vascular diseases such as pulmonary thromboembolism, in which the distribution of perfusion is altered. In contrast to right-to-left shunt, most patients with $\dot{V}/\dot{Q}$ mismatching respond dramatically to supplemental oxygen therapy. A clue to $\dot{V}/\dot{Q}$ mismatching, therefore, is that the $Pa{O_2}$ can be relatively easily brought up to acceptable values with administration of supplemental oxygen.

3. Diffusion limitation—The third mechanism of hypoxemia due to venous admixture is diffusion limitation of O_2 transfer. This is an unusual cause of hypoxemia, and the basis for this mechanism is often misunderstood. Normally, there is more than sufficient time for venous blood passing through the lungs to become fully equilibrated with the gases in the alveoli. Rarely, however, pulmonary capillary blood passes so quickly through the lungs that there is insufficient time for pulmonary capillary $P{O_2}$ to equilibrate with alveolar $P{O_2}$, resulting in hypoxemia. This is a form of venous admixture because the hypoxemia results from the influence of deoxygenated venous blood. Diffusion limitation resulting in hypoxemia can theoretically occur if $PA{O_2}$ is very low—so that the diffusion of oxygen across the alveolar-capillary barrier is slowed—or if the transit time for pulmonary capillary blood is very short. There are few diseases in which diffusion limitation for oxygen transfer is thought to be a major cause of hypoxemia. For example, hypoxemia in patients with pulmonary vascular disease may be due to diffusion limitation because of decreased mean transit time, especially if cardiac output is increased. Pulmonary alveolar proteinosis—a disease in which the alveolar spaces are filled with a homogeneous protein and lipid fluid—may slow diffusion of oxygen sufficiently to cause hypoxemia. In most other lung diseases presenting with hypoxemia, $\dot{V}/\dot{Q}$ mismatching and right-to-left shunt explain hypoxemia more often than diffusion limitation.

Clinical Features

Manifestations of hypoxemic respiratory failure are the result of a combination of features of arterial hypoxemia and tissue hypoxia (Table 12–1). Arterial hypoxemia increases ventilation by stimulation of carotid body chemoreceptors, leading to dyspnea, tachypnea, hyperpnea, and, usually, hyperventilation. The degree of ventilatory response depends on the ability to sense hypoxemia and the capacity of the respiratory system to respond. In hypoxemic patients with severe lung disease or ventilatory limitation, there may be little or no increase in ventilation and absence of hyperventilation. In patients who lack carotid body function, there will be no ventilatory response to hypoxemia. There may be cyanosis, especially marked in the distal extremities but also centrally prominent around the mucous membranes and lips. The degree of cyanosis depends on the hemoglobin concentration and the patient's state of perfusion.

Other effects attributable to hypoxemia are due to inadequate supply of oxygen to the tissues, or hypoxia. Hypoxia causes a shift to anaerobic metabolism, which is accompanied by generation of lactic acid. Increased levels of blood lactic acid may further stimulate ventilation. Mild early hypoxia may cause impaired mental performance, especially for complex tasks or abstract thinking. More severe hypoxia can cause much more severe alteration of mental status, including somnolence, coma, seizures, and permanent hypoxic brain damage. Sympathetic nervous system activity is increased, and this contributes to tachycardia, diaphoresis, and systemic vasoconstriction, leading to hypertension. More severe hypoxia, however, can lead to bradycardia, vasodilation, and hypotension as well as myocardial ischemia, infarction, arrhythmias, and cardiac failure.

Manifestations of hypoxemic respiratory failure are magnified in the presence of impaired tissue oxygen delivery. Patients with reduced cardiac output, anemia, or circulatory abnormalities in conjunction with arterial hypoxemia can be expected to have global and regional tissue hypoxia at less severe degrees of hypoxemia. Examples of this would be the increased risk of myocardial ischemia from hypoxemia in a patient with coexisting coronary artery atherosclerosis or a patient with hypovolemic shock who shows evidence of lactic acidosis in the presence of mild arterial hypoxemia.

OXYGEN DELIVERY & TISSUE HYPOXIA

Adequate O_2 delivery to the tissues is the most important function of the respiratory system, and this aspect requires normal function of the lungs, heart, and circulation. Recognition and treatment of compromised systemic O_2 delivery should be primary goals in management of respiratory failure in addition to correcting abnormalities of arterial blood gases.

Physiologic Considerations

A. Oxygen Delivery

Systemic O_2 delivery is the product of arterial O_2 concentration (mL O_2/L blood) and cardiac output (L/min). This calculation does not help determine whether the blood and O_2 are distributed to organs in proportion to their needs, so that even normal or high O_2 delivery may be insufficient under certain conditions such as shock, sepsis, or end-stage liver disease.

$$\frac{O_2\ \text{delivery}}{(\text{mL/min})} = \frac{\text{Arterial } O_2\ \text{content}}{(Ca{O_2},\ \text{mL } O_2/\text{L blood})} \times \frac{\text{Cardiac output}}{(Q,\ \text{L/min})}$$

where CaO_2, mL O_2/L blood = [O_2 saturation × hemoglobin, g/dL × 1.34 mL O_2/g hemoglobin + PaO_2, mm Hg × 0.003 mL O_2/mm Hg/dL] × 10.

In normal subjects at rest, normal arterial O_2 concentration is about 200 mL O_2/L blood (O_2 saturation 97%, hemoglobin 15 g/dL of blood, PaO_2 100 mm Hg). Resting cardiac output is about 5 L/min, resulting in normal O_2 delivery = 1000 mL O_2/min.

B. Causes of Decreased Oxygen Delivery

Factors included in the formula for O_2 delivery can be examined to determine pathologic states that result in potentially decreased O_2 delivery. First, arterial O_2 concentration can be reduced as the result of decreased O_2 saturation of hemoglobin from arterial hypoxemia (decreased PaO_2) or a rightward-shifted oxyhemoglobin dissociation curve (acidemia, hyperthermia, or hemoglobinopathy). Anemia is an important factor because O_2 concentration is largely the product of hemoglobin concentration and O_2 saturation. A decrease in hemoglobin from 12 g/dL to 8 g/dL by blood loss decreases O_2 concentration and O_2 delivery by 33%—considerably more than most changes in PaO_2 or O_2 saturation. Carbon monoxide, because of its high affinity for hemoglobin, displaces O_2 and reduces arterial O_2 concentration. In addition, the effect of carbon monoxide is to shift the oxyhemoglobin curve leftward, which, although it tends to increase O_2 concentration at any given PaO_2, causes problems in unloading O_2 at the tissue level.

Cardiac output is dependent on multiple factors, including adequate systemic venous return, right and left ventricular function, pulmonary and systemic resistance, and heart rate. Even in the absence of underlying intrinsic heart disease, patients with respiratory failure may have impaired or reduced cardiac output. Hypoxemia and acidosis have adverse effects on myocardial contractility or may result in tachycardia, bradycardia, or myocardial infarction. There is evidence that myocardial depression can be seen in conjunction with sepsis and septic shock, mediated through products of microorganisms or patient-produced cytokines, or other factors. Mechanical ventilation with positive pressure interacts in a number of ways with the heart and circulation. Although much of the decrease in cardiac output during positive-pressure ventilation is due to diminished systemic venous return, there is evidence that left ventricular diastolic compliance is altered, that pulmonary vascular resistance is increased, and that right and left ventricular afterload are affected. The degree and significance of interaction varies with the type and severity of respiratory failure and the type of mechanical ventilation.

C. Assessment of Oxygen Delivery

The assessment of adequacy of O_2 delivery remains a topic of debate. In normal subjects, total O_2 consumption of the body is independent of O_2 delivery over a wide range. Increasing or decreasing O_2 delivery (except at extremely low rates) by changing cardiac output or hemoglobin does not result in a parallel increase or decrease in O_2 consumption. However, in some patients with septic shock, ARDS, or other critical illness, O_2 consumption may become functionally dependent on O_2 delivery even when O_2 delivery is in the normal range. This finding has been taken to indicate that adequate O_2 delivery in a given patient cannot be assumed even when O_2 delivery is normal; an increase in O_2 consumption in response to increased O_2 delivery above normal indicates that the original O_2 delivery was in fact inadequate. To explain this finding, investigators have proposed that distribution of blood flow in the peripheral circulation is poorly matched to O_2 requirements of individual organs—a form of "distributive shock." In some studies, lactic acidosis has been associated with O_2 delivery dependency; this supports the concept of inadequate tissue oxygenation. In other studies, organ dysfunction is cited as evidence of hypoxia when O_2 consumption is no longer independent of O_2 delivery. On the other hand, some investigators believe that these findings are artifacts of measurements or do not reflect the responses of most patients with these disorders. There have been several studies suggesting that increasing O_2 delivery with resultant increased O_2 consumption has resulted in improved outcome from septic shock. Several other investigators, however, have been unable to find any difference in patient survival in critical illness by empirically increasing O_2 delivery. It is highly likely that this dependence of O_2 consumption on O_2 delivery is patient-specific. Therefore, attention should be paid to trying to identify evidence of inadequate O_2 delivery by monitoring renal, hepatic, cardiac, and other organ system functions.

TEMPERATURE & BLOOD GASES

The blood gas analyzer in the laboratory maintains the sample of blood at 37 °C while the PaO_2, $PaCO_2$, and pH are determined. For a given quantity of O_2 and CO_2 in an aliquot of blood, PaO_2 and $PaCO_2$ will change if the temperature of the blood changes. When the sample is cooled, PaO_2 and $PaCO_2$ decrease; when it is warmed, PaO_2 and $PaCO_2$ increase.

In patients with hypothermia or hyperthermia, some laboratories report "temperature-corrected" blood gases, ie, what the PaO_2 and $PaCO_2$ in the patient's blood would be if measured at the patient's actual temperature. These corrections are empirically determined and are easily derived from tables and nomograms or are automatically displayed by the analyzer.

However, temperature correction of a patient's blood gas results may lead to an incorrect clinical interpretation unless they are compared with temperature-corrected *normal* blood gas values. Arterial blood gases from a completely normal subject—free of lung disease or acid-base abnormalities—also change with temperature changes. For example, in a normal animal made hypothermic to 30 °C, the temperature-corrected PaO_2 and $PaCO_2$ decrease; and, because HCO_3^- remains constant, pH increases. If compared with customary normal values measured at 37 °C, interpretation of temperature-corrected PaO_2, $PaCO_2$, and pH would lead to an erroneous conclusion of hypoxemia and respiratory alkalosis. One approach to avoiding this problem is to use reference normal values at each temperature for comparison.

A preferable method is to report all blood gas values at the 37 °C at which the blood is analyzed regardless of the patient's actual temperature. These results can then be compared with normal values for PaO_2, $PaCO_2$, and pH determined at 37 °C. Interpretation using these values will be correct for both hypoxemia and acid-base status. Temperature correction of blood gases is unnecessarily complex and may be misleading if steps are not taken to provide corrected normal values.

Glenny R et al: Gas exchange in health: rest, exercise, aging. In: *Pulmonary and Peripheral Gas Exchange in Health and Disease.* Roca J, Rodriguez-Roisin R, Wagner PD (editors): Marcel Dekker, 2000.

Lumb AB: Distribution of pulmonary ventilation and perfusion. In: *Nunn's Applied Respiratory Physiology,* 5th ed. Lumb AB (editor). Butterworth Heinemann, 2000.

Roca J, Rodriguez-Roisin R: Distributions of alveolar ventilation and pulmonary blood flow. In: *Physiological Basis of Ventilatory Support.* Marini JJ, Slutsky AS (editors): Marcel Dekker, 1998.

Sassoon CSH, Mahutte CK: Work of breathing during mechanical ventilation. In: *Physiological Basis of Ventilatory Support.* Marini JJ, Slutsky AS (editors): Marcel Dekker, 1998.

West JB, Wagner PD: Ventilation, blood flow, and gas exchange. In: *Textbook of Respiratory Medicine,* 3rd ed. Murray JF, Nadel JA (editors): Saunders, 2000.

Williams AJ: ABC of oxygen. Assessing and interpreting arterial blood gases and acid-base balance. BMJ 1998;317:1213–6.

TREATMENT OF ACUTE RESPIRATORY FAILURE

Respiratory failure is treated by a combination of specific treatment directed at the underlying compromise of the respiratory system plus supportive care of oxygenation and ventilation. The general principles of support are similar regardless of the type of respiratory system disorder.

PHYSIOLOGIC BASIS OF TREATMENT

Hypercapnic Respiratory Failure

Because hypercapnia is synonymous with alveolar hypoventilation, supportive care restores alveolar ventilation to normal until the underlying disorder can be corrected. Alveolar ventilation can sometimes be improved by establishing an effective airway—suctioning to remove secretions, stimulation of cough, postural drainage, or chest percussion—or by establishing an artificial airway with an endotracheal tube or tracheostomy.

Mechanical assist devices may be necessary to achieve and maintain the desired alveolar ventilation until the primary problem is corrected. Although the mechanical ventilator can theoretically provide any desired amount of ventilation, care should be taken to correct hypercapnia judiciously in patients with chronic hypercapnia. This is because correction of $PaCO_2$ to normal in these patients can result in severe, life-threatening alkalemia since they have elevated serum bicarbonate levels as compensation.

Hypoxemia is often seen in patient with hypercapnic respiratory failure—especially those with lung disease—and administration of supplemental oxygen is often necessary. In some patients with hypercapnia, however, supplemental oxygen may be hazardous if not carefully adjusted and monitored. This group of patients with chronic lung disease (either obstructive or restrictive) or chest wall compromise (eg, kyphoscoliosis) appears to have particular insensitivity to hypercapnia as well as a dependence on hypoxemia to stimulate ventilation. If sufficient oxygen is given to overcome hypoxemia, ventilatory drive is subsequently blunted and the patient may hypoventilate further.

Patients with hypercapnic respiratory failure due to sedative drug overdose or botulism—and most patients with chest trauma—will improve with time, and treatment is largely supportive. Primary diseases associated with hypercapnia requiring specific treatment include myasthenia gravis, electrolyte abnormalities, obstructive lung disease, obstructive sleep apnea, and myxedema.

Hypoxemic Respiratory Failure

Oxygen supplementation is the most important therapy for hypoxemic respiratory failure. In severe disorders such as ARDS, mechanical ventilation, positive end-expiratory pressure (PEEP), and other types of respiratory therapy may be necessary. Although not a feature of most cases, hypercapnia may develop because the high work of breathing leads to respiratory muscle fatigue. Attention to oxygen transport is important, and severe anemia should be corrected and adequate cardiac output maintained. The underlying disease leading to hypoxemic respiratory failure must be addressed, especially if pneumonia, sepsis, or other cause is identified. Treatment may include diuretics, antibiotics, and bronchodilators as well as other measures.

In some patients with nonuniform lung disease involvement, dependent positioning of the uninvolved or less involved lung or lung areas may improve oxygenation. This is because gravity and the weight of the lungs increase perfusion and ventilation to dependent lung regions. Patients with severe hemoptysis or heavy respiratory secretions, however, should not be placed in this position because of the likelihood of aspiration of blood or secretions into uninvolved areas. In ARDS with diffuse noncardiogenic pulmonary edema, there has been considerable interest in placing the patient in the prone position. Patients who are prone rather than supine appear to have less tendency of dependent lung regions to collapse as well as smaller areas of the lungs to be compressed by the heart or abdominal contents. In some patients, improvement in arterial hypoxemia is transient after turning from supine to prone, but in many the effects persist for at least several hours.

AIRWAY

When upper airway obstruction is the patient's only problem, prompt restoration of an adequate airway is all that is required to reverse respiratory failure. In most patients, establishment of the airway is essential for ventilation, oxygenation, and delivery of respiratory medications.

Upper Airway Obstruction

Primary upper airway obstruction should be considered in all patients with respiratory difficulty—but especially if they present with any of the following: head and neck trauma, suspected malignancy of the larynx or trachea, acute dyspnea with wheezing (inspiratory, expiratory, or both), dysphagia, neurologic disease affecting motor or sensory function, speech difficulty, masses in the neck due to thyroid enlargement or lymphadenopathy, or pain, infection, or inflammation of the pharynx, larynx, or trachea. Patients with respiratory diseases such as asthma or COPD may also have upper airway obstruction from tracheal or subglottic stenosis if there is a history of recent or remote endotracheal intubation or tracheostomy. Acute respiratory distress, especially in the elderly and in children, should arouse suspicion of a foreign body in the airway. A frequent intermittent cause of upper airway obstruction is seen in obstructive sleep apnea syndrome (see below), in which obstruction occurs during certain stages of sleep. It is important to consider this not uncommon problem as a complicating factor in patients with respiratory failure from other causes.

Natural Airway

The normal natural airway permits speech, humidifies inspired gas, and protects against aspiration and infection; coughing is made effective and the mucociliary function of the trachea is maintained by the airway. When a decision is made to insert an artificial airway, the benefits and risks of the endotracheal tube must outweigh the benefits of the natural airway (Table 12–3). In patients with severe upper airway obstruction, the choice is usually easy. In other patients with

Table 12–3. Risks and benefits of the artificial airway.

Risks	Benefits
Trauma of insertion	Bypasses upper airway obstruction
Oro- or nasopharyngeal trauma due to chronic pressure	Route for oxygen and other medications
Tracheal damage (erosion, tracheomalacia)	Facilitates positive-pressure ventilation and PEEP
Impaired cough response	Route for respiratory medications
Increased aspiration risk	
Impaired mucociliary function	Facilitates suctioning of secretions
Increased infection risk	
No speech	Fiberoptic bronchoscopy route
Increased resistance and work of breathing	

acute respiratory failure, the decision rests primarily on whether oxygen, respiratory medications, and respiratory therapy via the natural airway will be adequate or whether an artificial airway would be preferable. A trial of aggressive treatment before intubation often provides useful information. Guidelines (Table 12–4) for selecting patients who need endotracheal intubation may be helpful, but clinical assessment of the response to therapy is usually more so. An important part of the decision to intubate is availability and the potential benefit of temporary positive-pressure ventilation provided without an endotracheal tube (noninvasive positive-pressure ventilation).

Endotracheal Tubes

Endotracheal tubes are usually made of relatively stiff plastic, with soft, low-pressure, easily deformable inflatable tracheal cuffs. Skilled practitioners should insert these tubes with proper attention to prevention of aspiration of gastric contents; adequate oxygenation during the procedure; avoidance of trauma to the mouth, tongue, nose, epiglottis, and vocal cords; and selection of an endotracheal tube of proper size for the patient. Experience with sedation using opioid analgesics or rapid-acting sedatives (eg, benzodiazepines such as midazolam) and muscle relaxants should be available for intubation of awake patients.

Nasotracheal intubation has the advantages of greater patient comfort, less severe positioning of the head and neck during placement, and somewhat better stabilization of the tube. However, the route of the tube and its smaller size can sometimes complicate suctioning and weaning from a mechanical ventilator. The smaller radius of curvature of the nasotracheal route has been linked to higher tube resistance compared with the same tube passed orally, but this finding has been questioned. The nasotracheal route is generally appropriate in patients who require intubation for reasons unrelated to lung disease, eg, sedative drug overdose. Otherwise, orotracheal intubation should be used, especially if a larger tube diameter is needed to facilitate airway suctioning or for subsequent fiberoptic bronchoscopy. Placing an orotracheal tube requires a laryngoscope for inspection of the vocal cords. Laryngoscopes with straight or curved blades to hold the tongue and other structures away are most often used, but small portable fiberoptic laryngoscopes have proved extremely useful for difficult intubations or special circumstances.

Small-diameter tubes impose less risk of trauma to the vocal cords and may be more comfortable for the patient. Larger tubes provide better access for tracheal suctioning, delivery of medications, and fiberoptic bronchoscopy if needed and will generally result in an adequate seal between the tube and the trachea with smaller cuff volume and pressure. Weaning from mechanical ventilation may be easier with a larger tube because of lower airflow resistance. Most women can accommodate endotracheal tubes 7.5–8 mm in inner diameter; men generally will accept tubes of 8.5 or 9 mm inner diameter. If the need for fiberoptic bronchoscopy is a consideration, a tube with at least 8 mm inner diameter is required, and 8.5 mm is preferable. Adequate ventilation during bronchoscopy through an endotracheal tube depends on the minute ventilation and flow requirements of the patient.

Table 12–4. Indications for intubation and mechanical ventilation.[1]

Physiologic

- Hypoxemia persists after oxygen administration
- $P_{CO_2} > 55$ mm Hg with pH < 7.25
- Vital capacity < 15mL/kg with neuromuscular disease

Clinical

- Altered mental status with impaired airway protection
- Respiratory distress with hemodynamic instability
- Upper airway obstruction[2]
- High volume of secretions not cleared by patient, requiring suctioning

[1]These are guidelines that must take into account the patient's clinical status and other factors.
[2]Consider need for tracheostomy if obstruction is above trachea. Approach endotracheal intubation with caution.

Care of the Artificial Airway

The intubated patient must be frequently suctioned because both the cough mechanism and the mucociliary clearance mechanism are impaired. The frequency of suctioning depends on the amount and nature of secretions. Although the artificial airway becomes rapidly colonized with bacteria, suctioning should be done using sterile technique to prevent introduction of additional organisms. A sealed system (suction catheter contained within a sheath in-line with the endotracheal tube) facilitates frequent suctioning and may minimize nosocomial contamination. For some patients, disposable suction catheters are more effective—especially those with bent or curved tips that can be directed into the right or left main bronchus as desired. It has become common practice to instill small aliquots of sterile normal saline into the endotracheal tube to facilitate suctioning of secretions, but this should be done only if increased amounts of secretions can be shown to be obtained.

Hypoxemia and tracheal trauma are the most common complications of suctioning. Minimal negative pressure should be used, and the suction catheter should be introduced gently. During suctioning, PaO_2 may fall rapidly, particularly if the patient is receiving high concentrations of inspired O_2 and suctioning is performed for more than 10–15 seconds. In patients with focal infiltrates or known collections of secretions in particular parts of the tracheobronchial tree, selective bronchial suctioning can be tried. By using bent-tip catheters and by positioning the patient's body or head, successful suctioning of the left main bronchus, for example, can often be accomplished.

In order to provide positive-pressure ventilation, the inflated tracheal cuff of the endotracheal tube exerts pressure on the interior of the trachea to create an effective seal. Almost all endotracheal tubes and tracheostomy tubes incorporate low-pressure, high-volume cuffs made of highly compliant rubber or plastic. These cuffs provide a tracheal tube seal after inflation to a relatively low pressure. If higher than normal pressures are needed to achieve a seal, damage to the trachea may occur, including erosion, inflammation, softening of the cartilage rings with tracheal dilation (tracheomalacia), and hemorrhage. Endotracheal cuff pressure must be monitored to anticipate these complications and to make certain that the least possible effective pressure and volume are used. The best way to do this is to slowly inflate the cuff with air, using a small syringe, until there is minimal leak around the cuff with inspiration and adequate tidal volume and ventilation are achieved. The pressure read on a manometer and the amount of air put into the cuff are recorded. The desired cuff pressure is the smallest possible that will maintain an adequate seal between the tube cuff and the trachea, and the pressure is ideally less than 15 cm H_2O. The incidence of tracheal complications rises when cuff pressures exceed 20–25 cm H_2O for prolonged periods.

Complications From Endotracheal Tubes

Complications from endotracheal tubes may be classified as early and late. Early complications are due to the trauma of tube insertion or to malpositioning of a tube into a main bronchus or in the esophagus. Physical examination and chest x-ray confirmation of the tube's position are essential. The tip of the tube should be in the center of the trachea and 3–5 cm above the carina, but head flexion or extension can cause 1–5 cm of movement of the endotracheal tube tip on chest x-ray. Analysis of expired CO_2 has been found to give reliable assurance of tracheal rather than esophageal placement; fiberoptic bronchoscopy can also be valuable for this purpose in selected patients.

Unplanned extubations are a complication of endotracheal intubation, occurring in 3–10% of cases. The endotracheal tube should be carefully secured, and the patient should be educated about the need for and importance of the tube. Agitation and patient movement have been found to be associated with extubation and sedation, and physical restraints should be used as necessary. Several studies have shown that unplanned extubations led to reintubation in about half of patients, but some patients can be carefully observed for respiratory distress and deterioration of arterial blood gases rather than immediate reintubation. Factors predictive of a high likelihood of the need for reintubation include the severity of the underlying disease, a high minute ventilation requirement during the preceding 24 hours, a high FIO_2 requirement, and altered mental status.

Aspiration of oral secretions or refluxed gastric secretions is a common problem in intubated patients. Contrary to common belief, the inflated tracheal cuff does not reliably protect against aspiration of secretions around the tube. Some investigators have found that continuous suction of secretions above the cuff decreased the incidence of nosocomial pneumonia; endotracheal tubes with a suction port at this point are available.

A randomized trial of orotracheal compared with nasotracheal intubation showed that there was a slightly greater frequency of radiographic sinusitis (by CT scan) in patients with nasotracheal intubation. Of note is the observation that the incidence was relatively high in both groups (30% nasotracheal and 22% orotracheal), indicating that this was a frequent complication in all patients needing endotracheal intubation for more than 7 days.

The majority of late complications arise from prolonged pressure of the tube against anatomic structures. The curve of the tube puts maximum pressure on the side of the mouth, the palate, and the posterior pharynx (from oral intubation) or the nasal turbinates and on the posterior pharynx (nasal intubation). The greatest pressure is exerted on the vocal cords, the narrowest part of the passage. Most late complications are due to laryngeal trauma, followed by the development of glottic injury and subglottic stenosis. The incidence of subglottic stenosis is estimated to be less than 5% of patients intubated for more than 10–14 days. A study of patients with translaryngeal intubation (orotracheal or nasotracheal) found that the extent of injury estimated by laryngoscopy was not predictive of late complications. The duration of translaryngeal intubation did not influence the ability of the larynx to heal without future ill effects.

Despite the inability to correlate late complications with the duration of intubation, early tracheostomy (within 5–7 days) is recommended if prolonged intubation is anticipated. Translaryngeal intubation for up to 10 days does not usually cause an appreciable increase in complications, and tracheostomy is preferred if intubation for 21 days or more can be anticipated. This conclusion is based on a similar incidence of complications from translaryngeal intubation and tracheostomy. Thus, translaryngeal intubation for as long as 21 days may be acceptable unless a longer need for an artificial airway is expected or whenever there is reason to suspect greater potential laryngeal trauma (patient movement, malnutrition, local or systemic infection). In such cases, earlier tracheostomy is advised.

Tracheostomy of course prevents or avoids laryngeal injury but does not prevent tracheal injury from the tracheostomy cuff. Attention to cuff pressure and cuff volume is essential for tracheostomy tubes as well as endotracheal tubes. Tracheostomy may be contraindicated if the patient has a bleeding disorder, local infection, or neck mass.

OXYGEN

Supplemental oxygen is required in almost all patients with respiratory failure. The amount of oxygen needed above that present in room air depends on the mechanism of hypoxemia; the type of oxygen delivery device depends on the amount of oxygen required, patient and physician preference, the potential for adverse effects of varying concentrations of oxygen, and the minute ventilation of the patient. Because high concentrations of oxygen are damaging to the lungs, efforts should be made to minimize the amount and duration of oxygen therapy.

Pa_{O_2} & $P(A-a)_{O_2}$

For normal subjects, the range for Pa_{O_2} during air breathing at sea level and at rest is 75–100 mm Hg, with a decline in Pa_{O_2} with age. One formula for calculating the average Pa_{O_2} decline with age in supine subjects is $Pa_{O_2} = 109 - 0.43 \times$ age (in years). Because the Pa_{CO_2} in normal subjects does not change appreciably with aging, the usual value for Pa_{CO_2} is about 40 mm Hg independent of age. Therefore, alveolar P_{O_2} during room air breathing at sea level is always about 100 mm Hg. Combining this with the predicted value for average P_{O_2}, the normal range for $P(A-a)_{O_2}$ is 0–30 mm Hg during air breathing, with the high end of the range seen in normal elderly subjects. $P(A-a)_{O_2}$ increases when breathing supplemental O_2 and can be as much as 100 mm Hg in normal subjects breathing 100% O_2. The increase in $P(A-a)_{O_2}$ reflects the small amount of physiologic right-to-left shunt found in normal subjects.

At different F_{IO_2} values, $P(A-a)_{O_2}$ does not remain constant and cannot be easily used as a measure of the severity of gas exchange or for predicting the response to a changed F_{IO_2}. Some authors have recommended comparing the ratio of Pa_{O_2}/PA_{O_2} rather than the difference between PA_{O_2} and Pa_{O_2} because the ratio tends to be more constant as F_{IO_2} is changed in a given patient. The physiologic behavior of Pa_{O_2} with respect to PA_{O_2}, however, shows that Pa_{O_2}/PA_{O_2} is often not sufficiently constant to predict Pa_{O_2} when F_{IO_2} is altered. Therefore, changes in F_{IO_2} must be followed by measurement of arterial blood gases. In recent years, the ratio Pa_{O_2}/PA_{O_2} has been found to be useful as a marker of the severity of gas exchange abnormality in hypoxemic respiratory failure and in the definition of refractory hypoxemia as seen in ARDS.

Oxygen Saturation & Oxygen Content

Oxygen saturation and oxygen content change little when Pa_{O_2} increases above about 60 mm Hg, though there is a small linear increase in O_2 content due to increased O_2 dissolved in the plasma (Figure 12–2). Oxygen saturation is about 92% when Pa_{O_2} is 60 mm Hg if the oxyhemoglobin curve is not shifted rightward or leftward by temperature or pH changes. The Pa_{O_2} at which hemoglobin is 50% saturated with oxygen (P-50) can be used to indicate the degree of shift of hemoglobin. With normal unshifted hemoglobin, increasing Pa_{O_2} above 60 mm Hg can only increase O_2 saturation

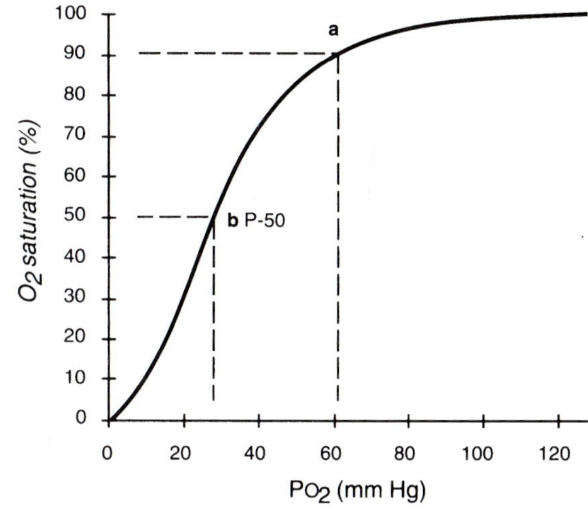

Figure 12–2. Normal oxyhemoglobin dissociation curve. At point *a*, $Pa_{O_2} = 60$ mm Hg results in O_2 saturation of about 90%. At point *b*, the saturation of hemoglobin is 50% ("P-50") at a Pa_{O_2} of about 26 mm Hg for hemoglobin at normal body temperature, pH, and 2,3-DPG. Increased temperature, decreased pH, and increased 2,3-DPG shift the curve to the right; decreased temperature, increased pH, decreased 2,3-DPG, and carbon monoxide shift the curve leftward.

from 92% to 100%. Therefore, for almost all purposes, an acceptable arterial PO_2 is 60 mm Hg or more, but little increase in O_2 content is seen with PaO_2 values above 60 mm Hg. Nevertheless, in most clinical situations, a higher PaO_2 is desired (80–100 mm Hg) in order to anticipate changes in lung gas exchange during suctioning or changes in the patient's condition. However, there is almost never a need for PaO_2 > 150 mm Hg unless the patient is anemic (prior to transfusion) or has carbon monoxide poisoning—or in some other special circumstances.

Inspired Oxygen Concentration

The mechanism of hypoxemia is what determines how much the arterial PaO_2 will increase with O_2 therapy. Figure 12–3 shows how the PaO_2 of patients with pure right-to-left shunts theoretically responds to increasing concentrations of inspired O_2 compared with patients who have $\dot{V}/\dot{Q}$ mismatching. Most patients with $\dot{V}/\dot{Q}$ mismatching will have a relatively large increase in PaO_2 for a small increase in inspired O_2 concentration; increasing FIO_2 from 0.21 to about 0.30–0.40 with O_2 masks, cannulas, or other devices will often raise PaO_2 to > 70–100 mm Hg in these patients. On the other hand, most patients who are hypoxemic due to right-to-left shunting are found to be refractory to O_2 therapy, demonstrating only a small increase in PaO_2 when the inspired O_2 concentration is increased from 0.21 to as much as 1.0. These patients will often require very high FIO_2 (> 0.60) to correct hypoxemia. In a patient with a right-to-left shunt, some venous blood (by definition) will always bypass alveolar spaces and fail to pick up O_2. Because only the blood exposed to the alveolar gas will pick up O_2, we can take advantage of this mechanism of hypoxemia to further distinguish right-to-left shunt from $\dot{V}/\dot{Q}$ mismatching. When given 100% O_2 (FIO_2 = 1.0) to breathe and after the alveolar spaces are completely washed out by O_2, patients with right-to-left shunting will always have some degree of reduced arterial PO_2, whereas patients with $\dot{V}/\dot{Q}$ mismatching will have an arterial PO_2 value close to that of normal subjects breathing 100% O_2. For clinical purposes, normal subjects and patients with $\dot{V}/\dot{Q}$ mismatching will have a PaO_2 > 550 mm Hg during 100% O_2 breathing; the PaO_2 of patients with right-to-left shunts will be less than 550 mm Hg (Table 12–2).

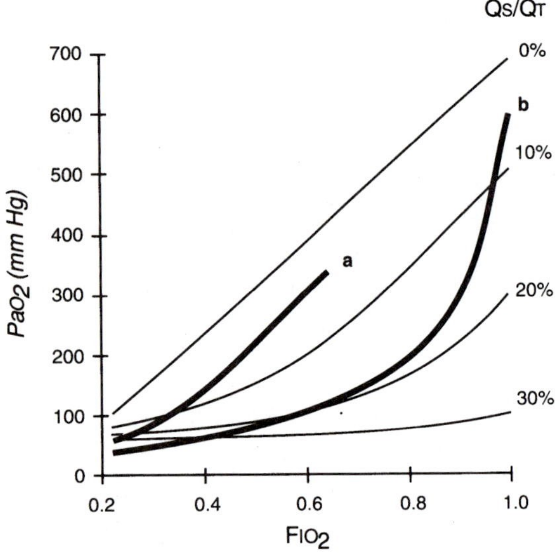

Figure 12–3. Relationship between PaO_2 and FIO_2 for pure right-to-left shunt ($\dot{Q}s/\dot{Q}t$) of 0%, 10%, 20%, and 30%. Line *a* shows a representative relationship of PaO_2 and FIO_2 for a patient with mild ventilation-perfusion ($\dot{V}/\dot{Q}$) mismatching. Line *b* demonstrates the relationship for severe $\dot{V}/\dot{Q}$ mismatching. With right-to-left shunt, PaO_2 remains < 550 mm Hg when breathing 100% oxygen, but the PaO_2 is > 550 mm Hg during 100% oxygen breathing even with severe $\dot{V}/\dot{Q}$ mismatching.

Patients with asthma, COPD, mild pneumonia, and pulmonary embolism usually can be given relatively low concentrations of supplemental O_2 (FIO_2 0.24–0.40) with a reasonable expectation that their PaO_2 will correct satisfactorily to a safe level. Hypoxemia in these patients, therefore, is due to $\dot{V}/\dot{Q}$ mismatching. Patients with more severe lung disease—especially those with pulmonary edema, collapse of lungs or lobes, severe lobar pneumonia, or ARDS—usually can be assumed to have right-to-left shunting as the mechanism of hypoxemia. These patients require higher inspired concentrations of O_2 (in the range of 0.50–1.0) to achieve the same PaO_2 goal.

Supplemental Oxygen Delivery Devices

Supplemental oxygen delivery devices are divided into low-flow and high-flow systems (Table 12–5). Low-flow O_2 devices include nasal cannulas and simple O_2 masks patients can use to draw small supplemental amounts of 100% O_2 while the bulk of the inspired tidal volume is provided by room air entrainment from around or outside the device. Because the flow of supplemental O_2 is constant, the inspired concentration of O_2 varies inversely with the patient's minute ventilation. Thus, at a constant flow of 2 L/min into nasal cannulas, a patient with a low minute ventilation will have a higher FIO_2 than another with a high minute ventilation who entrains a greater amount of room air per

Table 12–5. Oxygen delivery devices.

Device	O_2 Flow Rate (L/min)	FIO_2	Advantages	Disadvantages
Low-flow delivery devices				
Nasal cannula	2–6	0.24–0.35	Patient comfort	FIO_2 varies with $\dot{V}E$.
Simple mask	4–8	0.24–0.40	None	FIO_2 varies with $\dot{V}E$.
High-flow delivery devices				
Venturi mask	2–12[1]	0.25–0.50	Constant FIO_2 with $\dot{V}E$	Inadequate flow at high FIO_2.
Nonrebreathing mask	6–15	0.70–0.90	High FIO_2	Not comfortable; FIO_2 not adjustable.[2]
High-flow O_2 blender[3]	6–20	0.50–0.90	High FIO_2 at high total flow	

[1]The total inspiratory gas flow is the O_2 flow plus the amount of room air entrained. See specification for each model.
[2]FIO_2 can vary with O_2 flow rate set; however, the FIO_2 is most dependent on the amount of inadvertent room air entrained. In addition, total O_2 flow may be inadequate in patients with high inspiratory flow demand.
[3]O_2 is delivered from various types of "high-flow" O_2 blenders with room air entrainment. Different types of masks may be used.

minute. For a nasal cannula, the O_2 flow rate should be 0.5–4 L/min; for a simple mask, the O_2 flow should be a minimum of 4 L/min—in order to flush $PaCO_2$ out of the mask—and a maximum of 6–8 L/min.

High-flow oxygen delivery devices, including Venturi-type masks and nonrebreathing masks, generate the total air-oxygen mixture inhaled by the patient. Venturi-type masks direct O_2 through a constricted tube that increases gas velocity. The jet of O_2 exiting from the constriction generates sufficient negative pressure to draw a much higher volume of air into the breathing circuit. The relationship between O_2 flow, orifice size, and room air entrainment in Venturi-type masks is designed to generate a known total flow of gas at a relatively constant concentration of O_2. Different FIO_2 concentrations and different total flow amounts are generated by using a different-sized orifice or by changing the amount of air entrainment, depending on the design of the system. Venturi-type masks are ideal when a constant known FIO_2 in the range of 0.24–0.40 is needed. Maximum FIO_2 is usually considered to be about 0.50, and the total gas volume provided decreases as higher FIO_2 values are administered, making this type of mask less suitable for patients who have both minute ventilation requirements greater than 10–12 L/min and high FIO_2 requirements.

Another kind of high-flow device is the nonrebreathing mask, consisting of a bag reservoir that fills with 100% oxygen and one-way valves that permit inspiration only from the reservoir and prevent room air entrainment. The reservoir guarantees that even with vigorous inspiratory effort and high inspiratory flow, patients will inhale essentially 100% O_2. The nonrebreathing mask is used primarily for patients who require very high FIO_2 levels (in the range of 0.7–1.0). Limitations include inability to provide very high total gas volumes and patient discomfort. Because this mask is used in patients with severe hypoxemia requiring high inspired concentrations of O_2, a high percentage of them may have further deterioration and require other forms of treatment. Other high-flow oxygen delivery devices usually generate an oxygen-air mix similar to what is achieved with the Venturi-type masks but may be more reliably capable of providing a larger total flow and higher O_2 concentration. They can be used also to produce cool or warm aerosol along with high O_2 concentrations.

An air-oxygen blender provides oxygen during mechanical ventilation. The concentration can be varied from 0.21 to 1.0. Devices for intermittent positive-pressure breathing, continuous positive airway pressure (CPAP) masks, nasal CPAP, nebulizers for inhaled medications, and others can be provided with supplemental O_2 as needed in patients with hypoxemia.

Complications of Oxygen Therapy

Complications of oxygen therapy are not common. Aside from increased combustion risk from smoking or open flames, patients may occasionally have hypoventilation from loss of hypoxic drive and excessive drying of mucous membranes. On the other hand, more subtle toxic effects of O_2 and its metabolites are recognized as causing adverse changes.

Although O_2 itself is relatively nontoxic to biologic tissues, spontaneous and facilitated conversion into more reactive chemical relatives of O_2 has potential for damage to the lungs. The presence of inflammation and other biologic processes may increase the generation of more energetic and toxic oxygen moieties such as hydrogen peroxide, hydroxyl ion, and superoxide anion. In the presence of myeloperoxidase and hydrogen peroxide, chloride anion is converted to hypochlorous acid, which has potent biologic effects. The production of toxic products in a localized region of lung or other tissues is enhanced when PaO_2 is increased.

Toxicity from oxygen occurs primarily in the lungs in adults and is related not to its concentration nor to the arterial PO_2 but rather to the inspired oxygen partial pressure. Subjects at sea level given 100% oxygen to breathe have complained of chest pain, dry cough, and other discomfort after 6 hours. More severe oxygen toxicity has been demonstrated in humans and in experimental animals when 100% oxygen is given for 24–48 hours. In normal lungs, capillary leakage of fluid and protein has been demonstrated with accompanying increased $P(A–a)O_2$. Findings similar to those of ARDS, with exudative pulmonary edema, inflammatory changes, and subsequent fibrosis, have been attributed to oxygen toxicity, but the relationship to underlying disease requiring the high oxygen concentration is unclear.

Because of the potential adverse effects, it is advisable to limit high concentrations of oxygen ($FIO_2 > 0.5$) to short duration (< 72 hours) if possible. It is not known whether the presence and nature of coexisting lung injury enhances or protects against oxygen toxicity, but there is some evidence that viral pneumonia increases sensitivity to oxygen toxicity. It is highly likely that inflammatory cells—such as neutrophils—that encourage development of toxic oxygen products also increase the risk of oxygen toxicity. Infection, inflammation from any cause, and increased inflammatory cell function due to cytokine activation will probably correlate with potential oxygen-mediated tissue injury. A number of investigators have suggested that antioxidants (eg, vitamin A, vitamin E, acetylcysteine) and scavengers of toxic oxygen products (superoxide dismutase) may modulate lung damage from oxygen.

BRONCHODILATORS

Increased airway resistance is the major feature of asthma and other chronic obstructive pulmonary diseases. Resistance increases because of airway smooth muscle contraction, excessive secretions, airway inflammation and edema, and decreased lung elastic recoil. Bronchodilators affect directly only smooth muscle contraction, though some may have indirect effects on edema and inflammation. Bronchodilators are primary treatment for obstructive lung diseases, but increased airway resistance is a feature of many other kinds of lung diseases such as pulmonary edema, ARDS, and perhaps pneumonia. Bronchodilator drugs are often used in these and other respiratory failure settings. The benefits and risks of adverse effects must be considered when these drugs are prescribed.

There are five classes of bronchodilators: beta-adrenergic agonists, anticholinergics, methylxanthines, calcium antagonists, and a miscellaneous group of agents including magnesium sulfate. Calcium antagonists have been used as bronchodilators experimentally but are not approved for clinical use. Nifedipine, diltiazem, felodipine, verapamil, and other calcium antagonists are weak bronchodilators, and their primary value is that they can generally be safely used to treat hypertension, arrhythmias, and ischemic heart disease in patients with coexisting obstructive lung disease and respiratory failure.

Beta-Adrenergic Agonists

These drugs—also called sympathomimetics—are derivatives of naturally occurring epinephrine, with modifications to improve activity, specificity, dosing, and pharmacokinetic properties.

Identification of subclasses of adrenergic receptors using specific antagonists has led to designation of different drugs as having α-, β_1-, or β_2-adrenergic agonist activity. Stimulation of alpha-adrenergic receptors—present largely on systemic blood vessels—increases vascular tone and, in the presence of normal cardiac function, raises blood pressure. $Beta_1$-receptor stimulation leads to increased rate and force of cardiac contraction and peripheral vasodilation, whereas β_2-receptor agonists relax airway smooth muscle. In comparison with epinephrine and isoproterenol, newer agents such as albuterol and terbutaline have increased β_2-adrenergic activity with decreased β_1 activity, making these drugs more potent bronchodilators with fewer undesired cardiac effects.

A. Route of Administration

These agents are more effective when given by inhalation rather than when given orally or parenterally. For a given degree of bronchodilation, side effects are considerably less for the inhaled route, allowing a larger and longer-acting dose to be administered. Oral beta-adrenergic agonists are not as useful in acute respiratory failure as when the drugs are given by inhalation.

When given by inhalation, the onset of action of the beta-adrenergic agonists is rapid, and newer agents are metabolized slowly enough to allow for relatively long intervals between doses in most stable patients. Metered-dose inhalers (MDIs), if used properly, are as effective as gas-driven nebulizers or intermittent positive-pressure breathing for delivering bronchodilators. Most clinicians now recommend that patients use an MDI with a spacer device between the MDI and the mouth to facilitate correct use. For patients receiving mechanical ventilation, there are a number of devices that incorporate reservoirs in the ventilator circuit so that MDIs can be used. However, the comparative effectiveness of

MDIs and gas-driven nebulizers during mechanical ventilation is unclear. Either type of device can be used, and some objective measurement should be employed to determine whether effective bronchodilation is achieved in an individual patient. MDIs have previously used chlorofluorocarbons (CFCs) as propellants, but some manufacturers have switched to other agents such as hydrofluoroalkanes. There has been some evidence suggesting that these propellants are associated with improved distribution of the bronchodilator and greater clinical effectiveness.

B. Dose and Selection of Drug

Effective therapy may require two to four times the amounts of beta-adrenergic agonists than are usually recommended for patients with stable obstructive lung disease, so increased doses (more puffs from the MDI, increased quantity in nebulizer) and increased frequency of administration (up to every hour or by continuous nebulization) are often needed. Some protocols call for increasing amounts of beta-adrenergic agonists until a plateau in improved lung function is reached or until side effects such as tachycardia or muscle tremors are observed. Several studies have advocated use of continuous nebulization of beta-adrenergic agonists rather than frequent intermittent therapy (eg, every hour).

Selection of a particular beta-adrenergic agonist is based on potency, efficacy, ease of administration, and limitation of side effects. Albuterol—the most often used agent—can be given in a wide range of dosages as needed to treat bronchospasm. It has an early onset of action and is available in MDIs, in solution for nebulization, and in oral form. Levalbuterol is the (R)-albuterol isomer of racemic albuterol, thought to be the active beta-adrenergic agonist molecule. Some studies have linked increased bronchoreactivity to the (S)-isomer, but it is unclear if levalbuterol has any clinical advantage over the racemic mixture. Metaproterenol is available for inhalation and orally. Terbutaline can be given subcutaneously or orally, but there are no currently available parenteral forms of metaproterenol or albuterol.

Epinephrine is a potent beta-adrenergic agonist with strong cardiovascular effects due to its lack of specificity for β_2 receptors. In general, this drug offers no advantages for the treatment of bronchospasm when compared with more selective agents. A long-acting beta-adrenergic agonist, salmeterol, is useful for chronic treatment of asthma to prevent rather than treat bronchospasm. It is not recommended for acute bronchospastic attacks.

Albuterol can be given as two to four puffs from an MDI every 4–6 hours in stable patients with obstructive lung disease and bronchospasm. In patients with acute exacerbations of bronchospasm, the number of puffs can be increased to six to eight (or more, if tolerated) and the frequency to every 1–2 hours if needed. The response should be objectively measured, preferably by spirometry (FEV_1 or peak flow), to document the need for the higher dose; adverse effects should be carefully monitored, especially when the doses given exceed usual recommendations. Waiting 3–5 minutes between puffs improves the effectiveness of a given dose. A nebulized solution of 0.2–0.5 mL of albuterol (0.5%) or metaproterenol (5%) diluted in 2–3 mL of normal saline can be given by gas-powered nebulizer or intermittent positive-pressure breathing every 2–6 hours, but there is no evidence that this is more effective than administration by MDI. Individual patients may have a better response with certain routes of delivery, and poor response to one route does not rule out beneficial effects from another.

Patients receiving mechanical ventilation who require aerosolized beta-adrenergic agonist therapy have generally been treated by incorporating a nebulizer or aerosol generator in the ventilator circuit leading to the endotracheal tube. In recent years, MDIs have been successfully adapted for use with ventilators, but the type of adaptor and, most importantly, the dose of medication administered greatly affect the degree of bronchodilation. Patients who do not have the desired effect using a nebulizer or MDI should be considered for the alternative form of delivery, and the dose of beta-adrenergic agonist should be adjusted.

C. Adverse Effects

Side effects particularly important in the ICU and which may limit beta-adrenergic agonist use include tremors, tachycardia, palpitations, arrhythmias, and hypokalemia. Cardiac effects other than tachycardia may become important in patients with ischemic heart disease, but chest pain and ischemia are unusual. Tachycardia is sometimes more associated with respiratory distress and hypoxemia than with beta-adrenergic agonists and may resolve after bronchodilator therapy. Hypokalemia is exacerbated by thiazide diuretics and is probably caused by shifts of potassium from extracellular to intracellular compartments in response to beta-adrenergic stimulation.

An uncommon complication of beta-adrenergic agonists is worsening of hypoxemia from exacerbation of ventilation-perfusion mismatching. This may occur because these drugs oppose appropriate localized pulmonary artery vasoconstriction in areas of low ventilation-perfusion ratio; increased blood flow to these regions increases hypoxemia. Systemic side effects result largely from absorption through the mucous membranes of the mouth, and their incidence may be reduced by spacers or reservoirs that generate a mix of aerosol particles which more effectively reach the intrathoracic airways. Patients should be instructed to rinse the mouth after each inhalation of the medication.

Heavy use of beta-adrenergic agonist therapy in asthma has been associated with an increased risk of death and exacerbation of bronchospasm. The mechanism is unknown but may relate to side effects of the medications or, paradoxically, to their effectiveness as bronchodilators but not as drugs that address the underlying cause of asthma. These findings may or may not be relevant in the management of status asthmaticus or acute exacerbation of COPD in the ICU.

Beta-blockers are frequently used in ICU patients, including those with hypertension, ischemic heart disease, and arrhythmias. Beta-adrenergic agonists are less effective when receptors are blocked, and variable effects on both bronchodilation and the underlying cardiovascular condition are likely to be encountered. Caution should be exercised with beta-adrenergic agonists in patients with cardiac disease, hypokalemia, or other potential complicating factors.

Anticholinergics

The bronchodilator response to anticholinergic (parasympatholytic) drugs depends on the degree of intrinsic parasympathetic tone. These agents play a somewhat smaller role in asthma, a disorder in which the mechanism of airway obstruction relates to inflammation, than in chronic bronchitis, in which more parasympathetic tone appears to be present.

Ipratropium bromide is the available anticholinergic agent. Atropine sulfate should no longer be given as a bronchodilator because of its systemic toxicity, including decreased airway and salivary gland secretions, decreased gastrointestinal motility, tachycardia, decreased urinary bladder tone and function, pupillary dilation, and increased intraocular pressure. Toxic doses of atropine cause hyperthermia, vasodilation, altered mental status, and hypotension. On the other hand, ipratropium bromide given by inhalation is barely detectable in the blood and, because it is a quaternary ammonium compound, does not pass easily through lipid membranes, including the blood-brain barrier. Therefore, ipratropium's effects are strongly limited to bronchodilation, and only a very few complaints of other systemic parasympatholytic action have been encountered even when large doses are administered.

A. Indications

Anticholinergics are recommended primarily for bronchodilation in patients with chronic bronchitis. Some investigators have recommended ipratropium bromide as first-line therapy for this disorder when treated as an outpatient, but ipratropium should always be used in combination with beta-adrenergic agonists when treating respiratory failure. Because the effectiveness of anticholinergics depends on the degree of parasympathetically mediated increased smooth muscle contraction, other diseases in which airway secretions are prominent such as cystic fibrosis may respond well. Asthma usually responds better to other agents, but some studies support a benefit in acute exacerbations of asthma when added to beta-adrenergic agonists and corticosteroids.

B. Route and Dose

Ipratropium bromide is available in MDIs or in solution for nebulization. Each puff of the MDI provides 18 μg of the drug. The onset of action appears to be somewhat longer than that of beta-adrenergic agonists—approximately 30 minutes—and the peak effect occurs at around 60 minutes. The dose of ipratropium bromide recommended by some writers has increased with clinical experience from as few as two inhalations every 6 hours to as many as four to eight inhalations every 4 hours, with increasing effectiveness at the higher dose range in some cases. For nebulization of ipratropium, an effective dose appears to be 0.5 mg given every 6–8 hours, and the drug is available in unit dose vials containing 0.5 mg of ipratropium in 2.5 mL of normal saline. Even at the highest doses, side effects of ipratropium are minimal, and these doses appear to be safe. As with beta-adrenergic agonists given by MDIs, delivery appears to be more efficient with the aid of spacers or reservoirs. An MDI containing both ipratropium bromide and albuterol is available on prescription, but this agent is more likely to be helpful for stable ambulatory patients.

C. Adverse Effects

Very few adverse effects are reported—rarely, tachycardia, palpitations, and urinary retention.

Theophylline

Theophylline is an agent in the xanthine class of bronchodilators. It is somewhat less potent as a bronchodilator than the beta-adrenergic agonists. There is interest at present in evaluating the role of this drug and reassessing its risk-benefit ratio. Of particular interest are actions of theophylline other than bronchodilation, such as effects on respiratory muscles, the heart, and the immune system.

A. Mechanism of Action

Theophylline has a long history of use as a bronchodilator. Although for many years inhibition of phosphodiesterase action on cyclic AMP (cAMP) was thought to be its mechanism of action, therapeutic concentrations do not inhibit phosphodiesterase strongly, and it has been difficult to demonstrate a synergistic relationship with beta-adrenergic agonists, which stimulate cAMP production. Other proposed mechanisms of action of theophylline include effects on translocation of calcium, antagonism of adenosine, stimulation of beta-adrenergic receptors, and anti-inflammatory activity.

Theophylline has been relegated by some physicians to second-line therapy in obstructive lung disease because of the availability of potent beta-adrenergic agonists and other agents.

B. Pharmacokinetics

Theophylline is generally thought to be effective at a therapeutic level of 10–20 μg/mL; toxicity is increasingly likely when serum levels exceed 20–30 μg/mL, and severe toxicity is encountered above 40 μg/mL. The dose-response is curvilinear, with the increase in benefit being greatest when the theophylline level increases from 5 to 10 μg/mL and much less when the level increases from 15 to 20 μg/mL. About 90% of theophylline is metabolized by the liver to inactive products by the P450 cytochrome system. These enzyme systems are stimulated by tobacco or marijuana smoking and phenobarbital but are decreased in activity by cimetidine, erythromycin, oral contraceptives, and many other drugs. Theophylline metabolism is greatly reduced with fever, advanced age, cessation of smoking, or of a drug that enhances metabolism, liver disease, and heart failure. Hepatic failure and heart failure patients will often metabolize theophylline at less than 50% of normal rates.

C. Dose and Route of Administration

In the ICU, theophylline is usually given intravenously. Theophylline is available premixed in 5% dextrose in water at a concentration of 0.8 mg/mL. To achieve rapid therapeutic levels, intravenous loading is used, with 5 mg/kg of theophylline given over 20–30 minutes to patients who have not been receiving the drug. If the patient has been receiving theophylline during the last 24 hours, about 2 mg/kg should be given as the loading dose. This loading dose and the volume of distribution of theophylline are intended to achieve a serum level of about 10 μg/mL. Most studies have been based on actual rather than ideal body weight, but it is likely that the volume of distribution does not increase in proportion to increased body fat. Because metabolism of the drug begins immediately, a constant infusion is necessary to maintain this level. In the absence of factors that affect theophylline metabolism, the constant infusion is chosen to be 0.5–0.6 mg/kg/h, but this should be reduced to 0.1–0.2 mg/kg/h in patients with liver disease or heart failure or those who are taking cimetidine or erythromycin. Elderly patients have decreased clearance of theophylline, and a constant infusion of 0.2–0.4 mg/kg/h is recommended. When a steady state is reached after five half-lives have passed (about 18–36 hours), serum levels should be checked to adjust the infusion rate accordingly. Patients who are more likely to have theophylline toxicity should be checked earlier, and if the level is high the infusion rate should be lowered.

D. Adverse Effects

Tachycardia, nausea, and vomiting can occur even at therapeutic serum levels but are more common at levels over 20 μg/mL. More severe complications include cardiac arrhythmias, hypokalemia, altered mental status, and seizures, usually seen when theophylline levels exceed 35 μg/mL. Many drugs interfere with theophylline metabolism by hepatic enzymes, causing serum levels to rise (erythromycin, cimetidine and ranitidine, quinolones); and phenobarbital, rifampin, and smoking increase the rate of metabolism, sometimes causing serum levels to be low.

Magnesium Sulfate

Intravenous magnesium sulfate has been used as a bronchodilator in patients with asthma and chronic obstructive lung disease. The mechanism of action appears to be direct airway smooth muscle relaxation.

A. Indications

Clinical studies, including double-blind placebo-controlled trials, have used this drug in combination with beta-adrenergic agonists or other bronchodilators in asthmatics.

B. Route and Dose

Magnesium sulfate has been given as 1–2 g (8–16 meq) intravenously over 10–20 minutes. This dose can be repeated every 1–2 hours as long as the patient does not have renal insufficiency and does not develop signs of magnesium toxicity. Serum magnesium levels may be helpful in monitoring for toxicity.

C. Adverse Effects

Adverse effects are due to hypermagnesemia and include loss of deep tendon reflexes, bradycardia, hypotension, somnolence, muscle weakness, respiratory failure due to muscle weakness or paralysis, and cardiac arrest.

OTHER DRUGS

Corticosteroids

Although both corticosteroids and cromolyn have been used as anti-inflammatory drugs for respiratory diseases, there is little or no experience with the latter drug in acute respiratory failure in adults. The corticosteroids have been used for obstructive lung disease, including asthma and chronic bronchitis, to decrease airway obstruction from inflammation, edema, and airway lumen debris; and in ARDS in an effort to moderate its severity and prevent late fibrotic complications. Pharmaceutical preparations of corticosteroids have greater potency than cortisol, modified mineralocorticoid effects, a longer duration of action, different solubility and degree of systemic absorption, and different rates of metabolism. The precise mechanism of anti-inflammatory action of these agents is unknown, but they have effects on lymphocytes, cytokine production, interleukin release, macrophage function, immunoglobulin production, eosinophil activation and production, and other immune and allergic responses. The mechanism of corticosteroids in reducing airway inflammation is similarly unknown, but changes in inflammatory cell nature and number have been demonstrated after both systemic and topical administration.

A. Route of Administration

Corticosteroids used in asthma and COPD can be given orally, intravenously, or by aerosol. Aerosolized corticosteroids are useful for the treatment of stable mild to moderate asthma. The several available agents are designed to maintain activity at mucosal surfaces but have poor systemic absorption. In addition, any amount swallowed is rapidly and almost completely taken up by the liver and excreted. Comparison studies have found few differences between beclomethasone dipropionate, triamcinolone acetonide, and flunisolide. More potent anti-inflammatory corticosteroids such as budesonide and fluticasone are highly effective in chronic asthma and have been shown to have some value in selective patients with COPD.

Aerosolized corticosteroids are potentially poorly distributed in acute respiratory failure, and oral or parenteral forms are almost always used. Prednisone and methylprednisolone are given orally; methylprednisolone and hydrocortisone are given intravenously. Some studies have shown little difference between oral and intravenous administration, but comparisons are difficult because of different potencies of the agents used.

B. Dose

For treatment of obstructive lung disease with acute exacerbation, most investigators have recommended giving large doses initially and continuing for several days before tapering and discontinuing, if possible within 7–14 days. Others have suggested that tapering is not needed to avoid exacerbation of airway inflammation and that the practice unnecessarily prolongs treatment; they suggest that the corticosteroids can be stopped abruptly. Severe asthma and exacerbation of chronic bronchitis have been treated with 20–120 mg of methylprednisolone intravenously four times a day, usually in the range of 40–60 mg/dose. There is no evidence that higher doses achieve better outcomes or shorter duration of disease. Almost all patients can be switched to oral prednisone after 3–5 days of clinical response, usually in a dosage of 30–60 mg daily. There is evidence that oral prednisone and intravenous methylprednisolone are equally effective when given acutely to patients with moderately severe asthma, but the parenteral route is usually preferred. Inhaled corticosteroids are generally withheld during severe acute exacerbations.

C. Adverse Effects

Side effects of parenteral corticosteroids that are particularly important in the ICU include hyperglycemia, hypokalemia, sodium and water retention, acute steroid myopathy (especially at larger doses), impairment of the immune system, and psychiatric disorders. An association with gastritis and gastrointestinal bleeding has been suggested but is debated. Inhaled corticosteroids are relatively free of systemic side effects except for cough, perhaps provocation of bronchospasm, and oral and pharyngeal candidiasis. However, the more potent inhaled corticosteroids have long-term adverse effects on growth, osteoporosis, and cataract development. Prolonged muscle weakness affecting weaning from mechanical ventilation has been associated with simultaneous use of corticosteroids and nondepolarizing neuromuscular blocking drugs. Patients for whom corticosteroids are prescribed chronically are at risk for inhibition of the normal pituitary-adrenal axis; they may develop acute adrenal insufficiency with withdrawal of therapeutic corticosteroids.

Systemic corticosteroids should be discontinued as soon as possible to avoid side effects. However, too early and too rapid cessation can lead to exacerbation of disease. In most patients, close monitoring during this phase can identify potential problems, and selected patients can benefit from a longer course of corticosteroids. Corticosteroids are often started by inhalation if persistent airway inflammation is anticipated and the clinical course warrants continuation of this mode of therapy. Finally, some patients are unable to tolerate discontinuation of systemic corticosteroids; every effort should be made to reduce the dose to the lowest possible therapeutic level, and the risks and benefits of this therapy should be thoroughly reviewed.

Leukotriene Antagonists & Inhibitors

Leukotrienes are products of arachidonic acid metabolism and may have a role in certain kinds of asthma. In chronic asthma, inhibition of the effect of leukotrienes by leukotriene receptor antagonists (montelukast or zafirlukast) or inhibition of leukotriene production (zileuton, a 5-lipoxygenase inhibitor) has beneficial effects on the severity and course of the disease. There is no role for these agents in acute asthma exacerbations, but they can generally be continued in patients who are taking them already.

Expectorants & Nucleonics

There is little evidence that vigorous administration of fluids orally or intravenously improves either the volume or the characteristics of abnormal sputum except perhaps in patients who are volume-depleted. Oral potassium iodide may have some value in increasing the volume and thinning tenacious sputum. Iodinated glycerol has been shown to benefit stable COPD patients by increasing the force and frequency of coughing and thus perhaps aiding sputum clearance. The potential value of this drug in acute exacerbation of asthma or COPD is unknown. Other expectorants appear to be of little value, and cough suppressants such as codeine may be contraindicated when removal of secretions by coughing is desired.

Mucolytic agents can be applied directly to airway secretions, especially in patients with endotracheal tubes. Small amounts (3–5 mL) of normal saline, hypertonic saline, and hypertonic sodium bicarbonate can be instilled prior to suctioning and the results judged by the removal of greater amounts of secretions. Acetylcysteine disrupts disulfide bonds found in sputum proteins and can be a potent mucolytic agent. However, aerosolized acetylcysteine is relatively ineffective and may provoke bronchospasm in asthmatics. Small aliquots of acetylcysteine have been given by flexible bronchoscopic lavage into specific airways if necessary. Because some of the abnormal quality of sputum is due to DNA derived from cellular breakdown, enzymes that lyse DNA (DNAase) may have a beneficial role, but these agents are not approved for use in COPD or asthma.

Respiratory Stimulants

There is little indication for respiratory stimulant drugs. Most patients with respiratory failure have mechanical and gas exchange abnormalities that must be corrected, while very few patients lack sufficient ventilatory drive. In the small number of patients who could benefit from stimulation of the respiratory centers—such as those with central nervous system depression from sedative drug overdosage or immediately postanesthesia—temporary mechanical ventilatory support is effective and safe. Respiratory stimulants do not shorten the duration of mechanical ventilation.

Patients with acute or chronic hypoventilation syndromes (eg, obesity-hypoventilation) have been given methylphenidate, medroxyprogesterone, and doxapram hydrochloride with limited success and frequent side effects.

Sedatives & Muscle Relaxants

In patients not receiving mechanical ventilation, sedative drugs, including barbiturates and benzodiazepines, and drugs with respiratory depression potential, such as opioids, are contraindicated in most forms of respiratory failure. Attempts to attenuate but not eliminate respiratory drive with these agents in order to lessen dyspnea have not been successful. In patients with chest or abdominal pain from trauma or surgery limiting ventilation, analgesia is sometimes very important; tidal volume and minute ventilation may increase after treatment.

In patients who are receiving mechanical ventilation, sedation is often necessary, especially shortly after intubation and initiation of ventilatory support. Benzodiazepines such as diazepam and lorazepam are often used, and the dosage should be titrated as necessary. Lorazepam has the advantage of longer duration of action, which may be beneficial in patients requiring sedation for several days. All benzodiazepines will accumulate in body fat after repeated or prolonged use; they are metabolized by the liver, and hepatic dysfunction also prolongs their effect. Agitation caused by pain should be treated with analgesics such as morphine sulfate rather than increased doses of sedatives. Propofol, which must be given by continuous intravenous infusion, is an attractive sedative because awakening of the patient occurs 10–20 minutes after the infusion is stopped. This drug has a rapid onset of action and rapid termination of sedative effect, but only if the minimal infusion rate needed to achieve sedation is used. Many patients who might require muscle relaxants in order to tolerate mechanical ventilation can be successfully managed using propofol.

In an important randomized controlled trial, adult patients receiving mechanical ventilation had their sedation interrupted until they were awake every day. They were compared with a control group who had sedation stopped at the discretion of the physicians caring for them. The daily interruption group had a shorter median duration of mechanical ventilation and significantly shorter stays in the intensive care unit. No difference in complications, including those associated with extubation, was found. This study suggests that many mechanically ventilated patients require less sedation than is usually thought to be necessary.

In some patients, muscle relaxants are needed to facilitate oxygenation or ventilation. Because of the relatively long duration of relaxation generally needed, continuous intravenous infusion of pancuronium or atracurium is most often used. With these agents, great care is needed to ensure adequate sedation and maintenance of ventilation. These drugs should be used only by experienced physicians, and drug dosage should be carefully titrated using a peripheral nerve stimulator.

Because pancuronium has vagolytic effects and is associated with histamine release, it should be avoided in patients with unstable hemodynamics. Atracurium is metabolized in the plasma, and the duration of action is not affected by renal or hepatic insufficiency. These agents have been associated with prolonged neuromuscular weakness, especially when given in association with high dosages of corticosteroids in patients with respiratory failure.

CHEST PHYSIOTHERAPY

Chest physiotherapy is applied to the airways or to the outside of the chest. Techniques include incentive spirometry, intermittent positive-pressure breathing (IPPB), postural drainage, chest percussion, rotational therapy, and fiberoptic bronchoscopy.

Incentive Spirometry

Atelectasis is a common problem in postoperative patients and those with neuromuscular or chest wall disease. Because atelectasis in some patients appears to be due to repeated small inspirations, deeper breaths may be helpful. Incentive spirometers encourage expansion of the lungs as much as possible above spontaneous breathing; these have proved to be beneficial in controlled studies. Patients should be instructed to expand their lungs as much as possible for as long as they can rather than generate a high negative inspiratory pressure for a short time.

Intermittent Positive-Pressure Breathing

The benefit of intermittent positive-pressure breathing (IPPB) has been difficult to demonstrate in most patients. Although sometimes used to deliver bronchodilator medications, IPPB is usually intended to prevent or treat atelectasis. In objective studies, patients can improve atelectasis if and only if IPPB can increase the depth of breathing more than the patient alone can achieve. IPPB can be tried in patients with respiratory muscle weakness due to neuromuscular disease, those with chest wall abnormalities, and after abdominal surgery. In general, incentive spirometry should be tried first and IPPB used only when there is proof that larger inspired volumes can be reached with this technique.

Postural Drainage & Rotational Therapy

The patient may be placed in various positions to encourage drainage of airway secretions from specific segments or lobes of the lungs. This procedure may be particularly important in patients with lung abscess or bronchiectasis when large volumes of purulent secretions are present and one or a few regions of involvement can be identified. The objective measure of benefit is the increase in volume of expectorated secretions. It is less clear that patients with pneumonia are helped by postural drainage, but this measure might be tried to see if it encourages production of sputum. Patients with respiratory failure from diffuse airway disease are probably little benefited by postural drainage, and there is a risk that worsening of gas exchange may occur in some positions. Postural drainage and chest percussion should be withheld if there is no objective evidence that sputum expectoration is increased after treatment.

There are a number of different kinds of patient care beds that provide programmed rotation of the patient as well as vibration therapy or percussion to the chest wall. Of these modes, rotational therapy may be helpful in preventing or treating aspiration of secretions and pneumonia.

Chest Percussion

Chest percussion is often added to postural drainage and has the same indications. It should be discontinued if increased volume of secretions does not result. Chest percussion can cause worsening of hypoxemia, rib fractures, and skin abrasions. A recent study found that cardiac arrhythmia was a common complication of chest percussion and postural drainage, especially in the elderly and those with underlying heart disease. Patients with atelectasis and no evidence of increased airway secretions do not improve with chest percussion.

Fiberoptic Bronchoscopy

Fiberoptic bronchoscopy allows inspection of the airways out to several generations and provides a means of suctioning airway secretions. In respiratory failure, patients with segmental or lobar collapse due to mucous plugs who fail to respond to other forms of treatment may be helped by fiberoptic bronchoscopy; in these cases, the bronchoscope is essentially used as a visually directed suction catheter. Occasionally, unsuspected foreign bodies or airway tumors are found. Patients with atelectasis who have visible "air bronchograms" on chest x-rays appear to benefit less from bronchoscopy than those whose airways leading to the involved region are airless. The air bronchogram sign indicates that the airway is probably patent and not obstructed by secretions that can be removed by fiberoptic bronchoscopy. Because of cost and potential complications, fiberoptic bronchoscopy should not be the initial treatment of atelectasis or lobar collapse unless there is a strong likelihood of endobronchial obstruction. Likewise, routine fiberoptic bronchoscopy for postoperative patients should be discouraged.

Alexander E, Weingarten S, Mohsenifar Z: Clinical strategies to reduce utilization of chest physiotherapy without compromising patient care. Chest 1996;110:430–2.

Beckmann U, Gillies DM: Factors associated with reintubation in intensive care: an analysis of causes and outcomes. Chest 2001;120:538–43.

Boulain T: Unplanned extubations in the adult intensive care unit: a prospective multicenter study. Am J Respir Crit Care Med 1998;157:1131–7.

Diehl JL et al: Changes in the work of breathing induced by tracheotomy in ventilator-dependent patients. Am J Respir Crit Care Med 1999;159:383–8.

Epstein SK, Nevins ML, Chung J: Effect of unplanned extubation on outcome of mechanical ventilation. Am J Respir Crit Care Med 2000;161:1912–6.

Heffner JE: Timing of tracheostomy in ventilator-dependent patients. Clin Chest Med 1991;12:611–25.

Holzapfel L et al: Influence of long-term oro- or nasotracheal intubation on nosocomial maxillary sinusitis and pneumonia: results of a prospective, randomized, clinical trial. Crit Care Med 1993;21:1132–8.

Kress JP et al: Daily interruption of sedative infusions in critically ill patients undergoing mechanical ventilation. N Engl J Med 2000;342:1471–7.

Marik P, Hogan J, Krikorian J: A comparison of bronchodilator therapy delivered by nebulization and metered-dose inhaler in mechanically ventilated patients. Chest 1999;115:1653–7.

Ostermann ME et al. Sedation in the intensive care unit: a systematic review. JAMA 2000;283:1451–9.

Rumbak MJ et al: Significant tracheal obstruction causing failure to wean in patients requiring prolonged mechanical ventilation: a forgotten complication of long-term mechanical ventilation. Chest 1999;115:1092–5.

Stauffer JL, Olson DE, Petty TL: Complications and consequences of endotracheal intubation and tracheostomy. Am J Med 1981;70:65–76.

Stoller JK et al: Physician-ordered respiratory care vs physician-ordered use of a respiratory therapy consult service. Results of a prospective observational study. Chest 1996;110:422–9.

Sue DY: Acute Respiratory Failure. In: *Acute Emergencies and Critical Care in the Geriatrics Patient.* Yoshikawa TT, Norman DC (editors). Marcel Dekker, 2000.

Sugerman HJ et al: Multicenter, randomized, prospective trial of early tracheostomy. J Trauma 1997;43:741–7.

MECHANICAL VENTILATION

Mechanical ventilation in acute respiratory failure has been viewed as largely supportive in intention, but it is now clearly recognized that proper management of the patient-ventilator system can have a positive effect on outcome. The need for and the type of mechanical ventilatory support depend on the mechanism of respiratory failure. Potential complications of mechanical ventilation are also determined to some extent by the severity and mechanism of disease. The choice of ventilator, ventilator mode, and settings should be made by the critical care physician in consultation with respiratory care practitioners. Because changes in ventilator settings affect not only respiratory parameters but hemodynamic and other organ system functions as well, monitoring of the mechanically ventilated patient can be a complex task. Decisions to initiate and terminate mechanical ventilation require both physiologic understanding and clinical judgment. An important and relatively new recommendation is that the traditional physiologic goals of mechanical ventilation, such as $Pa{CO_2}$ or tidal volume, do not have to be in the normal range in order to benefit the patient. In addition, it is apparent that many complications of mechanical ventilation may be aggravated by attempting to restore physiologic variables completely to normal at a time when the lungs have abnormal structure or function.

The Patient-Ventilator System

The normal spontaneously breathing subject has an intact ventilatory control system, effective bellows (chest wall and diaphragm), and atmospheric gas exchanger (lung parenchyma and circulation). Feedback from chemoreceptors sensing $Pa{O_2}$ and pH (and indirectly $Pa{CO_2}$) and mechanoreceptors of the lung and chest wall provide input to a central integrator-controller that generates neural output at an appropriate frequency to signal the inspiratory effort. The bellows system produces negative intrathoracic pressure by contraction of the inspiratory muscles, thereby drawing gas into the lungs. The timing and amount of negative pressure determine the rate of inspiratory flow. The gas exchanger (lungs) distributes inspired gas in proportion to pulmonary blood flow, and O_2 and CO_2 move into and out of the circulation by diffusion. Exhalation occurs when the ventilatory control mechanism signals relaxation of the inspiratory muscles; there may or may not be active contraction of expiratory muscles. Exhalation is complete in the relaxed subject when passive mechanical forces of the lungs and chest wall equalize. The lung volume remaining is the functional residual capacity (FRC). The relative amounts of time spent during inspiration and expiration are determined by the magnitude of respiratory drive and the interactions between stimuli received by other receptors.

Important aspects of mechanical ventilation can be understood by comparing the parameters that must be chosen by the clinician during controlled-mode positive-pressure volume-cycled ventilation with the decisions made automatically by a spontaneously breathing normal person (Table 12–6). In this particular mode, the ventilator is set at a specific number of breaths per minute to be delivered to the patient. There is no negative or positive feedback from chemoreceptors or other sources that helps determine the respiratory rate. The clinician chooses the tidal volume on the ventilator control panel, and this volume is delivered each time the ventilator delivers a breath. The rate at which the tidal volume is delivered to the patient can be adjusted,

Table 12–6. Variables to be set during mechanical ventilation.[1]

Mode	How should each breath be initiated?
Tidal volume	What is the volume of each ventilator breath?
Respiratory rate	At what rate should the ventilator deliver breaths in the event of apnea?
FIO_2	What is the concentration of O_2 in the inspired gas?
Inspiratory flow	How fast should inspiratory flow be delivered?
PEEP	How much end-expiratory pressure is needed?
Peak pressure	At what peak airway pressure should inspiratory flow be stopped?
I:E ratio	What is the ratio of inspiratory:expiratory time?
Flow pattern	Should inspiratory flow be constant or follow some other pattern (descending or sinusoidal)?

[1]For volume preset (volume-cycled) ventilation.

and the inspiratory time is determined as the quotient of tidal volume divided by inspiratory flow rate. The amount of positive pressure generated by the ventilator depends on the inspiratory flow, the resistance of the airways, and the compliance of the lungs and chest wall. Passive exhalation begins immediately after the specified tidal volume has been delivered and lasts until the next inspiration begins. Consequently, the exhalation may or may not be completed before the next breath starts, resulting in air trapping and hyperinflation.

Respiratory Mechanics & Mechanical Ventilation

Lung compliance and airway resistance are the two most important physiologic concepts in understanding mechanical ventilatory support. Both are commonly altered from normal in patients with acute respiratory failure, especially lung compliance in ARDS, chest wall compliance in a variety of disorders, and resistance in asthma and COPD exacerbations. Mean airway pressure and extrinsic positive end-expiratory pressure (PEEP) are considered in managing patients during positive-pressure ventilation.

A. Compliance

When the lungs are expanded, elastic and structural tissues in the lungs and surface tension in the alveoli oppose expansion. At lung volumes near total lung capacity, the chest wall also exerts an opposing force. The amount of pressure needed to overcome these two forces, when related to a given change in lung or chest wall volume, is the respiratory system compliance (C_{rs}), the ratio of change in volume of the lungs or chest wall to the change in pressure ($\Delta V/\Delta P$). ΔP is the change of pressure measured between the inside and outside of the system, in this case alveolar pressure minus chest wall surface (usually atmospheric) pressure. Because pressure is needed to overcome both lung and chest wall elastic recoil, both lung compliance (C_l) and chest wall compliance (C_{cw}) are components of respiratory system compliance:

$$\frac{1}{C_{rs}} = \frac{1}{C_l} + \frac{1}{C_{cw}}$$

The pressure-volume relationship of the respiratory system is curvilinear (Figure 12–4). The individual components—lung compliance and chest wall compliance—can only be determined by measuring intrapleural pressure using an esophageal balloon. However, most often in the ICU the respiratory system as a whole is measured, and it is not partitioned into the two components.

All types of mechanical ventilators measure (proximal or circuit) airway pressure throughout the respiratory

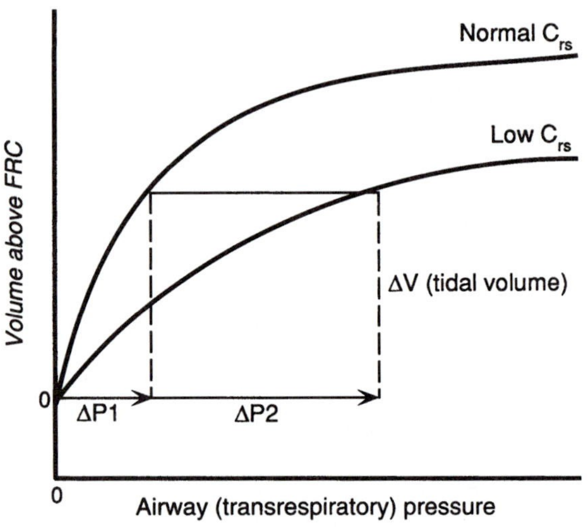

Figure 12–4. Hypothetical respiratory system pressure-volume curves during positive-pressure breathing. The normal curve is steeper at low lung volume than the curve for a patient with less compliant lung or chest wall (low C_{rs}). Mean respiratory system compliance for the tidal volume shown is $C_{rs} = \Delta V/\Delta P1$ (normal curve) or $C_{rs} = \Delta V/(\Delta P1 + \Delta P2)$ for the less compliant system.

cycle, but the following analysis assumes that a volume-cycled ventilator with a set tidal volume is being used. If, after the tidal volume is delivered to the patient by a positive-pressure ventilator, exhalation is delayed briefly and the patient makes no inspiratory or expiratory efforts, the pressure in the ventilator circuit ("inspiratory plateau pressure") equals the amount of pressure needed to distend the lungs and chest wall by the amount of tidal volume just delivered (Figure 12–5). Therefore, C_{rs} = tidal volume/(inspiratory plateau pressure − end-expiratory pressure). C_{rs} measured in this way is sometimes called static respiratory system compliance. Normal C_{rs} is approximately 100 mL/cm H_2O in the range of usual operational lung volume. Thus, for a tidal volume of 800 mL in a mechanically ventilated patient with normal chest wall and lung compliances, the inspiratory plateau pressure will be about 8–10 cm H_2O.

When a patient develops a higher than expected inspiratory plateau pressure for a given tidal volume (decreased C_{rs}), this means that there is decreased lung compliance (eg, pulmonary edema or interstitial fibrosis) or decreased chest wall compliance, such as in obesity, ascites, or kyphoscoliosis. Greater than normal inspiratory plateau pressures can also be found at extremes of lung volume. For example, at very low lung volume relative to total lung capacity, alveolar collapse leads to the tidal volume's being distributed over fewer lung units, resulting in a higher inspiratory plateau pressure. On the other hand, at high lung volumes relative to total lung capacity, lung units become overdistended and the lung is less compliant. Development of atelectasis, pulmonary edema, pleural effusions, acute changes in chest wall compliance, pneumothorax, and potentially dangerous overdistention of the lung can be suggested by a decrease in C_{rs}.

B. Resistance

Gas flows from a region of high pressure to a region of low pressure. Respiratory resistance arises from the loss of energy of gas moving through the airways from friction along the conduit walls. Resistance is a complex function of gas density and viscosity, velocity, the degree of turbulence, and the nature of the conduits, but resistance is always proportionate to the difference in pressure of the gas between upstream and downstream points. Resistance determines the rate of gas flow into or out of the lungs at a given pressure or the necessary pressure for a given flow. In mechanically ventilated patients, an estimate of relative airway resistance during inspiration can be made from the peak airway pressure during volume-cycled ventilation with constant inspiratory flow. More complex measurements are needed to determine airway resistance more accurately or under different circumstances.

In contrast to inspiratory plateau pressure—used above to estimate respiratory system compliance—peak airway pressure is the sum of the pressure needed both to expand the lungs and chest wall plus the pressure needed to push the gas through the airways. Thus, peak pressure always exceeds inspiratory plateau pressure by the amount needed to overcome airway resistance. A large difference between peak pressure and inspiratory

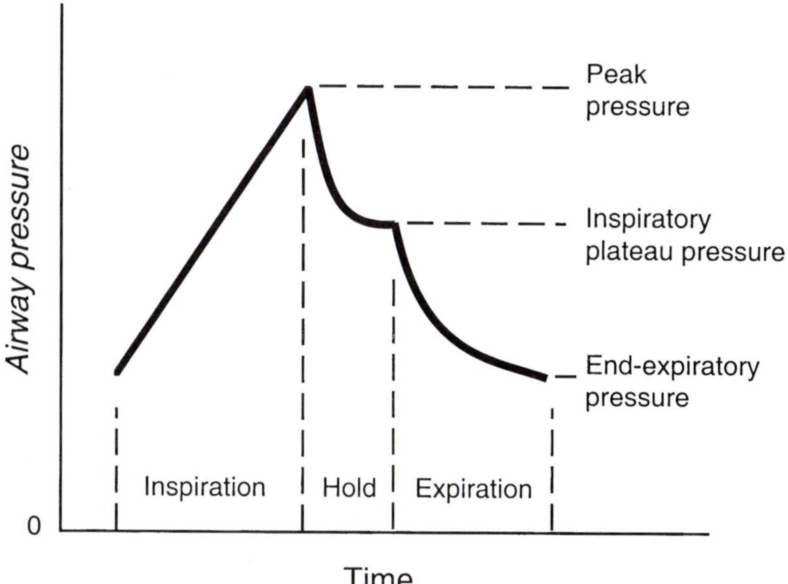

Figure 12–5. Airway pressure schematically shown during respiratory cycle for positive-pressure respiration. Peak airway pressure, pressure during inspiratory plateau, and positive end-expiratory pressure (PEEP) are shown. The difference between peak and inspiratory plateau pressures provides an indication of airway resistance. The tidal volume/(inspiratory plateau pressure – PEEP) is an estimate of respiratory system compliance.

plateau pressure (ie, > 5–10 cm H_2O) indicates that bronchospasm, airway secretions, or other causes of increased airway resistance are present. Dynamic respiratory system compliance is defined as the ratio of tidal volume to the difference between peak airway pressure and end-expiratory pressure. This variable reflects both lung compliance and airway resistance and may be useful in conceptualizing the work of breathing, but it is not strictly a measure of compliance.

C. Mean Airway Pressure

Mean airway pressure is the time-averaged pressure in the airway during the respiratory cycle. It reflects both the amount of pressure needed to overcome resistive and recoil forces during inspiration and any pressure imposed on the airway during expiration, eg, positive end-expiratory pressure. Mean airway pressure has been suggested as a measure of potential barotrauma to the lungs, as a predictor of impairment of cardiovascular function, and as a marker of improved distribution of ventilation. However, there is no agreement on how best to interpret this variable.

D. Dynamic Hyperinflation and Intrinsic PEEP

Inspired tidal volume in patients receiving positive-pressure ventilation is provided by increasing the pressure in the ventilator circuit, and gas flows from the ventilator into the patient. In contrast, expiration is passive and continues until the lung volume returns to the functional residual capacity (FRC). At this point, elastic inward recoil of the lungs and outward recoil of the chest wall are balanced, and—unless PEEP is set on the ventilator (see below)—alveolar pressure is equal to atmospheric pressure. By convention, pressures are expressed relative to atmospheric pressure, so alveolar pressure = 0 cm H_2O.

Dynamic hyperinflation occurs when the volume of gas in the lung at end-expiration is greater than the expected FRC. Among patients receiving mechanical ventilation, dynamic hyperinflation is most common with obstructive lung disease (asthma, COPD) who have slow expiratory airflow or in any patient who requires very large minute ventilation. In the latter case, the large minute ventilation requires either a high respiratory frequency, high tidal volume, or both. For either of these two reasons, there is a transient period where inspiratory tidal volume is greater than expiratory tidal volume, in effect "trapping" gas in the lung and increasing FRC.

Intrinsic PEEP, sometimes called "auto-PEEP," is the term used to denote the difference in pressure between the alveolar space at end-expiration and the pressure in the proximal airway or ventilator circuit. Intrinsic PEEP is seen in two common situations. First, intrinsic PEEP is associated with dynamic hyperinflation. This is evident because patients with dynamic hyperinflation continue to have expiratory flow right up to end-expiration, indicating a positive alveolar pressure relative to proximal airway pressure (hence, intrinsic PEEP). Second, any patient who actively contracts expiratory muscles at end-expiration develops positive alveolar pressure relative to external airway pressure. Note, however, that intrinsic PEEP in this situation is associated with normal or smaller FRC rather than with hyperinflation. Estimation of intrinsic PEEP is described below in the section on respiratory failure in COPD.

Dynamic hyperinflation can have marked consequences for the pulmonary and systemic circulations, resulting in hypotension and decreased cardiac output. It may also greatly increase the work of breathing and may be associated with barotrauma. Because alveolar pressure is elevated, dynamic hyperinflation makes it more difficult for patients to trigger mechanical ventilation in the assist-control or pressure support modes (see below). Dynamic hyperinflation and its marker, intrinsic PEEP, should be suspected in any patient with obstructive lung disease receiving mechanical ventilation—and in others with unexplained hypotension or worsening of gas exchange. Features suggesting dynamic hyperinflation include worsening of gas exchange with increasing minute ventilation, hypotension, presence of expiratory flow at end-expiration, high minute ventilation requirements (especially if > 15–20 L/min), and short expiratory time.

Common Methods of Mechanical Ventilation

The most common modes of mechanical ventilation (summarized in Table 12–7) include (1) volume-preset (volume-cycled), assist-control ventilation; (2) pressure-controlled ventilation; (3) pressure-support ventilation; and (4) intermittent mandatory ventilation. Other methods are used less often or are available only on a limited number of ventilators. Discussions of mechanical ventilation in patients with neuromuscular and chest wall disorders, ARDS, and obstructive lung diseases are found in the sections devoted to management of those disorders later in this chapter.

A. Classification of Mechanical Ventilators

A universally accepted classification of mechanical ventilators has not been developed. Historically, successive "generations" of ventilators have offered a variety of complex capabilities. First-generation volume-cycled ventilators were limited to providing ventilation in the assist-control mode only. Second-generation ventilators added intermittent mandatory ventilation (IMV), PEEP, and improved monitoring capabilities. Later machines used microprocessors to provide a broader

Table 12–7. Ventilator modes.

Mode	I-E Changeover	Independent Parameters	Dependent Variables	Secondary Modes	Advantages	Disadvantages	Application
Volume-cycled ventilation (VCV) (assist-control, volume-preset)	Set V_T delivered	V_T $\dot{V}_I$ (flow rate) Backup f	Peak Paw I:E ratio	PEEP; inverse I:E ratio (IRV)	Set V_T and backup rate always delivered.	May have high peak Paw when set V_T is delivered.	Primary ventilatory mode.
Pressure-controlled ventilation (PCV) (assist-control pressure-preset)	Set inspiratory time elapsed or set I:E ratio reached	Peak Paw T_I or I:E ratio	V_T $\dot{V}_I$ (flow rate)	PEEP; inverse I:E ratio (IRV)	Peak Paw cannot be exceeded; can set I:E ratio. Gas exchange may improve.	V_T, $\dot{V}_E$ may vary and not guaranteed; T_I and I:E ratio may conflict.	Primary ventilatory mode (ARDS).
Pressure-support ventilation (PSV)	Patient-determined	Pressure Support Pressure	V_T T_I I:E ratio f	PEEP	Patient-selected V_T, f T_I. May be better tolerated than other modes.	V_T, $\dot{V}_E$, f not guaranteed. Limited data on improve weaning of difficult patients.	Weaning: primary ventilatory mode.
Intermittent mandatory ventilation (IMV)	Ventilator breaths: Set V_T delivered (volume-cycled V_T)	Mandatory f and V_T	Peak Paw Spontaneous V_T, f	PEEP PSV	Mandatory backup V_T, f; spontaneous breaths interposed.	Fixed mandatory f, V_T, $\dot{V}_E$; spontaneous breaths may vary. Some ventilators have high work of breathing. Not shown to improve weaning.	Weaning; primary ventilatory mode.

Key:
V_T = Tidal volume
$\dot{V}_E$ = Minute ventilation
$\dot{V}_I$ = Inspiratory flow rate
Paw = Airway pressure
PEEP = Positive end-expiratory pressure
IRV = Inverse ratio ventilation
f = Respiratory rate
I:E ratio = Inspiratory:expiratory time ratio
T_I = Inspiratory time

range of options, including pressure-control and pressure-support modes, time- or volume-cycling, and various combinations. Some incorporate circuits that minimize the work of breathing and enhance monitoring capabilities with graphic displays. The newest mechanical ventilators have modes that allow patients to breathe spontaneously with pressure-support assistance and can provide additional ventilation to meet preset targets.

1. Inspiratory phase—A useful scheme divides mechanical ventilator methods into those in which the primary preset independent variable is tidal volume (volume-preset) or airway pressure (pressure-preset). The term "ventilator mode" has come to mean the method by which the patient-ventilator system initiates inspiration. Thus, the start of inspiration can be completely machine-controlled (control mode) or chosen by the patient (assist-control mode). The respiratory rate is set by the clinician, but in the assist mode, if the patient chooses to breathe at a faster rate, this overrides the set rate.

The method of changeover from the inspiratory to the expiratory phase is said to be how the ventilator is "cycled." The ventilator is either volume-cycled, time-cycled, or pressure-cycled depending on whether the inspiratory phase ends when a preset tidal volume, inspiratory time, or circuit pressure is reached, respectively. The inspiratory flow rate and pattern can be adjusted to provide an increasing, decreasing, or sinusoidal flow pattern during inspiration. Tidal volume, airway pressure, inspiratory flow rate, and inspiratory time are necessarily interactive. Thus, with different methods of mechanical ventilation, one or more variables are preset and independent while the others are dependent variables.

2. Expiratory phase—Exhalation is passive, occurring because lung recoil and chest wall recoil create positive pressure in the alveolar space relative to atmospheric pressure. If the exhalation is stopped before completion, end-expiratory lung volume rises and end-expiratory pressure is positive relative to atmosphere. This positive end-expiratory pressure (PEEP) is often selected to stabilize alveoli, prevent collapse of lung units, and improve hypoxemia in certain situations. All modes of positive-pressure mechanical ventilation described below can have PEEP added as necessary.

B. Volume-Preset Ventilation

Also called the volume-cycled assist-control mode, this is the most frequently used method of mechanical ventilatory support and is suitable for almost all types of respiratory failure. Basically, the ventilator delivers a preset tidal volume at a constant inspiratory flow at a respiratory frequency set on the machine; the patient may breath faster than that rate, ending up with a higher respiratory frequency.

In the assist-control mode, the physician chooses a minimum respiratory frequency. However, the assist-control mode allows the patient to initiate a ventilator-delivered breath by making an inspiratory effort. The ventilator senses this effort as a fall in ventilator circuit pressure. If the patient can make an inspiratory effort sufficient to "trigger" the ventilator at a frequency greater than the set respiratory frequency, the patient effectively determines the respiratory rate. If no inspiratory efforts are made or detected, the respiratory rate is equal to the preset rate. In general, the preset respiratory rate should be chosen to be slightly less than the patient's spontaneous rate, if any. This will guarantee that the patient will receive a relatively safe amount of ventilation in the event of patient apnea or hypopnea. The amount of patient effort needed to trigger the ventilator (sensitivity) can be adjusted on the ventilator. Sensitivity is usually chosen to be 1–2 cm H_2O less than the end-expiratory pressure. However, water condensed in the ventilator tubing, unavoidable delay in the triggering mechanism, and the presence of intrinsic PEEP may make it more difficult to trigger the ventilator.

Using volume-preset ventilation, the recommended tidal volume has for many years been as much as 10–12 mL/kg ideal body weight, but current recommendations are between 6 and 8 ml/kg ideal weight to minimize barotrauma and decrease lung injury. These tidal volumes should result in an inspiratory plateau pressure < 30 cm H_2O. The actual delivered tidal volume may be smaller or larger than what is selected. Patients who inspire vigorously along with the ventilator-delivered breath may draw additional volume from the ventilator. A smaller than expected tidal volume can occur if the pressure limit is reached while the inspired gas is delivered. The pressure limit is set by the operator and is intended to prevent injury to the patient if the chosen tidal volume would generate an excessively high pressure. For most patients, it is desirable to limit peak airway pressure to < 35–40 cm H_2O. Because the volume-preset ventilator will deliver the preset tidal volume and allow pressure to rise as necessary, when excessively high pressures are found, it may be necessary to decrease tidal volume if no reversible cause of increased airway resistance or decreased respiratory system compliance is found.

An inspiratory flow rate of about 1 L/s is set initially for most patients using volume-cycled ventilation, but higher flow rates may be necessary in patients with status asthmaticus or COPD or those with high minute ventilation. The flow can be adjusted according to the respiratory drive of the patient and the inspiratory time desired. Most volume-cycled ventilators used in the ICU are capable of constant inspiratory flow under most clinical conditions. This means that inspiratory flow will be constant even in patients with low lung or chest wall compliance or high airway resistance, and inspiratory flow will not decrease when a patient develops bronchospasm, airway secretions, atelectasis, or other conditions. Therefore, inspiratory time for a set tidal volume will remain relatively constant. In special circumstances such as severe hypoxemic respiratory failure, a decelerating inspiratory flow pattern may be helpful, and this pattern has been described as being similar to pressure-controlled ventilation.

Inspiratory time is usually chosen to be relatively short compared with expiratory time. An inspiratory time:expiratory time (I:E) ratio of 1:2–4 is most often used. An I:E ratio at or near 1:1 may improve oxygenation in selected patients. Inverse-ratio ventilation may be used with volume-preset ventilation (see below) in patients with ARDS. On the other hand, patients with high airway resistance need long expiratory times to complete exhalation; they may require an I:E ratio as high as 1:5–10.

Volume-preset, assist-control mechanical ventilation can be used to ventilate most patients with respiratory failure. The chief advantage of this mode is that a known tidal volume and—if the patient does not trigger the machine—a known respiratory frequency are provided. The tidal volume will not vary with changes in lung and chest wall mechanics. Another advantage is that clinicians are most often familiar with this mode.

C. Pressure-Controlled Ventilation

In pressure-controlled ventilation (PCV), maximum airway pressure is preset on the ventilator (rather than tidal volume), and tidal volume becomes a dependent variable. Although PCV is often thought of as a way of protecting the lungs from the effects of excessive airway and alveolar pressure and avoiding barotrauma, the major advantage of PCV is improved distribution of inspired gas with improved gas exchange. PCV should be considered strongly for patients with ARDS, for which most of the clinical experience has been gathered. It should not be used for mechanical ventilation of asthmatics or those with COPD.

With PCV the patient is provided with a preset constant positive pressure through the ventilator circuit throughout inspiration. The inspiratory flow pattern is complex and depends on the decreasing pressure gradient between airway and alveolar pressure during the inspiratory phase. The duration of inspiration is determined by setting either the inspiratory time or the I:E ratio and respiratory rate. Tidal volume is a function of the inspiratory flow pattern and inspiratory time. Pressure-controlled ventilation can be used in the assist-control mode, in which the respiratory rate is chosen either by the patient or, in the absence of sufficient respiratory drive, by the ventilator. In contrast to volume-cycled ventilation, in which tidal volume is preset, tidal volume is determined by inspiratory time and inspiratory flow. Airway pressure must be carefully chosen with respect to chest wall and lung compliance and airway resistance. In most patients, it is desirable to limit airway pressure with this mode to 30–40 cm H_2O, or a maximum tidal volume of 6–8 mL/kg ideal weight.

The potential advantages of pressure-controlled ventilation compared with volume-preset ventilation include reduced peak airway pressure and improved distribution of inspired gas. In theory, for the same tidal volume, peak airway pressure may not differ between the two modes. In practice, however, as the tidal volume is delivered during pressure-controlled ventilation, the difference between airway pressure and alveolar pressure falls, resulting in a progressive decline in flow rate—in contrast to constant flow during volume-preset ventilation. This mechanism is also responsible for the theoretical improvement in gas distribution. The highest flow and the largest proportion of tidal volume are delivered at the beginning of the breath, increasing the time available for gas to move to poorly ventilated lung regions. In several studies of patients with severe hypoxemia from ARDS, changing from conventional volume-preset ventilation to pressure-controlled ventilation was associated with improved PaO_2 and a decrease in inspiratory oxygen concentration.

Pressure-controlled ventilation has been frequently used with inverse-ratio ventilation (IRV), and some studies have not clearly distinguished each aspect's physiologic and clinical effects. IRV is set by choosing a prolonged inspiratory time (or shortened expiratory time) such that the time spent on each breath during inspiration exceeds expiratory time. That is, the I:E ratio varies from 2:1 to 4:1 rather than the conventional 1:2 to 1:4. Advocates of IRV argue that the shortened expiratory time increases end-expiratory volume, preventing or reducing atelectasis, while the lengthened inspiratory time improves inspiratory distribution of gas. However, increasing the time in which positive pressure is applied to the lungs should predictably impair cardiac output. IRV should be restricted to very careful use in selected patients with ARDS who demonstrate refractory hypoxemia when managed with other forms of treatment. IRV can also be used with more conventional volume-preset ventilation. One disadvantage of IRV is that patients usually require muscle relaxants or moderately heavy sedation.

D. Pressure-Support Ventilation

Pressure-support ventilation is the other major type of pressure-preset ventilation. This mode of ventilation provides a spontaneously breathing patient with a chosen amount of mechanical assistance during inspiration. Basically, when the patient initiates a breath, the pressure-support ventilator generates a preset positive pressure in the ventilator circuit. As long as the patient continues to inhale, the pressure is maintained at this constant level; when the patient stops inhaling, the pressure immediately falls to baseline. Thus, the patient's inspiratory effort is "supported" throughout inspiration. The net driving pressure is equal to the pressure-support pressure minus the alveolar pressure (negative) produced by the patient. The tidal volume is determined by the net driving pressure and the patient-selected duration of inspiration.

Pressure-support ventilation (PSV) allows the patient to inspire tidal volumes that might not be reached using only the patient's efforts, while the patient and not the ventilator selects the rate and tidal volume. PSV has been used both during weaning from mechanical ventilation and as a primary mode of ventilation. Potential advantages during weaning include the possibility that inspiratory muscles can contract to their accustomed length; respiratory rate may be slowed (because tidal volume is maintained); and patients may tolerate pressure support for prolonged duration. The respiratory muscles experience less afterload and therefore may be less prone to early fatigue. Pressure-support ventilation can be used as a primary ventilatory mode in suitable patients who are awake, alert, have adequate ventilatory drive, and who have moderately severe lung disease. The major advantage is that the patient and ventilator system often work more in synchrony, and in several studies patients have noted less discomfort and anxiety when pressure-support ventilation was used.

The level of PSV is chosen with consideration of respiratory system compliance, patient effort, desired tidal volume and minute ventilation, and severity of lung disease. Pressure-support pressure can be set to 10–15 cm H_2O as a starting point, and the tidal volume and rate measured can be used to decide on increasing or decreasing the pressure. Another method is to set pressure support at about two-thirds of the ventilator pressure needed during conventional mechanical ventilation to achieve a tidal volume of 6–8 mL/kg. Pressure-support pressure may also be set to achieve a selected minute ventilation or to provide enough support to inhibit accessory respiratory muscle contractions.

E. Intermittent Mandatory Ventilation (IMV)

In this mode, usually employed for weaning from mechanical ventilation but also occasionally for primary support, the ventilator provides tidal volume breaths at a preset fixed rate. In between ventilator-delivered breaths, the patient is able to breathe spontaneously through a parallel ventilator circuit at any rate, tidal volume, or pattern. In newer mechanical ventilators, the spontaneous breaths can be augmented by increased inspiratory pressure (ie, PSV) in combination with the ventilator-delivered breaths. For weaning purposes, the ventilator rate is reduced progressively as the patient's spontaneous rate and tidal volume are found to increase. The patient assumes an increasingly greater role in supplying the minute ventilation. As a primary support mode, it is believed by some investigators that the IMV mode is particularly well tolerated by patients who can, during the spontaneous breaths, adjust their minute ventilation and synchronize their breathing pattern more easily than with assist-control, volume-cycled mechanical ventilation. The benefit of IMV is unclear in patients who are difficult to wean from ventilatory support. There is no study supporting IMV as superior to other methods of weaning (see below). In addition, a high work of breathing may be engendered from the IMV breathing circuit in some mechanical ventilators that offer this mode.

F. Noninvasive Ventilation

As the name implies, noninvasive ventilatory support devices (ranging from negative pressure mechanical ventilators to positive pressure administered by a nasal or full face mask) have the advantage of not requiring an endotracheal or tracheostomy tube. As a result, patients are not subject to the potential complications associated with intubation, loss of airway defense mechanisms, and extubation. On the other hand, noninvasive modes do not provide the airway protection or access to respiratory secretions that are at hand when ventilation is delivered via the endotracheal route.

In addition, air leaks—which are common with all these devices—may be difficult to identify and correct and can result in a lower tidal volume or pressure level than what is desired or expected. Nevertheless, as experience with noninvasive ventilators (particularly the positive-pressure devices) grows, it has become clear that these devices can be useful in selected patients with acute or chronic respiratory failure.

1. Negative-pressure ventilation—Negative pressure ventilation may be successful in selected patients for temporary or long-term management, but this mode generally has limited use in the ICU. Tank-type negative pressure ventilators were used for poliomyelitis patients in the past, but current devices either use a shell fitted and sealed over the anterior chest (cuirass-type) or a pneumatic vest-like garment. A mechanical pump provides negative pressure to the outside of the chest wall. Suitable patients may be those with neuromuscular weakness who do not have high airway resistance, low respiratory compliance, or high ventilatory requirement. Negative pressure devices have the disadvantages of reducing patient mobility, causing skin irritation and breakdown, and limiting access to the chest or back for examination and routine nursing care. In addition, negative pressure mechanical ventilation has been implicated in the development of upper airway obstruction during sleep in some patients, presumably due to a lack of synchrony between upper airway dilator muscles and ventilator-initiated breaths.

2. Positive-pressure ventilation—These devices administer positive pressure to the airway via a nasal or nasal-oral circuit incorporating a nonrebreathing valve close to the patient to minimize added dead space. A wide variety of delivery circuits-ranging from snug-fitting nasal prongs to nasal, nasal-oral, and full face masks-are currently available in several sizes and shapes to accommodate most patients. Positive-pressure ventilation may be provided by certain conventional mechanical ventilators (those able to tolerate and compensate for air leaks) or, more commonly, by bilevel positive-pressure devices specifically designed for noninvasive use. Supplemental oxygen may be added using either a fixed liter-flow rate added to the inspiratory circuit (resulting in a potentially variable FIO_2) or, on newer models, via oxygen blenders capable of providing an FIO_2 as high as 1.0. Early bilevel machines were designed primarily for home use (for the treatment of obstructive sleep apnea) but very quickly found use in the ICU. Newer devices provide higher pressures (up to 35 cm H_2O) and better monitoring and alarm functions, making them better suited for use in the treatment of acute respiratory failure.

The success of these devices generally depends on having a cooperative patient and obtaining a proper fit of the circuit and attachment headgear (to maximize comfort and minimize potential air leaks). These devices are also best used in patients who do not require continuous or prolonged ventilatory support, since pressure sores can develop even with properly fitted masks. Other potential complications include nasal congestion, sinusitis, dry eyes, headaches, and gastric distention due to air swallowing. Compared with endotracheal mechanical ventilation, the use of noninvasive methods increases the level of care provided by nurses and respiratory therapists during the initiation of therapy (for mask fitting, monitoring, and ventilator adjustments). Administration of bronchodilators (or other treatments by inhalation) and eating generally require temporary removal of the circuit, further adding to the level of care required.

Nasal continuous positive airway pressure (nasal CPAP) is the treatment of choice for most patients with obstructive sleep apnea syndrome but may also be useful in the treatment of other ICU patients. CPAP administered via a nasal or nasal-oral mask (at pressures of 10–12.5 cm H_2O) can improve gas exchange in patients with pulmonary edema and has the added advantage of reducing left ventricular afterload and improving cardiac output in patients with congestive cardiomyopathies.

While the addition of a low level of CPAP may be helpful in treating other nonapneic causes of respiratory failure, noninvasive ventilatory support is usually more successful when the inspiratory and expiratory pressures can be adjusted independently, as with bilevel ventilatory support devices. Bilevel positive airway pressure devices offer the ability to titrate independently the inspiratory and expiratory positive airway pressure. When operating in the "spontaneous" mode, these devices can be thought of as being similar to inspiratory pressure support with PEEP. Airflow into the patient circuit is adjusted automatically to maintain the preset pressure levels. As a result, these devices are generally able to compensate for the air leaks inevitably seen with mask-delivery systems. Patient-initiated breaths are sensed as a demand for an increase in airflow into the patient circuit, which then triggers the switch to the higher IPAP level. IPAP is maintained until the required flow returns to a lower level, at which time the pressure returns to the set EPAP level. The actual tidal volume delivered during a given breath will depend on the differential pressure (IPAP–EPAP), the respiratory system compliance, and the amount of inspiratory effort generated by the patient. Some devices also offer a "timed" mode (similar to pressure-controlled IMV) and a "spontaneous or timed" mode (similar to pressure controlled IMV plus pressure support). However, these are generally less useful in treating patients with acute respiratory failure.

Noninvasive ventilation may also be given using a nasal or face mask connected to a conventional volume-cycled ventilator. This offers the potential advantages of allowing higher inspiratory pressures (bilevel positive airway pressure devices typically generate a maximum pressure of 20–35 cm H_2O) and having slightly more control over delivered tidal volume. Unlike ventilation through an endotracheal tube, however, positive pressure is sensed throughout the upper airway, often resulting in reduced patient tolerance and increased complications. In addition, inspiratory air leaks generally increase in proportion to the pressure delivered to the mask.

Noninvasive mechanical ventilation is often provided for obstructive sleep apnea patients unable to tolerate the CPAP levels required to maintain airway patency or in those with superimposed central hypoventilation. For these conditions, EPAP is increased until obstructive apneas are abolished and IPAP is titrated upward as necessary to reduce or eliminate hypopneas, oxygen desaturations, and snoring.

Noninvasive ventilation has also been shown to help selected patients with respiratory failure due to obstructive airway disease or restrictive lung disease. Several randomized, controlled studies in patients with acute exacerbation of COPD demonstrate that the early administration of noninvasive ventilatory support improves gas exchange, vital signs, and dyspnea scores and reduces the need for invasive mechanical ventilation. These studies also suggest that noninvasive mechanical ventilation may reduce morbidity and mortality rates as well as the number of both ICU and total hospital days. The mechanism of benefit is probably related both to the inspiratory assist provided by IPAP and the low levels of EPAP (3–6 cm H_2O) which reduce the amount of isometric contraction of inspiratory muscles needed to overcome intrinsic PEEP. Noninvasive ventilation has also been demonstrated to be helpful in treatment of acute respiratory failure caused by pneumonia and other disorders, with reported benefits including reduced intubation rates, fewer ICU days, and a decrease in nosocomial infections (as compared with endotracheal mechanical ventilation). Finally, noninvasive ventilation can be used to facilitate weaning from invasive mechanical ventilation resulting in higher overall weaning rates, shorter duration of ventilatory support, fewer ICU days, and improved 60-day mortality compared with routine weaning.

Patients most likely to benefit from noninvasive mechanical ventilation are those with moderate to severe dyspnea accompanied by tachypnea, accessory muscle use, paradoxic breathing, and gas-exchange abnormalities (eg, $PaCO_2 > 45$, $pH < 7.35$, or $PaO_2/FIO_2 < 200$). Severely ill patients (eg, respiratory arrest, hypotensive shock, uncontrolled arrhythmias, or ischemia) and those with excessive secretions or a loss of airway protection are better treated with intubation and mechanical ventilation. Furthermore, patients who are agitated or uncooperative and those with facial injuries or abnormalities interfering with mask fit are generally not candidates for noninvasive ventilation. After selecting and fitting the nasal mask, recommended initial settings are IPAP = 8–12 cm H_2O and EPAP = 3–5 cm H_2O. The IPAP is increased gradually as tolerated (generally to 10–20 cm H_2O) with therapeutic goals of dyspnea relief, good patient-ventilator synchrony, and improved gas-exchange. The EPAP may be increased if needed for alveolar recruitment (similar to PEEP changes in standard mechanical ventilation) but in patients with COPD should be kept below the level of intrinsic PEEP to avoid worsening hyperinflation. Supplemental oxygen is added to maintain O_2 saturation > 90%. Most patients benefit from ongoing encouragement and reassurance. Occasionally, light sedation is helpful in anxious and agitated patients; however, these medications have the potential for compromising airway patency, so close monitoring is essential.

G. Other Methods of Mechanical Ventilation

Less commonly used methods of mechanical ventilation in critical care areas include high-frequency ventilation, negative-pressure ventilation, and extracorporeal membrane oxygenation or CO_2 elimination. High-frequency ventilation uses very small tidal volume—sometimes less than anatomic dead space volume—and respiratory frequencies > 1/s (> 1 Hz). The tidal volume is provided by one of several means, including a high-velocity air-oxygen jet, a high-frequency inspiratory valve, or a mechanical or electromagnetic oscillator. The mechanism of gas movement is not known, though facilitation of gas diffusion has been postulated. Several years ago, there was considerable interest in these ventilators for severe hypoxemic respiratory failure, but several clinical studies failed to demonstrate advantages of these devices. A recent review of high-frequency ventilation in ARDS and acute lung injury concluded that high-frequency oscillation (HFO) may be promising but should still be considered experimental.

Negative-pressure ventilation may be successful in highly selected patients for temporary or long-term management, but this mode generally has limited use in the ICU. Tank-type negative pressure ventilators were used for poliomyelitis patients in the past, but current devices either use a shell fitted and sealed over the anterior chest (cuirass-type) or a pneumatic vest-like garment. A mechanical pump provides negative pressure to the outside of the chest wall. Suitable patients may be those with neuromuscular weakness who do not have high airway resistance, low respiratory compliance, or high ventilatory requirements. Negative pressure devices have the disadvantages of reducing patient mobility, causing skin irritation and breakdown, and limiting access to the chest or back for examination and routine nursing care. Negative pressure mechanical ventilation has also been implicated in the development of upper airway obstruction during sleep in some patients, presumably due to a lack of synchrony between upper airway dilator muscles and ventilator-initiated breaths.

Clinical Applications

The mode of mechanical ventilation and the settings to be used should be chosen in consultation with physicians and respiratory care practitioners who have experience in the management of respiratory failure. Some criteria for selection of modes in different types of respiratory failure are presented in Table 12–8, and further details are found in discussions of the various disorders. Proper monitoring of the patient-ventilator system greatly facilitates patient care as shown in Table 12–9.

Monitoring the Patient on Mechanical Ventilation

The patient-ventilator system warrants careful monitoring. After all, a patient's normal homeostatic and feedback mechanisms are no longer completely functioning, and extremes of inflation, arterial blood gases, and effects on hemodynamics are likely without the usual constraints. Some important monitoring principles and guidelines are included in Chapter 8.

Specific monitoring of mechanical ventilation can be divided into two categories. First, respiratory therapy departments and intensive care units have established routine monitoring standards for all patients on mechanical ventilation. These usually include hourly—or more frequent—measurement and documentation of peak and plateau airway pressure, minute ventilation, oxygen saturation by pulse oximetry, endotracheal tube cuff pressure and volume, tidal volume, and respiratory rate. The ventilator settings are charted, including mode, set tidal volume and rate, inspired concentration of oxygen, PEEP, and alarm settings and limits. Clinicians should review these data at least daily, and the data should be studied carefully if patients deteriorate suddenly, have difficulty with discontinuation of mechanical ventilation, develop new gas exchange problems, or show changes on chest x-rays.

A second category of mechanical ventilator monitoring involves more sophisticated measurements and calculations, and these are recommended for certain clinical situations. Intrinsic PEEP (auto-PEEP) can be automatically determined with some ventilators; in others, expiratory port occlusion (see below) is necessary. Intrinsic PEEP determination is essential in patients with COPD exacerbation and asthma. Respiratory system pressure-volume (PV) curves have been recom-

Table 12–8. Suggested ventilator strategies and tactics in respiratory failure.

Respiratory Failure	Strategy	Tactic
Neuromuscular or chest wall disorder	Avoid barotrauma. Minimize effects on cardiac output. Avoid hyperventilation. Prevent atelectasis and worsening Pao_2.	VT 6–8mL/kg; peak Paw < 40 cm H_2O Adjust $Paco_2$ to pH in presence of elevated HCO_3^- PEEP 3–5 cm H_2O
COPD, asthma	Improve gas exchange by avoiding hyperinflation. Decrease adverse effects on cardiac output. Decrease work of breathing.	Long expiratory time; high $\dot{V}$I (>1 L/s), low f, VT 6–8 mL/kg. Allow hypoventilation? Use muscle relaxants. PEEP < intrinsic PEEP?
ARDS	Improve arterial Pao_2. Decrease potential for O_2 toxicity. Meet ventilatory demand. Reduce potential for barotrauma. Limit adverse effects on cardiac output and O_2 delivery.	PEEP PCV or descending flow pattern (VCV) Use $FIO_2 < 0.50$ High VI, high f Low VT (6–8 mL/kg) Pplat < 30 cm H_2O PEEP < 10 cmH_2O

Key:
PCV = pressure-controlled ventilation
PC-IRV = pressure-controlled, inverse-ratio ventilation
PEEP = positive end-expiratory pressure
Pplat = inspiratory plateau pressure
$\dot{V}$T = tidal volume
$\dot{V}$I = inspiratory flow rate
f = respiratory rate

mended by some investigators, especially in Europe, in order to determine optimal PEEP settings and in limiting tidal volume in ARDS patients. Despite very important recent experimental information derived from PV curves, their clinical use has not become routine for a variety of technical reasons and problems of interpretation. Finally, esophageal pressure measurements during mechanical ventilation would provide important information about intrinsic PEEP, chest wall compared with lung compliance changes, and work of breathing. Once again, these measurements are not often made in the intensive care unit.

COMPLICATIONS

Some of the complications of mechanical ventilation are listed in Table 12–10. These can be divided into two categories: (1) complications and adverse effects of positive-pressure ventilation, and (2) complications of having a mechanical substitute for the natural ventilatory system. Because the vast majority of mechanically ventilated patients have endotracheal tubes or tracheostomy tubes, airway complications must also be considered under this heading.

A. BAROTRAUMA

Barotrauma is somewhat of a misnomer because it is now understood that lung injury from barotrauma occurs because of excessive and repeated stretching of the lungs regardless of the pressure. The degree of injury is related to stretching and volume change rather than pressure changes. Therefore, a patient with very stiff or noncompliant lungs may require high pressures to ventilate, but because the lungs are not particularly stretched, barotrauma is uncommon in this situation. On the other hand, a patient with very compliant lungs, such as are seen with bullous emphysema, requires very low pressures to stretch the lungs considerably. This type of patient is at high risk of barotrauma despite low pressure because of the large volume changes. Therefore, barotrauma might more properly be called volume trauma. Current recommendations to use smaller tidal volumes when mechanically ventilating patients with asthma, COPD, and ARDS have been associated with a reduced incidence of barotrauma.

Positive-pressure ventilation has been associated with several forms of barotrauma to the lungs. Most often appreciated is explosive barotrauma in which inspired gas under positive pressure ruptures an area of lung or airway. Air initially escapes into the interstitial spaces of the lungs and tracks along bronchovascular bundles toward the mediastinum. Therefore, at first the patient may have interstitial emphysema, which may be seen as thin air density lines only against a background of lung consolidation. Subsequently, the patient may

Table 12–9. Monitoring mechanical ventilation.

Variable or Ventilator Setting	Clinical Significance
Measured $\dot{V}_E$	Is patient breathing more than set V_T and f? Weaning may be feasible if $\dot{V}_E$ <12 L/min. High $\dot{V}_E$ relative to Pa_{CO_2} means high V_D/V_T or increased metabolic rate.
Peak airway pressure	High pressure at a given tidal volume suggests high airway resistance and/or low respiratory system compliance.
Inspiratory plateau pressure (see text)	High pressure suggests low respirator system compliance.
F_{IO_2}	Combined with Pa_{O_2}, indicates efficiency of oxygenation. Use F_{IO_2} to calculate $P(A–a)O_2$ or Pa_{O_2}/F_{IO_2} ratio.
Respiratory rate	During IMV, spontaneous rate and tidal volume indicate contribution of patient to total minute ventilation. During assisted ventilation, rate higher than set rate indicates patient has degree of respiratory drive.
Tidal volume	During pressure-support ventilation, comparison of V_T and support pressure assesses patient's contribution to total ventilation.
Intrinsic PEEP present?	See mechanical ventilator management of patients with respiratory failure from COPD. Useful in determining if gas exchange is compromised by dynamic hyperinflation.

develop evidence of air surrounding mediastinal structures or pneumomediastinum. If the air separates the lungs and pleura from the inner surface of the chest wall, an extrapleural pneumothorax can form. Another way in which pneumothorax can evolve is through rupture of the lung directly into space separating the visceral and parietal pleural surfaces. Positive-pressure ventilation, especially combined with PEEP, has been associated with explosive barotrauma, including interstitial emphysema and pneumothorax, but there continues to be debate about the relative contributions of underlying lung disease and positive-pressure ventilation. It is likely that both acute lung injury and some forms of chronic lung disease are associated with increased risk of barotrauma.

A more important and more common subtle form of barotrauma is manifested by evidence that positive-pressure ventilation and PEEP are associated with increased lung injury, leading to more severe gas exchange abnormalities and permanent histologic damage. Mechanical ventilation and PEEP in ARDS may damage the lungs in somewhat the same way supportive care for neonatal respiratory distress contributes to bronchopulmonary dysplasia. These considerations have led to recommendations that airway pressure and tidal volume should be limited in patients at risk. For example, in experimental animals, both the combination of low PEEP = 0 cm H_2O and high tidal volume of 39 mL/kg and the combination of high PEEP = 15 cm H_2O and low tidal volume of 7 mL/kg resulted in pulmonary edema. Current recommendations to use tidal volumes between 6 mL and 8 mL/kg ideal weight are based on a decreased likelihood of barotrauma, perhaps less lung injury, and improved patient outcomes.

B. Decreased Cardiac Output

Patients started on positive-pressure mechanical ventilation not infrequently become hypotensive, and this is largely because positive-pressure ventilation can compromise cardiac output. In normal subjects, negative pressure during spontaneous inspiration provides an additional impetus to venous return by exerting negative pressure on the intrathoracic venae cavae, the right atrium, and the right ventricle. Pulmonary vascular resistance falls during inspiration, allowing for improved emptying of the right ventricle.

Table 12–10. Complications of mechanical ventilation.

Complications of artificial airway

Complications of positive-pressure ventilation
Pneumothorax
Pneumomediastinum
Parenchymal barotrauma (lung injury)
Decreased cardiac output
Increased intracranial pressure
Impaired ability to monitor or interpret intrathoracic vascular pressures (pulmonary artery catheter)
Altered gas exchange (worsening of $\dot{V}/\dot{Q}$ mismatching)

Complications of artificial ventilation
Hypoventilation
Hyperventilation
Apnea
Oxygen toxicity
Mechanical or electrical failure or disconnection of ventilator
Increased risk of nosocomial pneumonia
Accidental thermal or chemical burns to airway
Aspiration and ventilator associated pneumonia
Psychologic dependence on ventilator

On the other hand, positive-pressure ventilation may have several adverse effects on cardiac output. First, positive pressure (rather than negative pressure) during inspiration tends to interfere with systemic venous return. Second, inflation of the lungs with positive pressure increases pulmonary vascular resistance and impedes right ventricular emptying. Third, there is evidence that positive-pressure ventilation and PEEP may decrease left ventricular compliance by causing the intraventricular septum to be less easily movable. There is little evidence of a negative inotropic effect of positive-pressure ventilation, and left ventricular afterload decreases during positive-pressure ventilation, potentially improving left ventricular function and ejection fraction. It is important to distinguish effects on cardiac output from effects on cardiac function; positive-pressure ventilation may improve cardiac function in some patients while reducing cardiac output in others.

Patients who become hypotensive or show evidence of decreased cardiac output while on positive-pressure ventilation should be assessed for volume depletion, the recent use of vasoactive drugs (including opioid analgesics and sedatives), excessively high tidal volume or airway pressure, and intrinsic PEEP, as well as other systemic causes of hemodynamic compromise. A trial of intravenous fluids is sometimes warranted while ventilator adjustments are considered.

C. Other Complications

Inadvertent hypoventilation and hyperventilation are not uncommon, because mechanical ventilators are unable to respond automatically to changes in blood gas partial pressures. Appropriate ventilation may not be delivered because of machine malfunction, disconnection from the patient, disconnection from electrical power, O_2, or compressed air, operator error, or obstruction of the ventilator circuit. A rare reported complication is injury from overheating of the humidifier used to warm and humidify inspired gas.

Ventilator circuits and humidifiers may become colonized with pathogenic bacteria or fungi, but changing and draining water and secretions from circuits has a beneficial effect on nosocomial infection. Nevertheless, nosocomial pneumonia is an important complication of mechanical ventilation. In a study of 264 patients admitted to a medical-surgical ICU who required mechanical ventilation for more than 48 hours, 22% developed bacterial pneumonia. Gram-negative bacilli were identified in 63% and *Staphylococcus aureus* in 23%. Forty-two percent of those with pneumonia died, compared with 37% of the same patients who did not develop nosocomial pneumonia. Although this difference in mortality rate was not statistically significant, pneumonia did increase the time spent in the ICU. The diagnosis of ventilator-associated pneumonia is very difficult. Some investigators have recommended that patients undergo invasive diagnostic testing using special fiberoptic bronchoscopic methods (eg, protected brush catheters with quantitative bacterial cultures); others suggest that these data do not improve diagnostic accuracy. Data suggest that decreasing the frequency of ventilator circuit changes is associated with fewer episodes of nosocomial pneumonia. Attention to careful suctioning, frequent draining of the condensate in the tubing, judicious use of antibiotics, and (if possible) avoiding prolonged mechanical ventilation may decrease the risk of nosocomial pneumonia.

Discontinuation of Mechanical Ventilation ("Weaning")

Once the need for it is corrected, mechanical ventilation can be discontinued easily and safely in the majority of patients, ie, those who do not have severe lung disease or neuromuscular weakness or who were electively placed on mechanical ventilation during surgery. In other patients—especially those with lung disease—mechanical ventilation must usually be discontinued gradually, with careful monitoring. The gradual reduction in ventilatory support has led to the use of the term "weaning" from the mechanical ventilator as the patient resumes spontaneous ventilation. Discontinuation of mechanical ventilation should be distinguished from discontinuation of endotracheal intubation or tracheostomy. Although the terms "intubation" and "ventilation" are often used synonymously, there are some patients in whom intubation is necessary but mechanical ventilation is not (eg, those with upper airway obstruction).

A. Physiologic Assessment

To be successfully taken off mechanical ventilation, the patient must have a sustained ventilatory capacity that equals or exceeds the ventilatory requirement. For most patients who fail to be weaned successfully, the ventilatory requirement (ie, how much minute ventilation is needed to maintain Pa_{CO_2}) is excessively high relative to ventilatory capacity (how much minute ventilation the patient is capable of providing without assistance) (Table 12–11). The ventilatory requirement is a function of the metabolic rate (oxygen uptake), CO_2 production, the set point for Pa_{CO_2}, and the efficiency of lung gas exchange (dead space:tidal volume ratio). Ventilatory capacity is determined primarily by the interaction of ventilatory drive, respiratory system mechanics, and inspiratory muscle strength and endurance.

Disuse of respiratory muscles leads to atrophy, earlier and easier fatigue, and possibly discoordination. In patients with increased airway resistance or decreased lung or chest wall compliance, respiratory muscles must generate relatively greater pressure for a given tidal vol-

Table 12–11. Factors contributing to difficult weaning: Increased ventilatory requirement or decreased ventilatory capacity.

Increased Ventilatory Requirement	Decreased Sustained Ventilatory Capacity
Fever	Respiratory muscle fatigue
Infection	Hypokalemia
Increased ventilatory drive	Hypophosphatemia
Metabolic acidosis	Decreased ventilatory drive
Excessive hyperalimentation (especially with carbohydrate?)	Bronchospasm
	Airway secretions
	Decreased lung or chest wall compliance
Liver disease	Neuromuscular weakness
	Malnutrition
	Small endotracheal tube
	Increased resistance of endotracheal tube or ventilator circuit

ume. Often these patients have an increased ventilatory requirement and, therefore, an increased pressure-time product—an index of muscle work and potential for fatigue. Factors associated with decreased muscle strength and endurance include electrolyte abnormalities (hypokalemia, hypophosphatemia), critical illness polymyopathy and polyneuropathy, high-dose corticosteroid therapy, malnutrition, and recent use of nondepolarizing muscle relaxants.

B. Predicting Successful Weaning

The underlying disease that caused a need for mechanical ventilation must be corrected first. The patient should have adequate gas exchange as assessed by an only moderate supplemental oxygen requirement (Pa_{O_2} > 60 mm Hg and F_{IO_2} < 0.5) and V_D/V_T < 0.50. The ventilatory requirement can be determined generally as the minute ventilation ($\dot{V}_E$) provided during mechanical ventilation. If gas exchange and the metabolic rate do not change, the patient will have to provide this amount of $\dot{V}_E$ to maintain Pa_{CO_2} at the preweaning level. Weaning is often unsuccessful when the $\dot{V}_E$ requirement is greater than 10–12 L/min, or about twice that of resting $\dot{V}_E$ in normal adults. Adequate ventilatory capacity is encouraged by ensuring normal electrolyte levels (especially phosphorus, magnesium, and potassium), discontinuing sedatives, and minimizing abnormal lung mechanics by treatment with bronchodilators and suitable patient positioning.

Assessment of ventilatory capacity has been addressed using a variety of "weaning parameters," some of which are shown in Table 12–12. Vital capacity, negative inspiratory pressure, spontaneous minute ventilation measured for 1 minute, and maximum voluntary ventilation measured for 8–10 seconds are used to estimate short-term ventilatory capacity. These variables have excellent predictive value in patients recovering from short-term general anesthesia, but their predictive value is only marginal in patients with acute or chronic lung diseases who require mechanical ventilation. This is largely because these parameters assess only ventilatory capacity and do not take into account the ventilatory requirement and work of breathing. In one study in which 58% of patients were successfully weaned, the following variables were found to be most closely correlated with success: days of mechanical ventilation before the weaning trial, respiratory frequency:tidal volume ratio, maximal inspiratory pressure, maximal expiratory pressure, and vital capacity. There were important differences between groups with COPD, neurologic respiratory failure, and other causes of respiratory failure; positive predictive values for successful weaning ranged from 74%–94%.

Indices that combine estimates of ventilatory requirement, work of breathing, and ventilatory capacity may be useful. For example, a spontaneous respiratory rate:tidal volume ratio (f/V_T) of less than 100/min/L may predict successful weaning because it is an index of requirement and capacity. This ratio, termed a shallow breathing index, proved to have greater sensitivity and specificity than other variables for prediction of weaning. However, a report of 52 patients undergoing weaning from mechanical ventilation indicated that 12 of 13 patients with a f/V_T > 105/min/L were successfully

Table 12–12. Some variables used to predict success during weaning from mechanical ventilation.

Ventilatory capacity

- $\dot{V}_E$ (on ventilator) < 10 L/min and $\dot{V}_E$ (spontaneous) = $\dot{V}_E$ (on ventilator)
- V_T > 5 mL/kg; VC > 10–15 mL/kg
- Spontaneous f < 25/min
- Maximum negative inspiratory pressure < –25 cm H_2O
- Maximal voluntary ventilation (MVV) > 2 x $\dot{V}_E$ (ventilator)

Ventilatory requirement

- Pa_{O_2} > 60 mm Hg with F_{IO_2} < 0.50
- V_D/V_T < 0.50

Combined indices

$$\frac{f\ (\text{breaths/min})}{V_T(\text{L})} < 100\ \text{breaths/min/L}$$

Successful 30-minute spontaneous breathing trial

weaned whereas only one patient who failed extubation had a ratio that high. Very low f/VT ratios have a high positive predictive value for successful weaning, whereas very high ratios would predict unsuccessful weaning. On the other hand, ratios between 70 and 110 may have less predictive value.

Nevertheless, prediction of successful or unsuccessful discontinuation of weaning continues to be poor. Because of this, a clinical trial of patients who have marginal or low likelihoods of successful weaning may be indicated. In one study, all patients using mechanical ventilation were given a daily spontaneous breathing trial unless they had contraindications such as apnea, hypopnea, severe hypoxemia, or high oxygen or minute ventilation requirements. Surprisingly, a higher proportion of patients than predicted by the patients' clinicians were able to be successfully discontinued from mechanical ventilation.

C. Weaning Methods

Patients who are easily weaned from mechanical ventilation are easily weaned regardless of the specific method used. Those who are difficult to wean for any reason will be difficult no matter which method is used. An explanation of the weaning procedure, including descriptions of possible discomfort and an assurance of close monitoring, should be provided to the patient before weaning is started.

Once weaning is attempted, signs that should lead to restarting mechanical ventilation or slowing the process of discontinuing ventilatory support include tachypnea, tachycardia (usually > 120/min), hypotension, severe anxiety, hypoxemia or a fall in pulse oximeter-estimated oxygen saturation, respiratory acidosis (pH < 7.30), arrhythmias, chest pain, or other signs of hemodynamic compromise. A study of a small number of patients showed that a fall in gastric intramural pH, suggesting tissue ischemia, was found in patients who failed weaning, whereas those who were successful had no change in gastric intramural pH. In any patient who has difficulty being weaned from mechanical ventilation, reassessment of ventilatory requirements and ventilatory capacity is indicated.

1. T tube—The ventilator circuit is disconnected from the endotracheal tube, and humidified oxygen is supplied by a tube connected across the endotracheal tube connection ("T tube") while the patient breathes spontaneously. The patient is carefully observed for signs of respiratory failure, discomfort, severe dyspnea, or other intolerance, and the duration of T tube sessions is increased depending on the patient's success. In between sessions, the patient is reconnected to the mechanical ventilator in the assist-control mode. In some patients, a T tube session may be as short as 5–10 minutes at first, with very gradual lengthening. The sessions may be repeated two to four times daily depending on patient tolerance. It is important to strike a balance between excessive respiratory muscle fatigue during the sessions and adequate time for the patient to assume some of the work of breathing.

A variation of the T tube weaning method uses the ventilator circuit and ventilator to provide the air-oxygen mixture during spontaneous breathing rather than a separate T tube. This method allows for monitoring and warning of low spontaneous tidal volume. Concern has been raised, however, that some ventilator circuits during spontaneous ventilation require much more patient effort than the conventional T tube. Some mechanical ventilators have systems that provide gas mixtures to spontaneously breathing patients with minimal work and effort.

2. Intermittent mandatory ventilation (IMV)—This mode is described above. The number of mechanical ventilator breaths each minute is gradually decreased over hours or days while the patient provides a progressively increasing share of the breaths taken each minute. The IMV mode in some mechanical ventilators requires that the patient do excessive work during the spontaneous breaths, and for that reason patients may tire easily. Despite encouraging data when IMV was first used in the 1970s, there is no evidence that using IMV facilitates weaning in patients with lung disease or in those who are difficult to wean. IMV has the advantage of providing good monitoring of the patient during weaning, with breath-by-breath spontaneous tidal volume and rate displayed by most ventilators. A combination of IMV and pressure support during the spontaneous breaths is often used.

3. Pressure-support ventilation—The theoretic advantages of pressure-support ventilation (PSV) are outlined above. During weaning by this technique, the pressure-support pressure is initially chosen to achieve a tidal volume of 6–8 mL/kg and a respiratory rate less than about 20/min. Pressure-support pressure is then gradually decreased until the patient's own tidal volume without pressure support is adequate. Mechanical ventilation can usually be discontinued when the pressure support is less than 7–10 cm H_2O.

When it is desired to rest the inspiratory muscles temporarily, either pressure-support pressure can be increased until tidal volume reaches the desired level with little or no patient effort or the patient can be ventilated using conventional mechanical ventilation. A few studies comparing pressure-support ventilation to T tube weaning and IMV have been completed, and T tube weaning and PSV seem to be similarly more successful than IMV weaning. It is likely that PSV and T tube weaning will both be useful depending on patient selection and clinician preference.

4. Noninvasive positive-pressure ventilation—Noninvasive positive-pressure ventilation has potential benefits in the weaning process, assuming that the patient is extubated. Some studies have suggested that patients who are marginal weaning candidates (COPD with high ventilatory requirements or low ventilatory capacity) may be successfully extubated with the use of face-mask noninvasive positive-pressure ventilation. The advantages might be decreased duration of intubation, fewer complications, and shorter hospital stays. Other studies have found that patients who have failed weaning or extubation might be temporarily supported using noninvasive positive-pressure ventilation rather than reintubation. Further studies are necessary to determine the precise role and outcome of noninvasive positive-pressure ventilation in weaning. If used, however, candidates should be carefully selected and closely monitored.

5. Other methods—Patients sometimes require prolonged nutritional support or require a long time to resolve a reversible neuromuscular disorder. Facilities that specialize in management and weaning of long-term ventilator-dependent patients may be a less costly alternative in selected patients. These patients may return to the ICU when weaning is more feasible. A number of specialized centers have reported considerable success in weaning patients after very prolonged mechanical ventilation.

Antonelli M et al: A comparison of noninvasive positive-pressure ventilation and conventional mechanical ventilation in patients with acute respiratory failure. N Engl J Med 1998;339:429–35.

Ely WE et al: Effect of the duration of mechanical ventilation on identifying patients capable of breathing spontaneously. N Engl J Med 1996;335:1864–9.

Ely EW, Evans GW, Haponik EF: Mechanical ventilation in a cohort of elderly patients admitted to an intensive care unit. Ann Intern Med 1999;131:96–104.

Esteban A et al: Effect of spontaneous breathing trial duration on outcome of attempts to discontinue mechanical ventilation. Am J Respir Crit Care Med 1999;159:512–8.

Girault C et al: Noninvasive ventilation as a systematic extubation and weaning technique in acute-on-chronic respiratory failure. Am J Respir Crit Care Med 1999;160:86–92.

Girou E et al: Association of noninvasive ventilation with nosocomial infections and survival in critically ill patients. JAMA 2000;284:2361–7.

Heffner JE, Hess D: Tracheostomy management in the chronically ventilated patient. Clin Chest Med 2001;22:55–69.

Heffner JE: Timing of tracheotomy in mechanically ventilated patients. Am Rev Respir Dis 1993;147:768–71.

Krishnan JA, Brower RG: High-frequency ventilation for acute lung injury and ARDS. Chest 2000;118:795–807.

McBibben AW, Ravenscraft SA: Pressure-controlled and volume-cycled mechanical ventilation. Clin Chest Med 1996;17:395–410.

Markowicz P et al: Multicenter prospective study of ventilator-associated pneumonia during acute respiratory distress syndrome. Incidence, prognosis, and risk factors. ARDS Study Group. Am J Respir Crit Care Med 2000;161:1942–8.

Mehta S, Hill NS: Noninvasive ventilation. Am J Respir Crit Care Med 2001;163:540–77.

Nava S et al: Noninvasive mechanical ventilation in the weaning of patients with respiratory failure due to chronic obstructive pulmonary disease: a randomized study. Ann Intern Med 1998;128:721–8.

Plant PK et al: Early use of noninvasive ventilation for acute exacerbations of chronic obstructive pulmonary disease on general respiratory wards: a multicentre randomised controlled trial. Lancet 2000;355:1931–5.

Sandur S, Stoller JK: Pulmonary complications of mechanical ventilation. Clin Chest Med 1999;20:223–47.

Slutsky AS: Mechanical ventilation. American College of Chest Physicians' Consensus Conference. Chest 1993;104:1833–59.

Tobin MJ: Advances in mechanical ventilation. N Engl J Med 2001;344:1986–96.

Tocino I, Westcott JL: Barotrauma. Radiol Clin North Am 1996;34:59–81.

Vallverdu I et al: Clinical characteristics, respiratory functional parameters, and outcome of a two-hour T-piece trial in patients weaning from mechanical ventilation. Am J Respir Crit Care Med 1998;158:1855–62.

ACUTE RESPIRATORY FAILURE FROM SPECIFIC DISORDERS

NEUROMUSCULAR DISORDERS

ESSENTIALS OF DIAGNOSIS

- *May present with decreased ventilation due to respiratory muscle weakness (usually high respiratory rate with low tidal volume) or decreased ventilatory drive (low respiratory rate and tidal volume).*
- *Pa_{CO_2} > 50 mm Hg.*
- *VC < 55% of predicted or < 1500 mL may be associated with hypercapnia.*
- *Neuromuscular disorders may be associated with atelectasis, aspiration, pneumonia, hypoxemia, and poor cough reflex.*
- *Suspect respiratory muscle weakness in all patients with neuromuscular weakness; general muscle strength does not always correlate with respiratory function.*

General Considerations

Respiratory failure from neuromuscular diseases results from respiratory muscle weakness or abnormal control of ventilation. Muscle weakness or paralysis can result from disease in any part of the nervous system involved with motor activity. Problems with control of ventilation arise in the course of diseases that affect the O_2 and CO_2 chemoreceptors, their connections to the central nervous systems, and the integrative and autonomic parts of the brain stem, primarily the medulla.

In addition to respiratory failure, neuromuscular disease can be associated with a number of other respiratory manifestations (Table 12–13). For critically ill patients, complications of underlying nonneurologic diseases and treatment may include neuromuscular weakness (electrolyte abnormalities, corticosteroid myopathy, and peripheral neuropathy) and depressed ventilatory drive (sedatives, opioid analgesics).

Pathophysiology

Respiratory failure in neuromuscular disease is due to weakness of the respiratory muscles: the intercostal muscles and the diaphragm. However, other factors contribute to abnormal gas exchange (Table 12–14). Acute weakness of inspiratory and expiratory muscles results in rapidly progressive decrease in vital capacity and progressive alveolar hypoventilation with hypoxemia. In most cases, the mechanical properties of the chest wall are altered but the lungs are normal unless complications occur. On the other hand, chronic manifestations of neuromuscular disease may cause long-term alteration of the lungs and chest wall. Other factors that contribute to differences in the presentation of respiratory failure include the age of the patient at onset of disease, the distribution of muscle weakness, the presence of a chronic or relapsing course, and underlying lung or heart disease.

Table 12–13. Respiratory complications of neuromuscular disease.

Hypercapnic respiratory failure
Hypoxemia
Pneumonia
Aspiration of gastric contents
Pulmonary edema
Abnormal ventilatory pattern
Upper airway obstruction
Atelectasis
Respiratory alkalosis
Pulmonary embolism

Table 12–14. Physiologic consequences of neuromuscular disease.

Decreased lung volumes
Alveolar hypoventilation
Decreased lung compliance
Increased chest wall compliance (acute weakness)
Decreased chest wall compliance (chronic spastic paralysis)
Abnormal abdominal wall mechanics
Ventilation-perfusion maldistribution
Atelectasis
Impaired cough effectiveness

A. Normal Respiratory Muscles

Respiratory muscles include the diaphragm, the intercostal muscles, muscles in the neck that can generate additional respiratory effort, and muscles of the abdominal wall. Other muscles play a key part in ventilation, including muscles in the upper airway and the smooth muscles of the lower airways. Respiratory muscles can be divided into inspiratory and expiratory muscles, though some are used during both parts of the respiratory cycle. The diaphragm is usually thought to generate negative intrathoracic pressure during contraction by pulling downward toward the abdomen. However, if abdominal wall muscles contract simultaneously with the diaphragm, the net effect is rather to pull the lower margins of the rib cage upward and outward, thereby expanding the thoracic volume. Muscles in the neck assist inspiratory efforts, especially when the work of breathing is increased, high ventilation is needed, the lungs are hyperinflated, or the diaphragm becomes fatigued. These accessory muscles include the sternocleidomastoids and scalenes.

Exhalation is usually passive, but normal subjects can increase expiratory flow by contracting expiratory muscles and generating higher positive intrathoracic pressures. Even passive exhalation is dependent on respiratory muscles, however, because passive expiratory flow is proportionate primarily to airway caliber and lung elastic recoil; both of these factors are maximized at high lung volumes, which require good inspiratory muscle strength to achieve.

B. Lung Volumes in Neuromuscular Disorders

Vital capacity (VC) and inspiratory capacity (IC) are diminished because of decreased ability to expand the lungs and chest wall voluntarily against passive inward recoil of those structures. While decreased IC contributes to decreased total lung capacity (TLC), the other component of TLC is the functional residual capacity (FRC), often considered to be determined by the passive balance between inward recoil of the lung and the outward recoil of the chest wall at relaxed end-expiration. But FRC does change with the onset of neuromuscular weakness. For example, normal volunteers given submaximal doses of muscle relaxants had about a 10% decrease in VC and TLC, but FRC decreased about 20% as a result of decreased stiffness of the chest wall. In a small number of patients with myasthenia gravis given pyridostigmine, an increase in FRC correlating with increase in respiratory muscle strength was found. One study of stable patients with moderate respiratory muscle weakness found that VC averaged about 50% of predicted from height and age, TLC about 67% of predicted, and FRC about 79% of predicted.

In chronic neuromuscular disease, both altered chest wall compliance and reduced lung compliance contribute further to decreased FRC. Patients with spinal cord injury and spastic paralysis of chest wall muscles may have chest wall compliances that are only 70% of normal. Decreased lung compliance results from small tidal volumes, perhaps adversely affecting surfactant distribution and perhaps stiffening and shortening of lung fibrous and elastic tissues after chronically reduced lung expansion.

C. Inadequate Cough

Inadequate cough, with retention of secretions and an increased tendency to pneumonia and atelectasis, is the most common and important problem seen in patients with neuromuscular weakness. Coughs are most effective in removing secretions from airways if large shear forces are generated by high-velocity gas movement in the airways. In normals, coughs are initiated at high lung volumes, depend on vigorous contraction of expiratory muscles to compress airways and generate high positive intrathoracic pressures, and are released explosively. The patient with neuromuscular weakness cannot produce effective cough if these three components are compromised.

Atelectasis results from the combination of low lung volume, impaired cough, and accumulation of secretions. At low lung volumes, alveoli are strongly influenced by surface forces generated at the interface between the alveolar gas and the wetted surface of the alveoli. This surface tension increases the tendency of the alveoli to collapse. Airway secretions will also contribute to atelectasis by obstructing inward airflow and allowing alveolar gas to be absorbed into the blood.

D. Abnormal Control of Ventilation

As described above, alveolar ventilation in normals is adjusted to regulate Pa_{CO_2}. Hypoxemia also stimulates respiration but does not usually play an active role in normals at sea level. Neurologic disorders that affect the central or peripheral chemoreceptors, the integrative centers in the brain stem, or the primary outputs to the respiratory muscles (phrenic nerves) may lead to inappropriate ventilation for the metabolic requirements of the patient. Both hypoventilation and hyperventilation may be seen depending on the site of the neurologic problem.

Clinical Features

Symptoms, signs, and laboratory findings depend on the type of neuromuscular disorder leading to respiratory failure (Table 12–15). Common to all forms of respiratory failure in neuromuscular diseases are hypoxemia, hypercapnia, atelectasis, poor cough, and risk of development of pneumonia and other complications. Patients who are immobilized by neuromuscular disease have an increased risk of developing deep venous thrombosis and pulmonary embolism. Occasionally, patients who have difficulty in weaning from mechanical ventilation are found to have an unsuspected primary or secondary neuromuscular disorder.

A. Disorders of Ventilatory Control

Impaired ventilatory control due to a primary neurologic disorder is a relatively unusual cause of respiratory failure. Patients can present with low respiratory rate and tidal volume, fluctuating uncoordinated breathing patterns, or markedly periodic breathing. Diseases that affect the medullary centers, including poliomyelitis and cerebral vascular disease, as well as depression by central nervous system drugs or hypothyroidism, can suppress the respiratory rhythm and output from the autonomic nervous system. In patients with impaired ventilatory control, clinical findings are related primarily to the effects of respiratory failure on gas exchange in addition to the consequences of the underlying disease. If central nervous system depression from opioid or sedative drugs is present, patients will often be lethargic or comatose. Other manifestations of autonomic dysfunction such as hypertension or hypotension and bradycardia or tachycardia can be seen in medullary infarction. Furthermore, infarction or ischemia of the medulla often results in characteristic effects on other neurologic pathways, including motor and sensory long tracts. A largely reversible disorder of ventilatory control may be seen in patients who have intermittent and transient hypoxemia, such as seen in those with severe sleep-disordered breathing or obstructive sleep apnea syndrome.

B. Neuromuscular Weakness

Respiratory failure from neuromuscular diseases with intact ventilatory control mechanisms usually presents

Table 12–15. Neuromuscular diseases associated with respiratory failure.

Medullary center injury or depression
- Poliomyelitis
- Cerebral vascular disease
- Hypothyroidism
- Narcotic and sedative drug overdosage

Primary muscle diseases
- Muscular dystrophy
- Myotonic dystrophy
- Polymyositis, dermatomyositis
- Drugs: corticosteroids
- Hypokalemia, hypophosphatemia
- Critical illness myopathy

Peripheral nerve diseases
- Peripheral neuropathies
- Guillain-Barré syndrome
- Vasculitis
- Diabetes
- Vitamin deficiency
- Toxin exposure
- Infection
- Infiltrative diseases
- Critical illness polyneuropathy

Neuromuscular junction diseases
- Myasthenia gravis and cholinergic crisis
- Botulism
- Tick paralysis
- Drugs: paralyzing agents, aminoglycosides

Spinal cord injury and disease
- Trauma
- Poliomyelitis
- Amyotrophic lateral sclerosis
- Malignancy
- Paraspinous or parameningeal abscess

Daiphragmatic paralysis

Cerebral cortical diseases
- Stroke
- Extrapyramidal disorders
- Neurogenic pulmonary edema

with low tidal volume and, because the responses to hypoxemia, hypercapnia, and lung and chest wall mechanoreceptors are intact, increased respiratory frequency. There are some differences between the clinical pictures depending on the particular disorder.

1. Muscle disease—Primary muscle diseases can be congenital or acquired. All can result in respiratory failure when severe, including the congenital muscular dystrophies; inflammatory muscle disorders such as polymyositis and dermatomyositis; drug-induced muscle weakness from such agents as corticosteroids; and muscle weakness caused by electrolyte and metabolic disturbances, including hypokalemia, hypophosphatemia, hypothyroidism and hyperthyroidism, and chronic renal failure. Muscle weakness may not affect all muscle groups equally. Proximal muscles may be more severely affected in some of the muscular dystrophies, and even when respiratory failure is developing there may be poor correlation between the strength of the extremity muscles and that of the respiratory muscles. Myotonic dystrophy, a rare disorder presenting with weakness and myotonic phenomena including impaired muscular relaxation, imposes the additional burden of a stiff chest wall and increased work of breathing.

The myopathic effects of corticosteroids can exacerbate the effects of the underlying disease for which the drug is administered, and corticosteroid-induced weakness in patients with asthma or interstitial pneumonitis can contribute substantially to respiratory impairment. A syndrome associated with use of neuromuscular junction blocking agents and corticosteroids can cause weakness and failure to wean from mechanical ventilation. In some of these patients, both evidence of myopathic changes on muscle biopsy and neuropathic changes evidenced by nerve conduction studies have been found. Hypokalemia and hypophosphatemia may also precipitate respiratory failure in ICU patients. Myxedema is associated with muscle weakness and elevated serum creatine kinase. Muscle weakness seen in thyroid disease is generally correlated with the severity of thyroid disease and corrects with treatment.

A variety of patients with critical illness have been reported to develop a syndrome called critical illness myopathy. This disorder has been associated with critical illness polyneuropathy but may occur alone. Clinically, these patients develop muscle weakness during treatment for serious illness though no specific cause of muscle injury can be identified. Histopathologic changes may include variation in muscle fiber size, fiber atrophy, angulated fibers, fatty degeneration, fibrosis, and single-fiber necrosis, but there are no inflammatory changes. There are structural differences between patients who receive corticosteroids and those whose muscles seem to be affected by some combination of cytokines and myotoxic substances. Common predisposing conditions include ARDS, pneumonia, liver and lung transplantation (possibly related to corticosteroids), liver failure, and acidosis. Because of common predisposing conditions, critical illness polyneuropathy should be distinguished from this syndrome. Both are associated with difficulty in weaning from mechanical ventilation and sometimes are not suspected until this stage of respiratory failure.

Primary muscle disorders often can be distinguished from peripheral neuropathy by the absence of sensory findings and by electromyography.

2. Peripheral neuropathies—Peripheral nervous system disorders can be divided into those that affect the neuromuscular junction and those that affect the peripheral nerves. Peripheral neuropathies, though seen in many disorders such as vasculitis, diabetes mellitus, vitamin deficiencies, toxin exposure (such as lead), infections, and infiltrative diseases, cause respiratory failure only rarely. For ICU patients, the most important disorders are acute polyradiculoneuritis (Guillain-Barré syndrome) and a recently described disorder called "critical illness polyneuropathy." Guillain-Barré syndrome is a demyelinating disease that is most often seen several weeks after a variety of nonspecific viral or other infectious illnesses, though the primary illness may be asymptomatic or difficult to pinpoint. Clinical findings of Guillain-Barré syndrome include ascending paralysis and sensory involvement initially of the lower extremities. In patients whose disease progresses over the course of about 2–4 weeks, involvement of the respiratory muscles, upper extremities, and trunk may contribute to the development of respiratory failure. Autonomic instability may further complicate diagnosis and management. Variants of Guillain-Barré syndrome may have different patterns of involvement, making diagnosis more difficult.

Critical illness polyneuropathy is seen in association with sepsis and multiple organ failure. Manifestations include muscle weakness and wasting and findings suggestive of peripheral neuropathy. Patients have flaccid weakness and loss of deep tendon reflexes. There is no evidence that metabolic or nutritional factors or inflammation plays a major role. The histologic appearance of primary axonal degeneration and denervation is consistent with widespread primary nerve injury. It has been speculated that the association with failure of other organ systems indicates that peripheral neuropathy is another marker of severe systemic illness. This disorder is associated with respiratory failure and difficulty in weaning from mechanical ventilation. As many as 70% of patients with sepsis and multiple organ failure have primary axonal degeneration of motor and sensory fibers, and 30% have difficulty in weaning from mechanical ventilation, limb muscle weakness, or diminished muscle reflexes. Electrophysiologic studies show reduction or absence of muscle and sensory action potentials, but slowing of nerve conduction or nerve conduction blocks is absent. Clinically, patients with critical illness polyneuropathy should be evaluated for botulism, Guillain-Barré syndrome, prolonged effects of muscle relaxants, and critical illness myopathy.

3. Neuromuscular junction disorders—Neuromuscular junction disorders include myasthenia gravis, an immunologic disease with antibodies to acetylcholine receptors; botulism, in which a specific neurotoxin produced by *Clostridium botulinum* is ingested; and drug-induced disorders, including pharmacologic blockade of the neuromuscular junction by paralyzing agents or inadvertent blockade by aminoglycosides and other drugs. Myasthenia gravis has occasionally gone unrecognized until it was severe enough to present with respiratory failure. Botulism should be suspected if there is descending paralysis and an appropriate clinical history. On occasion, botulism results from toxin produced by organisms infecting a wound, often in association with parenteral drug abuse. Weakness or difficulty in weaning in ICU patients should prompt a review of medications that can affect the neuromuscular junction. Rarely, these include calcium channel blockers, quinidine, procainamide, and lithium.

4. Spinal cord disorders—Acute cervical spinal cord injury resulting in quadriplegia may cause near-total respiratory muscle paralysis if above the C3 level, but some function of neck muscles may still be present. If injury is below C3–4, diaphragmatic activity may be preserved but respiratory failure may develop. In this setting, rib cage movement may be paradoxic, with inspiratory effort causing the chest wall to move inward because of flaccid paralysis of intercostal muscles. The mechanical efficiency of the diaphragm is also diminished as a result of flaccid paralysis of abdominal wall muscles, and cough effectiveness is greatly reduced. With time, the chest wall and abdominal wall become less compliant as muscle paralysis becomes spastic. In some patients, these changes may allow spontaneous efforts to become sufficient to maintain ventilation.

Other spinal cord diseases commonly presenting with respiratory failure include poliomyelitis and amyotrophic lateral sclerosis. Poliomyelitis has a variable prognosis, with both weakness and inability to protect the upper airway contributing to potential respiratory failure. Amyotrophic lateral sclerosis is progressive, and respiratory failure is inevitable and irreversible.

5. Diaphragmatic paralysis—Diaphragmatic paralysis from bilateral phrenic nerve injury or disease is rare. Vital capacity is usually less than 50% of predicted and worse when supine. The abdominal wall moves paradoxically inward during inspiration, increasing the work of breathing and making ventilation particularly inefficient for the other muscles of inspiration. Unilateral diaphragmatic paralysis is often well tolerated unless there is underlying lung disease or a requirement for increased work of breathing or minute ventilation during illness.

C. Diseases of the Cerebral Cortex

Patients with strokes have upper motor neuron paralysis but rarely present with primary respiratory failure. However, respiratory problems are the most common complications of stroke, including aspiration and lung infection due to generalized weakness, immobility, and aspiration. More recently, the respiratory complications of extrapyramidal disorders such as Parkinson's disease have become appreciated. The increased stiffness of the chest wall may have an adverse effect on work of breathing, and there are increased respiratory complications from immobilization. Isolated closed head injury of any kind requiring mechanical ventilation is commonly associated with pneumonia. In one study, 41% of these patients developed pneumonia and had a longer ICU stay compared with those without pneumonia.

A rare complication of cerebral injury is neurogenic pulmonary edema, seen in association with head injury, stroke, status epilepticus, and cerebral hypoxia. Although it can be indistinguishable from other forms of pulmonary edema, neurogenic pulmonary edema may appear and disappear rapidly despite causing severe gas exchange disturbances. The mechanism of neurogenic pulmonary edema is unknown but may be related to extreme changes in pulmonary vascular tone in response to autonomic stimuli. The pulmonary edema results both from changes in lung permeability and from increased regional lung hydrostatic pressures.

Among critically ill patients, neurologic status influences the ability to be weaned from mechanical ventilation. In one study, abnormal neurologic status was the major factor leading to prolonged mechanical ventilation, with reduced level of consciousness the most common cause. However, the underlying problem was more likely a systemic illness (drug toxicity or metabolic encephalopathy) rather than a specific primary central nervous system disease.

D. Laboratory Findings

Hypoxemia is common, and $PaO_2 < 70$ mm Hg on room air is likely. Hypercapnia with acute respiratory acidosis is the key marker of respiratory failure due to neuromuscular weakness or decreased ventilatory drive. Other laboratory findings are not particularly useful; but abnormal serum electrolytes, including decreased potassium, magnesium, calcium, and phosphorus, may contribute to muscle dysfunction. In patients with unexplained neuromuscular weakness, elevated serum creatine kinase suggests myopathy or myositis. Thyroid function tests may be useful even if the patient lacks the usual signs of hypothyroidism or hyperthyroidism. Diagnosis of specific neuromuscular disorders may be helped by electromyography, nerve conduction studies, or nerve biopsy.

E. Imaging Studies

Complications of neuromuscular diseases may be seen on chest x-ray. Atelectasis is a common finding—either as macroatelectasis, with focal linear, rounded, or other opacities visible on chest x-ray or evidence of segmental, lobar, or other collapse; or in some cases with no chest x-ray findings but only hypoxemia and an increased $P(A\text{–}a)O_2$. In one study, 95% of patients with neuromuscular disease requiring mechanical ventilation showed atelectasis at some time, most often as lobar atelectasis in the lower lungs. Pneumonia from aspiration is another common respiratory complication of neuromuscular diseases. Although dependent areas of the lungs are most often involved, new alveolar or interstitial infiltrates anywhere in the lungs suggest aspiration pneumonia.

When assessing neurologic disorders associated with respiratory failure, CT imaging is not often useful in evaluating the brain stem and has variable usefulness for spinal cord abnormalities. Magnetic resonance imaging (MRI) is highly effective for imaging these areas, but patients cannot undergo MRI while being supported with mechanical ventilation.

F. Assessing Respiratory Muscle Strength

Prediction of respiratory failure in these disorders primarily involves assessment of respiratory muscle strength. Adequate respiratory muscle function requires both inspiratory and expiratory strength, but neither maximum inspiratory pressure nor expiratory pressure strongly correlates with general muscle strength. In patients with polymyositis or other proximal muscle myopathies presenting with generalized weakness, mean maximum inspiratory and expiratory airway pressures averaged about 50% of normal in one study, while at the same time the average of maximum inspiratory plus maximum expiratory pressures was less than 70% of predicted in about two-thirds of patients. Arterial PCO_2 was inversely correlated with both respiratory muscle strength and vital capacity expressed as a percentage of predicted. Hypercapnia was especially likely when VC was less than 55% of predicted. In a study of patients with Guillain-Barré syndrome, one-half of a small group of patients developed respiratory failure. These had a mean VC when intubation was required of about 15 mL/kg compared with more than 40 mL/kg for nonintubated patients.

In patients with progressive neuromuscular weakness who are at risk of respiratory failure, a reasonable approach is to follow VC daily, or more often if necessary. If VC falls below about 20 mL/kg, is less than 55% of predicted, or decreases below 1500 mL in an adult, respiratory failure should be suspected and arterial blood gases should be obtained. Intubation and mechanical ventilation (or noninvasive ventilation if rapid reversal is expected) may be necessary if there is progressive hypercapnia. Although some investigators recommend using the mean or sum of maximum inspiratory and expiratory pressures rather than VC measurements, VC is usually more easily obtained in the intensive care unit.

Treatment

In most cases, treatment of respiratory failure due to neuromuscular disease is supportive, including airway protection and mechanical ventilation. The exceptions are the few diseases for which specific treatment is available. These treatable disorders include electrolyte abnormalities, myasthenia gravis, botulism, thyroid disease, and corticosteroid myopathy. It is essential to prevent respiratory complications when possible and to recognize and treat them promptly when they occur.

A. General Care

Patients with neuromuscular disorders should receive attention to airway protection, including examination of the swallowing mechanism and gag reflex, alteration of diet if necessary, careful feeding, and attention to body positioning. Feeding by mouth or by enteral feeding tubes should be monitored closely, especially because some neuromuscular diseases can affect gastric emptying and intestinal motility. In all neuromuscular disorders—even when stable—respiratory failure can be precipitated by stress from conditions such as pulmonary or other infections, concurrent illness such as heart failure, major surgery, medications, or electrolyte disturbances. General measures such as prophylaxis for gastritis and prevention of deep venous thrombosis should be instituted.

Prevention of atelectasis by mechanical means is controversial. Incentive spirometry is not as helpful in patients with neuromuscular weakness as in those with normal strength. Intermittent positive-pressure breathing (IPPB) seems attractive as a way of overcoming low lung volume during tidal breathing. However, results of studies have been mixed. Continuous positive airway pressure (CPAP) and bilevel noninvasive positive-pressure ventilation have also been tried without clear success. Some studies have shown that rotational therapy using special beds is helpful in decreasing atelectasis and pneumonia in immobile patients.

B. Treatment of Respiratory Failure

Treatment of respiratory failure in patients with neuromuscular disease includes airway protection and maintenance, oxygen, bronchodilators if necessary, and use of incentive spirometry to avoid atelectasis. Respiratory failure is usually of the hypercapnic variety unless there is atelectasis or consolidation from pneumonia. Mechanical ventilation is often necessary to perform the work of breathing in the patient with muscle weakness who develops hypercapnia.

If respiratory drive is inadequate, the assist-control mode is used with volume-preset ventilation. There is little rationale for IMV or pressure-control ventilation, and pressure-support ventilation cannot be used unless the patient can initiate and sustain inspiratory efforts. Lung compliance and resistance are normal in the absence of secondary pulmonary complications. Unless and until ventilation-perfusion maldistribution develops, high concentrations of supplemental oxygen are not needed. As in patients with obstructive or interstitial lung disease, tidal volumes should be limited to 6–8 mL/kg ideal body weight. Positive end-expiratory pressure (PEEP) may be quite helpful in decreasing atelectasis and for reducing the sense of dyspnea in some patients.

Patients with specific neuromuscular diseases may present with different needs. If respiratory muscle weakness is the primary problem but ventilatory control is intact, assist-control (volume- or pressure-preset) ventilation can be used, but pressure-support ventilation may be suitable. In some disorders, it may be desirable to rest the respiratory muscles entirely. The assist mode does not "rest" inspiratory muscles as much as the control mode—ie, if the patient initiates the breath, the inspiratory muscles continue to contract throughout inspiration; whereas if the ventilator initiates the breath, inspiration is completely passive on the patient's part. Pressure-support ventilation, though the inspiratory muscles are not completely rested, may have potential advantages of allowing some work to be done but with less effort.

In some patients, positive-pressure ventilation is needed only for some part of the day (at night, for example), and the patient can breathe well for long periods of time. Tracheostomy may be necessary in order to attach the ventilator at night, or noninvasive ventilation may be tried for intermittent use.

Bergofsky EH: Respiratory failure in disorders of the thoracic cage. Am Rev Respir Dis 1979;119:643–69.

Braun NMT, Arora NS, Rochester DF: Respiratory muscle and pulmonary function in polymyositis and other proximal myopathies. Thorax 1983;38:616–23.

Chevrolet JC, Deleamont P: Repeated vital capacity measurements as predicted parameters for mechanical ventilation need and weaning success in Guillain-Barré syndrome. Am Rev Respir Dis 1991;144:814–8.

Giostra E et al: Neuromuscular disorder in intensive care unit patients treated with pancuronium bromide. Chest 1994;106:210–20.

Gutmann L, Gutmann L: Critical illness neuropathy and myopathy. Arch Neurol 1999;56:527–8.

Hsieh AHH et al: Pneumonia following closed head injury. Am Rev Respir Dis 1992;146:290–4.

Hund E: Myopathy in critically ill patients. Crit Care Med 1999;27:2544–7.

Kelly BJ, Luce JM: The diagnosis and management of neuromuscular diseases causing respiratory failure. Chest 1991;99:1485–94.

Kelly BJ, Matthay MA: Prevalence and severity of neurologic dysfunction in critically ill patients. Chest 1993;104:1818–24.

Polkey MI, Moxham J: Clinical aspects of respiratory muscle dysfunction in the critically ill. Chest 2001;119:926–39.

Teener JW, Raps EC: Evaluation and treatment of respiratory failure in neuromuscular disease. Rheum Dis Clin North Am 1997;23:277–93.

Witt NJ et al: Peripheral nerve function in sepsis and multiple organ failure. Chest 1991;99:176–84.

THORACIC WALL DISORDERS

ESSENTIALS OF DIAGNOSIS

- *Chest wall anatomic deformity, chest wall stiffness, or severe obesity.*
- *Massive ascites, late stage pregnancy, recent abdominal or thoracic surgery, and large abdominal or pelvic masses may sometimes present with respiratory failure.*
- *Pa_{CO_2} > 50 mm Hg, usually with hypoxemia.*
- *Low tidal volume; usually, increased respiratory frequency.*
- *Primary lung disease absent but secondary complications frequent.*

General Considerations

Thoracic wall abnormalities other than those due to neuromuscular disease are relatively rare causes of respiratory failure. However, acquired and congenital abnormalities may result in distortion of the chest wall, mechanical disadvantage of the respiratory muscles, increased work of breathing, or limitation of chest wall expansion. Patients may develop chronic respiratory failure with hypoxemia, hypercapnia, and cor pulmonale but may also present with acute deterioration or exacerbations. The most common chronic disorders leading to respiratory failure in this category are severe obesity of the chest wall and abdomen, kyphoscoliosis and scoliosis, and ankylosing spondylitis. Massive ascites, late stage pregnancy, recent abdominal or thoracic surgery, and myotonic dystrophy may cause respiratory failure in a similar manner by limiting diaphragmatic excursion.

Pathophysiology

Thoracic cage abnormalities cause restriction of lung expansion. Vital capacity and total lung capacity are decreased. Functional residual capacity (FRC) is usually decreased except in most patients with spondylitis. Because of overall reduction in lung volumes, FEV_1 is also usually low, but the ratio of FEV_1 to VC is normal in the absence of obstructive lung disease. Respiratory failure results from a combination of increased work of breathing and ventilation-perfusion maldistribution due to restriction of expansion of the lungs and chest wall. The mechanics of the chest wall and the diaphragm are altered in ways unique to the type of disorder and the location of the abnormalities.

A. Chest Wall Deformity

Scoliosis and kyphosis may be idiopathic or due to poliomyelitis, tuberculosis, or other identifiable causes. Patients with scoliosis have an inverse relationship between the severity of scoliotic deformity and the compliance of the thoracic cage. Those who develop respiratory failure have the most severe thoracic deformity and lowest chest wall compliance. Patients with scoliosis breathe at low tidal volumes, presumably to minimize the work of breathing. Kyphosis alone rarely is associated with respiratory failure, but when seen together with scoliosis it may contribute to increased work of breathing and other abnormalities.

Ankylosing spondylitis limits rib cage expansion, and patients tend to breathe primarily by diaphragmatic movement as the thoracic cage becomes increasingly immobile. The contribution of thoracic cage expansion to tidal breathing may fall as minute ventilation increases. The position of the thoracic cage at end-expiration often becomes fixed at a volume larger than in normal subjects. The chest wall therefore exerts a greater than normal outward pull on the lungs, resulting in a normal or increased FRC despite low VC and TLC.

B. Obesity

1. Severe obesity—Severe obesity—in particular, predominantly central or truncal obesity—puts a heavy mechanical burden on the chest wall and the diaphragm during inspiration. Increased weight causes end-expiratory excursion of the chest wall and diaphragm to be more inward than normal. Thus, the amount of gas that can be maximally expired from the end-expiratory position (expiratory reserve volume; ERV) is reduced. On the other hand, the inspiratory capacity—the maximal amount of gas that can be inspired from the resting end-expiratory point—is normal or increased, at least in young obese adults with no underlying diseases. The work of breathing is increased, especially when minute ventilation increases. The larger mass of the chest wall and abdominal wall must be accelerated at each breath, and additional energy is expended to move them during tidal breathing. Small tidal volumes are usually selected by these patients, and the ability to increase minute ventilation can be limited and associated with severe dyspnea. It is likely that obesity associated with more peripheral distribution of added adipose tissue has less effect on respiratory function.

Obese patients are more prone to develop obstructive sleep apnea because of a greater amount of redundant soft tissue in the upper airway, potentiating airway obstruction during sleep-associated relaxation of upper airway muscles. A syndrome of obesity-hypoventilation has been described. The mechanism of this central hypoventilation is unclear but is probably associated with increased work of breathing, decreased responsiveness of the respiratory center, and chronic hypoxemia. These patients have daytime hypercapnia from a combination of depressed chemoresponsiveness, increased work of breathing, and abnormal pulmonary function. Patients with obesity-hypertension syndrome often have pulmonary hypertension and develop cor pulmonale.

C. Limitation of Diaphragmatic Excursion

Patients with massive ascites, late stage of pregnancy, recent abdominal or thoracic surgery, severe hepatomegaly, or large pelvic or abdominal tumors may occasionally present with respiratory problems. Most often they have basilar atelectasis, low tidal volumes, and mild hypoxemia. If diaphragmatic excursion is severely limited, these patients may develop hypercapnia. The underlying condition may contribute to additional problems. For example, patients with liver disease, ascites, or tumors may also have pleural effusions, further compromising lung function. Those with recent surgery may be unable or unwilling to take deep inspirations because of pain.

D. Gas Exchange and Pulmonary Hypertension

Patients with all types of chest wall abnormalities may have ventilation-perfusion maldistribution contributing to hypoxemia and hypercapnia. In obesity and limited diaphragmatic excursion, this finding has been attributed primarily to atelectasis at the bases of the lungs because of elevation of the diaphragm and low FRC. This is supported by observations that obese subjects have better gas exchange when standing than when supine and improvement in hypoxemia and reduced $P(A–a)O_2$ during exercise. Patients with ascites and abdominal fullness would be expected to be similar. In scoliosis and spondylitis, regional differences in ventilation can be explained by differences in expansion due to local chest wall stiffness in spondylitis or asymmetric deformity in scoliosis.

The combination of chronic hypoxemia and respiratory acidosis along with anatomic deformity of pulmonary vessels explains the pulmonary hypertension and cor pulmonale seen in some patients with severe chest wall abnormalities. For reasons that are not clear, cor pulmonale is often seen in chronic respiratory failure from scoliosis, sometimes in the absence of severe gas exchange abnormalities; it may be related to anatomic deformity or arrested development of pulmonary vessels.

Clinical Features

Some patients with thoracic wall abnormalities have chronic respiratory failure with chronic hypoxemia and hypercapnia. Decompensation leading to acute respiratory failure may be due to further abrupt worsening of the chest wall disease, development of a lung complication such as pneumonia or bronchospasm, or additional metabolic requirements imposed by surgical stress, infection, or other disease. The clinical history may reveal the cause of thoracic deformity, such as prior poliomyelitis or other disease, thoracic wall surgery or injury, tuberculosis of the spine, or surgery for pulmonary tuberculosis.

A. Symptoms and Signs

Dyspnea at rest and on exertion are common complaints, but some patients complain only of fatigue and weakness. Patients present usually with rapid, shallow tidal breathing unless there is a disorder of ventilatory control suggesting central hypoventilation. Physical examination can show obvious chest wall deformity or decreased range of motion of the chest wall or diaphragm, but the degree of abnormality may not be easily determined from examination alone. Wheezing, rhonchi, or stridor may be evidence of superimposed obstructive airway disease such as asthma, but kinking of large central and upper airways in scoliosis may be the cause. Other signs may be due to complications such as pneumonia, left heart failure, atelectasis, and pleural effusions. Findings of right heart failure, such as peripheral edema, elevated central venous pressure, and hepatic congestion, generally indicate chronic respiratory failure.

The likelihood of respiratory failure resulting from obesity is not well correlated with the degree of obesity. Lung volumes do not routinely decrease in proportion to excess weight, and no marker of obesity such as an excessive weight/height ratio or weight/height^2 (body mass index) is predictive of respiratory failure. For example, in otherwise normal subjects who are more than 160% of ideal weight, lung volumes and flows are usually found to be normal. Such normal lung function may not persist, however, as these patients age, and the decline in lung function with advancing age may be accelerated compared with nonobese subjects. In addition, obesity is associated with hypertension and cardiovascular disease, which may themselves contribute to decreased respiratory function. Central hypoventilation in obesity (obesity-hypoventilation syndrome) further dissociates the degree of obesity from the severity of hypercapnia, as does the high prevalence of basilar atelectasis causing hypoxemia.

Patients with ascites from liver disease and pregnancy frequently have increased ventilatory drive, probably because of hormonal changes. The severity of respiratory impairment from decreased diaphragmatic excursion is highly unpredictable, but most of the patients have some degree of hypoxemia and only rarely develop hypercapnia.

B. Laboratory Findings

Respiratory failure in these disorders is a result of insufficient minute ventilation to maintain CO_2 homeostasis. With mild thoracic wall disorders, patients can often maintain normal $Pa{CO_2}$ and $Pa{O_2}$. If the disorder progresses, the work of breathing increases. Compensation in the form of increased $Pa{CO_2}$ in exchange for decreased minute ventilation then occurs, resulting in chronic respiratory acidosis. The chronicity of respiratory failure can be confirmed by finding an elevated serum bicarbonate.

C. Imaging Studies

The likelihood of respiratory failure correlates with the severity of the deformity in scoliosis. Severe thoracic scoliosis is generally considered to be present when the angle of spinal curvature exceeds 70 degrees as measured on an x-ray film. This angle is measured as the angle between lines drawn perpendicularly to the longitudinal axis of two vertebral bodies, one above and one below the area of maximum deformity. The angle is 0 degrees in the absence of scoliosis and increases with increasing scoliosis. As many as 50% of patients with an angle greater than 80 degrees may be considered at risk for respiratory failure at some time in the future. An angle of 100 degrees seems to be associated with dyspnea on exertion and an angle greater than 120 degrees with alveolar hypoventilation.

Treatment

Care of the patient with respiratory failure from thoracic wall disorders is largely supportive. There may be a role for noninvasive positive-pressure ventilation to delay or prevent atelectasis, especially in severe obesity. Mechanical ventilation is initiated if the patient requires additional ventilatory support to overcome increased metabolic requirements or during an acute exacerbation due to infection or surgery. If concomitant central hypoventilation contributes to respiratory failure, patients will often respond after several days of correction of hypoxemia and respiratory acidosis by greatly improved respiratory drive. Respiratory stimulant drugs such as progesterone and almitrine are not helpful. Patients with limited diaphragmatic excursion are approached according to the type of problem. Those with severe ascites may benefit from large volume paracentesis or other efforts to decrease the volume of ascites. Pain management is critical in patients following abdominal or thoracic surgery.

Patients with right heart failure from cor pulmonale may have peripheral edema and hepatic congestion, but vigorous diuresis is not usually indicated and may be harmful. Patients with pulmonary hypertension may be sensitive to preload reduction and rapid decrease of intravascular volume. However, spontaneous diuresis as a response to improved oxygenation is a good sign. Patients with coexisting left heart failure may benefit from diuresis and decreased pulmonary edema.

The outlook for patients who present with respiratory failure from chest wall disorders is surprisingly favorable. In many cases, one or more precipitating factors can be identified and corrected. Other patients will respond with improved gas exchange after a short period of supplemental oxygen or mechanical ventilation. While there is little chance of improving the underlying pathophysiology in severe scoliosis or severe ankylosing spondylitis, weight reduction and treatment of obstructive sleep apnea in obesity can be highly effective.

Bergofsky EH: Respiratory failure in disorders of the thoracic cage. Am Rev Respir Dis 1979;119:643–69.

Goldstein RS: Hypoventilation: Neuromuscular and chest wall disorders. Clin Chest Med 1992;13:507–21.

Libby DM et al: Acute respiratory failure in scoliosis or kyphosis. Am J Med 1982;73:532–8.

Ray C et al: Effects of obesity on respiratory function. Am Rev Respir Dis 1983;128:501–6.

Weinberger SE, Schwartzstein RM, Weiss JW: Hypercapnia. N Engl J Med 1989;321:1223–31. JIM

CHRONIC OBSTRUCTIVE PULMONARY DISEASE

ESSENTIALS OF DIAGNOSIS

- *Chronic bronchitis or emphysema.*
- *Increased dyspnea and cough; decreased exercise tolerance.*
- *Increase in sputum amount, change in color to green or yellow, increased thickness.*
- *Respiratory muscle fatigue.*
- *Worsening hypoxemia or hypercapnia; new onset of hypercapnia.*

General Considerations

Chronic obstructive pulmonary disease (COPD) is the most common adult respiratory disorder leading to respiratory failure. Although asthma and cystic fibrosis are chronic obstructive diseases, COPD is usually considered to include chronic bronchitis and emphysema. Most patients with COPD have chronic respiratory failure, many with hypoxemia (some requiring home oxygen supplementation), a lesser proportion with chronic hypercapnia. Acute respiratory failure in COPD develops both in patients with and those without chronic respiratory failure. Although precipitated most often by exacerbation of airway obstruction from infection and increased sputum production, an important factor leading to acute respiratory failure is inspiratory muscle fatigue. Patients with COPD, because they have limited ventilatory reserve, may develop acute respiratory failure if they develop nonrespiratory disorders, including infection, heart failure, diabetes, or during or after major surgery.

A. Definition

Chronic bronchitis and emphysema have in common limitation of airflow caused by obstruction of intrathoracic airways, and airway obstruction is more marked during expiration. Chronic bronchitis is characterized by increased sputum production, chronic inflammation of the airways, hypertrophy of airway smooth muscles, increased number and size of airway mucus glands, and thickening of airway connective tissue. Patients with chronic bronchitis often have a history of cigarette smoking leading to hypertrophy of mucus glands. Chronic bacterial infection also plays a role.

Emphysema is characterized by destruction of alveoli and other tissues beyond terminal bronchioles. Decreased expiratory airflow in pure emphysema is not due to primary disease of the airways but results from decreased elastic recoil of the destroyed lung parenchyma. During expiration, a reduced pressure difference is found across the walls of conducting airways, lowering the distending pressure holding the airways open and leading to increased airway resistance. The pathogenesis of emphysema is not known. In some patients, deficiency of α_1-antiprotease has been identified, and these patients are thought to have destruction of lung elastic and connective tissue by unopposed action of leukocyte elastase. This accounts for a very small proportion of emphysema patients, and the mechanism of lung parenchymal destruction in the majority is unknown. Cigarette smoking, as well as some occupational exposures, is associated with development of emphysema. Many patients with emphysema have clinical features of chronic bronchitis.

B. Bacterial Infection and Sputum Changes

Acute respiratory failure in COPD is associated with episodes of worsening airway obstruction. Sputum production increases, and the characteristics of the sputum are altered in response to bacterial infection. Increased sputum and difficulty clearing sputum may provoke bronchospasm. Bacterial infection may also contribute to exacerbation by secondary infection following viral or mycoplasma infection. Of interest is that some of the evidence for the role of bacteria in causing exacerbation of COPD comes from serologic testing, but the most convincing data has been the demonstration of the beneficial effects of antibiotics in preventing exacerbation, shortening the course of acute deterioration, and decreasing the need for hospitalization.

COPD patients—even when stable—have bacteria colonizing the trachea and bronchi, whereas normal subjects do not have organisms in these sites. The most commonly found organisms from tracheal aspirates have been *Haemophilus influenzae* and *Streptococcus pneumoniae,* found in 30–60% of COPD patients, and during acute exacerbations there may be an increase in the numbers of these bacteria. Other bacterial pathogens, including *Moraxella catarrhalis,* are suspected of being an important cause of COPD exacerbation, but other bacteria capable of causing pneumonia, such as gram-negative aerobic bacilli, anaerobes, and staphylococci, do not seem to play a major role in exacerbation of COPD. There is debate about whether the type and number of bacteria are significantly different between chronic bronchitis with and without exacerbation. If the bacteria quantity and quality are only slightly different, then perhaps the host's response is the more important feature of acute exacerbation. For example, the number of inflammatory cells and the amount of other sputum components change during acute exacerbation. Sputum becomes thicker, more viscous, and more adherent to mucosal surfaces. A change from white to green or yellow reflects increased amounts of myeloperoxidase in neutrophils or an increase in the number of neutrophils. Increased amounts of protein, cellular and bacterial debris, and cellular DNA are responsible for mechanical changes in sputum. Disruption and inefficiency of the normal mucociliary clearance mechanisms results, with further worsening of airway obstruction.

C. Bronchospasm and Respiratory Failure

Bronchospasm is not a primary cause of airway obstruction in chronic bronchitis or emphysema as it is in asthma, but increased bronchomotor tone and airway smooth muscle contraction are present. In COPD, much of the airway smooth muscle contraction is mediated through the parasympathetic nervous system via the vagus nerve. Local irritation of the tracheobronchial mucosa from sputum, bacteria, and other debris stimulate the parasympathetic nervous system by way of vagal afferent pathways. Efferent fibers in the vagus nerve cause increased airway smooth muscle contraction and increased airway resistance. Patients with COPD will not infrequently have a heightened response to methacholine inhalation challenge, though not usually as marked as patients with asthma.

D. Lung Mechanics and Respiratory Muscles

As COPD patients develop increased airway resistance from secretions and bronchoconstriction, the work of breathing increases and the distribution of ventilation becomes more nonuniform. Normal ventilation requires increased respiratory muscle exertion. Several factors may prevent the patient with COPD from maintaining normal ventilation during an exacerbation. First, because of the increase in airway resistance, patients with severe COPD are unable to increase expiratory flow. To maintain minute ventilation, patients must either increase expiratory time by increasing the inspiratory flow rate (shortening inspiratory time) or breath at a relatively higher lung volume (with respect to TLC). Breathing at higher lung volumes is helpful because airway resistance is lower. Second, the work of breathing further increases. Increased airway resistance provides the major component of increased work, but hyperinflation displaces the tidal volume to a higher and flatter portion of the respiratory system's pressure-volume curve, resulting in increased elastic work of breathing as well. Although increased resistance is felt largely during expiration, it is the inspiratory muscles that provide compensation by having to generate faster inspiratory flow. The inspiratory muscles are disadvantaged by the decreased lung compliance accompanying hyperinflation. When the increased force needed exceeds the capacity of the inspiratory muscles, muscle fatigue ensues, and acute respiratory failure results from inability to maintain minute ventilation. Malnutrition, corticosteroids, hypophosphatemia, hypokalemia, and other factors may predispose patients to respiratory muscle fatigue.

E. Impaired Lung Gas Exchange

Patients with emphysema and chronic bronchitis have maldistribution of ventilation and perfusion even when stable, and gas exchange worsens during acute exacerbations of disease. Hypoxemia is generally responsive to oxygen therapy, but because of the increased V_D/V_T, hypercapnia may develop if patients are unable to sustain higher than normal minute ventilation.

F. Control of Ventilation

There has been considerable focus on the contribution of reduced ventilatory drive in acute respiratory failure in COPD, but this is not important in most patients, who appear to have normal or increased ventilatory drive. Chronic hypercapnia is found in many but not all patients with COPD; it is more common in chronic bronchitis compared to emphysema. Severity of COPD is not the major determinant of hypercapnia; decreased ventilatory response to CO_2 in family members of hypercapnic COPD patients, on the other hand, suggests that familial factors play a role.

In COPD patients with acute respiratory failure, the combination of severe hypoxemia and high Pa_{CO_2} and low pH depress central and peripheral chemoreceptor-mediated ventilatory drive. Hypoxic stimulation of the carotid bodies is thought to be relatively more preserved as a chemical stimulus for ventilation, and, when arterial hypoxemia is corrected by administration of supplemental oxygen, ventilatory drive may be suppressed and the patient's minute ventilation falls. However, this mechanism has been challenged by evidence suggesting that oxygen administration does not further depress minute ventilation acutely. Several recent studies have shown that breathing pattern and minute ventilation do not change appreciably after oxygen is given in the majority of COPD patients with acute exacerbations. Despite these data, high concentrations of oxygen should be given cautiously to COPD patients with hypercapnia or suspected hypercapnia (see below). Furthermore, because ventilation-perfusion mismatching is the largest contributor to hypoxemia, COPD patients will generally have adequate Pa_{O_2} with only small addition of supplemental oxygen.

Clinical Features

Features that warrant particular concern are listed in Table 12–16. These findings might suggest impending worsening of respiratory failure requiring close moni-

Table 12–16. Findings suggesting severe exacerbation of COPD.

Clinical
Pneumonia
Pneumothorax
Left ventricular failure
History of requiring mechanical ventilation
Nocturnal desaturation or apnea
Concurrent infection, renal insufficiency
Poor response to bronchodilators
Poor nutritional status
Paradoxic abdominal wall movement
Use of accessory muscles of respiration
Pulsus paradoxus
Severe pulmonary hypertension or cor pulmonale
Physiologic
pH < 7.25 with $P_{CO_2} > 60$ mm Hg
$Pa_{O_2} < 50$mm Hg
Respiratory muscle fatigue

toring, and potential need for endotracheal intubation and mechanical ventilation.

A history of chronic sputum production along with chronic cough, shortness of breath, a history of cigarette smoking, features of airway obstruction on pulmonary function tests, and lack of evidence of left heart failure will identify most patients with chronic bronchitis. The diagnosis of emphysema is made from an obstructive pattern on pulmonary function testing, decreased diffusing capacity for carbon monoxide, hyperinflation and abnormal lucency of lung fields on chest x-ray, and dyspnea. Emphysema patients do not have cough and sputum production as a primary feature but may develop these features similar to chronic bronchitis. The initial presentation of COPD is rarely acute respiratory failure, and it is highly likely that the patient will have had some symptoms of COPD even if a previous diagnosis has not been made. These symptoms usually include exertional dyspnea and chronic cough.

A. Symptoms and Signs

For the presentation of acute respiratory failure, patients will often have a variable history of increasing symptoms lasting hours to days, that may include low-grade fever, malaise, or upper respiratory symptoms leading to increased dyspnea, cough, inability to clear sputum from the airways, and decreased exercise tolerance. Some will report that prescribed home oxygen and bronchodilator drugs are less effective despite increased frequency and intensity of use. Sleeplessness because of dyspnea, sometimes for days, is a common complaint, and patients may state that they are unable to breathe when recumbent. On occasion, COPD exacerbations may present with evidence of severe right heart failure manifested by peripheral edema and ascites. A retrospective case-control study of patients admitted to an ICU with COPD exacerbation found that they had lower body weight, greater rate of deterioration of lung function over time, worse arterial blood gases and serum bicarbonate, and larger right ventricular diameter compared to those not requiring ICU admission. Numerous studies have confirmed a high prevalence of malnutrition in COPD patients (40–60%), and this is more marked in those who required mechanical ventilation for exacerbation of disease (74%) compared to those who did not need mechanical ventilation (43%).

The amount of sputum increases, but patients may be unable to cough up the sputum adequately. Sputum may change from white or clear to green or yellow and usually becomes thicker, more viscous and adherent, and produces longer strands. Blood-streaked sputum reflects increased airway inflammation but hemoptysis should raise concern about other processes as well.

Features of COPD can be found along with signs of acute respiratory failure. Increased anteroposterior diameter of the chest gives the appearance of a barrel chest, and on examination the hemidiaphragms are low and flat and move little even when the patient is stable; changes with impending respiratory failure may be difficult to discern. Clubbing and hypertrophic osteoarthropathy indicate severe chronic lung disease. Breath sounds are often difficult to hear, and low-pitched sonorous rhonchi rather than higher-pitched musical wheezes may be more common than in asthmatics. Especially in emphysema, but also in any patient with severe obstruction, breath sounds may be nearly inaudible. Signs of lung consolidation (pneumonia), decreased breath sounds with dullness to percussion (pleural effusions), and decreased breath sound with hyper-resonance to percussion (pneumothorax) are important in searching for contributing causes of acute decompensation. Especially in patients who have had prior tracheostomy or endotracheal intubation, acute respiratory failure could be due to upper airway obstruction. These patients may have loud stridor heard best over the tracheal during inspiratory efforts. Hypercapnic patients may be somnolent, stuporous, or comatose. Hypercapnia may be associated with asterixis.

It is essential to look for features on examination suggesting impending worsening of ventilatory function. These include use of accessory muscles of respiration (sternocleidomastoid contraction), intercostal retraction, and paradoxic abdominal wall motion (inward displacement of the anterior abdominal wall during inspiration)—all of which indicate high inspiratory work of breathing or impending inspiratory muscle fatigue. Patients who are unable to breathe while supine usually brace their arms on a table or the arms of a chair in order to facilitate inspiration using accessory muscles. On the other hand, while important, peripheral edema, hepatomegaly, ascites, a parasternal lift, and other features of right ventricular hypertrophy or cor pulmonale are not reliable predictors of severity of acute respiratory failure.

B. Laboratory Findings

Hypercapnia (Pa_{CO_2} > 45 mm Hg) with acute respiratory acidosis is often seen. In those who already have chronically elevated Pa_{CO_2}, serum bicarbonate is increased and the pH may be only mildly reduced. Therefore, the severity of acute hypercapnic respiratory failure is indicated by how low the pH is, not the degree of elevation of Pa_{CO_2}. Any patient with a pH < 7.30 should be considered to have severe acute hypercapnia.

Hypoxemia is due to both hypoventilation and $\dot{V}/\dot{Q}$ mismatching. Erythrocytosis, if present, is a marker of chronic hypoxemia. Electrolyte abnormalities may include hyponatremia caused by the syndrome of inappropriate antidiuretic hormone, and hypokalemia, especially in those receiving chronic corticosteroids or aggressive beta-adrenergic agonist therapy. Malnutrition contributing to respiratory failure is commonly observed, and the biochemical markers of decreased nutritional status such as serum albumin, prealbumin, and retinol-binding protein are often abnormally low.

C. Electrocardiography

The ECG may show right ventricular hypertrophy.

D. Imaging Studies

Chest x-ray findings range from essentially normal with a few increased linear bronchovascular markings and mild hyperinflation to severe hyperinflation with localized or diffuse bullae and cysts. The diaphragm is low and flat, especially as seen on lateral views, and there are often enlarged retrosternal and retrocardiac spaces. The chest x-ray should be carefully reviewed looking for pneumonia, pneumothorax, pleural effusions, evidence of pulmonary hypertension, evidence of left heart failure, and atelectasis.

E. Spirometry

Pulmonary function tests are rarely needed to diagnose obstructive lung disease during acute exacerbation. Peak flow measurements and FEV_1 are useful, however, in assessing the response to therapy and prognosis.

Differential Diagnosis

The differential diagnosis of respiratory failure from COPD includes asthma with acute exacerbation, upper airway obstruction, and left ventricular failure. Peripheral edema, weight gain, hepatomegaly, and other features of fluid overload may be due to cor pulmonale or left heart failure. Hyperinflation of the lungs on chest x-ray often makes the heart look smaller; some clinicians advise that a "normal-sized" heart be considered a sign of cardiomegaly in COPD.

Treatment

Treatment of acute respiratory failure in COPD consists of supportive care until the reason for exacerbation of airway obstruction is eliminated. Oxygen is usually needed for hypoxemia. Bronchodilators, corticosteroids, and antibiotics address airway obstruction and acute infection, but because of the importance of inspiratory muscle fatigue, the major therapeutic decision is when to start mechanical ventilation because the respiratory muscles are no longer able to maintain adequate ventilation.

A. Oxygen

Hypoxemia has several effects in COPD. Aside from the systemic effects of tissue hypoxia, hypoxemia is a respiratory stimulant. Patients may increase respiratory frequency, shortening expiratory time and developing further adverse hyperinflation. Increased ventilatory drive generates an increased inspiratory flow rate and may contribute to respiratory muscle fatigue.

Hypoxemia is due almost entirely to ventilation-perfusion mismatching. Therefore, small increases in inspired O_2 concentration usually lead to acceptable increases in PaO_2. An increase in FIO_2 to 0.24–0.35 is usually sufficient, and this can be provided by a Venturi-type mask or by nasal cannula (1–4 L/min). Oxygen therapy has been associated with worsening of hypercapnia and respiratory acidosis in occasional patients, and this has been attributed to loss of hypoxic drive with administration of O_2. While this particular mechanism has been questioned, caution in giving excessive O_2 is advised. However, this must be balanced with the very real danger of hypoxia if arterial O_2 saturation remains less than 90%. Patients with COPD and hypoxemia (PaO_2 < 55 mm Hg) when they are ready for discharge are candidates for home oxygen therapy. When given for 12–24 hours per day, long-term home oxygen improves prognosis.

B. Beta-Adrenergic Agonists

Response to these agents when given by aerosol is almost always achieved, though not usually as marked a response as in asthmatics. Because COPD patients are generally older and have more concurrent medical problems than asthmatics, side effects of hypokalemia, myocardial stimulation, tremor, effects on blood pressure, and drug interactions may be more significant. Therefore, in COPD patients, the drugs may be given in lower dosage and less often than in asthma. Oral beta-adrenergic agonists are of lesser value and may limit the amount of aerosolized drug that can be given.

C. Anticholinergics

Anticholinergic bronchodilators have become the primary therapy for chronic stable COPD, and are used in conjunction with beta-adrenergic agonists during acute exacerbations. Ipratropium bromide, in well-tolerated doses, has been shown to be superior to usual doses of beta-adrenergic agents in stable COPD, and a combination of modest doses of ipratropium, theophylline, and albuterol was better than ipratropium alone. Surprisingly, there is little evidence comparing the use of ipratropium with other bronchodilators during acute exacerbations. Nevertheless, because of the high level of safety of ipratropium and its potential as a bronchodilator in COPD, it should be included in pharmacologic regimens for management of COPD exacerbations. Effective doses can be as much as two or three times the dose usually recommended, but this is because this drug is very well tolerated with few if any side effects.

Ipratropium is available in metered-dose inhalers and in a solution for nebulization. Each puff from the metered-dose inhaler provides 18 μg of ipratropium inhaled solution; an effective starting dosage for stable COPD is two to four puffs every 6 hours. If the solution for nebulization is used, a roughly equivalent dosage of 500 μg is nebulized for inhalation every 6 hours. Because the effectiveness in acute exacerbation is not clear, both increased dosage and increased frequency may be necessary. Response to treatments should be closely monitored. A fixed-dose MDI containing a combination of albuterol and ipratropium is available; this is likely more suitable for chronic stable COPD patients.

D. Methylxanthines

Theophylline has a long history of use in COPD, but the degree of bronchodilation from theophylline has been called into question, and several studies in acute asthma have indicated that the addition of theophylline to beta-adrenergic agonists provides little or no benefit. Theophylline increases the rate and force of contraction of skeletal muscle and increases the force that can be generated by fatigued respiratory muscles. Myocardial effects, including increased contractility, may be beneficial. Theophylline has other effects unrelated to bronchodilator action, including evidence for immune modulation, alterations in calcium flux, diuretic action, and central respiratory stimulation. However, in chronic stable patients, several studies have found little or no benefit from addition of theophylline to regimens containing other bronchodilators. Other studies have demonstrated that theophylline can improve pulmonary gas exchange at rest, during exercise, and during sleep in patients with chronic severe COPD. In acute exacerbation of COPD, one controlled trial found no further improvement when aminophylline was added to a standard treatment regimen that included inhaled beta-adrenergic agonists and corticosteroids. These studies, plus the narrow therapeutic range for theophylline coupled with its dangerous toxic effects, have decreased its use as a primary bronchodilator. On the other hand, one study of patients with asthma and COPD presenting to an emergency room found that, despite no significant difference in FEV_1 after aminophylline administration, there was a threefold reduction in the hospital admission rate in the treated group.

As in all patients, theophylline should be used carefully in COPD patients, and only when maximum therapy with other bronchodilators proves inadequate. Advanced age, heart disease, liver disease, and concomitant drugs (including some antibiotics such as erythromycin and fluoroquinolones) decrease theophylline clearance. Severe COPD by itself may be a factor increasing the incidence of theophylline toxicity. Moderate therapeutic levels of theophylline should be sought—10–12 μg/mL—in most patients. Theophylline toxicity must be considered in patients with unexplained tachycardia, arrhythmias, hypokalemia, or gastrointestinal or central nervous system symptoms.

E. Corticosteroids

Corticosteroids have an undisputed role in management of acute exacerbation of asthma, and recent data support their use in COPD patients. In one controlled study during acute exacerbation of COPD, slightly more rapid improvement was seen in patients given methylprednisolone compared with placebo. Several recent studies of systemic corticosteroids in acute exacerbation of COPD found improvement in lung function, decreased symptoms, and better outcome. Subsequent exacerbations were not affected, as would be expected. Studies of stable COPD patients have reported mixed results, with several indicating that those with features of asthma such as sputum eosinophilia, greater bronchodilator response, and fluctuation of pulmonary function had a greater benefit from corticosteroids.

Severe acute exacerbations of COPD should be treated with corticosteroids, but it is likely that some subgroups will benefit more than others. These might include those with predominant bronchospasm and those with increased numbers of blood or sputum eosinophils. The optimal dose and duration of corticosteroid treatment in COPD exacerbation is unknown, and the likelihood of complications from these drugs in COPD patients is high. Therefore, somewhat smaller doses and earlier withdrawal of corticosteroids have been recommended. An appropriate starting dose would be 20–40 mg of methylprednisolone intravenously (or of prednisone orally) three or four times daily. These dosages should be given for approximately 3 days, then tapered rapidly and withdrawn, if possible, within 7 days. However, some recent data suggest that 10 days of corticosteroids was better than 3 days of treatment. Although there are no data supporting rapid withdrawal, metabolic complications from corticosteroids (hyperglycemia, hypokalemia) and corticosteroid myopathy may be avoided.

F. Antibiotics

Antibiotics are given routinely for acute exacerbations of COPD, though benefit has not been clearly established in all patients. The goals of treatment are to shorten the duration of exacerbation and decrease the degree of severity in those with little pulmonary reserve. Long-term goals of prolonging time between exacerbations, slowing progression, and modifying bacterial flora may or may not be achieved. A large randomized trial found that patients who had all three of increased volume of sputum, increased dyspnea, and increased purulence of sputum were the most likely to improve with antibiotic therapy. Patients without these changes are statistically more likely to have viral infection and not improve with antibiotics.

Broad-spectrum drugs are usually used, aimed at *H influenzae, S pneumoniae,* and other organisms commonly found in sputum of COPD patients. However, one published chronic bronchitis guideline has recommended selecting the type of antibiotic based on age, number of exacerbations, and lung function. Simple chronic bronchitis (age < 65, fewer than 4 exacerbations per year, and mild impairment in lung function) should have therapy directed against *H influenzae, S pneumoniae,* and *M catarrhalis.* Those with complicated chronic bronchitis (age over 65, more exacerbations, and poorer lung function) may have other gram-negative bacilli involved, and therapy should be adjusted accordingly.

Because of the emergence of β-lactamase-producing haemophilus and *M catarrhalis,* second-generation cephalosporins, amoxicillin-clavulanic acid, extended spectrum macrolides, or trimethoprim-sulfamethoxazole are now often prescribed for simple chronic bronchitis exacerbation. For complicated exacerbations, second- or third-generation cephalosporins or fluoroquinolones may be more efficacious. The clinical significance of penicillin-resistant *S pneumoniae* is unknown in patients with COPD (although it is known for other infections with these organisms). Comparison studies often do not clearly support the efficacy of one agent over another, and cost, availability, and drug toxicity are important factors. Individual agents all have their advantages and disadvantages.

Antibiotics previously used may be ineffective. Erythromycin is not active against haemophilus, and ampicillin and amoxicillin are destroyed by beta-lactamases and have no activity against atypical bacteria. Extended-spectrum macrolides, azithromycin and clarithromycin, are effective against common organisms in COPD exacerbations, as are fluoroquinolones such as levofloxacin. Clinicians at each hospital and intensive care unit should be aware of local bacterial sensitivities, the frequency of resistance, and local efforts to reduce development of resistant organisms (eg, restricted use of antibiotics).

In patients with COPD who are found to have pneumonia, antibiotic therapy should be intensified. Use of agents with particular efficacy against *S pneumoniae,* aerobic gram-negative bacilli, *Mycoplasma pneumoniae,* and *Legionella pneumophila* should be considered, and intravenous antibiotics are probably indicated at least initially until the patient has shown clinical response.

G. Mechanical Ventilation

Patients with COPD and acute respiratory failure who require mechanical ventilation either have very severe obstruction, or encounter fatigue of respiratory muscles and inability to maintain adequate minute ventilation. Hypercapnia and respiratory acidosis are the most common reasons for starting mechanical ventilation; hypoxemia is not often the primary problem and can usually be satisfactorily treated by supplemental oxygen alone. Although mechanical ventilation is frequently administered to patients with acute exacerbations of COPD, a subset of patients has been identified who have poorer prognosis. These patients are more likely to have pulmonary infiltrates on chest radiographs, lower serum albumin, and lower baseline lung function. In several studies, mortality from acute exacerbation of COPD requiring mechanical ventilation ranges from 30–50%.

1. Volume-preset ventilation—The volume-preset (volume-cycled) mode is most often used in COPD patients and is generally well tolerated. Because of increased resistance in intrathoracic airways, exhalation of the tidal volume is prolonged in COPD. Thus, sufficient expiratory time during mechanical ventilation must be allowed to avoid "air trapping" or hyperinflation. Tidal volume is generally limited to 6–8 mL/kg; inspiratory time is kept relatively short by choosing high inspiratory flow (at least 1 L/s, often 1.25–1.5 L/s); and expiratory time is kept relatively long by seeking a slow respiratory rate. The I:E ratio should be at least 1:3. If patients have chronic hypoventilation with compensatory elevation of plasma bicarbonate, minute ventilation should be chosen to avoid causing acute alkalemia by correcting Pa_{CO_2} to normal. High concentrations of supplemental oxygen during mechanical ventilation rarely are required, and most patients have satisfactory Pa_{O_2} when the inspired O_2 fraction is 0.3–0.5. A need for higher inspired oxygen concentrations suggests atelectasis or consolidation rather than airway obstruction alone.

An inspiratory plateau pressure (see above) greater than 35 cm H_2O is likely to be associated with barotrauma and hyperinflation; pressures greater than this should be avoided by prolonging expiratory time as much as possible. As in asthmatics, lower tidal volume (6–8 mL/kg) during mechanical ventilation is recommended to decrease barotrauma and other complications. Pa_{CO_2} is allowed to rise (permissive hypercapnia) as long as pH remains above 7.25–7.30. Smaller tidal volume also has a beneficial effect by reducing intrinsic PEEP.

The finding of an increased peak airway pressure (rather than inspiratory plateau pressure) should prompt an examination of the patient for pneumothorax, bronchospasm, or airway obstruction with mucus or foreign body rather than hyperinflation.

If patients are able to contribute some efforts to ventilation, the pressure-support mode may be useful. With this mode patients can choose the rate and depth of breathing while having some of the inspiratory work of breathing taken on by the mechanical ventilator. This mode may be particularly helpful during weaning. The pressure-controlled mode should not be used in COPD exacerbations because the inspiratory flow rate, tidal volume, and I:E ratio cannot be maintained consistently.

2. Intrinsic PEEP—In any situation in which a high ventilatory requirement or severe airway obstruction is present, expiration may not be completed by the onset of the next inspiration. Because expiratory flow persisting right up to "end-exhalation" indicates that there is a positive-pressure gradient between alveoli and atmosphere at end-expiration, alveolar positive end-expiratory pressure (PEEP) must be present. PEEP generated in this way is termed intrinsic PEEP, or "auto-PEEP." The most accurate method of estimating the magnitude of intrinsic PEEP is to use an esophageal balloon connected to a pressure transducer to measure intrathoracic pressure. The change in intrathoracic pressure between end-exhalation and the onset of inspiratory gas flow into the lungs is approximately equal to the intrinsic PEEP (provided that there is minimal or no active expiratory muscle contraction at end-exhalation). For clinical purposes, another method is to occlude the expiratory port of the ventilator circuit just at the end of expiration. An increase in pressure displayed on the ventilator manometer indicates the presence and degree of intrinsic PEEP (Figure 12–6). This method may underestimate the degree of intrinsic PEEP in patients with severe obstruction, especially those with heterogeneous distribution of increased resistance.

High levels of intrinsic PEEP adversely affect lung compliance, work of breathing, and cardiovascular function and dominate gas exchange by affecting distribution of ventilation. COPD patients who develop intrinsic PEEP while undergoing mechanical ventilation may have worsening of hypoxemia and hypercapnia. In this common clinical scenario, Pa_{CO_2} can paradoxically worsen when minute ventilation is increased, leading to rapid deterioration. Lowering respiratory frequency and tidal volume instead in this situation improves gas exchange, reducing Pa_{CO_2}. Clinicians should be aware of this potential problem and act accordingly.

Another effect of auto-PEEP is an increase in the work of breathing when assisted mechanical ventilation is used. In this mode, the ventilator initiates inspiratory flow when it senses negative pressure in the circuit, but if alveolar end-expiratory pressure is positive, inspiratory muscle contraction will not immediately generate pressure that is negative with respect to atmospheric pressure. Thus, additional work of breathing is performed by the patient. Some investigators have added PEEP (extrinsic PEEP) to the ventilator circuit in this situation in order to change the absolute pressure at which the ventilator initiates inspiratory flow. Ideally, the small amount of PEEP reduces the work of breathing but does not worsen hyperinflation. The use of PEEP in this situation is debated, but the usual recommended amounts of "extrinsic" PEEP are small (75–85% of estimated intrinsic PEEP) and probably do not cause adverse effects if carefully monitored.

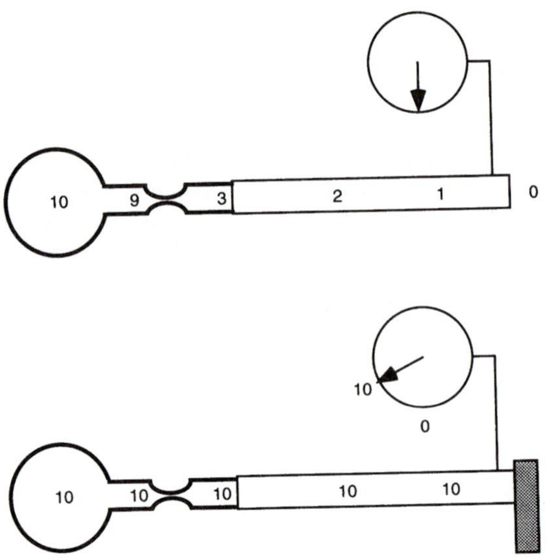

Figure 12–6. Demonstration of "intrinsic PEEP" in a patient with obstructive lung disease. In the top figure, increased airway resistance slows expiratory airflow so that the lung is still emptying until the start of the next inspiration. Alveolar pressure at end-expiration is positive (+10 cm H_2O in this example). Because of the high downstream resistance, a large pressure drop occurs before the pressure manometer site, and manometer pressure reads 0 cm H_2O despite positive alveolar pressure. If, however—as shown in the bottom figure—at end-expiration, the expiratory port is occluded, stopping flow, pressure equalizes throughout the system. The manometer now reads a positive pressure that approximates "intrinsic PEEP." Some mechanical ventilators can make this measurement automatically. In patients with very heterogeneous distribution of airway resistances and compliances, the occlusion method may underestimate the level of intrinsic PEEP.

3. Noninvasive ventilation—In the last several years, studies have shown a benefit of noninvasive positive-pressure ventilation for acute respiratory failure in selected patients with COPD. Theoretically, the use of a face mask or nasal interface can provide positive-pressure ventilation to the patient without endotracheal intubation. In selected patients, only short-term support may be needed until the reversible problem leading to exacerbation can be corrected. A further attraction is obviation of the need for prolonged weaning after intubation and conventional mechanical ventilation. Some studies have used noninvasive ventilation on a continuous basis for 24–48 hours or more; in other studies, patients are placed on noninvasive ventilation for 8–20 h/d with interspersed spontaneous breathing periods. Patients who are poor candidates for noninvasive positive-pressure ventilation include those with apnea, concurrent unstable medical problems, swallowing dysfunction, impaired cough, poor fit of the mask, upper airway narrowing, or those unable to cooperate fully.

For COPD exacerbations, several forms of noninvasive positive-pressure ventilation have been used. First, low levels of continuous positive airway pressure (CPAP) alone has been given. The CPAP theoretically acts by reducing the work of breathing in patients who have developed intrinsic PEEP and hyperinflation. Other patients have been administered bi-level positive pressure, with a small expiratory pressure (3–5 cm H_2O) and a time-cycled or patient-initiated larger inspiratory pressure (8–15 cm H_2O). In this mode, the expiratory pressure acts to overcome intrinsic PEEP, while the inspiratory pressure support provides assistance during inspiration without providing enough pressure to deliver the entire tidal volume. Success of noninvasive ventilation has been measured by rate of subsequent endotracheal intubation and improvement in arterial blood gases. Success rates of 40–60% have been reported, but most studies have been on selected patients who are cooperative, do not have excessive airway secretions, and who can tolerate a face mask or nasal interface. If noninvasive ventilation is used in a patient with exacerbation of COPD, very careful monitoring is recommended.

H. Respiratory Stimulants and Depressants

In the past, acute respiratory failure in COPD was considered to be partly due to insufficient ventilatory drive, and respiratory stimulant drugs were often administered. Increasing ventilatory drive makes little sense if respiratory muscle fatigue and hyperinflation are exacerbated, and stimulants should rarely be used. Acetazolamide, a carbonic anhydrase inhibitor, is occasionally given to enhance excretion of bicarbonate accumulated as compensation for hypercapnia, but its indications are not clear. It should be considered only in patients in whom the precipitating factors have been reversed and there is obvious "metabolic alkalosis" as a consequence of compensation for chronic respiratory acidosis. Most patients who benefit from acetazolamide will have known chronic hypercapnia and a know steady-state serum bicarbonate level as a target value.

Respiratory depressant drugs, including sedatives and opioids, should be avoided in COPD exacerbations while patients are spontaneously breathing. These drugs are useful, however, in patients during mechanical ventilation. On occasion, muscle relaxants are essential to avoid hyperinflation.

I. Other Therapy

A published guideline developed following an extensive critical review of the literature recently concluded that there was no benefit from chest physiotherapy and mucolytic medications in patients with COPD exacerbation.

Bach PB et al: Management of acute exacerbations of chronic obstructive pulmonary disease: a summary and appraisal of published evidence. Ann Intern Med 2001;134:600–20.

Barr RG et al: Methyl-xanthines for exacerbations of chronic obstructive pulmonary disease (Cochrane Review). In: *The Cochrane Library,* Issue 1, 2001. Oxford: Update Software.

BTS guidelines for the management of chronic obstructive pulmonary disease. The COPD Guidelines Group of the Standards of Care Committee of the BTS. Thorax 1997;(Suppl 5): S1–28.

Connors AF Jr, McCaffree R, Gray BA: Effect of inspiratory flow rate on gas exchange during mechanical ventilation. Am Rev Respir Dis 1981;124:537–43.

Derenne JP, Fleury B, Pariente R: Acute respiratory failure of chronic obstructive pulmonary disease. Am Rev Respir Dis 1988;138:1006–33.

Grossman RF et al: A 1-year community-based health economic study of ciprofloxacin vs. usual antibiotic treatment in acute exacerbations of chronic bronchitis. Chest 1998;113:131–41.

Hill NS. Noninvasive ventilation in chronic obstructive pulmonary disease. Clin Chest Med 2000;4:783–797.

Niewoehner DE et al: Effect of systemic glucocorticoids on exacerbations of chronic obstructive pulmonary disease. N Engl J Med 1999;340:1941–47.

Saint S et al: Antibiotics in chronic obstructive pulmonary disease exacerbations: a meta-analysis. JAMA 1995;108: 43S-52S.

Sayiner A et al: Systemic glucocorticoids in severe exacerbations of COPD. Chest 2001;119;726–30.

Sethi JM, Siegel MD: Mechanical ventilation in chronic obstructive lung disease. Clin Chest Med 2000;4:799–818.

Sherk PA, Grossman RF: The chronic obstructive pulmonary disease exacerbation. Clin Chest Med 2000;4:705–21.

Snow V, Lascher S, Mottur-Pilson C: Evidence base for management of acute exacerbations of chronic obstructive pulmonary disease. Ann Intern Med 2001;134:595–9.

ACUTE RESPIRATORY DISTRESS SYNDROME

ESSENTIALS OF DIAGNOSIS

- *Appropriate clinical situation.*
- *Hypoxemia that responds poorly to increased inspired oxygen concentration (refractory hypoxemia).*

- *Bilateral, diffuse pulmonary infiltrates.*
- *Absence of clinical evidence of hydrostatic or cardiogenic pulmonary edema.*

General Considerations

Acute respiratory distress syndrome (ARDS) is a disorder of severe hypoxemic respiratory failure that occurs in association with a variety of critical situations including trauma, aspiration, shock, and pulmonary and extrapulmonary infection. Other terms used to describe this syndrome may be more descriptive of its pathophysiology, such as noncardiogenic or exudative pulmonary edema with acute lung injury. ARDS deserves considerable attention because of its high mortality rate and the interest it has aroused in the mechanism of acute lung damage from apparently different causes. Because of superficial similarity to neonatal respiratory distress syndrome, ARDS has frequently stood for "adult" respiratory distress syndrome. However, consistent with the original definition and the recommendation from recent consensus conferences, ARDS should be understood to mean "acute" respiratory distress syndrome.

Although the term ARDS was first used in 1967, it is not a new disease. Well-documented descriptions of hypoxemic respiratory failure after severe trauma were reported during World War II, and there were even earlier reports of pulmonary edema associated with severe infection. The last 25 years have shown a remarkable increase in recognition of this syndrome, and there is general agreement that the outcome from ARDS remains relatively poor. Nevertheless, there is very encouraging prognostic information that reflects improved understanding of the pathophysiology and response to therapy of ARDS.

The major change in the management of ARDS has been the recognition that a low tidal volume strategy (6–8 ml/kg ideal weight) can lead to decreased mortality. This important finding has a strong basis in pathophysiology and has markedly changed the supportive treatment of this disorder.

Definition

ARDS can be defined as the clinical syndrome resulting from the severe end of the spectrum of acute lung injury. In acute lung injury, variable inflammation, disruption of normal lung architecture by tissue destruction and repair processes, and increased lung permeability to capillary fluids are seen. By definition, acute lung injury does not result primarily from elevated left atrial or pulmonary capillary pressure (although elevated pressures may be found coincident to the lung injury). The acute nature of both the lung injury and ARDS generally require the syndromes to evolve over hours to days, rather than weeks to months.

The clinical syndrome of ARDS includes clinical features, radiographic findings, and physiologic derangements, and the association with one of several clinical situations. Table 12–17 lists criteria for ARDS. Older criteria had required lung compliance measurement to establish increased lung stiffness, pulmonary artery wedge pressure measurement to exclude cardiogenic pulmonary edema, and the presence of a known clinical disorder likely to cause lung injury. The North American-European Consensus Committee statement requires only refractory hypoxemia (Pa_{O_2}/F_{IO_2} < 200 regardless of PEEP), diffuse pulmonary infiltrates on chest roentgenogram, and absence of clinical features suggestive of heart failure. These criteria have a very high degree of concordance with other definitions. It should be emphasized that criteria for ARDS are designed primarily to facilitate comparison of patients in research studies. On the basis of appropriate clinical judgment, an individual patient may be diagnosed as having ARDS and treated accordingly without meeting all criteria.

Pathophysiology

ARDS results from a combination of acute lung injury, pulmonary edema from increased permeability of the alveolar epithelium (noncardiogenic pulmonary edema), and fibroproliferation with collagen deposition. The first two mechanisms had been known, but the contribution of fibrosis to ARDS treatment and outcome has become better appreciated.

A. Acute Lung Injury

One of the intriguing aspects of ARDS is the variety of clinical situations associated with acute lung injury, both direct and indirect. Lungs can be injured directly, such as from severe bacterial, viral, or other infectious

Table 12–17. Criteria for diagnosis of acute respiratory distress syndrome.

Refractory hypoxemia
$Pa_{O_2}/F_{IO_2} < 200$
Diffuse bilateral pulmonary infiltrates (< 7 days old)
Absence of heart disease
PA wedge < 18 mm Hg or
No evidence of left ventricular failure

pneumonia; aspiration of gastric contents; near drowning; inhalation of toxic gases, such as smoke, chemicals, or poison gas; or blunt trauma to the lungs. Other disorders cause indirect lung injury, such as bacterial or fungal sepsis, severe nonthoracic trauma, fat embolism after orthopedic injury, pancreatitis, hemodynamic shock, and drugs; these probably damage the lung through circulating mediators.

It has been proposed that ARDS occupies the severe end of a spectrum of lung injury seen in many clinical contexts, with the histologic hallmark of diffuse alveolar damage as the common feature of inflammatory, toxic, infectious, or other processes that injure the lung parenchyma. Diffuse alveolar damage consists of disruption of normal alveolar architecture, replacement of type I with type II alveolar epithelial cells, damage to pulmonary capillaries, increased collagen deposition, exudative pulmonary edema, and a variable amount and variety of inflammatory cells. Evidence of both ongoing acute and chronic processes may be found. This disorder is seen in other clinical situations such as cytotoxic drug exposure, as a complication of severe pulmonary infections, and may be idiopathic, but the severity, quantity of lung involved, and acute onset determine its connection with ARDS.

An approximate time course for diffuse alveolar damage has been proposed. Early in the course (1–7 days), lung injury is coincident with exudative pulmonary edema, variable inflammation, platelet-fibrin thrombi, and disappearance of type I alveolar epithelial cells. This is followed by a proliferative phase (days 7–21) in which there is histologic evidence of type II alveolar cell proliferation and the beginning of organization and fibrosis (see below). The fibrotic phase occurring later may be indistinguishable from the various forms of idiopathic interstitial pneumonitis, especially idiopathic pulmonary fibrosis.

In ARDS, every potential mediator that could lead to diffuse alveolar damage has been implicated, including neutrophils and lymphocytes and their cytokines, prostaglandins, leukotrienes, platelets, coagulation factors, adhesion molecules, and immunoglobulins, as well as exogenous substances such as endotoxin and other products of bacteria and fungi. Endogenous cell products have received the most attention—some as mediators of injury, such as oxygen radicals and proteolytic and elastolytic enzymes; but others as amplifiers of inflammation and injury, such as interleukins, platelet activating factor, complement, and other substances that are chemotactic, bronchoreactive, or vasoreactive. These may be active in the early, middle, or late phases of lung injury. A role for injury from oxygen radicals is supported by the finding of reduced alveolar fluid glutathione in patients with ARDS. The coagulation system has been suggested by some investigators as having a central function in lung injury, perhaps by linking intravascular events to direct injury to the endothelium and by activation of inflammatory sequences. Elevated serum levels of tumor necrosis factor (TNF) are found in some patients with ARDS but also in those with sepsis and other systemic disorders. A potent cytokine, TNF has a variety of systemic effects some of which could cause or potentiate lung damage. The finding of multiple elevated cytokines in ARDS suggests the possibility of common regulatory factors being involved. One factor, NF-κB, regulates production of TNF, IL-1, IL-6, and IL-8. This hypothesis is attractive because of the frequent association of IL-6, TNF, and IL-8 with lung injury.

A key role for polymorphonuclear leukocytes in lung injury is supported by finding neutrophils in large numbers in the lungs of ARDS patients; the finding that neutrophils are primed to release potentially toxic substances from their granules; an increase in neutrophil chemotactic factors and activators; and, in some animal models, attenuation of lung injury after neutrophil depletion. For example, neutrophil activating protein/interleukin-8 (NAP-1/IL-8) was found in high concentrations in alveolar fluid and there was a correlation between levels and the number of neutrophils. High concentrations of NAP-1/IL-8 was also associated with poor clinical outcome. On the other hand, neutropenic cancer patients may develop ARDS indistinguishable from that observed in nonneutropenic patients, and diffuse alveolar damage in some animal models does not require the presence of neutrophils.

Levels of both cytokines and modulators of cytokine function are highly variable in ARDS, and it is clear that cytokines taken individually or as patterns of response are not able to predict development or prognosis of ARDS. In parallel with the diversity of clinical conditions associated with diffuse alveolar damage and acute lung injury, it is highly likely that different conditions in different patients explains why consistent findings cannot be identified. While this makes a single common causative mechanism unlikely (as well as a single common therapy), this hypothesis helps explain why so many conditions can result in very similar histologic and physiologic features. Nevertheless, there is now ample evidence that persistent elevation of inflammatory cytokines in blood or alveolar fluid is associated with poor outcome in ARDS in all forms of this disorder.

Patients may develop secondary bacterial or fungal pneumonia during the course of ARDS, further confusing the picture. Administration of high concentrations of inspired oxygen contribute to lung injury, and high airway pressure and relatively high tidal volume during mechanical ventilation are closely linked to worsening pulmonary edema and fibrosis.

B. Noncardiogenic Pulmonary Edema

Normal lungs are very dry to permit efficient gas exchange, and the structure and activity of the lungs maintain only a small amount of fluid in the lungs. Normal lungs have tight junctions between alveolar epithelial cells, an extensive lymphatic system, low hydrostatic pressure in the pulmonary capillaries, and other mechanisms to avoid pulmonary edema. However, lung injury from any number of insults can promote pulmonary edema by damaging these mechanisms.

Pulmonary edema is a major clinical manifestation of ARDS. The pulmonary edema fluid contains a high concentration of protein. This is in marked contrast to pulmonary edema due to elevated pulmonary venous pressure (hydrostatic pulmonary edema) or to decreased plasma albumin concentration (hypo-oncotic pulmonary edema), in which the edema fluid is a low-protein transudate. ARDS has been also called exudative or noncardiogenic pulmonary edema, reflecting the increased permeability of the injured lung to water, solute, and protein. Exudative pulmonary edema forms in the absence of elevated pulmonary artery wedge pressure, and the ratio of edema fluid protein to plasma protein is high. Edema fluid accumulates both in the pulmonary interstitium and in the alveoli, and, because of potential fluid pathways, lung lymphatics and bronchovascular spaces (surrounding the bronchioles, bronchi, and pulmonary arteries) may become engorged. Pulmonary edema removal by the pulmonary circulation and lymphatics is severely impaired because of the acute lung injury.

C. Chronic Lung Injury

Diffuse alveolar damage seen in ARDS may follow several courses and may resolve entirely with little or no evidence of chronic damage after weeks or months. However, other patients develop mild to severe pulmonary fibrosis. One of the most interesting findings in ARDS is evidence of very early deposition of type III collagen (procollagen III peptide in alveolar fluid) in the lung, sometimes within 24 hours of the onset of diffuse alveolar damage. Evidence for early fibrosis has been associated with poorer long term prognosis, stressing the potentially inappropriate role of remodeling and repair in late lung injury. These findings have challenged the time course of acute lung injury leading to irreversible fibrosis only at a later date.

Attraction and activation of fibroblasts may be mediated by various substances such as platelet-activating factor that are increased in blood and pulmonary edema fluid. Oxygen toxicity may play a role, especially if patients require very high inspired oxygen to treat hypoxemia. Another potential contributor to chronic lung damage is recognized to be overdistention of the lungs by high tidal volume, high PEEP, or high airway pressure.

In chronic lung injury, variable amounts of collagen are laid down into the alveolar and interstitial spaces with distortion and disruption of the normal lung parenchyma, resulting in restrictive lung disease, reduced exercise capacity, and hypoxemia. Histologic findings may be indistinguishable from idiopathic pulmonary fibrosis. Particularly sensitive findings are the PaO_2 and $P(A–a)O_2$ during exercise. Recent data show that survivors with more severe early ARDS had worse late stage pulmonary function than those with less severe acute disease. Lung function as assessed by spirometry, total lung capacity, and diffusing capacity for carbon monoxide averaged about 80% of predicted in these survivors. The greatest degree of improvement was seen in the first 3 months and there was little additional improvement between 6 months and 1 year.

The relationship of collagen deposition, severity of lung injury, and outcome provides some possibilities for intervention. These include potential inhibition of chemotactic or activating factors for fibroblasts, removal of some forms of collagen during tissue repair phases, and limitation of lung injury by controlling inflammation, oxygen toxicity, and ventilator-induced lung injury.

D. Physiologic Manifestations

1. Refractory hypoxemia—Hypoxemia in ARDS is primarily due to right-to-left shunt and $\dot{V}/\dot{Q}$ mismatching resulting from atelectasis and filling of alveolar spaces with edema fluid. $\dot{V}/\dot{Q}$ mismatching may also result from nonuniform changes in airway resistance, decreases in regional lung compliance, and primary and secondary alterations of lung blood flow. Hypoxemia is usually severe and not easily corrected even when the patient is given high concentrations of inspired O_2, termed "refractory hypoxemia" (Figure 12–7). As part of the definition of ARDS, the ratio of PaO_2 to FIO_2 is less than 200.

Studies comparing CT lung imaging with changes in PEEP in ARDS patients have shown that a majority of lung is completely airless, with small proportions having either normal inflation or potential for recruitment. These findings suggest that right-to-left shunting plays the major role in refractory hypoxemia, while the use of PEEP walks a fine line between recruitment of atelectatic lung and overdistention of normal lung.

2. Altered static lung mechanics—Lung compliance is severely decreased and airway resistance increased in ARDS. Decreased lung compliance results from a combination of interstitial pulmonary edema, collapse of lung units, airway obstruction, and inactivation of alveolar surfactant. Ineffective surfactant in ARDS may be due to reduced pool sizes, alteration in surfactant proteins, altered metabolism, or inactivation by plasma proteins, oxygen radicals, or phospholipases exuding into the alveolar spaces. In later stages, lung compliance is reduced because of accumulation of collagen.

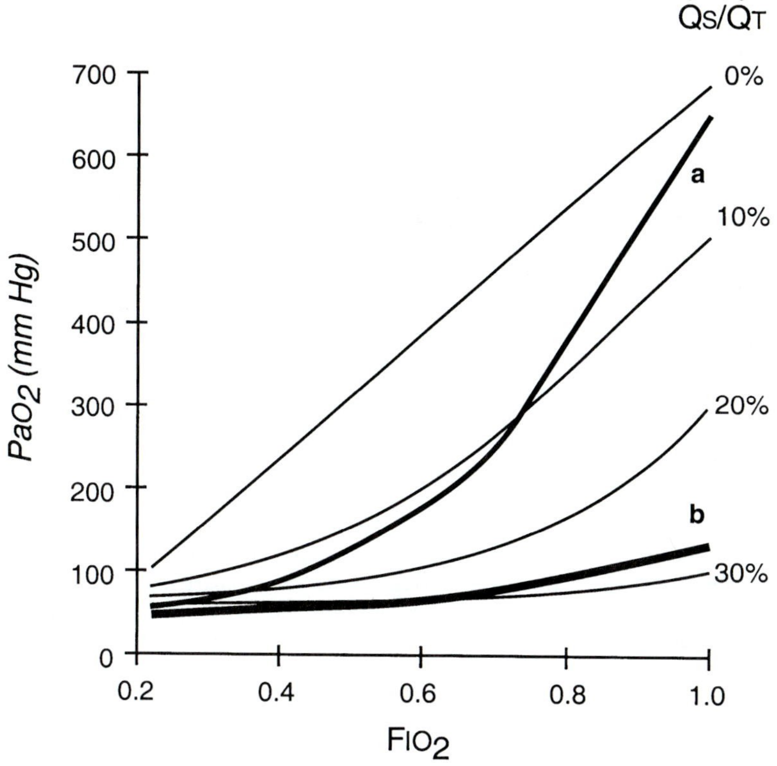

Figure 12–7. Lines showing Pa_{O_2} versus FI_{O_2} for various constant shunt fractions ($\dot{Q}s/\dot{Q}T$) between 0% and 30%. Superimposed are typical responses in patients with ARDS (lines *a* and *b*). Line *b* shows severe hypoxemia with a response suggesting severe right-to-left shunt as the primary mechanism of hypoxemia. Line *a* demonstrates severe hypoxemia but with Pa_{O_2} increasing more rapidly with increasing FI_{O_2} than with pure right-to-left shunt. The mechanism of hypoxemia is probably severe ventilation-perfusion mismatching.

As pointed out above, studies correlating regional radiographic lung volume change and inflation pressure have suggested that disease involvement in ARDS is much less uniform than formerly thought. Most lung regions are extensively involved and completely airless, some participate variably in gas exchange, and other small uninvolved regions accept the bulk of ventilation. These latter regions have been shown to have normal specific lung compliance, indicating that the primary cause of decreased overall lung compliance is overdistention of these small uninvolved regions of the lung rather than diffuse involvement of the entire lung. This finding has major implications for how patients with ARDS should be mechanically ventilated, notably the use of a low tidal volume strategy.

The pressure-volume (PV) curve of the lungs in ARDS is shifted downward and rightward (Figure 12–8). The lungs require greater pressure to inflate, and the work of breathing is increased. An increase in lung compliance may indicate improvement of the disease or recruitment of atelectatic lung, especially with the application of PEEP. Some investigators have noticed that the respiratory system compliance curve, which considers both lung and chest wall mechanics, is altered in ARDS. Patients with nonpulmonary causes of ARDS (abdominal sepsis, trauma, post surgery) had greater response to PEEP, suggesting that the "pulmonary ARDS" patients (mostly those with pneumonia) had more severe and less recruitable lung consolidation while the nonpulmonary ARDS patients had more atelectasis.

The shape of the PV curve has been stressed by a number of clinicians. The curve has been divided into sections, including a flat initial response of volume to increasing pressure, a lower inflection point after which compliance (slope) increases, an upper inflection point, and then another region of low compliance (flat slope). The regions of the PV curve may have important implications for adjusting PEEP (see below) and limiting tidal volume.

3. Increased airway resistance—Increased airway resistance is described in ARDS patients, probably due to edema in the bronchovascular spaces surrounding the bronchi, but there may be inflammatory mediators that can induce bronchoconstriction. Another cause may be the normal increase in airway resistance in areas of decreased pulmonary perfusion in response to ventilation-perfusion mismatching. The increased airway resistance, as much as sixfold compared with normals, contributes

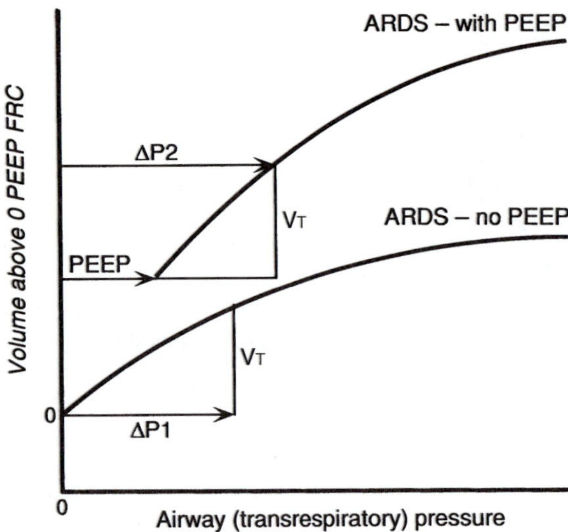

Figure 12–8. Hypothetical respiratory system pressure-volume curves for a patient with ARDS showing a flatter than normal relationship (decreased respiratory system compliance, C_{rs} = VT/ΔP1). With addition of PEEP, a shift to a more compliant curve may occur such that C_{rs} = VT/(ΔP2 – PEEP) increases. The change in compliance may represent recruitment of poorly ventilated or nonventilated lung units with application of PEEP and may be correlated with improved oxygenation and gas exchange.

to higher airway pressure and work of breathing. In one study, increased resistance correlated positively with both peak airway pressure and the severity of gas exchange abnormality.

E. Multiple Organ System Failure

Although often viewed as a primary lung disorder, ARDS is clearly associated with multiple organ system dysfunction and failure. Subtle evidence of organ system dysfunction is very common in both survivors and nonsurvivors of ARDS, and renal failure, liver failure, central nervous system failure, heart failure, thrombocytopenia, and gastrointestinal bleeding and malabsorption contribute greatly to mortality and morbidity. In fact, of those who died with ARDS, respiratory failure has been estimated to be the primary cause in as few as 16%. Sepsis and nonrespiratory failure accounted for the remainder.

The cause of multiple organ system failure in ARDS remains poorly understood. There are three major theories. First, some investigators believe that the same systemic process that damages the lungs injures other organs as well; ARDS is simply the most obvious and earliest manifestation. For example, one study found that ARDS patients had increased urinary myoglobin and β_2-microglobulin during development of pulmonary edema, and there was a correlation between pulmonary edema and the amount of these proteins in the urine. This mechanism of multiple organ failure may be particularly likely in patients with sepsis and shock. Circulating factors such as endogenous cytokines or endotoxin are likely mediators of multiple organ failure in this hypothesis.

Another hypothesis is that hypoxemia and inadequate O_2 delivery are the causes of multiple organ failure. Some studies of ARDS patients suggest that tissue oxygen consumption is dependent on systemic oxygen delivery even when oxygen delivery is normal or elevated. Thus, a small decrease in oxygen delivery can cause oxygen consumption to fall, resulting in tissue hypoxia and potential organ damage. Such a dependent relationship could theoretically be caused by mismatching of organ perfusion and oxygen consumption, impaired diffusion of oxygen from the capillaries, or impaired unloading of oxygen from hemoglobin. This picture is very closely related to distributive shock. The view that oxygen consumption is closely linked to oxygen delivery has been challenged by those who argue that the relationship can be entirely explained by mathematical coupling. Studies undertaken to test the hypothesis that increasing oxygen delivery will meet higher targets have not been shown to raise oxygen consumption consistently and have not shown improved outcomes.

A final consideration in multiple organ system failure is the effect of therapy of ARDS. Positive-pressure ventilation and positive end-expiratory pressure are important parts of the supportive care of ARDS, but these can have adverse effects on cardiac output and oxygen delivery. Invasive monitoring, artificial airway, and other devices contribute to infection and sepsis. This theory is attractive because retrospective data have shown that mortality, while still high, is less often related to respiratory failure than to nonrespiratory organ dysfunction and sepsis. Recent clinical studies provide circumstantial support for this theory. For example, use of a low tidal volume strategy reduces mortality in ARDS patients by close to 25%. Because there was no difference in the degree of obvious barotrauma, a beneficial effect on nonrespiratory organ system function cannot be excluded.

Clinical Features

A. Predisposing Condition

More than 100 clinical situations have been reported to be associated with development of ARDS. Prospective studies have helped to identify the most common conditions, and it appears that 60–80% of cases of ARDS can be accounted for by sepsis, trauma, diffuse pulmonary infection, and aspiration of gastric contents, with other conditions being much less frequent (Table 12–18).

The overall attack rate of ARDS is relatively low. In one study, only 8% of patients at risk with any of the nine most frequently associated predisposing conditions developed ARDS, though the incidences ranged from 6–50% for individual risks. In those with multiple predisposing conditions, the incidence of ARDS increases substantially, with an average incidence of 42% for two or more risks for ARDS compared with 19% for those with a single risk in one study—though 41% of patients with sepsis alone developed ARDS.

1. Sepsis—Sepsis is present in as many as 50% of ARDS patients. In medical patients, sepsis is the most common ARDS association; in trauma patients, sepsis is the most common association in ARDS developing 48 hours or more after admission. A distinction can sometimes be made between pneumonia leading to ARDS and infection from a nonlung site leading to ARDS. In severe pneumonia, gas exchange abnormalities and chest x-ray features of ARDS are sometimes seen prior to or in the absence of other characteristics of systemic infection, suggesting that much of the lung injury is due to the infectious agent and local response to infection within the lung. Pathogens include bacteria, fungi, viruses, *Pneumocystis carinii,* and rickettsiae. On the other hand, a nonpulmonary primary site of infection can often be identified in ARDS patients, including the gastrointestinal tract, urinary tract, heart, or soft tissues. Although gram-negative enteric bacilli are most often encountered, ARDS can result from systemic infection with any bacterial, viral, or fungal pathogen. Sepsis is of particular interest because it appears that circulating mediators, including interleukins and other responses to infection, are largely responsible for ARDS, hypotension, and multiorgan system failure in addition to the microbial organisms themselves. ARDS seen as a complication of sepsis has a higher than average mortality rate, especially if the source of infection is not readily identified and treated.

2. Aspiration of gastric contents—Aspiration of gastric contents leading to ARDS is defined as an observed aspiration during intubation or witnessed vomiting in a patient with impaired airway protective mechanisms. Although acidic gastric fluid is thought to be the primary cause of lung injury, studies support a contributory role for bacteria, partially digested food particles, gastric enzymes, and other noxious substances. Neutralization of gastric acid prior to aspiration does not prevent or moderate development of acute lung injury. Other syndromes of aspiration, including necrotizing pleuropulmonary infection and lung abscess, can lead to ARDS if there is severe lung injury response or sepsis. Aspiration of gastric contents is particularly common in medical patients of advanced age, those who have neurologic diseases resulting in paralysis or impaired swallowing, or those who have advanced organ system failure. However, in other ICU patients, including surgical and obstetric patients, aspiration potential is increased by administration of sedatives, muscle relaxants, general anesthesia, or local anesthesia to the pharynx and larynx; during endotracheal intubation; during enteral feeding; and in diabetics or others with impaired gastrointestinal motility. In a sizeable number of patients, aspiration of gastric contents can only be presumed because predisposing factors are absent and there is no observed aspiration event.

3. Trauma—Trauma is a common predisposing condition to ARDS, but the precise mechanism is uncertain. Direct trauma to the thoracic wall may result in lung contusion, with hemorrhage into the lung resulting in abnormal gas exchange, atelectasis, and further lung injury.

Nonthoracic trauma is also associated with an increased incidence of ARDS. In some of these patients, lung injury results from fat embolism syndrome, a disorder seen in fractures of long bones, or pancreatitis from blunt or sharp abdominal trauma. However, in others, investigators have found correlation with both

Table 12–18. Some predisposing conditions associated with ARDS.

Infection
- Pneumonia: bacteria, fungi, viruses, *Pneumocystis carinii*
- *Nonpulmonary:* Sepsis from gram-negative bacilli, staphylococci, other gram-positive cocci, candida

Aspiration of gastric contents

Trauma
- Thoracic: lung contusion
- Nonthoracic
  - Hemorrhagic shock
  - Head trauma
  - Burns
  - Blunt abdominal trauma and pancreatitis
- Orthopedic: fat embolism syndrome, severe fracture

Other conditions
- Drugs: opiate or salicylate overdose
- Pancreatitis
- Toxic: smoke or gas inhalation
- Amniotic fluid embolism
- Central nervous system pulmonary edema
- Near-drowning
- Multiple transfusions of blood and blood products
- Collagen vascular disease, including vasculitis and pulmonary hemorrhage

hypotension and shock and with the amount of blood and blood products transfused, suggesting that the nature and extent of trauma may have something to do with the development of ARDS. Hypotension and shock have the potential to cause release of systemic mediators, and tissue damage has been shown to release a variety of agents that could result in lung injury. Although the number of blood transfusions administered seems to correlate with the development of ARDS, the requirement for transfusions is usually closely tied to the severity of trauma. On the other hand, medical patients with heavy transfusion requirements and without trauma have an increased risk of ARDS.

4. Risk modifiers—Cigarette smoking has been associated with increased likelihood of permeability pulmonary edema and alveolar hemorrhage. With similar acute risk for ARDS development, a higher proportion of chronic alcoholics will have ARDS. Although risk balancing is difficult, elderly patients seem to be at somewhat higher risk of developing ARDS, and outcome has been reported to be poorer.

B. Symptoms and Signs

Patients have severe dyspnea and respiratory distress. Findings on examination include features of hypoxemia, such as cyanosis, tachycardia, and tachypnea, but rales and wheezes are the only features on chest examination. Although the lungs are fluid filled, sputum production is rare except in those with bacterial pneumonia. Evidence of the underlying problem leading to ARDS may be found, including fever, hypotension, trauma, or findings of organ system dysfunction. Features of congestive heart failure are notably absent. Early in ARDS, symptoms and signs are limited to the lungs. If multiple organ system failure develops, then clinical features of hepatic, renal, or central nervous system failure may become evident.

C. Laboratory Findings

A key feature of ARDS is refractory hypoxemia. Arterial PO_2 is severely reduced even when the patient is given supplemental oxygen. Even 100% O_2 may not raise PaO_2 above 60–100 mm Hg. Arterial pH may be high, normal, or low, depending on the success of the patient in maintaining $PaCO_2$ with severe lung disease and the presence of hypotension and metabolic acidosis.

Other laboratory findings reflect the clinical condition leading to ARDS and the multiorgan system dysfunction seen as a consequence of this disorder. Renal and hepatic failure and electrolyte disturbances are frequent complications.

D. Imaging Studies

At disease onset, the chest x-ray shows diffuse bilateral infiltrates consistent with pulmonary edema. Unless there is coexisting heart disease, cardiomegaly is absent, and there is a lack of the central perihilar prominence of edema seen in congestive heart failure. In fact, some have pointed out that ARDS is associated with predominantly peripheral distribution of infiltrates. Nevertheless, distinguishing cardiogenic from noncardiogenic pulmonary edema is never perfect. In patients with severe pneumonia leading to ARDS, there may be focal infiltrates. In later stages of ARDS, the original dense opacification may change to a pattern of reticular densities consistent with the proliferative and fibrotic stages of lung injury. CT scans have been reported to show patchy as well as diffuse infiltrates, reflecting the recently recognized nonhomogeneous distribution of lung injury.

Chest x-rays are essential in monitoring patients for complications of ARDS, including barotrauma. Early evidence of air leaking into the lung interstitium may sometimes be found as linear low density streaks of air surrounding bronchovascular bundles. Occasionally this finding is seen as a lucency surrounding a pulmonary artery and bronchus. Air may track to the mediastinum (pneumomediastinum) or into the pleural space (pneumothorax).

Differential Diagnosis

Cardiogenic pulmonary edema is the most important disorder to be distinguished from ARDS (Table 12–19). This may be particularly difficult when ARDS is seen in conjunction with fluid overload or concomitantly with congestive heart failure. Septic shock may confound this distinction because circulating endotoxin or cytokines may exert myocardial depressant activity.

Treatment

Treatment of ARDS centers on management of severe hypoxemia, correction of the underlying disease that led

Table 12–19. **Distinguishing cardiogenic from noncardiogenic pulmonary edema.**

Cardiogenic	Noncardiogenic (ARDS)
Prior history of heart disease	Absence of heart disease
Third heart sound	No third heart sound
Cardiomegaly	Normal-sized heart
Central distribution of infiltrates	Peripheral distribution of infiltrates
Widening of vascular pedicle (increased width of mediastinum at level of azygos vein)	Normal width of vascular pedicle
Elevated pulmonary artery wedge pressure	Normal or low pulmonary artery wedge pressure
Positive fluid balance	Negative fluid balance

to ARDS, and supportive care to prevent complications. Four major concepts have evolved. First, almost all types of therapy shown to benefit patients with ARDS—including oxygen, positive end-expiratory pressure, and positive-pressure ventilation—have potentially severe adverse effects. Second, although ARDS is often considered primarily respiratory failure, multiple nonpulmonary organ system failure and infection contribute greatly to its outcome. Third, careful management of mechanical ventilation, especially tidal volume, is associated with fewer complications and improved survival. Finally, prognosis is especially poor if the underlying process is not identified or is poorly treated.

A. Oxygen

Treatment of hypoxemia in ARDS is begun almost always using 100% oxygen (F_{IO_2} 1.0), and the concentration of O_2 is reduced with the goal of maintaining Pa_{O_2} > 60 mm Hg (arterial O_2 saturation about 90%). The Pa_{O_2} increases little with administration of increasing concentrations of inspired oxygen (refractory hypoxemia) even when 100% O_2 is given, reflecting severe right-to-left shunt or $\dot{V}/\dot{Q}$ mismatching. A very few patients can be managed using a nonrebreathing oxygen mask, but most patients will be given oxygen via mechanical ventilation, because patients are unable to tolerate the increased work of breathing without mechanical support. The response to administration of O_2 in ARDS is shown in Figure 12–7, and examining the changes in venous admixture as O_2 is given and other types of therapy are administered can be helpful. The F_{IO_2} should be lowered as soon as possible to less than 0.5 to reduce the risk of lung damage from oxygen toxicity. In most patients, lowering F_{IO_2} is helped by using positive end-expiratory pressure (PEEP) or other mechanical ventilation methods to improve lung gas exchange. Because both PEEP and high F_{IO_2} both have the potential for complications, a compromise between high F_{IO_2} and high PEEP must often be chosen.

B. Positive End-Expiratory Pressure (PEEP)

PEEP includes both positive end-expiratory pressure provided with mechanical ventilation and spontaneously breathing patients who are given continuous positive airway pressure (CPAP). During exhalation, alveolar pressure is higher than atmospheric pressure, providing a pressure gradient. When PEEP is applied, a pneumatic or other valve stops exhalation when the pressure in system decreases to a value set by the clinician. This PEEP is termed extrinsic PEEP. The effective PEEP is the sum of extrinsic and intrinsic or auto-PEEP (see above).

1. Mechanism—The mechanism of action of PEEP is not known, but PEEP probably works by counteracting the tendency of alveoli to collapse in the face of pulmonary edema, low lung volume, and loss of surfactant. Gas transfer, especially oxygenation of pulmonary capillary blood, improves in areas of low $\dot{V}/\dot{Q}$.

PEEP does not decrease the rate of pulmonary edema formation nor speed the rate of water reabsorption. It is also unlikely that PEEP is able to force open collapsed alveoli directly by application of positive pressure to the conducting airway leading to the collapsed airspace. Some investigators have found that PEEP may affect the distribution of pulmonary artery blood flow away from poorly ventilated areas and toward better-ventilated regions, resulting in improved arterial oxygenation. Finally, some studies have indicated that PEEP may have a beneficial effect on the amount or nature of lung injury.

If alveoli that would otherwise be collapsed are recruited by PEEP to participate in gas exchange, each tidal volume will be delivered into a larger number of lung units. Lung compliance should increase as PEEP as added, and the increase in compliance should parallel improvement in arterial oxygenation (Figure 12–8). On the other hand, if PEEP simply distended alveoli that are already participating in tidal gas exchange, then lung compliance would remain constant or, if the lung units become overdistended, lung compliance would decrease. An upward shift in the position of the pressure-volume curve indicates recruitment of lung units; movement along the original pressure-volume curve suggests that no recruitment occurred and gas exchange will not be improved.

2. PEEP and the PV curve—In patients with early acute phase ARDS, the pressure-volume curve (Figure 12–9) is flat at lung volumes near the end-expiratory volume. In this region, compliance is abnormally low. As airway pressure is raised—eg, during a tidal volume breath given with positive-pressure ventilation—many patients will demonstrate a region of steeper slope or higher compliance. In theory, the region of higher compliance can only be explained by recruitment of additional lung units. These units must have been previously completely collapsed, but open when the airway pressure exceeds the units' critical opening pressures. The changeover point between the low compliance and higher compliance regions on the PV curve has been called the lower inflection point. In theory, PEEP should be chosen to be just above the lower inflection point to maximize recruitment and minimize lung overdistention and other complications of PEEP.

Some investigators have also stressed giving sufficient PEEP to prevent having the patient breathe in the low lung volume region below the lower inflection point. At lung volumes near the end-expiratory volume, alveoli are highly prone to collapse. As the tidal volume

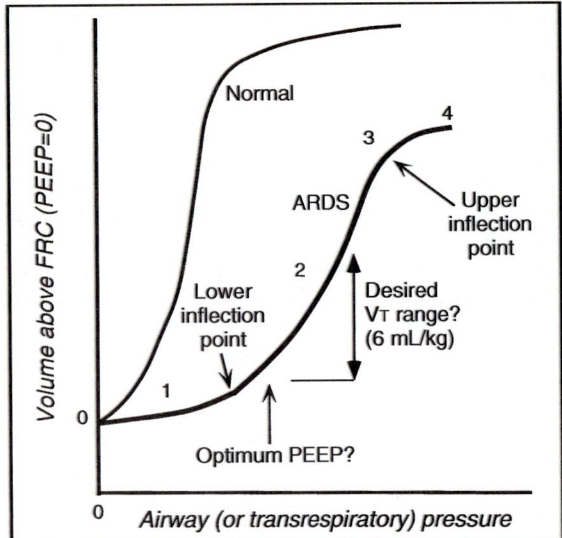

Figure 12–9. Hypothetical PV curves shown for normal and ARDS. Regions on the ARDS PV curve include (1) a region of low compliance at low lung volume—a lower inflection point; (2) a region with a steeper slope showing higher compliance—an upper inflection point; and (3) a region with a flatter slope (poorly compliant). In theory, PEEP might be chosen to be above the lower inflection point to maximize recruitment and minimal shear stress on the lungs. Tidal volume should be adjusted to stay within region (2) to avoid overdistention. This concept has been challenged because of evidence that recruitment occurs throughout the PV curve and is not restricted to the area around the lower inflection point. See text.

is administered, recruited alveoli are repeatedly exposed to large shear stress as they change from completely closed to completely open. Such damage occurs in small airways and bronchioles leading to the atelectatic lung units. Lung injury from this mechanism may be moderated if sufficient PEEP is given to raise the end-expiratory lung volume high enough to prevent cyclical lung unit collapse.

On the other hand, selecting an optimal PEEP value using the lower inflection point remains controversial for several reasons. First, some patients with ARDS will demonstrate PV curves that have no inflection points and no regions of increasing compliance. This configuration has been associated with later stages of ARDS during which lung units are poorly or not recruited at higher lung volume, and improvement of PaO_2 in response to PEEP is generally poor. Second, some ARDS patients whose respiratory PV curves have been partitioned into the lung and chest wall PV curves have shown no inflection point on the lung PV curve but only on the chest wall PV curve. This finding challenges the notion of lung recruitment with PEEP. Next, the lower inflection point in ARDS patients may be as high as 15–18 cm H_2O, or considerably higher than many clinicians believe is necessary. It is likely that a more modest level of PEEP in conjunction with a low tidal volume strategy will have the most physiologic and clinical benefit. Finally, some workers have not found that the linear segment of the PV curve is associated with constant compliance, implying that the lower inflection point is not sharply defined.

3. Adverse effects—Adverse effects of PEEP include reduced cardiac output that, in turn, decreases systemic oxygen delivery. There have been several postulated mechanisms of decreased cardiac output from PEEP, including, among others, (1) decreased systemic venous return, (2) impaired ventricular performance, (3) increased pulmonary vascular resistance, and (4) decreased left ventricular compliance. It may be important to distinguish between decreased cardiac output and decreased cardiac function, however, because positive-pressure ventilation and PEEP can support ventricular function, especially in severe pump failure and cardiogenic shock. Decreased cardiac output lowers systemic oxygen delivery, the product of cardiac output and arterial oxygen content.

PEEP has been associated with barotrauma, including pneumothorax and lung injury, with exacerbation of pulmonary edema, interstitial fibrosis, and inflammation. Debate continues about whether the underlying lung disease that led to the use of PEEP contributes to barotrauma or whether barotrauma is solely related to PEEP. It is clear that the degree of lung distention rather than the PEEP or airway pressure is the important variable. Large end-inspiratory lung volume rather than high distending pressure appears to be most important in causing barotrauma. In experimental animals, high end-inspiratory lung volumes were reached using either low PEEP and very high tidal volume or very high PEEP and low tidal volume. Both groups showed evidence of barotrauma. The relationship of PEEP to barotrauma is clearly related to tidal volume, and the low tidal volume strategy will influence the incidence of lung injury from PEEP.

Patients in whom PEEP is poorly tolerated generally may have hypotension, tachycardia, and decreased cardiac output as the earliest manifestations. Hemodynamic intolerance may be signs of volume depletion, severe pulmonary hypertension, or ventricular dysfunction. A pulmonary artery catheter may be helpful, and volume expansion or vasopressor drugs may be necessary. In other patients, PEEP may improve PaO_2 only slightly, suggesting that they have few recruitable lung units. PEEP is generally contraindicated in very asymmetric or localized lung disease with hypoxemia. In ARDS patients with a patent foramen ovale, PEEP has been shown to worsen $Pa{O_2}$. In 39 patients with ARDS given PEEP 10 cm H_2O, mean $P(A–a)O_2$ improved and only seven patients had an increase in shunt fraction, but in seven patients with patent foramen ovale, six had an increase in shunt fraction and little or no improvement in $P(A–a)O_2$. A failure to improve oxygenation with PEEP may be due to increased right-to-left shunting of blood due to an increase in pulmonary vascular resistance mediated by PEEP.

4. Application of PEEP—In patients with ARDS, many clinicians prefer to give oxygen at FIO_2 1.0 initially, then decrease as much as possible consistent with adequate $Pa{O_2}$ and O_2 saturation while PEEP is titrated upwards. As described above, to avoid the lowest lung volume range at which additional stress-induced lung injury may occur, a minimum PEEP of 5 cm H_2O should probably be given, but the minimum PEEP defined by the lower inflection point may be substantially higher in some patients. An alternative strategy is to use predetermined combinations of PEEP and FIO_2 (Table 12–20) with a clear target for $Pa{O_2}$ and O_2 saturation.

PEEP should be adjusted incrementally, with close monitoring of respiratory mechanics (especially inspiratory plateau pressure), arterial blood gases, and hemodynamic variables. An initial PEEP of 5 cm H_2O is almost always well tolerated, but blood pressure, heart rate, and pulse oximetry should be checked immediately before and after the addition. If the patient is stable, allow 10–20 minutes before arterial blood gases and cardiac output are determined. If desired goals are not met, PEEP can be increased by 2–3 cm H_2O at a time. In some patients, changes in $Pa{O_2}$ may not occur until several hours after PEEP is changed. These patients cannot be easily identified, but clinicians should be aware that changes in blood gases and hemodynamics may occur both immediately and long after a change is made in PEEP.

The goal of PEEP is to facilitate oxygen transfer across the lungs without impairing systemic oxygen delivery. In most this is achieved by using the lowest PEEP consistent with adequate arterial O_2 saturation (> 90%). For some time, the concept of "best PEEP" has been promoted, variously described as the PEEP level applied to an individual patient with ARDS that results in the best balance between tissue oxygenation and adverse effects. Most now agree that the optimal PEEP is the least that achieves predetermined objectives of patient management rather than some theoretically

Table 12–20. Lower tidal volume strategy for ARDS.[1]

Step 1: Calculate predicted body weight (PBW) in kg.	0.91 x (height, cm – 152.4) + 50 (for men) or 45.5 (for women).			
Step 2: Set ventilatory mode (volume-cycled assist/control) and tidal volume.	a. Initial tidal volume = 6 mL/kg PBW (if higher, then lower 1 mL/kg/h). b. Measure inspiratory plateau pressure (Pplat) with 0.5 s pause every 4 hours and after every change in PEEP or tidal volume. c. Adjust tidal volume based on inspiratory plateau pressure. If Plat > 30 cm H_2O, decrease tidal volume to 4–5 mL/kg. If Pplat < 25 cm H_2O and tidal volume < 6 mL/kg, increase tidal volume by 1 mL/kg.			
Step 3: Adjust respiratory rate.	a. Initial respiratory rate to maintain same minute ventilation. b. Adjust to keep pH 7.30–7.45. c. Do not exceed rate > 35/min, or increase rate if $Pa{CO_2}$ < 25 mm Hg.			
Step 4: Adjust FIO_2 and PEEP to maintain $Pa{O_2}$ 55–80 mm Hg using only these combinations. Minimize both FIO_2 and PEEP	<u>FIO_2</u> 0.3–0.4 0.4 0.5 0.6	<u>PEEP</u> 5 8 8, 10 10	<u>FIO_2</u> 0.7 0.8 0.9 1.0	<u>PEEP</u> 10, 12, 14 14 16, 18 18–25
Step 5: Manage acidosis or alkalosis as needed.	pH < 7.30, increase rate (see Step 3) pH < 7.30 and rate = 35, consider bicarbonate influsion pH < 7.15, consider increase in tidal volume (even if limited in Step 2) pH > 7.45 and no patient triggering, decrease rate (keep > 6/min)			

[1]Modified from The Acute Respiratory Distress Syndrome Network. Ventilation with lower tidal volumes as compared with traditional tidal volumes for acute lung injury and the acute respiratory distress syndrome. N Engl J Med 2000;342:1301–8.

ideal value. Thus, PEEP should be titrated until PaO_2, arterial oxygen content, and oxygen delivery are increased to acceptable levels as long as adverse effects are minimized. In practice, most clinicians prefer PEEP levels between 5 and 12 cm H_2O and rarely exceed this range because of fear of barotrauma and decreased cardiac output. There are little data to support higher PEEP levels except in rare patients with persistent hypoxemia. Although respiratory system pressure-volume curves can be determined, most clinicians adjust PEEP using a combination of response of arterial blood gases, hypothetical maximum and minimum PEEP values, and hemodynamic response.

Withdrawal or reduction of PEEP has received some attention. Despite concern about worsening of hypoxemia and difficulty in returning patients to their baseline state, decreasing PEEP in appropriate patients by decrements of 2–4 cm H_2O with careful monitoring is usually safe.

C. Mechanical Ventilation

1. Low tidal volume strategy—The most important development in the management of ARDS has been the demonstration that mechanical ventilation with lower tidal volume than conventionally used is associated with improved clinical outcome. This has been termed a "low tidal volume" or "lung protective" strategy. In experimental animals, overdistention of lung regions causes increased epithelial permeability and a histologic picture of diffuse alveolar damage. In ARDS, a retrospective study showed that limiting peak inspiratory pressure with low tidal volume during mechanical ventilation was associated with a 16% mortality rate in ARDS, in contrast to a predicted mortality rate of 40%. However, a recent NIH study found that mortality decreased from 40% (12 mL/kg predicted body weight) to about 31% in a group whose tidal volume was targeted at 6 mL/kg predicted body weight, or even lower if inspiratory plateau pressure was > 30 cm H_2O. A protocol for adjusting the mechanical ventilation using a low tidal volume strategy is summarized in Table 12–20.

Reducing tidal volume is associated with little or no change in the dead space/tidal volume ratio and may result in improved O_2 delivery. Because lung injury is associated with inspiratory lung volume, higher levels of PEEP may be safer if tidal volume is limited. Studies have shown little or no adverse effects of low tidal volume, as long as PEEP is given, but $PaCO_2$ may increase as minute ventilation is decreased with the lower tidal volume. Low tidal volume ventilation with elevated $PaCO_2$ has been termed "permissive hypercapnia." Acute respiratory acidosis with permissive hypercapnia has been shown to be surprisingly well tolerated in several clinical trials, and the benefits of low tidal volume strategy in improved outcome have been demonstrated in acute asthma and ARDS. However, there may be more subtle effects of respiratory acidosis on nonpulmonary system function, including renal and neurologic, that are not yet appreciated.

There is not yet agreement on the mechanism of improved clinical outcome with a low tidal volume strategy. No differences in pneumothorax (explosive barotrauma) were reported, but there were small differences in the rate of nonpulmonary organ dysfunction. An attractive hypothesis is that acute lung injury is enhanced by lung overdistention, and low tidal volume moderates this "ventilator-associated lung injury." For example, the levels of a variety of proinflammatory cytokines in blood and alveolar fluid have been found to be lower in randomized ARDS patients treated with low tidal volumes. It is likely that the severe regional heterogeneity of lung involvement is important because overdistention would predominate in the most compliant portions of the lungs (Figure 12–10).

2. Volume-preset ventilation—Most ARDS patients are ventilated using conventional volume-preset (volume-cycled) positive-pressure ventilators. Initial tidal volume is set at 6 mL/kg ideal body weight, and peak inspiratory flow rate is generally at least 1–1.2 L/s owing to the high demand for inspiratory flow. Adjustments in tidal volume depend on the level of the inspiratory plateau pressure (Pplat) as shown in Table 12–20. PEEP is given as necessary for refractory hypoxemia and in order to lower the FIO_2 to levels regarded as nontoxic.

It has been shown that volume-preset ventilation using a high peak flow and a descending inspiratory flow pattern may have characteristics similar to those of pressure-controlled ventilation (PCV). In theory, these settings may improve distribution of ventilation to poorly ventilation lung regions, improving hypoxemia without increased PEEP or FIO_2.

3. Pressure-controlled ventilation—Pressure-controlled ventilation (PCV) might seem like a very attractive option in the management of ARDS, largely because the preset maximum positive airway pressure cannot be exceeded. However, this feature does not automatically provide the same benefit as a low tidal volume strategy unless the maximum pressure is adjusted to also limit tidal volume. On the other hand, PCV does have the theoretical advantage of generating maximum inspiratory flow at the beginning of the inspired breath. In some patients, distribution of ventilation may be enhanced, especially to the most poorly ventilated lung regions. Some investigators believe that the characteristics of PCV make it the optimal mode for almost all patients with ARDS, but others do not find any advantages over volume-preset ventilation.

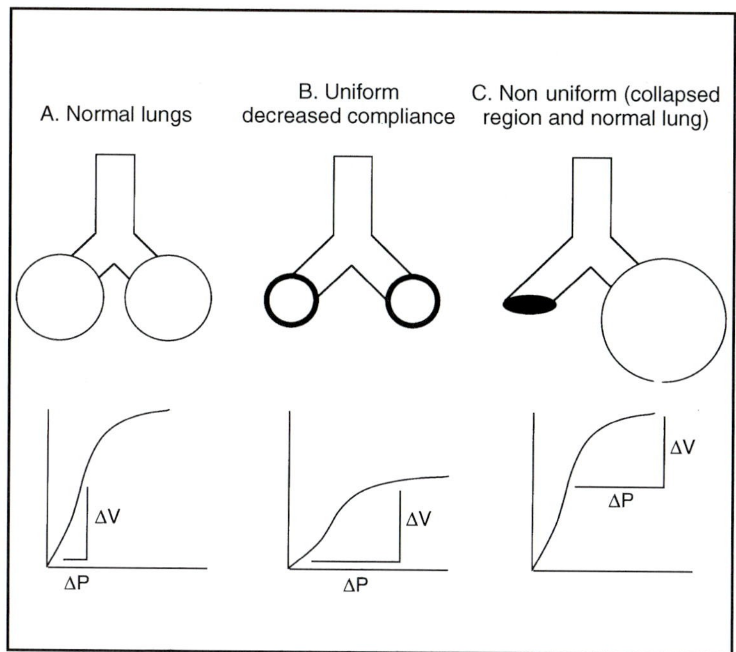

Figure 12–10. Schematic illustrating heterogeneity of lung injury in ARDS and effect on respiratory system compliance for the same tidal volume (ΔV) in all three examples. Normal lungs with uniformly normal compliance are shown in *a*. A representative PV curve is shown with a small ΔP change as the tidal volume is delivered (ΔV). In *b*, there is uniformly decreased compliance of the lungs. The flatter slope of the PV curve results in a larger ΔP required to deliver the same tidal volume (ΔV). ARDS is now recognized to have nonuniform lung involvement *(c)*, and the decreased respiratory system compliance arises from collapse of the majority of lung units and overdistention of remaining normal units. In *c* the same tidal volume is delivered to a smaller region of normal lung so that ΔP is large for the same ΔV. The overall compliance shown in *c* (ΔV/ΔP) is the same as in *b*.

A few studies have shown that PCV compared with conventional volume-preset ventilation may result in increased PaO_2, decreased mean and peak airway pressure, and less impairment of cardiac output. Other studies have shown no appreciable differences. Careful adjustment of inspiratory time may be needed to optimize tidal volume and minute ventilation. PCV with pressure limited to 30–40 cm H_2O might be considered in ARDS patients with severe hypoxemia unresponsive to PEEP with conventional volume-preset ventilation or in those who require excessively high airway pressures or PEEP with conventional ventilation. Because PCV uses a fixed airway pressure, tidal volume will vary with changes in airway resistance, respiratory system compliance, and patient efforts. Minute ventilation will vary correspondingly.

4. Inverse ratio ventilation—In ARDS patients with refractory hypoxemia, inverse ratio ventilation (IRV) has been used. In contrast to conventional ventilation, inspiratory time is made longer than expiratory time by decreasing the inspiratory flow rate, holding inspiration for a preset time before allowing for exhalation, or, if a time-cycled ventilator is used, directly increasing inspiratory time. How IRV improves oxygenation is not clear. There may be improved distribution of inspired gas resulting from the longer time allowed for gas movement during the inspiratory phase. The shortened expiratory time, on the other hand, may result in dynamic hyperinflation, raising end-expiratory volume and improving gas exchange in a manner similar to intrinsic PEEP.

Inverse ratio ventilation can be used with either volume-preset ventilation or PCV. When initiated, an I:E ratio of 1:1 should be tried first, and blood pressure, heart rate, and pulse oximetry should be closely monitored. If needed, I:E ratio can be further altered to 1.5:1, 2:1, or more. Because of shortened expiratory time, end-expiratory pressure may rise, and PEEP may have to be adjusted downward. It is unusual for I:E ratios of greater than 3:1 or 4:1 to improve gas exchange.

Increased time spent during inspiration and dynamic hyperinflation can cause severely reduced cardiac output and hypotension. Prolonged inspiratory time may be very uncomfortable to the patient, and sedation or muscle relaxants are always needed. Monitoring of IRV is complex because I:E ratio, peak airway pressure, and PEEP do not adequately reflect all the essential parameters and because the pattern of inspiratory pressure and flow in IRV differs depending on how IRV is produced. Monitoring mean airway pressure has been suggested, but this value does not correlate with gas exchange or hemodynamic compromise in IRV.

There have been no controlled clinical trials demonstrating improved outcome with IRV. This method should be reserved for the rare patient with refractory hypoxemia unresponsive to PEEP and oxygen therapy.

5. Other modes of mechanical ventilation—A lung protective strategy is the basis for several other modes of mechanical ventilation. Carrying low tidal volume to extreme is extracorporeal membrane oxygenation and

CO_2 removal, in which the lungs are completely rested. Clinical trials have been unable to demonstrate improved clinical outcomes from this practice. High frequency ventilation has been used for more than 20 years. With this method, very small tidal volumes (1–2 mL/kg or less) at respiratory rates as high as several hundred per minute are administered by a high-velocity jet or an oscillating membrane. High frequency oscillation has been successful in neonatal respiratory distress, but scaling up to larger patients has not been uniformly feasible. Gas exchange can often be maintained or improved, but no difference in clinical outcome has been demonstrated. Another lung protective method is tracheal gas insufflation, in which a 4–6 L/min flow of fresh gas is provided into a small catheter placed in the lower trachea. The effect is to reduce the apparent dead space and achieve improved gas exchange with lower tidal volume and pressure. As such, it may be an adjunct to low tidal volume methods.

A more radical method of ventilation is undergoing clinical trials. With partial liquid ventilation (PLV), the lungs are filled with a perfluorocarbon, a substance in which oxygen is highly soluble. Conventional volume-preset ventilation is used but gas movement through the lungs is almost entirely by diffusion. PLV has the potential advantages of overcoming loss of surfactant, recruiting lung units without increased airway pressure, and avoiding further lung injury.

While not a ventilatory mode, a number of investigators have advocated placing the patient into the prone position during mechanical ventilation for ARDS. Several studies have demonstrated improvement in Pa_{O_2} in 50–75% of patients turned from supine to prone, with many patients having prolonged benefit. The mechanism of prone positioning appears to depend on the smaller volume of lung that is compressed by the abdominal contents and heart in the prone position and by more uniform lung distention in that position. Hypoxemia is more likely to improve in patients with early stage ARDS with pulmonary edema than after significant fibrosis develops. Because the prone position may allow adequate gas exchange with lower values of PEEP, tidal volume, and F_{IO_2}, this technique might also be considered a lung protective strategy.

D. Supportive Care

Patients with ARDS often require prolonged mechanical ventilation and long duration of stay in the ICU, putting them at risk for complications of ICU monitoring and therapy, infection, and prolonged bed rest. Attention must be paid to maintaining nutrition, preventing deep venous thrombosis and gastrointestinal bleeding, and preventing other complications. However, recognizing that deaths in patients with ARDS often result from infection and nonrespiratory system failure, supportive care focuses especially on minimizing cardiovascular compromise and preventing infection.

E. Treatment and Prevention of Infection

Infection is a major prognostic factor in ARDS, either as the primary cause of ARDS or secondarily as a cause of death. In one study, the mortality rate was 78% in patients who developed ARDS during bacteremia and 60% in those with nosocomial pneumonia. In another study, infection was absent in two-thirds of survivors but present in two-thirds of nonsurvivors. The major infection sites were the lungs or pleura, the abdomen, soft tissues, and other locations, and about 5% had multiple sites of infection. Gram-negative bacilli made up 57% of 177 isolates causing infection in ARDS in one series, while gram-positive cocci were found in 36% and other organisms in 7%. Of pneumonias, gram-negative organisms were found in 58% and were related to endotracheal intubation and prolonged need for ventilatory support. The finding of gram-negative pathogens in ARDS patients with pneumonia assumes particular importance because those patients had only a 12% survival rate despite appropriate in vitro sensitivity of bacteria to administered antibiotics, whereas patients with ARDS associated with gram-negative bacillary abdominal infections had a 59% survival rate.

Sepsis or severe pneumonia should be suspected as the cause of ARDS in all cases unless a highly likely alternative is present. A primary infection site may be easily identified, but in doubtful cases occult lung and abdominal sources must be investigated. Antibiotics should be selected on the basis of clinical findings and epidemiologic data. Some important considerations include the likelihood of gram-negative bacilli, staphylococci, and candidemia in hospitalized patients, previous antibiotic use, the possibility of infection with anaerobic organisms, immunologic competence of the patient, gastric antacid administration, and other host and local ICU factors. Ventilator-associated pneumonia is a common complication of ARDS with prolonged mechanical ventilation. The diagnosis is difficult to confirm, but new or changing infiltrates, fever, purulent sputum, and worsening gas exchange usually make the diagnosis. The finding of bacteria in sputum cultures from intubated patients should not automatically lead to a diagnosis of pneumonia. However, a variety of protected brush cultures, quantitative culture of bronchoalveolar lavage fluid, and other techniques may be helpful.

F. Pharmacologic Therapy

There are at present no established pharmacologic therapies for ARDS, but drug treatment has been attempted in several ways. A large number of studies have attempted to intervene in the early stages of acute lung injury by interruption of cytokine pathways (antagonists, receptor antagonists), inhibition of endotoxin (monoclonal antibodies), reduction of nonspecific inflammation (corticosteroids, prostaglandin and leukotriene inhibitors), and prevention of oxidant damage (antioxidants such as acetylcysteine, vitamin C, superoxide dismutase). None have proved to be successful. Inhaled nitric oxide has been given to patients with ARDS. This gas is a potent endogenous vasodilator that selectively dilates pulmonary vessels in well-ventilated regions of the lung when given by inhalation, and it is rapidly inactivated before reaching the systemic circulation. Clinical trials have shown improvement in gas exchange, probably because of improved distribution of pulmonary perfusion. No large study has concluded that nitric oxide improves clinical outcome.

Diuretics such as furosemide should be given to ARDS patients who show evidence of volume overload and are judged to have adequate systemic volume. Diuretics should be used judiciously to avoid volume depletion and compromise of right and left ventricular filling.

Corticosteroids are attractive in ARDS because of potential roles for cytokine and inflammation mediated lung injury, and these drugs are potent inhibitors of these processes. Several large studies have shown that high-dose corticosteroids are unable to affect the incidence, severity, or outcome in the acute phases of ARDS. However, one group of investigators has found that administration of high-dose corticosteroids in the later phases of ARDS (after day 10) was associated with improved survival, better gas exchange, and less organ dysfunction. Further study is needed to determine the role of corticosteroids in ARDS. The role of nonsteroidal anti-inflammatory drugs, antioxidants, and other drugs such as ketoconazole and pentoxifylline remains unclear despite small studies showing potential benefit. There is some interest in surfactant replacement therapy, largely because of the availability of synthetic agents and its successful use in neonatal respiratory distress. However, compared with neonates, surfactant is not absent in ARDS but rather less active, probably from inhibition by serum proteins in the exudative pulmonary edema fluid. If successful, surfactant replacement may improve lung compliance and gas exchange and lessen barotrauma and duration of mechanical ventilation. The dose, delivery, type of surfactant, and clinical value of this therapy are unknown.

Prognosis

In the first description of the syndrome of ARDS, 12 patients were described of whom 7 died. Despite improvement in care, the mortality rate has changed only slightly. Nevertheless, recent studies have been encouraging. In one study from Seattle, mortality was 50–60% in the mid 1980s, but fell to 30–40% in the late 1990s. The large NIH sponsored trial using low tidal volumes reported mortality of 30–40% as well.

A. Respiratory Failure and Outcome

Previously, patients with ARDS often died early in the course of the disease from intractable hypoxemic respiratory failure. Hypoxemia could not be corrected adequately by administration of high concentrations of oxygen, and survival was often less than 3 days after onset. Accordingly, treatment focused on reversing hypoxemia with positive end-expiratory pressure, changes in ventilator management, and extracorporeal membrane oxygenation. Despite clear improvement of hypoxemia in significantly more patients, these measures have had little or no effect on outcome. One retrospective study found that unmatched patients who did not receive PEEP had no higher mortality than those who were given PEEP, though the PEEP group died later in their course. Other studies indicate that the severity of respiratory failure at the onset of ARDS correlates poorly with mortality rate. Comparison of survivors and nonsurvivors of ARDS showed that gas exchange variables such as PaO_2, $P(A{-}a)O_2$, and dead space/tidal volume ratio were not different at the onset of disease. In another analysis of 49 variables in 88 patients, the number of neutrophils and lack of acidosis were associated with survival, whereas the severity of respiratory failure and lung mechanics, response to PEEP, wedge pressure, blood pressure, and cardiac output were not predictive. On the other hand, a few studies do find a correlation between outcome and severity of respiratory failure, but more closely with initial response to therapy. That is, those patients who have a marked improvement in oxygenation with initial therapy (oxygen and PEEP) at 24 hours do significantly better than those with a poorer response.

B. Nonrespiratory Organ Failure and Outcome

Respiratory failure has been reported to be an unusual cause of death in ARDS. In one study, death associated with ARDS was due to irreversible respiratory failure in only 16%, and most of these died in the first 3 days of being studied. In contrast, of the 68% of deaths in this series, most were due to sepsis, with others resulting from cardiac, central nervous system, and hepatic failure. In another study, multiple organ system dysfunction was found in almost all patients with sepsis and ARDS but much less frequently in those with ARDS who showed no evidence of infection. The kidneys are the most commonly affected nonpulmonary organ in ARDS, with renal failure developing and contributing to morbidity and mortality data in 30–50%. In a European multicenter report, the overall mortality rate from ARDS was 59%, but death occurred in 38% of cases of ARDS following trauma and 68% of those with intra-abdominal sepsis. Probably because of decreased organ system reserve, patients over age 70 in this report had a mortality rate of 82%. A study of the importance of multiple organ failure in ARDS found that nonsurvivors had more severe thrombocytopenia than survivors as well as lower blood pH, more liver dysfunction, and higher serum creatinine concentrations. However, a prospective study of 215 ARDS patients found that the cause of death (53% of total) was progressive respiratory failure in 40%, although sepsis and multiple organ system failure were also commonly causes of death. The authors speculated on several reasons for differences, but the most likely explanation is that a greater proportion of their patients had primary pulmonary infection as the underlying cause of ARDS.

Current Controversies & Unresolved Issues

A. Fluid Management

Whether intravascular volume should be reduced or increased in ARDS remains a controversial issue. Because of increased lung permeability, pulmonary edema is generated and maintained at pulmonary capillary hydrostatic pressures that are normal or low. It is argued that resolution of pulmonary edema would be facilitated by further lowering of microvascular hydrostatic pressure with diuretics and fluid restriction. On the other hand, there is concern about oxygen delivery to the tissues in the face of intravascular volume depletion. Positive-pressure ventilation and PEEP tend to reduce cardiac output and oxygen delivery, and cardiac output is maintained to a large degree by ensuring adequate intravascular fluid volume. Sepsis and shock, major factors in ARDS, often require massive addition of fluid because of hypotension and decreased tissue perfusion. These factors suggest that volume expansion may be needed and that diuretics and negative fluid balance should be avoided.

In favor of volume expansion and maintenance of intravascular fluid volume, some investigators have shown that oxygen consumption varies directly with oxygen delivery in patients with ARDS. In normal subjects, the metabolic rate of the body determines oxygen consumption ($\dot{V}O_2$), and O_2 delivery is adequate enough so that even a large decrease in O_2 delivery does not decrease $\dot{V}O_2$ until O_2 delivery is severely reduced. Increased O_2 delivery does not increase $\dot{V}O_2$. In ARDS patients, however, increasing O_2 delivery sometimes does increase $\dot{V}O_2$, suggesting that O_2 delivery was initially insufficient to meet metabolic demands even when the O_2 delivery rate was in the normal range. This circumstance has been termed O_2 delivery-dependent oxygen consumption and may be a contributing cause of multiorgan system failure. A number of investigators, however, have attributed O_2 delivery-dependent oxygen consumption to an artifact of mathematical coupling. Studies designed to test the hypothesis have not found that increasing oxygen delivery results in better clinical outcome.

Retrospective evidence indicates that net negative fluid balance is desirable in ARDS. Reduction of pulmonary microvascular pressure decreases lung water despite severe lung injury and cumulative net negative fluid balance and weight loss are significantly higher in survivors compared with nonsurvivors of ARDS. These trials have the problem of self-selecting patients with better prognoses, but they nonetheless suggest that fluid balance may be an important determinant of outcome. In one study, increased survival in ARDS patients was found in those who had at least a 25% reduction in pulmonary capillary wedge pressure compared with those who did not, and survivors of ARDS were found to have lower wedge pressures and body weights compared with nonsurvivors, and the mean number of days of mechanical ventilation and days of ICU care were less in those who gained less than 1 L of fluid over the first 36 hours. There was a lack of detrimental effect on nonpulmonary organ system function despite low fluid intake.

In a prospective study of 52 critically ill patients, those with extravascular lung water > 7 mL/kg ideal body weight were given diuretics and, even if hypotensive, fluid restriction. The other group was given diuretics only if normotensive and wedge pressure was over 10 mm Hg. Extravascular lung water fell more markedly, and ventilator days, ICU days, and cumulative positive fluid balance were significantly less in those whose lung water was measured. The authors concluded that negative fluid balance, especially in those with pulmonary edema, was clinically beneficial.

Given these conflicting data about fluid balance, a reasonable approach is to monitor the patient carefully and administer as little fluid as necessary to maintain adequate oxygen delivery. In the absence of lung water determination, pulmonary artery wedge pressure should probably not be allowed to be as low as 5–8 mm Hg if that level is associated with a fall in cardiac output or blood pressure. On the other hand, excessive fluid administration should be avoided when pulmonary artery wedge pressures exceed 12–14 mm Hg. With lack of evidence of inadequate systemic O_2 delivery (stable renal function, absence of lactic acidosis), there is increasingly supportive data for trying to achieve net negative fluid balance by fluid restriction and diuretics. It should be emphasized, however, that wedge pressure and cardiac output measurements should not be considered in absolute terms and should be interpreted with full appreciation of their possible inaccuracy in patients with lung disease and positive-pressure ventilation.

B. Periodic Lung Recruitment

The PV curve of the lungs, both in normals and those with ARDS, shows hysteresis, or a different curve during inflation and deflation. Because the inflation limb requires higher pressures at the same lung volume than the deflation limb, it appears that a relatively high transpulmonary pressure may be needed initially to "open" lung units. Subsequently, the amount of pressure needed is considerably less. This finding has led to the recommendation for periodic "recruitment maneuvers" superimposed on conventional ventilatory techniques.

Some investigators have suggested that patients with ARDS should have the airway pressure increased to 30–45 cm H_2O and held constant for 30 seconds while ventilator cycling is inhibited. This can be done by using the continuous positive airway pressure (CPAP) mode, but the patient must be heavily sedated or paralyzed. Successful recruitment is marked by subsequent increase in lung compliance (lower inspiratory plateau pressure at the same tidal volume) and lower oxygen requirements. The frequency, magnitude, safety, and clinical benefit of aggressive lung recruitment is not established.

C. Routine Use of PV Curves

Pressure-volume curves have been recommended for determining optimal PEEP and tidal volume levels to avoid ventilator-associated lung injury. There is no doubt that careful PV curve determination has been instrumental in enhancing our understanding of lung and chest wall mechanics in ARDS, but routine use is not practical for a combination of technical and clinical reasons.

Artegas A et al: The American-European Consensus Conference on ARDS, part 2. Ventilatory, pharmacologic, supportive therapy, study design strategies, and issues related to recovery and remodeling. Acute respiratory distress syndrome. Am J Respir Crit Care Med 1998;157:1332–47.

Bernard GR et al: The American-European Consensus Conference on ARDS. Definitions, mechanisms, relevant outcomes, and clinical trial coordination. Am J Respir Crit Care Med 1994;149:818–24.

Brower RG, Fessler HE: Mechanical ventilation in acute lung injury and acute respiratory distress syndrome. Clin Chest Med 2000;3:491–510.

Esteban A et al: Prospective randomized trial comparing pressure-controlled ventilation and volume-controlled ventilation in ARDS. Chest 2000;117:1690–6.

Gattinoni L et al: Acute respiratory distress syndrome caused by pulmonary and extrapulmonary disease: different syndromes? Am J Respir Crit Care Med 1998;158:3–11.

Gattinoni L et al: Effects of positive end-expiratory pressure on regional distribution of tidal volume and recruitment in adult respiratory distress syndrome. Am J Respir Crit Care Med 1995;151:1807–14.

Harris RS, Hess DR, Venegas JG: An objective analysis of the pressure-volume curve in the acute respiratory distress syndrome. Am J Respir Crit Care Med 2000;161:432–39.

Hudson LD: Protective ventilation for patients with acute respiratory distress syndrome. N Engl J Med 1998;338:385–7.

Meade MO et al: Agreement between alternative classifications of acute respiratory distress syndrome. Am J Respir Crit Care Med 2001;163:490–3.

Milberg JA et al: Improved survival of patients with acute respiratory distress syndrome (ARDS): 1983–1993. JAMA 1995;273:306–9.

Nakos G et al: Effect of the prone position on patients with hydrostatic pulmonary edema compared with patients with acute respiratory distress syndrome and pulmonary fibrosis. Am J Respir Crit Care Med 2000;161:360–8.

Parsons PE: Mediators and mechanisms of acute lung injury. Clin Chest Med 2000;3:467–76.

Tobin MJ: Advances in mechanical ventilation. N Engl J Med 2001;344:1986–96.

Ventilation with lower tidal volumes as compared with traditional tidal volumes for acute lung injury and the acute respiratory distress syndrome. The Acute Respiratory Distress Syndrome Network. N Engl J Med 2000;342:1301–8.

Ware LB, Matthay MA: The acute respiratory distress syndrome. N Engl J Med 2000;342:1334–9.

OBSTRUCTIVE SLEEP APNEA & OBESITY-HYPOVENTILATION SYNDROME

ESSENTIALS OF DIAGNOSIS

- *Excessive daytime somnolence with evidence of upper airway obstruction during sleep (obstructive sleep apnea syndrome).*
- *Impaired ventilatory response to CO_2 and hypoxemia (obesity-hypoventilation syndrome).*
- *May have cor pulmonale, hypertension, and left ventricular dysfunction.*

General Considerations

The obstructive sleep apnea syndrome is a common condition (affecting 5% of adult men and approximately half that number of women) closely associated with snoring, which is characterized by repeated episodes of upper airway collapse during sleep with resulting acute hypercapnia, hypoxemia, sleep disruption, and hemodynamic alterations. Severely affected patients may develop respiratory failure and present to the ICU with marked hypercapnia, polycythemia, altered mental status, and pulmonary hypertension with cor pulmonale. Alternatively, obstructive sleep apnea may be observed in ICU patients admitted for other indications (eg, unstable angina pectoris or cardiogenic pulmonary edema); in such cases, the recognition and treatment of the sleep-disordered breathing may be a critical component of the overall ICU therapy. It should be noted, however, that most patients with obstructive sleep apnea do not have daytime hypoventilation and therefore do not have respiratory failure in the usual sense.

A. Normal Breathing During Sleep

For the purpose of this chapter, sleep may be separated into two main types—rapid eye movement (REM) sleep and non-REM sleep—which differ considerably in their effects on breathing and upper airway resistance. Although REM and non-REM sleep stages alternate throughout the night, the majority of REM sleep is normally concentrated during the latter half of the sleep period.

In normal awake individuals, the control of breathing is influenced not only by chemical and mechanical stimuli but also by inputs from higher cortical centers. With the transition to sleep (usually light nonREM sleep), volitional influences are lost and, in addition, the responsiveness of the central respiratory center to increasing $PaCO_2$ is blunted relative to the awake state. Upper airway caliber is also reduced due to both gravitational effects (related to the supine position) and a decrease in the tonic activity of upper airway dilator muscles which, during wakefulness, prevent inspiratory narrowing due to negative intra-airway pressures. The net effects of these changes in ventilatory drive and airway caliber are a slight increase in inspiratory upper airway resistance and mild hypoventilation ($PaCO_2$ 42–44 mm Hg at sea level) relative to the awake state.

During REM sleep, ventilation is irregular and appears to be under the control of behavioral processes activated during this dreaming state. Ventilatory responsiveness to chemical stimuli is markedly reduced and there is a profound suppression of skeletal muscle tone (including the intercostal muscles and other accessory muscles of respiration). Although brief central apneas and hypopneas can result in transient mild arterial O_2 desaturation, these are clinically unimportant in normal individuals.

B. Obstructive Sleep Apnea Syndrome

In contrast to mild narrowing of the upper airway found in normal persons, an exaggerated response is seen in obstructive sleep apnea syndrome, with episodic partial (hypopnea) or complete (apnea) obstruction of the upper airway during sleep. These events may last from 10 seconds to 90 seconds and are terminated by arousal from sleep, resulting in sleep fragmentation. The site of obstruction can occur at any point along the airway above the level of the glottis and often more than one site is involved. A strong association of obstructive sleep apnea with obesity in men suggests that small upper airway caliber is an important predisposing factor, though obstructive sleep apnea is found in nonobese individuals as well. Other potential factors include adenotonsillar hypertrophy or other anatomic abnormalities, increased collapsibility of the upper airway, inflammation or edema of these structures, and abnormal neural reflexes. The degree of respiratory drive plays a role, as does the amount of nasal airway resistance; both of these factors tend to increase the amount of intraluminal negative pressure and, thereby, the tendency to collapse the pharyngeal airway during inspiration.

Patients with obstructive sleep apnea syndrome tend to experience most of their problems during the wake-to-sleep transition (when ventilatory control is relatively unstable) and during REM sleep (when respiratory muscle hypotonia and chemical insensitivity combine to produce frequent and prolonged apneas). Because the threshold for arousal is relatively low during lighter non-REM sleep (stages 1 and 2), patients with obstructive sleep apnea may alternate between these sleep stages and wakefulness throughout the entire night and never reach the more restorative non-REM stages 3 or 4. For similar reasons, REM sleep is also typically fragmented and reduced in quantity. While the severity of daytime sleepiness generally correlates with the frequency of obstructive breathing events, some patients may have minimal sleepiness in spite of severe disruption of breathing during sleep (defined as more than 30 apneas or hypopneas per hour).

Hemodynamic abnormalities during sleep are common in patients with obstructive sleep apnea. Hypoxemia and high levels of circulating catecholamines contribute to increase both systemic and pulmonary vascular resistance. Blood pressure peaks immediately after arousal when a sudden increase in cardiac output meets these high vascular resistances. The markedly negative intrathoracic pressures during obstructed inspiratory efforts raise the transmural myocardial pressure, further increasing both right and left ventricular afterload. In addition to apnea-related fluctuations in blood pressure, obstructive sleep apnea increases the risk of daytime hypertension. This effect has been shown to be independent of obesity, age and gender and is thought to be related to a "resetting" of the carotid baroreceptors as a result of repeated hypoxemia. Left ventricular hypertrophy is common in patients with obstructive sleep apnea and left ventricular diastolic dysfunction (more often than systolic abnormalities) may result in cardiogenic pulmonary edema in these patients. Increased myocardial O_2 requirements combined with apnea-related hypoxemia can precipitate myocardial ischemia and present as nocturnal angina in patients with underlying coronary artery disease. Cardiac arrhythmias—including bradycardias and pauses up to 13 seconds during apneas and ventricular ectopy associated with severe desaturation—may be seen in the most severe cases.

Obstructive sleep apnea has also been strongly associated with coronary artery disease and stroke, although a direct causal relationship has yet to be shown. Suggested pathophysiologic mechanisms include the hemodynamic abnormalities described earlier as well as increases in platelet activation and plasma fibrinogen that have been reported in patients with untreated obstructive sleep apnea.

C. Obesity-Hypoventilation Syndrome

Obesity-hypoventilation syndrome is an uncommon condition in which usually massively obese individuals develop hypercapnic respiratory failure from a combination of depressed response to CO_2 and hypoxia, increased work of breathing, and possibly abnormal heart and lung function. Obesity-hypoventilation syndrome has a variable relationship to obstructive sleep apnea, perhaps because of the association of each with obesity, but most obesity-hypoventilation syndrome patients have obstructive sleep apnea. Obesity-hypoventilation patients have daytime hypercapnia and decreased response to hypercapnia—in contrast to the majority of obstructive sleep apnea patients, who while awake maintain normal $Pa{CO_2}$ and have a normal ventilatory response to CO_2. Patients with obesity-hypoventilation syndrome often have pulmonary hypertension leading to cor pulmonale.

Clinical Features

A. Symptoms and Signs

Patients with obstructive sleep apnea may complain of daytime hypersomnolence, a history of heavy snoring, awaking gasping for breath, and unrefreshing sleep. Bed-partners (if available) often provide more reliable information and will describe repeated periods of apnea terminated by loud snorts and gasping. Systemic hypertension is common. These patients may be seen occasionally in the ICU for severe nocturnal hypoxemia, cardiac arrhythmias, cardiac ischemia, or altered mental status. Patients with obesity-hypoventilation syndrome often have severe right and left heart failure with dyspnea and pulmonary and peripheral edema.

On examination of the obstructive sleep apnea patient, periodic breathing may be noted during sleep. Unlike the "Cheyne-Stokes" breathing pattern seen in severe heart failure, however, the patient with obstructive sleep apnea will have little or no air flow in spite of the increasing respiratory efforts. After a time varying from seconds to minutes, the patient arouses, may awaken briefly, and opens the airway to the accompaniment of snoring and upper respiratory noises. During the apnea, the patient may demonstrate use of accessory muscles, intercostal retractions and paradoxical inspiratory chest wall movements, and movement of the neck toward the thoracic inlet during inspiratory maneuvers. The findings are characteristic of obstruction of the upper airway while respiratory efforts are being made. Pulsus paradoxus is not uncommon during apneic events.

Those with respiratory failure associated with obstructive sleep apnea or those with obesity-hypoventilation syndrome may have acute respiratory acidosis, which may be severe enough to cause lethargy or coma. Other patients may seek medical attention primarily for severe peripheral edema and massive weight gain because of right ventricular failure from pulmonary hypertension. Dyspnea or wheezing suggests a component of obstructive lung disease or pulmonary edema. Most, but not all, patients with severe sleep apnea will show evidence of hypersomnolence.

B. Laboratory Findings

Most patients with obstructive sleep apnea have few abnormal laboratory findings when awake. Erythrocytosis is unusual in obstructive sleep apnea alone and suggests superimposed obesity-hypoventilation or other causes of sustained hypoxemia. In patients seen in the ICU who present with respiratory failure, hypercapnia and hypoxemia are seen. Chronic CO_2 retention leads to elevated serum bicarbonate (chronic respiratory acidosis). Electrocardiography may show evidence of left sided or biventricular hypertrophy, tachycardia or bradycardia in association with apneic events, and rarely ventricular ectopy. The chest x-ray is usually not helpful except for confirming cardiomegaly, pulmonary edema from left ventricular failure, or enlarged pulmonary arteries in patients with pulmonary hypertension. Patients with obesity-hypoventilation syndrome have abnormally low ventilatory response to CO_2 and hypoxia.

C. Confirmatory Testing

Traditionally, confirmation of obstructive sleep apnea has been made by polysomnography. Measurements made during sleep demonstrate episodic upper airway obstruction by showing periods of absence of airflow despite evidence of inspiratory effort. Arterial hypoxemia or O_2 desaturation proves that obstruction is causing significant gas exchange abnormalities. In the sleep laboratory, the number, nature, severity, and duration of sleep-disordered breathing events (apneas, hypopneas) are carefully measured and counted. Other measurements include electroencephalography and electrocardiography. Portable cardiorespiratory recorders (four to six channels including, at a minimum, airflow, respiratory effort, saturation, and heart rate) are better suited for use in the ICU and generally provide the information needed to guide treatment. In some patients presenting to the ICU, diagnostic testing may not be feasible and a presumptive diagnosis of obstructive sleep apnea may have to be made prior to confirmatory testing. In these patients, direct observation of the sleeping patient and pulse oximetry trends demonstrating an episodic ("sawtooth") pattern of desaturations in the ICU can be used to initiate and titrate therapy.

Differential Diagnosis

Obstructive sleep apnea syndrome may coexist with other lung diseases. Both obstructive sleep apnea and COPD are common in men, and these diseases complicate each other. Severe cardiomyopathy and central nervous system disease may present with periodic breathing, dyspnea, and hypersomnolence. Obesity is associated with hypoxemia from atelectasis. Weight gain, edema, heart failure, and hypoventilation may be seen with hypothyroidism. Thyroid function should be determined in all patients considered to have obesity-hypoventilation syndrome.

Treatment

A. Mild Obstructive Sleep Apnea

Patients with mild obstructive sleep apnea are unlikely to be seen in the ICU for this problem alone, but this syndrome is common and may be seen in those admitted with other diseases. In these patients, apneic episodes occur relatively infrequently during sleep onset and REM sleep, and daytime hypercapnia is not a problem. Treatment is directed at weight reduction, abstinence from alcohol, treatment of nasal disease (if present) and avoidance of a supine body position during sleep. Nocturnal nasal CPAP can be used if necessary. Additional treatment options include mouthpieces which displace the mandible anteriorly during sleep (thereby pulling the tongue away from the posterior pharyngeal wall) and, rarely, pharyngeal surgery. Successful management should result in reduced daytime somnolence and improvement of such neuropsychiatric symptoms as may be present.

B. Severe Obstructive Sleep Apnea

Severe obstructive sleep apnea may require aggressive relief of nocturnal upper airway obstruction. Tracheostomy is very effective because of unequivocal reversal of upper airway obstruction, but this is very rarely required even in severe sleep apnea.

1. Nasal CPAP—Nasal continuous positive airway pressure (CPAP) has become the treatment of choice for this disorder. By providing positive pressure to the collapsible portion of the upper airway during sleep, nasal CPAP effectively prevents airway obstruction during inspiration.

Nasal CPAP is generally provided by a blower attached to flexible tubing leading to a small mask placed over the nose or small soft nasal prongs. A sufficient continuous flow of air is blown into the system and, via a controllable vent, continuous positive pressure in the range of 12–20 cm H_2O can be maintained. The appropriate level of nasal CPAP is best determined during polysomnography; however, rough approximations may be made in the ICU by direct observation of the patient during sleep and upward titration of CPAP until apneas, snoring, and desaturations are eliminated. Newer "auto-titrating" devices that adjust pressure based on the shape of the inspiratory flow profile can also help identify optimal pressures. Most patients in whom it is tried, at least for the short term, tolerate nasal CPAP, but not all patients can be successfully managed in this way. For those unable to tolerate the required CPAP pressures, bi-level nasal ventilation (see above) may be more comfortable and effective while allowing a lower expiratory pressure level.

Nasal CPAP has a variable role in patients with obstructive sleep apnea who present with respiratory failure to the ICU. In many, nasal CPAP is sufficient to restore and maintain upper airway patency and normalize gas exchange during sleep. These patients probably have only mild respiratory center depression from hypoxemia and hypercapnia. Some patients are improved by the combination of nasal CPAP and oxygen. On the other hand, some obstructive sleep apnea patients with respiratory failure have little immediate response to nasal CPAP, which suggests that upper airway obstruction is no longer the only factor. In these patients, nasal CPAP can be tried, but if satisfactory results are not quickly obtained, more definitive efforts at restoring ventilation and oxygenation must be made.

Effective treatment with nasal CPAP is often accompanied by a "rebound" of sleep, which gradually returns to more normal quantities over several days. A spontaneous diuresis is also commonly seen and is the result of a reduction in hypoxia-induced pulmonary vasoconstriction and a lowering of left ventricular afterload. Hypertension may resolve (or at least be more easily controlled) with effective nasal CPAP therapy.

2. Oxygen—Oxygen is given to correct hypoxemia—sometimes alone but usually combined with nasal CPAP or positive-pressure ventilation in the setting of respiratory failure with obstructive sleep apnea. Hypoxemia is a serious complication of this syndrome, with potential for arrhythmias, altered mental status, and further deterioration of ventilatory drive. However, oxygen therapy alone typically prolongs apnea duration, resulting in worsening hypercapnia and respiratory acidosis.

In patients with acute respiratory failure, however, hypoxemia is often very severe and may cause hypoxic inhibition of central respiratory neural output and marked hypoxia of the brain, heart, and other organs.

The goal is to raise arterial P_{O_2} to at least 60–70 mm Hg for at least several days. Oxygen should be given with careful monitoring of mental status, vital signs, respiratory rate, and arterial blood gases. Increased hypercapnia indicating worsening of respiratory failure with oxygen administration should suggest the need for initiating or increasing ventilatory support rather than discontinuing oxygen.

3. Other treatment—Endotracheal intubation or tracheostomy is highly effective. In patients with localized obstruction due to adenotonsillar hypertrophy or nasal polyps, surgical excision may be curative but should not be done until the patient has been stabilized medically. Other surgical treatments (including uvulopalatopharyngoplasty and mandibular osteotomy with hyoid suspension) have even less of a role since these procedures tend only to reduce the severity of the obstruction and the results are difficult to predict. Diuretic administration may be helpful if elimination of obstructive breathing events and desaturations is insufficient to induce a spontaneous diuresis. Pulmonary edema is often the result of left ventricular diastolic dysfunction and beta-blockers may be more effective than afterload-reducing medications. There is no role for respiratory stimulants or carbonic anhydrase inhibitors in the treatment of obstructive sleep apnea syndrome. The use of sedative-hypnotic agents is contraindicated in patients with obstructive sleep apnea syndrome since they suppress the arousal response and therefore tend to lengthen apneas and cause more severe O_2 desaturations.

C. Obesity-Hypoventilation Syndrome

Patients often benefit from diuresis in response to oxygen and diuretics. Because of coexisting obstructive sleep apnea, maintenance of upper airway patency is essential. Mechanical ventilation may be necessary. Left ventricular failure is treated with diuretics with beta-blockers or afterload reduction added as indicated clinically based on estimates or objective measures of LV function.

Mechanical ventilation should not be withheld until gas exchange becomes severely abnormal. More often, mechanical ventilation is required as a temporizing measure while oxygen and other treatment correct the acute physiologic derangement. Mechanical ventilation is sometimes necessary so that oxygen can be safely given in patients who have decreased ventilatory drive. After a few days of improved arterial P_{O_2} (Pa_{O_2} > 70–80 mm Hg), many patients will have improved ventilatory drive and marked attenuation of hypercapnia. Patients will often regain significant ventilatory responsiveness to CO_2.

Some patients can be successfully ventilated using noninvasive nasal ventilation with bilevel positive-pressure ventilation. This procedure requires careful monitoring and observation, because minute ventilation and airway patency cannot be guaranteed as with conventional mechanical ventilation using an endotracheal tube. Bilevel positive-pressure ventilation is much like inspiratory pressure support ventilation, with increased pressure maintained at a preset level throughout inspiration. Although back-up rates can be added (similar to pressure-controlled IMV), they generally add little to spontaneous ventilation in these patients due to the limited ability of inspiratory pressure applied noninvasively to counteract forces produced by the weight of the chest and abdomen.

Medroxyprogesterone acetate may have a beneficial effect in patients with chronic obesity-hypoventilation, but its usefulness in acute respiratory failure is unclear. In the long term, weight loss is of substantial benefit.

Faccenda JF et al: Randomized placebo-controlled trial of continuous positive airway pressure on blood pressure in the sleep apnea-hypopnea syndrome. Am J Respir Crit Care Med 2001;163:344–8.

Mohensin V: Sleep-related breathing disorders and risk of stroke. Stroke 2001;32:1271–8.

Naughton MT, Bradley TD: Sleep apnea in congestive heart failure. Clin Chest Med 1998;19:99–113.

Shahar E et al: Sleep-disordered breathing and cardiovascular disease: cross-sectional results of the Sleep Heart Health Study. Am J Respir Crit Care Med 2001;163:19–25.

Tkacova R et al. Effects of continuous positive airway pressure on obstructive sleep apnea and left ventricular afterload in patients with heart failure. Circulation 1999;98:2269–75.

Renal Failure

13

Andre A. Kaplan, MD, FACP

ACUTE RENAL FAILURE

Acute renal failure can be defined as a precipitous impairment of kidney function without regard to etiology or mechanism. It can occur as a result of many causes, but clinical findings, complications, and some forms of treatment are the same in all cases. The causes can be divided into three main groups: "prerenal," resulting from rapidly reversible renal hypoperfusion; "postrenal," due to obstruction to urine flow; and "intrinsic," due to lesions directly involving the renal parenchyma. In most patients, intrinsic renal failure can be considered a diagnosis of exclusion once pre- and postrenal causes are eliminated.

Clinical Features

Investigations useful in determining the cause and severity of acute renal failure are listed in Table 13–1.

A. History

Noting the time of onset of renal problems helps differentiate between acute renal failure and the natural progression of chronic renal disease. The most common causes of chronic renal failure are diabetes, hypertension, chronic glomerulonephritis, and polycystic kidney disease. The patient's drug history should seek to identify those medications known to cause renal dysfunction, including nonsteroidal anti-inflammatory drugs (NSAIDs), angiotensin-converting enzyme (ACE) inhibitors, and antibiotics (Table 13–2). Exposure to hydrocarbons (carbon tetrachloride), ethylene glycol (antifreeze), or radiologic contrast agents can also cause acute renal failure.

B. Symptoms and Signs

Acute renal failure is rarely associated with flank pain or dysuria, exceptions being conditions characterized by severe renal inflammation, crystalluria, acute obstruction, intrarenal hemorrhage, and arterial embolization. Most of the symptoms associated with acute renal failure are the result of renal dysfunction. Salt and water overload, resulting in edema, hypertension, and pulmonary congestion, is most often the result of inadequate diuresis. Manifestations associated with acute retention of uremic toxins include anorexia, nausea, hiccuping, vomiting, hematemesis, impaired hemostasis, neuromuscular irritability, asterixis, lethargy, coma, and seizures. Conditions more often seen after prolonged uremia include pruritus, pericarditis, and anemia. Spontaneous bone fractures due to secondary hyperparathyroidism and altered vitamin D metabolism are ***not*** associated with acute renal failure, and their presence argues strongly for chronic uremia as the cause. Hyperkalemia due to impaired renal excretion can cause cardiac arrhythmias. Uremic acidosis may elicit Kussmaul respirations.

Evaluation of intravascular volume status and degree of hydration should include measurement of orthostatic blood pressure and heart rate, assessment of mucosal hydration and skin turgor, and inspection for the presence or absence of edema (peripheral and sacral), jugular venous distention, pulsus paradoxus, cardiac rubs or gallops, pulmonary rales, or effusions and ascites. Equally informative are signs of associated morbidity, including those of congestive heart failure, cirrhosis, or systemic vasculitis.

C. Laboratory Findings

1. Serum creatinine and glomerular filtration rate—Creatinine is made in the muscle and released into the circulation at a rate of 15–25 mg/kg/d for a middle-aged man and 10–20 mg/kg/d for a middle-aged woman. Under conditions of severe muscle damage (rhabdomyolysis), leakage of creatinine into the serum can exceed the above estimates. Creatinine is excreted primarily by glomerular filtration, with only a small percentage (10%) secreted by the tubules and virtually none reabsorbed. The normal glomerular filtration rate (GFR) must be reduced by about half before there is a substantial increase in serum creatinine levels (> 1 mg/dL). As a result, serum creatinine is not a reliable guide to modest decreases in renal function. In contrast, preexistent increases in serum creatinine support the diagnosis of chronic renal disease.

When creatinine levels are relatively stable over several days, a crude estimate of the prevailing GFR can be made using the following formula:

$$\text{GFR} = \frac{[140-\text{age}][\text{wt(kg)}]}{72 \times \text{Serum creatinine (mg/dL)}}$$

Table 13–1. Renal assessment.

History
Physical examination
Serum chemistries
Urea, creatinine, electrolytes, abnormal serologic tests (see text)
Urine chemistries
Na, FE_{Na}, urea, FE_{Ur}, creatinine
24-hour clearance: creatinine, urea, protein
Urinalysis
Dipstick determinations
Microscopy
Sulfosalicylic acid
Urine culture/Gram stain
Hemodynamic monitoring
Ultrasound imaging
Radiography
KUB, IVP, tomography, CT scan, MRI
Invasive radiography
Renal arteriography (selective, digital subtraction)
Retrograde pyelography
Percutaneous antegrade pyelography
Nuclear scanning
Split function studies and renal flow (DTPA, MAG-3)
Gallium scan
Renal biopsy

The result (in mL/min) is multiplied by 0.85 for a female.

This calculation is useful in providing a quick estimate of renal function but is potentially misleading if there are subsequent changes in the serum creatinine level. In order to validate the calculation, a 24-hour urine collection for creatinine is required.

During bouts of severe renal failure, serum creatinine increases by 1–2 mg/dL/d. More rapid increases in serum creatinine suggest rhabdomyolysis. Spurious increases in serum creatinine can occur without declines in GFR when certain cephalosporins or ketones (acetoacetate) interfere with the colorimetric reaction used for its identification. Likewise, cimetidine and trimethoprim-sulfamethoxazole can compete for tubular secretion and result in increases in serum creatinine unrelated to decreased GFR.

2. Urea—Urea is the major nitrogen-containing metabolite of protein catabolism and is excreted primarily by the kidneys. Normally, 35–50% of filtered urea is reabsorbed by the tubules. Under conditions of decreased renal blood flow, tubular reabsorption of urea can increase to 90% or more. Since creatinine is not reabsorbed, serum urea increases more rapidly than serum creatinine under these conditions, as seen in prerenal renal failure. In general, when measured as blood urea nitrogen (BUN) in mg/dL, the normal ratio of BUN to serum creatinine is 10:1. If it rises to levels of 20:1 or more, one should suspect prerenal azotemia. In addition to variations in renal handling, blood urea concentrations are also subject to the state of protein catabolism. Six grams of protein yields approximately 1 g of urea nitrogen. Under most clinical conditions there is a direct relationship between the amount of protein ingested and urea nitrogen production. Under conditions of stress, inadequate caloric intake, or corticosteroid administration, endogenous protein catabolism results in enhanced urea production. Gastrointestinal hemorrhage and the resulting absorption of blood proteins—approximately 200 g of protein in 1 L of whole blood—can also increase urea production.

3. Plasma electrolytes—Abnormalities of plasma sodium, potassium, bicarbonate, calcium, magnesium, and phosphate are common in acute renal failure, and their determination and monitoring are an integral part of the diagnosis and management of acute renal failure.

4. Serologic markers—A search for abnormal serologic markers, such as various autoantibodies, is part of the basic workup of immunologically mediated renal disease, including glomerulonephritis.

5. Urine electrolytes—Evaluation of random urine samples provides quick information about the current state of renal function. The fractional excretion of sodium (FE_{Na}) is the best means of differentiating between prerenal azotemia and acute tubular necrosis and can be calculated as follows:

$$FE_{Na} = \frac{\text{Urine Na (meq/L)}}{\text{Urine Cr (mg/dL)}} \times \frac{\text{Serum Cr (mg/dL)}}{\text{Serum Na (meq/L)}} \times 100$$

In the context of oliguria (urine output < 500 mL/d), an FE_{Na} less than 1% is most commonly associated with prerenal azotemia, but it may also be seen with acute glomerulonephritis. Under similar oliguric conditions, an FE_{Na} greater than 1% is probably related to acute tubular necrosis. Unfortunately, the potential usefulness of this test is often lost if diuretics are given prior to collection of the urine sample.

The fractional excretion of urea (FE_{Ur}) can also be useful and is similarly calculated as follows:

$$FE_{Ur} = \frac{\text{Urine Ur (mg/dL)}}{\text{Urine Cr (mg/dL)}} \times \frac{\text{Serum Cr (mg/dL)}}{\text{Serum Ur (mg/dL)}} \times 100$$

Normal values in well-hydrated individuals are between 50% and 65%. Values below 35% are most

Table 13–2. Drugs associated with acute renal failure.

Drug	Mechanism of Nephrotoxicity
Antibiotics	
Abacavir	AIN
Acyclovir	Crystalluria
Aminoglycosides	ATN; electrolyte-wasting
Amphotericin B	ATN; electrolyte-wasting, renal tubular acidosis
Cephalosporins	AIN, spurious increased creatinine
Cidofovir	ARF
Ciprofloxacin	AIN
Dapsone	ATN
Foscarnet	ATN, electrolyte-wasting, hypocalcemia
Ganciclovir	ARF
Indinavir	Nephrolithiasis, crystalluria, pyuria, obstruction
Meropenem	ARF
Penicillins	AIN
Pentamidine	ATN
Polymyxin B	ATN (may occur when given orally)
Quinolones	AIN?
Rifampin	AIN
Sulfadiazine	ARF, crystalluria
Sulfamethoxazole	AIN, crystals, decreased creatinine secretion
Sulfisoxazole	Crystalluria
Valacyclovir	ARF
Immunosuppressive agents	
Cisplatin	ATN, HUS, Glomerular capillary thrombosis
Cyclosporine	Intrarenal vasoconstriction
Daclizumab	ATN, renal dysfunction?
Ifosfamide	ARF
Interferon	Prerenal azotemia? ATN?
Interleukin-2	Shock-like syndrome, prerenal azotemia
Methotrexate	Crystalluria (high-dose IV)
Mitomycin	HUS
Tacrolimus	Intrarenal vasoconstriction
Diuretics	
All	Prerenal azotemia
Mannitol	Osmotic nephrosis

(*continued*)

Table 13–2. Drugs associated with acute renal failure. (continued)

Drug	Mechanism of Nephrotoxicity
Antihypertensives	
ACE inhibitors	Hemodynamic compromise (most common with bilateral renal artery stenosis), AIN
Angiotensin receptor blockers	Hemodynamic compromise (most common with bilateral renal artery stenosis)
Anti-Inflammatory drugs	
Celecoxib	AIN
Diclofenac	AIN
Fenoprofen	AIN, nephrotic syndrome
Ibuprofen	AIN
Indomethacin	AIN, nephrotic syndrome
Ketorolac	AIN
Nabumetone	AIN
Naproxen	AIN, nephrotic syndrome
NSAIDs (all)	Prerenal azotemia (especially in CHF, cirrhosis, nephrosis, chronic renal failure, volume depletion), ATN
Rofecoxib	AIN
Sulindac	AIN, nephrotic syndrome
Tolmetin	AIN
Antiplatelet agents	
Clopidogrel	HUS
Ticlopidine	Nephrotic syndrome, HUS
Miscellaneous agents	
Allopurinol	AIN
Cimetidine	AIN, decreased creatinine secretion
Disopyramide	Obstructive uropathy
Immune globulin intravenous	Prerenal azotemia with filtration failure due to hyperoncotic plasma
Lithium	AIN
Omeprazole	AIN
Phenindione	AIN
Phenytoin	AIN
Ranitidine	AIN
Radiocontrast agents	
All	ATN (especially with volume depletion or advanced diabetic nephropathy)

Key: ACE = angiotension-converting enzyme, AIN = allergic interstitial nephritis, ATN = acute tubular necrosis, CHF = congestive heart failure, HUS = hemolytic uremic syndrome, NSAID = nonsteriodal anti-inflammatory drug. (See Table 13–6.)

compatible with renal hypoperfusion and are not affected by loop diuretics such as furosemide. A markedly diminished FE_{Ur} cannot distinguish between a rapidly reversible prerenal azotemia and more definitive ischemic damage, such as occurs in acute tubular necrosis. Nonetheless, values below 35% are very useful in identifying renal hypoperfusion in patients taking diuretics, as is most often the case in decompensated congestive heart failure. Osmotic diuresis resulting from administration of mannitol or acetazolamide or from diabetic ketoacidosis increases the fractional excretion of urea despite the existence of volume depletion.

Twenty-four-hour urine collections for determinations of creatinine, urea, and protein are the most reliable means of assessing renal function and determining nitrogen balance. Creatinine or urea clearance can be calculated as follows:

$$\frac{\text{Creatinine clearance}}{\text{(mL/min)}} = \frac{\text{Urine Cr (mg/dL)} \times \text{Urine volume (mL/min)}}{\text{Serum Cr (mg/dL)}}$$

$$\frac{\text{Urea clearance}}{\text{(mL/min)}} = \frac{\text{Urine Ur (mg/dL)} \times \text{Urine volume (mL/min)}}{\text{Serum Ur (mg/dL)}}$$

When serum levels of creatinine or urea are increasing rapidly, the mean of the pre- and postcollection values is used in the denominator. Timed collections less than 24 hours are reasonably accurate for creatinine but are less useful for assessing proteinuria or urea production.

Modest amounts of proteinuria (< 1 g/d) are common in many forms of acute renal failure, but proteinuria in the nephrotic range (> 3.5 g/d) is most often related to glomerular disease except when associated with low-molecular-weight proteins, such as Bence Jones protein in multiple myeloma. Urine protein electrophoresis performed on a 24-hour urine collection will distinguish between these two disorders.

6. Urinalysis–Routine urinalysis consists of rapid dipstick tests and microscopic examination. Dipstick determinations measure pH and can reveal the presence of hemoglobin (positive for intact red cells, free hemoglobin, and myoglobin), protein, glucose, and ketones. Microscopic analysis can suggest infection (white cells, white cell casts, bacteria), nephritis (red and white cells, with or without cellular casts), or nephrosis (granular casts, oval fat bodies). Red cell casts are most commonly associated with glomerulonephritis but may be occasionally seen with other types of acute glomerular injury such as cholesterol emboli or with malignant hypertension. White cell casts are most often seen with infectious pyelonephritis, but, when associated with sterile urine, may be a sign of immunologically mediated interstitial nephritis. Tubular epithelial cells can be found with interstitial nephritis or acute tubular necrosis. When associated with muddy-brown casts, acute tubular necrosis is a more likely diagnosis. Eosinophiluria, demonstrable on smears of urine sediment stained with Wright's or Hansel's stain, can occur in drug-induced allergic interstitial nephritis.

The urine dipstick test for protein is most sensitive for albumin, while sulfosalicylic acid added to the urine causes precipitation of all proteins. When the urine dipstick is negative or only modestly positive for protein and the sulfosalicylic acid precipitation is markedly positive, Bence Jones proteinuria should be suspected.

Urine culture and Gram staining should be performed on any urine containing white cells. Sterile pyuria is often a sign of drug-induced interstitial nephritis, but renal tuberculosis should also be considered.

7. Assessment of intravascular volume–Central venous pressure monitoring can be accomplished with subclavian, internal jugular, or femoral catheterization. A low central venous pressure is most compatible with decreased intravascular volume; elevated central venous pressure may be secondary to intravascular expansion or pulmonary hypertension. Pulmonary artery catheterization is the most reliable means of assessing optimal fluid status by determination of cardiac output and left ventricular filling pressure.

8. Renal biopsy–Renal biopsy is most often helpful when inflammatory nephritis (glomerulonephritis, allergic interstitial nephritis, etc.) is suspected. However, in patients suspected of having acute tubular necrosis in whom renal failure fails to resolve in 6–8 weeks, renal biopsy may be indicated to diagnose irreversible causes of renal failure (cholesterol emboli, cortical necrosis, etc.).

D. Imaging Studies

Renal **ultrasound** provides an accurate means of measuring renal size (small kidneys are evidence of chronic renal disease) and determining the existence of hydronephrosis. Because potentially nephrotoxic contrast agents are not required, ultrasound has become the first choice in the evaluation of ureteral obstruction. In very rare cases, tumor infiltration or retroperitoneal or perirenal fibrosis may inhibit the expansion of the renal pelvis, thus yielding a falsely negative result.

The plain **abdominal x-ray** can demonstrate the presence of radiopaque kidney stones but is often more valuable in evaluation of associated disease processes. **Intravenous pyelography (IVP)** most reliably identifies the site of renal obstruction provided creatinine levels are not excessively elevated (≤ 4 mg/dL). **Retrograde pyelography** can image both the ureters and the bladder. **Percutaneous pyelography** can determine the site of renal obstruction when retrograde pyelography is unsuccessful. **CT scanning** can evaluate the site of obstruction (extrinsic versus intrinsic obstruction) and assess for associated morbidity. Selective **renal angiography with digital subtraction** is the best way to assess the renal vasculature for stenosis or hemorrhagic leak.

The potential for radiocontrast nephrotoxicity should always be considered. Risk factors include volume depletion, low cardiac output, preexisting renal disease, large contrast load or multiple exposures to contrast, a history of contrast-induced acute renal failure, multiple myeloma, and, most significantly, advanced diabetic nephropathy. Patients with diabetic nephropathy and creatinine levels above 4 mg/dL have a 90% probability of developing some degree of renal dysfunction. In some of these patients, renal failure may be irreversible. Patients at increased risk should be well hydrated prior to and immediately after exposure to radiocontrast dyes, and every effort should be made to limit the amount of contrast administered. The newer low-osmolality agents may be preferable. Other means of minimizing the risk of contrast-induced renal damage include oral administration of the antioxidant acetylcysteine and infusions of the dopamine agonist fenoldopam.

Radionuclide scanning provides the only noninvasive means of assessing the relative percentage of renal function from each kidney ("split function studies"). Renal blood flow can be assessed with DTPA (diethylenetriamine pentaacetic acid), which is excreted by glomerular filtration and may demonstrate renal vascular stenosis. Repeat examination after administration of captopril increases this test's sensitivity. Gallium scans can identify any type of renal inflammation and are most valuable in assessing unilateral lesions or identifying a renal origin of pyuria. Gallium scans may also be positive in patients with nephrosis. MAG3 (technetium ^{99m}Tc mercaptoacetyltriglycine) is both filtered and secreted and is the radionuclide imaging agent of choice for patients with substantial renal failure.

Magnetic resonant imaging is not yet widely employed in the evaluation of acute renal failure, but it may be of value in the diagnosis of renal vein thrombosis. Gadolinium-enhanced magnetic resonance angiography is emerging as an accurate means for assessing renal artery stenosis without the risks of catheterization or the contrast used for percutaneous angiography.

Complications

The complications of acute renal failure are listed in Table 13–3. Cardiovascular problems are most often due to fluid overload and electrolyte abnormalities. Pericarditis is probably the result of retained uremic toxins. Insufficient erythropoietin may cause decreased red cell production and anemia, but this mechanism is more commonly observed in patients with chronic renal failure. In contrast, platelet dysfunction, clinically diagnosed on the basis of prolonged bleeding time, is a

Table 13–3. Complications associated with acute renal failure.[1]

Cardiovascular
Edema
Anasarca
Hypertension
Congestive heart failure
Pulmonary edema
Arrhythmias
Myocardial infarction
Pericarditis
Hematologic
Anemia
Platelet dysfunction
Gastrointestinal bleeding
Inadequate wound hemostasis
Infectious
Septicemia
Pneumonia
Catheter-related infections
Urinary tract infections
Wound infections
Metabolic
Hyperkalemia
Hyponatremia
Hypocalcemia
Hyperphosphatemia
Hypophosphatemia (parenteral hyperalimentation)
Hypermagnesemia
Hypomagnesemia
Acidosis
Alkalosis (vomiting, nasogastric tube losses)
Hypoglycemia (decreased insulin catabolism)
Neurologic
Neuromuscular irritability
Somnolence
Coma
Convulsions
Gastrointestinal
Nausea
Vomiting
Gastritis

[1]Modified from Brezis M, Rosen S, Epstein FH: Acute renal failure. In: *The Kidney*, 4th ed. Brenner B, Rector FC (editors). Saunders, 1991.

common consequence of acute renal failure. Infections represent an important cause of morbidity and death in acute renal failure—especially urinary tract infections, which are particularly difficult to eradicate because of inadequate urine concentrations of antibiotics. Electrolyte and acid-base abnormalities are common, the most serious being hyperkalemia. Hypoglycemia may result from decreased renal catabolism of exogenously administered insulin. Neurologic abnormalities include somnolence, coma, and convulsions and are often compelling indications for initiation of dialysis. Gastrointestinal hemorrhage in acute renal failure is due to the combination of uremic coagulopathy and gastritis, but in chronic renal failure, arteriovenous malformations are the most common causes.

Choudhury D, Ahmed Z: Drug-induced nephrotoxicity. Med Clin North Am 1997;81:705–17.

Ghantous VE et al: Evaluating patients with renal failure for renal artery stenosis with gadolinium-enhanced magnetic resonance angiography. Am J Kidney Dis 1999;33:36–42.

Kaplan AA, Kohn OF: Fractional excretion of urea as a guide to renal dysfunction. Am J Nephrol 1992;12:49–54.

Mathur VS et al: The effects of fenoldopam, a selective dopamine receptor agonist, on systemic and renal hemodynamics in normotensive subjects. Crit Care Med 1999;27:1832–7.

Mindell JA, Chertow GM: A practical approach to acute renal failure. Med Clin North Am 1997;81:731–48.

Tepel M et al: Prevention of radiographic-contrast-agent-induced reductions in renal function by acetylcysteine. N Engl J Med 2000;343:180–4.

PRERENAL RENAL FAILURE

ESSENTIALS OF DIAGNOSIS

- *BUN:creatinine ratio > 20:1.*
- *Decreased urine output (unless renal losses are primary).*
- *FE_{Na} < 1% and FE_{Ur} < 35%.*
- *Urine sediment may show a few granular casts but absence of inflammatory cells and red and white cell casts.*
- *No evidence of urinary tract obstruction.*

General Considerations

Prerenal azotemia can be defined as a state of renal hypoperfusion that can be rapidly reversed with proper management. All causes of renal hypoperfusion stimulate renal autoregulatory mechanisms that function to maintain glomerular filtration despite decreasing renal blood flow. Central in this response is the balance between vasoconstricting angiotensin II and vasodilating renal prostaglandins. Angiotensin II causes vasoconstriction of both the afferent and the efferent glomerular arterioles, but resistance in the efferent arteriole is higher. As a result, glomerular hydrostatic pressure increases, filtration fraction rises, and unfiltrable serum proteins are concentrated. The resulting increase in efferent arteriolar oncotic pressure stimulates water and urea reabsorption from the proximal tubule, thus decreasing the fractional excretion of urea and increasing the BUN:creatinine ratio. Furthermore, angiotensin II acts directly on the proximal tubule to stimulate sodium reabsorption, thus decreasing the fractional excretion of sodium.

The causes of prerenal failure can be classified as shown in Table 13–4. A decrease in cardiac output can be the result of primary cardiac disease or insufficient end-diastolic filling pressures. Volume depletion can occur along obvious routes such as the gastrointestinal or urinary system, via surgical drains, or via more occult mechanisms, including diaphoresis and retroperitoneal hemorrhage. Redistribution of fluid out of the intravascular space with insufficient circulating volume can occur with hypoalbuminemia, vasodilatory shock with capillary leak (sepsis), or intra-abdominal accumulation (peritonitis, ascites, pancreatitis). Crush injury with massive tissue damage can cause sufficient localized edema to result in intravascular depletion. Rarely, overzealous administration of vasodilators decreases effective circulating volume and can mimic endogenous causes of vasodilatory shock.

Intrarenal vasoconstriction can be mediated by several mechanisms, including an imbalance between vasoconstrictive angiotensin II and vasodilating prostaglandins (most often seen when prostaglandin synthetase inhibitors are given to patients with nephrosis, cirrhosis, congestive heart failure, preexisting renal disease, or volume depletion). Renal artery stenosis, preeclampsia, malignant hypertension, scleroderma with severe hypertension and renal failure, and intravenous cyclosporine may be associated with intrarenal vasoconstriction mediated by angiotensin II or endothelin. Finally, obstruction to blood flow to or from the kidney can result from renal artery stenosis or emboli to the renal arteries, related to valvular heart disease or in patients with atrial or ventricular mural thrombi; can occur from valvular heart disease or arrhythmias; or can occur as a complication of percutaneous renal angioplasty. Renal vein thrombosis in adults is most often seen in the context of nephrotic syndrome and is considered to be the result of its associated hypercoagulable state.

Table 13–4. Causes of prerenal renal failure.

Decreased cardiac output
Myocardial infarction
Cardiomyopathy
Pericarditis (constrictive or cardiac tamponade)
Arrhythmias
Valvular dysfunction
Pulmonary embolus
Pulmonary hypertension
Mechanical ventilation (especially with PEEP)
Trauma
Extracellular volume depletion
Dehydration
GI losses (vomiting, NG suction, diarrhea, ostomy output)
Renal losses (diuretics, osmotic diuresis, nonoliguric ATN, adrenal insufficiency)
Peritoneal losses (surgical drains)
Skin losses (burns, diaphoresis)
Hemorrhage (gastrointestinal, intra- and retroperitoneal)
Redistribution of fluid
Hypoalbuminemia (nephrosis, cirrhosis, malnutrition)
Vasodilatory shock (sepsis, hepatic failure)
Peritonitis
Pancreatitis
Crush injury
Ascites
Vasodilators
Primary intrarenal vasoconstriction
NSAID (prostaglandin inhibition)
Hepatorenal syndrome
Preeclampsia
Malignant hypertension
Scleroderma
Cyclosporine
Renovascular obstruction
Renal artery (intravascular stenosis, embolus, laceration, thrombus)
Renal vein (intravascular thrombosis, tumor infiltration, extravascular compression)

Clinical Features

A. Symptoms and Signs

Patients may present with a history of excessive fluid losses from diarrhea, high urine output, or sweating, and this may be compounded by low fluid intake. They may complain of lightheadedness or syncope and may have tachycardia, hypotension, and diaphoresis. Often, postural decrease in blood pressure and increase in heart rate are present in patients with significant volume depletion. Although prerenal azotemia is most commonly associated with volume depletion, patients with congestive heart failure, systemic vasodilation, or hypoalbuminemia may have substantial peripheral edema yet still have insufficient cardiac output or intravascular volume to maintain adequate renal perfusion. Conversely, a severely hypoalbuminemic patient who appears euvolemic is likely to be intravascularly depleted.

Thromboembolic diseases, including renal artery embolization and renal vein thrombosis, decrease renal perfusion but are distinct in their symptomatology and diagnostic workup. Renal artery embolization is most often associated with cardiac valvular disease and can present with nausea, vomiting, flank pain, and hematuria.

Renal vein thrombosis in adults is most often associated with nephrotic syndrome, but it may also result from extrinsic compression by tumor. Acute thrombosis can present with flank pain, hematuria, and increased proteinuria and may be misdiagnosed as a kidney stone. Chronic thrombosis may be asymptomatic except for an ipsilateral varicocele when the thrombosis is in the left renal vein.

B. Laboratory Findings

Considering these confusing clinical presentations, evaluation of serum and urine chemistries is required to confirm the diagnosis. Although both serum creatinine and urea nitrogen increase, low tubular flow results in increased reabsorption of urea. Therefore, the serum BUN:creatinine ratio increases usually to > 20:1, and the FE_{Ur} is less than 35%. Because renal tubular function is normal in early prerenal azotemia, avid sodium reabsorption in the face of volume depletion causes FE_{Na} to be very low, usually less than 1%. Urinary sediment is usually normal except for the finding of a few granular casts; white blood cells and red and white cell casts are absent.

C. Imaging Studies

The diagnosis of thromboembolic disease may be suspected with the demonstration of decreased function on IVP or absent flow on radionuclide scan. The definitive diagnosis and a judgment about the advisability of operation are best arrived at by renal angiography (the presence of collateral circulation suggests a better surgical outcome). Renal venography is the most definitive diagnostic test for renal vein thrombosis but risks dislodging the thrombus, with resulting pulmonary embolization. Digital subtraction renal angiography with evaluation of the venous phase, CT scan, and MRI are safer alternatives.

Treatment

(See also Chapter 2.)

Prerenal azotemia caused by volume depletion should be treated by correction of decreased extracellular fluid volume. Most often, normal saline is given intravenously in an amount sufficient to replete volume, but in some patients blood or colloid solutions are needed. The total volume of replacement should be estimated as in most cases 10–25% of extracellular fluid volume (ie, 2–4 L) but the amount actually given should be carefully titrated by monitoring urine output, blood pressure, and heart rate. Elderly patients and those with heart failure should be given fluid cautiously, usually with central venous pressure or pulmonary artery pressure monitoring. Fluid replacement should also take into account continued losses from the gastrointestinal tract and other sources of fluid loss.

Prerenal azotemia associated with cardiac failure usually responds to standard drugs and procedures for improving cardiac output, including loop diuretics, vasodilators, inotropic agents, and oxygen. Low-dose dopamine (< 5 μg/kg/min) has become a popular means of initiating diuresis in resistant cases and is sometimes remarkably effective. However, its use is still considered controversial and unsupported by large randomized studies. If diuresis is associated with increasing BUN, angiotensin-converting enzyme inhibitors may be beneficial in decreasing renal resistance. When successful, this approach yields an increase in the fractional excretion of urea, which can be followed on a daily basis and used as a guide to further treatment. The management of pericarditis, arrhythmias, pulmonary emboli, and pulmonary hypertension is discussed elsewhere. One should note that positive end-expiratory pressure for treatment of respiratory failure can spuriously elevate pulmonary wedge pressure, thus making it a misleading measure of intravascular volume.

Volume repletion should be tailored to the patient's cardiopulmonary reserve. The hypoalbuminemic states associated with cirrhosis or malnutrition can be corrected with intravenous albumin, but worsening of associated ascites may occur in one-third of patients. In contrast, albumin infusions are futile in patients with ongoing nephrotic syndrome.

Treatment of vasodilatory shock often requires a combination of fluids and vasoconstrictors. Crush injury represents a particular case where intravascular volume depletion combines with the potential nephrotoxicity of myoglobin to yield a toxic acute tubular necrosis. Proper prevention of myoglobin nephrotoxicity can be accomplished with aggressive intravascular volume expansion (see below).

Primary intrarenal vasoconstriction by prostaglandin synthetase inhibitors reverses spontaneously after cessation of these drugs. Prevention of hepatorenal syndrome involves restoration of intravascular volume despite increasing ascites or edema (see below). Preeclamptic renal failure must be treated by delivery or termination of pregnancy. Malignant hypertension and renal crises associated with scleroderma can be successfully treated with ACE inhibitors. Patients with refractory hypertension may require nitroprusside, but prolonged use of this agent in renal failure may predispose to thiocyanate toxicity. Intrarenal vasoconstriction resulting from high doses of intravenous cyclosporine is reversed by decreasing or discontinuing the drug.

Renal artery stenosis can be treated by percutaneous angioplasty or surgery. Massive renal artery embolization resulting from cardiac sources can be managed with anticoagulation and thrombolytic therapy but may require operative management. Renal vein thrombosis is treated with long-term anticoagulation with heparin and warfarin but may respond to either intravenous or intra-arterial thrombolytic therapy.

Corwin HL, Lisbon A: Renal dose dopamine: Long on conjecture, short on fact. (editorial) Crit Care Med 2000;28:1657–8.

Ichai C et al: Comparison of the renal effects of low to high doses of dopamine and dobutamine in critically ill patients. A single-blind randomized study. Crit Care Med 2000;28: 921–8.

Markowitz GS et al: Renal vein thrombosis treated with thrombolytic therapy: case report and brief review, Am J Kidney Dis 1995;25:801–6.

Witz M et al: Renal vein occlusion: a review. J Urol 1996; 155:1173–9.

POSTRENAL RENAL FAILURE

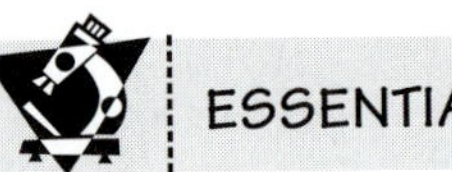

ESSENTIALS OF DIAGNOSIS

- *Dilated renal pelvis on ultrasound.*
- *Enlarged, palpable bladder (if obstruction to bladder outflow).*

General Considerations

Demonstrable changes in renal function occur only if both kidneys are involved or if there is preexisting kidney disease involving the contralateral kidney. It is important to keep in mind that obstruction to urine flow decreases tubular sensitivity to antidiuretic hormone, leading to nephrogenic diabetes insipidus. Thus, the presence of a high urine volume does not rule out the possibility of partial obstruction.

Obstruction to urine flow can occur anywhere along the urinary tract and may be secondary to extrinsic compression or intrinsic blockage (Table 13–5). Causes include tumors, stones, blood clots, and sloughed renal papillae—the result of papillary necrosis, a condition known to occur with analgesic abuse, diabetes, recurrent infections, and sickle cell anemia. Although sloughed renal papillae usually cause unilateral obstruction, blockage of the bladder neck can cause bilateral obstruction and acute-onset oliguria. In men, the most common cause of postrenal renal failure is prostatic hypertrophy.

Clinical Features

A. Symptoms and Signs

Obstruction to urine flow resulting in renal failure may be accompanied by symptoms and signs related to unilateral ureteral obstruction or urethral or bladder obstruction. Occasionally, obstruction is not associated with any symptoms or signs.

Acute ureteral obstruction may be painful, with the patient complaining of severe flank and mid back pain, especially when caused by renal stones or blood clots. Examination may indicate localized tenderness, especially to percussion. Urethral obstruction, especially in prostatic hypertrophy, will cause bladder distention and inability to urinate. Although urine output is very often low or absent, partial obstruction may cause renal failure without oliguria or anuria.

B. Laboratory Findings

Elevated serum creatinine and BUN are indicative of renal insufficiency, and serum electrolytes reflect the severity of renal failure. In patients with renal stones or blood clots, hematuria without red blood cell casts is a prominent feature, but ureteral or urethral obstruction from extrinsic compression such as tumors will not be associated with abnormal urinary sediment.

Table 13–5. Causes of postrenal renal failure.

Ureteral obstruction (bilateral or unilateral single kidney)
- ***Extrinsic***
  - Tumors (endometrial, cervix, lymphoma, metastatic)
  - Retroperitoneal fibrosis or hemorrhage
  - Accidental surgical ligation
- ***Intrinsic***
  - Stones, blood clots, sloughed papillae (papillary necrosis), tumors (transitional cell, etc.)

Bladder or urethral obstruction
- Prostatic hypertrophy or tumor
- Bladder carcinoma
- Uterine prolapse
- Stones, blood clots, sloughed papillae
- Neurogenic bladder (functional or iatrogenic)
- Obstructed Foley catheter

C. Imaging Studies

The existence of postrenal obstruction, regardless of the site or cause, can almost always be determined by renal ultrasound examination. In very rare cases, however, tumor infiltration of the renal parenchyma or perirenal fibrosis may inhibit dilation of the renal pelvis and yield a falsely negative ultrasound examination. Minimal or absent caliceal dilation may also occur during the first few hours after an acute obstruction. Radiologic procedures requiring potentially nephrotoxic radiocontrast agents are most helpful in determining the site and nature of the obstruction. Intravenous pyelography is most often employed in the context of suspected kidney stone, but imaging is poor if serum creatinine levels are elevated. Retrograde pyelography performed through a cystoscope avoids intravenous contrast and offers a direct view of the bladder and the possibility of a corrective urologic procedure. Percutaneous pyelography demonstrates the site of obstruction and offers rapid relief of obstruction if the catheter is left in situ. CT scans and MRI are most helpful for determining the extrinsic or intrinsic nature of the obstruction. Radionuclide scanning can be valuable in cases of suspected obstruction when dilation of the renal pelvis can be identified but the severity of the blockage is in doubt.

Treatment

Acute ureteral obstruction with a kidney stone or sloughed papillae is most often managed with aggressive hydration and control of pain. Treatment of other causes of ureteral obstruction, such as tumors, depends on the location and extent of obstruction and may require surgical relief of the obstruction. Percutaneous nephrostomy is a reasonable alternative for short-term correction of obstruction of the kidney. Bladder obstruction or dysfunction can be treated initially with insertion of a Foley catheter, but in some patients this may be difficult to perform without special urologic instruments. An infected, obstructed kidney is a medical emergency that cannot be adequately managed with antibiotic therapy alone. Rapid relief of obstruction is essential.

Klahr S: Obstructive uropathy. In: *Current Therapy in Nephrology and Hypertension,* 4th ed. Glassock RJ (editor). Mosby Year Book, 1998.

INTRINSIC RENAL FAILURE

Intrinsic renal failure is often a diagnosis of exclusion after prerenal and postrenal causes have been eliminated or treated. Cases of intrinsic acute renal failure can be categorized as follows (Table 13–6): (1) those involving the glomeruli (glomerulonephritis), (2) those involving the interstitium (interstitial nephritis), (3) those leading to microcapillary or glomerular occlusion, (4) acute tubular necrosis, and (5) cortical necrosis.

1. Glomerulonephritis

ESSENTIALS OF DIAGNOSIS

- *Nephritic urine sediment with red cells, white cells, and red cell casts.*
- *Proteinuria (variable, sometimes in nephrotic range: ≥ 3.5 g/d).*
- *Kidney size normal or increased, no evidence of obstruction.*
- *Hypertension (variable).*
- *Evidence for immunologic disease: antinuclear antibodies, antistreptolysin O, cryoglobulins, antineutrophil cytoplasmic antibodies (ANCA), antiglomerular basement membrane (anti-GBM) antibodies, IgA levels, hepatitis B antigen, HIV, decreased C3 and C4.*
- *Renal biopsy to confirm diagnosis.*

Table 13–6. Causes of intrinsic acute renal failure.

Acute glomerulonephritis
Postinfectious: streptococcal, bacteria, hepatitis B, HIV, visceral abscess
Systemic vasculitides: systemic lupus erythematosus, Wegener's granulomatosis, polyarteritis nodosa, Henoch-Schönlein purpura, IgA nephritis, Goodpasture's syndrome
Membranoproliferative glomerulonephritis
Idiopathic
Acute interstitial nephritis
Drugs: penicillins, NSAIDs, ACE inhibitors, allopurinol, cimetidine, H_2 blockers, proton pump inhibitors
Infectious: streptococcal infections, diphtheria, leptospirosis
Metabolic: hyperuricemia, nephrocalcinosis
Poisons: ethylene glycol (calcium oxalate)
Autoimmune disease: systemic lupus erythematosus, cryoglobulinemia
Microcapillary/glomerular occlusion
Thrombotic thrombocytopenic purpura, hemolytic uremic syndrome, disseminated intravascular coagulation, cryoglobulinemia, cholesterol emboli
Acute tubular necrosis
Drugs: aminoglycosides, cisplatin, amphotericin B
Ischemia
Septic shock
Intratubular obstruction: rhabdomyolysis, hemolysis, multiple myeloma, uric acid, calcium oxalate
Poisons: radiopaque contrast media, carbon tetrachloride, ethylene glycol, heavy metals
Cortical necrosis

Key: ACE = angiotensin-converting enzyme; NSAID = nonsteroidal anti-inflammatory drug

General Considerations

Table 13–6 lists several glomerulonephritides that are most commonly associated with acute renal failure. Most—perhaps all—are immunologically mediated as a result of recent or ongoing infections, systemic vasculitis, or idiosyncratic autoimmune reactions. Histologic evaluation is most often positive for immune deposits in varying locations within the glomerular structures. In "pauci-immune" glomerulonephritis, such as is found with Wegener's granulomatosis or polyarteritis, no immune deposits are found but the presence of antineutrophil cytoplasmic antibodies may stimulate leukocytes to release their enzymes, thus mediating an intraglomerular inflammatory reaction.

Clinical Features

A. Symptoms and Signs

Patients with acute glomerulonephritis may present with edema (especially in periorbital distribution), hypertension, fatigue, and possibly pulmonary congestion. They may note smoky, rusty-colored, or grossly bloody urine. These findings are common to glomerulonephritis due to any cause. Other clinical features reflect the underlying disease causing glomerulonephritis. Postinfectious glomerulonephritis presents about 10 days after acute infection, usually a streptococcal pharyngitis or skin infection. Symptoms and signs of systemic vasculitis are highly variable and depend on the distribution of involvement and the size of the vessels involved. They may include arthralgias and arthritis, fever, rash, myalgias and muscle tenderness, hypertension, abdominal pain, nausea, vomiting, diarrhea, headache, and other features that are manifestations of organ system involvement, including the heart, gastrointestinal tract, kidneys, central nervous system, peripheral nerves, lungs, pleura, and pericardium. In some situations, the clinical presentation may strongly suggest a given diagnosis, such as one of the pulmonary-renal syndromes.

B. Laboratory Findings

The most compelling finding suggestive of acute glomerulonephritis is the presence of red cell casts in the urine. These casts are the result of leakage of red cells past damaged glomeruli into the tubular lumen, and they must be carefully distinguished from granular pigmented casts. The absence of red cell casts does not rule out the diagnosis of glomerulonephritis, however, and they are occasionally found in other disorders such as acute interstitial nephritis and cholesterol emboli. Other urinary abnormalities include varying degrees of proteinuria and pyuria in the absence of urinary infection. A history of symptoms suggestive of systemic vasculitis can be confirmed by serologic testing, including antinuclear antibodies, anti-GBM antibodies, IgA levels, antistreptolysin O antibodies, cryoglobulins, antineutrophil cytoplasmic antibodies, antibodies and markers for hepatitis B or human immunodeficiency virus, and decreased levels of the third and fourth components of complement (C3, C4).

Since therapy of glomerulonephritis often entails long-term risk, renal biopsy should usually be performed to confirm the diagnosis.

Treatment

Most cases of acute glomerulonephritis are treated with aggressive immunosuppressive medications, including high-dose corticosteroids and cyclophosphamide. Recent reports suggest that mycophenolate mofetil may be an effective alternative to cyclophosphamide in some cases. Since therapy is likely to be prolonged, with the possibility of substantial morbidity, consultation with a nephrologist is strongly suggested prior to initiation of treatment. On the other hand, poststreptococcal glomerulonephritis is treated with supportive therapy alone, including prevention of fluid overload and control of hypertension.

Glomerulonephritis associated with infective endocarditis responds to appropriate antibiotics. Goodpasture's syndrome and cryoglobulinemia often require plasma exchange.

Chan TM et al: Efficacy of mycophenolate mofetil in patients with diffuse proliferative nephritis. Hong Kong-Guangzhou Nephrology Study Group. N Engl J Med 2000,343:1156–62.

Kaplan AA: Therapeutic plasma exchange for the treatment of rapidly progressive glomerulonephritis. Ther Apher 1997;1:255–9.

Kunis CL et al: Intravenous "pulse" cyclophosphamide therapy of crescentic glomerulitis. Clin Nephrol 1992;37:1–7.

2. Acute Interstitial Nephritis

ESSENTIALS OF DIAGNOSIS

Interstitial nephritis:

- *History of drug sensitivity, infection, or toxin ingestion.*
- *Flank pain (occasionally).*
- *Kidney size normal or increased.*

Allergic interstitial nephritis:

- *Fever, rash, peripheral blood eosinophilia.*
- *Sterile pyuria, hematuria, white cell casts, tubular epithelial cells, eosinophiluria.*
- *Positive renal gallium scan with prolonged renal uptake.*

General Considerations

Several drugs are capable of eliciting an autoimmune attack on the renal interstitium, resulting in allergic interstitial nephritis (Table 13–2). Direct invasion by infection is less common. Acute urate nephropathy results from the intratubular precipitation of uric acid and is most often associated with the chemotherapeutic treatment of large lymphomas or leukemias, with serum levels of uric acid often above 20 mg/dL. The metabolism of ethylene glycol, ingested accidentally or deliberately, results in calcium oxalate deposition within the interstitium and may result in irreversible renal damage. Autoimmune diseases such as systemic lupus erythematosus or cryoglobulinemia may cause a "pure" interstitial nephritis but more often present with concomitant glomerular disease.

Clinical Features

A. Symptoms and Signs

Drug-induced allergic interstitial nephritis is often associated with a history of drug hypersensitivity and classically presents with a triad of fever, rash, and peripheral blood eosinophilia. Unfortunately, the triad is complete in only one-third of cases. The rash is usually symmetric and widespread, appears suddenly, and is usually not pruritic. In the case of NSAID toxicity, nephrotic syndrome with glomerular involvement may be present in addition to evidence of interstitial involvement.

B. Laboratory Findings

Further evidence for interstitial nephritis includes sterile pyuria, white cell casts, and, occasionally, eosinophiluria. Hematuria and varying degrees of proteinuria are usually present as well. Infectious causes of interstitial nephritis can be identified by blood or urine cultures. Acute urate nephropathy should be anticipated whenever aggressive chemotherapy is initiated in a patient with a large lymphoma or acute leukemia. In these patients, serum uric acid is often above 20 mg/dL, and urinalysis reveals flat, rhomboid crystals of uric acid or needle-shaped crystals of sodium urate. Autoimmune diseases are best identified by finding serologic evidence of specific diseases.

C. Imaging Studies

A gallium scan positive for prolonged renal uptake (> 72 hours) supports the diagnosis of allergic interstitial nephritis.

Treatment

Drug-induced acute interstitial nephritis usually reverses spontaneously after cessation of the offending agent, but patients may benefit from a course of corticosteroids if renal failure is severe or prolonged. In anticipation of aggressive chemotherapy for lymphomas or leukemias, the risks of acute urate nephropathy can be greatly reduced by pretreatment with allopurinol and forced alkaline diuresis designed to keep urine pH > 7.0. Alkalinization of the urine can be accomplished by administration of 5% dextrose in water to which approximately 100–150 meq/L of sodium bicarbonate has been added. Acetazolamide may be added to stimulate bicarbonate excretion.

Infectious causes of interstitial nephritis are treated with antibiotics selected for urinary tract bacterial pathogens and adjusted on the basis of urine and blood cultures. Ethylene glycol-induced renal failure may require hemodialysis.

Michel DM, Kelly CJ: Acute interstitial nephritis. J Am Soc Nephrol 1998;9:506–15.

3. Microcapillary & Glomerular Occlusion

ESSENTIALS OF DIAGNOSIS

- *Hematuria.*
- *Proteinuria (variable).*
- *In thrombotic thrombocytopenic purpura-hemolytic uremic syndrome and disseminated intravascular coagulation: thrombocytopenia and microangiopathic hemolytic anemia.*
- *In cryoglobulinemia: cryoglobulin present in serum, purpura (variable), and hypertension (variable).*
- *In cholesterol embolization: hypertension, signs of peripheral vascular occlusive disease (claudication), skin discoloration (livedo reticularis, purple toes), eosinophilia, and a history of recent intra-aortic catheterization.*

General Considerations

These disorders have in common obstruction of the various parts of the renal circulation or glomerular vascular pole. Thrombotic thrombocytopenic purpura (TTP), hemolytic uremic syndrome (HUS), and disseminated intravascular coagulation (DIC) have the potential to deposit thrombi of fibrin and platelets in the glomerular capillary lumen. Cryoglobulins can precipitate in glomerular capillaries but may also cause an immunologically mediated glomerulonephritis. Microscopic cholesterol emboli may occur spontaneously in patients with severe atherosclerotic disease but are most often seen after catheterization of the aorta for diagnostic purposes. Cholesterol emboli are of varying size and may block intrarenal arteries, preglomerular arterioles, or the vascular pole of the glomerulus.

Clinical Features

A. TTP and HUS

Thrombotic thrombocytopenic purpura and hemolytic uremic syndrome can be suspected when severe thrombocytopenia is associated with microangiopathic hemolytic anemia in the presence of normal prothrombin time and partial thromboplastin time. Symptoms include jaundice, renal disease, and varied neurologic manifestations.

B. DIC

Disseminated intravascular coagulation is often associated with sepsis and is diagnosed by a combination of thrombocytopenia, increased fibrin split products, and elevated prothrombin time and partial thromboplastin time. Owing to the ongoing coagulopathy, renal biopsies are only rarely performed in these diseases.

C. Cryoglobulinemia

Cryoglobulinemia is often associated with purpura and hypertension and is confirmed by identification of serum cryoglobulins. It has now been established that many cases of cryoglobulinemia are associated with hepatitis C infection.

D. Cholesterol Embolization

A syndrome of microvascular embolization with livedo reticularis, purple toes, signs of peripheral vascular disease, and occasionally eosinophilia will lead to a suspicion of cholesterol embolization. Renal biopsy, however, is the only confirmatory test.

Treatment

Thrombotic thrombocytopenic purpura requires aggressive plasma exchange with fresh frozen plasma. Hemolytic uremic syndrome may respond to intravenous immune globulin or plasma exchange. Disseminated intravascular coagulation is best treated by management of the inciting cause. Cryoglobulinemia may respond to immunosuppressive therapy or plasma exchange. If there is an associated hepatitis C infection, long-term management may include interferon. Renal failure associated with cholesterol embolization is irreversible. However, on occasion, renal failure from cholesterol emboli may be associated with an element of acute tubular necrosis due to vascular occlusion. In these patients, some improvement may occur. On theoretical grounds, anticoagulation is contraindicated since it may be a precipitating factor.

Bueno D Jr, Sevigny J, Kaplan AA: Extracorporeal treatment of thrombotic microangiopathy: a ten year experience. Ther Apher 1999;3:294–7.

D'Amico G: Renal involvement in hepatitis C infection: Cryoglobulinemic glomerulonephritis. Kidney Int 1998;54:650–71.

Gupta BK et al: Cholesterol crystal embolization-associated renal failure after therapy with recombinant tissue-type plasminogen activator. Am J Kidney Dis 1993;21:659–62.

Kaplan AA: Therapeutic apheresis for renal disorders. Ther Apher 1999;3:25–30.

Rock GA et al: Comparison of plasma exchange with plasma infusion in the treatment of thrombotic thrombocytopenic purpura. N Engl J Med 1991;325:393–7.

Venkatesan J, Henrich WL: Atheroembolic renal disease. In: *Current Therapy in Nephrology and Hypertension,* 4th ed. Glassock RJ (editor). Mosby Year Book, 1998.

4. Acute Tubular Necrosis

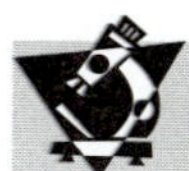

ESSENTIALS OF DIAGNOSIS

- *History of exposure to nephrotoxic drugs or hypotension.*
- *Oliguria in ischemic ATN but absence of oliguria in toxic ATN.*
- *FE_{Na} > 1%.*
- *Urinalysis: tubular epithelial cells, red cells, and "muddy brown" casts.*

General Considerations

The most common form of hospital-acquired intrinsic acute renal failure is referred to as acute tubular necrosis (ATN). This designation is somewhat misleading because in many cases there is more tubular dysfunction than necrosis. In general, the pathogenesis involves direct toxicity to the tubular epithelium, resulting in inability to reabsorb glomerular filtrate properly and massive sodium wasting, intrarenal vasoconstriction, and tubular blockage with necrotic cellular debris and proteinaceous material. The most common causes are ischemia, exogenous toxins including drugs (Table 13–2) and radiocontrast agents, and endogenous toxins such as myoglobin, hemoglobin, light chains of immunoglobulins, or crystals (Table 13–6). Any cause of prerenal azotemia (Table 13–4), if sufficiently severe or prolonged, can cause ischemic tubular damage and lead to this disorder. Furthermore, all conditions of renal hypoperfusion increase the likelihood of toxicity from exogenous or endogenous toxins. In many cases, a combination of noxious stimuli can be identified.

Clinical Features

Ischemic acute tubular necrosis is most often encountered after an identifiable episode of hemodynamic compromise or after prolonged ischemia during aortic surgery. The presentation is that of acute onset of oliguria with an FE_{Na} > 1% and a urine rich with cellular and proteinaceous debris, including red cells, white cells, tubular epithelial cells, and "muddy-brown" casts. In this setting, correction of identifiable prerenal factors and a renal ultrasound examination excluding obstruction are often sufficient to make the diagnosis on clinical grounds, and renal biopsy is usually reserved for patients in whom renal failure is abnormally prolonged (6–8 weeks).

Acute tubular necrosis from toxic causes is often nonoliguric, and the urine sediment may be unremarkable. A history of toxin exposure (aminoglycosides, radiocontrast agents, etc.) and the exclusion of prerenal and postrenal causes are often sufficient for a clinical diagnosis. Urinalysis with dipstick positive for blood in the absence of identifiable red cells is suggestive of rhabdomyolysis or hemolysis.

Treatment

Although several experimental treatments have been designed to enhance recovery (anti-endothelin antibodies, ATP, $MgCl_2$, thyroxine, growth factors, etc.), none are currently applied in clinical practice. Experimentally, infusions of atrial natriuretic peptide have been shown to increase creatinine clearance and decrease the need for dialysis, but currently available treatment strategies are limited to prevention and management. Preventive measures include ensuring adequate hydration when nephrotoxic agents are unavoidable (radiocontrast or necessary nephrotoxic antibiotics) and proper dosing of nephrotoxic drugs with special attention to changing renal function and daily measurements of toxic drug levels. Recent evidence suggests that pretreatment with acetylcysteine or infusions of fenoldopam may help prevent contrast-induced nephropathy.

In the early stages of oliguric acute tubular necrosis, a short course of mannitol or furosemide may decrease the tendency toward tubular obstruction. Mannitol has the theoretical advantage of stimulating an osmotic diuresis originating in the proximal tubule, with the possibility of increasing tubular flow throughout the nephron. Unfortunately, when mannitol is given without resulting diuresis, it may precipitate intravascular volume expansion, which may be poorly tolerated. If diuresis is not established after 24 hours of treatment with furosemide or mannitol, further attempts at diuretic therapy will be futile and potentially harmful.

Mathur VS et al: The effects of fenoldopam, a selective dopamine receptor agonist, on systemic and renal hemodynamics in normotensive subjects. Crit Care Med 1999;27:1832–7.

Star RA: Treatment of acute renal failure. Kidney Int 1998;54:1817–31.

Tepel M et al: Prevention of radiographic-contrast-agent-induced reductions in renal function by acetylcysteine. N Engl J Med 2000;343:180–4.

5. Cortical Necrosis

Cortical necrosis is the result of severe and prolonged renal hypoperfusion and has been most often associated with the hemodynamic catastrophes of pregnancy, including eclampsia, abruptio placentae, and postpartum hemorrhage. The diagnosis is usually suspected when an episode of acute renal failure fails to resolve in 6–8 weeks. Renal biopsy is often required for definitive diagnosis. Renal damage is irreversible.

COMMON SYNDROMES ASSOCIATED WITH ACUTE RENAL FAILURE

1. Pigment Nephropathy: Rhabdomyolysis & Hemolysis

ESSENTIALS OF DIAGNOSIS

- *Urine dipstick positive for heme in the absence of red cells.*
- *In rhabdomyolysis: elevated creatine kinase and aldolase; decreased BUN:creatinine ratio.*
- *In hemolysis: elevated serum free hemoglobin, decreased haptoglobin; elevated LDH.*

General Considerations

Rhabdomyolysis is commonly associated with acute renal failure, especially in the context of traumatic crush injury. Hemolysis is usually more insidious and less likely to cause renal failure except when severe, such as with major transfusion incompatibilities.

In the case of rhabdomyolysis, intravascular volume depletion promotes intratubular precipitation of myoglobin and is probably the most important comorbid factor in the initiation of nephrotoxicity. Hemoglobin-related toxicity seems to be enhanced by the presence of fragmented red cell membranes. Several etiologic factors in the development of rhabdomyolysis and hemolysis are listed in Table 13–7.

Table 13–7. Causes of pigment nephropathy: hemolysis and rhabdomyolysis.

Rhabdomyolysis
- Physical trauma: crush injury, heat stress, electrocution, exercise, hypothermia, malignant hyperthermia, neuroleptic malignant syndrome
- Anoxic injury: arterial occlusion, seizures, tetanus, compartment syndrome
- Metabolic: hypokalemia, hypophosphatemia, diabetic ketoacidosis, myxedemia, carnitine deficiency, hereditary muscle enzyme deficiency
- Infections: influenza-like viral infections, gas gangrene, pyomyositis
- Inflammation: polymyositis, dermatomyositis
- Poisons and toxins: ethanol, amphetamine, cocaine, snake and spider venom.

Hemolysis
- Transfusion reactions
- Drug toxicities: quinine sulfate, hydralazine, etc.
- Poisons and toxins: benzene, aniline, fava beans, snake and spider venom, etc.
- Mechanical trauma: valvular prosthesis, extracorporeal circulation, march hemoglobinuria
- Enzyme deficiencies: glucose-6-phosphate dehydrogenase deficiency
- Osmotic stress: intoxication with hypotonic fluids: drowning, transuretheral prostatectomy, incorrect priming of extracorporeal circulation
- Infections: malaria
- Autoimmune: drugs, systemic lupus erythematosus

Clinical Features

A. Symptoms and Signs

Patients may note dark-colored red or brown urine. Symptoms and signs in rhabdomyolysis may be due to crush injury and other associated trauma and may be focal or diffuse. However, patients with rhabdomyolysis due to inflammatory muscle disorders such as polymyositis may complain of muscle pain, tenderness, and weakness. Patients with hemolysis-induced renal failure will have symptoms related to severe anemia. Other clinical findings are due to renal failure and associated complications.

B. Laboratory Findings

In the absence of detectable red cells in the urine, a urinalysis dipstick positive for heme is virtually diagnostic of hemoglobinuria or myoglobinuria. Similarly, a highly positive heme reaction (3+ or 4+) in the face of minimal hematuria (3–5 red cells/hpf) is equally suspicious. Since myoglobin is sufficiently small to be filtered, patients with myoglobinuria have brown urine, but the serum is clear. In contrast, hemoglobinuria may also produce a dark brown urine, but the spun serum sample is pink, since haptoglobin-bound hemoglobin is a complex which is too large to be filtered. Further confirmation of the diagnosis is seen in serum chemistry values. Rhabdomyolysis is associated with elevated creatine kinase (CK) and other muscle-derived enzymes released into the circulation, including aspartate aminotransferase (AST), lactic dehydrogenase (LDH), and aldolase. Of these, aldolase is specific for muscle damage. Occasionally, creatinine released from damaged muscle leads to an abnormally low BUN:creatinine ratio (< 10:1). Severe hemolysis capable of producing renal failure is usually associated with detectable free hemoglobin levels above 25 mg/dL and a marked decrease in free haptoglobin. As with rhabdomyolysis, elevated LDH and AST may be present; thus, these abnormalities do not permit distinction between the two disorders.

C. Imaging Studies

Imaging studies are not helpful in diagnosis of pigment nephropathy other than in evaluating the extent of injury in patients with traumatic rhabdomyolysis. In patients with serious trauma with renal failure, however, injury to the kidneys, ureters, bladder, or urethra should be considered, and ultrasound, CT, or IVP may be helpful in distinguishing direct injury from rhabdomyolysis.

Treatment

The single most important therapeutic maneuver is to restore circulating volume rapidly and initiate diuresis. If oliguria is present, a single dose of mannitol, 12.5 g intravenously, can be given to promote diuresis. If successful, mannitol can be continued as a 5% infusion. Alternatively, furosemide, 40–200 mg intravenously, can be given and repeated every 6 hours if necessary. Forced diuresis with aggressive hydration should strive for a urine output of at least 100 mL/h and should be maintained until levels of creatine kinase or haptoglobin begin to normalize. Alkalinization of the urine is recommended by some, but there is no definitive evidence that it is necessary.

Rhabdomyolysis is commonly associated with several potentially troublesome electrolyte disorders. Hypocalcemia may be seen early, probably as a consequence of precipitation of calcium salts due to associated hyperphosphatemia. Despite extremely low levels of serum calcium, tetany is uncommon, perhaps due to the associated acidosis. Severe hyperuricemia may also be encountered. Hyperkalemia, sometimes extremely difficult to control, may be encountered with both rhabdomyolysis and hemolysis.

Better OS, Stein JH: Early management of shock and prophylaxis of acute renal failure in traumatic rhabdomyolysis. N Engl J Med 1990;322:825–9.

Knochel JP: Rhabdomyolysis and acute renal failure. In: *Current Therapy in Nephrology and Hypertension,* 4th ed. Glassock RJ (editor). Mosby Year Book, 1998.

2. Pulmonary Renal Syndromes

Any type of acute renal failure can present with fluid overload and pulmonary edema, but there are several conditions in which simultaneous involvement of both lung and kidneys is a common presentation or an intrinsic part of the basic pathogenesis (Table 13–8). Of these, two are of particular importance since their rapid identification and subsequent treatment can be lifesaving: Goodpasture's syndrome and paraquat intoxication.

Goodpasture's Syndrome

Goodpasture's syndrome is an autoimmune disease characterized by the formation of anti-glomerular basement membrane antibodies that attack both the pulmonary capillary and the glomerulus. The classic clinical presentation is that of a young male smoker with signs of acute glomerulonephritis (hematuria, proteinuria, red cell casts) and hemoptysis associated with bilateral pulmonary infiltrates. Iron deficiency anemia is also a frequent finding.

The diagnosis of Goodpasture's syndrome can be made by detecting serum levels of anti-GBM antibodies or by linear immunofluorescence of the glomerular basement membrane on renal biopsy. Unfortunately, availability of these confirmatory tests may be delayed, and rapid initiation of treatment often depends on a high de-

Table 13–8. Pulmonary renal syndromes causing acute renal failure.

Disease	Renal Involvement
Goodpasture's syndrome	RPGN
Wegener's granulomatosis	RPGN
Systemic lupus erythematosus	RPGN
Churg-Strauss syndrome	RPGN
Sarcoidosis	Interstitial nephritis
Scleroderma	Hypertensive renal crisis
Pulmonary embolism	Prerenal azotemia
Pneumonia	Prerenal azotemia
Poisons (paraquat)	Actue tubular necrosis
Congestive heart failure	Prerenal azotemia
Adult respiratory distress syndrome	Acute tubular necrosis, prerenal azotemia

Key: RPGN = rapidly progressive glomerulonephritis; ATN = acute tubular necrosis

gree of suspicion. Early initiation of treatment is essential, since therapeutic success in reversing renal failure is rare if the therapy is started after the onset of oliguria. Aside from smoking, genetic predisposition and hydrocarbon exposure have been identified as associated risk factors.

Both life-threatening hemoptysis and rapidly progressive renal failure can be successfully treated with a combination of corticosteroids, cyclophosphamide, and 2 weeks of daily plasma exchange.

Paraquat Poisoning

Paraquat is a herbicide used in concentrated solutions. Ingestion is highly corrosive for the oral and esophageal mucosa, and net absorption results in pulmonary edema and anuria. Effective treatment involves gastric lavage and aggressive use of charcoal adsorbents. Charcoal hemoperfusion and continuous hemofiltration may also be successful.

Hoffman GS et al: Wegener's granulomatosis: An analysis of 158 patients. Ann Intern Med 1992;116:488–98.

Weber MF et al: Antineutrophil-cytoplasmic antibodies and antiglomerular basement membrane antibodies in Goodpasture's syndrome and Wegener's granulomatosis. J Am Soc Nephrol 1992;2:1227–34.

Winchester JF: Paraquat and the bipyridyl herbicides. In: *Clinical Management of Poisoning and Drug Overdose.* Haddad LM, Winchester JF (editors). Saunders, 1990.

3. Hepatorenal Syndrome

Conditions associated with combined hepatic and renal failure include infections (sepsis, hepatitis, leptospirosis), drug toxicity (acetaminophen, allopurinol, rifampin, methoxyflurane), poisons (rodenticide, carbon tetrachloride), and autoimmune disorders (systemic lupus erythematosus, vasculitis, cryoglobulinemia). More common, however, is prerenal azotemia associated with cirrhosis. Patients presenting with this combination often have signs of advanced liver disease, hypoalbuminemia, and ascites. Under these conditions, if prerenal azotemia becomes unresponsive to intravascular volume replacement, a diagnosis of "hepatorenal syndrome" becomes appropriate. This syndrome is a condition of severe renal vasoconstriction presenting with extremely low urinary sodium (< 10 meq/L), decreased FE_{Ur} (< 20%), an extremely high urine:plasma creatinine ratio, and a relatively unimpressive urine sediment showing bile-pigmented casts.

Since hepatorenal syndrome is considered to be almost universally fatal, prevention is the only feasible management option. Most patients with hepatorenal syndrome develop the problem during hospitalization. Gastrointestinal hemorrhage, bacterial peritonitis, and the overzealous use of diuretics to control ascites have all been shown to precipitate hepatorenal syndrome. Thus, it is crucial that all patients presenting with liver disease and prerenal azotemia receive aggressive volume repletion. In many cases, pulmonary edema and ascites may be limiting factors in repletion; central venous pressure or pulmonary artery catheterization may be required to judge adequately how much fluid can be safely administered. With increasing central venous pressure, there will also be the increased risk of variceal hemorrhage. In patients with peripheral edema associated with hypoalbuminemia, albumin infusions can successfully mobilize fluid into the intravascular space, but ascites formation increases in approximately one-third of patients. In the same vein, high-volume paracentesis should be performed in conjunction with intravenous albumin infusions in order to minimize the tendency for intravascular volume depletion.

Although hepatorenal syndrome is considered to be almost universally fatal, liver transplantation has been associated with return of renal function. Most recently, there have been reports in Europe of successful treatment of hepatorenal syndrome with albumin-based dialysis (MARS: molecular adsorbent recycling system).

Epstein M: Hepatorenal syndrome: emerging perspectives. Semin Nephrol 1997;17:563–75.

Kaplan AA, Epstein M: Extracorporeal blood purification in the management of hepatic failure. Semin Nephrol 1997; 17:576–82.

Gines A et al: Randomized trial comparing albumin, dextran 70, and polygeline in cirrhotic patients with ascites treated by paracentesis. Gastroenterology 1996;111:1002–10.

Mitzner SR et al: Improvement of hepatorenal syndrome with extracorporeal albumin dialysis MARS: results of a prospective, randomized, controlled clinical trial. Liver Transpl 2000;6: 277–86.

4. Renal Failure in AIDS

Acute renal failure occurs in more than 50% of hospitalized patients with AIDS. The combination of volume depletion, nephrotoxic medications, and sepsis accounts for most cases (Table 13–9), but most AIDS patients presenting with acute renal failure can recover renal function and be discharged from the hospital.

Intravascular volume depletion can result from poor fluid intake, fever, and gastrointestinal disturbances or may be secondary to hypoalbuminemia due to nephrotic syndrome or malnutrition. Enlarged periaortic lymph nodes can obstruct lower extremity venous return, resulting in severe leg edema but insufficient central venous pressure. Careful attention to restoring intravascular volume not only reverses prerenal azotemia but will serve to reduce substantially the risk of nephrotoxicity associated with medications and radiocontrast agents. In many cases of drug-induced renal failure, renal function may return rapidly after termination of exposure to the drug, such as can be seen with nonsteroidal anti-inflammatory drugs and the crystalluria associated with indinavir and acyclovir. In other cases, a full-blown syndrome of acute tubular necrosis may develop; this disorder may require dialytic therapy before recovery.

A renal syndrome that seems to be unique to patients with AIDS is rapidly progressive focal segmental glomerulosclerosis. This syndrome is most common in blacks and is associated with nephrotic-range proteinuria (> 3 g/d), enlarged, hyperechogenic kidneys on renal ultrasound, and—in contrast to focal segmental glomerulosclerosis in the non-AIDS population—normotension. Progression of this type of renal disease can be explosive, reaching a stage of irreversible renal failure in weeks or months. Recent experience, however, suggests that the new highly active antiretroviral therapeutic (HAART) regimens can slow the progression of this type of AIDS nephropathy.

Standard precautions during hemodialysis are employed to limit transmission of HIV and hepatitis B. In addition, HIV has been identified in peritoneal dialysate from patients with AIDS, and this effluent should be handled with appropriate precautions.

Krishnan M et al: Acute renal failure in an HIV-positive 50 year old man. Am J Kidney Dis 2000;36:1075–8.

Rao TK: Acute renal failure syndromes in human immunodeficiency virus infection. Semin Nephrol 1998;18:378–95.

Winston JA, Burns GC, Klotman PE: Treatment of HIV-associated nephropathy. Semin Nephrol 2000;20:293–8.

Table 13–9. Causes of acute renal failure associated with AIDS.

Prerenal azotemia
Volume depletion, hypoalbuminemia, nonsteroidal anti-inflammatory drugs

Acute tubular necrosis
Pentamidine, amphotericin B, aminoglycosides, foscarnet, acyclovir, radiocontrast agents, sepsis, shock

Allergic interstitial nephritis
Trimethoprim-sulfamethoxazole, phenytoin

Rapidly progressive focal segmental glomerulosclerosis

Obstructive uropathy
Sulfadiazine-related crystalluria, lymphoma, retroperitoneal fibrosis

Nephrolithiasis
Indinavir-induced crystalluria

Thrombotic thrombocytopenic purpura/hemolytic uremic syndrome

Renal edema
Hypoalbuminemia with massive proteinuria

Multiple myeloma

Acute glomerulonephritis

5. Renal Failure in the Renal Transplant Recipient

Acute renal failure in the transplant recipient can be arbitrarily defined as being early (less than 10 days after transplantation) or late (more than 10 days). In the early period, acute renal failure may be due to ischemic acute tubular necrosis of the transplanted graft, acute or hyperacute immunologic rejection, or technical problems related to the surgery (obstruction, leak, or infection of the renal artery or vein or of the ureter). Acute drug toxicity from cyclosporine can present as prerenal azotemia associated with hypertension and is most often encountered with relatively elevated intravenous dosing.

Acute renal failure in the late period may be the result of acute rejection, cyclosporine toxicity, ureteral obstruction, renal artery stenosis, or recurrence of the original renal disease. Acute rejection may present with fever, graft tenderness, and swelling where the kidney is implanted into the iliac fossa, but concurrent immunosuppressive therapy with steroids or cyclosporine may mask these signs. If the history, physical examination, and imaging studies (ultrasound, nuclear flow scans) cannot distinguish the cause of renal failure, renal biopsy may be required. In any event, prompt and continued consultations with the patient's transplant surgeon and nephrologist are essential to proper management.

The intensivist is often in a position to identify potential organ donors. Acceptable donors for renal transplantation are aged 6 months to 60 years with no identifiable renal disease, no active infection, and no malignancy (except brain tumors). Physicians working in the intensive care unit should familiarize themselves with local laws and policies regarding the procurement of organs and the criteria for brain death.

Kasiske BL et al: Recommendations for the outpatient surveillance of renal transplant recipients. American Society of Transplantation. J Am Soc Nephrol 2000;11(Suppl 15):S1–86.

Silkensen JR. Long-term complications in renal transplantation. J Am Soc Nephrol 2000;11:582–8.

NONDIALYTIC THERAPY FOR ACUTE RENAL FAILURE

FLUID BALANCE

Achieving the appropriate fluid balance in the setting of an intensive care unit involves two potentially conflicting goals: providing sufficient volume to ensure adequate renal perfusion and avoiding volume overload with resulting pulmonary congestion. In some patients, when decreased renal perfusion is suspected in the context of pulmonary compromise, only a pulmonary artery catheter will yield sufficient information to guide appropriate therapy. Optimum fluid management for acute renal failure can be arbitrarily divided into three periods: (1) the prevention phase, during the initial onset of oliguria; (2) the oliguric phase, once renal failure is well established; and (3) the recuperative phase, often heralded by relative polyuria. Not all episodes of acute renal failure pass through each of these phases, but a discussion of their management is a useful guide to overall treatment goals.

Prevention Phase

On initial presentation, the onset of oliguria should call for prompt evaluation of the type of renal dysfunction. If volume depletion is suspected, rapid restoration of circulating volume may prevent ischemic damage. Restoration of adequate circulating volume can be achieved by administration of crystalloid or colloid. If simple fluid repletion is required, normal saline usually suffices. In the context of hypoalbuminemia and edema, intravenous albumin can serve to draw excess extravascular fluid into the circulation.

If oliguria persists despite adequate fluid replacement and acute tubular necrosis is suspected, a short trial of diuretic therapy may offer some benefit in limiting renal damage. A single intravenous 12.5-g dose of mannitol may initiate diuresis and has the theoretical advantage of limiting epithelial cell swelling and intratubular precipitation of cellular debris. If initially unsuccessful, further mannitol administration is potentially harmful in that it may lead to poorly tolerated intravascular expansion. Alternatively, furosemide may be given intravenously at a dose of 200 mg (1-hour infusions are preferable to more rapid injection) and may be safely repeated within 6 hours. Dosages above 1 g/d have been associated with ototoxicity. If, despite the above maneuvers, oliguria persists more than 24 hours, diuretics should be discontinued, and the physician should be prepared to manage a potentially prolonged period of oliguria.

Oliguric Phase

The oliguric phase of acute renal failure may persist for several weeks. During this period, especially in the critical care setting, the patient may require enormous amounts of intravenous fluids, including hyperalimentation, vasopressors, and antibiotics. Every effort should be made to minimize the volume of these infusions. Continuous infusions of vasopressors should be maximally concentrated, and antibiotics should be given in minimum volumes of fluid. When given in adequate amounts, parenteral hyperalimentation always requires 1–2 L/d. Thus, enteral alimentation is always preferred when possible.

Proper maintenance of fluid balance requires careful attention to all avenues of fluid intake and output, including surgical drains, nasogastric suction, and diarrhea. Normal insensible losses can equal 1000 mL/d but can increase substantially in the presence of fever, burns, or exfoliative dermatitis. Increased minute ventilation enhances water loss from the lungs even if the inspired gas is humidified. On the other hand, metabolism of carbohydrate and fat yields approximately 500 mL/d of metabolically produced water. Thus, unless insensible losses are increased, an anuric patient requires only 500 mL/d of water.

Finally, despite meticulous monitoring of fluid input and output, there can be no substitute for daily weight measurements.

Recuperative Phase

In many patients with acute renal failure, the oliguric phase is followed by a period of relative polyuria, heralding the beginning of tubular recuperation. During this period, serum urea nitrogen and creatinine may remain elevated, and renal dysfunction persists. One must bear in mind that the urine produced is not appropriately concentrated and that reabsorption of sodium and other ions is inadequate. During this phase, it is the goal of management to replace lost volume and electrolytes. Urinary sodium and potassium should be measured and replaced in appropriate amounts. Abnormalities of magnesium, calcium, and phosphate should also be anticipated.

Monitoring Fluid Balance

In the presence of active pulmonary disease such as pneumonia, acute respiratory distress syndrome (ARDS), or pulmonary edema and suspected prerenal azotemia, aggressive fluid replacement may worsen pulmonary gas exchange. Furthermore, in patients with vasodilatory shock or hypoalbuminemia, substantial edema may be present and still the patient has insufficient circulating volume. In these settings, intravascular pressure monitoring becomes invaluable. Although central venous pressure can be easily monitored via subclavian, internal jugular, or femoral vein catheterization, a more definitive assessment of optimum cardiac filling pressures can be obtained with pulmonary artery catheterization. This is because central venous pressure can be increased by pulmonary hypertension or central venous thrombosis or occlusion even in a volume-depleted patient. Similarly, positive-pressure ventilation and, especially, positive end-expiratory pressure may spuriously elevate pulmonary capillary wedge pressure.

ACID-BASE BALANCE

Uremic acidosis occurs as a result of the slow accumulation of phosphates and sulfates and is related to protein catabolism. Approximately 1 meq of acid is retained for every gram of protein catabolism. Thus, a 70-g protein diet yields approximately 70 meq of acid, which, when distributed into the total body water compartment, consumes approximately 2 meq of bicarbonate per liter per day. Replacement of this amount of bicarbonate is relatively easy and can be in the form of intravenous sodium bicarbonate, orally administered sodium or potassium citrate, or as acetate in hyperalimentation solution (1 meq of acetate converts to 1 meq of bicarbonate, plus some energy). The patient's tolerance for the associated sodium and potassium load should be considered.

Patients with prolonged uremia may present with a substantial buffer deficit (serum bicarbonate < 15 meq/L), Kussmaul respirations, and associated hypocalcemia. In this situation, bicarbonate replacement relieves the dyspnea by correction of acidosis, but the rapid increase in serum pH may precipitate tetany. Under these conditions, after determination of serum calcium and phosphate, it may be prudent to administer one ampule of calcium gluconate after the first 50–100 meq of bicarbonate. However, if phosphate levels are particularly elevated, there is a theoretical risk of metastatic calcifications with calcium administration.

Lactic acidosis is potentially a more difficult problem. In the presence of insufficient tissue oxygenation, lactic acid production can exceed 50 meq/h. This amount of acid lowers serum bicarbonate at a rate of 1–2 meq/L/h. In the face of oliguria, replacement of this amount of bicarbonate would risk intravascular fluid overload and hypernatremia and may require dialytic therapy. Therefore, in lactic acidosis, an aggressive effort to restore adequate tissue perfusion is the mainstay of treatment.

Metabolic alkalosis is an uncommon complication of acute renal failure, but it may occur as a result of massive losses from gastric suctioning. Decreasing net acid loss can be achieved by raising gastric pH with H_2 blockers such as cimetidine or ranitidine or with proton pump inhibitors such as omeprazole or lansoprazole. If these efforts fail, acid can be given carefully as arginine hydrochloride or dilute hydrochloric acid. These treatments can produce severe life-threatening hyperkalemia and must be given with vigilant monitoring of potassium levels.

ELECTROLYTES

Sodium

Sodium balance in acute renal failure is maintained by evaluation and matching of sodium losses. Urinary losses are best measured with 24-hour collections but can be reasonably assessed by random sampling and multiplication of sodium concentration by the day's total urine volume. After diuretic administration, urinary sodium will be increased for several hours and may not reflect a constant excretion rate. Gastrointestinal losses must be either measured (nasogastric suction) or estimated (diarrhea) (Table 13–10).

Table 13–10. Sodium content: intake and output.

Sodium Content of Intravenous Infusion Fluids	Sodium Content of Body Fluids
1 g Na^+ = 43 meq Na^+	Gastric fluid = 30–90 meq Na^+ per liter
1 g NaCl = 17 meq Na^+	Diarrhea = 50–110 meq Na^+ per liter
1 L of 0.9% NaCl = 154 meq Na^+	Small bowel ostomy = 70–150 meq Na^+ per liter
1 L of 0.45% NaCl = 77 meq Na^+	Biliary drainage = 120–170 meq Na^+ per liter
1 L of Ringer's lactate = 130 meq Na^+	Sweat = 20–100 meq Na^+ per liter
50 mL of 7.5% $NaHCO_3$ = 44 meq Na^+	

In oliguric renal failure, hyponatremia is the most common electrolyte abnormality and is almost always the result of excessive free water administration. Since most fluid losses are lower in sodium when compared with serum (Table 13–10), a reasonable initial approach is to add 50 meq of sodium to each liter of infused fluid, most notably the hyperalimentation fluid. Daily monitoring of serum sodium allows for readjustment of water and sodium administered as necessary.

Potassium

Hyperkalemia is the most serious electrolyte abnormality associated with acute renal failure. Cardiotoxicity, however, does not correlate strictly with the measured serum potassium, and may be encouraged by acidosis, serum calcium concentration, and medications. The most rapid and reliable means for assessing cardiotoxicity is to obtain an ECG, which may show hyperkalemia in the form of peaked T waves, a prolonged PR interval, diminished to absent P waves, widening of the QRS complex, prolongation of the QT interval, and ultimately a sine wave pattern. Immediate management requires medications designed to stabilize the myocardial membrane and promote intracellular movement of potassium. Infusion of calcium, bicarbonate, and insulin with glucose temporarily improves the electrocardiographic abnormalities. Definitive procedures for removing potassium should be initiated as soon as possible.

In oliguric patients unresponsive to diuretic therapy, exchange resins of sodium polystyrene sulfonate are the most efficient means of extracorporeal potassium removal. Administration can be either orally or by retention enema for at least 30 minutes (orally: 50 g of resin in 150 mL of 20% sorbitol; by enema: 50 g of resin in 200 mL of tap water to avoid sorbitol-induced colonic irritation). These doses can be repeated every hour as necessary. Each potassium ion removed will be exchanged for a sodium ion—a situation that may be poorly tolerated in the hypernatremic or fluid-overloaded patient. In addition, to avoid the possibility of forming intraluminal concretions, sodium polystyrene sulfonate should never be given concurrently with aluminum hydroxide (used as a phosphate binder or antacid). When these measures are poorly tolerated because of fluid overload or hypernatremia—or when the gastrointestinal tract is not available for use—dialytic therapy should be considered.

Maintaining potassium balance requires evaluation of renal and extrarenal losses (Table 13–11). A normal diet contains approximately 70–100 meq of potassium per day, and dietary potassium restriction to 2 g (50 meq) per day is reasonable for patients with oliguric renal failure.

Table 13–11. Potassium content: intake and output.

2 g K^+ in diet = 50 meq
Gastric fluid = 4–12 meq K^+/L
Diarrhea = 10–30 meq K^+/L
Abdominal drainage = approximately the serum level
Urine = 5–150 meq K^+/L
Sodium polystyrene sulfonate (Kayexalate) = 1 meq K^+/g of retained absorbent per hour
Sorbitol-induced diarrhea = 30–40 meq K^+/L
Peritoneal dialysis (2 L/h), CAVH (1 L/h) = 5–10 meq K^+/h[1]
Hemodialysis = 40–60 meq K^+/h[1]

[1]Assuming serum [K^+] = 5 meq/L

Key: CAVH = continuous arteriovenous hemofiltration

Calcium

Hypocalcemia often accompanies chronic renal failure and is the result of hyperphosphatemia and altered vitamin D metabolism. In acute renal failure, hypocalcemia may be associated with the hyperphosphatemic phase of rhabdomyolysis or may occur during administration of the antiviral agent foscarnet. Hypercalcemia is seen in multiple myeloma or hyperparathyroidism. Urinary calcium losses are minimal during acute renal failure. Frank tetany is rare and is usually the result of overly aggressive correction of acidosis. Since hypoalbuminemia and acid-base disturbances are common in the critically ill patient, ionized calcium levels, when available, are preferred to total serum calcium.

Magnesium

Magnesium excretion is limited during renal failure, and magnesium-containing antacids such as Maalox and Mylanta should be avoided. Magnesium wasting may occur with amphotericin-induced renal failure or during the polyuric recuperative phase of acute tubular necrosis.

Phosphate

Hyperphosphatemia results from insufficient renal excretion and secondary hyperparathyroidism. Avoiding hyperphosphatemia limits the risk of metastatic calcifications and helps maintain normal levels of ionized calcium. Diets should be limited to 800 mg/d of phosphorus, but even at this level oral phosphate binders are required to limit gastrointestinal absorption. When serum phosphorus exceeds 6 mg/dL, aluminum hydroxide antacid is given at a dosage of 30 mL with each meal and at night. Sevelamer at a dose of 806–1612 mg with each meal can also be used as an effective phosphate binder and has the advantage of not having the potential for aluminum toxicity or the constipation associated with aluminum hydroxide.

When levels are controlled below 6 mg/dL, calcium carbonate can be used at an initial dose of 500 mg with each meal and at night. Intravenous hyperalimentation should be prepared without phosphate until levels are normalized. However, once normal phosphorus levels are reached, intravenous hyperalimentation solutions should contain approximately 100–250 mg of phosphorus per day (5–10 meq of sodium or potassium phosphate). In the presence of renal failure, hypophosphatemia is almost always the result of prolonged parenteral nutrition devoid of phosphate.

NUTRITION

Nitrogen Balance

Several studies have suggested that appropriate nutritional support can promote renal recovery and improve overall survival in patients with acute renal failure. Unfortunately, there is often conflict between giving adequate protein replacement while at the same time limiting the production of nitrogenous wastes. Under ideal conditions, an adequate diet should include 1 g/kg/d of protein and 35–40 kcal/kg/d as carbohydrates and fats. There is no definitive evidence that diets with substantially more than 1.2 g/kg/d of protein enhance survival rates or reduce morbidity, with the possible exception of the patient with extensive burns. Overly aggressive protein feeding (> 2 g/kg/d) is unwarranted and can lead to abnormally high amino acid levels and an unnecessary increase in retained nitrogen wastes. In the very stable patient with minimal net negative nitrogen balance (< 5 g/d), protein intake can be limited to 0.6 g/kg/d. In the nonoliguric patient, this may reduce the need for dialysis, but careful attention to nitrogen balance is required.

Nitrogen balance can be easily evaluated by measuring the rate of urea production, commonly referred to as the urea nitrogen appearance (UNA). The daily UNA can be measured by obtaining a 24-hour urine for urea nitrogen measurement and evaluating the change in blood urea nitrogen occurring at the beginning and end of the 24-hour collection. The UNA can then be calculated using the following formula:

$$\text{UNA (g/d)} = \frac{\text{BUN}_2 - \text{BUN}_1}{100} \times \text{Total body water} + \text{UUN}$$

where UNA equals the daily urea nitrogen appearance in grams per day; BUN_1 and BUN_2 are the levels of blood urea nitrogen in mg/dL at the beginning and end of the 24-hour urine collection; total body water in liters is estimated as 60% of lean body mass plus the amount of any extra edema fluid; and UUN is the urine urea nitrogen expressed as grams per day.

Under conditions of nitrogen balance, UNA is dependent on protein ingestion and can be calculated as follows:

$$\text{UNA (g/d)} = \frac{\text{Protein intake (g/d)}}{6.25} - \text{Nonurea nitrogen (g/d)}$$

It is assumed that every 6.25 g of protein contains 1 g of nitrogen and that the production of nonurea nitrogen is 30 mg/kg/d of lean body mass. The minimum amount of urea clearance required to remove a given amount of UNA can be calculated using the following formula:

$$\frac{\text{Urea clearance}}{\text{(L/d)}} = \frac{\text{UNA (g/d)}}{\text{BUN (mg/dL)}} \times 100$$

When the above formulas are used, a 70-kg patient receiving 1 g/kg/d of protein will receive 11 g of nitrogen (70 g ÷ 6.25). On balance, approximately 2 g of nitrogen will become nitrogenous wastes other than urea; the remaining 9 g will form urea.

On the other hand, many patients with acute renal failure present with a degree of hypercatabolism. Under these conditions, urea production is greatly enhanced owing to the catabolism of endogenous proteins, and UNA can greatly exceed that predicted from exogenous protein administration alone. For example, under conditions of severe stress, endogenous protein breakdown can generate 30 g or more of urea nitrogen per day, representing the catabolism of approximately 200 g of protein. In addition to enhanced proteolysis accompanying hypercatabolism, increased urea production is often the result of gastrointestinal bleeding, with the ultimate breakdown and absorption of the blood and its proteins. There are approximately 200 g of protein per liter of whole blood.

Treatment of endogenous hypercatabolism and the negative nitrogen balance that results is controversial. Although adequate nutrition is essential, it is often not sufficient to match the ongoing catabolism. Several studies have demonstrated that increased protein catabolism associated with stress is mediated by hormones (glucagon, catecholamines, and cortisol) and cytokines (interleukins, tumor necrosis factor, etc). For this reason, overly aggressive protein administration is not only futile but yields unnecessary amounts of nitrogenous waste, thereby increasing the need for dialysis therapy. Until specific therapy for cytokine neutralization is available, the most successful strategy will be to administer the majority of needed calories in the form of carbohydrates, thus allowing for the maximum administration of "anticatabolic" insulin.

Calories

Adequate caloric intake is essential to minimize negative nitrogen balance and to improve overall survival. In the critically ill patient with acute renal failure, approximately 35 kcal/kg/d is a reasonable goal. Hyperglycemia resulting from administration of large amounts of carbohydrate can be managed with insulin.

Vitamins & Trace Elements

There is no evidence that patients with acute renal failure have unique requirements for either vitamins or trace elements. Thus, daily minimum requirements should be adequate. Once dialysis is initiated, replacement of water-soluble vitamins should be assured. In most situations, a standard multivitamin preparation suffices with the possible exception of folic acid, which should be replaced at a dosage of at least 1 mg/d.

Fournier A et al: The crossover comparative trial of calcium acetate versus sevelamer hydrochloride (Renagel) as phosphate binders in dialysis patients. Am J Kidney Dis 2000;35:1248–50.

Feinstein EI et al: Total parenteral nutrition with high or low nitrogen intakes in patients with acute renal failure. Kidney Int 1983;26(Suppl 16):S319–23.

Woolfson AM, Heatley RV, Allison SP: Insulin to inhibit protein catabolism after injury. N Engl J Med 1979;300:14–7.

DIALYTIC THERAPY FOR THE CRITICALLY ILL PATIENT

Renal replacement therapy can provide homeostasis of fluid, electrolyte, acid-base, and nitrogen balance. Consequently, the initiation of renal replacement therapy should be considered whenever any of these factors cannot be controlled with other therapy. At present, three types of renal replacement treatment are available for the patient with acute renal failure: intermittent hemodialysis, peritoneal dialysis, and continuous renal replacement therapy (CRRT) (Table 13–12). The particular therapy chosen is often dictated by the patient's condition (massive fluid overload, hypercatabolism, vascular instability) and associated morbid states (respiratory compromise, hemorrhagic risks, abdominal surgery). Aside from these needs, the patient's baseline

Table 13–12. Renal replacement therapies: Urea clearance and protein losses.[1]

		Time-Averaged			
		Urea Clearance			Protein Loss
Treatment	Prescription	mL/min	L/d	L/wk	g/d[2]
Hemodialysis[3]	3 × 4 h/wk 7 × 4 h/wk	14.3 33.3	21 48	144 336	6 15
Peritoneal dialysis	2 L/h	26.7	24	168	30
CAPD	2 L/6 h[4]	6.9	10	70	10
CAVH	14 L/d	9.7	14	98	15
CAVHD	1–2 L/h	19–35	29–51	189–357	11
CVVH	1–3 L/h	17–50	24–72	168–504	18–36
CVVHD	1–3 L/h	19–52	27–75	189–525	18–36

[1]Modified from Kaplan AA: Dialysis and other extracorporeal therapy for acute renal failure. In: *Current Therapy in Nephrology and Hypertension*, 4th ed. Glassock RJ (editor). Mosby, 1998.
[2]Includes amino acids and peptides. Published data have been adjusted to account for increased porosity of currently available dialyzers.
[3]Assumes average urea clearance of 200 mL/min.
[4]Assumes 3 L/d net filtrate.

Key: CAPD = chronic ambulatory peritoneal dialysis
CAVH = continuous arteriorvenous hemofiltration
CAVHD = continuous arteriorvenous hemodialysis
CVVH = continuous venovenous hemofiltration
CVVHD = continuous venovenous hemodialysis/hemodiafiltration

requirements for fluid and solute removal depends on nutritional intake and residual renal function.

Using conventional techniques, machine-driven hemodialysis is best suited for the hemodynamically stable patient in whom solute balance is the major concern and rapid fluid removal is well tolerated. Peritoneal dialysis is preferred in the patient with significant hemorrhagic risk and in whom vascular access is difficult to obtain. Continuous hemofiltration and its related techniques are best for providing fluid removal in the patient with vascular instability or massive fluid overload. Despite these generalizations, with appropriate technical modifications, adequate renal replacement therapy can be provided by any of these methods.

INDICATIONS FOR DIALYTIC THERAPY

Fluid Overload

Poorly tolerated volume overload is the most evident indication for initiating renal replacement therapy. In general, the need to relieve pulmonary vascular congestion is the most pressing issue. It should be noted that even massive amounts of peripheral edema may be appropriate for the patient's condition (hypoalbuminemia, vasodilatory shock), and fluid removal may cause intravascular volume depletion, hampering the return of endogenous renal function. When hypotension is associated with edema and apparent pulmonary congestion, pulmonary artery catheter monitoring can be invaluable in determining the amount of fluid that can be safely removed.

In the hemodynamically stable patient, intermittent hemodialysis can provide the most rapid removal of fluid by easily removing 1–2 L of fluid per hour by ultrafiltration. In patients with vascular instability, one of the continuous therapies is more appropriate, since modest rates of fluid removal can proceed steadily throughout the day. For example, peritoneal dialysis can provide for the gentle removal of the 2–3 L/d necessitated by intravenous medications and hyperalimentation. Excessive net fluid removal (> 5–10 L/d), however, may lead to hypernatremia, since fluid removed by peritoneal dialysis is hyponatric when compared with plasma. In patients presenting with massive fluid overload, continuous hemofiltration offers the best-tolerated treatment, since the ultrafiltrate is isosmotic. A reasonable combination of treatments would employ several days of continuous hemofiltration to achieve normovolemia followed by intermittent hemodialysis to provide maintenance therapy.

Electrolyte Abnormalities

Electrocardiographic changes caused by hyperkalemia should be initially treated with nondialytic therapy (calcium, glucose, and insulin). The only renal replacement therapy capable of rapid potassium removal is machine-driven hemodialysis, providing clearance rates of 150–250 mL/min or more (Table 13–11). Neither continuous hemofiltration nor peritoneal dialysis can achieve potassium clearance rates much above 20–40 mL/min, and both of these continuous therapies are best reserved for normalization of modest levels of hyperkalemia or for maintaining potassium balance.

Toxic serum levels of calcium, magnesium, or phosphate are also most rapidly corrected with machine-driven hemodialysis. Once normal levels are achieved, any of the renal replacement therapies can maintain homeostasis if nutritional intake is limited and magnesium-containing phosphate binders are avoided. Renal replacement therapies utilizing dialysate (hemodialysis, peritoneal dialysis, continuous hemodialysis) may contain calcium concentrations of 3.5 meq/L (1.75 mmol/L of ionized calcium) in the dialysate. Therefore, successful and rapid treatment of hypercalcemia requires lower dialysate calcium concentrations of 2.5 meq/L (1.25 mmol/L) or less. Severe hypophosphatemia may complicate all renal replacement therapies, especially in patients being maintained on intravenous hyperalimentation devoid of phosphate.

Acid-Base Abnormalities

Uremic acidosis rarely generates more than 50–100 mmol of acid per day and can be easily corrected by any of the renal replacement techniques. Severe uremic acidosis is most often encountered as a presenting abnormality of unattended chronic renal failure. Under these conditions, hemodialysis can provide the most rapid correction of acidosis, but aggressive hemodialysis may precipitate a dysequilibrium syndrome. Despite associated hyperkalemia, the dialysate bath composition should include at least 2 mmol/L of potassium, since correction of acidosis causes a substantial lowering of serum potassium concentration. Consideration should also be given to a relatively low-calcium bath (2.5 meq/L), because overly aggressive correction of longstanding hypocalcemia may precipitate nausea, vomiting, muscle cramping, and hypertension.

Lactic acid may be produced at rates of up to 50 mmol/h and is usually associated with severe hemodynamic instability. Although daily hemodialysis can provide adequate replacement of lost bicarbonate, the patient may be left with rapidly worsening acidosis during the interdialytic period. Continuous hemofiltration can provide continuous correction of acidosis and may be best for managing the fluid overload often associated with shock and its treatment. Replacement solutions containing 150 mmol/L of bicarbonate can provide as much as 100 mmol/h of continuous buffer replacement, but required calcium replacement must be administered in a separate solution. Peritoneal dialysis, with exchanges at 2 L/h, can provide approximately 25 mmol of buffer per hour. Dialytic solutions containing lactate should be avoided, since conversion to bicarbonate may be slowed in patients with circulatory impairment.

Uremia

Although urea is not universally accepted as a uremic toxin, its levels are most commonly used to judge the degree of uremic toxicity. Several studies suggest that maintaining predialysis BUN at or below 120 mg/dL (43 mmol/L) is beneficial for overall survival, and it is no longer acceptable to tolerate excessively high urea levels prior to initiation of renal replacement therapy. There is good or better evidence to suggest that proper protein-calorie nutrition is also beneficial. Thus, it is inappropriate to withhold adequate nutrition in order to avoid the associated increase in nitrogen and fluid intake. On empiric grounds, when pericarditis, encephalopathy, or hemorrhage is associated with BUN levels above 100 mg/dL, it is hard to argue that such symptoms are not at least partially the result of retained uremic toxins. With the above considerations in mind, it is reasonable to initiate renal replacement therapy when BUN is above 100 mg/dL (36 mmol/L). Nonetheless, if rapid return of renal function is anticipated (prerenal azotemia, obstructive uropathy), levels of 150 mg/dL (54 mmol/L) or more may be tolerated for a limited period.

Specific indications for dialytic therapy for complications of uremia include uremic encephalopathy, pericarditis, and uremic platelet dysfunction. Slowed mentation, somnolence, and convulsions are part of the uremic syndrome and are usually associated with other neuromuscular manifestations, including asterixis, myoclonus, and muscle twitching. In general, these symptoms respond within several days after the start of dialytic therapy.

Despite the existence of massive pericardial effusions, patients with uremic pericarditis may present with hypertension and pulmonary congestion. The treatment of uremic pericarditis often presents two distinct problems: removal of fluid in the face of potentially compromised hemodynamics and the definitive treatment of the pericardial inflammation. Initial rapid fluid removal with hemodialysis may be well tolerated, but as volume removal proceeds, intravascular pressures may become inadequate to maintain intracardiac filling, and severe hypotension may result. Thus, normovolemia should be achieved with gentle fluid removal and anticipation of rapid declines in blood pressure. Although the toxins responsible for uremic pericarditis have not been identified, it has been shown empirically that aggressive solute removal can lead to resolution of pericarditis. Hemodialysis performed five times weekly is recommended, but means to limit anticoagulation should be employed in order to minimize the risk of hemopericardium. In patients with large pericardial effusions, early use of pericardiotomy may be recommended, since aggressive hemodialysis may be associated with a high mortality rate. In one retrospective report, peritoneal dialysis was found to be superior to hemodialysis in avoiding the need for surgical drainage. Peritoneal dialysis also avoids the risk of anticoagulation.

Uremic platelet dysfunction is most often identified with prolongation of the bleeding time. In general, bleeding times will normalize along with lowering of serum urea. Acutely, rapid correction of platelet dysfunction can be achieved with infusions of desmopressin at a single dose of 0.3 μg/kg.

DRUG DOSING DURING RENAL REPLACEMENT THERAPY

Many renally excreted medications require dosage modification in order to account for the amount removed by a given renal replacement therapy. Unfortunately, most of the published data are of questionable accuracy as a result of variability between patients and the great differences in clearance rates achievable with each technique. Four factors govern the removability of a given drug: molecular weight, degree of protein binding, volume of distribution, and endogenous plasma clearance. In general, hemodialysis can offer the most rapid clearance rates for a low-molecular-weight drug (< 500). Continuous hemofiltration—but not continuous hemodialysis—will efficiently remove drugs with molecular weights as high as 10,000 or more. Peritoneal dialysis will eliminate drugs in the range of MW 500 to MW 10,000. Highly protein-bound medications are not substantially removed by any of the renal replacement techniques, with the possible exception of peritoneal dialysis. In addition, modifications of the major techniques may profoundly alter clearance rates, since most of the published data were obtained with more conventional methodology. For example, it has recently been shown that the most modern "high-flux" dialyzers can offer substantial removal of relatively high-molecular-weight drugs (> 1500), thus greatly changing their dosing requirements as compared with previous recommendations.

Aronoff GR et al: *Drug Prescribing in Renal Failure: Dosing Guidelines for Adults,* 4th ed. American College of Physicians, 1999.

Golper TA et al: Drug dosing in dialysis patients. In: *Replacement of Renal Function by Dialysis,* 4th ed. Jacobs C et al (editors). Kluwer Academic, 1996.

STOPPING DIALYSIS

Owing to the availability of chronic dialysis, irreversibility of renal failure is not an acceptable indication for stopping treatment. Instead, the patient's wishes and overall clinical status should be the only considerations in discontinuing therapy. In general, withholding of dialysis may be considered when there is evidence of irreversible vital organ failure or severe cerebral damage. Most forms of acute renal failure reverse within 8 weeks. If renal failure persists beyond this period, one should initiate plans for maintenance dialysis therapy.

SPECIFIC TYPES OF RENAL REPLACEMENT THERAPY IN ACUTE RENAL FAILURE

1. Hemodialysis

Intermittent hemodialysis is the most widely used technique for acute renal failure. The method of treatment chosen varies depending on the rate of generation of nitrogenous wastes and the patient's tolerance for fluid overload. In general, 4-hour treatments performed three times weekly are sufficient to provide adequate replacement in the oliguric or anuric patient. Patients with significant residual renal function may require fewer treatments per week, especially if renal failure is nonoliguric. Conversely, the patient with severe hypercatabolism and poorly tolerated fluid overload may require daily treatments.

The major advantage of hemodialysis is its highly efficient solute removal, thus limiting treatment time and making the patient available for other procedures and treatments. Disadvantages include relatively rapid fluid removal, which may be poorly tolerated, and the need for large-bore hemoaccess. The need for anticoagulation is another drawback, but this difficulty can be moderated in several ways.

EFFECTIVENESS OF HEMODIALYSIS

Solute clearance and ultrafiltration rates are variable depending on the blood flows obtained and the dialyzers chosen. Most modern dialyzers provide 150–250 mL/min of urea clearance with blood flows between 200 and 300 mL/min. More rapid solute clearance can be obtained with the newer more porous filters, especially when operated at blood flows of up to 400 mL/min. Currently available dialyzers can also produce between 1 L and 3 L of ultrafiltrate per hour, usually limited by the patient's hemodynamic stability. "High-flux" dialyzers provide the most rapid solute clearance, but their use requires dialysis equipment with volumetric control of fluid removal.

In general, urea removal during hemodialysis follows first-order kinetics and assumes that urea is distributed throughout total body water. Under normal operating conditions, a 4-hour dialysis will lower pretreatment urea levels by approximately 50–70%. Factors that may decrease treatment efficiency include inadequate blood flow to the dialyzer, access recirculation, and dialyzer clotting.

Vascular Access

Efficient hemodialysis requires blood flows of at least 200–300 mL/min and a relatively large-bore vascular access. In the acute setting, the most widely used method is the percutaneous cannulation of either the femoral or the subclavian vein with double-lumen catheters. Regardless of placement site, the use of double-lumen catheters may allow a certain percentage of dialyzed blood leaving the efferent lumen to reenter the afferent lumen. This process is known as recirculation and may reach values of 50% or more, resulting in extremely inefficient dialysis treatment.

Percutaneous placement of a double-lumen catheter in the **femoral vein** is the most widely used method for achieving rapid access for hemodialysis. Extensive experience has shown this method to be safe and well tolerated despite the necessity for repeated punctures. A disadvantage is that the catheter limits the patient's mobility, and an unresolved issue is the length of time a single catheter can be safely left in place. Ideally, the catheter should be removed after every procedure; however, this is often impractical or impossible. In any event, catheters should never be left in place for more than 3–5 days. When alternative access sites are unavailable, catheters may be replaced over a guidewire and the removed catheter tip sent for culture. Careful attention to sterile technique during placement and meticulous care of the access site are essential. The most serious complications of femoral vein access are retroperitoneal hemorrhage and pulmonary embolism. Retroperitoneal hemorrhage may result from iliac vein rupture and has been associated with difficult guidewire placement. Pulmonary emboli are the result of catheter-related thrombi and are most apt to occur with catheters left in situ for prolonged periods. Other complications include hematomas, thrombophlebitis, arteriovenous fistulas, sepsis, and access site infection.

Subclavian vein access allows for unhindered patient mobility, and catheters in the subclavian vein have been safely left in place for prolonged periods. The major disadvantage is the increased risk of life-threatening complications during placement. Radiologic evaluation for catheter placement is required prior to the first treatment. Sharp angulations of the distal catheter tip necessitate catheter repositioning to avoid vessel rupture. Massive hemothorax and pericardial tamponade are among the most serious complications. These complications can occur even after previously successful treatments. Cardiac arrhythmias, thrombophlebitis, sepsis, air embolism, pneumothorax, and access site infection are other complications. Recently, it has been demonstrated that prolonged cannulation can lead to significant subclavian vein stenosis, thus rendering the ipsilateral arm incapable of supporting subsequent permanent hemoaccess. Given this risk, use of this access site is to be avoided in those patients for whom there is a high probability of permanent renal failure (eg, diabetic patient with preexisting renal dysfunction suffering from subsequent acute renal injury).

The **right internal jugular vein** offers an alternative to subclavian cannulation. A potential advantage of this method is that the catheter's route is relatively straight, thus avoiding the sharp angulations associated with the subclavian route. Nonetheless, retrograde cannulation of the subclavian vein is possible, and radiologic evaluation of placement is required. A drawback to this technique is the relatively awkward placement and the difficulty of access site care. "Tunneled" access to the internal jugular is becoming more popular and allows for much easier access site care.

Anticoagulation

The need for anticoagulation can be the most significant disadvantage associated with hemodialysis. Several methods have been proposed for reducing hemorrhagic risks. Regional heparinization is performed by infusing heparin into the blood before it reaches the filter with continuous neutralization with protamine into the blood after the filter, but this procedure has fallen out of favor because of the "heparin rebound" effect, which may appear up to 10 hours after treatment.

Low-dose heparin (10–20 units/kg/h) and bedside monitoring of coagulation status have been shown to be superior to regional heparinization in controlling hemorrhagic risks. Low-molecular-weight heparin has been proposed because of its limited effect on platelet function. Unfortunately, these low-molecular-weight fragments have a prolonged half-life (18 hours) and are not neutralized by protamine.

Citrate anticoagulation has been used successfully but requires careful attention to dialysate calcium concentration and may require substantial amounts of sodium and fluid infusions.

Because of their short half-life, prostacyclin and its derivatives have been used. Although successfully employed in stable patients, prostacyclin may be inappropriate for the critically ill. Aside from a considerable list of potentially troublesome secondary effects, including flushing, nausea, headache, and abdominal pain, the antiplatelet action of prostacyclin is still demonstrable up to 2 hours after cessation of infusion, and there is no known method for reversing the effect.

An increasingly popular approach is to completely avoid anticoagulation by using high blood flows and frequent saline flushes of the filter (200 mL every 20 minutes). The new, more porous dialyzers have ultrafiltration capabilities that will easily remove the excess fluid administered.

Complications

Although hemodialysis is performed by specially trained nursing personnel and is directed by a nephrologist, complications may occur in the intensive care setting when the intensivist is the first physician to evaluate the situation. During treatment, the most commonly encountered complication is hypotension. Other complications include cardiac arrhythmias, hypoxemia, hemorrhage, air embolism, pyrogenic reactions, and dysequilibrium syndromes.

A. Hypotension

Poorly tolerated fluid removal is the most obvious cause of hypotension, but several more subtle mechanisms may play a role in some patients. Relative intolerance to acetate can cause hypotension, and bicarbonate-based dialysates are now commonly used for any patient in whom vascular instability is considered a potential difficulty. The relative bioincompatibility of cuprophane- and cellulose-based membranes can, in rare cases, cause enhanced activation of complement and the acute onset of severe respiratory distress and hypotension resistant to volume replacement. This constellation of symptoms has been called the "first-use syndrome" and has been managed with intravenous aminophylline or subcutaneous epinephrine. Once a patient's susceptibility is established, the syndrome will occur at the initiation of every treatment with an unused dialyzer, usually within 15–20 minutes. Definitive management consists of switching to a more biocompatible membrane.

More recently, a similar anaphylactoid type syndrome has been described involving the use of polyacrylonitrile dialyzers (AN-69) in patients treated with angiotensin-converting enzyme inhibitors. Regardless of the cause, symptomatic hypotension during dialysis should be initially treated by lowering the transmembrane pressure, decreasing the blood flow, evaluating for cardiogenic causes, and administering normal saline, albumin, or hypertonic glucose. If significant wheezing is present, the first-use syndrome should be suspected.

B. Cardiac Arrhythmias

Several abnormalities increase the risk of cardiac arrhythmias during dialysis. Of these, the best-established is digitalis toxicity initiated by the rapid lowering of serum potassium levels. Many dialysate baths contain 2 mmol/L of potassium or less; dialysate baths containing 3.5 mmol/L of potassium have been shown to reduce the risk of digitalis toxicity. Other causes of arrhythmias include abnormalities of magnesium or calcium, hypoxia, pericarditis, myocardial infarction, acetate toxicity, and complications of subclavian catheterization.

C. Hypoxemia

The hemodialysis procedure can induce hypoxemia by at least two mechanisms. The more benign of these involves the loss of CO_2 through the dialyzer with subsequent decrease in respiratory drive. This complication occurs with acetate-buffered dialysate solutions, which are currently being replaced with bicarbonate-based solutions. When this type of hypoxia does occur, it can be easily managed with supplemental oxygen. A more ominous cause involves the first-use syndrome (see above), with rapid activation of complement leading to leukoagglutination in the lung and severe bronchospasm. This presentation calls for termination of treatment and the potential need for aminophylline or epinephrine. Subsequent treatments must be performed with a more biocompatible membrane.

D. Hemorrhage

If serious hemorrhage occurs during dialysis, previously administered heparin should be neutralized with protamine. A rational starting dose would be 1 mg of protamine for every 100 units of heparin administered. If possible, protamine infusions should be limited to no more than 15 mg over 5 minutes in order to minimize the risk of anaphylactoid reactions. There is considerable individual variation in protamine requirements, and normalization of the partial thromboplastin time should be sought. There is also the possibility of a "heparin rebound" effect occurring up to 10 hours after successful neutralization.

E. Dialysis Dysequilibrium

This syndrome of headache, nausea, muscle irritability, obtundation, and delirium or seizures may be associated with rapid correction of severe uremia. To decrease the risk, short, gentle treatments (blood flows < 200 mL/min) should be prescribed until BUN levels approach 100 mg/dL (36 mmol/L).

Beathard GA: Management of bacteremia associated with tunneled-cuffed hemodialysis catheters. J Am Soc Nephrol 1999;10:1045–9.

Brunet P et al: Anaphylactoid reactions during hemodialysis and hemofiltration: Role of associating AN69 membrane and angiotensin I converting enzyme inhibitors. Am J Kidney Dis 1992;19:444–7.

Mujais SK, Ing T, Kjellstrand CM: Acute complications of dialysis In: *Replacement of Renal Function by Dialysis,* 4th ed. Jacobs C et al (editors). Kluwer Academic, 1996.

2. Peritoneal Dialysis

Peritoneal dialysis offers the best method of renal replacement for the patient in whom it is difficult or impossible to obtain adequate hemoaccess. In contrast, patients with recent abdominal surgery may be poor candidates owing to the risks of abdominal wound dehiscence and infection of recently implanted vascular grafts. In patients with previous abdominal surgery, intraperitoneal adhesions may limit dialysate distribution, thus causing decreased ultrafiltration and decreased solute removal. A major advantage of this technique is that no anticoagulation is required. Disadvantages include substantial protein loss (Table 13–12), risks of peritonitis, drainage difficulties, compromised pulmonary function due to elevated diaphragms, hydrothorax, glucose and electrolyte abnormalities, and a relatively immobile patient.

Capabilities

Solute removal with this technique depends mostly on dialysate volume and how long the dialysate is allowed to stay in the peritoneal space before drainage (dwell time). A reasonably aggressive schedule incorporates 2-L exchanges every hour. Assuming a 50% equilibration between serum and dialysate urea levels during a 2-hour dwell time, this schedule provides 24 L of urea clearance per day. A more modest schedule would be similar to that of chronic ambulatory peritoneal dialysis (CAPD), with 2-L exchanges every 4–6 hours. Assuming a 100% equilibration of urea after a 6-hour dwell time, four 2-L exchanges yield 8 L of urea clearance per day. Associated net filtration of approximately 2 L/d will add to these predicted values. Peritonitis hastens equilibration between serum and dialysate, thus yielding greater solute clearance during the more rapid exchange schedules.

Fluid removal is directly dependent on the concentration of glucose in the dialysate and the dwell times allowed. With 1.5% dextrose solution, a 2-L exchange performed every hour can extract 100–200 mL of fluid. A 4.25% solution provides 500 mL of filtrate per hour. Prolonging dwell times decreases net filtration rate because of an increasing equilibration of dialysate glucose with serum levels, thus decreasing the osmotic drive for fluid removal. The onset of peritonitis markedly limits ultrafiltration because of rapid absorption of dialysate glucose.

Access

There are two widely used methods for obtaining access to the peritoneal cavity. Bedside placement of a stiff Teflon catheter is the most rapid means of access. Complications include bowel perforation, bladder perforation, pericatheter leakage, hemorrhage, and infection. Foley catheter placement to ensure bladder decompression prior to insertion is strongly recommended. A major drawback is that the patient must be bedridden, and drainage problems are not uncommon. Patients with previous abdominal surgery may have adhesions of bowel to the abdominal wall, thus increasing the risk of perforation. Bowel perforation may sometimes be successfully managed by repositioning the catheter and initiating empiric antibiotic therapy in the dialysate (Table 13–13). Abdominal wall infection should be considered a contraindication to catheter placement.

The surgical placement of a pliable Silastic catheter (Tenckhoff type) is the safest method of obtaining access. Drawbacks are catheter malposition, abdominal pain, and delays in catheter placement. When initiating treatment, low-volume exchanges may limit the risk of suture line dehiscence.

Complications

The most common complication of peritoneal dialysis is failure to drain or insufficient drainage. Identification of the cause can often be aided by determining if the ability to infuse fluid through the catheter is maintained. If fluid infusion is obstructed, the catheter may suffer from intrinsic blockage, and an attempt at declotting may be appropriate with saline flushes or thrombolysis with urokinase or tissue plasminogen activator. If declotting is impossible, catheter replacement is necessary. A catheter that allows unimpeded fluid infusion but not outflow may be malpositioned or may be suffering from a "ball valve" effect caused by omentum wrapped around its pores. Initial management of this problem consists of having the patient move from side to side or be placed in the Trendelenburg position. On occasion, an enema may yield dramatic results. If these initial efforts fail, catheter position must be determined by radiographic technique and repositioned, either with an intracatheter guidewire or by surgical revision.

Peritonitis most often arises from contamination during bag exchanges, though intraperitoneal contamination can also occur as a result of intra-abdominal disease. Clinical signs of peritonitis include abdominal pain, nausea, cloudy dialysate effluent, and loss of ultrafiltration (decreased fluid output per exchange). As opposed to spontaneously occurring peritonitis, peritoneal infection in the context of peritoneal dialysis may be successfully managed with intraperitoneal antibiotics (Table 13–13). A reasonable diagnostic plan would include evaluation of white blood cell count in the effluent (with peritonitis, > 100 granulocytes/μL) and Gram staining, and empiric treatment until the results of culture of the effluent are reported. Common antibiotic regimens are listed in Table 13–13. Treatment should be continued for at least 10 days. Fungal peritonitis most often requires removal of the catheter and is best treated with cessation of peritoneal dialysis.

In the immediate period after catheter placement, the dialysate effluent can be blood-tinged. The intraperitoneal administration of heparin (500–1000 units per 2-L bag) may limit the formation of fibrin clots but is unlikely to cause systemic anticoagulation. Open drainage systems are associated with a high rate of peritonitis, and a closed system, with bag-to-bag connections similar to those used in chronic ambulatory peritoneal dialysis, is preferred. Spent dialysate should be monitored daily for cell count. If granulocyte counts begin to increase above 100/μL, empiric antibiotic therapy should be initiated pending culture results. Massive protein losses are associated with peritonitis but may also occur without infection (Table 13–12).

Table 13–13. Intraperitoneal doses of antibiotics for dialysis-related peritonitis.[1]

Organism	Initial Dose (per 2 L)	Maintenance Dose (per 2 L)[2]
Staphylococcus epidermidis	Vancomycin 1 g Cefazolin 1 g	1 g every 5 days × 3 500 mg per exchange x 14 days
Staphylococcus aureus	Vancomycin 1 g	1 g every 5 days × 3
Escherichia coli	Ampicillin 500 mg	100 mg per exchange × 14 days
Pseudomonas aeruginosa	Gentamicin 70–100 mg	15 mg per exchange × 14 days

[1]Modified from Holley JL, Piraino BM: Complications of peritoneal dialysis: Diagnosis and management. Semin Dialysis 1990;3:245–48.
[2]Dosing appropriate for four exchanges per day.

These losses should be measured, and protein intake should be upwardly adjusted. Substantial glucose absorption can lead to hyperglycemia and can be controlled with intraperitoneal insulin. A reasonable starting dose would be 5–10 units per 2-L dialysate bag.

Goldberg L et al: Initial treatment of peritoneal dialysis peritonitis without vancomycin with a once-daily cefazolin-based regimen. Am J Kidney Dis 2001;37:49–55.

Keane WF et al: Adult peritoneal dialysis-related peritonitis treatment recommendations: 2000 update. Perit Dial Int 2000;20:396–411.

Mion C: Continuous peritoneal dialysis In: *Replacement of Renal Function by Dialysis,* 4th ed. Jacobs C et al (editors). Kluwer Academic, 1996.

3. Continuous Renal Replacement Therapy (CRRT)

The term CRRT (continuous renal replacement therapy) has been applied to a wide array of extracorporeal techniques for supporting the critically ill patient with acute renal failure. Originally proposed as a simple method of filtration powered by arteriovenous circuits and known as CAVH (continuous arteriovenous hemofiltration), filtrate outputs provided by a patient's unstable blood pressure were found to be inadequate for removing the large amounts of nitrogenous wastes associated with the hypercatabolic patient. In an attempt to deal with this inadequacy, several technical modifications have been developed to enhance the efficiency of the treatment. These include the addition of a diffusive component to solute removal, known as CAVHD (continuous arteriovenous hemodialysis), and the development of specialized machines for providing continuous pumped filtration—allowing for a new set of extremely efficient techniques that do not require arterial access and that are no longer dependent on the variability of the patient's changing blood pressure—CVVH (continuous venovenous hemofiltration), CVVHD (continuous venovenous hemodialysis), and CVVHDF (continuous venovenous hemodiafiltration).

The continuous therapies have several potential advantages over intermittent dialytic techniques. The most obvious is that the treatment is continuous, allowing for a constant readjustment of fluid and electrolyte therapy and the administration of large amounts of parenteral nutrition without the risk of interdialytic volume overload. Second among the advantages—at least for the hemofiltration-based treatments (CAVH, CVVH)—is its convective mode of solute transport, known to increase middle molecule clearance when compared with diffusion-based dialytic techniques. When compared with peritoneal dialysis, CRRT is not contraindicated in patients with prior abdominal surgery and offers isovolumetric fluid removal without the risk of peritonitis. The major drawbacks are the need for continuous anticoagulation and that the patient must remain bedridden during the treatment.

Issues that arise when considering the application of CRRT include the amount of solute clearance required, the type of replacement fluid or dialysate to administer, the type of anticoagulation to be employed, the amount of nutrition to be infused, the amount of nutrients lost in the filtrate or dialysate, and the impact of the treatment on drug dosing and the complications likely to be encountered. Each of these issues may have a substantial impact on outcome. For example, a recent study demonstrated that patients receiving filtration rates of 35 mL/kg/h (approximately 2.5 L/h) had a significantly increased survival when compared with patients receiving filtration rates of 20 mL/kg/h (approximately 1 L/h). One must also consider who is going to monitor the treatment and how these personnel are trained.

The following techniques for continuous renal replacement therapy are available. Each technique has advantages and disadvantages, and some are more practical or effective in patients with hypotension, those requiring large volume of fluid removal, or those needing dialysis as well as ultrafiltration.

Continuous Arteriovenous Hemofiltration (CAVH)

The standard CAVH circuit allows blood to flow from an arterial access through a tubing circuit to a low-resistance hemofilter and back to a venous access. Filtrate, which is relatively protein-free, is produced at a rate of several hundred milliliters per hour and is collected into a bag connected to the ultrafiltrate port of the filter. In the postdilution mode, the replacement fluid is infused into the venous tubing. Continuous anticoagulation is administered through a prefilter tubing connection.

Management of the circuit and maintenance of its patency are subject to a variety of procedural choices such as how often to rinse the system with saline, how often to change the filters and tubing, and how to achieve hemoaccess. These issues will often depend on the clinical setting and the type of system components being employed. A manual endorsed by the American Association of Critical Care Nurses is available from the American Nephrology Nurses' Association.

Slow Continuous Ultrafiltration (SCUF)

Blood pressure-driven filtration is a means of providing continuous isoosmotic fluid removal for aid in the management of oliguric patients. The circuit is similar to that of CAVH, but no replacement fluid is administered. Although insufficient for adequate solute removal, this technique has been found useful as a means of maintaining fluid balance in patients intolerant of aggressive fluid removal and in those with cardiodynamic instability such as may be seen during aortic balloon pumping or during open heart surgery.

Continuous Arteriovenous Hemodialysis & Hemodiafiltration (CAVHD)

The circuit is essentially the same as that for CAVH but with the addition of a constant infusion of dialysate passing through the filtrate compartment of the filter. At the relatively slow blood flow rates encountered with an arteriovenous circuit, complete blood to dialysate equilibrium of urea is achieved, and clearance rates increase linearly with dialysate flow rates up to 33.3 mL/min (2 L/h). Further increases in dialysate flow up to 4 L/h can yield urea clearances approaching 50 mL/min. In most clinical situations, the dialysate flow rate is set at 1 L/h, resulting in 17 mL/min of urea clearance by diffusion. The major advantage of this system is the enhanced solute clearance, which has allowed the technique to be applied to certain intoxications.

An interesting issue common with all the diffusion-based CRRT techniques (CAVHD, CVVHD) is the amount of back filtration that can occur. About 60% of the dialysate's glucose is absorbed through the membrane. At the common flow rate of 1 L/h, a standard 1.5% dextrose-containing dialysate (such as is commonly used for peritoneal dialysis) produces a net glucose transfer averaging 120 mg/min (175 g/d), while a 4.25% solution yields approximately 415 mg/min (600 g/d). This amount of carbohydrate must be accounted for when considering the patient's nutritional and insulin requirements.

Continuous Venovenous Hemofiltration (CVVH)

This circuit requires a blood pump and an air detector and is often equipped with arterial and venous pressure monitors. Equipment especially designed for this treatment is available. This technique has the clear advantage of avoiding the potential complications of arterial access and is capable of providing a substantial amount of convection-based clearance. Common output rates are between 1 L/h and 2 L/h, replaced with the appropriate replacement solution. Blood flow rates between 100 and 150 mL/min allow for a decreased tendency of filter clotting and limit the dosage requirements for anticoagulants.

Continuous Venovenous Hemodialysis or Hemodiafiltration (CVVHD/F)

The addition of a diffusive component to the CVVH system allows for the maximum clearance capabilities of any of the continuous therapies. The basic circuit resembles that of CVVH but allows a variable amount of dialysate to flow past the filtrate compartment of the filter as with CAVHD. The machines utilized are similar to those employed for CVVH.

Hemoaccess

The blood pressure-driven treatments (CAVH, CAVHD) require large-bore arterial and venous access. The most widely used is the combined cannulation of the femoral artery and vein. Hemoaccess for pump-driven continuous therapies (CVVH, CVVHD) does not require arterial catheterization and utilizes the same access as for machine-driven hemodialysis (see above).

Femoral artery and femoral vein cannulation is the most widely used method for obtaining an arteriovenous circuit. Adequate blood flows are best obtained with large-bore catheters (0.3 cm luminal diameter) with minimal taper and no side holes. Standard hemodialysis catheters are often inadequate. Despite the apparent risk of arterial cannulation, the reported complication rate is low. The successful use of these catheters may be due to the common practice of restricting their insertion to the well-trained, experienced operator. Furthermore, access site care is enhanced because of the constant monitoring of the filter circuit. Potential complications include retroperitoneal hemorrhage, vascular occlusion, sepsis, access site infection, and hematomas.

Anticoagulation

The need for continuous anticoagulation is a major drawback to all methods of continuous therapy and has led to a high incidence of hemorrhagic complications. It may be helpful to use regional heparinization with the slow continuous postfilter infusion of protamine. Starting dosage is usually 10 units/kg/h of heparin, with a neutralizing dose of protamine initially at 1 mg/h for every 100 units/h of heparin. Dosages should be adjusted to provide partial thromboplastin times of 150 seconds or more in the postheparin circuit and approximately 50 seconds in the postprotamine circuit. After establishing required dosing, the partial thromboplastin time should be monitored three times daily to determine the need for further adjustments. In a patient with a severe preexisting coagulopathy, reasonable filter life may be achievable without any anticoagulation. The prefilter infusion of replacement fluid may also help to prolong filter life. Varying protocols for citrate anticoagulation have been proposed. These techniques have been shown to provide sufficient and safe anticoagulation, but alkalemia, hypernatremia, and the risk of systemic hypocalcemia must be addressed for each of the different protocols. Both prostacyclin and low-molecular-weight heparin have been tried, but their use retains the same drawbacks noted for hemodialysis—notably, prolonged duration of action with no method for rapid neutralization.

Predilution

The infusion of replacement fluid into the prefilter tubing segment of the circuit dilutes the intraplasmatic urea concentration and promotes the transfer of intraerythrocytic urea into the plasma compartment where it is available for removal in the filtrate. The predilution technique also limits the hemoconcentration that occurs at the venous side of the hemofilter. The potential advantages of the predilution mode include enhanced urea clearance and the possibility of increasing filter patency by the prefilter dilution of hematocrit, clotting factors, and platelets. Disadvantages include the increased cost of replacement fluid and inability to estimate plasma electrolyte concentrations from analysis of the filtrate.

Replacement Fluids & Dialysate

All hemofiltration-based techniques (CAVH, CVVH) require large volumes of sterile, pyrogen-free replacement fluid. A physiologic and relatively inexpensive formulation consists of two easily prepared solutions given in alternating fashion. The first solution is prepared by adding one 10-mL ampule of 10% calcium gluconate to 1 L of 0.9% NaCl. The second solution is prepared by adding 50 meq of sodium bicarbonate to 1 L of 0.45% NaCl. When these two solutions are given alternately, the net result is an electrolyte solution containing sodium 141 meq/L, chloride 101 meq/L, bicarbonate 25 meq/L, and calcium 4 meq/L. Diffusion-based treatments (CAVHD, CVVHD) require dialysate solutions with adequate buffering capacity. Common practice has been to employ peritoneal dialysis solutions, but several premixed solutions are now being marketed.

Careful attention to fluid balance is essential and can be aided by connecting the filtrate output to a volumetric pump or a balancing scale designed to match inputs and outputs. Regardless of the CRRT technique employed, volume outputs and inputs can easily attain 25–50 liters per day or more. Thus, even small percentage errors in fluid balance can lead to substantial changes in the patient's volume status. Evaluation with daily weights is essential.

Kaplan AA: Continuous renal replacement therapies in the intensive care unit. J Intensive Care Med 1998;13:85–105.

Ronco C: Effects of different doses in continuous veno-venous haemofiltration on outcomes of acute renal failure: a prospective randomised trial. Lancet 2000;356:26–30.

Tolwani AJ et al: Simplified citrate anticoagulation for continuous renal replacement therapy. Kidney Int 2001;60:370–4.

CRITICAL ILLNESS IN PATIENTS WITH CHRONIC RENAL FAILURE

Patients receiving maintenance dialysis often require treatment in the critical care unit. Cardiac disease, gastrointestinal hemorrhage, and infections are the most common comorbid conditions. Standard treatment options often must be modified for dialysis patients. Unresponsiveness to standard diuretic regimens means that fluid removal for pulmonary edema or severe hypertension calls for ultrafiltration by dialytic means. For upper gastrointestinal hemorrhage, magnesium-containing antacids are best avoided and H_2 blockers may require dosage adjustments. Antibiotic treatment may actually be facilitated in that antibiotics normally cleared by the kidney may have more prolonged therapeutic levels and the nephrotoxicity of certain medications is no longer a major consideration.

In general, however, management of the patient on dialysis is similar to that of the patient with acute renal failure with the exception of several special considerations as outlined below.

NUTRITION & FLUIDS

Fluid & Electrolyte Restrictions

Normal fluid restriction for a patient receiving maintenance hemodialysis (three times weekly) is often dependent on the patient's tolerance for aggressive fluid removal during each treatment. In general, fluid restriction should be 1–1.5 L/d and is dictated by the patient's tendency to develop hypertension or pulmonary congestion in the interdialysis period. A certain degree of pedal edema is tolerated as long as hypertension or pulmonary congestion is not present. A patient maintained on chronic ambulatory peritoneal dialysis can often tolerate a more liberal fluid restriction, since dialysate glucose concentrations can be adjusted to achieve greater fluid removal on an ongoing basis. A restriction of 1.5–2 L/d of fluid intake is often well tolerated, and that amount is easily removed with the ongoing dialysis.

Nitrogen Balance & Caloric Requirements

Nitrogen balance studies in hemodialysis patients suggest that protein requirements are between 1 and 1.2 g/kg/d. The caloric requirement to maintain neutral nitrogen balance is 37 kcal/kg/d. Patients receiving chronic ambulatory peritoneal dialysis lose a substantial amount of protein in the dialysate (approximately 10 g/d), and their protein requirements approach 1.4 g/kg/d. Glucose absorption from the dialysate is substantial but depends on the dialysate glucose concentration and the length of the dialysate dwell time. A gross estimate of the absorbed glucose can be calculated by measuring the glucose concentration of the dialysate effluent and comparing this figure with the infused concentration.

VASCULAR ACCESS IN HEMODIALYSIS PATIENTS

The hemodialysis patient's permanent vascular access is the lifeline to adequate treatment, and these surgically implanted access sites must be treated with care. There are two commonly used means for creating a subcutaneous arteriovenous connection: surgical anastomosis of an artery and vein, often in the wrist ("primary" arteriovenous fistula); and placement of a polytetrafluoroethylene graft between artery and vein in the brachial fossa. The primary arteriovenous fistula is more resistant to infection and thrombosis, but it requires up to 6 weeks to mature, and its placement is surgically impossible in many patients with inadequate distal vasculature. Polytetrafluoroethylene grafts are available for use within 1–2 weeks but are more prone to infection and pseudoaneurysm formation. A properly functioning graft or fistula will have a palpable thrill and a bruit audible with a stethoscope. These findings should be checked daily. In general, the sites should not be used for routine venipuncture, and blood pressure readings should be taken on the contralateral arm. It is not uncommon for a prolonged period of hypotension to result in a thrombosed access. If an access site is found to be clotted (inaudible bruit), vascular surgical consultation should be sought immediately. In some cases, thrombolytic therapy with urokinase or tissue plasminogen activator may avoid the necessity for surgical revision. Angioplasty by interventional radiology may also be successful.

Infection of the vascular access route is the most common infectious complication in the hemodialysis population. Erythema and tenderness over the site are the most common signs; however, occult septicemia can result from an apparently unaffected site. Access site infection should be suspected in all cases of systemic infection. Blood cultures from the access site are a reasonable first step in diagnosing infection. As opposed to other infections with implantable grafts, successful treatment without removal of the graft is possible with prolonged administration of antibiotics. Most antibiotic regimens for access site infections include vancomycin, since that agent is poorly dialyzable, and a single dose can maintain adequate serum levels for 3–5 days.

Nassar GM, Ayus JC: Infectious complications of the hemodialysis access. Kidney Int 2001;60:1–13.

CHRONIC AMBULATORY PERITONEAL DIALYSIS PATIENTS

Chronic ambulatory peritoneal dialysis (CAPD) commonly involves four 2-L exchanges per day. Net fluid removal is dependent on the rate of exchange and the dialysate glucose concentration (1.5%, 2.5%, or 4.25%). Peritoneal dialysis catheters are surgically placed Silastic tubing with direct connections to the intraperitoneal space. Strict sterility should be maintained whenever the connection between the catheter and the dialysate tubing is interrupted. Drainage problems are not uncommon and may respond to moving the catheter or turning the patient. On occasion, an enema may cause sufficient intra-abdominal movement to produce adequate drainage. Standard intraperitoneal antibiotic therapy for peritonitis is outlined in Table 13–13.

RENAL TRANSPLANT PATIENTS

The differential diagnosis of acute renal failure in the transplanted kidney is discussed above. Other commonly encountered problems in the transplant recipient include infections, gastrointestinal complications, and hypertension.

Infections

Renal transplant patients require continuous immunosuppressive therapy that may include varying combinations of corticosteroids, azathioprine, cyclosporine, mycophenolate mofetil, and tacrolimus. The type of infection likely to occur as a result of the immunocompromised state has been noted to be somewhat bimodal in distribution. Whereas common bacterial pathogens, including streptococci, staphylococci, and gram-negative bacteria, seem to predominate in the immediate posttransplant period, common opportunistic infections with viral, protozoal, or fungal organisms seem to occur 1 month or more after surgery. It is important to note that the classic signs of infection, including fever, may be masked by the anti-inflammatory corticosteroids. In general, if a life-threatening infection is identified, it is often prudent to discontinue immunosuppressive medication temporarily despite the risk of graft rejection. In any event, close consultation with the patient's nephrologist or transplant surgeon is essential.

Gastrointestinal Complications

Peptic ulcer disease, colonic perforation, and pancreatitis are the most common gastrointestinal complications in the renal transplant patient. Bleeding or perforation of a peptic ulcer carries a particularly high morbidity, and prophylactic use of H_2 antagonists, proton pump inhibitors, or antacids has been found to be effective. Colonic perforations are uncommon but are apt to be lethal if not quickly identified. Pancreatitis is believed to be a result of long-term use of corticosteroids, and severe sequelae including hemorrhagic pancreatitis and pseudocyst formation have been reported.

Hypertension

Hypertension can complicate up to 50% of all renal transplants. Possible causes include renal artery stenosis of the native or transplanted kidneys, allograft dysfunction, cyclosporine, and recurrence of the original renal disease. Renal artery stenosis of the grafted kidney may be successfully treated by percutaneous angioplasty. Cyclosporine-induced hypertension may result from the intrarenal vasoconstriction associated with endothelin and may respond to a decrease in dosage. In contrast, allograft dysfunction related to ongoing infection may require increased immunosuppression.

Kasiske BL et al: Recommendations for the outpatient surveillance of renal transplant recipients. American Society of Transplantation. J Am Soc Nephrol 2000;11(Suppl 15):S1–86.

Silkensen JR: Long-term complications in renal transplantation. J Am Soc Nephrol 2000;11:582–8.

Gastrointestinal Failure in the ICU 14

Gideon P. Naude, MD

This chapter addresses the common causes that fall under the broad category of gastrointestinal failure. Pancreatitis, bowel obstruction, paralytic ileus, diarrhea, and malabsorption are discussed here. Gastrointestinal hemorrhage and specific gastrointestinal diseases are presented in other chapters. For an overview of abdominal pathology, the reader is referred to Chapter 32, which discusses the acute abdomen.

PANCREATITIS

ESSENTIALS OF DIAGNOSIS

- *Severe abdominal pain, usually radiating to the back.*
- *Nausea and vomiting.*
- *Hemodynamic and respiratory compromise in severe cases.*
- *Elevated serum levels of pancreatic enzymes.*
- *Pancreatic enlargements on CT scan.*

General Considerations

Acute inflammation of the pancreas has a wide clinical spectrum, from mild (acute edematous pancreatitis) to very severe (necrotizing pancreatitis). Most patients have a benign course, and recovery is uncomplicated. In approximately 30% of cases, the inflammatory process is aggressive and associated with a mortality rate that approaches 50%. In the latter group, management within the ICU is required. Aggressive early resuscitation may prevent the onset of lethal multisystem organ failure.

Acute pancreatitis is frequently precipitated by gallstone obstruction of the pancreatic duct. Although identification of a persisting stone within the common bile duct itself (choledocholithiasis) is unusual, careful straining of stools identifies a gallstone in up to 90% of patients who have had an attack of pancreatitis within the preceding 10 days. Pathogenesis may be related to obstruction of the pancreatic duct during passage of the stone, which results in ductal hypertension and causes breakdown of intracellular compartmentalization, leading to zymogen activation.

In the United States, alcohol consumption is responsible for about 40% of cases of pancreatitis. Acute pancreatitis may occur at any time in the course of ongoing excessive consumption, though commonly the initial attack comes after several years of alcohol abuse. The initial episode may be followed by further attacks. The usual pattern is a severe first attack followed by subsequent attacks that are less dramatic, presumably because of the loss of active pancreatic tissue. Alcohol is the etiologic factor most commonly associated with chronic pancreatitis, and microscopic examination of the gland at first acute presentation often demonstrates evidence of chronicity such as scarring and replacement of acinar elements with fibrous tissue. This may have implications for pancreatic endocrine function during subsequent acute attacks.

The mechanism of pancreatic damage by alcohol is incompletely understood and may be idiosyncratic. Alcohol has been shown to have ultrastructural effects on acinar cells. It may also cause spasm of the sphincter of Oddi, producing ductal hypertension.

Postoperative pancreatitis is most commonly seen following operations on the biliary tree. The onset of atypical pain or unexpected ileus following surgery raises the possibility of pancreatitis. Because postoperative pancreatitis often lacks the usual clinical features, early detection may be difficult. Acute pancreatitis following endoscopic retrograde cholangiopancreatography (ERCP) is seen in approximately 2% of cases and may be severe.

Acute pancreatitis may occur in conjunction with elevations of serum calcium, including transient hypercalcemic states that may occur with intravenous infusions. Other metabolic causes include hyperlipidemia, hypothermia, protein deficiency, and diabetes.

Drugs and toxins probably account for more cases of pancreatitis than is usually suspected. Common drugs include furosemide, azathioprine, estrogen-containing contraceptives, tetracyclines, and corticosteroids. Scorpion envenomation is a common cause in tropical environments such as the Caribbean.

Blunt trauma may be associated with acute pancreatitis, particularly if there is acute ductal obstruction caused by hematoma. More commonly, chronic pancreatitis, pseudocyst formation, or pancreatic fistulas result from blunt injury.

Pancreas divisum, ductal abnormalities, and pancreatic carcinoma have all been suggested as etiologic factors for acute pancreatitis. When pancreas divisum is present, the narrow opening of the minor papilla may obstruct the flow of pancreatic secretions. Unfortunately, sphincteroplasty of the minor ampulla has mixed results.

Less common causes of acute pancreatitis include infectious agents such as paramyxovirus (mumps), Epstein-Barr virus, mycoplasma species, hepatitis virus, and ascaris; and autoimmune disorders, including systemic lupus erythematosus, necrotizing angiitis, and thrombotic thrombocytopenic purpura. In some patients, the etiologic factor is never discovered.

Pathophysiology

The pancreas produces a wide variety of digestive enzymes that have the potential for causing serious cellular and biologic disruption. Proteases such as trypsin, chymotrypsin, and elastase have been shown to activate proenzymes in the inflammatory and complement cascades. Lipases such as phospholipase A_2 can liberate phospholipid remnants. These particles perpetuate the inflammatory response and may have direct cellular toxicity. Normally, intrapancreatic enzyme control is achieved by secretion of inactive proenzymes (zymogens), intracellular enzyme inhibitors, and compartmentalization by storage of zymogens and enzyme activators in separate cytosol granules. Once the integrity of this protective process is breached, autodigestion initiates an inflammatory process that is self-sustaining.

Acinar damage quickly disrupts normal organ function, resulting in almost immediate cessation of exocrine secretion and alteration of endocrine secretion. For this reason, ongoing formation and leakage of pancreatic enzymes is probably only a minor factor in the perpetuation of acute pancreatitis following the initial insult. Factors contributing to progressive disease with severe inflammation and necrosis are unknown, but organ ischemia and infection are likely to be important.

Systemic toxicity and functional impairment of other organ systems are related to the release of inflammatory mediators such as interleukin-1, arachidonic acid metabolites, kinins, and tumor necrosis factor. There are profound changes in immune competence and inappropriate activation of lymphocytes and polymorphonuclear neutrophils.

Clinical Features

Clinical evaluation of acute pancreatitis consists of confirmation of the diagnosis, estimation of severity, determination of prognosis, and identification of pancreatic necrosis.

A. Symptoms and Signs

Pain is the most constant symptom, though its nature and severity are variable. Radiation to the back is observed in 50% of patients, but no pattern can be considered typical. The intensity of the pain does not correlate with the degree of pancreatic inflammation. Occasionally, other clinical features such as vomiting are dominant. The diagnosis should be considered in all patients with abdominal pain of recent onset, especially if associated with physiologic compromise such as hypotension or hypoxia.

Various clinical signs have been described. Abdominal distention and tenderness are common, but peritonitis is rare. Abdominal findings do not indicate the severity of the retroperitoneal process. If the inflammatory process has extended beyond the pancreas, erythema around the flanks may occur. The classic signs of hemorrhagic pancreatitis—ecchymoses in the flank (Grey Turner's sign) or umbilicus (Cullen's sign)—are not commonly present.

Signs of respiratory compromise may indicate incipient respiratory failure. Tachypnea greater than 20 breaths/min and a limited chest expansion on inspiration are important. Clinical evidence of bilateral pleural effusion is commonly found in patients with severe pancreatic inflammation.

B. Laboratory Findings

Elevation of enzyme markers such as amylase and lipase was traditionally considered diagnostic, but the sensitivity and specificity of these tests are generally inferior to those of CT. A normal serum amylase level does not exclude the diagnosis, and enzyme elevation may be observed in a variety of other conditions, including perforated or penetrating peptic ulcer, ruptured ectopic pregnancy, and bowel obstruction or infarction. Measurement of the renal clearance of amylase does not enhance the sensitivity of this variable.

C. Imaging Studies

Organ imaging has replaced serum biochemical analysis as the diagnostic modality of choice in acute pancreatitis. In all but the mildest cases, imaging the pancreas by CT or ultrasonography should be the initial investigation. Demonstration of organ enlargement confirms the diagnosis. Enzyme levels frequently return to normal within a few days, whereas pancreatic radiologic derangement persists for at least a week. Therefore, organ imaging is also valuable in the retrospective diagnosis of this condition. Very early in the disease, however, CT scan may be unhelpful since macroscopic changes may take hours to develop. During this brief period, measurement of enzyme markers is preferable.

The value of CT scan versus ultrasonography is debated. Actually, the procedures are complementary, and both should be used. With the interference of bowel gas, examination of the retroperitoneum by ultrasonography is often limited initially. However, valuable information concerning the biliary tree may be obtained. CT scans have low sensitivity for the detection of gallstones but are generally superior to ultrasonography for the delineation of retroperitoneal disease processes.

D. Estimation of Severity and Determination of Prognosis

Determination of the severity of acute pancreatitis based on clinical evaluation alone is accurate in only 35–40% of patients. A number of scoring methods have been devised for objective assessment of the severity and prediction of morbidity and mortality. These scoring techniques are useful in ensuring early institution of appropriate management and in tracking physiologic progress. However, sickness scoring systems are of limited use in making management decisions for individual patients. Their most valuable contribution in acute pancreatitis may be in assessment of new treatment strategies and evaluation of quality assurance.

Initial scoring systems for acute pancreatitis were developed prior to the widespread availability of CT scanning and are based on multiple clinical and biochemical parameters. They include Ranson's Early Prognostic Signs, Imrie's Prognostic Criteria, Simplified Prognostic Criteria, the Glasgow Criteria, and the APACHE (Acute Physiology and Chronic Health Evaluation) scoring system. These systems have various drawbacks. Most are complex and difficult to remember; extensive data collection and computation are required; and lack of data on all parameters occurs frequently. Completed scores may not be available during initial management.

Ranson's method (Table 14–1) is the standard against which other scoring systems are judged. A score of less than 2 based on Ranson's criteria indicates mild disease with a good prognosis. A score greater than 6 correlates with a mortality rate of 20% and a complication rate of 80%. Imrie's system is a simplification of the original Ranson criteria and is popular in the Commonwealth countries. The Simplified Prognostic Criteria (SPC) with only four parameters is easier to remember. Two SPC signs are the equivalent of six or more Ranson signs. As a general guideline, all patients with more than three of Ranson's criteria or APACHE II scores greater than 8 should be managed the ICU.

With the advent of routine organ imaging in acute pancreatitis, scoring systems based on the CT appearances of the primary disease process have been developed. These are at least as good predictors of severity and outcome as any of the physiologic scoring systems and have the advantage of immediate availability. Multiple scans may be necessary to ensure the accuracy of this technique, as the CT appearance may change with time.

Table 14–1. Ranson's criteria of severity of acute pancreatitis.[1]

Criteria present initially
Age > 55 years
White blood cell count > 16,000/μL
Blood glucose > 200 mg/dL
Serum LDH > 350 IU/L
AST (SGOT) > 250 IU/dL
Criteria developing during first 24 hours
Hematocrit fall > 10%
BUN rise > 8 mg/dL
Serum Ca^{2+} < 8 mg/dL
Arterial Po_2 < 60 mm Hg
Base deficit > 4 meq/L
Estimated fluid sequestration > 600 mL

[1]Morbidity and mortality rates correlate with the number of criteria present. Mortality rates correlate as follows: 0–2 criteria present = 2%; 3 or 4 = 15%; 5 or 6 = 40%; 7 or 8 = 100%.

Another system, based on the quality and quantity of peritoneal fluid that can be recovered by lavage, has also been described. It has the disadvantage of requiring an invasive procedure and is not widely used except by clinicians who favor peritoneal lavage as a treatment measure in acute pancreatitis.

E. Identification of Pancreatic Necrosis

The most serious local complication of acute pancreatitis is pancreatic necrosis, which, if infection occurs and treatment is not provided, carries a 100% mortality rate. Following initial resuscitation, identification and delineation of this process are the primary aims of management, since timely operation will significantly reduce the mortality rate.

Clinical signs include increasing pain and abdominal distention. Progressive physiologic derangement and increasing systemic toxicity are observed with necrosis. Physiologic monitoring by repeated objective scoring assessments may be useful to record progressive deterioration at this stage.

Identification and assessment of pancreatic necrosis are based on a combination of clinical appraisal, sickness scoring, measurement of serum factors, organ imaging, and fine-needle aspiration biopsy of the pancreas. Several serum factors can be correlated with pancreatic necrosis. Biochemical parameters include a fall in α_2-macroglobulin and C3 and C4 complement factors and a rise in α_2-antiprotease, C-reactive protein, and pancreatic ribonuclease. These parameters lack absolute sensitivity and at best only complement other methods.

CT scanning is becoming established as the best means of assessment of pancreatic necrosis. Enhanced physiologic imaging using high-resolution contrast-enhanced scanning techniques increases the sensitivity and specificity of this technique and has been reported to clearly establish the presence and extent of pancreatic necrosis. The initial CT scan should be performed for diagnosis and estimation of disease severity. Repeated scanning is necessary in all but the mildest cases to monitor local progression of disease. Subsequent scans may be scheduled after 1 week if the clinical course gradually improves. Patients who fail to respond after adequate initial resuscitation or show evidence of worsening clinical status require earlier evaluation and are candidates for scanning with dynamic vascular enhancement in an attempt to establish the presence and extent of the necrosis.

F. Needle Aspiration

Needle aspiration of pancreatic and peripancreatic collections under CT control is becoming accepted as a means of identification of superinfection. At least 40% of necrotic collections are found to be infected at the time of initial management. The most common organism is *E coli,* but a wide variety of gram-positive and gram-negative aerobic and anaerobic organisms (as single or mixed cultures) have been isolated. Aspiration culture results may be used as a guide to antibiotic selection.

G. Systemic Considerations

Respiratory failure is common in patients with moderate to severe acute pancreatitis. Indium-labeled leukocyte scintiscans demonstrate early margination of the leukocytes in the lungs. The quantitative deposition correlates with other prognostic indicators. This is identical to the pattern seen in sepsis-related ARDS. Assessment of ventilation and gas exchange should be included in the initial evaluation. Patients may have clinical evidence of bilateral pleural effusion with or without evidence of underlying atelectasis. It is often useful to include a few CT images of the lung bases at the same time as the pancreatic scanning. Such lung sections clearly demonstrate the pulmonary involvement, which may be more significant than the chest x-ray suggests. In the more fulminant cases, the clinical picture is one of typical ARDS. A marked rise in liver aminotransferase (AST > 1000 units/L) suggests the possibility of ischemic hepatitis. This diagnosis should be included in the differential in evaluation of a patient suspected of having gallstone pancreatitis and persistent choledocholithiasis. In its more severe form, ischemic hepatitis may be associated with other metabolic derangements, including a rise in bilirubin. Gradual recovery can usually be expected.

A low Glasgow coma score may be observed for several reasons in patients with severe acute pancreatitis. The use of sedation and opioids for pain relief may modify cerebral function, and catastrophic illness is often associated with acute organic brain syndrome. Pancreatic encephalopathy has also been described as a separate entity. It is attributed to the release of pancreatic lipases, but the evidence for this view is inconclusive. MRI demonstrates patchy white matter abnormalities that resemble plaques seen in multiple sclerosis.

Treatment

Critical care of the patient with acute pancreatitis consists essentially of maintaining adequate perfusion and oxygen delivery to essential organs during resolution of the primary disease process. Early and aggressive resuscitation reduces the mortality rate by reducing the incidence of multisystem organ failure.

A. Fluid Resuscitation and Physiologic Monitoring

The degree of intravascular fluid depletion is difficult to gauge accurately in patients with acute pancreatitis. Tissue fluid shifts related to systemic release of vasoactive toxins and severe retroperitoneal losses may be dramatic. As much as 10–20 L of replacement fluid may be required in the first 24 hours. Replacement by crystalloid has no clear advantage over colloid. In cases where the albumin is less than 3.0 g/L, the use of albumin replacement may be considered. Depending on the clinical severity, blood transfusion should be considered when the hemoglobin is less than 10 g/dL. The use of fresh frozen plasma for systemic deactivation of proteases has provided apparent benefit in empiric trials. Controlled studies, however, have failed to provide objective evidence of an improvement in outcome, and routine use of fresh frozen plasma should await further evaluation.

As in any shock state, adequacy of fluid replacement is assessed by measurement of central venous or pulmonary arterial wedge pressure, aiming for values at least 10 mm Hg above the intrathoracic pressure. In cases where positive-pressure ventilation is being used, the systemic venous pressure or the pulmonary arterial wedge pressure should be at least 10 mm Hg higher than the ventilatory positive end-expiratory pressure.

The adequacy of fluid replacement can be further assessed by measurement of the response to repeat fluid challenges with 250–500 mL of balanced salt solution. If central filling pressures are sufficient, such challenges will be followed by a sustained rise in central venous pressure of 3–5 mm Hg. Once filling pressures are optimized, the increment in cardiac output in response to further fluid replacement is minimal, and the patient should be kept stable at this level.

Successful fluid resuscitation should be accompanied by improved peripheral perfusion as indicated by limb temperature, peripheral pulse volume, arterial blood pressure, urinary output, and mixed venous oxygen. Low mixed venous oxygen tension ($P\bar{v}O_2 < 40$ mm Hg) indicates that the perfusion state is inadequate. If central filling pressures have been optimized, myocardial dysfunction should be suspected.

B. Inotropic Support

Echocardiographic evaluation is useful for differentiation of the hypovolemic state from the hypocontractile state. In the former, heart size is normal or less than normal and there is evidence of vigorous wall motion. In the latter, there is usually discernible chamber enlargement and segmental or global hypokinesia.

If myocardial hypocontractility is diagnosed, inotropic support should be instituted. Strict guidelines for choice of inotropic agents are not available. In general, however, for patients in whom persistent hypotension dominates, an incrementally increased infusion of dopamine titrated against blood pressure is the preferred initial strategy. In situations where tissue perfusion remains poor despite adequate arterial pressures, inotropic agents without prominent alpha-adrenergic effects such as dobutamine may be preferable. Irrespective of the agent used, the clinical objective is improvement of organ perfusion, and mixed venous oxygenation should be specifically evaluated rather than relying solely on monitoring of arterial blood pressure.

C. Respiratory Support

Patients with significant hypoxia ($PaO_2 < 60$ mm Hg) despite high inspired oxygen or clinical evidence of compromised ventilation (respiratory rate of > 30/min or dyskinetic breathing pattern) should be considered for early intubation and mechanical ventilatory support. Sedation, analgesia, and mechanical ventilation improve overall cardiopulmonary performance.

D. Renal Support

Impaired renal function—indicated by rising serum urea nitrogen and creatinine or oliguria with frank acute tubular necrosis—is often seen in severe acute pancreatitis. Early and adequate fluid replacement minimizes the risk, but renal function may continue to deteriorate despite adequate hemodynamic resuscitation. Low-dose dopamine may increase renal blood flow, minimizing the ischemic insult.

Fortunately, the prognosis for renal function is good, and in most cases temporary hemodialysis or hemofiltration will maintain adequate homeostasis until renal function returns.

Once acute tubular necrosis has become established, it is important to avoid secondary ischemic insults, which may result in acute cortical necrosis and permanent loss of renal function.

E. Nutrition

Acute pancreatitis is a hypermetabolic state similar to sepsis. Retroperitoneal edema may contribute to prolonged small bowel dysfunction and make enteral nutritional support impossible. This, along with ongoing negative nitrogen balance, mandates the institution of total parenteral nutrition. While early institution of total parenteral nutrition is theoretically desirable, these patients are variably intolerant of the high metabolic loads. The degree of insulin resistance is often extreme, with high-dose insulin infusions required to stabilize serum glucose levels at less than 150 mg/dL. Early institution of total parenteral nutrition is not critical, and in the hemodynamically unstable patient, delayed introduction is advised.

It has been proposed that hyperlipidemia may in itself stimulate the pancreas and help perpetuate the inflammatory process. For this reason, total parenteral nutrition regimens with reduced fat content have been advocated. There is, however, no objective evidence that patients with acute pancreatitis are adversely affected by customarily used lipid regimens, and the use of nutritional formulas low in lipids is a matter of personal choice.

Evidence of the benefit of total parenteral nutrition for modification of the disease process within the pancreas is not yet available. Nor is there real evidence to suggest the superiority of any particular regimen for the maintenance of basic nutrition.

Patients with acute pancreatitis do appear to have a heightened susceptibility to intravenous line infections, and meticulous care of catheters is required. Dedicated ports exclusively for total parenteral nutrition infusions—with meticulous care during line changes—may help reduce infection rates.

F. Other Modalities

Little can be done to substantially modify the inflammatory process within the pancreas. Various interventions have been proposed, but none have been shown to have substantial value. Steroids are not indicated. Inhibitors of pancreatic function such as glucagon and octreotide have been used without demonstrable benefit. Antiproteases such as aprotinin have also lacked obvious therapeutic effect and have now been largely abandoned.

The nature and extent of surgery are dependent on appraisal of the radiologic appearance of the pancreas and the physiologic status of the patient. Peritoneal lavage, manipulation of the biliary tree, and pancreatic procedures as well as operative management of complications all have a place in the operative management of severe acute pancreatitis. Optimal timing of any procedure is critical and is based largely on clinical judgment.

Once the patient with severe acute pancreatitis is resuscitated, efforts must be directed toward the detection and management of pancreatic necrosis. Dynamic contrast-enhanced CT scanning is the most accurate method for evaluating pancreatic ischemia and can also aid in planning operative treatment.

1. Peritoneal lavage—This relatively noninvasive procedure was first advocated in 1965 and widely adopted thereafter. However, subsequent controlled trials and standardization of patient selection showed no significant difference in overall mortality rates. A more recent trial of therapeutic peritoneal lavage for 7 days reported a reduction in both the incidence and the mortality rate of pancreatic sepsis in patients with severe acute pancreatitis. Some now advocate continuous lavage with 2-L exchanges performed every hour. A modified balanced salt solution is usually used.

2. Biliary procedures—Overwhelming evidence of the association of choledocholithiasis with gallstone pancreatitis prompted evaluation of the role of removal of common bile duct stones in the management of acute pancreatitis. Up to 95% of patients with gallstone pancreatitis pass a gallstone in the feces during the course of the illness. Choledocholithiasis can be demonstrated in approximately 70% of these patients within the first 48 hours after presentation, with the rate of stone detection falling off rapidly thereafter.

Initial experience with urgent cholecystectomy or cholecystostomy with choledochostomy in acute pancreatitis demonstrated a 72% common duct stone retrieval rate and a 2% mortality rate. However, these results were difficult to replicate and were reported prior to the general use of scoring systems to standardize illness severity and prognosis in the management of patients with acute pancreatitis. Early definitive surgery in the acute phase of acute pancreatitis carries an unacceptable morbidity and mortality rate. However, results suggest that early ERCP and endoscopic sphincterotomy may have a favorable impact on survival in patients with severe disease. Patient selection for ERCP and the inherent risks and timing of this procedure in the very sick patient need to be considered prior to adoption of this policy. Ascending cholangitis in association with acute pancreatitis is ideally treated by ERCP and sphincterotomy. Most surgeons would advocate semielective cholecystectomy once the patient has recovered from the acute event—ideally, during the same hospital admission.

3. Necrosectomy—This operation, involving empiric debridement of devitalized pancreatic tissue, has gradually become the treatment of choice in patients with severe necrotizing pancreatitis. It has replaced formal pancreatic resection, which carries a persistently high mortality rate. The nonanatomic basis of this approach makes the outcome of surgery particularly dependent on optimal timing of operation. Clinically detectable separation of necrotic and viable tissue is best seen after 7 days, and patients in whom the initial operation can be delayed that long have an overall lower mortality rate. Minimal debridement should be planned if earlier operation is mandated by deteriorating condition of the patient.

In many cases, several operations are required for complete debridement, as demarcation progresses over a period of time. Attempted resection of nondemarcated tissue to avoid multiple laparotomies is associated with increased morbidity and perhaps increased mortality rates. The use and placement of drains and the value of pancreatic bed lavage are matters of personal preference, though posterior drainage is gaining in popularity. Pancreatic fistulas should be managed by external drainage in the acute setting.

Management of the abdominal wall in the intervals between multiple, closely timed laparotomies is also a matter of choice for the surgeon. Vertical incisions with the use of zipper closure techniques or horizontal incisions with isolation of the supracolic compartment and an open wound have been advocated. If the abdomen is left open, paralysis of the patient is mandatory to prevent evisceration until early adhesions contain the abdominal contents.

4. Enteric fistulas—The massive retroperitoneal inflammation associated with acute pancreatitis may lead to vascular complications. These include thrombosis and aneurysm formation, with the former being the most common. The middle colic vessels supplying the transverse colon are especially at risk, though gastric, duodenal, and small bowel fistulas have also been described. If necrosectomy is required, consideration should be given to examination of the transverse colon. If evidence of ischemia is present, elective terminal ileostomy at the time of first laparotomy may be valuable. Other enteric fistulas are investigated and managed in routine fashion. *One must be alert to this possibility to avoid dangerous delays in diagnosis.*

5. Bleeding—Catastrophic bleeding is difficult to manage surgically because the inflamed pancreatic bed makes delineation of anatomy and accurate dissection hazardous. Embolization of the bleeding vessel by angiographic techniques is probably the treatment of choice. Bleeding from erosion into the splenic artery or other vessels may be life-threatening.

6. Pancreatic abscess—Pancreatic abscess occurs with delayed infection of limited pancreatic necrotic tissue that has progressed beyond demarcation to liquefaction and isolation. It is differentiated from infected necrosis by its delayed presentation (4–6 weeks). Abscesses are best diagnosed by CT scan. The value of percutaneous CT-guided catheter drainage in comparison with laparotomy has not been established.

7. Pancreatic pseudocyst—Pancreatic pseudocysts form by one of two mechanisms. Following acute pancreatitis, extravasation of pancreatic enzymes produces necrosis of surrounding tissues and forms a sterile collection of fluid that is not reabsorbed as the inflammatory process subsides. If the fluid collection becomes infected, a pancreatic abscess results. If not, the fluid is retained by the surrounding organs as a pseudocyst. The second mechanism typically follows trauma and is caused by ductal obstruction that leads to a retention cyst. Pseudocysts occur in about 2% of all cases of acute pancreatitis, and over 85% are singular. Pseudocyst formation presents several weeks after the episode of acute pancreatitis, making de novo presentation in the ICU somewhat uncommon. However, patients are frequently readmitted to a critical care facility when increased epigastric pain, fever, and amylase elevation occur after initial therapy for pancreatitis. Pain is the most common finding, but a few patients have a palpable mass, jaundice, or weight loss. A CT scan is the procedure of choice for establishing the diagnosis, though serial ultrasonography is useful for determining changes in the size of the pseudocyst. Infection, rupture, and hemorrhage are the major complications of pancreatic pseudocysts. Many resolve spontaneously, though internal drainage via cystoenterostomy may be required. Critical care management is similar to that for acute pancreatitis, with particular requirements for parenteral nutritional support and treatment of infectious complications.

Acosta JM, Ledesma CL: Gallstone migration as a cause of acute pancreatitis. N Engl J Med 1974;290:484–7.

Acosta JM: Early surgery for acute gallstone pancreatitis: Evaluation of a systematic approach. Surgery 1978;83:367–70.

Agarwal N, Pitchumoni CS: Assessment of severity in acute pancreatitis. Am J Gastroenterol 1991;86:1385–91.

Balthazar EJ et al: Acute pancreatitis: Value of CT in establishing prognosis. Radiology 1990;174:331–6.

Beger HG et al: Necrosectomy and postoperative local lavage in necrotizing pancreatitis. Br J Surg 1988;75:207–12.

Blamey SL et al: Prognostic factors in acute pancreatitis. Gut 1984;25:1340–6.

Block S et al: Identification of pancreas necrosis in severe acute pancreatitis: Imaging procedures versus clinical staging. Gut 1986;27:1035–42.

Boon P et al: Pancreatic encephalopathy: A case report and review of the literature. Clin Neurol Neurosurg 1991;93:137–41.

Cotton PB: Pancreas divisum. Pancreas 1988;3:245–7.

De Coninck B et al: Scintigraphy with Indium–labelled leukocytes in acute pancreatitis. Acta Gastroenterol Belg 1991;54:176–83.

Di Carlo V et al: Hemodynamic and metabolic impairment in acute pancreatitis. World J Surg 1981;5:329–39.

Fink AS et al: Indolent presentation of pancreatic abscess. Arch Surg 1988;123:1067–72.

Freeny PC: Angio–CT diagnosis and detection of complications of acute pancreatitis. Hepatogastroenterology 1991;38:109–15.

Friedman AD et al: Pancreatic enlargement in alcoholic pancreatitis: Prevalence and natural history. J Clin Gastroenterol 1991;6:666–72.

Imrie CW et al: A single–centre double–blind trial of Trasylol therapy in primary acute pancreatitis. Br J Surg 1978;65:337–41.

Imrie CW et al: Arterial hypoxia in acute pancreatitis. Br J Surg 1977;64:185–8.

Kivisaari L et al: A new method for the diagnosis of acute haemorrhagic–necrotizing pancreatitis using contrast enhanced CT. Gastrointest Radiol 1984;9:27–30.

Kloppel G et al: Human acute pancreatitis: Its pathogenesis in the light of immunocytochemical and ultrastructural findings of acinar cells. Virchows Arch [A] 1986;409:791–803.

Larvin M, Chalmers AG, McMahon MJ: Dynamic contrast enhances computed tomography: A precise technique for identifying and localizing pancreatic necrosis. Br Med J 1990; 300:1425–8.

Leese T et al: Multicentre clinical trial of low volume fresh frozen plasma in acute pancreatitis. Br J Surg 1987;74:907–11.

Malfertheiner P, Kemmer TP: Clinical picture and diagnosis of acute pancreatitis. Hepatogastroenterology 1991;38:97–100.

McKay AJ et al: Is an early ultrasound scan of value in acute pancreatitis? Br J Surg 1982;69:369–72.

Meyer P et al: Role of imaging technics in the classification of acute pancreatitis. Dig Dis 1992;10:330–34.

Moulton JS: The radiologic assessment of acute pancreatitis and its complications. Pancreas 1991;6(Suppl 1):S13–22.

Neoptolemos JP et al: ERCP findings and the role of endoscopic sphincterotomy in acute gallstone pancreatitis. Br J Surg 1988;75:954–60.

Neoptolemos JP et al: The role of clinical and biochemical criteria and endoscopic retrograde cholangiopancreatography in the urgent diagnosis of common bile duct stones in acute pancreatitis. Surgery 1987;100:732–42.

Pemberton JH et al: Controlled open lesser sac drainage for pancreatic abscess. Ann Surg 1986;203:600–4.

Pisters PWT, Ranson JHC: Nutritional support for acute pancreatitis. Surg Gynecol Obstet 1992;175:275–84.

Pitchumoni CS, Agarwal N, Jain NK: Systemic complications of acute pancreatitis. Am J Gastroenterol 1988;83:597–606.

Planche NE et al: Effects of intravenous alcohol on pancreatic and biliary secretion in man. Dig Dis Sci 1982;27:449–53.

Ranson JH et al: Prognostic signs and non-operative peritoneal lavage in acute pancreatitis. Surg Gynecol Obstet 1976;143:209–19.

Ranson JH et al: Prognostic signs and the role of operative management in acute pancreatitis. Surg Gynecol Obstet 1974;139:69–81.

Ranson JH et al: Respiratory complications in acute pancreatitis. Ann Surg 1974;179:557–66.

Safrany L, Cotton PB: A preliminary report: Urgent duodenoscopic sphincterotomy for acute gallstone pancreatitis. Surgery 1981;89:424–8.

Saluja AK et al: Pancreatic duct obstruction in rabbits causes digestive zymogen and lysosomal enzyme colocalization. J Clin Invest 1989;84:1260–6.

Schmidt E, Schmidt FW: Advances in the enzyme diagnosis of pancreatic diseases. Clin Biochem 1990;23:383–94.

Stanten R, Frey CF: Comprehensive management of acute necrotizing pancreatitis and pancreatic abscess. Arch Surg 1990; 125:1269–74.

Steer ML: How and where does acute pancreatitis begin? Arch Surg 1992;127:1350–3.

Vincent JL, De Backer D: Initial management of circulatory shock as prevention of MSOF. Crit Care Clin 1989;5: 369–78.

BOWEL OBSTRUCTION

ESSENTIALS OF DIAGNOSIS

- *Colicky abdominal pain.*
- *Emesis.*
- *Dehydration.*
- *Peristaltic "tinkles and rushes" on abdominal auscultation.*
- *Air-fluid levels on abdominal x-ray.*

General Considerations

Bowel obstructions are common among critically ill patients and may be the underlying reason for ICU admission or may develop as part of another disease process. Obstructions of the small bowel may be mechanical or paralytic. Mechanical obstructions occur when a physical impediment to the aboral progress of intestinal contents is present. Paralytic ileus (functional obstruction) occurs when an underlying disease process interferes with normal peristalsis. Metabolic derangements, neurogenic causes, drug effects, and peritonitis are the most common causes of paralytic ileus. Mechanical obstruction can be divided into simple obstructions, involving only the bowel lumen; and strangulated obstructions, which impair blood supply and lead to necrosis of the intestinal wall. A simple obstruction takes place at just one location. When the bowel lumen is occluded in two or more locations, a closed-loop obstruction is created. Closed-loop obstructions are often associated with strangulation because blood supply may be compromised.

Adhesions from previous abdominal surgery are the most common cause of small bowel obstruction. Onset is usually insidious, with abdominal bloating and crampy abdominal pain. External hernias through the abdominal wall that become incarcerated are the second most common cause of small bowel obstruction. Internal hernias can also occur at the obturator foramen, through the diaphragm, or at the foramen epiploicum (Winslow). Defects caused by surgery such as those adjacent to stomas also are potential sites for the formation of internal hernias.

Neoplasms within or extrinsic to the small bowel may produce obstruction directly or by mass effect. Such tumors may serve as the lead point for an intussusception. Although rare in adults, intussusception may occur without a lesion serving as a lead point. An invagination occurs in which one loop of bowel folds into another and produces colicky pain, passage of blood per rectum, and a palpable abdominal mass.

Volvulus is produced when mobile bowel rotates around a fixed point. This is frequently the consequence of congenital abnormalities or acquired adhesions. Obstruction typically occurs abruptly and leads to intestinal strangulation if not relieved quickly. Sigmoid and cecal volvulus of the colon is significantly more common than small bowel volvulus.

Other less common causes of small bowel obstruction include gallstone ileus, ingested foreign bodies, inflammatory bowel disease, stricture due to radiation therapy, cystic fibrosis, and posttraumatic hematoma. Gallstone ileus occurs in patients with cholelithiasis who develop a fistula between the gallbladder and a loop of small bowel, typically the duodenum. As the gallstone progresses distally, it produces a pattern of intermittent small bowel obstruction at different levels, referred to as "tumbling" obstruction. Air in the biliary tree on abdominal x-ray is the key to the diagnosis.

When the small bowel is obstructed, distention with gas and fluid occurs proximally. Swallowed air is the major cause of distention. This is due to the high nitrogen content in room air, which is not well absorbed by the mucosa. Bacterial fermentation produces other gases also, such as methane. Inflammation leads to transudation of fluid from the extracellular space into the bowel lumen and peritoneal cavity. As the proximal lumen distends and fluid accumulates, the bidirectional flow of salt and water is disrupted and secretion is enhanced. Other substances such as prostaglandins and endotoxins released by bacterial proliferation in the static lumen further the process. Fluid losses may be so severe that hypotension results and may ultimately lead to cardiovascular collapse unless recognized and treated expeditiously.

Vomiting usually accompanies small bowel obstruction and becomes progressively more feculent as the illness progresses. Peristaltic "rushes" are the auscultatory hallmark of this problem. Aspiration of vomitus may lead to severe pneumonia and respiratory distress. Respiration is adversely affected by abdominal distention and impaired diaphragmatic excursion.

Closed-loop obstruction is a feared consequence of complete mechanical obstruction. When it occurs, no outlet for the accumulated intraluminal contents exists, and perforation of the bowel may occur. Strangulation rarely results from progressive distention, though venous outflow becomes significantly impaired as the bowel and mesentery continue to distend. This ultimately results in intestinal gangrene and intraluminal bleeding. Free perforation occurs as a consequence of gangrene, releasing the highly toxic stagnant intraluminal mixture of bacterial products, live bacteria, necrotic tissue, and blood. There are no specific historical, physical, or laboratory findings that exclude the possibility of strangulation in complete small bowel obstruction, which occurs in approximately one-third of cases. The early appearance of shock, gross hematemesis, and profound leukocytosis suggests the presence of a strangulated obstruction.

Clinical Features

A. Symptoms and Signs

Obstruction of the proximal small bowel usually presents with vomiting. The extent of associated abdominal pain is variable and is usually described as intermittent or colicky with a crescendo-decrescendo pattern. When the obstruction is located in the mid or high small bowel (jejunum and proximal ileum), the pain may be more constant. As the site of involvement progresses distally, poorly localized crampy pain and abdominal distention become more common (Figure 14–1).

In the early stages of obstruction, vital signs are normal. As loss of fluid and electrolytes continues, dehydration occurs, manifested as tachycardia and postural hypotension. Body temperature is usually normal but may be mildly elevated. Abdominal distention is minimal or absent initially. It is more pronounced with distal obstruction and when more proximal lesions have been allowed to progress without decompression. Dilated loops of small bowel may be visible beneath the abdominal wall in thin patients. Characteristic peristaltic rushes, gurgles, and high-pitched tinkles may be audible and occur in synchrony with cramping pain.

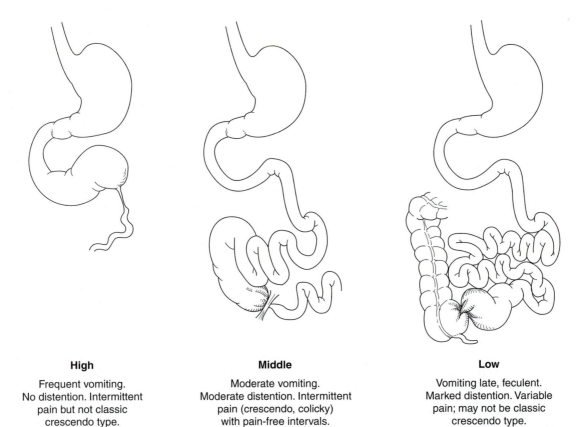

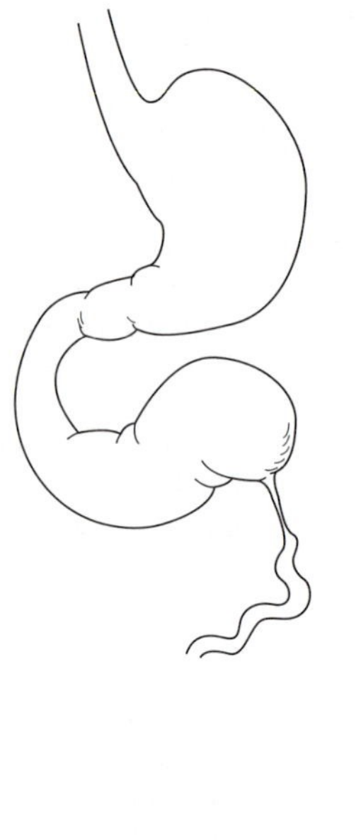

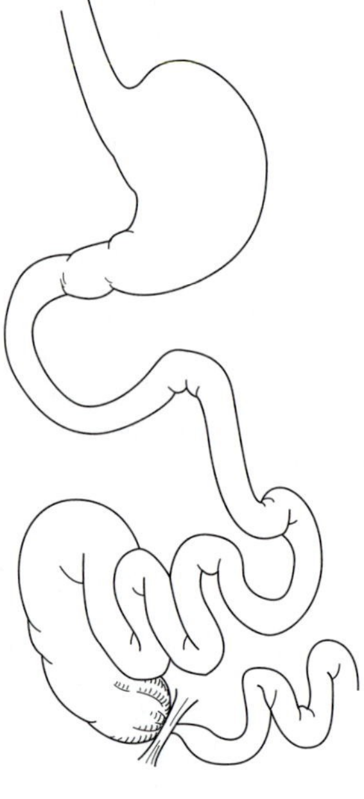

Middle
Moderate vomiting.
Moderate distention. Intermittent
pain (crescendo, colicky)
with pain-free intervals.

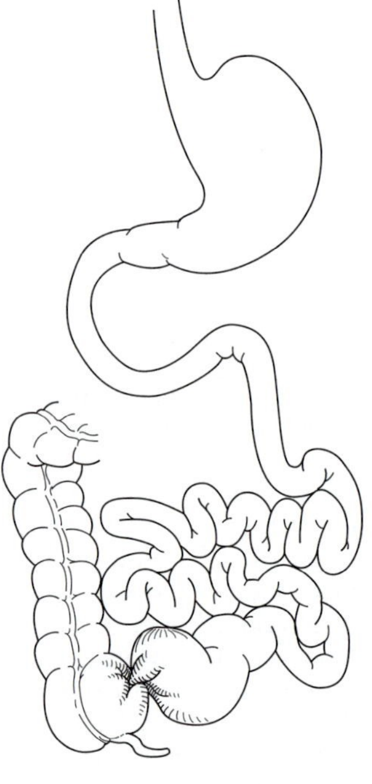

Figure 14–1. Small bowel obstruction. Variable manifestations of obstruction depend upon the level of blockage of the small bowel. (Reproduced, with permission, from Way LW, Doherty GM (editors): *Current Surgical Diagnosis & Treatment,* 11th ed. McGraw-Hill, 2002.)

Rectal examination is usually normal. Abdominal wall hernias should be sought.

B. Laboratory Findings

Early in the process, laboratory findings are normal. With progression, there is hemoconcentration, leukocytosis, and electrolyte abnormalities whose extent and nature depend in part upon the level of obstruction present. Increases in serum amylase are common.

C. Imaging Studies

On plain abdominal films, a ladder-like pattern of dilated small bowel loops and air-fluid levels will be noted, particularly in distal obstruction. The colon may not contain gas. If a gallstone precipitated the event, it may be noted on the film, or air may be seen in the biliary tree. When strangulation and necrosis occur, loss of mucosal regularity, gas within the bowel wall, and "thumbprinting" of the bowel wall occur. On rare occasions, gas may be seen within the portal vein. Free air on an upright chest x-ray is highly suggestive of intestinal perforation.

Contrast studies are usually not required and should not be performed because of the risk of barium peritonitis if a perforation is present. However, in patients with high-grade partial obstructions who are poor surgical risks, administration of a dilute barium mixture through the nasogastric tube can be used to determine whether a residual lumen is still present for the passage of gas and liquid contents.

Differential Diagnosis

Ileus is a prominent feature of the differential diagnosis. It can be caused by a number of intra-abdominal and retroperitoneal processes, including intestinal ischemia, ureteral colic, pelvic fractures, and back injuries. It may occur after routine abdominal surgery. If paralytic ileus is present, the pain is usually not as severe and tends to be more constant.

Obstipation and abdominal distention characterize obstruction of the large intestine. Vomiting seldom occurs, and the pain is less colicky. The diagnosis is usually made on the basis of x-ray findings that show colonic dilation proximal to the point of obstruction.

Small bowel obstruction can be confused with acute gastroenteritis, acute appendicitis, and acute pancreatitis. Strangulating obstructions may be mimicked by acute pancreatitis, ischemic enteritis, or mesenteric vascular occlusion due to venous thrombosis.

Paralytic ileus must be differentiated from mechanical obstruction. Radiographic findings usually show a more diffuse pattern of air-fluid levels without a distinct cutoff point. These patients may be very ill with other systemic diseases or may be apparently well with seemingly minor electrolyte abnormalities. Pseudo-obstruction is particularly common among patients with diabetes who are recovering from an episode of ketoacidosis or who have recently undergone intra-abdominal surgery. Treatment of pseudo-obstruction is directed at the disease process causing the ileus. Metoclopramide may be helpful once the presence of mechanical obstruction has been excluded.

Treatment

A. Supportive Measures

Partial small bowel obstructions may be treated with intravenous hydration and nasogastric suction if the patient continues to pass stool and flatus. Fluid and electrolyte losses are corrected with balanced salt solutions. Isotonic solutions should be used to treat hemoconcentration. The extent of fluid resuscitation is best guided by urine output, though in elderly patients or those with cardiopulmonary disease a pulmonary artery flotation catheter is advisable. If strangulation is suspected, broad-spectrum antibiotics should be administered promptly.

B. Surgery

Planning for surgery should be started concurrently with fluid and electrolyte therapy because the patient must be fully resuscitated before operation commences. If obstruction is due to a simple obstructing band or adhesion, lysis is usually all that is required. When closed-loop and strangulated obstructions are present, intestinal resection may be necessary. The major problem at surgery is distinguishing viable from necrotic bowel. In severe cases, patients may have to be returned to the operating room within 24–48 hours for a "second-look" procedure to make certain that all remaining bowel is viable.

Prognosis

The mortality rate for simple obstruction is almost 2%. It increases to about 8% if strangulation is present and surgery is performed within 36 hours after presentation—and to 25% if operation is delayed beyond that point.

Cheadle WG, Garr EE, Richardson JD: The importance of early diagnosis of small bowel obstruction. Am Surg 1988;54:565–9.

Frazee RC et al: Volvulus of the small intestine. Ann Surg 1988;208:565–8.

Pain JA, Collier D S, Hanka R: Small bowel obstruction: Computer-assisted prediction of strangulation at presentation. Br J Surg 1987;74:981–3.

Pickleman J, Lee RM: The management of patients with suspected early postoperative small bowel obstruction. Ann Surg 1989;210:216–9.

OBSTRUCTION OF THE LARGE BOWEL

ESSENTIALS OF DIAGNOSIS

- *Constipation or obstipation.*
- *Abdominal distention and tenderness.*
- *Abdominal pain.*
- *Nausea and vomiting (late).*
- *Characteristic x-ray findings.*

General Considerations

About 15% of intestinal obstructions involve the large bowel. The sigmoid colon is most commonly involved. When complete obstruction is present, carcinoma is usually the cause. Other causes include diverticular disease, volvulus, inflammatory disorders, benign tumors, and fecal impaction. Obstructive bands from adhesions and intussusception are rare causes of large bowel obstruction.

If obstruction occurs at the level of the cecum, the signs and symptoms will be similar to those of small bowel obstruction. With more distal colonic obstruction, physical findings will depend on the competence of the ileocecal valve. A form of closed-loop obstruction will occur if the colon cannot decompress itself in retrograde fashion through the ileocecal valve into the small bowel.

Colonic distention is a progressive process in which intraluminal pressures can reach very high levels that can impair the circulation and lead to gangrene and perforation.

Clinical Features

A. Symptoms and Signs

Patients typically complain of a deep-seated cramping pain referred to the hypogastrium. Lesions of fixed portions of the colon (cecum, hepatic flexure, and splenic flexure) radiate anteriorly. Pain from obstruction of the sigmoid colon usually radiates to the left lower quadrant. Severe continuous pain suggests intestinal ischemia. When a progressive process is responsible, the obstruction may develop insidiously, though careful questioning often reveals signs of chronic disease such as a change in stool caliber, frequency of defecation, and dark or black feces.

The usual feature of complete obstruction is constipation or obstipation. Vomiting is a late finding and may not occur if the ileocecal valve does not allow contents to reflux back into the small intestine. Feculent vomiting is a late manifestation.

Abdominal distention with peristaltic waves radiating across the abdominal wall may be observed if the patient is thin. On auscultation, high-pitched metallic tinkling and associated rushes and gurgles can be heard. Localized tenderness or a nontender palpable mass may indicate a strangulated closed loop. Occult blood on rectal examination may be due to carcinoma, while fresh blood is characteristic of diverticular disease and intussusception.

B. Endoscopy

Sigmoidoscopy and colonoscopy are often beneficial in establishing the diagnosis and may be therapeutic if sigmoid volvulus is present. Care must be exercised when advancing the endoscope to prevent accidental perforation of an attenuated colonic wall.

C. Imaging Studies

Plain abdominal x-rays reveal a distended colonic segment. With low sigmoid or rectal obstructions, the entire colon may be dilated. If the ileocecal valve is incompetent, retrograde decompression will cause distention of the terminal ileum.

The diagnosis is confirmed by barium enema. Water-soluble contrast medium should be used if strangulation or perforation is suspected. Barium is contraindicated in the presence of suspected colonic perforation.

Differential Diagnosis

It is important to differentiate small bowel obstruction from colonic obstruction. With the latter, onset is typically slower and there is less pain. Vomiting is very unusual with colonic obstruction despite considerable abdominal distention. Plain abdominal x-rays are essential to the differential diagnosis, and adjunctive contrast studies are sometimes helpful.

Treatment

The primary goal of therapy is decompression of the obstructed segment and prevention of perforation. Operation is almost always required in cases of mechanical obstruction. The surgical procedure depends upon the lesion present, the status of the patient, the extent of colonic dilation, and whether there is evidence of perforation. In general, proximal diversion (colostomy) is required to decompress the dilated colon. Simultaneous or subsequent excision of the obstructing lesion is required before colonic continuity can be reestablished.

Prognosis

The prognosis is dependent upon the age and general condition of the patient as well as the extent of vascular impairment of the bowel, the presence or absence of perforation, the cause of obstruction, and the promptness of surgical management. Mortality rates are about 20% overall. If the cecum perforates, mortality rates of 40% can be expected. In the case of colonic obstruction secondary to carcinoma, the prognosis is worse.

Buechter KJ et al: Surgical management of the acutely obstructed colon: A review of 127 cases. Am J Surg 1988;156:163–8.

Gosche JR, Sharpe JN, Larson GM: Colonoscopic decompression for pseudo-obstruction of the colon. Am Surg 1989;55:111–5.

Harig JM et al: Treatment of acute nontoxic megacolon during colonoscopy: Tube placement versus simple decompression. Gastrointest Endosc 1988;34:23–7.

Sloyer AF et al: Ogilvie's syndrome: Successful management without colonoscopy. Dig Dis Sci 1988;33:1391–6.

ADYNAMIC (PARALYTIC) ILEUS

ESSENTIALS OF DIAGNOSIS

- *Continuous abdominal pain.*
- *Vomiting.*
- *Abdominal distention.*
- *Obstipation.*
- *Precipitating factor.*
- *Radiographic evidence of gas and fluid in the small or large bowel.*

General Considerations

Adynamic ileus is often associated with neurogenic or muscular impairment of small or large bowel function. This may be due to a variety of causes such as alimentary tract surgery, a ruptured viscus, hemorrhage, pancreatitis, or peritonitis. Other causes include anoxic injury, anticholinergic medications, opioids, vertebral fractures, renal colic, injuries of the spinal cord, severe infections of either the thoracic or the abdominal cavity, uremia, diabetic coma, and electrolyte abnormalities.

Recent abdominal surgery is a principal cause of adynamic ileus among critical care patients. In the 24 hours following surgery, motility within the small bowel returns to normal while gastric function will return after approximately 24 hours. The colon requires several days to regain normal motility. The pain associated with ileus is constant but not severe or colicky, as it is with mechanical obstruction. Mild abdominal tenderness is noted along with distention. If this is due to an intraperitoneal inflammatory process, signs and symptoms of that disorder are usually present. Plain films of the abdomen are extremely helpful.

Similar to paralytic ileus of the small bowel, pseudo-obstruction (Ogilvie's syndrome) of the colon may occur. This is a severe form of ileus that often arises in bedridden patients who have serious systemic illnesses. The abdomen is usually silent, and abdominal cramping is not present. Tenderness may be noted. Plain films show a dilated colon that may reach alarming proportions. The entire colon may contain gas, but the distention is typically localized to the right colon with cutoff at the splenic flexure. Contrast studies may be required to prove the absence of obstruction, but instillation of radiopaque material must be stopped as soon as the dilated colon is reached. The risk of cecal perforation is very high in patients with pseudo-obstruction. Decompression of the colon should be attempted as quickly as possible, using a fiberoptic colonoscope. Recurrence rates are as high as 20%. Initial colonoscopic decompression is successful in 90% of patients. Percutaneous cecostomy is reserved as an option for decompression if colonoscopy fails.

Clinical Features

A. Symptoms and Signs

Mild to moderate abdominal pain is usually present. It is continuous rather than colicky and is often associated with emesis, which may become feculent. Symptoms of the underlying condition may also be present, such as prostration from a ruptured viscus. Dehydration is usually present as a consequence of fluid translocation into distended loops of bowel.

Massive abdominal distention and localized tenderness are common. Bowel sounds are absent or decreased.

B. Laboratory Findings

Hemoconcentration and electrolyte deficits occur with prolonged vomiting. Elevated serum amylase levels and leukocytosis are usually present.

C. Imaging Studies

The specific radiographic finding noted on flat plate upright abdominal films is gas-filled loops of intestine. Air may even be present in the rectum. Air-fluid levels in the distended bowel are common. A contrast enema or barium swallow with subsequent small bowel "follow-through" films may be helpful in differentiating adynamic ileus from mechanical obstruction.

Differential Diagnosis

Idiopathic pseudo-obstruction is usually seen in teenagers or young adults and is characterized by symptoms of small bowel obstruction that recur but never produce evidence of organic obstruction on x-ray. Treatment is with nasogastric intubation and suction.

Intravenous fluids and parenteral nutrition are required. Occasionally, colonoscopic decompression or cecostomy is useful. The variant known as chronic pseudo-obstruction is associated with cramping abdominal pain, abdominal distention, and vomiting. There may be involvement of the esophagus, the stomach, the small bowel, the colon, or the urinary bladder. All or some of these patients have abnormal motility with sparing of some portions of the alimentary tract. Metoclopramide is often helpful.

Treatment

A. Supportive Measures

Most cases of ileus in the postoperative period respond to restriction of oral intake and nasogastric suction. Fluid and electrolyte replacement is essential.

B. Decompression

When colonic dilation is present, colonoscopy may be valuable. Use of a rectal tube was common practice at one time but has now been largely abandoned.

C. Surgery

If there is a failure of conservative therapy, surgery may be necessary. Operation is performed to decompress the bowel either by enterostomy or by cecostomy and to exclude mechanical obstruction. Bowel biopsy may be performed to identify neurogenic causes.

Prognosis

The initiating disorder will often dictate the prognosis. Adynamic ileus may resolve without specific therapy. Decompression usually helps return bowel function to normal.

Current Controversies & Unresolved Issues

Recent studies have reported the use of new agents in the treatment of adynamic ileus. Cisapride, 1 mg/kg/d in four divided doses, has been used with good success for colonic pseudo-obstruction. Erythromycin has also been investigated as a potential agent for shortening the period of postoperative ileus after intra-abdominal surgery. A prospective study comparing placebo with erythromycin (250 mg intravenously every 8 hours for nine doses) found no effect of the drug in reducing time to passage of flatus, first bowel movement, or total hospital stay. Intravenous lidocaine has also been found to shorten the duration of paralytic ileus, presumably by suppressing inhibitory gastrointestinal reflexes. Additional trials of all of these agents are required before they can be either recommended or discredited.

Bonacini M et al: Effect of intravenous erythromycin on postoperative ileus. Am J Gastroenterol 1993;88:208–11.

Dorudi S, Berry AR, Kettlewell MG: Acute colonic pseudo-obstruction. Br J Surg 1992;79:99–103.

Jetmore AB et al: Ogilvie's syndrome: Colonoscopic decompression and analysis of predisposing factors. Dis Colon Rectum 1992;35:1135–42.

MacColl C et al: Treatment of acute colonic pseudoobstruction (Ogilvie's syndrome) with cisapride. Gastroenterology 1990;98:773–6.

Rimback G, Cassuto J, Tollesson PO: Treatment of postoperative paralytic ileus by intravenous lidocaine infusion. Anesth Analg 1990;70:414–9.

Vantrappen G: Acute colonic pseudo-obstruction. Lancet 1993; 341:152–3.

DIARRHEA & MALABSORPTION

Critically ill patients often develop diarrhea from a number of causes including overly aggressive enteral feeding, infectious diarrhea, and malabsorption. After gastrointestinal resection, short gut syndromes and exocrine insufficiency may contribute. These common causes are discussed in the next several sections.

PANCREATIC INSUFFICIENCY

Following pancreatic surgery, pancreatectomy, or pancreatitis, pancreatic exocrine insufficiency can develop. Varying degrees of insufficiency may be present without overt symptoms. Following total pancreatectomy, malabsorption of 70% of dietary fat is common. However, in the face of a normal pancreatic remnant, some resections have little or no effect on fat absorption.

Patients with pancreatic insufficiency have increased fecal fat and decreased serum cholesterol. Steatorrhea manifests itself as frequent bulky light-colored stools. A loss of 90% of pancreatic exocrine function is required before such findings appear. If the patient retains 2–10% of normal pancreatic function, steatorrhea is mild to moderate. If less than 2% of normal function remains, steatorrhea is severe.

Pancreatic insufficiency affects fat absorption more than that of proteins or carbohydrates. Malabsorption secondary to fat loss or vitamin deficiency is rarely a problem. B vitamins, which are water-soluble, are absorbed through the small intestine. Fat-soluble vitamins depend on bile salt micelle formation for solubilization and do not require pancreatic enzymes for absorption. Vitamin B_{12} deficiency occurs rarely but, when present, is an indication for exogenous enzyme replacement.

Diagnosis

A. Secretin or Cholecystokinin Test

The duodenum is intubated and pancreatic juice recovered after intravenous injection of synthetic or purified secretin or cholecystokinin. Optimally, pancreatic fluid bicarbonate should exceed 80 meq/L and bicarbonate production should be greater than 15 meq every 30 minutes.

B. Pancreolauryl Test

A meal containing fluorescein dilaurate is ingested, and the subsequent urinary excretion of fluorescein is measured. Pancreatic esterase is responsible for the absorption and release of fluorescein. The test is both specific and sensitive and is the best modality for testing pancreatic exocrine function.

C. PABA Excretion (Bentiromide Test)

The synthetic peptide bentiromide is administered (1 g orally), and the urinary excretion of aromatic amines is measured. Patients with chronic pancreatitis excrete about 50% of the normal amount of the amines.

D. Fecal Fat (Balance) Measurement

A diet containing 75–100 g of fat—measured and given in the same amount each day—is ingested daily for 5 days. Excretion of less than 7% of the ingested fat is normal. Fat excretion of more than 25% of the total daily intake suggests significant steatorrhea.

Treatment

The diet should provide 3000–6000 kcal daily. Patients with steatorrhea may not have diarrhea. Dietary fat restriction is intended primarily to control diarrhea. If a patient does have diarrhea and is restricted to 50 g of fat, the daily allotment of fat should be increased until the diarrhea reappears.

Pancreatic enzyme replacement can be accomplished with exogenous extracts. With these formulations, 30,000–50,000 units of lipase can be distributed over several feedings during the day. If malabsorption does not improve with enzymes alone, the difficulty is usually due to destruction of the administered lipase by gastric acid. To alleviate this problem, an H_2 receptor-blocking agent is given and an enteric-coated lipase formulation provided. When lipase is administered in this form, the gastric pH is less likely to affect the enzyme.

Caloric supplementation may be given in the form of powder or as an oil containing medium-chain triglycerides (MCTs). The fatty acids are more readily absorbed in this preparation than when long-chain triglycerides are used. The MCT oil is associated with bloating, diarrhea, nausea and vomiting, and very poor patient acceptance.

2. Lactase Deficiency

Lactase deficiency is a common problem among critically ill patients. The symptoms are variable and can range from minor abdominal bloating to distention, flatulence, and cramping pain. Some patients, however, have severe diarrhea in response to only a small amount of lactose. Although a lactose tolerance test is available, clinical suspicion and relation of the diarrhea to the time of refeeding usually suggests the diagnosis. Some illnesses such as gastroenteritis may injure the microvilli and lead to a temporary lactase deficiency. Several congenital defects of disaccharidase have been described. Most patients will give a history of dietary problems with milk products, but the difficulties occasionally surface at times of physiologic stress. They include sucrose-isomaltose and glucose-galactose intolerance. Disaccharide deficiency secondary to short bowel syndrome, celiac disease, giardiasis, ulcerative colitis, cystic fibrosis, and postgastrectomy problems may be noted. In all cases, removal of lactose from the diet and use of a non-lactose-based enteral nutritional supplement usually solves the problem.

Choosing and using a pancreatic enzyme supplement. Drug Ther Bull 1992;30:37–40.

Gillanders L et al: Dietary management of the patient with massive enterectomy. N Z Med J 1990;103:322–3.

Hammer HF et al: Carbohydrate malabsorption: Its measurement and its contribution to diarrhea. J Clin Invest 1990; 86:1936–44.

Nightingale JM et al: Short bowel syndrome. Digestion 1990; 45:77–83.

Romano TJ, Dobbins JW: Evaluation of the patient with suspected malabsorption. Gastroenterol Clin North Am 1989;18: 467–83.

DIARRHEA

Diarrhea is defined as an increase in the fluidity, frequency, or quantity (> 200 g/d) of bowel movements. Several factors to be considered in the evaluation of diarrhea may influence the frequency or even the fluidity of bowel movements. Malabsorption or excessive secretion of water usually results in passage of stools that contain excess water and are therefore considered as diarrhea. The best index is daily stool weight. Therefore, one may have small-volume diarrhea, large-volume diarrhea, and other variants that depend on the content of blood, mucus, or exudate. The various types of diarrhea are listed in Table 14–2. Common causes of diarrhea among patients in an ICU include psychogenic

Table 14–2. Classification of diarrhea.

I. Diarrhea secondary to excessive fecal water:
  A. Secretory diarrhea: Produced by excessive secretion by the mucosal cells of the intestine. **Causes:** cholera, toxigenic *Escherichia coli* infections, Zollinger-Ellison syndrome, and VIPoma.
  B. Osmotic diarrhea: Produced by an excess of water-soluble molecules in the lumen of the bowel, which cause osmotic retention of intraluminal water. **Causes:** Abuse or surreptitious use of laxatives, administration of magnesium hydroxide, or undigested disaccharides.
  C. Exudative disease: Produced by intestinal loss of serum proteins, blood, mucus, or pus due to abnormal mucosal permeability.
  D. Accelerated transport: Impaired contact between intestinal chyme absorbing surface, which results in rapid transport. Common in short bowel syndromes.
  E. Motility disturbances: Causes: Amyloidosis, scleroderma, diabetes mellitus, and bacterial overgrowth.
II. Diarrhea not secondary to excessive fecal water:
  A. Small, frequent, and painful evacuations caused by partial obstruction of the left colon or rectum.

disorders, drugs (especially antacids, antibiotics, and metoclopramide), intestinal infections, cholestatic syndromes (hepatitis, bile duct obstruction, steatorrhea), malabsorption (short bowel syndrome, afferent loop syndrome), diabetic neuropathy, hyperthyroidism, and immunodeficiency.

Diagnosis

In general, diarrheal episodes are self-limiting, and diagnostic testing is not necessary. However, in patients with unexplained severe or chronic diarrhea, etiologic evaluation may become necessary. Review of the patient's chart, evaluation of drugs being used, and physical examination are often all that are needed to establish the cause. Examination of stool for polymorphonuclear cells and parasites and culture for bacterial pathogens may be required. A sample for culture is best obtained with the sigmoidoscope. Rectal biopsy may be helpful and even necessary, especially when *Entamoeba histolytica* infection is suspected. Assays of stool for *Clostridium difficile* toxin are highly accurate and establish the diagnosis of pseudomembranous enterocolitis.

Treatment

Before specific therapy for diarrhea is begun, it is important to make certain that fluid losses have been replaced and electrolyte imbalances corrected. Malnutrition should be managed with parenteral nutrition.

Antidiarrheal agents should be used with great caution and attention to the patient's critical care history. The antidiarrheal agent most commonly used is bismuth subsalicylate. This can be given in liquid or tablet form. The usual dose is 30 mL up to eight times a day. Opioid analogs are also popular; the most frequently prescribed form is diphenoxylate with atropine, one tablet three or four times daily as needed. This drug is contraindicated in patients with jaundice or pseudomembranous or endotoxin colitis and must be used with caution in patients with advanced liver disease or those who are addiction-prone. Concurrent use of this medication with monoamine oxidase inhibitors may precipitate a hypertensive crisis. A secondary drug is loperamide, 4 mg initially and then 2 mg for each loose stool to a maximum dose of 16 mg/d. Loperamide is effective in both acute and chronic diarrhea. Opioids such as paregoric and codeine phosphate were popular in the past but have little role in critically ill patients.

Clonidine, when administered as a 1-mg patch, is useful in patients who have diabetes or cryptosporidiosis. Octreotide acetate is useful when diarrhea is due to carcinoid tumors, VIPoma, or AIDS. It is usually started at a dose of 50 μg subcutaneously once or twice daily. For carcinoid and VIPomas, the required dose may be higher but averages 300 μg/d in two to four divided doses.

Grube BJ, Heimbach DM, Marvin JA: *Clostridium difficile* diarrhea in critically ill burned patients. Arch Surg 1987; 122:655–61.

Pesola GR et al: Hypertonic nasogastric tube feedings: Do they cause diarrhea? Crit Care Med 1990;18:1378–82.

Tibibian N: Diarrhea in critically ill patients. Am Fam Phys 1989;40:135–40.

Infections in the Critically Ill 15

Mallory D. Witt, MD, & Laurie Anne Chu, MD

The management of infected critically ill patients is a challenge for ICU physicians and staff. Patients admitted with symptoms prior to hospitalization are considered to have community-acquired infections, and those who develop infection more than 48 hours following admission are considered to have hospital-acquired, or nosocomial, infections. Seriously ill patients presenting with fever must be quickly evaluated for possible infection, since most are treatable. However, drug fever, hypersensitivity reaction, collagen-vascular disease, neoplastic disease, pulmonary embolism, trauma, burns, pancreatitis, hypothalamic dysfunction, and other noninfectious causes of fever must be considered in the differential diagnosis.

In contrast, some patients may appear to be stable but nonetheless have serious infections. Elderly patients, uremic patients, and patients with end-stage liver disease or those receiving corticosteroids will often fail to mount a significant febrile response even to serious infection. In addition, some infections are notorious for presenting with minimal symptoms—these include infective endocarditis, spontaneous bacterial peritonitis, intra-abdominal abscess, endophthalmitis, and meningitis. In the absence of other symptoms and signs, fever in the asplenic patient, the neutropenic or immunosuppressed patient, the intravenous drug user or alcoholic, and the elderly patient requires a rapid and thorough diagnostic evaluation.

The infectious syndromes that may require direct admission and immediate therapy in the ICU—sepsis, community-acquired pneumonia, urosepsis, infective endocarditis, intra-abdominal infections, and necrotizing soft tissue infections—will be described in the following sections. Special hosts such as patients with diabetes, asplenia, or neutropenia as well as corticosteroid-treated individuals will be discussed, they often have unique presentations and complications. Care of the HIV-infected patient is discussed in another chapter.

This chapter will also focus on other nosocomially-acquired infections that are of great concern to the critical care physician, either because of a high mortality rate, diagnostic challenge, frequency of occurrence, contagiousness, or acquisition of antimicrobial resistance. Two unique disease entities—botulism and tetanus—will also be discussed in this chapter.

SEPSIS

ESSENTIALS OF DIAGNOSIS

- *Wide spectrum of clinical findings ranging from fever, hypothermia, tachycardia, and tachypnea to profound shock and multi-organ failure.*
- *Severe or complicated sepsis: lactic acidosis, ARDS, acute renal failure, DIC, shock, central nervous system dysfunction, or hepatobiliary disease.*
- *May present with altered mental status, unexplained hyperventilation, or tachycardia alone.*
- *Often an identifiable site of infection.*
- *Predisposing risk factors for infection: organ system failure, bed rest, invasive procedures, any antibiotic use, immunocompromised state.*

General Considerations

To avoid ambiguity in interpreting the results of clinical trials and to facilitate communication among clinicians, it has been recommended that specific terminology be used when referring to sepsis and sepsis syndromes. The systemic inflammatory response syndrome (SIRS) is the body's response to various insults, both infectious and noninfectious. Patients with two or more of the following criteria are considered to have SIRS: (1) temperature > 38 °C or < 36 °C, (2) heart rate > 90 beats per minute, (3) respiratory rate > 20 breaths per minute or $PaCO_2$ < 32 mm Hg, (4) white blood cell count > 12,000 cells/μL, < 4000 cells/μL, or > 10% immature (band) forms. Sepsis is defined as the SIRS in response to infection. Severe sepsis is defined as sepsis associated with organ dysfunction, hypoperfusion, or hypotension. Septic shock is the presence of hypotension (despite adequate fluid resuscitation) plus hypoperfusion or perfusion abnormalities. Multiple organ dysfunction syndrome is defined as the presence of altered organ function such that homeostasis cannot be maintained without intervention. The vague terms "sepsis syndrome" and "septicemia" should no longer be used.

Sepsis, severe sepsis, and septic shock can be considered points on a continuum describing increasing severity of an individual patient's systemic response to infection. A prospective observational study demonstrated that, among hospitalized patients meeting the criteria for SIRS, 26% subsequently developed sepsis, 18% developed severe sepsis, and 4% developed septic shock. The interval from SIRS to severe sepsis and septic shock was inversely correlated with the number of SIRS criteria met. The mortality rates of sepsis, severe sepsis, and septic shock were 16%, 20%, and 46%, respectively.

Sepsis and septic shock are common problems encountered in ICUs. Septic shock with multiple organ failure is the most common cause of death in intensive care units. There are currently over 500,000 new episodes of sepsis each year in the United States, as copmared with 1979, when approximately 200,000 cases were reported. The greatest increases occurred in persons over 65 years of age, but increases were noted in all age groups. This increase is due to more aggressive support of seriously ill patients, the care of more immunocompromised patients, utilization of more mechanical and invasive devices (eg, bladder catheters, endotracheal tubes, intravascular catheters) in ICUs, and increased longevity of patients with susceptibility to infection, and increasing numbers of resistant organisms. Given the increasing use of invasive maneuvers in critically ill patients, there is no reason to expect that the number of cases will decrease in the future. The mortality rate from sepsis ranges from 30–50% in published studies, with 100,000–150,000 patients dying each year. The immediate cause of death is usually septic shock or multiple organ failure. Approximately 25% of patients develop at least one of the major morbid responses attributable to sepsis.

Pathophysiology

The complex pathophysiology of sepsis is not completely understood. Sepsis begins with colonization and proliferation of microorganisms at a tissue site. Various host characteristics and organism virulence factors determine both invasiveness and subsequent intensity of the local inflammatory response. Replicating microorganisms release numerous exogenous enzymes and toxins which in turn trigger the release of endogenous mediators, resulting in both local and systemic inflammatory responses. The exogenous substances differ by type of microorganism. In the case of gram-negative bacilli, endotoxin (lipid A) contained in the outer cell membrane is the chief toxic substance that initiates the cascade of events clinically recognized as sepsis or septic shock. Endotoxin activates the complement cascade and Hageman factor, leading to initiation of both coagulation and fibrinolysis. Prekallikrein is converted to kallikrein, resulting in the production of bradykinin, a mediator of hypotension.

Endotoxin, after binding and activation of macrophages, also initiates the production of numerous endogenous cytokines. The biologic effects of these mediators are amplified, causing host injury by way of endothelial inflammation, abnormalities in vascular tone, altered regulation of coagulation, and myocardial depression. Many of these endogenous mediators have been identified: tumor necrosis factor, platelet activating factor, interleukins, interferon, prostaglandins, thromboxane, leukotrienes, complement components C3a and C5a, and others have been shown to mediate and trigger the pathophysiologic events.

Tumor necrosis factor (TNF), probably the key endogenous mediator, acts on a variety of cells and stimulates the production of other cytokines involved with sepsis and septic shock. Plasma TNF concentrations are elevated in both gram-negative and gram-positive sepsis. While endotoxin triggers TNF production in gram-negative sepsis, the stimulus for release of TNF in gram-positive sepsis is unknown. However, recent studies have shown that mediators other than endotoxin can induce TNF production, including IFN-alpha, prostaglandin E_2, immune complexes, and colony-stimulating factors.

Pathophysiologic factors in gram-positive bacterial sepsis are not clearly defined. In the case of *S aureus* strains that cause toxic shock syndrome, toxic shock syndrome toxin-1 (TSST-1) is the principal exogenous mediator. Some virulent strains of group A beta-hemolytic streptococci produce similar toxins.

Microbiologic Etiology

Virtually any microorganism can cause sepsis or septic shock, including bacteria, viruses, protozoa, fungi, spirochetes, and rickettsiae. Bacteria are the most common etiologic agents.

Gram-negative sepsis cannot be distinguished from gram-positive sepsis on the basis of clinical characteristics alone. However, certain epidemiologic, host, and clinical factors increase the likelihood of particular organisms. For example, *E coli* is the most frequently demonstrated etiologic agent of sepsis, largely because the urinary tract is the most commonly recognized source of infection. The incidence of infection caused by other gram-negative bacteria, staphylococci, streptococci, anaerobes, candida, and other organisms is largely determined by epidemiologic and host factors that may be identified by a thorough history and physical examination.

Clinical Features

A. Symptoms and Signs of Sepsis

Sepsis can present with a spectrum of clinical features ranging from fever, tachycardia, and tachypnea to profound shock and multi-organ failure. The challenge to the critical care specialist is to make the diagnosis early in the course of the disease to increase the likelihood of a successful outcome. Early in sepsis, the diagnosis may not be obvious. Moreover, debilitated patients may not exhibit significant symptomatology at the onset of sepsis.

Implicit in the term "sepsis" is a documented site of infection along with systemic signs and symptoms of fever (or hypothermia), tachycardia, and tachypnea (Table 15–1). In more severe or complicated sepsis, there is also impaired organ system function, including lactic acidosis, acute respiratory distress syndrome (ARDS), acute renal failure, disseminated intravascular coagulation (DIC), central nervous system dysfunction, and shock. A systolic blood pressure less than 90 mm Hg or a decrease from baseline of over 40 mm Hg signifies septic shock. Septic shock can be further subclassified into responsive and refractory shock states. Patients who do not respond to aggressive administration of fluid and who require dopamine at a rate of more than 6 μg/kg/min (or other vasopressor agents) are considered to be in refractory shock, which implies a very poor prognosis.

Table 15–1. Consensus Conference Group definitions of stages of sepsis.[1]

Stage	Characteristics
I	Systemic inflammatory response syndrome (SIRS). Two or more of the following: 1. Temperature > 38° C or < 36° C 2. Heart rate > 90 per minute 3. Respiratory rate > 20 per minute 4. White blood cell count > 12,000/μL or < 4000/μL or > 10% bands
II	Sepsis SIRS plus a culture-documented infection
III	Severe sepsis Sepsis plus organ dysfunction, hypotension or hypoperfusion (lactic acidosis, oliguria, hypoxemia, or acute alteration in mental status)
IV	Septic shock Hypotension (despite fluid resuscitation) plus evidence of hypoperfusion

[1]American College of Chest Physicians/Society of Critical Care Medicine Consensus Conference: Definitions for sepsis and organ failure and guidelines for the use of innovative therapies in sepsis. Crit Care Med 1992;20:864–74.

Patients with clinical features of sepsis must be carefully evaluated, with particular attention paid to their immune status, clinical condition, and the presence of specific epidemiologic factors. The main purpose of the physical examination in the septic patient is to identify the source of infection and to note the presence of major morbid states or shock. In particular, a search for a focus of infection that may require surgical drainage should be undertaken, as these patients are unlikely to respond to antibiotics alone.

B. Laboratory Findings

Patients suspected of having sepsis should have relevant cultures obtained to document the infection and laboratory testing to identify the presence of any major morbid states. No single laboratory test is specific for sepsis. An elevated white blood cell count is nonspecific and cannot differentiate infection from other inflammatory or otherwise pathologic states. However, an increase in immature polymorphonuclear white blood cells ("bands") strongly suggests infection. Routine serum electrolytes, blood urea nitrogen, serum creatinine, and liver function tests may assist in determining the site of infection as well as identifying complications of sepsis such as acute renal failure or hepatobiliary dysfunction. Arterial blood gases, plasma lactate, and coagulation tests may demonstrate respiratory insufficiency, metabolic acidosis, and DIC, respectively.

Although most septic patients are intermittently bacteremic or fungemic, only 40% have a pathogen identified by blood cultures. Nevertheless, blood cultures should be obtained in every patient suspected of having sepsis. The laboratory may use special procedures and blood culture equipment to enhance growth and isolation of fungi, including candida. Two sets of blood cultures as well as urine, respiratory secretions, and wound exudates for Gram staining and culture should be collected. If indicated by clinical findings, cerebrospinal fluid, pleural fluid, ascites fluid, and joint fluid should be analyzed as well.

C. Imaging Studies

A chest radiograph may serve to identify pneumonia or ARDS; other studies such as ultrasonography, CT, or MRI may be necessary to identify the site of infection. They are not useful in making an initial diagnosis of sepsis or septic shock.

Differential Diagnosis

Many clinical conditions can resemble sepsis, septic shock, and multiple organ dysfunction syndrome. Patients with severe burns, multiple trauma, severe hemorrhagic or necrotizing pancreatitis, pulmonary emboli, acute myocardial infarction, and various metabolic and hematologic abnormalities may have features that mimic sepsis and its complications.

Treatment

Despite modern therapy, the mortality rate in sepsis is still unacceptably high, ranging from 30–50%; mortality approaches 100% in patients with septic shock or failure of three or more organ systems. However, the mortality rate can be reduced by early diagnosis and prompt initiation of appropriate therapy. Any delay permits the pathophysiologic events in sepsis to proceed, with a concomitant increase in morbidity and mortality.

A. Supportive Care

Treatment of sepsis begins with oxygen and ventilatory support as needed. The PO_2 should be maintained above 60–65 mm Hg with oxygen delivered by cannula, mask, or respirator if necessary.

The administration of intravenous fluids, whether crystalloid or colloid, expands the intravascular volume to correct the relative deficit resulting from vasodilation due to bacterial products or host responses. Several liters of intravenous fluids are usually required over the first 2–6 hours. If cardiogenic pulmonary edema is a concern, pulmonary arterial catheterization and monitoring will clarify the issue and guide the appropriate amount of fluid administration. Hypotension may persist despite fluid replacement because of very low systemic vascular resistance; in some patients, decreased myocardial contractility may contribute. Vasopressor agents should be used to maintain systolic blood pressure above 90 mm Hg. Dopamine is usually chosen, beginning with 3–5 μg/kg/min and increased as necessary. Patients not responding to dopamine may require the addition of norepinephrine in low dosage or other pressor agents. Vasopressors are not effective when fluid replacement has been inadequate.

B. Antibiotics

The next therapeutic challenge is the choice of appropriate antibiotics. All available clinical, epidemiologic, and laboratory data should be considered in making this decision. Rarely is the causative microorganism known at the time treatment for sepsis is initiated, but if the source can be determined and a Gram-stained smear of infected material (eg, sputum, urine, purulent drainage) examined, the long list of possible microorganisms can often be shortened. The following sections will provide a guide to initial antimicrobial selection depending on the potential source of infection. Importantly, these intravenous antibiotics must be given without delay and in appropriate doses. Adjustments for age and for renal and hepatic function are not required for the starting dose of antibiotics.

C. Surgical Drainage

Significant collections of purulent material must be drained and necrotic tissue excised in order to treat sepsis. Surgeons may be reluctant to operate because of the coexistence of acute renal failure, ARDS, or other organ system failure, but the pathophysiologic consequences of sepsis will probably continue unless surgical drainage is initiated.

D. Adjunctive Therapy

Two large studies have concluded that corticosteroids have no role in treatment except when sepsis is complicated by adrenal insufficiency. Naloxone has been shown to transiently increase blood pressure, but administration of this competitive antagonist to opioids and endorphins does not change the outcome of sepsis and septic shock.

A recent large trial comparing monoclonal antibodies to recombinant human activated protein C (drotrecogin alfa [activated]) with placebo in patients with sepsis showed a statistically significant decrease in mortality in the treatment group. Adjunctive treatment with activated protein C should be considered in patients with severe sepsis, defined as evidence of end-organ dysfunction with shock, acidosis, oliguria, or hypoxemia. The mechanism of action is unknown, but activated protein C may modulate coagulation and inflammation associated with severe sepsis.

Current Controversies & Unresolved Issues

A. Antiendotoxin Antibodies

Clinical trials using different antiendotoxin monoclonal antibodies in patients with gram-negative sepsis and septic shock have been published. The agents were given in conjunction with the usual standard aggressive therapy in randomized, placebo-controlled, double-blind fashion. It appears that while some studies showed improved outcome in subsets of patients with gram-negative bacteremia, other trials did not confirm these results, and some trials showed a possible detrimental effect on patients without gram-negative bacteremia. The challenge is to identify very early which patients are truly septic from gram-negative bacilli and which patients are most likely to benefit from antiendotoxin therapy. Antiendotoxin antibodies are not available for clinical purposes.

B. Granulocyte Colony-Stimulating Factor (G-CSF; Filgrastim)

The use of filgrastim has been proposed in an attempt to augment the immune response in sepsis. A multicenter double-blind, placebo-controlled trial in patients with bacterial community-acquired pneumonia using filgrastim versus placebo showed that patients who received filgrastim had more rapid resolution of chest radiograph infiltrates and developed sepsis-related organ failure less frequently. Both of these findings were statistically significant. In another very small placebo-controlled trial of patients with severe pneumonia and sepsis, patients who received filgrastim had a significantly decreased mortality compared with the placebo group. Further studies are needed to identify the patient population that will benefit most from this adjunctive therapy and to determine the optimal dose and timing of administration.

C. Anti-inflammatory Agents

Various nonglucocorticoid anti-inflammatory agents—interleukin-1 receptor antagonists, bradykinin antagonists, platelet-activating factor antagonists, monoclonal antibodies against tumor necrosis factor, soluble tumor necrosis factor receptors, and prostaglandin antagonists—have been investigated in an attempt to abort the systemic inflammatory response. From these various studies, the only conclusions that can be drawn are as follows: In high doses, these anti-inflammatory agents can be harmful in sepsis, and any beneficial effects are likely to be very small. Thus, trials with large numbers of patients to identify possible subgroups of patients who could benefit from such intervention will be needed to show statistically significant improvements in outcome.

American College of Chest Physicians/Society of Critical Care Medicine Consensus Conference: definitions for sepsis and organ failure and guidelines for the use of innovative therapies in sepsis. Crit Care Med 1992;101:1644–55.

Balk RA: Severe sepsis and septic shock: definitions, epidemiology, and clinical manifestations. Crit Care Clin 2000;16:179–92.

Bernard GR et al: Efficacy and safety of recombinant human activated protein C for severe sepsis. N Engl J Med 2001; 344:699–709.

Bone RC: Why sepsis trials fail. JAMA 1996;276:565–6.

Rangel-Frausto MS et al: The natural history of the systemic inflammatory response syndrome (SIRS). JAMA 1995;273: 117–23.

Root RK, Dale DC: Granulocyte colony-stimulating factor and granulocyte-macrophage colony-stimulating factor: comparisons and potential for use in the treatment of infections in nonneutropenic patients. J Infect Dis 1999;179(Suppl 2): S342–52.

Task Force of the American College of Critical Care Medicine, Society of Critical Care Medicine. Practice parameters for hemodynamic support of sepsis in adult patients in sepsis. Crit Care Med 1999;27:639–60.

Vincent JL: New therapies in sepsis. Chest 1997;112(6 Suppl): 330S–38S.

Wheeler AP, Bernard GR: Treating patients with severe sepsis. N Engl J Med 1999;340:207–14.

Zeni F, Freeman B, Natanson C: Anti-inflammatory therapies to treat sepsis and septic shock: a reassessment. Crit Care Med 1997;25:1095–1100.

COMMUNITY-ACQUIRED PNEUMONIA

ESSENTIALS OF DIAGNOSIS

- *Patients present with cough, fever, and occasionally pleuritic chest pain.*
- *Chest x-ray shows pulmonary infiltrates.*
- *Most common cause of community-acquired pneumonia is* Streptococcus pneumoniae.

General Considerations

Community-acquired pneumonia accounts for a large number of hospitalizations each year and is the fifth or sixth leading cause of death in industrialized communities. Mortality ranges from 5–36%, the latter number reflecting the death rate in patients with community-acquired pneumonia requiring critical care. It is crucial for the physician to be able to recognize the high-risk patient, to initiate diagnostic procedures, and to begin appropriate and prompt antimicrobial therapy.

A variety of risk factors for community-acquired pneumonia have been identified and include increasing age, alcoholism, immunosuppression, institutionalization, and underlying cardiac, pulmonary, or neurologic disease. A meta-analysis evaluating outcomes of patients with community-acquired pneumonia revealed eleven statistically significant factors associated with mortality: male sex, diabetes mellitus, underlying neurologic or neoplastic disease, pleuritic chest pain, hypothermia, tachypnea, hypotension, leukopenia, multilobar infiltrates, and bacteremia. Increasing age and bacterial etiology of the infection were strongly associated with mortality as well. Patients with infections due to *Pseudomonas aeruginosa, Staphylococcus aureus,* and enteric gram-negative rods are at particularly high risk for increased morbidity and mortality.

Microbiologic Etiology

The most common cause of community-acquired pneumonia requiring intensive care hospitalization is *S pneumoniae,* implicated in up to 66% of cases where an etiologic diagnosis is made. *Haemophilus influenzae* is typically the second most common cause, accounting for about 9% of cases, and usually occurs in persons with chronic obstructive pulmonary disease. *Moraxella catarrhalis* is similarly seen in patients with preexisting lung disease. *Staphylococcus aureus* can cause severe pneumonia, with disease acquired either by aspiration or by hematogenous spread. The former is seen in patients with decreased local host defenses (post-influenza, laryngectomy, bronchiectasis, or cystic fibrosis) or generalized decrease in immunity (eg, malnutrition, immunosuppression). Hematogenous disease is typically seen in injection drug abusers or patients with indwelling intravascular catheters. Aerobic gram-negative rods such as *Escherichia coli* and klebsiella species are uncommonly implicated as pathogens in community-acquired pneumonia, but they can cause severe pulmonary disease in patients with advanced age and underlying illness who are colonized with these enteric organisms. Therefore, when enteric organisms are recovered from sputum samples, it can be difficult to tell if their presence is pathogenic or simply reflects colonization. *Pseudomonas aeruginosa* is traditionally considered a nosocomial pathogen, though it can cause severe community-acquired pneumonia. The physician should consider this organism in a patient who was recently hospitalized, has recently received or is currently receiving broad-spectrum antibiotics, or is a resident of a nursing home.

Atypical pathogens, especially legionella species, can cause severe community-acquired pneumonia. Legionellae are implicated in 2–6% of cases of community-acquired pneumonia. More than half of these are caused by *L pneumophila* subgroup 1. *Chlamydia pneumoniae* and *Mycoplasma pneumoniae* typically cause tracheobronchitis or mild pneumonia and only occasionally severe pneumonia.

Respiratory tract viruses are not commonly thought of as agents of community-acquired pneumonia. However, influenza virus, respiratory syncytial virus, adenovirus, and parainfluenza virus have all been associated with severe pneumonitis. In the appropriate host, varicella-zoster virus, cytomegalovirus, and hantavirus should be considered.

In patients with episodes of altered level of consciousness caused by seizures, other neurologic diseases, and substance abuse, an aspiration syndrome should be considered. Aspiration of gastric contents can cause a chemical pneumonitis—with or without a polymicrobial pneumonia—that can lead to an anaerobic lung abscess if left untreated.

Other less common causes of community-acquired pneumonia include *Pneumocystis carinii* in the patient with risk factors for HIV infection or receiving immunosuppressive therapy. The physician should maintain a high level of suspicion for *Mycobacterium tuberculosis* in the appropriate host. In patients with a history of travel to the appropriate areas, organisms causing endemic mycoses *(Histoplasma capsulatum, Blastomyces dermatitidis, Coccidioides immitis)* should be considered. Infection with *Coxiella burnetii,* the agent of Q fever, can present as a community-acquired pneumonia in a patient with a history of exposure to infected cattle, sheep, goats, or parturient cats. *Chlamydia psittaci* likewise should be considered if a history of exposure to psittacine birds is elicited. Despite aggressive diagnostic efforts, no etiologic agent is identified in over 30% of cases of community-acquired pneumonia.

Clinical Features

The diagnosis of community-acquired pneumonia and the choice of empiric antibiotics depends on results of a detailed history and physical examination of the patient, microbiologic analysis of the sputum, and review of the chest radiograph.

A. Symptoms and Signs

Patients with severe community-acquired pneumonia may report fever, chills, cough (either dry or productive), dyspnea, and pleuritic chest pain. Nonspecific symptoms, such as diarrhea, headache, myalgias, or nausea and vomiting, are often present. On physical examination, the typical patient with severe community-acquired pneumonia will have either fever or hypothermia accompanied by tachycardia, tachypnea, abnormal breath sounds, and possibly egophony or other evidence of lung consolidation. If a pleural effusion is present, the patient may have decreased breath sounds with dullness to percussion in the involved hemithorax. The physical examination may provide some clues that will help guide empiric therapy. The presence of thrush or oral hairy leukoplakia may suggest an undiagnosed HIV infection. Poor dentition, caries, and gingival disease are often seen in patients with aspiration pneumonia. Bullous myringitis is occasionally seen with *Mycoplasma pneumoniae* infection and may occur also in patients with viral infection. The finding of a new right-sided heart murmur would be consistent with right-sided endocarditis. The skin should be examined carefully for any lesions that may suggest one of the endemic mycoses.

B. Laboratory Findings

Routine laboratory studies are essential, such as a complete blood count; serum electrolytes, urea nitrogen, and creatinine; arterial blood gas determinations; and chest x-ray. Because of their high degree of specificity, blood cultures should be obtained on all patients; 25% of patients with pneumococcal pneumonia will be bacteremic. Pleural fluid collections, when present, should be sampled in order to differentiate between a parapneumonic effusion and a complicated effusion or empyema, the latter of which would require definitive drainage. Pleural fluid should be submitted for Gram stain, culture, cell count, pH, total protein, and LDH concentration.

The Gram-stained smear of sputum may be the most immediately helpful tool in deciding on empiric antibiotic therapy. To ensure an adequate specimen, the stain should have 10 or fewer squamous epithelial cells and more than 25 polymorphonuclear cells per high-power field. Table 15–2 provides a guide to the probable pathogen based on the Gram-stained smear of sputum (and other stains) that can be done in an expeditious fashion. Legionella urinary antigen is 90% sensitive and 90% specific for *Legionella pneumophila* group 1 and should be determined in appropriate settings.

Other more invasive methods of diagnosis are used in special situations. Fiberoptic bronchoscopy with bronchoalveolar lavage may assist in the diagnosis of pneumonia caused by *Pneumocystis carinii, Mycobacterium tuberculosis,* and certain fungi. However, routine bacterial culture is not specific for diagnosis of pneumonia caused by bacteria that can colonize the respiratory tract. The specificity of this procedure can be increased by quantitative cultures and cytologic examination of the specimen for intracellular bacteria. The specificity of bronchoscopy cultures may be increased by use of the protected brush technique with quantitative cultures. Bronchoscopy allows for direct inspection of the airways and sampling from the site of infection. Percutaneous fine-needle lung aspiration has been performed in some situations. This procedure is the most sensitive and specific of all diagnostic maneuvers; however, complications include bleeding and pneumothorax, which can increase patient morbidity.

Table 15–2. Sputum-guided potential pathogens for severe community-acquired pneumonia.

Staining Characteristic	Potential Pathogen
Gram-positive diplococci Gram-positive cocci in clusters	*Streptococcus pneumoniae* *Staphylococcus aureus*
Gram-negative coccobacilli	*Haemphilus influenzae* *Moraxella catarrhalis*
Gram-negative bacilli	Enteric gram-negative rods *(Escherichia coli, Klebsiella penumoniae, Pseudomonas aeruginosa)*
Mixed bacteria	Oral contamination Mixed aerobes and anaerobes
No organisms present	Viruses *Mycoplasma penumoniae* *Chlamydia pneumoniae* *Coxiella burnetii* Legionella species
Acid-fast stain-positive	*Mycobacterium pneumoniae* Nocardia species
KOH/Calcofluor White stain-positive	*Coccidioides immitis* *Histoplasma capsulatum* *Blastomyces dermatitidis* *Cryptococcus neoformans*
Silver stain-positive	*Pneumocystis carinii*

Differential Diagnosis

The differential diagnosis of severe community-acquired pneumonia is extensive. In addition to the many infectious causes of pneumonia, diseases that can mimic community-acquired pneumonia include cardiogenic pulmonary disease, adult respiratory distress syndrome, pulmonary emboli with infarction, pulmonary hemorrhage, and lung cancer. Other less common diseases are pneumonitis due to collagen-vascular diseases, radiation or chemical pneumonitis, hypersensitivity pneumonitis, sarcoidosis, pulmonary alveolar proteinosis, and occupational lung disease.

Treatment

A. Empiric Antibiotic Therapy

Because it is impossible to cover all pathogens empirically, the physician must use all available data to make an informed decision regarding therapy. Table 15–3 provides a guide for treatment of pneumonia according to pathogen. In most situations involving hospitalized patients, when no clues to etiologic agent can be obtained from history, physical examination, or laboratory data, empiric antibiotic therapy should consist of a third-generation cephalosporin in combination with a macrolide or a quinolone.

B. Resistance Issues and Therapeutic Implications

Streptococcus pneumoniae is the most common cause of community-acquired pneumonia, and the emergence of penicillin-resistant strains of this pathogen is thus of concern when choosing empiric therapy for critically ill patients. There is marked geographic variation in the rates of penicillin resistance, ranging from 2% to as high as 50%. In general, the levels of beta-lactam antibiotics that can be achieved in the lung and in the blood with intravenous therapy far exceed the MIC for pneumococci with intermediate and high levels of resistance (as long as the MIC is < 4 μg/dL). Thus, in most cases, a third-generation cephalosporin is adequate. Few data are available regarding pneumococcal infections when the organism's MIC is < 4 μg/dL. Some authorities suggest using vancomycin, imipenem, or one of the newer quinolones such as levofloxacin if infection with such a strain is suspected. Risk factors for drug-resistant *S pneumoniae* include extremes of age, recent antimicrobial therapy, coexisting illnesses, immunodeficiency or HIV-infection, attendance at a day care center or family member of a child attending a day care center, and institutionalization.

Table 15–3. Empiric antibiotic therapy for community-acquired pneumonia in hospitalized patients.

Patient Category	Most Likely Causative Organisms	Empiric Antibiotic Choices[1]
Hospitalized patient without cardiopulmonary disease	*S pneumoniae* *H influenzae* *M pneumoniae* *C pneumoniae* Mixed infections Miscellaneous	Second- or third-generation cephalosporin *plus–* Intravenous azithromycin or doxycycline (if macrolide-intolerant) *or–* Antipneumococcal fluoroquinolone[2]
Hospitalized patient with cardiopulmonary disease	*S pneumoniae* *H influenzae* *M pneumoniae* *C pneumoniae* Mixed infections Enteric gram-negative rods Anaerobes Miscellaneous	Third-generation cephalosporin[3] *plus* intravenous azithromycin *or–* Antipneumococcal fluoroquinolone[2]
Intensive care unit patient without risk for *Pseudomonas aeruginosa*	*S pneumoniae* Legionella species *H influenzae* *M pneumoniae*	Third-generation cephalosporin[3] *plus* either intravenous azithromycin or antipneumococcal fluoroquinolone[2]
Intensive care unit patient with increased risk for *Pseudomonas aeruginosa* (recent antibiotic use or hospitalization)	*S pneumoniae* Legionella species *H influenzae* *C pneumoniae* Enteric gram-negative rods *P aeruginosa* *S aureus* Miscellaneous	Antipseudomonal beta-lactam[4] *plus* antipseudomonal quinolone[5] *or–* Antipseudomonal beta-lactam[4] *plus* aminoglycoside plus either intravenous azithromycin or antipneumococcal fluoroquinolone[2]

[1]Initial enteric therapy. Subsequent changes should be based on results of microbiologic studies, clinical response, and ability to receive oral antibiotics.
[2]Fluoroquinolone with increased activity against *S penumoniae:* eg, levofloxacin, sparfloxacin, gatifloxacin, moxifloxacin.
[3]Third-generation cephalosporin: eg, ceftriaxone, cefotaxime.
[4]Antipseudomonal beta-lactam: eg, ceftazidime, cefipime, peperacillin-tazobactam, imipenem, meropenem.
[5]Antipseudomonal fluoroquinolone: eg, ciprofloxacin.

Bartlett JG et al: Practice guidelines for management of community-acquired pneumonia in adults. Clin Infect Dis 2000;31:347–82.

Campbell GD, Silberman R: Drug-resistant Streptococcus pneumoniae. Clin Infect Dis 1998;26:1188–95.

Fine MJ et al: Prognosis and outcomes of patients with community-acquired pneumonia. JAMA 1995;274:134–41.

Marrie TJ: Community-acquired pneumonia: Epidemiology, etiology, treatment. Infect Dis Clin North Am 1998;12:723–40.

Ortqvist A: Initial investigation and treatment of the patient with severe community-acquired pneumonia. Semin Respir Infect 1994;9:166–79.

UROSEPSIS

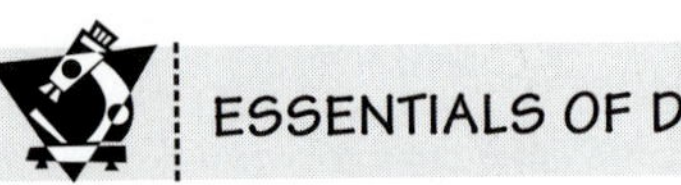

ESSENTIALS OF DIAGNOSIS

- *The patient may be asymptomatic.*
- *Flank or abdominal pain.*
- *Pyuria and white blood cell casts.*
- *Positive urine culture.*

General Considerations

Approximately 250,000 episodes of acute pyelonephritis occur in the United States each year. Most cases can be managed in the outpatient setting. However, if hospitalization is required, the physician must be alert for complications such as underlying immunosuppression, urinary tract obstruction, and intrarenal or perinephric abscess formation. When hypotension or other signs of sepsis are present, patients should be admitted to the intensive care unit for appropriate hemodynamic monitoring and management.

Pathophysiology

There are two primary routes by which bacteria invade the urinary system. In by far the most common route of infection, bacteria gain access to the bladder via the urethra. Urinary tract infections are common in women, as the relatively short female urethra allows retrograde passage of bacteria into the bladder. In contrast, urinary tract infection in men is a rare event in the absence of a urethral catheter or unless there is obstruction of the urethra (eg, prostatic hyperplasia), preventing adequate bladder drainage. Once bacteria have entered the bladder, they may under some circumstances ascend the ureters to the renal pelvis and parenchyma. This process is facilitated by the presence of vesicoureteral reflux. For example, in the renal transplant patient, the transplanted kidney is placed in the pelvis with the ureter surgically implanted in the bladder; as a result, simple cystitis frequently leads to acute transplant pyelonephritis.

Infection of the urinary tract by hematogenous spread is a much less common occurrence. Staphylococcal bacteremia or endocarditis can lead to seeding of renal parenchyma with subsequent abscess formation. However, experimentally produced gram-negative bacteremia rarely leads to acute pyelonephritis.

Microbiologic Etiology

The majority (70–95%) of cases of community-acquired, acute urinary tract infections are caused by *E coli,* with staphylococcus species, enterococci, proteus, klebsiella, and enterobacter identified in most of the remaining cases. The list of etiologic agents is modified by factors such as use of indwelling urinary catheters, residence in an institutionalized setting, urinary tract instrumentation, immunosuppression, or recent broad-spectrum antibiotic administration. In any of these settings, multidrug-resistant gram-negative bacilli, coagulase-negative staphylococci, or candida species may be responsible for infection.

Clinical Features

A. Symptoms and Signs

Patients with urinary tract infections as the source of sepsis may present with localizing symptoms such as flank pain or dysuria. However, many patients have nonspecific complaints, such as nausea, vomiting, abdominal pain, fever, and chills. Physical examination may be helpful if flank tenderness is present. An indwelling bladder catheter should trigger a prompt evaluation of the urinary tract for the source of sepsis.

B. Laboratory Findings

Routine laboratory tests, such as a complete blood count and chemistry panel, should be obtained. Microscopic evaluation of a urine specimen is the most important diagnostic test, typically revealing hematuria, proteinuria, and pyuria ($\geq$ 10 leukocytes/μL of urine), often with white cell casts. Gram stain of the urine should be performed: The presence of one organism per oil immersion field correlates with $\geq 10^5$ bacteria per milliliter of urine, with a sensitivity and specificity approaching 90%. The presence of five or more organisms per oil immersion field increases the specificity to 99%. Additionally, determining the morphology of the infecting bacteria (ie, gram-negative bacillus or gram-positive cocci) may be used to direct empiric therapy. Identification of the pathogen and the results of antimicrobial susceptibility testing are usually available within 48 hours, allowing tailoring of antimicrobial therapy. Any patient sick enough to warrant hospitalization should have blood cultures sent. A renal ultrasound examination or an abdominal CT scan should be obtained in any patient with suspected urinary tract obstruction.

C. Complications

Possible complications of acute pyelonephritis include urosepsis, perinephric abscess, intrarenal abscess, urinary tract obstruction, and emphysematous pyelonephritis. In general, any patient who appears toxic or has persistent fever or positive blood cultures beyond the third day of appropriate therapy should undergo investigation for obstruction, abscess, or other complications.

Perinephric abscesses usually are confined to the perinephric space by Gerota's fascia but may extend into the retroperitoneum. Thirty percent of patients with perinephric abscess have a normal urinalysis, and up to 40% have a sterile urine culture. Intrarenal abscess is usually a complication of systemic bacteremia; thus, the etiologic agent is often a staphylococcus. A plain film of the abdomen may reveal an abdominal mass, an enlarged indistinct kidney shadow, or loss of the psoas margin. Rapid diagnosis of perinephric or intrarenal abscess can be made by renal ultrasound, CT, or MRI. Renal ultrasound can detect an abscess once it reaches 2–3 cm in size, while CT scan and MRI are more sensitive, detecting abscesses as small as 1 cm in diameter. Definitive treatment requires drainage of larger abscesses, either by percutaneous access or open surgical drainage, with concomitant antimicrobial therapy.

Emphysematous pyelonephritis is a rare complication of urinary tract infections. The typical patient is an elderly female with diabetes and chronic urinary tract infections and underlying renal vascular disease. The infecting organism is typically *E coli.* Mortality approaches 70% despite appropriate antimicrobial therapy. Diagnosis is easily made with a plain film or with the more sensitive CT scan of the abdomen; both will reveal gas in the renal parenchyma.

Treatment

In all patients, initial antimicrobial therapy should target the organism seen on the Gram-stained smear of the urinary sediment. In the absence of an identified organism on Gram stain, empiric therapy should consist of an aminoglycoside, an extended-spectrum penicillin (such as mezlocillin, azlocillin, or piperacillin), a third-generation cephalosporin, or a fluoroquinolone depending on the severity of the infection, the patient's renal function and risk for renal insufficiency, and other factors. For emphysematous pyelonephritis, immediate nephrectomy is usually required.

Hooton TM, Stamm WE: Diagnosis and treatment of uncomplicated urinary tract infection. Infect Dis Clin North Am 1997;11:551–81.

Pappas PG: Laboratory in the diagnosis and management of urinary tract infections. Med Clin North Am 1991;75:313–25.

Ronald AR, Harding GK: Complicated urinary tract infections. Infect Dis Clin North Am 1997;11:583–92.

Sobel JD, Kaye D: Urinary tract infections. In: *Principles and Practice of Infectious Diseases,* 5th ed. Mandell GL, Bennett JE, Dolin R (editors). Churchill Livingstone, 2000.

INFECTIVE ENDOCARDITIS

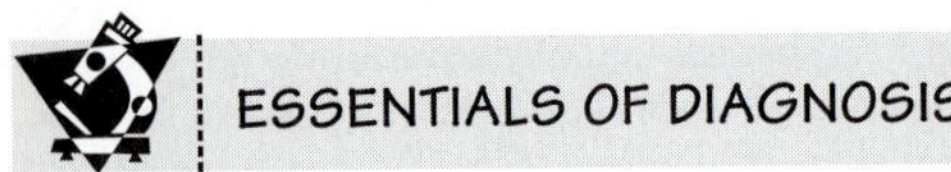
ESSENTIALS OF DIAGNOSIS

- *Clinical presentation varies depending on infecting organism.*
- *Patients with* S aureus *infective endocarditis typically present with a short prodrome and a sepsis syndrome*
- *Clues to the diagnosis of subacute infective endocarditis include a new regurgitant murmur, Roth spots, Osler nodes, Janeway lesions, splinter hemorrhages, hematuria, and splenomegaly.*
- *Blood cultures are needed for diagnosis.*

General Considerations

The incidence of infective endocarditis in the general population is estimated to be 1.7–4 cases per 100,000 persons. It is the fourth leading cause of life-threatening infectious disease. Risk factors include underlying valvular abnormalities. Congenital or rheumatic heart disease, mitral valve prolapse (particularly when regurgitation or thickened, redundant valve leaflets are present), calcific valvular heart disease, or prosthetic valves are implicated in a large percentage of cases. Another increasingly important risk factor is injection drug use. Among injection drug users, the presentation of infective endocarditis is usually acute, reflecting the virulent nature of *Staphylococcus aureus,* the pathogen most commonly associated with infective endocarditis in this population.

Pathophysiology

The first step in infective endocarditis is the establishment of bacteremia. This can occur during a dental or other medical procedure, as a complication of injection drug use, or from minor trauma. However, in most cases no initiating event is identified. The organism attaches to the abnormal endothelial surface of the cardiac valve and the vegetation propagates with further bacterial proliferation. The complications which then arise are the result of either (1) direct local invasion (eg, periannular abscess formation), (2) systemic embolization (eg, splenic, renal, or cerebral embolic), or (3) immunologic phenomena (eg, glomerulonephritis or vasculitis).

Microbiologic Etiology

The microbiologic etiology of infective endocarditis has undergone a shift in the past 3–4 decades. In the 1960s and 1970s, viridans streptococci and enterococci accounted for about 80% of cases and staphylococci for approximately 15%. In more recent series, the viridans streptococci and enterococci still account for 50% of cases, but staphylococci are now implicated in approximately 50% of cases of acute infective endocarditis.

The most common bacterial cause of native valve infective endocarditis remains the viridans streptococci group. As noted above, *S aureus* infective endocarditis usually occurs in injection drug users and diabetics who tend to have skin and nasal colonization with the organism. Other less common pathogens include *Streptococcus pneumoniae,* group A, B, C and G streptococci, *Listeria monocytogenes, Pseudomonas aeruginosa, Serratia marcescens,* and, rarely, *Neisseria gonorrhoeae.* In cases of culture-negative endocarditis, the HACEK group of microorganisms *(Haemophilus parainfluenzae, Haemophilus aphrophilus, Actinobacillus actinomycetemcomitans, Cardiobacterium hominis, Eikenella corrodens,* and *Kingella kingae),* nutritionally variant streptococci (now abiotrophia species), brucella, legionella, and bartonella species, *Coxiella burnetii,* and fungi should all be considered. The most common reason for culture-negative infective endocarditis is prior antibiotic therapy.

Clinical Features

A. Symptoms and Signs

The clinical presentation of infective endocarditis varies dramatically depending on the infecting organism. Patients with *S aureus* infective endocarditis typically present with a short prodrome and a sepsis syndrome. Only rarely are the immunologic phenomena associated with subacute infective endocarditis present. Among injection drug users, the disease is usually right-sided, involving the tricuspid valve. Thus, pulmonary manifestations predominate, which may be manifested as multiple parenchymal infiltrates, cavities, pleural effusion, or empyema. A murmur may not be readily appreciated. The less virulent organisms, such as the viridans streptococci, typically present with the classic subacute infective endocarditis syndrome. Nonspecific symptoms such as fatigue, malaise, or back pain have usually been present for weeks. Clues to the diagnosis of subacute infective endocarditis include a new regurgitant murmur, Roth spots, Osler nodes, Janeway lesions, splinter hemorrhages, hematuria, and splenomegaly.

Complications of subacute infective endocarditis, such as congestive heart failure or central nervous system emboli, may necessitate admission to an intensive care unit.

B. Laboratory and Radiographic Findings

The first clue to the diagnosis of infective endocarditis is often a blood culture yielding growth of an appropriate organism. In the patient with suspected infective endocarditis who presents with subacute symptoms, three separate sets of blood cultures should be obtained up to 24 hours apart prior to initiating empiric antimicrobial therapy. A complete blood count may reveal only leukocytosis in a patient with acute *S aureus* infective endocarditis; however, evidence of anemia of chronic disease may be present in a patient with subacute infective endocarditis. Urinalysis may reveal hematuria, proteinuria, or pyuria. A chemistry panel may demonstrate renal insufficiency (the result of renal infarction), septic emboli, or immune complex glomerulonephritis. Patients may have other nonspecific indicators of acute inflammation, such as an elevated erythrocyte sedimentation rate or C-reactive protein, hypergammaglobulinemia, or a positive test for rheumatoid factor. Chest x-ray may reveal multiple pulmonary infiltrates, cavitary lesions, pleural effusion in right-sided disease, or pulmonary edema in left-sided disease. A 12-lead electrocardiogram should be obtained on all patients to look for intracardiac conduction delay, manifested as a new first-, second-, or third-degree heart block, suggesting the presence of an aortic ring abscess. Any patient with neurologic symptoms should undergo brain CT to look for embolic events or intracranial hemorrhage from rupture of a mycotic aneurysm.

Diagnosis of infective endocarditis is aided by use of the Duke criteria (Table 15–4). Echocardiography should be obtained on all patients in whom the diagnosis is entertained, as it provides both diagnostic and prognostic information. The sensitivity of the transthoracic echocardiogram for demonstrating valvular vegetations is only about 50–60%, and for that reason the procedure cannot exclude infective endocarditis entirely. On the other hand, transesophageal echocardiography has a sensitivity and specificity approaching 90% and is particularly useful in detecting periannular aortic abscess formation.

C. Complications

Because the most seriously ill patients with infective endocarditis are admitted to the intensive care unit, this population is likely to have a high rate of complications. Thus, it is important for the physician to remain vigilant for these potential life-threatening events.

Congestive heart failure is the most common complication of acute infective endocarditis. It may occur acutely as a result of perforation of a valve leaflet or rupture of a chorda tendinea, from valvular outlet obstruction due to large vegetations, from creation of fistulous tracts leading to high-output failure, or from prosthetic valve dehiscence. Congestive heart failure may also present insidiously as a result of progressive valvular insufficiency or ventricular dysfunction. Congestive heart failure that is refractory to medical management necessitates valve replacement.

Systemic embolization occurs in 20–50% of patients with infective endocarditis. Risk factors for embolic events include vegetation size greater than 1 cm on the transesophageal echocardiogram, vegetation location on the anterior leaflet of the mitral valve, increasing vegetation size during appropriate antimicrobial therapy, and infection with *S aureus,* candida species, one of the HACEK group, or the abiotrophia species. There is general agreement that the occurrence of two or more

Table 15–4. Duke criteria for diagnosis of infective endocarditis (IE).[1]

Major Criteria 1. Positive blood culture for IE	A. Typical microorganism for infective endocarditis from two separate blood cultures: i. Viridans streptococci, *Streptococcus bovis,* or HACEK group (haemophilus, antinobacillus, cardiobacterium, eikenella, kingella) ii. Community-acquired *Staphylococcus aureus* or enterococci in the absence of a primary focus B. Microorganisms consistent with IE from persistently positive blood cultures defined as – i. More than two positive blood cultures drawn more than 12 hours apart, or — ii. All of three or a majority of four or more separate cultures of blood (with first and last samples drawn 1 hour or more apart).
2. Evidence of endocardial involvement	A. Positive echocardiogram for IE, defined as— i. Oscillating intracardiac mass on valve or supporting structures, in the path of regurgitant jets, or implanted material in the absence of an alternative anatomic explanation, or— ii. Abscess, or— iii. New partial dehiscence of prosthetic valve, or— B. New valvular regurgitation (worsening or changing of preexisting murmur not sufficient)
Minor Criteria	1. Predisposition: predisposing heart condition or intravenous drug use 2. Fever: temperature ≥ 38° C 3. Vascular phenomena: arterial embolism, septic pulmonary infarcts, mycotic aneurysm, intracranial hemorrhage, conjunctival hemorrhages, Janeway lesions 4. Immunologic phenomena: glomerulonephritis, Olser nodes, Roth spots, rheumatoid factor 5. Microbiologic evidence: positive blood culture but not meeting major criterion as noted above (excludes single positive cultures for coagulase-negative staphylococci and organisms that do not cause endocarditis). 6. Echocardiogram: findings consistent with IE but do not meet a major criterion as noted above.
Definite IE	Pathologic criteria Microorganisms: demonstrated by culture or histology in a vegetation, or in a vegetation that has embolized, or in an intracardiac abscess, or— Pathologic lesions: vegetation or intracardiac abscess present, confirmed by histology showing active endocarditis
	Clinical criteria, using specific definitions above Two major criteria, or— One major and three minor criteria, or— Five minor criteria
Possible IE	Findings consistent with IE that fall short of "definite" but not "rejected"
Rejected	Firm alternative diagnosis explaining evidence of infective endocarditis, or— Resolution of endocarditis syndrome, with antibiotic therapy for 4 days or less antibiotic or— No pathologic evidence of infective endocarditis at surgery or autopsy after antibiodic therapy for 4 days or less.

[1]Adapted from Durack DT, Lukes AS, Bright DK: New criteria for diagnosis of infective endocarditis. Am J Med 1994;96:200–9.

serious embolic events while on appropriate antimicrobial therapy is an indication for valve replacement.

Periannular extension of infection occurs in 10–40% of cases of native valve infective endocarditis and 55–100% of cases involving a prosthetic valve. Periannular abscess formation is more common when the aortic valve is involved. The infection spreads from the aortic ring and can rupture through the membranous septum to involve the atrioventricular node; thus, the finding of a new intracardiac conduction delay is often a first clue to this life-threatening complication. Creation of an intracardiac shunt can also occur. Periannular extension of infection is best diagnosed by transesophageal echocardiography, which has a sensitivity of 76–100% and a specificity of 55%. In most cases, periannular abscess formation requires valve replacement.

In a patient with infective endocarditis who has persistent bacteremia, fever, or sepsis in the setting of appropriate antimicrobial therapy, the possibility of a splenic or renal abscess should be considered. Splenic infarction occurs in about 40% of cases of left-sided endocarditis; of these, 5% develop into an abscess. Abdominal CT or MRI may be useful for diagnosis. Most renal abscesses will require drainage in conjunction with appropriate antimicrobial therapy. Splenectomy is the definitive treatment for splenic abscess.

One of the most feared complications of infective endocarditis is a mycotic aneurysm. The most common site of involvement is the intracranial arteries, followed by the visceral bed and the upper and lower extremities. The incidence of intracranial mycotic aneurysms in patients with infective endocarditis is about 1.2–5%. The overall mortality of this complication is 60% —30% without rupture and 80% with rupture. The diagnostic method of choice is four-vessel cerebral angiography. Therapy, including potential surgery, should be individualized to the patient.

Treatment

The spectrum of initial antimicrobial therapy in a critically ill patient with suspected infective endocarditis should be broad, directed at those pathogens most commonly implicated in this disease. Initial therapy should include a semisynthetic penicillin with activity against *S aureus,* a penicillin with activity against streptococci and enterococci, and an aminoglycoside for synergy against these organisms. When faced with a patient with a history of a serious allergic reaction to penicillin, the physician should substitute vancomycin. Subsequent antibiotic therapy must be tailored once the infecting organism and its drug susceptibility pattern are known.

Bayer AS et al: Diagnosis and management of infective endocarditis and its complications. Circulation 1998;98:2936–48.

Bayer AS: Infective endocarditis. Clin Infect Dis 1993;17:313–22.

Cunha BA, Gill MV, Lazar JM: Acute infective endocarditis: diagnostic and therapeutic approach. Infect Dis Clin North Am 1996;10:811–34.

Wilson WR et al: Antibiotic treatment of adults with infective endocarditis due to streptococci, enterococci, staphylococci and HACEK microorganisms. JAMA 1995;274:1706–13.

NECROTIZING SOFT TISSUE INFECTIONS

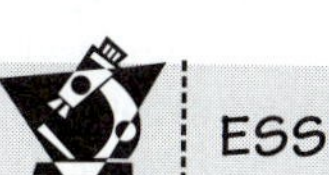

ESSENTIALS OF DIAGNOSIS

- *Patients complain of pain out of proportion to findings.*
- *Essential to differentiate a necrotizing soft tissue infection from a simple cellulitis.*
- *Metabolic acidosis, renal insufficiency, and other signs of organ dysfunction may be present.*

General Considerations

The true incidence of necrotizing soft tissue infections is difficult to quantify, as they are not reportable. Necrotizing fasciitis is an uncommon soft tissue infection caused by a variety of toxin-producing bacteria. There is fascial necrosis, often with less marked involvement of overlying skin and underlying muscle, and marked systemic toxicity. The true incidence of necrotizing soft tissue infections is difficult to quantify since they are not reportable. Necrotizing fasciitis can result from a large number of associated conditions, including trauma, surgical procedures, and relatively benign local infections of the skin or soft tissues. The mortality rate is approximately 20–30% in most series, with some studies reporting mortality rates of over 75%. Risk factors for necrotizing soft tissue infections include diabetes mellitus (the most common pre-existing condition), peripheral vascular disease, alcoholism, injection drug use, obesity, malnutrition, and immunosuppression. The multitude of terms used to describe soft tissue infections may be confusing to the reader: hemolytic streptococcal gangrene, progressive synergistic bacterial gangrene, necrotizing erysipelas, suppurative fasciitis, acute dermal gangrene, Fournier's gangrene, and progressive postoperative bacterial synergistic gangrene have all appeared in the literature. Distinguishing between the various categories of necrotizing soft tissue infections is not always necessary, as prognosis and treatment of these conditions are quite similar.

Pathophysiology

In the pathogenesis of necrotizing soft tissue infections, bacteria are typically introduced into the skin or soft tissues by trauma, either inadvertent or iatrogenic. Inciting events that have been reported to lead to soft tissue infections include surgery, blunt or penetrating trauma, insect bites, varicella infection, injection drug use, perforated viscus, perineal abscess, diverticulitis, percutaneous drainage of intra-abdominal abscess, renal calculi, dental infection or procedure, pharyngitis, and exposure to sea water. Hematogenous introduction of the bacteria into soft tissue has been documented with *Streptococcus pyogenes* and, less commonly, *Staphylococcus aureus.*

Once bacteria gain entry into the host tissues, bacterial toxins and endogenous cytokines act synergistically to produce tissue damage. Both exotoxin A and exotoxin B have been identified in invasive group A streptococcal infections. Histopathologic examination of involved tissue typically reveals widespread necrosis of the fascia and subcutaneous fat and thrombosis and endarteritis of small vessels. Occasionally, myonecrosis of underlying skeletal muscle will be observed.

Microbiologic Etiology

There are three predominant types of necrotizing fasciitis, with distinctions based on microbiologic etiology. Type 1 is polymicrobial infection, with a combination of non-group A streptococci, anaerobes, and facultative anaerobes, usually Enterobacteriaceae. Among persons developing type 1 necrotizing fasciitis, certain host factors are associated with infection by specific bacteria. For example, diabetics tend to become infected with bacteroides species, *Staphylococcus aureus,* and the Enterobacteriaceae. Immunosuppressed patients may become infected with *Pseudomonas aeruginosa* and other Enterobacteriaceae. Clostridium species are more commonly seen following trauma. On average, four different species of bacteria are identified by culture in patients with type 1 necrotizing fasciitis.

Type 2 necrotizing fasciitis is defined by infection with group A beta-hemolytic streptococci, occurring either alone or in combination with staphylococcus. Type 3 necrotizing fasciitis is characterized by infection with marine vibrios following exposure to sea water. This group of gram-negative rods consists of *Vibrio vulnificus, V parahaemolyticus, V damsela,* and *V alginolyticus; V vulnificus* is considered to be the most virulent.

Clinical Features

A. Symptoms and Signs

The typical patient presents with a history 5–7 days or fewer of localized pain, redness, and swelling. On physical examination, the patient may be tachycardiac or tachypneic (in compensation for metabolic acidosis). Fever is not uniformly present, with up to 50% of patients being afebrile. An area of what initially appears to be a simple cellulitis may be noted, with localized warmth, erythema, and tenderness of the skin and soft tissues. An important clue to the diagnosis of necrotizing fasciitis is the presence of pain out of proportion to physical findings. Rapid progression of soft tissue involvement is typical, with the evolution of a smooth, tense, and edematous lesion to blister and bulla formation with an underlying dusky blue hue. With progression of soft tissue involvement, the subcutaneous nerves are destroyed, resulting in anesthesia of overlying skin. However, physical findings may be nonspecific, with 75% of patients presenting only with pain, swelling, and cutaneous erythema. Specific findings suggestive of invasive soft tissue involvement, such as crepitus and blistering, are present in less than 40% of patients.

B. Laboratory Findings

Complete blood count, a chemistry panel, and liver enzymes should be obtained on all patients. Leukocytosis with left shift is typically present; blood chemistries may reveal metabolic acidosis, renal insufficiency, and other evidence of organ dysfunction. Creatine kinase may be elevated, reflecting myonecrosis. One retrospective study identified a white blood cell count > 14,000/μL, serum sodium < 135 mmol/L, and serum urea nitrogen > 15 mg/dL as useful in distinguishing patients with necrotizing fasciitis from patients with cellulitis. Plain films occasionally reveal gas in the soft tissue, a finding that is specific for necrotizing fasciitis. MRI may be a more sensitive tool in differentiating a necrotizing soft tissue infection from simple cellulitis; however, this diagnostic modality is not readily available at all centers. Diagnosis requires surgical exploration of the involved soft tissue—the hallmark of necrotizing fasciitis is nonadherence of fascia to underlying muscles on blunt dissection. In some cases, a full-thickness biopsy with immediate frozen section will reveal fascial necrosis. Surgically debrided tissue should be submitted for aerobic and anaerobic bacterial cultures to allow appropriate tailoring of antibiotic therapy. Gram stain of an aspirate from the necrotic center of the lesion has been shown to correlate well with culture results.

Differential Diagnosis

The differential diagnosis of necrotizing fasciitis includes cellulitis, erysipelas, thrombophlebitis, myositis, and compartment syndrome. In many cases, the differentiation of these entities from necrotizing fasciitis can be made on clinical grounds.

Treatment

A. Empiric Antibiotic Therapy

Empiric antimicrobial treatment of necrotizing fasciitis should include coverage of aerobic gram-positive cocci, aerobic gram-negative rods, and anaerobes. Initial antimicrobial choices could include a penicillin or a first-generation cephalosporin, along with an aminoglycoside and either clindamycin or metronidazole. If *Streptococcus pyogenes* is suspected, the treatment of choice is high-dose penicillin. In this setting, there are animal data to support the addition of clindamycin; in the presence of a high inoculum of organisms in a stationary phase of growth, penicillin-binding proteins are not fully expressed, reducing the efficacy of penicillin. Furthermore, clindamycin acts as a protein synthesis inhibitor at the ribosome, which may suppress streptococcal toxin production. If vibrio infection is suspected, tetracycline should be added to the regimen. When clostridial myonecrosis is a consideration, high-dose penicillin with or without clindamycin should be initiated.

B. Surgery

Because of the large amount of tissue hypoxia, necrosis, and blood vessel thrombosis, antibiotics alone should never be considered definitive therapy for necrotizing fasciitis. Early debridement of all necrotic tissue is imperative for control of infection. The goal of surgery is twofold: to render a prompt diagnosis and to perform definitive debridement. Patients require frequent reevaluation of the surgical site—at least every 24 hours. Repeat debridement is often necessary.

C. Adjunctive Therapies

Supportive care is critical, with appropriate fluid resuscitation and nutritional support to promote wound healing. The issue of adjunctive hyperbaric oxygen therapy is controversial; however, the data to support its use consist of retrospective studies, case reports, and animal studies. If hyperbaric oxygen is readily available, its use can be considered. However, it should never be considered an alternative to adequate surgical debridement.

Prognosis

The mortality rate associated with necrotizing fasciitis is high. Risk factors for mortality have been identified as age over 60 years, female sex, extent of infection on presentation, delay in surgical debridement, elevated creatinine, elevated blood lactate, white blood cell count > 30,000/μL, presence of bacteremia, and degree of organ dysfunction on admission. The physician should maintain a high level of suspicion when evaluating patients with soft tissue infections, as early diagnosis with prompt surgical debridement remains the most important modifiable determinant of prognosis.

Chapnick EK, Abter EI: Necrotizing soft-tissue infections. Infect Dis Clin North Am 1996;10:835–55.

Elliott D, Kufera JA, Myers RA: The microbiology of necrotizing soft tissue infections. Am J Surg 2000;179:361–66.

Elliot DC, Kufera JA, Myers RAM: Necrotizing soft tissue infections: risk factors for mortality and strategies for management. Ann Surg 1996;224:672–83.

Green RJ, Dafoe DC, Raffin TA: Necrotizing fasciitis. Chest 1996;110:219–29.

Hill MK, Sanders CV: Skin and soft tissue infections in critical care. Crit Care Clin 1998;14:251–62.

Rahmouni A et al: MR imaging in acute infectious cellulitis. Radiology 1994;192:493–6.

Wall DB et al: Objective criteria may assist in distinguishing necrotizing fasciitis from nonnecrotizing soft tissue infection. Am J Surg 2000;179:17–21.

INTRA-ABDOMINAL INFECTIONS

ESSENTIALS OF DIAGNOSIS

- *Symptoms may be nonspecific, with patients reporting vague abdominal pain, anorexia, and fever.*
- *Abdominal examination may reveal absent or diminished bowel sounds, with peritoneal signs.*
- *Laboratory findings are nonspecific in patients with intra-abdominal sepsis.*

General Considerations

Intra-abdominal infections rank among the four most serious infectious diseases requiring admission to an intensive care unit. However, the actual incidence of intra-abdominal infections is difficult to quantify, as this category includes a wide range of diagnoses.

Pathophysiology

See Table 15–5.

Microbiologic Etiology

See Table 15–5. The majority of intra-abdominal infections are polymicrobial in nature, caused by Enterobacteriaceae, anaerobes, or streptococci. The organisms isolated from a given intra-abdominal infection reflect the flora native to the involved region of the gastrointestinal tract. The normal flora of the stomach, duodenum, and proximal small bowel consist of small numbers of viridans streptococci and other microaerophilic streptococci. The distal small bowel is populated with larger numbers of Enterobacteriaceae, enterococci, and anaerobes. The colon is estimated to contain up to 10^{12} organisms per gram of feces. The predominant flora consists of anaerobes, Enterobacteriaceae, and enterococci. Candida species colonize the gastrointestinal tract in approximately 50% of individuals, which may contribute to intra-abdominal infection in these patients. The normal microbiologic flora of the gastrointestinal tract are altered dramatically by antibiotic therapy, selecting for increased colonization with candida species,

Table 15–5. Intra-abdominal infections: pathophysiology, microbiology, and treatment.

Intra-abdominal Infection	Pathophysiology	Microbiologic Etiology	Diagnostic Tests	Empiric Antimicrobial Therapy
Intraperitoneal abscess	Complication of spontaneous or secondary peritonitis	Enterobacteriaceae, anaerobes, streptococci, candida species	CT scan, ultrasound Perhaps radionuclide scan	Aminoglycoside + metronidazole or clindamycin *or–* Third-generation cephalosporin + metronidazole or clindamycin *or–* Beata-lactam–beta-lactamase inhibitor *or–* Imipenem
Pancreatic abscess	Complication of pancreatitis (biliary, ethanol, postsurgical, or posttraumatic)	Enterobacteriaceae, anaerobes, streptococci, enterococci, candida species	CT scan or ultrasound	Aminoglycoside + metronidazole or clindamycin *or–* Third-generation cephalosporin + metronidazole or clindamycin *or–* Beta-lactam—beta-lactamase inhibitor *or–* Imipenem
Hepatic abscess	Local spread from contiguous infection or hematogenous seeding of the liver	Mixed facultative and anaerobic species (most common), unless biliary tract source (enteric gram-negative bacilli and enterococci). Consider *Entamoeba histolytica*	CT scan or ultrasound	Aminoglycoside + metronidazole or clindamycin *or–* Third-generation cephalosporin + metronidazole or clindamycin *or–* Beta-lactam–beta-lactamase inhibitor *or–* Imipenem
Peritonitis (spontaneous)	Translocation of bacteria across gut lumen in cirrhosis	*E coli* (most frequent), *K pneumoniae, S pneumoniae,* sreptococci, enterococci	Paracentesis (neutrophils > 250/μL, positive Gram stain or culture)	Third-generation cephalosporin (preferably cefotaxime or ceftriaxone)
Peritonitis (secondary)	Perforation of viscus	Enterobacteriaceae, anaerobes, streptococci, enterococci, candida species	Paracentesis (polymicrobial Gram stain or culture). Plain films or CT showing free peritoneal air.	Aminoglycoside + metronidazole or clindamycin *or–* Third-generation cephalosporin + metronidazole or clindamycin *or–* Beta-lactam–beta-lactamase inhibitor *or–* Imipenem

enterococci, and other relatively resistant gram-negative bacilli such as pseudomonas and enterobacter species.

Intra-abdominal infections may be caused by pathogens not typically associated with gastrointestinal flora. In patients with particular risks (ie, suspected exposure or immunocompromised) the following organisms should be considered: *Mycobacterium tuberculosis, Neisseria gonorrhoeae, Chlamydia trachomatis, Coccidioides immitis, Yersinia enterocolitica,* and actinomyces.

Clinical Features

A. Symptoms and Signs

The symptoms and signs of intra-abdominal sepsis not only vary among patients but also depend on the underlying etiology of the infection. Symptoms may be nonspecific, with patients reporting vague abdominal pain, anorexia, or subjective fever. Patients may be febrile or hypothermic; tachycardia is common, and tachypnea may be present in compensation for an underlying metabolic acidosis. Abdominal examination may reveal absent or diminished bowel sounds, with peritoneal signs. Patients who are morbidly obese, elderly, neutropenic, or receiving steroids or other immunosuppressive agents are more likely to have nonspecific complaints. Moreover, they may have relatively benign abdominal findings on physical examination even in the presence of severe intra-abdominal pathology. Thus, the physician must maintain a high level of suspicion when evaluating these patient populations.

B. Laboratory Findings

Laboratory findings are nonspecific in patients with intra-abdominal sepsis. Peripheral leukocytosis is common, though leukopenia may be seen in some patients perhaps due to intra-abdominal sequestration of white blood cells. Metabolic acidosis may be present and should prompt consideration of bowel ischemia. Elevation of liver aminotransferases, though relatively common, is a nonspecific finding in intra-abdominal infection and only rarely heralds a focal intrahepatic infection. Elevation of serum alkaline phosphatase and total bilirubin mandates prompt investigation of the biliary tree to rule out cholecystitis, cholangitis, or an obstructing mass. An elevated serum amylase or lipase may point to pancreatitis, though an abnormal serum amylase may also be seen with bowel infarction or perforation. If ascites is present, a diagnostic paracentesis should be performed, with fluid submitted for cell count, protein, albumin, Gram stain, and culture.

C. Imaging Studies

Supine and upright films of the abdomen may reveal free air if viscus perforation is present. Other diagnostic clues may be present on plain radiographs, such as an elevated hemidiaphragm from a possible intra-abdominal abscess. Abdominal ultrasound is another radiographic diagnostic tool that is often readily available and relatively inexpensive to perform. Abdominal ultrasonography is particularly useful in detecting pathology of the right upper quadrant, retroperitoneum, and pelvis, where its sensitivity is about 90%. However, it is less sensitive in the interloop areas, and the presence of large amounts of bowel gas may limit the utility of ultrasonography. CT of the abdomen is more sensitive than ultrasound in the diagnosis of intra-abdominal pathology; however, it is more expensive and requires administration of intravenous and oral contrast. MRI may be a useful diagnostic tool as it avoids the need for intravenous contrast administration; however, it is costly, not readily available in all centers, and may not be usable in all patients (eg, those needing mechanical ventilation).

Treatment

Most intra-abdominal infections are caused by polymicrobial enteric flora; thus, empiric therapy should be targeted toward the facultative gram-negative bacilli and the anaerobes. An aminoglycoside is traditionally recommended as first-line therapy against gram-negative bacilli and is the standard against which all other regimens are compared. In patients unable to tolerate an aminoglycoside, alternative agents include third-generation cephalosporins, aztreonam, a fluoroquinolone, or an extended-spectrum penicillin. Either metronidazole or clindamycin should be added for anti-anaerobic coverage. Increasing prevalence of clindamycin-resistant *Bacteroides fragilis* may render this agent less useful in some areas. Metronidazole resistance among *B fragilis* is rare. The combination of metronidazole and aztreonam is not recommended because of the lack of gram-positive coverage. Monotherapy options include imipenem-cilastatin, meropenem, or a beta-lactam with a beta-lactamase inhibitor (such as ticarcillin-clavulanate or piperacillin-tazobactam). The decision to add an antifungal agent should be individualized. Immediate empiric antifungal therapy is rarely indicated unless a primary fungal process is suspected. If, during the course of therapy, candida is isolated from blood or peritoneal cultures or if histopathologic evidence of fungal tissue invasion is obtained, initiation of antifungal therapy is appropriate. In addition to empiric antimicrobial therapy, surgical consultation should be obtained for all patients with suspected intra-abdominal sepsis.

Cooper GS, Shales DM, Salata RA: Intraabdominal infection: differences in presentation and outcome between younger patients and the elderly. Clin Infect Dis 1994;19:146–8.

Levison ME, Bush LM: Peritonitis and other intra-abdominal infections. In: *Principles and Practice of Infectious Diseases,* 5th ed. Mandell GL, Bennett JE, Dolin R (editors). Churchill Livingstone, 2000.

McClean KL, Sheehan GJ, Harding GKM: Intraabdominal infection: a review. Clin Infect Dis 1994;19:100–16.

INFECTIONS IN SPECIAL HOSTS

Many patients have underlying diseases that render them more susceptible to specific pathogens. Included among these are patients with neutropenia, organ transplant recipients, diabetics, asplenic individuals, patients on chronic corticosteroid therapy, and HIV-infected patients. Knowledge of an underlying condition may lead a physician to modify or broaden empiric antibiotic therapy when such a patient is admitted to the intensive care unit with infection or suspected infection. The physician should also keep in mind that relative immunosuppression may alter or minimize presenting symptoms and physical findings. Patients with HIV-infection represent a population with specific management issues (see Chapter 27). In general, immunocompromised patients who require intensive care for an infectious process should have an infectious disease consultant involved in their care.

The Neutropenic Patient

Advances in the fields of oncology and hematology have led to increasing numbers of patients with hematologic or solid organ malignancies undergoing intensive chemotherapy regimens. One of the major complications of such therapy—and an important cause of morbidity and mortality—is supervening infection. The febrile neutropenic patient has a greater than 60% chance of being infected; however, only 30–50% of these episodes can be documented microbiologically. Because these patients have a diminished immune response to infection due to their neutropenia, it often happens that no obvious signs of infection such as purulent drainage, erythema, or edema are present. Fever is usually the only sign. Empiric antimicrobial therapy of the febrile neutropenic patient is the standard of care.

Using the IDSA guidelines, neutropenia is defined as < 500 neutrophils/μL or < 1000 neutrophils/μL with an anticipated decline to < 500 neutrophils/μL. Fever is defined as a single oral measurement of > 38.3 °C or ≥ 38 °C over a period of 1 hour. A thorough history and physical examination should be performed in patients with neutropenia and fever, with scrutiny of the skin, oropharynx, and perirectal areas to localize a source of infection. Blood cultures for bacteria and fungi, a chest radiograph, liver enzymes, a complete blood count, and a chemistry panel should be obtained. Once such tests have been performed, empiric antimicrobial therapy should be initiated without delay. Typical pathogens identified in febrile neutropenic patients are aerobic gram-negative bacilli of enteric origin. The most common organisms isolated from blood cultures are *E coli,* klebsiella species, and *Pseudomonas aeruginosa.* An increasing incidence of bacteremia due to gram-positive organisms such as *Staphylococcus epidermidis, Staphylococcus aureus,* and beta-hemolytic streptococci has been documented in recent years, thought to be the result of increased use of indwelling intravenous catheters, administration of chemotherapeutic regimens that induce mucositis, and use of antimicrobial agents with broad gram-negative coverage.

Initial empiric therapy should be targeted against gram-negative bacilli, using an anti-pseudomonal beta-lactam antibiotic (such as piperacillin or ceftazidime) in conjunction with an aminoglycoside. Other possible regimens include a combination of two beta-lactam agents or monotherapy with ceftazidime or a carbapenem. The decision to add vancomycin to initial empiric therapy should be individualized: If an indwelling catheter is the obvious source of infection or there is reason to think that a gram-positive infection is likely, then vancomycin may be added to the initial regimen. However, it has been demonstrated that patients do not suffer increased morbidity or mortality if vancomycin is withheld until there is clinical or microbiologic evidence for such an infection.

Once results of blood and other body fluid cultures become available, antimicrobial therapy may be directed at specific organisms identified. If, however, the patient remains febrile after 5–7 days of broad-spectrum antimicrobial therapy and no source of infection has been found, empiric antifungal therapy should be added. Amphotericin B is usually the antifungal agent of choice in this setting. Approximately one-third of neutropenic patients who remain febrile for 1 week or more on broad-spectrum antimicrobial therapy will be found to have a systemic fungal infection, usually with candida or aspergillus species.

Organ Transplant Recipients

Organ transplant recipients, because of the nature of their immunosuppressive therapy, are particularly vulnerable to infectious complications. Susceptibility to specific infectious complications in the transplant host varies with time in the post-transplant setting. A patient's risk of acquiring a particular infection is determined by their net state of immunosuppression as well as individual epidemiologic exposures, both in the community and hospital (eg, Mycobacteria tuberculosis, Legionella). In the first month after transplantation, 90% of infectious complications are typical hospital-acquired infections, such as transplant wound infection, pneumonia, urinary tract infection, or catheter-related infections. Rarely a systemic infection may be transmitted along with the allograft, or more commonly, an underlying latent infection in the transplant recipient may recrudesce with immunosuppression. One to six months following transplantation, organ transplant recipients are particularly vulnerable to viral infections, especially cytomegalovirus (CMV). In the absence of an environmental exposure to a specific pathogen, other opportunistic infections are rare during this time period. Six months after transplantation, an individual's risk of infection depends on the clinical course and health care status. In the 80% of patients who have experienced an uneventful posttransplant course, infectious complications are typically the same as those of the community at large. Another approximately 10% of patients will suffer from chronic or progressive viral infections such as CMV, hepatitis B virus, hepatitis C virus, or Epstein-Barr virus. In the remaining 10% of patients, chronic or recurrent rejection requires repeated courses of high-dose immunosuppressive therapy. This population is particularly susceptible to opportunistic infections with *Pneumocystis carinii, Listeria monocytogenes, Nocardia asteroides, Cryptococcus neoformans,* and aspergillus.

Asplenic Patients

The spleen serves a critical function in antibody synthesis, microbial filtration, and opsonin production. Patients with asplenia are therefore uniquely susceptible to overwhelming infection with encapsulated organisms such as *Streptococcus pneumoniae, Neisseria meningitidis,* and *Haemophilus influenzae.* Other less common pathogens seen in the asplenic host include *Klebsiella pneumoniae, Streptococcus agalactiae, E coli, Capnocytophaga canimorsus,* and *Staphylococcus aureus.* They are also prone to severe infection with intracellular parasites such as babesia and plasmodium. When one is attempting to identify at-risk patients, a history of surgical splenectomy can be obtained from the patient or physical examination will reveal the presence of a surgical splenectomy scar. However, a functional asplenic state may be overlooked. Conditions that can lead to functional asplenia include congenital hyposplenism, sickle cell disease, graft-versus-host disease, rheumatoid arthritis, systemic lupus erythematosus, amyloidosis, ulcerative colitis, celiac disease, and chronic alcoholism. A clue to asplenia is the presence of Howell-Jolly bodies on peripheral blood smear, as these inclusions are typically removed by a functioning spleen. In an asplenic patient with overwhelming sepsis, high-grade bacteremia is often present; thus, Gram stain of the buffy coat will often reveal the infecting organism. Empiric antimicrobial therapy should include coverage for the encapsulated organisms; a third-generation cephalosporin is a reasonable choice.

The Patient on Chronic Corticosteroid Therapy

Impaired cell-mediated immunity is usually seen in patients maintained on a dosage of prednisone ≥ 40–60 mg/d. In addition to having increased susceptibility to community-acquired pathogens, patients on chronic steroid therapy are particularly vulnerable to intracellular pathogens. Examples include salmonella species, legionella species, *Listeria monocytogenes, Mycobacterium tuberculosis,* and various viruses (eg, herpesviruses). Other organisms that must be considered when evaluating a steroid-treated patient with clinical evidence of severe infection are candida species, aspergillus species, *Cryptococcus neoformans,* nocardia species, *Toxoplasma gondii,* and *Pneumocystis carinii.*

Patients With Diabetes Mellitus

Patients with diabetes mellitus often have more severe manifestations of infectious disease than other hosts. In addition, there are specific disease entities that more commonly occur in diabetics than in other hosts. For example, rhinocerebral mucormycosis should be considered in any patient with diabetic ketoacidosis and facial pain, ocular complaints, or neurologic symptoms. Physical examination may reveal a black eschar on the hard palate or nasal mucosa. Definitive diagnosis of this life-threatening infection is made by tissue biopsy, which will reveal fungal elements invading tissues. Therapy consists of surgical debridement, with adjunctive high doses of intravenous amphotericin B. Diabetics are also uniquely susceptible to urinary tract infections. In addition, serious complications of the urinary tract infection may occur, such as emphysematous pyelonephritis, which require surgical therapy along with antimicrobial therapy. Emphysematous cholecystitis may occur in the diabetic host, usually the result of an anaerobic infection with clostridia. Emphysematous cholecystitis should be suspected when gas is seen on abdominal plain film or CT scan. Emergent cholecystectomy is indicated for this condition. Because of impaired vascular perfusion, patients with diabetes mellitus are prone to more severe necrotizing soft tissue infections, necessitating a high degree of vigilance for these life-threatening infections, with rapid diagnosis and immediate surgical debridement.

Cunha BA: Infections in nonleukopenic compromised hosts (diabetes mellitus, SLE, steroids, and asplenia) in critical care. Crit Care Clin 1998;14:263–82.

Fishman JA, Rubin RH: Infection in organ-transplant recipients. N Engl J Med 1998;338:1741–51.

Hathorn JW, Lyke K: Empirical treatment of febrile neutropenia: evolution of current therapeutic approaches. Clin Infect Dis 1997;24(Suppl 2):S256–65.

Hughes WT et al: 1997 Guidelines for the use of antimicrobial agents in neutropenic patients with unexplained fever. Clin Infect Dis 1997;25:551–73.

Joshi N et al: Infections in patients with diabetes mellitus. N Engl J Med 1999;341:1906–12.

Smitherman KO, Peacock JE: Infectious emergencies in patients with diabetes mellitus. Med Clin North Am 1995;79:53–77.

PRINCIPLES OF ANTIBIOTIC USE IN THE INTENSIVE CARE UNIT

The choice of antimicrobial agents to be used in established or strongly suspected bacterial or other infections must be based on an assessment of what organisms are most likely to be involved. Initial empiric therapy should be dictated, whenever possible, by the results of Gram-stained smears of properly collected specimens such as sputum, urine, aspirated purulent material, or body fluids (blood, cerebrospinal fluid, peritoneal fluid, synovial fluid, pleural fluid, or pericardial fluid).

Epidemiologic factors, site of infection, and the clinical status of the patient must also be considered in selecting antibiotics. The results of pretreatment cultures can provide a definitive microbiologic diagnosis, and in vitro antibiotic susceptibility testing, if appropriate, can be performed. Interpretation of microbiologic cultures obtained after initiation of antimicrobial therapy is difficult; in this setting, the presence of sterile cultures may be misleading.

Some general guidelines may be helpful in selecting therapy. Certain pathogens have a predilection for causing infection at certain sites, eg, *Streptococcus pneumoniae* (pneumonia, meningitis) and *Escherichia coli* (urinary tract infections, bacteremia). Certain antimicrobials have predictable activity against specific organisms, eg, penicillins for streptococci and vancomycin for staphylococci and streptococci, including methicillin-resistant strains. However, an increasing number of microorganisms are manifesting resistance to standard antimicrobials (Table 15–6). Therefore, obtaining cultures in conjunction with susceptibility testing is imperative.

Despite the availability of numerous antimicrobial agents most pathogens are optimally treated with to only a few drugs. Antimicrobial therapy should be as specific, nontoxic, and inexpensive as confirmatory cultures and susceptibility tests allow. Used wisely, antimicrobials rarely fail; regimens should not be changed haphazardly in a random search for an effective agent. Changes should be based on a complete and logical data base, which usually includes results of standardized susceptibility testing performed in a reliable laboratory. In the ICU patient, the choice of antibiotics may be dictated by the presence of hepatic or renal dysfunction. In addition, the dosages of some agents must be modified in patients with impaired excretion of the drugs because of decreased kidney or liver function.

This section describes some of the newer antimicrobial agents with the goal of establishing general guidelines for their use. It is important to keep in mind that the choice of a specific agent should be based on the nature of the infection as well as patient factors; the newest antimicrobial drug is often not the best choice.

Table 15–6. Emerging resistance to antibiotics.

Organisms With Emerging Resistance	Antibiotics
Streptococcus pneumoniae	Beta-lactams, macrolides, quinolones
Staphylococcus aureus	Methicillin, aminoglycosides, quinolones, glycopeptides (vancomycin, teicoplanin)
Enterococcus	Aminoglycosides, penicillin, glycopeptides (vancomycin, teicoplanin)
Haemophillus influenzae	Ampicillin (beta-lactamase-negative), chloramphenicol
Pseudomonas aeruginosa (including other group 1 beta-lactamase-producing gram-negative bacilli)	Aminoglycosides, beta-lactams, carbapenems, quinolones
Enterobacteriaceae	Beta-lactams
Acinetobacter baumanii	Beta-lactams, carbapenems, quinolones, aminoglycosides
Bacteroides fragilis	Clindamycin

Since the development and use of the sulfonamides in the 1930s and penicillin in the 1940s, numerous effective antibacterial and antifungal agents—and, more recently, antiviral agents—have become available. The similarities of many of these antibiotics are more striking than their differences. Nonetheless, many antibiotics have special roles in the treatment of the infected patient.

Penicillins

Mezlocillin is more active in vitro than carbenicillin or ticarcillin against Enterobacteriaceae and contains less sodium, but evidence for greater clinical efficacy is lacking. Some strains of enteric gram-negative bacilli are resistant to mezlocillin; thus, these agents should generally be used in combination with an aminoglycoside or other antimicrobial agent with gram-negative activity until the antimicrobial susceptibility of the infecting organism is known. Mezlocillin is not the drug of choice for any gram-positive infection because of its limited spectrum of activity.

Azlocillin is equivalent to carbenicillin in its activity against Enterobacteriaceae. In vitro, it is more active against *Pseudomonas aeruginosa* than all extended-spectrum penicillins with the exception of piperacillin, but evidence for greater clinical efficacy is lacking. Azlocillin is no longer available for use in the United States. Piperacillin has greater in vitro activity than all extended-spectrum penicillins against *P aeruginosa* and more activity against many Enterobacteriaceae than carbenicillin or ticarcillin. It also contains less sodium than carbenicillin or ticarcillin.

Mezlocillin, azlocillin, and piperacillin are not the agents of choice for infection with any gram-positive organisms.

Cephalosporins

The cephalosporins constitute a large group of antibacterial agents that have undergone considerable chemical modification over the years. For convenience, they have been divided into "generations" that distribute the drugs according to similarities of antibacterial activity as well as date of introduction and release. In general, first-generation cephalosporins are more active against gram-positive cocci than the second-generation or third-generation agents, whereas the third-generation cephalosporins (cefotaxime, cefoperazone, and ceftriaxone) are most active against gram-negative bacilli. However, only two third-generation cephalosporins, ceftazidime and cefoperazone, have sufficient in vitro activity against *P aeruginosa* to justify their use when this organism is suspected or identified. Cefoxitin, cefotetan, and ceftizoxime are active against anaerobic bacteria.

Cefepime is a new antimicrobial agent that has been referred to as a fourth-generation cephalosporin. It has excellent activity against the Enterobacteriaceae, enterobacter species, *P aeruginosa,* and *Streptococcus pneumoniae,* moderate activity against *Staphylococcus aureus,* and limited antianaerobe activity.

Carbapenems

Imipenem and meropenem are the two carbapenems currently available for use. The presence of the carbapenem ring increases the potency and antibacterial spectrum of these agents. In place of an acylamino side group off the beta-lactam ring—found in the penicillins and cephalosporins—imipenem has a short hydroxyethyl side chain that protects the ring from degradation by bacteria-produced beta-lactamases. The alkylthio side chain attached to the carbapenem nucleus increases activity against *P aeruginosa* and other gram-negative bacteria. The carbapenems inhibit bacterial cell wall synthesis by binding preferentially to one of the penicillin-binding proteins, PBP-2. The carbapenems are active against most aerobic and anaerobic gram-positive and gram-negative organisms. Imipenem is available only in combination with cilastatin sodium; the latter is added to prevent renal metabolism of the imipenem, which decreases nephrotoxicity. Imipenem-cilastin sodium has been associated with adverse central nervous system reactions, including seizures. Slight structural modifications have rendered meropenem resistant to degradation by the dehydropeptidases of the renal brush border while conferring slightly greater activity against aerobic gram-negative bacilli but slightly less activity against aerobic gram-positive cocci—and have decreased the epileptogenic potential of the drug.

Monobactams

Aztreonam is the only clinically useful member of the class of beta-lactam antibiotics referred to as monobactams. It has minimal activity against gram-positive bacteria and anaerobes but is extremely active against aerobic gram-negative bacilli, including *P aeruginosa.* The drug is highly resistant to enzymatic hydrolysis by beta-lactamases and is a poor inducer of chromosomal beta-lactamases. The narrow spectrum of aztreonam may allow maintenance of host-defensive microflora and may reduce the emergence of resistant bacteria.

Aminoglycosides

Netilmicin has in vitro antibacterial activity similar to that of gentamicin and tobramycin but is more active than other aminoglycosides against pseudomonads other than *P aeruginosa.* Amikacin has greater activity against a wider spectrum of gram-negative bacilli than other aminoglycosides. Aminoglycoside levels and renal function studies should be monitored closely in patients receiving these agents. Patients with normal and stable renal function can be monitored once or twice weekly after the correct aminoglycoside dosing has been established. Patients with abnormal but stable renal function should be monitored two to four times weekly. Finally, patients with fluctuating renal function, including many critically ill patients with sepsis, may require daily monitoring, with dosage adjustment to avoid nephrotoxicity or ototoxicity.

Aminoglycosides exert a postantibiotic effect against gram-negative bacteria; growth of these bacteria is inhibited for 4–6 hours beyond any measurable aminoglycoside in the serum or tissue. The postantibiotic effect has led to recommendations to increase the dosing interval for gentamicin and tobramycin from every 8 hours to every 24 hours and for amikacin from every 12 hours to every 24 hours.

Quinolones

The quinolones are a relatively new class of antimicrobial agents that have expanded significantly in recent years. Quinolones act by binding to bacterial DNA gyrase and topoisomerase IV, thus preventing DNA replication. Resistance occurs via accrual of mutations at the enzyme target or by active efflux of the drug out of bacterial cells. The earlier quinolones (norfloxacin, ciprofloxacin, ofloxacin, lomefloxacin, and enoxacin) have activity primarily against gram-negative organisms and staphylococci, with limited activity against streptococci and anaerobes. The newer agents (levofloxacin, sparfloxacin, grepafloxacin, gatifloxacin, and moxifloxacin) have greater potency against streptococci, particularly *Streptococcus pneumoniae,* including penicillin-resistant *S pneumoniae.* Some of the newer agents have significant anaerobic activity. All quinolones have activity against atypical pneumonia pathogens, including legionella, *Chlamydia pneumoniae, Mycoplasma pneumoniae, Chlamydia trachomatis,* and some mycobacteria.

In general, the quinolones have excellent bioavailability and may be given either orally or intravenously. Side effects include nausea, vomiting, photosensitivity, central nervous system symptoms, and a prolonged QT interval.

Beta-Lactamase Inhibitors

Beta-lactamases are bacterial enzymes that can inactivate beta-lactam antibiotics such as penicillins and cephalosporins. However, beta-lactam antibiotics can be protected from enzymatic cleavage by steric hindrance of the beta-lactam ring or by coupling the antibiotic with a beta-lactamase inhibitor. The inhibitor effectively acts as a decoy, binding the enzyme that prevents it from inactivating the antibiotic. Three beta-lactamase inhibitors are now available for clinical use: sulbactam, clavulanate, and tazobactam. All three are administered in fixed combination with beta-lactam antibiotics. Sulbactam is available in combination with ampicillin, clavulanate with amoxicillin or ticarcillin, and tazobactam with piperacillin. In general, the beta-lactamase inhibitors demonstrate activity against the beta-lactamases of *Neisseria gonorrhoeae, K pneumoniae, S aureus, H influenzae, M catarrhalis,* bacteroides species, *E coli,* and other Enterobacteriaceae. They have little to no activity against chromosomally based beta-lactamases such as those found among enterobacter, citrobacter, serratia, pseudomonas, and morganella species. These beta-lactam–beta-lactamase inhibitor combinations may have a special niche in the treatment of patients with polymicrobial infections.

Triazoles

The triazoles are fungistatic drugs, which inhibit the fungal cytochrome P450 enzyme to block the transformation of lanosterol to ergosterol, the major sterol in the fungal cell membrane. The result is osmotic instability and loss of integrity of the fungal cell wall. There are currently two available triazoles. Fluconazole is available in both oral and parenteral forms, and essentially equivalent blood levels are achieved by either route. Fluconazole has a wide volume of distribution, achieving high levels in urine, sputum, saliva, peritoneal fluid, vaginal secretions, bile, cerebrospinal fluid, skin, liver, and prostate. Achievable cerebrospinal fluid levels are about 60–80% of serum levels. Fluconazole is 80% excreted unchanged in the urine, and doses do need to be adjusted for renal insufficiency. Fluconazole is active against *Candida albicans, Candida tropicalis, Candida parapsilosis, Coccidioides immitis,* and *Cryptococcus neoformans.* It has been shown to be effective in the treatment of hematogenous, mucosal, and end organ candidal infection. Caution should be used when treating infection with certain non-*albicans* species such as *Candida krusei* and *Candida glabrata,* as these organisms are less sensitive to fluconazole.

Itraconazole is the other triazole that is available for clinical use. A parenteral form has recently become available. Oral formulations have inconsistent absorptions and so should be avoided in the critically ill patient. Compared with fluconazole, itraconazole has greater activity against aspergillus, *Blastomyces dermatitidis, Histoplasma capsulatum,* and *Sporothrix schenkii.*

Amphotericin B Lipid Formulations

Amphotericin B desoxycholate has long been the standard for treatment of severe mycoses. It is a fungicidal drug that binds to ergosterol in the cell wall and causes osmotic instability and cell death. The major weakness of amphotericin B desoxycholate has been its numerous adverse effects, especially nephrotoxicity. The new lipid formulations of amphotericin B have the advantage of causing less nephrotoxicity. There are currently three formulations available: amphotericin B lipid complex, amphotericin B colloidal dispersion, and liposomal amphotericin B. They are approved for use in patients with invasive fungal infections who are intolerant of amphotericin B desoxycholate. Liposomal amphotericin B has an additional indication for empiric therapy in febrile patients with neutropenia. There are some data, mostly from retrospective comparisons and a few prospective trials, suggesting improved response rates with lipid formulations and a lower incidence of nephrotoxicity. Due to the significant cost differential between the lipid formulations of amphotericin B and amphotericin B desoxycholate, use of the lipid formulations is generally reserved for specific subgroups of patients. For example, in high-risk patients such as marrow transplant recipients with suspected invasive aspergillosis, earlier use of the lipid formulations may be warranted in an attempt to improve response rates and to decrease renal toxicity.

Macrolides

The three macrolides available for clinical use in the United States are erythromycin, clarithromycin, and azithromycin. In comparison with erythromycin, the latter two have greater activity against *Haemophilus influenzae, Chlamydia trachomatis, Mycobacterium avium* complex, and other nontuberculous mycobacteria. The role of these agents in the critically ill patient is limited to treatment of patients suspected of having atypical pneumonias. All three agents possess good activity against *Mycoplasma pneumoniae, Chlamydia pneumoniae,* and legionella species. Erythromycin and azithromycin are available in a parenteral formulation, while clarithromycin is available only in an oral form.

Quinupristin/Dalfopristin

Quinupristin/dalfopristin is a formulation of two bacteriostatic antimicrobial agents which, when combined, are bactericidal. Its antimicrobial activity is the result of inhibition of protein synthesis at the 50S ribosome. Quinupristin/dalfopristin is available for intravenous use only. Its spectrum of activity is similar to that of vancomycin and includes *Streptococcus pneumoniae,* other streptococcus species, *Staphylococcus aureus,* and coagulase-negative staphylococci. It is bacteriostatic for *Enterococcus faecium* and has no activity against *Enterococcus faecalis.* The niche for quinupristin/dalfopristin is in the treatment of vancomycin-resistant *Enterococcus faecium* and possibly glycopeptide-insensitive *Staphylococcus aureus.*

Linezolid

Linezolid belongs to the class of drugs known as oxazolidinones. These drugs block bacterial protein synthesis at the ribosome at a very early stage. Because of its novel mechanism of action, linezolid does not share cross-resistance with other antimicrobial agents. Linezolid's spectrum of activity is essentially identical to that of vancomycin. Much like quinupristin/dalfopristin, the major indications for use of this agent is the treatment of vancomycin-resistant enterococcus and glycopeptide-insensitive *Staphylococcus aureus* infections. Linezolid is approved for treatment of pneumonia, bacteremia, and skin and soft-tissue infections due to gram-positive organisms. Linezolid is available in both an oral and parenteral formulation, with excellent oral bioavailability.

Alvarez-Elcoro S, Enzler MJ: The macrolides: erythromycin, clarithromycin, and azithromycin. Mayo Clin Proc 1999; 74:613–34.

Dix SP, Andriole VT: Lipid formulations of amphotericin B. Curr Clin Top Infect Dis 2000;20:1–23.

Edson RS, Terrell CL: The aminoglycosides. Mayo Clin Proc 1999;74:519–28.

Hellinger WC, Brewer NS: Carbapenems and monobactams: imipenem, meropenem, and aztreonam. Mayo Clin Proc 1999;74:420–34.

Lundstrom TS, Sobel JD: Antibiotics for gram-positive bacterial infections: vancomycin, quinupristin/dalfopristin, and linezolid. Infect Dis Clin North Am 2000;14:463–74.

Marshall WF, Blair JE: The cephalosporins. Mayo Clin Proc 1999;74:187–95.

Plouffe JF: Emerging therapies for serious gram-positive bacterial infections: a focus on linezolid. Clin Infect Dis 2000;31 (Suppl):S144–9.

Talan DA: Clinical perspectives on new antimicrobials: focus on fluoroquinolones. Clin Infect Dis 2001;32(Suppl 1):S64–71.

Terrell CL: Antifungal agents. Part II. The azoles. Mayo Clin Proc 1999;74:78–100.

Wright AJ: The penicillins. Mayo Clin Proc 1999;74:290–307.

EVALUATION OF THE INTENSIVE CARE UNIT PATIENT WITH NEW FEVER

The evaluation of new fever in the ICU setting involves consideration of diagnoses much different FROM those encountered in patients in a community setting. There are many noninfectious causes of fever that must be considered and ruled out in order to avoid missing important diagnoses and perhaps administering antimicrobial agents unnecessarily.

Clinical Features

A. History and Examination

When eliciting a history, special attention should be paid to the quality and quantity of respiratory secretions, changes in the patient's tolerance to oral intake, the condition of the patient's skin, and the presence or absence of diarrhea. Because many patients in an intensive care unit will be unable to provide a history, information should be elicited from family members or caregivers, and a thorough physical examination should be performed.

It is recommended that temperatures be taken using an electronic probe in the mouth, rectum, or external auditory canal. Axillary temperature measurements may be spuriously low and so should not be used. Sinusitis should be considered in patients with nasotracheal or nasogastric tubes—which block the sinus ostia, thus predisposing to infection. Careful auscultatory examination should be performed to look for new pulmonary findings that may indicate a nosocomial pneumonia or a new or changing murmur that may indicate endocarditis. Abdominal examination should be performed to assess the presence of focal tenderness and the presence or absence of bowel sounds. All intravascular catheter sites should be scrutinized for signs of inflammation at the catheter exit site or along the subcutaneous tunnel. The patient's skin requires careful inspection for any lesions that may indicate hematogenous seeding (either bacterial or fungal), rashes that may indicate a drug reaction, and decubitus ulcers or surgical wounds that may become infected.

B. Laboratory and Imaging Studies

Laboratory evaluation should include a complete blood count, routine chemistries with liver enzymes, and urinalysis. Cultures of blood and urine should be obtained routinely. Other evaluations should be directed by the results of the history and physical examination. A chest radiograph and sputum sample for culture should be obtained when nosocomial pneumonia is suspected. Stool specimens for *C difficile* toxin should be collected from patients who develop diarrhea while hospitalized. Routine stool cultures and stool for ova and parasites are not useful in evaluation of new fever in a patient in the critical care unit. Any wounds that appear infected should be debrided, and any purulent material obtained should be cultured. If the abdominal examination or the liver enzymes suggest an intra-abdominal process, a right upper quadrant ultrasound or CT scan of the abdomen and pelvis may be requested. If sinusitis is suspected, CT or MRI of the sinuses may be helpful.

Treatment

Empiric therapy will depend on the results of the physical examination and initial laboratory data.

O'Grady NP et al: Practice guidelines for evaluating new fever in critically ill adult patients. Clin Infect Dis 1998;26:1042–59.

NOSOCOMIAL PNEUMONIA

ESSENTIALS OF DIAGNOSIS

- *Fever, tachypnea, tachycardia, and abnormal breath sounds.*
- *Risk factors include altered mental status, lung disease, endotracheal tube or tracheostomy.*
- *Change in volume or appearance of sputum.*
- *Infiltrates or other changes on chest x-ray.*
- *Hypoxemia or worsening arterial blood gases.*

General Considerations

It is estimated that at least 5% of hospitalized patients will develop a nosocomial infection, and nosocomial pneumonia is responsible for 15% of all nosocomial infections. Pneumonia is the second most common nosocomial infection after urinary tract infections and is the leading cause of death due to hospital-acquired infection. The mortality rates range from 5–20% when pneumonia is due to gram-positive cocci, from 30–50% with enteric gram-negative bacilli, and up to 70% with *P aeruginosa.*

Pathophysiology

Pneumonia develops from one of three mechanisms: (1) inhalation of an aerosol containing infectious microorganisms, (2) hematogenous seeding of microorganisms in the lung, or (3) aspiration of oropharyngeal flora.

A. Inhalational Pneumonia

Infectious particles less than 3–5 μm in diameter are capable of reaching the terminal bronchi and alveoli during inhalation. *Mycobacterium tuberculosis,* legionella, and influenza virus—as well as many fungi—are known to cause nosocomial pneumonia by this route of spread. Contaminated respiratory equipment has been recognized as a source of infected aerosols and a cause of gram-negative bacillary necrotizing pneumonia. Hospital policies and procedures requiring rigorous, frequent changing and disposal of equipment have markedly decreased the incidence of inhalation pneumonia in the hospital setting.

B. Hematogenous Pneumonia

Pneumonia caused by the hematogenous seeding of infection is uncommon. Patients predisposed to hematogenous pneumonia are those with *S aureus* or candidal infections associated with infected intravenous catheters, septic thrombophlebitis, or endocarditis of the right side of the heart. Pneumonia develops as a consequence of infected thrombi forming within the intravascular space and traveling through the bloodstream to reach the pulmonary circulation (septic pulmonary emboli).

C. Aspiration Pneumonia

Aspiration of oropharyngeal bacterial flora is the most common mechanism responsible for nosocomial pneumonia. Although all individuals aspirate microscopic quantities of oropharyngeal secretions, certain factors increase the risk of pneumonia. These include (1) high frequency and large volume of secretions aspirated, (2) aspiration of particularly virulent bacterial species, (3) the presence of particulate matter in the aspirate, and (4) abnormalities of the lower airway and alveolar defense mechanisms. Aerobic enteric gram-negative bacilli are not usually part of the flora colonizing the oropharynx in normal, healthy, nonhospitalized individuals. However, oropharyngeal colonization by gram-negative bacilli increases with the duration of hospital stay, so that by day 10 over half of ICU patients will have oropharyngeal colonization by such flora. Patients receiving antibiotics develop gram-negative colonization more rapidly.

Prophylaxis of stress ulcers with the use of antacids or H_2-receptor antagonists has been considered a risk factor for gram-negative aspiration pneumonia via gastric acid neutralization, allowing subsequent overgrowth of enteric gram-negative bacilli. However, a prospective study evaluating cultures of the oropharynx, tracheal aspirates, and gastric aspirates—followed by culture of lower respiratory tract secretions by the protected bronchoscopic technique in the event of development of nosocomial pneumonia—failed to note a correlation between the culture results from the gastric aspirates and the respiratory tract secretions. This study suggests that stomach contents are not necessarily an important source of pathogens in nosocomial pneumonia. Similarly, the use of selective decontamination of the digestive tract is not recommended on a routine basis.

Microbiologic Etiology

The microbiology of pneumonia in hospitalized patients is significantly different from that of pneumonia acquired outside the hospital. The most common pathogen in nosocomial pneumonia is *P aeruginosa,* followed by *S aureus, H influenzae,* klebsiella species, Enterobacteriaceae, and *E coli.* Other important causes of nosocomial pneumonia include acinetobacter species, other nonfermenting gram-negative bacilli, and viridans streptococci. Approximately 20–40% of nosocomial pneumonias are polymicrobial in etiology. Anaerobic bacteria are not considered an important pathogen in nosocomial pneumonia. Legionellae are common causes of nosocomial pneumonia in some hospitals.

Clinical Features

The diagnosis of pneumonia depends on physical examination findings, microbiologic analysis of lower respiratory secretions, and review of the chest x-ray. Although risk factors for development of pneumonia should be considered in assessing the likelihood of pneumonia, any critically ill patient—especially one with underlying heart or lung disease—should be considered at risk for nosocomial pneumonia. Studies have identified many different risk factors in the development of nosocomial pneumonia. Among the most important of these are neurologic impairment, witnessed aspiration, mechanical ventilation (with increasing risk associated with prolonged need for mechanical ventilation), underlying chronic lung disease, the presence of acute respiratory distress syndrome, increasing age, use of a nasogastric tube, enteral feeding, low endotracheal cuff pressure, severity of underlying illness, need for tracheostomy, and supine position of the patient.

A. Symptoms and Signs

Patients with suspected nosocomial pneumonia require prompt assessment prior to the initiation of therapy. The clinical features of pneumonia in hospitalized patients are subtle and variable, and in occasional cases there may be no symptoms or examination findings. Use of clinical and radiographic features alone to diagnose nosocomial pneumonia will lead to the misclassification of many disorders as nosocomial pneumonia. Some diagnostic clues include altered mental status, fever, tachypnea, tachycardia, and abnormal breath sounds. Physical findings commonly include crackles or rales rather than evidence of lung consolidation. Wheezing may be present, and localized wheezing may suggest aspiration of a foreign body. The presence of preexisting abnormal lung findings may make the diagnosis difficult. Patients with a tracheostomy or endotracheal tube may first manifest a lower respiratory tract infection by a change in gross appearance of the respiratory secretions or an increase in oxygen requirement. The physician should ask the respiratory therapist or nurse about the quantity and appearance of these secretions. The development of purulence or an increase in the quantity of secretions suggests heavy bacterial colonization or infection, often prior to the development of a radiographic infiltrate.

B. Laboratory Findings

Most patients in the ICU are too debilitated to produce an adequate sputum sample; samples of respiratory secretions may in such cases be obtained by endotracheal suctioning or fiberoptic bronchoscopy. It is clear that endotracheal aspirates alone are often inaccurate in diagnosing the etiologic agent of a nosocomial pneumonia. Quantitative endotracheal aspirates, a protected specimen brush, or bronchoalveolar lavage will often provide more useful information. However, most diagnostic modalities for nosocomial pneumonia are neither sensitive nor specific. Respiratory cultures obtained by any means must be interpreted with caution, as airways of hospitalized patients are almost always colonized with various potentially pathogenic bacteria. In various studies, the sensitivity of cultures from endotracheal aspirates, protected specimen brush, and bronchoalveolar lavage were 52–100%, 65–100%, and 80–100%, respectively, with specificities of 29–100%, 60–100%, and 75–100%, respectively. The large variation in sensitivity and specificity is due to differences in patient population (eg, previous antibiotic therapy) and the diagnostic criteria used. In the few studies that have evaluated changes in clinical outcome based on the results of invasive sampling of respiratory secretions, no change in mortality was seen despite modification of antibiotic treatment. The presence of more than five cells with intracellular organisms in bronchoalveolar lavage fluid increased the sensitivity of this sampling technique to 91% and the specificity to 89%. A Gram stain of the sputum may help identify the etiologic agent and suggest appropriate empiric therapy. A sputum Gram stain that reveals 10 or fewer squamous epithelial cells and more than 25 polymorphonuclear cells per high-power field can be considered an adequate specimen. Typically, the Gram stain may be more helpful than the culture in patients already receiving antimicrobial agents that may inhibit bacterial growth in culture.

A complete blood count, blood cultures, and a chest x-ray are essential. The chest x-ray may reveal an infiltrate, but nonspecific findings such as atelectasis may be the only findings. Patients with prior pulmonary disease often have preexisting abnormalities on chest x-ray that make it difficult to identify new infiltrates. Blood cultures, when positive, should be considered definitive for the etiologic agent. However, only 20% of pneumonias caused by gram-negative organisms are associated with a positive blood culture. Pleural fluid, if present, should be obtained by thoracentesis for Gram stain, culture for aerobic and anaerobic organisms, and determination of cell count, pH, total protein, and LDH concentration. Serologic studies are seldom useful in determining the cause of nosocomial pneumonia.

Differential Diagnosis

The differential diagnosis of nosocomial pneumonia includes virtually all processes associated with pulmonary infiltrates. Acute respiratory distress syndrome, pulmonary emboli with infarction, cardiogenic pulmonary edema, lung cancer, and atelectasis are often difficult to differentiate from an infectious lung process. Less common diseases to be considered include collagen-vascular disease, pulmonary hemorrhage, radiation pneumonitis, hypersensitivity pneumonitis, sarcoidosis, occupational lung diseases, and pulmonary alveolar proteinosis.

Treatment

A. Antibiotics

Empiric antimicrobial therapy for nosocomial pneumonia should be based on clinical features, epidemiologic and host factors, and results of an initial Gram stain. Surveillance data relating to local nosocomial flora leading to pneumonia in the ICU should be reviewed. Antibiotic therapy should be administered intravenously and should target a broad spectrum of bacteria. The possibility of resistant microorganisms should be considered in the hospitalized patient with nosocomial pneumonia.

Cefipime, meropenem, or an extended-spectrum penicillin provides the broadest coverage for infections with most Enterobacteriaceae, *P aeruginosa,* and *S aureus* as well as *S pneumoniae* and *H influenzae.* If the prevalence of methicillin-resistant *S aureus* strains is high and staphylococcal pneumonia is a consideration, vancomycin should be included in the initial drug regimen. Quinolones have excellent activity against most Enterobacteriaceae as well as *H influenzae* but possess less activity against streptococci and staphylococci (except for levofloxacin and the newer quinolones) and little to none against most anaerobes.

B. Supportive Care

Patients with pneumonia require suctioning of respiratory secretions, postural drainage, and, occasionally, fiberoptic bronchoscopy. Coughing is the most effective way to clear the large airways of respiratory secretions. In patients with endotracheal tubes or tracheostomies, use of appropriate suctioning must substitute for cough. Postural drainage and chest percussion may be useful in selected patients, but only if it can be demonstrated that removal of respiratory secretions is improved. In certain patients, fiberoptic bronchoscopy can be helpful in identifying endobronchial obstruction, and this technique may aid in suctioning secretions from particular airways. Most patients with pneumonia are given bronchodilators, but the effectiveness of these agents in patients without obstructive lung disease is not known.

Prevention

Prevention of nosocomial pneumonia is of utmost importance in decreasing morbidity and mortality rates and controlling the costs of hospital care. Recognition of the aspiration-prone patient is essential. Patients with nasogastric tubes for enteral feeding should have the head of the bed elevated 30–45 degrees during feeding. All patients should be turned frequently, if possible. Appropriate disposal, disinfection, or sterilization of respiratory equipment is critical for prevention of contamination and subsequent inhalation pneumonias. Nurses, physicians, and respiratory therapists must use sterile techniques for endotracheal suctioning. Meticulous hand washing before and after patient examination and wearing gloves when appropriate will help decrease the overall incidence of nosocomial infections in the ICU. Other interventions that may help in prevention of nosocomial pneumonia include placing patients in the semirecumbent position, avoidance of prolonged nasal intubation (which may lead to nosocomial sinusitis), and subglottic suctioning.

Bonten MJ et al: The stomach is not a source of colonization of the upper respiratory tract and pneumonia in ICU patients. Chest 1994;105:878–84.

Chastre J et al: Evaluation of bronchoscopic techniques for the diagnosis of nosocomial pneumonia. Am J Respir Crit Care Med 1995;152:231–40.

Cook DJ et al: Incidence of and risk factors for ventilator-associated pneumonia in critically ill patients. Ann Intern Med 1998;129:433–40.

Cook DJ, Kollef MH: Risk factors for ICU-acquired pneumonia. JAMA 1998;279:1605–6.

Cunha BA: Nosocomial pneumonia: diagnostic and therapeutic considerations. Med Clin North Am 2001;85:79–114.

Kollef MH: The prevention of ventilator-associated pneumonia. N Engl J Med 1999;340:627–34.

Lode HM et al: Nosocomial pneumonia in the critical care unit. Crit Care Clin 1998;14:119–33.

Mayer J: Laboratory diagnosis of nosocomial pneumonia. Semin Respir Infect 2000;15:119–31.

Mayhall CG: Nosocomial pneumonia: diagnosis and prevention. Infect Dis Clin North Am 1997;11:427–57.

URINARY CATHETER-ASSOCIATED INFECTIONS

ESSENTIALS OF DIAGNOSIS

- *Although the patient may be asymptomatic, suprapubic tenderness suggests lower tract infection; fever and flank pain suggest upper tract infection.*
- *Pyuria and white blood cell casts.*
- *Positive urine culture*

General Considerations

A urinary (bladder) catheter provides a portal of entry into the urinary tract for microorganisms. Urinary catheter-associated infections account for up to 40% of all nosocomial infections. Less than 5% of patients who develop bacteriuria will develop bacteremia; however, owing to the great frequency of nosocomial bacteriurias, they account for 15% of all nosocomial bacteremias. The mortality from urosepsis ranges from 25–60%. Thus, early recognition and appropriate treatment of urinary catheter-associated infections can significantly reduce morbidity and length of stay in the ICU.

The urinary catheter allows transit of microorganisms colonizing the perineum and the urethral meatus to pass through the urethra and enter the bladder. Most catheter-associated bacteriuria occurs by extraluminal ascent of bacteria via the mucous film coating the outer surface of the catheter, presumably the result of contamination of the urine in the collection bag. Bacteriuria occurs in catheterized patients at a rate of 5–10% per catheter day, with bacteremia and sepsis occurring in 2–4%. By the tenth day of catheterization, nearly 100% of patients will have bacteriuria, either symptomatic or asymptomatic. Colonization of the bladder may lead to lower or upper urinary tract infections or urosepsis.

The most common microorganisms causing infection in short-term catheterized patients in the ICU include *E coli, K pneumoniae, Proteus mirabilis, P aeruginosa,* Enterobacteriaceae, *S epidermidis, S aureus,* and enterococci. Polymicrobial infections occur in up to 15% of catheterized patients. Anaerobic infections are extremely rare. Candiduria is common in patients receiving corticosteroids or antibiotics and in those with diabetes mellitus. Urinary tract infections with candida species or *S aureus* should raise the question of hematogenous spread, as occasionally a urinary tract infection with one of these organisms is a marker of disseminated disease.

Risk factors for catheter-associated bacteriuria include prolonged duration of catheterization, lack of a urinometer, diabetes mellitus, absence of systemic antibiotic use, female sex, microbial colonization of the urinary drainage bag, an indication for catheterization other than surgery or output measurement, abnormal serum creatinine, errors in catheter care, and periurethral colonization with potential uropathogens. Once bacteriuria has occurred, it is difficult to prevent subsequent infection; thus, prevention of the initial bacteriuria is critical. The only two factors shown to decrease the risk of nosocomial catheter-associated bacteriuria are maintenance of a closed catheter system and early removal of the urinary catheter.

Clinical Features

A. Symptoms and Signs

Diagnosis of catheter-related urinary tract infection is straightforward even though most patients with catheter-associated urinary tract infections are asymptomatic. Up to 30% of patients will have fever or other symptoms of urinary tract infection. Fever or other systemic signs of infection, as well as pain localized to the flank, suggest upper tract infection.

B. Laboratory Findings

The white blood cell count may be elevated with serious infection. Definitive diagnosis is based on urinalysis and results of urine culture. Direct examination of the urine continues to be valuable for early diagnosis of bacterial infections of the genitourinary tract. Pyuria and white blood cell casts indicate the presence of urinary infection rather than simple bacterial colonization of the urine. The presence of white blood cell casts suggests upper tract disease. The presence of one or two leukocytes per high-power field (400 ×), or bacteria seen under oil immersion

(1000 ×) in unspun urine has a 95% correlation with the presence of more than 100,000 CFU/mL of urine. Thus, microscopy is useful for identification of urinary tract involvement with a high urine bacterial count.

The presence of bacteria in a concentration greater than 100,000 CFU/mL with accompanying pyuria is consistent with infection. In catheterized patients, bacterial counts of > 1000 CFU/mL, if untreated, will increase to > 100,000 CFU/mL within 24–48 hours. Urine culture for bacteria and fungi must be submitted to the laboratory, with prompt processing. Alternatively, specimens may be refrigerated at 4 °C, where bacterial counts will remain stable for up to 24 hours. Urine left at room temperature for over 2 hours after collection has been shown to have significantly higher urine bacterial colony counts, thereby confounding the diagnosis of urinary tract infection.

Most microbiology laboratories routinely identify and perform antimicrobial susceptibility tests on microorganisms present in numbers $\geq 10^4$ CFU/mL. If polymicrobial bacteriuria is anticipated (eg, chronic indwelling catheter or neurogenic bladder), the laboratory should be alerted to this possibility.

C. Imaging Studies

Seriously ill patients presenting with a urinary tract infection, whether catheter-related or not, who have high fever, flank pain, or urosepsis require further evaluation for upper tract disease. Ultrasonography is useful to assess the anatomy of the genitourinary tract and to rule out an obstructed ureter. Further studies, including an intravenous pyelogram, retrograde pyelogram, or CT scan, may be necessary to diagnose renal abscess, perinephric abscess, or nephrolithiasis.

D. Complications

Complications of bladder and kidney infections are common and potentially serious. The urinary tract is the most common site of origin of gram-negative bacteremia and sepsis. Acute pyelonephritis, chronic pyelonephritis, emphysematous pyelonephritis, renal abscess, and urosepsis may complicate an untreated urinary tract infection.

Differential Diagnosis

Urinary tract infections should be differentiated from asymptomatic bacteriuria, urethritis, prostatitis, sexually transmitted diseases, pelvic inflammatory disease, diverticulitis, intra-abdominal abscess, and peritonitis.

Treatment

A. Asymptomatic Patient With Bacteriuria

Antibiotic therapy in the asymptomatic bacteriuric patient with an indwelling catheter and an unremarkable urinalysis is discouraged, as bacteriuria will recur when treatment is discontinued and selection of antibiotic-resistant organisms is likely.

B. Patient With Abnormal Urinalysis and Bacteriuria

In patients with abnormal urinalysis and bacteriuria, the urinary catheter should be removed and antibiotics initiated. If the patient requires an indwelling catheter for bladder drainage, a new catheter can be reinserted. In general, empiric therapy should be directed against nosocomial gram-negative pathogens; an aminoglycoside, a cephalosporin, or a quinolone given intravenously is usually appropriate initial antibiotic treatment. Therapy may be discontinued in uncomplicated cases at 7 days. However, more seriously ill patients with prolonged fever, suspected upper tract involvement, positive blood cultures, renal insufficiency, or sepsis require a longer course of intravenous antibiotics and further evaluation for upper tract disease.

C. Candiduria

Asymptomatic candiduria in immunocompromised patients or symptomatic candidal urinary tract infections in all patients require antifungal treatment. Oral fluconazole, a short course of intravenous amphotericin B, or amphotericin B bladder irrigation is effective for candidal infections confined to the bladder. Upper tract infection requires systemic treatment with oral or intravenous fluconazole or intravenous amphotericin B; complications such as fungal ball, renal or perirenal abscess, or hematogenous dissemination should be considered. In all cases, the catheter should be removed or changed. Asymptomatic candiduria in most patients without immunocompromise will usually clear once the indwelling catheter has been removed and antimicrobial therapy discontinued.

Current Controversies & Unresolved Issues

The appropriate course of action to take with a hospitalized patient who develops asymptomatic nosocomial bacteriuria associated with a urinary catheter remains controversial. The literature suggests that the treatment of bacteriuria in an attempt to avoid complications is not useful. One approach is to remove the catheter as soon as possible after discovery of bacteriuria, with a repeat urinalysis and urine culture 3–5 days later. If the urinalysis is normal and the urine culture is sterile, it is likely that the infection has cleared. If bacteriuria persists, the patient must be monitored for resolution or be treated with a short course of antibiotic therapy. Exceptions to the above rule would be the presence of bacteriuria with organisms that have a high predilection for causing subsequent bacteremia (eg, *Serratia marcescens*) and bacteriuria in patients at risk for serious complications (eg, neutropenic or pregnant patients).

Questions about the value of screening tests for bacteriuria in patients who have urinary catheters are unresolved. Several tests correlate reasonably well with bacteriuria of ≥ 100,000 CFU/mL. The leukocyte esterase-nitrate test has a sensitivity of about 85% in detecting bacteria at ≥ 10^5 CFU/mL. However, the predictive value of a positive test is much lower (25–50%) than that of a negative test.

Attempts to decrease the incidence of bacterial colonization by use of silver-alloy coated urinary catheters have been investigated. It appears that such catheters can decrease the incidence of bacteriuria, but by how much varies widely in different studies. It remains to be seen which population of patients will benefit most from these catheters and whether the use of such catheters will prevent the emergence of antimicrobial-resistant organisms.

Paradisi F, Corti G, Mangani V: Urosepsis in the critical care unit. Crit Care Clin 1998;14:165–80.

Rosser CJ, Bare RL, Meredith JW: Urinary tract infections in the critically ill patient with a urinary catheter. Am J Surg 1999;177:287–90.

Saint S et al: The efficacy of silver alloy-coated urinary catheters in preventing urinary tract infection: a meta-analysis. Am J Med 1998;105:236–41.

Tambyah PA, Halvorson KT, Maki DG: A prospective study of pathogenesis of catheter-associated urinary tract infections. Mayo Clin Proc 1999;74:131–6.

Warren JW: Catheter-associated urinary tract infections. Infect Dis Clin North Am 1997;11:609–22.

INTRAVENOUS CATHETER-ASSOCIATED INFECTIONS

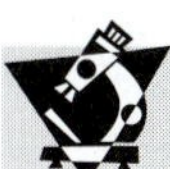

ESSENTIALS OF DIAGNOSIS

- *Exit site infection: erythema, tenderness, induration, and exudate at cutaneous exit site.*
- *Tunnel infection: induration, erythema, tenderness at least 1 cm deep to the skin exit site and without purulent drainage through the exit site.*
- *Catheter sepsis: fever, tachypnea, and tachycardia with positive blood cultures with no other site of infection identified.*

General Considerations

"Short-term" central intravenous and arterial access with indwelling catheters are an integral part of the monitoring and management of patients in the ICU. These catheters are required for administration of antimicrobial therapy, blood products, fluids and electrolytes, and monitoring of hemodynamic status. "Short-term" catheters may be metal needles or Teflon or other synthetic catheters inserted into vessels with only a short distance between skin and intravascular space. These include radial, dorsalis pedis, and femoral artery catheters, intravenous catheters inserted into superficial veins on the extremities, and large-bore central venous catheters inserted into subclavian or internal jugular veins in the neck. The wide-lumen catheters through which pulmonary artery catheters and temporary transvenous cardiac pacemakers are placed are also considered "short-term" catheters.

Patients requiring "long-term" central venous catheters, used primarily for administration of cancer chemotherapy or for total parenteral nutrition, are often admitted to the ICU. It is estimated that over 400,000 Hickman or Broviac type catheters have been implanted in the United States alone. These long-term catheters have in common a subcutaneous tunnel through which the catheter passes after entering the skin and before entering the vein. The presence of a Dacron cuff just inside the exit site of the catheter stimulates growth of the surrounding tissue, thus preventing microorganisms from entering the catheter tract. This permits long-term use of the catheter with a greatly decreased incidence of catheter-related infection.

Two recent additions to the armamentarium of long term venous access catheters are the midline catheters and the peripherally inserted central venous catheters (PICCs). The midline catheter is inserted into the proximal basilic or cephalic vein or into the distal subclavian vein via the antecubital fossa. The PICCs are inserted into the superior vena cava via the antecubital fossa as well. This method of venous access is associated with fewer mechanical complications lower rates of phlebitis and bloodstream infection and is easier to maintain. It appears that the PICC can be left in for a long duration, the specifics are not yet known.

Pathophysiology

Infection of intravascular catheters typically results from one of four events. The most common mechanism of infection is migration of cutaneous colonizing organisms from the insertion site to the catheter tip, frequently seen with short-term catheters. Inadvertent contamination of the catheter hub by the physician or nurse at the time of insertion or by frequent device manipulation can also lead to infection and is an important factor in long-term catheter infection. Contamination of the infusate and hematogenous seeding of the intravascular device from another primary site of infection are less common problems.

Microbiologic Etiology

Gram-positive organisms—most commonly coagulase-negative staphylococci, followed by *Staphylococcus aureus* —and enterococci are implicated in most bloodstream infections due to intravenous devises. The incidence of nosocomial infections due to candida species, especially *C albicans,* has increased dramatically in recent years. Bloodstream infection due to gram-negative bacilli (*E coli,* klebsiella, enterobacter, pseudomonas) are usually related to pressure monitoring systems or contamination of intravenous solutions. It is important to remember that virtually any organism can cause intravenous catheter infection in an immunocompromised host.

Clinical Features

A. Symptoms and Signs

When evaluating a patient with a possible catheter-related infection, several syndromes need to be considered. If an intravascular catheter is removed, growth of ≥ 15 colony-forming units (semiquantitative) or ≥ 10^3 organisms (quantitative culture) from a distal or proximal segment of the intravascular catheter in the absence of accompanying clinical symptoms defines bacterial colonization of the catheter. An exit site infection is characterized by the presence of erythema, tenderness, induration, and purulence within 2 cm of the exit site of the catheter. A tunnel infection is manifested by erythema, tenderness, and induration in the tissues over the catheter and more than 2 cm from the exit site. Finally, a catheter-related bloodstream infection is defined as isolation of the same organism from both the catheter tip and from peripherally drawn blood cultures in the appropriate clinical setting with no other source of infection identified.

It is important to distinguish patients with severe granulocytopenia and catheter-related infections from their immunocompetent cohorts. These patients may not manifest typical inflammatory changes at the site of infection—especially notable is the lack of purulent drainage. However, erythema is still present with infection, and patients may complain of local tenderness, either of which should alert the physician to the probability of infection.

Complications that may occur as a result of catheter-related infections include septic thrombophlebitis and endocarditis. Associated risk factors for catheter-related infections include extremes of age, altered host defenses (especially skin diseases), severity of the underlying disease, use of a multi-lumen catheter, and the presence of infections remote from the catheter site. However, the most important hospital-related risk factor is the duration of use of a particular catheter site. Total parenteral nutrition has also been identified as a risk factor, perhaps because of the length of time the catheter is required to remain in place and the fact that TPN solutions may act as a culture medium to promote the growth of various organisms. Location of the central venous catheter influences the risk of infection. Femoral catheters are most prone to infection, followed by internal jugular catheters; the latter is probably the result of contamination with oropharyngeal secretions and difficulty with immobilization. Subclavian catheters are least prone to infection.

B. Laboratory Findings

Local catheter-related infections (exit site or tunnel infections) may be associated with few or no laboratory abnormalities. Culture of drainage fluid or exudate associated with the exit site may be helpful in determining a causative organism.

Bacteremia (positive blood cultures) may be related to intravascular devices and may occur with or without sepsis. Device-related bacteremia has been defined using quantitative blood culture techniques. A device-related bacteremia is defined as (1) a greater than tenfold increase in colony-forming units of bacteria per milliliter of blood obtained through the device compared with blood drawn from a distant peripheral vein; (2) in the absence of positive peripheral blood cultures, more than 1000 CFU/mL in blood obtained through the device; or (3) organisms isolated from a catheter tip upon removal in the appropriate clinical setting. When no other clinical source of infection is evident, resolution of fever upon removal of the device is also suggestive of catheter-related infection.

Differential Diagnosis

Exit site, catheter tunnel, or catheter infection must be differentiated from chemical phlebitis, which can cause erythema, tenderness, and induration of the vessel wall and overlying skin. Fever may also be present in chemical phlebitis, but systemic symptoms and signs consistent with sepsis syndrome are absent, and exudate cannot be expressed from the exit site. Thrombophlebitis may complicate catheter-related infection. Pain, tenderness, and erythema at the infected site as well as edema distal to the site are common presenting signs. Thrombosis of a central venous catheter can cause edema proximal to the site of thrombosis, but tenderness, erythema, and fever are typically absent. Catheter tip sepsis usually presents with no symptoms or signs of local infection and must be differentiated from infection from any other source.

Treatment

A. Exit Site Infections

Short-term catheters suspected of being infected should be removed. However, there is increasing interest in maintaining long-term catheters in the presence of certain infections. Few data are available to assist in developing recommendations regarding removal or maintenance of an infected long-term catheter. From the published data that do exist, it appears that treatment of an infected catheter with antibiotics alone is successful in about 50% of cases. Thus, in some settings, it may be reasonable to attempt to eradicate a long-term catheter exit site infection with local care plus intravenous antibiotics. Empiric therapy should include vancomycin to cover coagulase-negative staphylococci and *S aureus,* as well as an aminoglycoside or cephalosporin with activity against *P aeruginosa* and other gram-negative bacilli. Definitive therapy can be selected using culture results. If there is no response within a few days or if the exit site infection appears to be progressing to involve the catheter tunnel—or if fungi or resistant bacteria are isolated—the catheter should be removed.

B. Tunnel Infections

Patients with tunnel infections require removal of the catheter for definitive therapy. The tunnel itself may require surgical incision and debridement. Empiric antibiotic therapy should consist of vancomycin to cover coagulase-negative staphylococci and *S aureus* and a third-generation cephalosporin or an aminoglycoside to treat gram-negative bacilli.

C. Catheter Tip Sepsis

Short-term catheters should be removed and antibiotics administered. For a long-term catheter, catheter tip sepsis may be treated initially with intravenous antibiotics while leaving the catheter in place. However, if the patient is in septic shock, the long-term catheter should be removed immediately. Vancomycin in conjunction with a third-generation cephalosporin or aminoglycoside is appropriate initial therapy. Definitive therapy should be guided by the results of the blood culture. Patients should be treated for a total of 2–3 weeks. Catheter tip sepsis in certain patient populations mandates immediate removal of a long-term catheter. These include patients with neutropenia, severe immunocompromise, persistent bacteremia or sepsis despite appropriate antibiotics, septic thrombosis, and patients whose catheters are infected with *S aureus,* candida or other fungi, or antibiotic-resistant bacteria.

Management decisions must be based on the clinical circumstance. The intravascular device should be removed immediately in any patient in whom rapid resolution of the signs of infection does not occur. It should be emphasized that neutropenic patients may not develop the classic local signs of infection; therefore, the diagnosis of catheter-associated infection in these patients may be difficult.

Finally, the risk of catheter-related infection may be significantly reduced by appropriate care of the catheter and by observing strict hand washing, dressing, and glove precautions.

Current Controversies & Unresolved Issues

A. Prevention of Catheter-Related Infection

The challenge of preventing intravenous catheter infections in the ICU while providing reliable access for intravenous antimicrobial therapy, total parenteral nutrition, hemodynamic monitoring, or temporary hemodialysis is daunting. Many recommendations have been put forward for prevention of catheter-related infections, but only a few are supported by data. Only some include use of full barrier precautions during catheter insertion, subcutaneous tunneling of short-term catheters placed in the internal jugular or femoral veins, use of contamination shields for pulmonary artery catheters, application of povidone-iodine ointment at hemodialysis catheter insertion sites, use of antiseptic-filled hubs, and use of specialized nursing teams to care for patients with short-term peripheral catheters.

Recently, the use of antibiotic impregnated catheters has been proposed in an attempt to decrease the incidence of catheter site colonization and subsequent bloodstream infection. A meta-analysis showed that central venous catheters impregnated with chlorhexidine and silver sulfadiazine seemed to be effective in decreasing catheter-related bacteremia in patients at high risk for infection (ie, patients who require short-term catheters and multi-lumen catheters). However, the impact of these catheters on the development of subsequent antimicrobial resistance is not clear.

The cost associated with catheter tip sepsis has been estimated to be about $6000 per bacteremic episode. Adopting these advances and other approaches to decrease catheter infection reduce morbidity and the costs of care.

B. Diagnosis of Catheter-Related Bacteremia

The laboratory diagnosis of catheter-related bacteremia continues to be controversial. Semiquantitative culture of the external surface of the catheter tips is the method most often used to detect catheter colonization and device-related bacteremia. However, this method may fail to detect significant colonization of the internal lumens of catheters. Several quantitative methods have been described, but their sensitivities and specificities are not yet known, and a definitive cutoff level for a positive result remains to be established.

C. Duration of Intravascular Catheter Use

Recent studies have attempted to clarify the utility of routine change of the catheter site and the safety of exchanging a central venous catheter over a guidewire. Pulmonary artery catheters—despite the need for manipulation of the catheter during measurements—can be left in place unless there is unexplained fever, positive blood culture, or evidence of skin site infection. However, a maximum of 4–6 days at a given site would appear to be a reasonable limit. Central venous catheters may be left in place without a predetermined duration of placement; they should be removed in the presence of a positive blood culture, an infected insertion site, suspicion of catheter-related infection, or when there is no further need for the catheter. It does not appear that routine replacement of central venous catheters is indicated.

Microorganisms most commonly cause catheter-related infection by migrating along the outer site of the catheter from the skin surface to the tip. Despite this fact, exchange of a central venous or pulmonary artery catheter at the same site using a guidewire has become accepted practice in many ICUs, perhaps because several studies have documented little or no increase in infection rates when this technique was used to replace catheters suspected of exit-site infection or nonfunctional catheters. A recent meta-analysis suggested that central venous catheter exchange over a guidewire leads to a trend toward decreased mechanical complications, but a trend toward increased bacterial colonization of the catheter, catheter site infection, and catheter-related bacteremia was noted.

Cook D et al: Central venous catheter replacement strategies: a systematic review of the literature. Crit Care Med 1997;25:1417–24.

Cunha BA: Intravenous line infections. Crit Care Clin 1998;14:339–46.

Mayhall CG: Diagnosis and management of infections of implantable devices used for prolonged venous access. Curr Clin Top Infect Dis 1992;12:83–110.

Mermel LA et al: Guidelines for the management of intravascular catheter-related infections. Clin Infect Dis 2001;32:1249–72.

Mermel LA: Prevention of intravascular catheter-related infections. Ann Intern Med 2000;132:391–402.

Pearson ML: Guideline for the prevention of intravascular-device-related infections. Hospital Infection Control Practices Advisory Committee. Infect Control Hosp Epidemiol 1996;17:438–73.

Pittet D, Tarara D, Wenzel RP: Nosocomial bloodstream infection in critically ill patients: excess length of stay, extra costs, and attributable mortality. JAMA 1994;271:1598–1601.

Raad I: Management of intravascular catheter-related infections. J Antimicrob Chemother 2000;45:267–70.

Veenstra DL et al: Efficacy of antiseptic-impregnated central venous catheters in preventing catheter-related bloodstream infection: a meta-analysis. JAMA 1999;281:261–7.

CLOSTRIDIUM DIFFICILE-ASSOCIATED DIARRHEA

ESSENTIALS OF DIAGNOSIS

- *Watery diarrhea and low-grade fever.*
- *Previous or current treatment with antibiotics—but may occur as long as 6 weeks after antibiotic has been stopped.*
- *Presence of* C difficile *toxin in stool*
- *Sigmoidoscopy may reveal white or yellow plaques of pseudomembranous colitis*

General Considerations

Diarrhea developing in an ICU patient can be due to infectious or noninfectious causes. The most important infectious cause of nosocomial diarrhea is infection with *Clostridium difficile.* Nosocomial gastroenteritis caused by salmonella, shigella, *E coli,* and campylobacter is exceedingly rare and should only be considered in outbreak situations.

At least two things must occur for a patient to develop *C difficile*-associated diarrhea: acquisition of or colonization with *C difficile* and administration of an inducing agent. More than 20% of patients hospitalized for over a week are colonized with *C difficile.* The risk of acquisition of *C difficile* increases with length of hospital stay, reaching 50% in patients hospitalized over 1 month. It appears that the administration of certain antibiotics or chemotherapeutic agents induce the organisms to elaborate toxins: toxin A, an enterotoxin; and toxin B, a cytotoxin. The spectrum of disease encountered with this disorder ranges from simple diarrhea to pseudomembranous colitis, rarely complicated by toxic megacolon, which can result in colonic perforation and death.

The most common antibiotics implicated in the development of *C difficile*-associated diarrhea are ampicillin, clindamycin, and the cephalosporins. Antibiotics uncommonly associated with the disorder include trimethoprim-sulfamethoxazole, the quinolones, aztreonam, the carbapenems, and metronidazole. Vancomycin, erythromycin, tetracycline, and the aminoglycosides rarely cause *C difficile*-associated diarrhea. Although the disorder is usually self-limited, resolving when antibiotics are stopped and treatment is initiated, severe complications may occur.

Clinical Features

A. Symptoms and Signs

C difficile typically produces watery diarrhea and low-grade fever with or without abdominal pain. Diarrhea may develop after a single dose of an antibiotic or may be delayed as long as 6 weeks following the last dose of the antimicrobial agent. If the patient develops pseudomembranous colitis, sigmoidoscopy may reveal characteristic white or yellow plaques or pseudomembranes. Patients may become seriously ill, with fluid and electrolyte imbalance, toxic megacolon, and colonic perforation.

B. Laboratory Findings

It is recommended that diarrheal stools of patients who have been hospitalized for more than 72 hours with a history of prior antibiotic use be evaluated for *C difficile*-associated diarrhea. The diagnosis rests on the identification of *C difficile* toxin in the stool. The most sensitive and specific test for this disorder is a tissue culture assay for toxin B cytotoxicity, with a sensitivity of 94–100% and a specificity of 99%. However, this test is cumbersome to perform and takes 1–3 days to complete. Enzyme-linked immunoassays for identification of toxins A and B have a sensitivity of 71–94% and a specificity of 92–98%. In 20% of patients, toxin assays on multiple stool samples may be required to demonstrate the presence of the toxin.

Identification of fecal leukocytes is neither sensitive nor specific for *C difficile*-associated diarrhea. Nosocomial acquisition of enteric pathogens such as salmonella, shigella, and *Campylobacter jejuni* is extremely rare; thus, performing routine stool cultures is not cost effective in hospitalized patients with diarrhea.

Differential Diagnosis

Noninfectious causes of nosocomial diarrhea include medication administration, enteral feeding, inflammatory bowel disease, ischemic colitis, gastrointestinal bleeding from a variety of lesions, and systemic illness. Antimicrobial administration can cause diarrhea by altering normal bowel flora (ceftriaxone, tetracycline, amoxicillin-clavulanic acid) or by bowel irritation (erythromycin). Infectious causes of nosocomial diarrhea are rare and include enteric pathogens and cytomegalovirus colitis in the immunocompromised host.

Treatment

If antibiotic-associated colitis develops in patients receiving antibiotic therapy, improvement often occurs with discontinuation of antibiotics. Specific antimicrobial therapy should be administered to those with persistent diarrhea or in patients with severe illness. Asymptomatic carriers of *C difficile* should not be treated, since doing so may prolong the carrier state. Oral vancomycin and metronidazole are equally effective. Metronidazole is less expensive and does not exert selective pressure for vancomycin-resistant enterococci—and is thus the agent of first choice. It should be given at a dose of 500 mg orally three times a day for 10–14 days. In patients unable to tolerate oral medications, intravenous metronidazole at a dose of 500 mg every 8 hours can be used as initial therapy. Vancomycin is recommended at a dosage of 125–250 mg orally every 6 hours for 10–14 days in the event of treatment failure or for persistent symptoms. As many as 20% of patients will relapse within the first 2 weeks after completing a course of treatment, but most of these will respond to a second course of metronidazole. Risk factors for relapse include chronic renal failure, multiple previous episodes of *C difficile*-associated diarrhea, continuation of other antimicrobial therapy, community-acquired *C difficile*-associated diarrhea, and high white blood cell counts.

Patients diagnosed with or suspected of having *C difficile*-associated diarrhea should be managed with enteric precautions. The organism is particularly well suited to survive for prolonged periods on a variety of surfaces and has been cultured from hospital carpeting, beds, and walls. It is easily transmitted by the hands of hospital personnel from patient to patient. Therefore, appropriate isolation precautions are essential when caring for these patients.

It has become clear that *C difficile* is a significant nosocomial pathogen; thus, prevention and control in the hospital setting are crucial. *C difficile*-associated diarrhea has been strongly associated with use of certain antimicrobial agents, so that alteration of patterns of antimicrobial use may be helpful in reducing its incidence.

Given the high recurrence rate of *C difficile*-associated diarrhea, various nonantimicrobial approaches have been employed to allow the bowel to reestablish its normal flora, such as oral administration of *Saccharomyces boulardii,* lactobacilli, or normal fecal flora. However, these strategies have not been adequately studied to support formal recommendations.

Cunha BA: Nosocomial diarrhea. Crit Care Clin 1998;14:329–38.

Johnson S, Gerding DN: *Clostridium difficile*-associated diarrhea. Clin Infect Dis 1998;26:1027–36.

Kelly CP, Pothoulakis C, Lamont JT: *Clostridium difficile* colitis. N Engl J Med 1994;330:257–62.

Mylonakis E, Ryan ET, Calderwood SB: *Clostridium difficile*-associated diarrhea: a review. Arch Intern Med 2001;161: 525–33.

HEMATOGENOUSLY DISSEMINATED CANDIDIASIS

ESSENTIALS OF DIAGNOSIS

- *Fever despite broad-spectrum antibacterial therapy and negative bacterial blood cultures.*
- *Possible skin manifestations.*
- *Consider in neutropenic hosts and patients with long-term vascular access.*

General Considerations

According to the National Nosocomial Infections Surveillance System Survey, candida was the fourth most common nosocomial pathogen recovered from blood in the United States during the period 1990 through 1992. This trend of increasing prevalence of candidal infections appears to be similar in other developed countries. Data from outcome studies have shown that the attributable mortality of candidemia approaches 35%, with prolongation of hospital stay by up to 30 days.

The typical distribution of candidemia among hospitalized patients is 25% from the surgical intensive care unit, 25% from the bone marrow transplant unit, 20% from the medical intensive care unit, 10% from the hematology and oncology wards, and 20% from the general medical wards. The incidence of candidemia is much lower on pediatric, newborn, obstetric, and gynecology wards. Patients at increased risk for hematogenously disseminated candidiasis include those with extensive burns, indwelling venous catheters, broad-spectrum antibiotic exposure, immunosuppression (especially neutropenia), severe mucositis, previous surgical procedures (particularly gastrointestinal surgery), total parenteral nutrition, concomitant bacteria or other infections, and mucosal colonization by candida species. Mortality from candidemia is highest among those patients with high APACHE II scores, rapidly fatal underlying disease, and persistent candidemia despite appropriate antifungal therapy.

Microbiologic Etiology

Candida albicans is the species most commonly isolated from blood cultures; however, recent emergence of non-*albicans* species has been noted. *C albicans* accounts for approximately 50% of all cases of nosocomial candida bloodstream infections; *C tropicalis, C glabrata, C parapsilosis,* and *C krusei,* in decreasing order, make up the remainder of cases. Why non-*albicans* species are being increasingly isolated is not entirely clear. However, the widespread use of empiric fluconazole may exert selective pressure leading to the emergence of candida species less sensitive to the triazoles.

Fungemia caused by *C tropicalis* usually occurs as a result of endogenous infection, though cases of nosocomial transmission have also been documented. Most isolates of *C tropicalis* are sensitive to amphotericin B, flucytosine, and the triazoles. *C glabrata,* a pathogen with decreased susceptibility to fluconazole, is the third most common species isolated in nosocomial bloodstream infections. An increased incidence of infection with this pathogen has been noted in transplant patients receiving antifungal prophylaxis with fluconazole or in patients receiving empiric antifungal therapy with fluconazole. *C parapsilosis* infection occurs almost exclusively in the presence of indwelling venous catheters, prosthetic devices, or invasive devices and is not usually a member of the patient's endogenous flora. This organism is usually susceptible to both amphotericin B and fluconazole. *C krusei* is considered to be resistant to fluconazole and is seen most commonly in neutropenic patients, especially those receiving fluconazole for antifungal prophylaxis or empiric therapy.

Clinical Features

A. Symptoms and Signs

Most patients with hematogenously disseminated candidiasis have no systemic symptoms or signs of infection other than persistent fever in the setting of broad-spectrum antibiotics. Careful physical examination should be performed to assess the presence of skin lesions characteristic of candidemia. Three types of lesions have been described with hematogenously disseminated candidiasis: The classic lesion is macronodular, erythematous, and 0.5–1 cm in diameter. Lesions resembling ecthyma gangrenosum and purpura fulminans have also been described. In all three types of lesions, the organisms are readily seen on histopathologic examination of punch biopsy specimens. Any new neurologic symptom should prompt a CT scan or MRI of the brain, since candidal micro- and macroabscesses of the central nervous system have been described in patients with candidemia. Patients should undergo daily physical examination looking for new cardiac murmurs, bone or joint findings, and hepatosplenomegaly. Endocarditis, osteomyelitis, arthritis, and hepatosplenic candidiasis are all documented complications of candidemia. All patients should have a thorough ophthalmoscopic examination to rule out candidal endophthalmitis, typically appearing as white "cotton ball" lesions that may extend into the vitreous.

B. Laboratory Findings

Laboratory findings in hematogenously disseminated candidiasis are nonspecific. The rate of premortem diagnosis of disseminated candidemia is typically low, in the range of 10–40%. With the development of new blood culturing techniques such as the BACTEC system, the yield of positive blood cultures for candida has increased, though IT is still less than 50%. Thus, the diagnosis is made on mainly clinical grounds. Appropriate imaging studies should be obtained when there is suspicion of end-organ dissemination; biopsy of suspicious lesions should be pursued to look for histopathologic evidence of invasive candidal infection.

Treatment

A. Empiric Antifungal Therapy

The diagnosis of hematogenously disseminated candidemia is typically made on clinical grounds, and patients are often treated empirically based on the presence of multiple risk factors or evidence for mucosal colonization with candida species. A critical intervention in the treatment of candidemia is the removal of all potentially infected venous catheters, especially in neutropenic patients.

The antifungal agent of choice depends upon the clinical status of the patient and the physician's knowledge of the possible infecting candida species. In the pretriazole era, amphotericin B was used exclusively in all patients with suspected or documented fungal infection. However, there are now data to suggest that in a nonneutropenic patient who is hemodynamically stable, fluconazole will provide response rates of 60–100%. Factors that may prompt the physician to use amphotericin B as empiric therapy include hemodynamic instability or known colonization of the patient with non-*albicans* candida species, such as *C glabrata* or *C krusei.* There is general agreement that a neutropenic patient with suspected invasive fungal infection should receive amphotericin B as the agent of choice. Flucytosine may be used in combination with either amphotericin B or fluconazole in severe infections. Itraconazole is available in an intravenous formulation; however, formal studies to support recommendations for its use have not been completed.

Edwards JE: Candida species. In: *Principles and Practice of Infectious Diseases,* 5th ed. Mandell GL, Bennett JE, Dolin R (editors). Churchill Livingstone, 2000.

Edwards JE et al: International conference for the development of a consensus on the management and prevention of severe candidal infections. Clin Infect Dis 1997;25:43–59.

Pfaller MA: Nosocomial candidiasis: emerging species, reservoirs, and modes of transmission. Clin Infect Dis 1996;22(Suppl 2):S89–94.

Rex JH et al: Practice guidelines for the therapy of candidiasis. Clin Infect Dis 2000;30:662–78.

Uzun O, Anaissie EJ: Problems and controversies in the management of hematogenous candidiasis. Clin Infect Dis 1996; 22(Suppl 2):S95–101.

Wenzel RP: Nosocomial candidemia: risk factors and attributable mortality. Clin Infect Dis 1995;20:1531–4.

ANTIMICROBIAL RESISTANCE IN THE INTENSIVE CARE UNIT

Critically ill patients often receive broad-spectrum antimicrobial therapy during their hospitalization; thus, the ICU is fertile ground for the emergence of antimicrobial resistance. In the following section, specific resistance problems encountered in the ICU will be reviewed, including vancomycin-resistant enterococci, methicillin-resistant *S aureus,* glycopeptide-insensitive *S aureus,* gram-negative bacilli with extended-spectrum beta-lactamases, gram-negative bacilli that produce group 1 beta-lactamases, and *Acinetobacter baumanii.*

Vancomycin-Resistant Enterococci

A. Incidence

Enterococci are normal inhabitants of the gastrointestinal tract and are generally considered to be organisms of low virulence. Patients with serious nosocomial infections caused by enterococci have high morbidity and mortality rates due to their underlying disease. In the past, most enterococcal infections were caused by *Enterococcus faecalis,* and only about 5–10% of infections due to enterococci were due to *E faecium.* However, the emergence of glycopeptide-resistant *E faecium* has led to a shift in the relative frequency of infection with this species. The most common site of origin of enterococcal infection is the urinary tract, followed by intra-abdominal or pelvic infection as part of a polymicrobial process. Bacteremia usually occurs as a complication of one of the above or may result from infection of an indwelling venous catheter or prosthetic device.

National nosocomial surveys have demonstrated an increase in the prevalence of vancomycin-resistant enterococci among enterococcal isolates to levels of 20% or greater. Case-control studies have identified several risk factors for acquisition of vancomycin-resistant enterococci. Host factors include advanced age, severity of underlying disease, hematologic malignancy, neutropenia, cirrhosis, hemodialysis, recent intra-abdominal surgery, prior nosocomial infection, the presence of pressure sores, prolonged hospitalization, invasive procedures, contact with another person colonized or infected with vancomycin-resistant enterococci, and previous antimicrobial therapy (especially with a third-generation cephalosporin and vancomycin). Patients in certain health care settings, including long-term care facilities, outpatient dialysis units, intensive care units, and oncology or transplant wards, have the highest prevalence of vancomycin-resistant enterococci carriage.

B. Mechanism of Resistance

Enterococci become vancomycin-resistant through acquisition of genes conferring resistance; these genes are specified as *vanA* or *vanB*. The most common phenotype, *vanA*, is transmitted by a transposon, and confers high-level resistance to vancomycin and teicoplanin. The *vanB* phenotype is chromosomally-based, and confers variable resistance to vancomycin, while maintaining susceptibility to teicoplanin. Both phenotypes are easily transferable among different enterococci via conjugation. The mechanism of resistance involves a change in the cell wall building block, D-alanine-D-alanine, the target site for vancomycin, to D-alanine-D-lactate.

C. Therapy

Treatment of serious vancomycin-resistant enterococcal infections is difficult. Many strains are resistant to ampicillin and aminoglycosides, so the remaining options are few in number and antienterococcal activity is limited. Carbapenems, fluoroquinolones, tetracyclines, chloramphenicol, rifampin, novobiocin, and nitrofurantoin have all been used in various combinations in an attempt to treat infection with vancomycin-resistant enterococci. Quinupristin/dalfopristin and linezolid are both drugs recently licensed in the United States that include vancomycin-resistant enterococci in their spectrum of activity. Urinary tract infections may be treated successfully with nitrofurantoin and removal of the urinary catheter. Mixed infections, such as intra-abdominal abscesses or skin and soft tissue infections, should undergo aggressive debridement. Indwelling venous catheters and prosthetic devices should be removed whenever possible. Treatment of serious vancomycin-resistant enterococcal infection should include at least two antimicrobial agents to which the organism is susceptible, and one of these should be an aminoglycoside unless contraindicated.

D. Prevention

In the United States, most carriage of vancomycin-resistant enterococci and outbreaks of infection are due to patient-to-patient spread. Thus, strict infection control measures are necessary to prevent spread and persistence of the organisms. Strict contact isolation should be observed for any patient infected or colonized with the organism. In addition, the use of empiric vancomycin for the treatment of hospitalized patients should be limited to those with clear indications.

Methicillin-Resistant *Staphylococcus aureus* (MRSA)

A. Incidence

The National Nosocomial Infection Surveillance surveys have demonstrated an increase in the percentage of MRSA from about 2–3% of all *S aureus* isolates in 1975 to over 34% between 1997 and 1999. The incidence of community-acquired MRSA is also increasing, accounting for as many as 25% of all *S aureus* isolated from bloodstream infections in 1999. Risk factors for community acquisition of MRSA include injection drug use, chronic antimicrobial therapy, and hemodialysis. The major route of spread of MRSA is direct patient-to-patient contact or via the hands of medical personnel. Common sites of MRSA colonization include the anterior nares, wounds, burns or other areas of decreased skin integrity, the perineal area, the upper respiratory tract, and the skin adjacent to invasive devices, gastrostomy tubes, and tracheostomies. Risk factors for both colonization and infection with MRSA include previous hospitalization, prolonged hospital stay, hospitalization in a burn unit or intensive care unit, chronic prior antimicrobial therapy, exposure to a colonized health care worker or patient, the presence of surgical wounds or burns, and the use of invasive devices.

B. Mechanism of Resistance

Resistance of *S aureus* to methicillin is transmitted chromosomally via the *mecA* gene. Acquisition of this gene results in altered penicillin-binding protein 2A. Presence of the *mecA* gene is also associated with resistance to other antibiotics, including all beta-lactams, aminoglycosides, macrolides, tetracycline, rifampin, and fluoroquinolones.

C. Therapy

Most strains of MRSA are sensitive to the glycopeptides vancomycin and teicoplanin. In the United States, vancomycin is the drug of choice for serious infections with MRSA. There may be a role for quinupristin/dalfopristin and linezolid in the treatment of infections with this organism. Eradication of MRSA carriage may be attempted with either topical or systemic antimicrobials or by bathing with antiseptic soaps. The efficacy of any of these approaches to eradication is inconsistent and often incomplete.

Glycopeptide-Insensitive *S aureus* (GISA)

A. Incidence

The emergence of GISA is probably the most disturbing development to occur in the antibiotic era. Glycopeptide insensitivity among *S aureus* is defined as an MIC to vancomycin of 8–16 μg/mL. The first reported case of infection with this organism occurred in Japan in May of 1996. There have been six cases reported in the United States to date. Most of these patients were on hemodialysis, and most had had recurrent MRSA bacteremias that were treated with prolonged courses of vancomycin.

B. Mechanism of Resistance

The mechanism of vancomycin insensitivity is not clear. It is known, however, that the mechanism through which enterococci become resistant to vancomycin is not responsible for staphylococcal insensitivity to glycopeptide. Scanning and transmission electron microscopy of the insensitive organisms show a thickened bacterial cell wall. A fully vancomycin-resistant *S aureus* strain has been created in vitro, demonstrating a similarly thickened bacterial cell wall. It is hypothesized that decreased vancomycin access to the target sites may occur as a result of sequestration of the drug in the cell wall.

C. Therapy

Therapy of GISA infection is not standardized. Antimicrobial therapy should be based on the organism's susceptibility profile. Preliminary in vitro data suggest that as the bacteria becomes more resistant to vancomycin, they become more susceptible to oxacillin. Thus, there may be a role for combination therapy with vancomycin and oxacillin. A role for quinupristin/dalfopristin and linezolid in the treatment of these infections is a possibility also.

Gram-Negative Bacilli Producing Extended-Spectrum Beta-Lactamases (ESBLs)

A. Incidence

Bacterial strains with ESBLs were first identified in the mid 1980s. Most are strains of *Klebsiella pneumoniae* or *Escherichia coli.* ESBL production has been noted in other species of Enterobacteriaceae as well but with much lower frequency. The actual incidence of ESBL-producing strains is difficult to quantify, as surveillance and reporting are incomplete. Most strains are isolated from hospitalized patients. Risk factors for acquisition include prolonged hospital stay; admission to an intensive care unit, oncology unit, or nursing home; recent surgical or invasive procedures; urinary catheterization; and prior extended-spectrum cephalosporin use. Notably, outbreaks with ESBL-producing strains have been linked to heavy ceftazidime use within a hospital.

B. Mechanism of Resistance

The ESBLs are descendants of the beta-lactamases responsible for ampicillin resistance in *E coli* and penicillin resistance in *K pneumoniae.* This plasmid-mediated gene confers resistance not only to the extended-spectrum cephalosporins but also to aztreonam. The gene may also encode resistance to aminoglycosides, tetracyclines, trimethoprim-sulfamethoxazole, or chloramphenicol. The plasmids bearing these genes are stable and are easily transmissible from bacteria to bacteria.

C. Therapy

Most laboratories do not test for ESBL-producing strains. On routine susceptibility testing, ESBL-producing strains may appear to be sensitive to the extended-spectrum cephalosporins and aztreonam. Clues to the presence of an ESBL-producing strain are (1) clinical failure in the setting of "appropriate" antimicrobial therapy; (2) presence of resistance to certain other antibiotics, such as aminoglycosides, tetracyclines, trimethoprim-sulfamethoxazole, or chloramphenicol, which are often transmitted on the same plasmid as the ESBL; and (3) diminished susceptibility to ceftriaxone, ceftazidime, or aztreonam. (If this pattern is seen, resistance to all extended-spectrum cephalosporins and aztreonam should be assumed.) ESBL-producing organisms usually display susceptibility to cephamycins (cefotetan and cefoxitin) and the carbapenems, with variable susceptibility to the beta-lactam–beta-lactamase inhibitor combinations. Carbapenems are the mainstay of therapy in the seriously ill patient infected with an ESBL-producing organism, as cases of cephamycin resistance have been reported to emerge during the course of cephamycin therapy.

Gram-Negative Bacilli Producing Group 1 Beta-Lactamases

A. Incidence

Group 1 beta-lactamases are chromosomally based beta-lactamases. The most commonly encountered organisms with group 1 beta-lactamase production are enterobacter species, *Pseudomonas aeruginosa,* citrobacter species, *Serratia marcescens,* and *Morganella morganii.* According to the National Nosocomial Infection Surveillance System, infections due to these organisms have been increasing in incidence. This recent trend is of concern given the resistance of these pathogens to extended-spectrum cephalosporins, with documented cepha-losporin resistance developing even while on appropriate therapy. Risk factors for acquisition of these pathogens include prior therapy with ceftizoxime, cefotaxime, or ceftazidime and perhaps with extended-spectrum penicillins—as well as length of previous antimicrobial therapy.

B. Mechanism of Resistance

The mechanism of resistance of group 1 beta-lactamase-producing organisms is induction of a chromosomally based gene that encodes for production of a group beta-lactamase (a cephalosporinase), which inactivates all cephalosporins.

C. Therapy

Therapy should be based on antimicrobial susceptibility data for a given strain. These organisms usually retain their sensitivity to the carbapenems and the fluoroquinolones. Emergence of resistance in the setting of ongoing antimicrobial therapy occurs in approximately 5% of patients. It is more likely to occur with use of a third-generation cephalosporin rather than an aminoglycoside or an extended-spectrum penicillin. Whether combination therapy will decrease the risk of emerging resistance is not yet known. At this time, it appears that monotherapy with an extended-spectrum cephalosporin should be avoided when treating infection caused by group 1 beta-lactamase-producing organisms.

Acinetobacter baumanii

A. Incidence

A baumanii is a gram-negative coccobacillus that may occur as a normal skin colonizer. It is considered to be relatively nonvirulent; however, the emergence of this organism has been increasingly noted in the nosocomial setting. In a critically ill patient, the presence of *A baumanii* bacteremia adds an attributable mortality of about 20%. The treatment challenge with this organism results from its inherent resistance to a wide array of antimicrobial agents. Risk factors for infection include underlying illness and prior colonization with the organism.

B. Mechanism of Resistance

The mechanism of resistance to the beta-lactam drugs is the production of a plasmid-mediated penicillinase. Resistance to cephalosporins occurs as a result of overproduction of a chromosomal cephalosporinase.

C. Therapy

As with most multidrug-resistant pathogens, therapy should be based on available susceptibility data. However, pending this information, one of the carbapenems can be considered for empiric therapy, as these agents tend to retain their activity against *A baumanii.*

Infection Control Concepts

The specter of antimicrobial-resistance increasingly threatens physicians' ability to treat bacterial infections. Numerous studies have demonstrated a stepwise increase in incidence of drug resistance from the community to the general inpatient ward to the intensive care unit. Control of antimicrobial resistance is the responsibility of every critical care physician. This can be broken down into two critical components: (1) prevention of emergence of new resistance mechanisms or resistant species and (2) prevention of spread of organisms from patient to patient.

A. Prevention of Emergence of Resistance

The central component of prevention is reducing selection pressure for resistance by judicious use of antimicrobials. It has been shown in several studies that even though overuse of antibiotics can foster antimicrobial resistance, changes in antibiotic use can result in recovery of susceptibility. Judicious antimicrobial use includes careful consideration of which patients are appropriate candidates for antimicrobial therapy, when such therapy should be initiated, which antimicrobial agents should be administered, and for what duration. The goal of antimicrobial therapy in the intensive care unit is to rapidly identify and treat a seriously ill patient with suspected or confirmed infection with the correct agents. The physician should make every attempt to differentiate between true bacterial infection and simple colonization. Moreover, it should be kept in mind that not all fever is the result of infection, and when no source of infection can be identified, noninfectious causes of fever should be considered (Table 15–7). Prophylactic use of antimicrobial agents should be avoided in the absence of a clear indication.

There is much controversy over the empiric use of combination therapy (eg, a beta-lactam plus an aminoglycoside) in a patient suspected of being infected with an aerobic gram-negative bacillus. Some in vitro data suggest that combination therapy may decrease the emergence of chromosomally mediated resistance, though it

Table 15–7. Some noninfectious causes of fever in the ICU.

Common causes
Drug fever
Malignancy
Deep venous thrombosis
Posttransfusion
Postoperative (atelectasis)
Thrombophlebitis
Chemical aspiration pneumonitis
Less common causes
Hyperthyroidism
Adrenal insufficiency
Transplant rejection
Alcohol withdrawal, drug withdrawal
Pancreatitis
Pulmonary embolism
Hematoma

may actually worsen plasmid-mediated resistance. While it is acceptable to use broad-spectrum empiric antimicrobial therapy initially, antibiotics should be tailored once culture data become available. In addition, focal collections of purulent material should be drained whenever possible to decrease inoculum size, thereby improving the outcome of antimicrobial therapy. Prolonged courses or inappropriately broad-spectrum antibiotics should be avoided.

B. Prevention of Spread of Infection

Prevention of spread of infection involves prompt identification of patients colonized or infected with multidrug-resistant organisms plus rapid institution of appropriate isolation procedures. Even in wards or intensive care units not known to have patients colonized or infected with multidrug-resistant organisms, routine hand washing with antiseptic soaps by all personnel should be the rule.

Archibald L et al: Antimicrobial resistance in isolates from inpatients and outpatients in the United States: increasing importance of the intensive care unit. Clin Infect Dis 1997;24:211–5.

Chow JW et al: Enterobacter bacteremia: clinical features and emergence of antibiotic resistance during therapy. Ann Intern Med 1991;115:585–90.

Cisneros JM et al: Bacteremia due to *Acinetobacter baumanii:* epidemiology, clinical findings, and prognostic factors. Clin Infect Dis 1996;22:1026–32.

Diekema DJ et al: Survey of infectious due to *Staphylococcus* species: frequency of occurrence and antimicrobial susceptibility of isolates collected in the United States, Canada, Latin America, Europe, and the Western Pacific region for the SENTRY Antimicrobial Surveillance Program, 1997–1999. Clin Infect Dis 2001;32(Suppl 2):S114–32.

Fridkin SK: Vancomycin-intermediate and -resistant *Staphylococcus aureus:* what the infectious disease specialist needs to know. Clin Infect Dis 2001;32:108–15.

Hayden MK: Insights into the epidemiology and control of infection with vancomycin-resistant enterococci. Clin Infect Dis 2000;31:1058–65.

Jacobson KL et al: The relationship between antecedent antibiotic use and resistance to extended-spectrum cephalosporins in group I β-lactamase-producing organisms. Clin Infect Dis 1995;21:1107–13.

Leclercq R, Courvalin P: Resistance to glycopeptides in enterococci. Clin Infect Dis 1997;24:545–56.

Mainardi JL, Carlet J, Acar J: Antibiotic resistance problems in the critical care unit. Crit Care Clin 1998;14:199–219.

Martin MA: Methicillin-resistant *Staphylococcus aureus:* the persistent resistant nosocomial pathogen. Curr Clin Top Infect Dis 1994;14:170–91.

Moellering RC: Vancomycin-resistant enterococci. Clin Infect Dis 1998;26:1196–9.

Pitout JD, Sanders CC, Sanders WE Jr: Antimicrobial resistance with focus on β-lactam resistance in gram-negative bacilli. Am J Med 1997;103:51–9.

Sieradzki K et al: The development of vancomycin resistance in a patient with methicillin-resistant *Staphylococcus aureus* infection. N Engl J Med 1999;340:517–23.

Sirot D: Extended-spectrum plasmid-mediated β-lactamases. J Antimicrob Chemother 1995;36(Suppl A):19–34.

Smith TL et al: Emergence of vancomycin resistance in *Staphylococcus aureus.* N Engl J Med 1999;340:493–501.

Thomson KS, Prevan AM, Sanders CC: Novel plasmid-mediated β-lactamases in Enterobacteriaceae: emerging problems for new β-lactam antibiotics. Curr Clin Top Infect Dis 1996; 16:151–63.

Tilley PA, Roberts FJ: Bacteremia with *Acinetobacter* species: risk factors and prognosis in different clinical settings. Clin Infect Dis 1994;18:896–900.

BOTULISM & TETANUS

Patients with botulism and tetanus have primarily neurologic complications that almost always require management in an intensive care unit. Both disorders are caused by toxins produced by clostridia. In tetanus, patients have traumatic or surgical wounds contaminated by *C tetani.* Most cases of botulism are due to ingestion of preformed food-borne toxin; rarely, botulism may result from toxin produced by cutaneous infection with *C botulinum.*

BOTULISM

ESSENTIALS OF DIAGNOSIS

- *Nausea, vomiting, dysphagia, diplopia, dilated and fixed pupils.*
- *Sudden weakness in a previously healthy person.*
- *Cranial nerves affected first (except I and II), followed by descending symmetric paralysis or weakness.*
- *Autonomic nervous system involvement: paralytic ileus, gastric dilation, urinary retention, and orthostatic hypotension.*
- *Absence of sensory or mental status changes.*
- *Botulism toxin isolated from serum, stool, or other body fluid.*

General Considerations

Botulism is an acute neurologic disorder caused by the production of a neurotoxin produced by *Clostridium botulinum.* Improperly canned or home-prepared foods are common sources of the toxin. There are three clinical forms of botulism: food-borne botulism, wound botulism, and infant botulism. Infant botulism results from the ingestion of botulism spores, which germinate in the intestine and produce toxin. Most infants recover with supportive care only. Food-borne and wound botulism are generally more serious illnesses.

A. *C botulinum* and Botulism Toxins

C botulinum is an anaerobic gram-positive rod that survives in soil and marine sediment by spore formation. Under anaerobic conditions that permit germination, toxin production occurs. Although boiling for 10 minutes will kill bacteria and destroy toxins, spores are heat-resistant and can survive boiling for 3–5 hours. Food contaminated by botulism toxin may have no detectable change in appearance or taste.

Botulism toxin is the most potent toxin known on a per weight basis. Eight immunologically distinct toxins have been described: A, B, Cα and Cβ, D, E, F, and G. Each strain of *C botulinum* can produce only a single toxin type. Toxins A, B, and E have been the most common causes of human disease. Toxins A and B are the most potent; even small tastes of food contaminated with these toxins have resulted in full blown disease.

Specific *C botulinum* toxins appear to be geographically distributed throughout the world. In the United States, toxin A is found predominantly west of the Mississippi, while toxin B is found in the eastern states. Toxin E is found in the Great Lakes region and in Alaska, where one of the highest rates of botulism worldwide is seen.

Toxins produced by *C botulinum* block acetylcholine release at peripheral neuromuscular and autonomic nerve junctions, resulting in weakness, flaccid paralysis, and sometimes respiratory failure. Toxin binding is irreversible.

B. Food-Borne Botulism

Botulism toxins are large proteins. In food-borne botulism, ingested preformed toxin is absorbed in the stomach and upper small intestine. Toxins are reduced in size by proteolytic enzymes, but their activity is unchanged. Pancreatic trypsin may actually enhance the toxicity of some toxin strains. In addition to improperly home-canned foods, outbreaks of botulism have been traced to noncanned foods such as eviscerated dried fish, yogurt flavored with hazelnut conserve, a garlic-in-oil product, homemade salsa, cheese sauce, baked potatoes sealed in aluminum foil, and sautéed onions stored under a layer of butter.

C. Wound Botulism

Wound botulism is a rare condition that results when *C botulinum* grows and produces toxin in traumatized, devitalized tissue. The wound may appear insignificant. Toxin production is followed by onset of symptoms after an incubation period of 4–14 days. Many cases of wound botulism have occurred in teenagers, children, and injection drug users. Sinus infection with *C botulinum* has been reported after intranasal cocaine use; evidence suggests that botulism toxin can be inhaled or inoculated through the eye. In recent years, there has been an increase in the number of cases of wound botulism linked to the subcutaneous injection of impure "black tar" heroin imported from Mexico.

D. Adult Infectious Botulism

While most cases of adult botulism are the result of ingested preformed toxin, there have been cases of botulism in patients with documented *C botulinum* colonization of the intestinal tract. Risk factors include abdominal surgery, gastrointestinal tract abnormalities, and recent antibiotic administration, all of which presumably alter the normal gastrointestinal flora.

Clinical Features

The diagnosis of food-borne botulism should be considered when an acute illness with gastrointestinal or neurologic manifestations affects two or more persons who have shared a meal during the preceding 72 hours. Wound botulism presents with similar neurologic symptoms but without gastrointestinal complaints.

A. Symptoms and Signs

An initial pentad of signs and symptoms has been described in botulism: nausea and vomiting, dysphagia, diplopia, dilated and fixed pupils, and an extremely dry mouth unrelieved by drinking fluids. Over 90% of patients have at least three of these signs or symptoms. Symptoms can occur as early as 2 hours or as late as 8 days after toxin ingestion but usually occur within 18–36 hours. Onset of symptoms can be abrupt or may evolve over several days. Abnormalities of cranial nerve motor functions are followed by descending symmetric paralysis or weakness. Respiratory muscle weakness may be subtle or may progress rapidly to respiratory failure. Somatic musculature is affected last. Patients may develop autonomic nervous system manifestations, including constipation from paralytic ileus, gastric dilation, urinary retention, and orthostatic hypotension.

Notably absent in patients with botulism are sensory disturbances, changes in sensorium, and fever. Cranial nerves I and II are spared. Deep tendon reflexes may be intact, diminished, or absent, but pathologic reflexes cannot be demonstrated. In addition, the heart rate may be normal or slow unless secondary infection is present.

B. Laboratory Findings

The diagnosis of botulism is confirmed by isolating botulism toxin through a mouse neutralization bioassay. Toxin may be identified in samples of serum, stool, vomitus, gastric aspirate, and suspected foods. *C botulinum* may be grown on selective media from samples of stool or foods. Specimens for toxin analysis should be refrigerated, but culture samples for *C botulinum* should not. Because the toxin may enter the bloodstream through the eye or a small break in the skin, only experienced personnel, preferably immunized with botulinum toxoid, should handle specimens.

Electromyography may be useful in establishing a diagnosis of botulism but can be nonspecific and nondiagnostic even in severe cases. Low-amplitude and short-duration motor unit action potentials, small M wave amplitudes, and posttetanic fasciculation may be seen. A modest increment in M wave amplitude with rapid repetitive nerve stimulation may help to localize the disorder to the neuromuscular junction. Single-fiber electromyography may be a more useful and sensitive method for the rapid diagnosis of botulism intoxication, particularly when signs of general muscular weakness are absent. Cerebrospinal fluid is normal.

Differential Diagnosis

Differentiating botulism from other diseases is critical to early implementation of appropriate therapy. Table 15–8 lists diseases that must be differentiated from botulism.

Treatment

A. Supportive Care

Meticulous supportive care is essential for patients with all forms of botulism. If respiratory failure has not already occurred at the time of diagnosis, the patient should be hospitalized in a monitored setting and closely followed with serial measurements of vital capacity. Respiratory failure can occur with unexpected suddenness. Pulmonary infections are a common complication of botulism, often the result of aspiration of oropharyngeal secretions or a complication of atelectasis. The development of fever should prompt an evaluation of possible pneumonia. Improvement in ventilatory and upper airway muscle strength in patients who develop respiratory failure is most significant over the first 12 weeks, but recovery may not be complete for up to a year.

Wound botulism requires thorough debridement of the infected wound and administration of penicillin in addition to antitoxin therapy.

Table 15–8. Differential diagnosis of botulism.

Myasthenia gravis
Tick paralysis
Poliomyelitis
Guillain-Barré syndrome (Miller-Fisher variant)
Psychiatric disorder
Stroke (brain stem)
Rabies
Diphtheria
Eaton-Lambert syndrome

B. Botulism Antitoxin

Botulism antitoxin should be administered to all patients with food-borne or wound botulism. Because only equine antitoxin is available, all patients must first undergo testing for hypersensitivity to equine serum. Twenty percent of patients will experience some degree of hypersensitivity, and anaphylaxis can also occur. Trivalent antitoxin for toxins A, B, and E is distributed through the Centers for Disease Control and Prevention. Polyvalent antitoxin for toxins A, B, C, D, E, and F is also available for specific outbreaks.

Antitoxin should be given as soon as available, but it may be beneficial even when given several weeks after toxin ingestion, since circulating toxin can be detected in serum up to 30 days after intoxication. Antitoxin will not neutralize toxin already bound to neuromuscular junctions, and, though it can slow disease progression, it has no effect on established neurologic impairment. Two vials of the appropriate antitoxin should be given, one intramuscularly and one intravenously. This regimen may be repeated after 2–4 hours.

Because of the risk of adverse reactions, prophylactic antitoxin is not recommended for those who have been exposed to botulism toxin but have no symptoms. If recognized early enough, patients may undergo gastric lavage or induced vomiting in an attempt to eliminate the toxin prior to absorption.

Current Controversies & Unresolved Issues

Administration of antibiotics to patients with food-borne botulism is controversial, but some physicians give penicillin to eradicate potential bowel carriage of the organism. The benefit of this approach is uncertain.

Guanidine hydrochloride is thought to increase acetylcholine release from terminal nerve endings and is advocated by some in the treatment of botulism. Reports of its efficacy are conflicting.

Critchley EM, Mitchell D: Human botulism. Br J Hosp Med 1990;43:290–92.

Kudrow DB et al: Botulism associated with *Clostridium botulinum* sinusitis after intranasal cocaine abuse. Ann Intern Med 1988;109:984–85.

Lecour H et al: Food-borne botulism: a review of 13 outbreaks. Arch Intern Med 1988;148:578–80.

Shapiro RL, Hatheway C, Swerdlow DL: Botulism in the United States: a clinical and epidemiologic review. Ann Intern Med 1998;129:221–8.

Wilcox PG, Morrison NJ, Pardy RL: Recovery of the ventilatory and upper airway muscles and exercise performance after type A botulism. Chest 1990;98:620–6.

TETANUS

ESSENTIALS OF DIAGNOSIS

- *Generalized weakness or stiffness, with trismus ("lockjaw") and severe generalized spasms.*
- *Opisthotonos and abdominal rigidity.*
- *Respiratory failure, tachycardia, hypertension, fever, and diaphoresis may be present.*

General Considerations

Although entirely preventable by appropriate vaccination, tetanus still occurs in developing countries and infrequently in developed countries. An estimated 1 million cases occur worldwide each year. In 1995 through 1997 in the United States, fewer than 50 cases were reported annually.

Patients who have never received a primary immunization series with tetanus toxoid are at risk for the development of tetanus. Many elderly patients and patients born or raised in developing countries have not been vaccinated and are at risk. Elderly women may be at higher risk than elderly men, since many men were vaccinated during military service. Male gender and black race are risk factors in the United States, perhaps because of the higher incidence of trauma in these groups. Injection drug users, particularly "skin poppers," are predisposed to tetanus. Tetanus is more frequent in warmer climates and months, in part because of the greater frequency of contaminated wounds. Tetanus is not transmitted from person to person.

A. *Clostridium tetani* and Tetanospasmin

The clinical syndrome of tetanus is caused by a potent neurotoxin, tetanospasmin, released from *C tetani.* A slender, motile, gram-positive nonencapsulated anaerobic rod, *C tetani* is a spore-forming organism that is commonly found in nature. Spores may be found in soil and dust but are particularly common in areas contaminated with human or animal excreta. Spores may remain viable for years and then germinate when they are introduced into an appropriate anaerobic environment such as devitalized tissue. The presence of other bacterial organisms appears to enhance the reversion of spores to vegetative forms and the release of tetanospasmin.

B. Pathophysiology

Tetanospasmin migrates into the central nervous system either transsynaptically along peripheral motor nerves or by hematogenous or lymphatic routes. It binds to the presynaptic inhibitory neurons and prevents the release of acetylcholine from nerve terminals in muscle. The functional loss of these inhibitory neurons allows lower motor neurons to increase muscle tone, producing rigidity and spasm of both agonist and antagonist muscles. Once tetanospasmin is fixed to nervous tissue, it cannot be neutralized by antitoxin. Tetanospasmin also binds to cerebral gangliosides, which may be the cause of seizures seen in tetanus. Disturbances of the autonomic nervous system are common, manifested by sweating, fluctuating blood pressure, tachycardia and cardiac arrhythmias, and increased production of catecholamines.

Clinical Features

Tetanus may occur in the neonate in the first month of life or as one of three patterns in adult patients. Generalized tetanus is the most common adult presentation. Local tetanus and, even more rarely, cephalic tetanus are manifested by local muscle spasms in areas contiguous with an infected wound. Both local and cephalic tetanus may progress to generalized tetanus. Tetanus is a diagnosis of exclusion. If the diagnosis is not considered, the opportunity for early treatment will be lost.

A. Introduction of *C tetani*

The wound into which *C tetani* has been introduced may appear insignificant. However, particularly high-risk wounds include those contaminated with dirt, feces, soil, or saliva as well as any puncture wound, crush wound, burn, decubitus ulcer, or frostbite injury. Tetanus has also been reported following elective and emergency surgical procedures, particularly those involving the gastrointestinal tract. The postpartum uterus is also susceptible to *C tetani* infection. Thus, tetanus should be considered in the postoperative patient who develops crampy abdominal pain and abdominal wall rigidity with no history of tetanus vaccination. *C tetani* may be harbored in the middle ear (chronic otitis media) and in wounds of the head, predisposing a patient to cephalic tetanus.

B. Symptoms and Signs

Tetanus can present 1–54 days following a puncture or other wound, but an incubation period shorter than 14 days is most common. Longer incubation periods are generally related to injury sites farther away from the central nervous system. Generalized weakness or stiffness is a frequent initial symptom, with trismus ("lockjaw") being the most common complaint. As symptoms progress over 1–7 days, severe generalized reflex spasms develop. Opisthotonos, abdominal rigidity, and a grotesque facial expression called risus sardonicus are classic signs. Spasms may be precipitated by minor disturbances such as a draft or noise or by jarring the bed. In the absence of seizures, the patient's sensorium is usually clear. Involvement of the respiratory muscles may lead to hypoventilation. Autonomic dysfunction may occur, causing tachycardia, hypotension, fever, and diaphoresis, and can be difficult to manage.

Complications of tetanus include pneumonia, venous thrombosis, pulmonary embolism, and long bone and spine fractures from severe sustained muscle contractures. The mortality rate from tetanus ranges from 21–31% in the United States and may be as high as 52% in patients over 60 years of age. Poor outcome is associated with autonomic disturbances such as blood pressure lability, with cardiac arrhythmias and rate disturbances, and with hyperglycemia, hyperthermia, and anticoagulation therapy.

Some studies have suggested a poor prognosis when patients present with short incubation periods and heavily contaminated wounds. A better prognosis is suggested if there is no demonstrable focus of infection.

C. Laboratory Findings

The wound in a patient suspected of having tetanus should be cultured anaerobically for *C tetani.* However, the etiologic confirmation is infrequently made in this manner, and the diagnosis usually is based on the absence of detectable tetanus toxoid antibody and the exclusion of other diseases.

Differential Diagnosis

The differential diagnosis of tetanus includes a list of rather unusual diseases not commonly encountered in the ICU (Table 15–9).

Table 15–9. Differential diagnosis of tetanus.

Meningoencephalitis (viral, bacterial)
Phenothiazine overdose
Peritonsillar abscess
Hypercalcemic tetany
Retropharyngeal abscess
Retroperitoneal hemorrhage
Dental abscess
Epilepsy
Mandibular fracture
Opioid withdrawal
Tonsillitis
Strychnine poisoning
Diphtheria
Rabies
Mumps
Perforated peptic ulcer
Trichinosis
Septicemic spondylitis
Mandibular osetomyelitis

Treatment

A. Tetanus Immune Globulin

Patients who present with tetanus should receive tetanus immune globulin as early as possible to neutralize unbound toxin. Delay in treatment may result in a poorer prognosis. The optimal dose of tetanus immune globulin has not been established, but a single dose of 500–3000 units intramuscularly can be given. It is advised that some of the dose be injected into the area of the presumed injury. Some researchers have advocated doses as high as 10,000 units or more.

B. Supportive Care

Penicillin G, 10–20 million units/d, should be given intravenously for 10–14 days. Far more importantly, wounds should be properly debrided. In patients with wounds that continue to be infected, it may be necessary to repeat passive immunization with tetanus immune globulin after 3–4 weeks, since toxin production may continue and antibiotic therapy will not eradicate the spores.

Tracheostomy should be performed in all but very mild cases to allow for prolonged respiratory assistance with a ventilator. Problems arising from cardiovascular instability should be treated appropriately.

Analgesics should be used relieve pain from muscle contractions. Benzodiazepines—particularly diazepam—may be effective in reducing muscle spasms. Inadequate muscle relaxation or inadequate control of seizure activity can lead to complications such as long bone and vertebral fractures. Benzodiazepines may not prevent reflex spasms, however, and effective respiration may require neuromuscular blockade.

Patients require nutritional support and meticulous attention to the prevention of decubiti and flexion contractures. Consideration should be given to subcutaneous heparin therapy, particularly in injecting drug users and elderly patients, who appear to be at highest risk for pulmonary embolism. Constipation is common, and an initial cleansing enema is helpful. A rectal tube helps to control abdominal distention. Nosocomial infections may develop and should be considered if a patient with tetanus develops more than a moderate elevation in temperature.

C. Immunization

Patients who develop tetanus are not subsequently immune to the infection. Tetanospasmin is toxic in such minute quantities that it appears to escape reaction by the immune system, and protective antibody is not produced. Therefore, active immunization with a primary immunization series with tetanus toxoid should be administered to all patients during the convalescent phase of illness—usually a period of several weeks.

Current Controversies & Unresolved Issues

Many controversies remain in the management of patients with tetanus, particularly with respect to cardiovascular complications. Suggested therapeutic modalities occasionally are based on single case reports.

Clonidine has been reported to control sympathetic overactivity in severe tetanus. More recently, the beta-blocker esmolol was reported to be effective in controlling autonomic instability. Patients with severe tetanus who failed to respond to beta blockade and low doses of ganglionic blocking agents had dramatic suppression of cardiovascular instability when given continuous spinal anesthesia with bupivacaine, which provided complete blockade of sympathetic and parasympathetic portions of the autonomic nervous system.

Intrathecal therapy with tetanus antibody (antitetanus equine serum or tetanus immune globulin) has also been of interest. A meta-analysis of clinical trials has suggested a possible benefit from the use of antitetanus equine serum, but the authors concluded that neither antitetanus equine serum nor tetanus immune globulin should be given except in the context of a well-designed controlled trial. The addition of systemic corticosteroids to intrathecal immune globulin was suggested to improve survival in one study.

Another area of interest in the treatment of tetanus is the control of the severe spasms without sedation and artificial ventilation. Intrathecal baclofen and intravenous magnesium sulfate have both been used for control of spasms due to tetanus. In patients treated with these modalities, it appears that less autonomic instability is encountered, and spasms are controlled while preserving spontaneous ventilation.

Abrutyn E, Berlin JA: Intrathecal therapy in tetanus: a meta-analysis. JAMA 1991;266:2262–7.

Attygalle D, Rodrigo N: Magnesium sulphate for control of spasms in severe tetanus: can we avoid sedation and artificial ventilation? Anaesthesia 1997;52:956–62.

Bleck TP et al: Tetanus: pathophysiology, management, and prophylaxis. Dis Mon (Sept) 1991;27:545–603.

Dressnandt J et al: Intrathecal baclofen in tetanus: four cases and a review of reported cases. Intensive Care Med 1997;23: 896–902.

Fleshner PR, Hunter JG, Rudick J: Tetanus after gastrointestinal surgery. Am J Gastroenterol 1988;83:298–300.

Gregorakos L et al: Management of blood pressure instability in severe tetanus: the use of clonidine. Intensive Care Med 1997;23:893–5.

Jagoda A, Riggio G, Durguieres T: Cephalic tetanus: a case report and review of the literature. Am J Emerg Med 1988; 6:128–30.

King WW, Cave DR: Use of esmolol to control autonomic instability of tetanus. Am J Med 1991;91:425–8.

Luisto M: Outcome and neurological sequelae of patients after tetanus. Acta Neurol Scand 1989;80:504–11.

Richardson JP, Knight AL: The prevention of tetanus in the elderly. Arch Intern Med 1991;151:1712–7.

Shibuya M et al: The use of continuous spinal anesthesia in severe tetanus with autonomic disturbance. J Trauma 1989; 29:1423–9.

Stair TO et al: Tetanus immunity in emergency department patients. Am J Emerg Med 1989;7:563–6.

Surgical Infections

16

James A. Murray, MD, & Howard Belzberg, MD

Infection is a persistent problem in the intensive care unit. Many patients present to the ICU with existing infectious processes. Patients in the ICU are at increased risk of developing an infection during this period of critical illness. When patients die in the ICU, it is more often due to sepsis and the resulting organ failure than to the underlying problem. Sepsis is responsible for more than 500,000 deaths annually in the United States.

The manifestations of infections in critically ill patients can be quite variable. Because of the variety of syndromes and the frequency of infections, the critical care physician must be able to evaluate patients in timely fashion and provide immediate and appropriate interventions. In many cases, even a delay of 1–2 days in instituting appropriate therapy may lead to fatal outcomes. The variable and frequently atypical presentations of infections in the ICU demand that the physician be astute in recognizing early signs of infections and be aggressive in evaluating and treating these severely ill patients.

SURGICAL SITE INFECTIONS

ESSENTIALS OF DIAGNOSIS

- *Typically appear between postoperative days 4 and 8.*
- *Fever.*
- *Wound tenderness and erythema.*
- *Edema or fluctuance.*
- *Gross purulence.*
- *Separation of the wound.*

General Considerations

The concepts and definitions of surgical wound infections have recently evolved. They have been standardized to include infections of the incision as well as infections deep to the incision. Surgical site infections are divided into those involving the incision and those involving the organ or space entered during the operation. Infections of the incision are further divided into superficial (skin and subcutaneous tissues) and deep (deeper soft tissues of the incision) compartments. Specific criteria have been established to improve consistency in diagnosing and reporting surgical site infections.

Surgical site infections account for about 15% of all nosocomial infections. Among surgical patients, site infections account for 38% of nosocomial infections. Two-thirds are confined to the wound, and one-third involve the space or cavity accessed during the operative procedure. These infections prolong hospitalization and increase medical expenses. The physical, psychologic, and economic costs associated with wound infections make it imperative that aggressive prophylactic measures be instituted and that wound infection rates be closely monitored.

Surgical wounds are classified into one of four categories based on the type of operative procedure performed and the associated risk for a surgical site infection. This takes into account the extent of contamination encountered during the operative procedure (Table 16–1). Antibiotic prophylaxis and the incidence of wound infections can be determined based on this classification of the operation. For most surgical site infections, the source of microbes is the endogenous flora of the patient's skin, mucous membranes, or hollow viscus entered at the time of surgery. Antibiotic prophylaxis should be directed at the organism colonizing the surfaces or contents of the tissues involved in the operation.

Risk Factors Influencing Infection Rates

The incidence of wound infections is also influenced by the patient's overall status, surgical technique, and the timing of prophylactic antibiotic administration as well as numerous other factors. Many patient-related factors have been identified that contribute to the risk of postoperative wound infections. (Table 16–2). Coincident remote-site infection and very young or old age are significant risk factors. Significant increases in postoperative wound infection rates have been noted when an elective operation is performed in the presence of a remote infection. It is essential that treatment be provided for the remote infection for at least 48 hours before proceeding with the elective operation.

Table 16–1. Wound infection stratification scheme.

Class	Name	Definition
I	Clean	An uninfected operative wound in which no inflammation is present and the respiratory, alimentary, genital, or uninfected urinary tract is not entered. Clean wounds are closed primarily.
II	Clean-contaminated	An operative wound in which the respiratory, alimentary, genital, or urinary tracts are entered under controlled conditions and without unusual contamination. Specifically, operations involving the biliary tract, appendix, vagina, and oropharynx are included in this category provided no evidence of infection or major break in technique is identified.
III	Contaminated	Open, fresh accidental wounds. Operations with major breaks in sterile technique or with gross spillage from the gastrointestinal tract and incisions in which acute, nonpurulent inflammation is encountered are included in this category.
IV	Dirty-infected	Old traumatic wounds with retained devitalized tissue and those that involve existing clinical infection or perforated viscera. This definition suggests that the organisms causing postoperative infection were present in the operative field before operation.

Although diabetes has not been shown to be an independent risk factor, poor glucose control (> 200 mg/dL) in the early postoperative period (48 hours) is associated with an increased risk of infection. Nicotine has been shown to delay wound healing and impair blood supply, increasing the risk for surgical site infections. Steroid use and malnutrition have been associated with increased risk of surgical site infections in most studies. A prolonged period of preoperative hospitalization has been associated with a higher incidence of nosocomial colonization, infection, and surgical site infections. This may be a marker for the patient's severity of illness and comorbidities.

Surgical antimicrobial prophylaxis is the administration of a brief course of antibiotics just prior to the operative procedure. It assumes that no established infection or inflammation is present at the time of operation. Preoperative antimicrobial prophylaxis is indicated for operations that entail entry into a hollow viscus under controlled circumstances. Prophylaxis should be provided also in clean cases where a prosthetic material is being incorporated whenever an infection would pose catastrophic risk. Administration of antibiotics in contaminated wound and dirty wound cases is considered therapeutic.

The ideal antimicrobial agent used should be safe, inexpensive, and provide the most specific coverage for the organisms anticipated to be the most probable intraoperative contaminants. Administration of antibiotic prophylaxis should be completed shortly before the skin incision. This provides for optimal tissue levels at the time of the incision. Therapeutic levels should be maintained through the course of the operation. If the operation is longer than 3 hours, an additional dose of antibiotics should be given depending on the half-life of the antibiotic. For patients requiring massive transfusions or resuscitation, additional doses of antibiotics should be considered because of the significant dilution effect.

Clinical Features

A. Symptoms and Signs

Surgical site infections typically present between postoperative days 4 and 8. The signs and symptoms associated with surgical site infections have been noted since ancient times and described in terms that have become traditional: *calor* (heat), *odor* (foul smell), *dolor* (pain), *rubor* (redness). The clinical manifestation of these four signs varies by location. Infections of the incision are more likely to produce local findings and can present with systemic symptoms in severe cases. The findings of localized tenderness, pain, and warmth can be noted. It is difficult to differentiate normal postoperative incisional pain from pain secondary to an infection. In the

Table 16–2. Patient-related risk factors for surgical site infections.

Age
Nutritional status
Diabetes
Smoking
Obesity
Coexistent remote infection
Bacterial colonization
Altered immune response
Length of preoperative hospital stay

presence of infection, the pain may be greater than would be expected, or notably increased over what was noted during previous examinations. The wound may also demonstrate new or progressive edema, erythema, crepitance, fluctuance, or purulence. The patient is often febrile. While the source of postoperative fever is most often due to causes other than the wound, the wound should be closely inspected. If a wound infection is suspected even though the clinical signs are minimal, the area of concern—or even the entire wound—should be opened. Any fluid expressed from the wound should be cultured.

Some aggressive forms of wound infections can appear within 48 hours after an operation and must be considered in patients with significantly elevated temperatures in the early postoperative phase (> 38.8 °C). These are typically clostridial or beta-hemolytic streptococcal infections. These patients appear acutely toxic with rapid progression of the infection. All layers of the wound can be involved. A rapid diagnosis is critical. This is usually based on clinical presentation and Gram stain results.

LABORATORY FINDINGS

Leukocytosis and left shift are usually present. A falling platelet count is often an early finding. Gram stain and cultures should be obtained from wounds with purulent discharge or wounds that have been opened due to concern about infection.

Differential Diagnosis

The differential diagnosis of a wound infection includes inadequate pain control, atelectasis, thrombophlebitis, aspiration, and drug reaction as well as the other causes of postoperative fever. It must be remembered that wound separation and drainage of fluid from the wound may be due to an intra-abdominal abscess in communication with the wound or to fascial dehiscence. Failure to consider these possible underlying causes of wound infection early may lead to significant problems.

Treatment

Adequate opening of the wound to allow drainage is the most essential aspect of therapy for surgical site infections involving the incision. Infections of the space or organ require drainage either through percutaneous techniques or operative procedures. The presence of necrotic tissue or foreign bodies requires debridement upon opening. The wound should be packed and dressing changes initiated. Once an infected wound is opened, the clinician can decide to allow healing by secondary intention or to attempt delayed primary closure in a few days. Quantitative cultures may be beneficial in such cases. If less than 10^5 organisms are present, the wound may be closed with a high likelihood of success.

Antibiotic therapy is typically not required for uncomplicated surgical site infections limited to the incision. Opening of the wound and providing adequate drainage are usually sufficient. In cases of aggressive infections, extensive cellulitis, or tissue necrosis—or if the patient has preexisting comorbidities or is immunocompromised—adequate antimicrobial therapy should be initiated promptly.

Current Controversies & Unresolved Issues

Current opinion about antimicrobial prophylaxis is tending toward minimizing its use (fewer doses and less broad-spectrum). The supplemental administration of oxygen during and shortly after operation was recently demonstrated to significantly reduce the incidence of wound infections in elective colorectal operations. Patients were provided with an FIO_2 of 0.80 during the operation and for 2 hours postoperatively. The incidence of wound infections was dramatically reduced.

Emori TG, Gaynes RP: An overview of nosocomial infections including the role of the microbiology laboratory. Clin Microbiol Rev 1993;6:428–42.

Supplemental perioperative oxygen to reduce the incidence of surgical-wound infection. Grief R et al for the outcomes research group. N Engl J Med 2000;342:161–7.

Luna CM et al: Impact of BAL data on the therapy and outcome of ventilator-associated pneumonia. Chest 1997;111:676–85.

Platt R et al: Perioperative antibiotic prophylaxis for herniorrhaphy and breast surgery. N Engl J Med 1990;322:153–60.

NECROTIZING SOFT TISSUE INFECTIONS

ESSENTIALS OF DIAGNOSIS

- *Edema beyond area of erythema.*
- *Subcutaneous crepitance.*
- *Skin vesicles or bullae.*
- *Absence of lymphangitis.*

General Considerations

Necrotizing soft tissue infections are a group of clinically diverse diseases characterized by rapidly spreading necrosis involving the skin, subcutaneous tissue, fascia, or muscle. Although uncommon, they are associated with a high morbidity and mortality. They are caused by endogenous aerobic and anaerobic bacteria. These infections can involve any part of the body and commonly affect the extremities, perineum, groin, and abdomen. Rapid diagnosis, use of appropriate antibiotics, and aggressive operative debridement are essential. Aggressive surgical debridement, repeated every 1–2 days, is the most important part of the therapy.

Necrotizing soft tissue infections can be primary or secondary. Primary infections, which are those occurring in the absence of a portal of entry for bacteria, are uncommon. Secondary infections can be due to post-operative infections, post-traumatic infections, or complications of unrecognized or inadequately treated infections. Patients typically have associated conditions (such as diabetes or vascular disease) that compromise their ability to contain the infection and predispose them to the development of tissue necrosis.

Necrotizing soft tissue infections can be subclassified into categories such as cellulitis, fasciitis, and myonecrosis depending on the deepest layer of involvement. Necrotizing soft tissue infections can be caused by a single organism, but more likely are due to polymicrobial infections. Polymicrobial infections are often caused by the synergistic activity of facultative aerobic and anaerobic bacteria. Bacterial synergism is typically associated with a more virulent infection. This group of diseases can also be classified according to causative organism, eg, clostridial or nonclostridial, monomicrobial or polymicrobial, synergistic gangrene or streptococcal gangrene. The rapid onset and progression of these infections is due to the production of toxic proteolytic enzymes that account for the tissue damage and necrosis.

Necrotizing skin infections are more likely to occur in patients with impaired host defenses, such as are present with advanced age, diabetes mellitus, malignancy, peripheral vascular disease, chronic alcoholism, and chronic renal failure; or in patients receiving immunosuppressive agents. Typically, these factors are present along with extensive contamination, devitalized tissue, or foreign bodies. Although these infections may present as primary necrotizing infections, the majority occur as secondary infections with violation of the skin and underlying tissues. A combination of virulent organisms and impaired host defenses allows them to develop.

Clinical Features

A. Symptoms and Signs

The diagnosis of necrotizing skin infections is primarily clinical and should be made on the basis of the history and physical examination. These lesions may initially appear small and trivial. But even under close observation they can progress rapidly. Characteristic features include edema and tenderness beyond the zone of erythema, vesicles or bullae, palpable crepitus or air on radiographic studies, and the absence of lymphangitis or lymphadenitis. Fever, tachycardia, and hypotension are typically present.

Should the clinical diagnosis not be certain, fine-needle aspiration or incisional biopsy should be performed. These may demonstrate organisms on Gram stain or evidence of necrosis. If an incisional biopsy is performed, the tissues should be thoroughly inspected for evidence of necrosis. The fascial planes can be probed with forceps to determine if the fascia is intact. Easy passage through the fascial plane or a grayish appearance of the fascia is consistent with necrotizing infection.

B. Laboratory Findings

Along with leukocytosis, patients may have profound anemia due to intravascular hemolysis. Disseminated intravascular coagulopathy may occur. Rhabdomyolysis may be seen, which can contribute to renal failure or exacerbate renal dysfunction due to ongoing sepsis or underlying disease.

C. Imaging Studies

Soft-tissue radiographs may demonstrate subcutaneous emphysema. Subcutaneous crepitus and radiographic findings occur late in the clinical course. Plain radiographs are helpful if positive but are rarely diagnostic in patients with necrotizing soft tissue infections.

Treatment

A. Operative Treatment

The successful management of necrotizing soft tissue infections depends on early diagnosis and immediate operative debridement. Delays in operation are associated with a significant reduction in survival. Operative debridement must be aggressive and extensive. Amputation of an affected extremity is often required to prevent the infection from spreading to the torso. Because infection often spreads well beyond the margins of the cutaneous manifestations, failure to adequately debride all tissues will lead to further spreading of necrosis. All margins of the wound must appear healthy and viable. Marginal areas should be assumed to be infected and excised. Wound drainage or exudates should be sent for culture.

Once debridement is complete, the wound should be lightly packed and dressed with moistened gauze. Planned reoperation every 24–48 hours is required to examine the wound edges and ensure that ongoing tissue necrosis is not present.

Intravenous antibiotic therapy is required. Broad-spectrum coverage can be provided with a single agent or multiple agents. Coverage should provide adequate aerobic and anaerobic activity. It is important to initially provide adequate coverage of the potential organisms with broad-spectrum antibiotics and then taper therapy once culture results have been returned.

B. Adjuvant Therapy

Topical antimicrobial agents may provide higher tissue concentration at the site of contamination. Once the soft tissue infection has been controlled, extensive reconstruction and aggressive rehabilitation are required. Reconstruction and coverage of wounds may be done with simple skin grafts, but complex tissue transfers are often needed to provide coverage of exposed bones, tendons, nerves, and other anatomic features.

Current Controversies & Unresolved Issues

Hyperbaric oxygen has been advocated for extensive necrotizing soft tissue infections, especially those due to clostridial infections. While some studies support the use of hyperbaric oxygen, others do not. Operative debridement should be performed immediately, without delay for transfer to facilities where hyperbaric oxygen can be used. This therapy does neutralize toxins already present and promotes healing in areas of marginal viability. However, hyperbaric oxygen should not be used as a substitute for aggressive debridement of infected necrotic tissue.

Bilton BD et al: Aggressive surgical management of necrotizing fasciitis serves to decrease mortality: a retrospective study. Am Surg 1998;64:397–400.

Korhonen K, Kuttila K, Ninikoski J: Tissue gas tensions in patients with necrotizing fasciitis and healthy controls during hyperbaric oxygen: a clinical study. Eur J Surg 2000;166:530–4.

Nichols RL, Florman S: Clinical presentations of soft-tissue infection and surgical site infections. Clin Infect Dis 2001; 33(Suppl);S84–93.

PERITONITIS & INTRA-ABDOMINAL ABSCESS

ESSENTIALS OF DIAGNOSIS

- *Abdominal pain.*
- *Absent or diminished bowel sounds.*
- *Abdominal tenderness, guarding, or rigidity.*
- *Leukocytosis.*
- *Fever.*

General Considerations

Peritonitis can be classified as primary, secondary, or tertiary. Primary peritonitis occurs from hematogenous or lymphatic seeding of the peritoneal cavity with bacteria from a remote site. Secondary peritonitis is due to contamination of the peritoneal cavity from a hollow viscus within the abdominal cavity. Tertiary peritonitis is a persistent intra-abdominal infection that did not respond to previous operative efforts.

The severity of illness following peritoneal contamination from a hollow viscus perforation is highly variable. The factors involved include the site of perforation, the contents spilled, the quantity and virulence of bacteria within the inoculum, the duration of contamination, and the patient's ability to respond to the insult.

Clinical Features

A. Symptoms and Signs

The diagnosis of peritonitis is suggested by the history and physical findings. Abdominal pain is a constant finding. Involuntary guarding, rigidity, and increased pain with slight movements are all signs of significant peritoneal irritation. The abdomen may be distended. Bowel sounds are absent. Fever along with signs of hypovolemia due to fluid sequestration may be seen.

B. Laboratory Findings

Leukocytosis with a shift to the left is usually present. In severe cases, leukopenia may be present.

C. Imaging Studies

Radiographic studies may demonstrate free air or extravasation of contrast. Ultrasonography and especially CT may help localize an abscess. CT may also demonstrate subtle findings of free extraluminal air or free air anterior to the liver, which may be missed by plain films. Other signs of peritonitis on CT scan include bowel wall thickening and mesenteric stranding.

Treatment

A. Operative Treatment

Early diagnosis and prompt intervention are required to minimize the systemic effects and limit the ongoing inflammatory process. The exact cause of peritonitis is not always obvious prior to operative exploration. Localized peritonitis is more amenable to operative resection and surgical drainage. In stable patients with localized tenderness and hemodynamic stability, percutaneous drainage of a localized fluid collection may be sufficient. Control of ongoing spillage from the gastrointestinal tract is necessary. Diffuse suppurative peritonitis is a more difficult situation to manage. Despite adequate control of spillage, these patients tend to be critically ill in the postoperative period.

B. Adjunctive Treatment

Antimicrobial coverage with broad-spectrum antibiotics is required. Cultures of the peritoneal fluid should be obtained. The results of these cultures should be used in tailoring antibiotics to the patient. Antifungal therapy has been demonstrated to reduce the incidence of fungal sepsis in some critically ill patients undergoing reoperation.

Current Controversies & Unresolved Issues

Routine reexploration and irrigation of the abdominal cavity for patients with peritonitis has been advocated. Irrigation of the abdominal cavity to reduce the bacterial load is often done to prevent abdominal abscesses. However, this practice causes an increase in inflammatory cytokines and may result in a significant second inflammatory stimulus to the patient.

Barie PS: Serious intra-abdominal infections. Curr Opin Crit Care 2001;7:263–7.

Bohnen JM et al: Guidelines for clinical care: anti-infective agents for intra-abdominal infection—a Surgical Infection Society policy statement. Arch Surg 1992;127:83–9.

CATHETER-RELATED INFECTION

Intravascular catheters are essential devices in the intensive care unit. Nevertheless, they are frequently associated with local and systemic complications. Catheter-related infections—particularly bloodstream infections—are associated with increased morbidity and mortality, prolonged hospitalization, and increased medical costs.

An estimated 200,000 nosocomial bloodstream infections occur each year. Most are related to the use of an intravascular device. Bloodstream infections are considerably more common in patients with indwelling intravascular catheters than among patients without them. Intravascular devices can be classified as long-term or short-term. This discussion will describe the management and infectious complications associated with short-term central venous catheters.

Temporary central venous catheters account for about 90% of all bloodstream infections due to intravascular catheters. Multiple risk factors have been identified for infection. These include the number of lumens and the site of insertion. The multilumen catheter may increase the risk of infection in two ways. First, each lumen serves as a portal of entry and therefore contributes to the risk. Second, patients with multilumen catheters are generally more acutely ill than patients with single-lumen catheters. A higher level of acuity means more interventions. The number of times an intravenous infusion system is opened (eg, to draw a sample or give a medication) correlates positively with the risk of contamination and subsequent infection.

The site of insertion has a significant impact on the incidence of catheter-related infectious complications. The internal jugular artery is more frequently associated with infections than the subclavian vein. This may be due to the increased motion at the internal jugular site or its proximity to oropharyngeal secretions.

Other factors associated with central-venous-catheter-related infections include repeated catheterization, the presence of an infectious process elsewhere in the body, exposure of the catheter to bacteremia, absence of systemic antibiotic therapy, duration of catheterization, type of dressing, and the technique and experience of personnel placing the catheter.

Pulmonary artery catheters differ from central venous catheters in that they are inserted through an introducer sheath and the duration of use averages less than 3 days. Most pulmonary artery catheters are heparin-bonded. This reduces catheter thrombosis and microbial adherence to the catheter. Risk factors reported for catheter-related infections in patients with a pulmonary artery catheter are duration of catheterization longer than 3 days, colonization of the skin insertion site, introducer being left in place for more than 5 days, and catheter insertion in the operating room with suboptimal barrier precautions.

Diagnosis

Diagnosis typically relies on both clinical and laboratory criteria, both of which have significant limitations. In order to increase the sensitivity and specificity of culture techniques, semiquantitative and quantitative methods have been introduced. Growth of more than 15 colony-forming units or more than 10^3 organisms, respectively, are considered indicative of a catheter infection.

Catheter-related bloodstream infection is defined as isolation of the same organism by either semiquantitative or quantitative cultures and from the blood cultures. The patient should have accompanying clinical symptoms of bloodstream infection. Removal of the catheter typically results in rapid resolution of symptoms. In the absence of laboratory confirmation, resolution of symptoms following removal is considered indirect evidence of catheter-related bloodstream infection.

Prevention of catheter-related bloodstream infections is essential. Because of the high frequency of catheter use and the impact on patient outcome, measures of prevention must be implemented. Strict adherence to hand washing and aseptic technique is crucial. For central venous catheters, the subclavian vein site has a lower risk of infection than the internal jugular or femoral vein sites. Fewer technical complications are associated with insertion at the internal jugular site.

Barrier precautions must be maximized. The use of gowns, gloves, masks, and large drapes results in a significantly lower rate of infection and should be enforced. The fenestrated drape provided in central venous catheter kits is associated with a higher infection rate than sterile sheets.

The timing and method of catheter placement also influence infection rates. Lines placed under emergent conditions have a much higher rate of infection and should be removed within 24 hours after insertion. Although duration of catheterization is a risk factor for infection, routine line exchanges and removal based on days of catheterization do not reduce the risk of infection. Guidewire exchanges are acceptable as long as the site of insertion does not show signs of inflammation or infection.

Antimicrobial or antiseptic impregnated catheters have led to a reduction in infectious complications associated with short-term central venous catheters. Coating the catheters has reduced bacterial adherence and biofilm formation and thus colonization of the catheters.

Treatment

If catheter-related bloodstream infection is suspected, the catheter should be removed. The venous access site may be preserved by changing the wire over a guidewire as long as the catheter site shows no signs of inflammation or purulence. If the cultures from the line removed are negative, the new catheter may be preserved. If the cultures are positive, the catheter should be removed and a new site used for insertion of a new catheter.

Management of a catheter-related bloodstream infection requires antimicrobial therapy to cover the suspected organisms. Because of the high frequency of staphylococcal infections, it may be reasonable to use vancomycin as empiric therapy. Once culture and sensitivity results have been obtained, antibiotic therapy can be more selective.

Over the past two decades, the microbiologic profile of pathogens reported as nosocomial bloodstream infections has changed remarkably. Four significant pathogens have been reported as increasingly more prevalent during the past decade. These organisms are coagulase-negative staphylococci, candida species, *Staphylococcus aureus,* and enterococci.

Coagulase-negative staphylococci have become the most frequently isolated pathogens in catheter-related infections and account for 25–30% of all nosocomial bloodstream infections. This increased prevalence can be attributed to an increased use of prosthetic and indwelling devices, improved survival of premature infants and the increased use of lipids in these patients, and the recognition of coagulase-negative staphylococci as a significant nosocomial pathogen. *S aureus,* which had been the most frequently reported pathogen prior to 1986, may be complicated by metastatic foci of infection requiring prolonged antibiotic therapy (eg, endocarditis and osteomyelitis).

Enterococci are another emerging pathogen with a significant resistance potential. Vancomycin-resistant enterococcus accounts for about 3–5% of all enterococcal bloodstream infections. The use of indwelling devices, the use of vancomycin and cephalosporins, and prolonged hospitalization are just three of the risk factors associated with vancomycin resistance. Although endogenous sources of enterococcus are important, health care workers, patient care equipment, and contaminated environmental surfaces are more common sources.

Fungal infections represent an increasing proportion of catheter-related bloodstream infections. *Candida albicans* was the predominant species initially, but other species such as *Candida glabrata* and *Candida torulopsis* are becoming more prevalent and challenging the practices of the intensive care physician. These species are resistant to the azoles, particularly fluconazole.

With the use of broad-spectrum antibiotics, the role of gram-negative bacteremia related to indwelling catheters has increased. The source of these infections is often endogenous, typically due to seeding of the catheter from a remote infection. Infection could also be due to sources such as contaminated pressure-monitoring equipment.

Pearson ML: Guideline for prevention of intravascular-device-related infections. Hospital Infection Control Practices Advisory Committee (HICPAC). Infect Control Hosp Epidemiol 1996;17:438–73.

VENTILATOR-ASSOCIATED PNEUMONIA

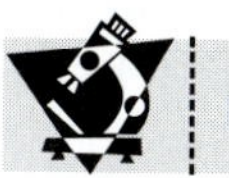

ESSENTIALS OF DIAGNOSIS

- *Fever.*
- *Leukocytosis.*
- *New or progressive infiltrate on chest x-ray.*
- *Purulent sputum.*

General Considerations

Nosocomial pneumonia has become more common than surgical site infections in postsurgical patients. Ventilator-associated pneumonia is a major problem in intensive care units. It must be distinguished from other nosocomial pneumonias because the diagnosis, treatment, prognosis, and outcome differ significantly.

Numerous risk factors have been identified that predispose critically ill patients to the development of ventilator-associated pneumonia. Among them are gastric neutralization, recumbent positioning, the presence of a nasogastric tube, frequent changes of ventilator tubing, abdominal or thoracic surgery, and the immunocompromised state. The more severe the illness (as demonstrated by increasing APACHE scores), the higher the risk of ventilator-associated pneumonia. The risk also increases by up to 3% per day of mechanical ventilation.

The standard clinical criteria for diagnosis of ventilator-associated pneumonia typically have included two or three findings—fever, leukocytosis, purulent sputum—in association with a new or progressive infiltrate on chest radiographic studies. Unfortunately, fever and leukocytosis are nonspecific and are typically present in patients in the ICU as part of the inflammatory response associated with the underlying disease. Radiographic studies of the chest can be abnormal due to ARDS, aspiration, pulmonary contusions, effusions, atelectasis, etc. When all four criteria are present, specificity in diagnosis of pneumonia increases but sensitivity is less than 50%.

As a result of these difficulties, additional measures have been employed to diagnose ventilator-associated pneumonia. Since the endotracheal tube and upper airways become colonized following intubation, the presence of bacteria in specimens obtained by aspiration from the upper airway may be unreliable. The presence of PMNs (> 25 per low-power field) and the absence of epithelial cells (< 10 per low-power field) signifies an adequate specimen with evidence of purulence. Because of contamination of the specimen by organisms colonizing the endotracheal tube and the upper airway, many culture results will in fact be falsely positive. Patients receiving systemic antibiotics at the time the culture specimen was obtained can have falsely negative culture results.

As a result of the difficulties noted from the clinical and microbiologic evaluation of these patients, invasive methods were developed to assist in the diagnosis of ventilator-associated pneumonia. Bronchoalveolar lavage and protected specimen brushings with quantitative culture technique have been used to improve the sensitivity and specificity of the diagnosis of ventilator-associated pneumonia. Because of the invasive nature of these procedures, complications may develop. Skilled personnel are required to perform the test reliably to make certain that an adequate specimen is obtained.

Bronchoalveolar lavage has a sensitivity of 70–100% depending on the method of comparison. Most studies agree that a result of greater than 10^4 organisms per microliter is considered a positive result. Again, the quantitative cultures may be adversely affected if the patient was receiving systemic antibiotics. The major risk of bronchoalveolar lavage is the reduction in arterial oxygenation, which may take hours to return to pre-lavage levels.

Collection of protected specimen brushings is an invasive procedure. It requires skilled personnel and incurs substantial costs. The results may not be reproducible in up to 25% of patients. The sensitivity and specificity are better, however, than those of clinical diagnostic criteria.

The one distinct advantage of these two invasive techniques is that a negative result has been shown to allow cessation or reduction of antibiotic use without an increase in ventilator days or mortality.

Treatment

The microbiologic profile of each ward or ICU must be known so that early effective therapy can be provided as soon as ventilator-associated pneumonia is suspected. Cases that present on or after day 5 are typically caused by enteric organisms, with occasional gram-positive organisms such as *S aureus.* These organisms are more virulent and have a broader resistance pattern.

The one factor that has been shown to improve outcome in treating patients with ventilator-associated pneumonia is timing. Early administration of appropriate antibiotics is crucial. Antibiotic therapy should be instituted as soon as the diagnosis is suspected. Patients who receive early appropriate therapy have lower mortality. Patients in whom antibiotic therapy is not started until culture results are available and patients who receive inappropriate antibiotics early—even if antibiotic therapy is adjusted when culture results are available—have a significantly higher mortality.

Antonelli M et al: Risk factors for early onset pneumonia in trauma patients. Chest 1994;105;224–8.

Guidelines for prevention of nosocomial pneumonia. Centers for Disease Control and Prevention. MMWR Morb Mort Wkly Rep 1997;46(RR-1):1–79.

Khuri SF et al: Risk adjustment of the postoperative mortality rate for the comparative assessment of the quality of surgical care: Results of the National Veterans Affairs Surgical Risk Study. J Am Coll Surg 1997;185:315–27.

Kollef M: Ventilator-associated pneumonia. JAMA 1993;270: 1965–70.

Kollef MH: The prevention of ventilator-associated pneumonia. N Engl J Med 1999;340:627–34.

Bleeding & Hemostasis 17

Elizabeth D. Simmons, MD

Bleeding is a common problem in critically ill patients in the intensive care unit. A rational approach to diagnosis and treatment of bleeding requires an understanding of the major elements of the hemostatic system, currently available laboratory tests of hemostatic function, and specific disorders of hemostasis. Bleeding disorders are generally categorized into defects of coagulation and fibrinolysis, defects of platelets, and defects of vascular integrity, but critically ill patients who are bleeding may have defects in multiple arms of the hemostatic system. Furthermore, defective hemostasis may result in thrombosis as well as bleeding.

Normal Hemostasis & Laboratory Evaluation

A. Normal Hemostasis

The major elements of hemostasis are outlined in Table 17–1. A complex interaction of vascular endothelium, platelets, red blood cells, coagulation factors, naturally occurring anticoagulants, and fibrinolytic enzymes results in formation of blood clot at the site of vascular injury and activation of repair mechanisms to promote healing of the injured blood vessel. Vascular injury results in platelet adhesion and aggregation, activation of coagulation factors ultimately resulting in cleavage of fibrinogen to fibrin, and formation of a stable blood clot consisting of cross-linked fibrin polymers, platelets, and red blood cells. Simultaneously, naturally occurring anticoagulants and fibrinolytic enzymes are activated, a process that limits the amount of clot formed and degrades clot once the vessel is repaired. The latter aspects of hemostasis serve to confine clot formation to the site of vascular injury while permitting continued blood flow through the affected blood vessel. The precise factors that regulate the balance between clot formation and breakdown are not well understood.

B. Laboratory Tests of Hemostasis (Table 17–2)

There are several generally available laboratory tests for evaluation of the function of the hemostatic system. Currently available screening laboratory tests detect clinically significant defects (quantitative and qualitative) of most but not all of the important elements of hemostasis. The history should dictate the choice of tests to determine the adequacy of hemostatic function. A highly suggestive history for a bleeding disorder calls for sophisticated or specialized laboratory testing, whereas abnormal test results may not be predictive of future risk of bleeding in the absence of a significant bleeding history.

1. Tests of coagulation—Calcium and phospholipid are required for normal coagulation to occur. In the laboratory, measurement of coagulation times (eg, prothrombin time and partial thromboplastin time) involves mixing decalcified plasma (collected in citrate) and a phospholipid substitute (thromboplastin), adding calcium, and determining the time for visible clot formation using an automated system. Different phospholipid reagents activate different parts of the coagulation cascade, and an activating agent is added for performance of the activated partial thromboplastin time (aPTT). Prothrombin time (PT) is generally reported as the international normalized ratio (INR), which compares observed results against a reference thromboplastin to minimize interlaboratory variability due to differing sensitivities of thromboplastin reagents. The thrombin time is performed by adding excess thrombin to decalcified plasma (phospholipid is not required).

Standard coagulation times are not prolonged until factor activities drop to less than 20–50% of normal (depending upon the specific factor deficiency). Therefore, a mixture of patient plasma with normal plasma in equal quantities ("1:1 dilution") should normalize a prolonged coagulation time if due solely to one or more factor deficiencies. Failure of a prolonged coagulation time to correct after 1:1 dilution with normal plasma implies the presence of a circulating inhibitor of coagulation, including heparin.

In vitro assessment of coagulation depends on the action of factor XII, high-molecular-weight kininogen, and prekallikrein (the contact factors), whereas in vivo hemostasis appears to occur normally even with complete deficiency of any of these proteins. Factor XI likewise is essential for in vitro coagulation, but factor XI deficiency generally is associated with a very mild bleeding tendency. Specific coagulation factor deficiencies can be identified using known deficient plasma in a modification of the 1:1 dilution test when clinically indicated.

Standard screening coagulation tests (prothrombin time, partial thromboplastin time, and thrombin time) do not detect mild coagulation factor deficiencies, factor

Table 17–1. Normal hemostasis.

Element	Participation in Hemostasis
Endothelium	
Procoagulant	Release of vWF, factor VIII, tissue factor, plasminogen activator inhibitor, and platelet activating factor in response to injury; maintains tight interendothelial junctions to prevent blood extravasation.
Anticoagulant	Negative charge repels platelets and coagulation factors; produces prostacyclin; releases tissue plasminogen activator in response to vessel injury; provides thrombomodulin for thrombin-mediated activation of protein C; provides heparin-like molecules which interact with antithrombin III and accelerate its inactivation of thrombin and other serine proteases.
Platelets	Adhere to exposed subendothelium via vWF and aggregate in response to activation (via fibrinogen-glycoprotein IIb/IIIa interaction); secrete agonists which stimulate further platelet aggregation; provide phospholipid for production of thromboxane A_2 and for coagulation reactions; provide surface on which coagulation reactions are localized; secrete coagulation factors (V, vWF), which increase local concentration; provide contractile machinery for clot retraction; perhaps maintain interendothelial tight junctions by secretion of metabolically active substances.
Coagulation factors	
Proenzymes	In response to vascular injury, sequential activation (VII, IX, X, II) results in generation of thrombin and cleavage of fibrinogen to fibrin.
Thrombin	In addition to cleavage of fibrinogen, activates platelets, factors V, VIII, and XIII, and protein C.
Fibrinogen	Cleaved by thrombin to fibrin, which polymerizes to insoluble fibrin clot.
Factor XIII	After activation by thrombin, cross-links fibrin polymers to stabilize clot.
Cofactors	Factors V and VIII, both activated by thrombin, act as cofactors for X and IX, respectively.
Tissue factor	Integral membrane constituent of vascular endothelial cells and stimulated monocytes; acts as receptor for factor VII; initiates blood coagulation.
Calcium, phospholipid	Necessary for several steps in coagulation.
Contact factors	Factor XII, HMW kininogen, and prekallikrein are important for in vitro hemostatsis only.
Anticoagulants[1]	
Protein C	Vitamin K-dependent anticoagulant, inactivates factors V and VIII after activation by thrombin bound to thrombomodulin on endothelial surfaces.
Protein S	Vitamin K-dependent cofactor for protein C.
Thrombomodulin	Receptor for thrombin, initiates activation of protein C pathway.
Antithrombin III (AT III)	Inactivates thrombin and other serine proteases of the coagulation cascade.
Tissue factor pathway inhibitor (TFPI)	Inhibits tissue factor/factor VIIa complex.
Fibrinolytic system	
Tissue plasminogen activator	Cleaves fibrin-bound plasminogen to plasmin.
Urokinase	Plasminogen activator found in urine and in plasma when fibrinolysis is stimulated.
Plasminogen	Once activated to plasmin, lyses fibrin and fibrinogen.
Plasminogen activator inhibitor-1 (PAI-1)	Prevents activation of plasminogen by tissue plasminogen activator.
Alpha$_2$-antiplasmin	Inactivates circulating plasmin and prevents lysis of fibrin and fibrinogen.
Blood elements and rheology	Laminar flow prevents contact of cellular elements with endothelium; free flow prevents accumulation of factors at uninjured sites and dilutes concentration of activated factors; dislodges platelet plugs if not firmly attached to subendothelium; provides inhibitory plasma proteins other than antithrombin to inactivated coagulation factors.

[1]Precise physiologic role in hemostasis not well defined: Other serine proteinase inhibitors (Serpin): alpha$_2$-macroglobulin, alpha$_1$-proteinase inhibitor, C1 esterase inhibitor, protein C inhibitor, heparin cofactor II.

Table 17–2. Tests of hemostatic function (average normal values given).

Test (normal range)	Significance of Abnormal Test
Coagulation	
Prothrombin time (PT) (10–13 seconds) International normalized ratio (INR) (1.0)	Deficiencies of or inhibitors to extrinsic and common pathway factors: VII, X, V (< 50%), II (< 30%), fibrinogen (< 100 mg/dL).
Activated partial thromboplastin time (aPTT) (25–40 seconds)	Deficiencies of or inhibitors of contact factors, intrinsic and common pathway factors: XII, HMW kininogen, prekallikrein, XI (< 50%), VIII, IX (< 20%), X, V, II (< 30–50%), fibrinogen (< 100 mg/dL). Decreased value may indicate increased concentration of factor (especially VIII) or hypercoagulable condition.
Thrombin time (TT) (10 seconds)	Deficiency or defect of fibrinogen, inhibitors of thrombin action (heparin), or inhibitors of fibrin polymerization (FDP, myeloma proteins).
Reptilase time	Similar to thrombin time but unaffected by heparin.
Stypven time (Russell viper venom time)	Differentiate factor X from factor VII deficiency (abnormal in factor X deficiency).
1:1 dilution test (corrects to normal)	Failure to correct consistent with inhibitors to specific factors or to phospholipid; heparin effect. Correction to normal consistent with factor deficiency.
Factors assays (60% to > 100%)	Deficiencies of one or more coagulation factors.
5 M urea clot stability	Deficiency of factor XIII.
Platelets	
Platelet count (150,000–400,000/μL)	Quantitative abnormalities of platelets.
Bleeding time (< 7 minutes)	Impaired platelet function, thrombocytopenia, severe anemia, improper technique.
Aggregation (qualitative)	Impaired platelet aggregation in response to platelet agonists; can localize defect based on pattern of abnormal aggregation.
Ristocetin cofactor assay	Decreased quantity or function of vWF in patient plasma.
Fibrinolysis	
Fibrin(ogen) degradation products (FDP) (< 10 μg/mL)	Accelerated fibrinolysis.
Fibrinogen (150–400 mg/dL)	Deficiency of fibrinogen.
Euglobulin lysis time (> 2 hours)	Accelerated fibrinolysis.
Protamine sulfate test	Positive test indicates presence of circulating fibrin monomers.
D-dimer test	Positive test indicates presence of cross-linked FDP, formed only if activation of factor XIII has resulted in cross-linkage of fibrin polymers.

XIII deficiency, defects in fibrinolysis, or abnormalities of platelets, blood vessels, or supporting connective tissue. They are not useful for determining deficiencies of the naturally occurring anticoagulants or for evaluating patients with thrombotic disorders (except for patients with lupus anticoagulants and contact factor deficiencies). Coagulation times shorter than normal occur frequently, particularly if there are higher than normal levels of any of the factors measured by the test (especially factor VIII) and may mask deficiencies of other factors.

2. Platelets—The platelet count can be determined by automated cell counter or by estimation on a peripheral blood smear (normal, 10–20/hpf). The bleeding time is an in vivo test of platelet function. Bleeding time is affected by platelet number, platelet function, position and depth of the incision, maintenance of constant pressure above the site of the incision, medications, hemoglobin concentration, and renal function. In thrombocytopenic patients, the bleeding time varies as a function of the cause as well as the degree of thrombocytopenia. Although the bleeding time is useful in diagnosis of disorders of platelet function, it may not be reliable as a predictor of clinical bleeding. Other tests of platelet function include in vitro platelet aggregation in response to various agonists (eg, thrombin, epinephrine, adenosine diphosphate, ristocetin) for evaluation of patients suspected of having significant disorders of platelet function rather than number.

3. Fibrinolysis—Elevated fibrin and fibrinogen degradation products and decreased fibrinogen concentration may reflect excessive intravascular fibrinolysis, but these measurements are not specific. The protamine sulfate test and the D-dimer test may be useful to confirm the presence of disseminated intravascular coagulation as the cause of elevated fibrin degradation products. The euglobulin lysis time, which measures the action of plasminogen activators and plasmin in blood, may be useful for confirming the presence of excessive fibrinolysis. Specific assays for elements of the fibrinolytic system are available if clinically indicated.

INHERITED COAGULATION DISORDERS

ESSENTIALS OF DIAGNOSIS

- *Personal and family history of bleeding disorder.*
- *Abnormal screening coagulation tests.*
- *Abnormal specific factor assays.*

General Considerations

Inherited coagulation disorders result from a decrease in quantity or function of a single coagulation factor, though there are some cases of familial multiple coagulation factor deficiencies. The inheritance pattern may be autosomal or X-linked, dominant or recessive, or may be the result of a new mutation, so a negative family history does not preclude the presence of an inherited disorder of coagulation. A personal history of bleeding may be absent if the defect is mild or if there has been no prior challenge to the hemostatic system (eg, major surgery or trauma). In addition, some coagulation defects are variable over time, with fluctuations both in bleeding manifestations and in laboratory abnormalities. Nevertheless, most of the inherited disorders of blood coagulation result in a typical clinical bleeding history accompanied by characteristic reproducible laboratory abnormalities (Table 17–3).

Von Willebrand's disease is the most common inherited bleeding defect in humans, but prevalence figures vary widely because of variable expression and penetrance of the genetic abnormality. The disease results from inheritance of an autosomal dominant (rarely, autosomal recessive) decrease in the quantity or function of von Willebrand factor. Von Willebrand factor is essential in platelet adhesion and serves as a carrier for the procoagulant factor VIII protein. Clinical manifestations typically reflect impaired platelet function, with epistaxis, easy bruising, menorrhagia, and excessive bleeding after surgery, trauma, or dental procedures. Severe deficiencies (< 1% activity) are rare and may result in bleeding similar to that seen in hemophilia A. Von Willebrand's disease is heterogeneous in severity and is subject to variability over time and within families. During pregnancy, von Willebrand factor levels increase, often sufficiently to permit adequate hemostasis at childbirth.

Hemophilia A, which accounts for 80% of all hemophilia, results from inheritance of an X-linked recessive mutation in the factor VIII gene, giving rise to severe (< 1% activity), moderate (1–5% activity), or mild (> 5% activity) factor VIII deficiency. The incidence of hemophilia A is approximately 1:5000 men. Hemophilia A does occur in women, due either to early X chromosome inactivation of the normal X in a heterozygous female or to inheritance of two abnormal X chromosomes (one from an affected father and one from a carrier mother).

Clinical manifestations depend upon the severity of the deficiency (70% of patients have severe deficiency) but typically include lifelong spontaneous hemarthroses and soft tissue hematomas, hematuria, and, if severe, increased epistaxis, gum bleeding, and ecchymoses. Postoperative or dental bleeding is severe and prolonged. Central nervous system hemorrhage occurs in about 3% of cases and may be fatal. The severity of the deficiency is generally constant within a family and over time in an individual, but it varies between families.

Hemophilia B results from inheritance of an X-linked recessive mutation in the factor IX gene. The pathophysiology and clinical manifestations are virtually identical with those of hemophilia A, though severe deficiency is present in only 50%. Hemophilia B is much less common than hemophilia A, with an estimated incidence of 1:50,000 men.

Inherited deficiencies of all the other coagulation factors have been reported (Table 17–3), but these are rare. All are autosomally inherited, usually recessive,

Table 17–3. Clinical manifestations of inherited coagulation factor deficiencies.

	Factor Deficiency										
	vWF	**VIII**	**IX**	**II**	**V**	**VII**	**X**	**XI**	**XIII**	**Fibrinogen**	**Dysfibrinogenemia**
Inheritance	AD/AID /AR	XR	XR	AR	AR	AR	AIR	AR	AR	AR	AD
Incidence	1:100	1/10 K	1/40 K	Rare	Rare	Rare	Rare	Rare[1]	1/1 mil	Rare	Rare
Clinical manifestations Severity (most cases)	Mild	70% severe	50% severe	Mild	Mild, variable	Moderate	Moderate	Mild	Severe	Mild	Mild
Easy bruising	+	(+)	(+)	(+)	+	+	+	(+)	+		+
Epistaxis	+	(+)	(+)	(+)	+	+	+	(+)	+	+	+
Menorrhagia	+			(+)	+	+	+	(+)	+	+	+
Soft tissue hematomas		+	+	(+)	(+)	+	+	(+)	+		
Hemarthrosis	•	+	+	(+)	(+)	+	+		+	(+)	
Intracranial hemorrhage		+	+		•	+	+		+	+	
Gastrointestinal hemorrhage		+	+		(+)	+	+			+	
Bleeding with trauma, surgery, or dental procedures	+	+	+	+	+	(+)	(+)	(+)	+	•	(+)
Umbilical stump bleeding		•	•	+					+	•	(+)
Spontaneous abortions									+	+	+
Male infertility									+		
Poor wound healing		(+)	(+)						+		+
Thromboembolic complications						+				+ (with rx)	+

(continued)

Table 17–3. Clinical manifestations of inherited coagulation factor deficiencies. (continued)

	Factor Deficiency										
	vWF	**VIII**	**IX**	**II**	**V**	**VII**	**X**	**XI**	**XIII**	**Fibrinogen**	**Dysfibrinogenemia**
Laboratory abnormalities											
PT prolonged				+	+		+			+	+
aPTT prolonged		+	+	+	+	+	+	+		+	(+)
Thrombin time prolonged										+	+
Bleeding time prolonged	+				(+)		(+)			(+)	
Other laboratory tests						Stypven time	Stypven time		5 M urea		Reptilase Euglobulin lysis

[1]Factor XI deficiency much more common in Ashkenazic Jews (5–11% heterozygous).

Key:

Inheritance: AD, autosomal dominant; AR, autosomal recessive, XR, X-linked recessive; AIR, autosomal incompletely recessive; AID, autosomal incompletely dominant

Frequency of clinical manifestations: + common; (+) occasional; • rare

and often result from consanguineous parentage. Clinical severity correlates with the degree of factor deficiency but is typically milder and more variable than in hemophilias A and B. Combined deficiencies of multiple coagulation factors are rare. Deficiencies of factor XII, prekallikrein, and high-molecular-weight kininogen cause prolongation of the aPTT but are not associated with excessive bleeding or thrombosis.

Clinical Features

A. Symptoms and Signs

Bleeding may occur spontaneously, but patients will sometimes give a history of bleeding only after surgery, trauma, or dental extractions. In those with von Willebrand's disease, platelet function is affected, so that easy bruising and menorrhagia may be prominent complaints. On the other hand, patients with hemophilia often have spontaneous hemarthroses, soft tissue hematomas, and hematuria. Physical findings may reflect recent bleeding or may show evidence of chronic bleeding such as decreased range of joint motion.

B. History

A detailed personal and family history of bleeding will often uncover the nature of the coagulation disorder and suggest its inheritance pattern. A family history of consanguinity is pertinent for the rare autosomal recessive disorders, and Ashkenazic Jewish ancestry may suggest the possibility of factor XI deficiency.

C. Laboratory Findings

Laboratory abnormalities may suggest an underlying hereditary bleeding disorder, but it is important to remember that not all prolonged coagulation tests indicate a bleeding diathesis, and some inherited bleeding disorders are associated with normal coagulation tests. There may be variability over time in some disorders, such as von Willebrand's disease. The extent of laboratory evaluation for an inherited coagulation disorder should be determined by the clinical history. Table 17–3 outlines the typical laboratory features of the inherited coagulation disorders. Functional assays for factors II, V, VII, VIII, IX, X, XI, and XII using known deficient plasma in a modification of the 1:1 dilution test confirm specific factor deficiencies. Clot stability in 5 M urea with and without the addition of normal plasma is the test of choice for diagnosis of factor XIII deficiency. The diagnosis of von Willebrand's disease is based on finding a low von Willebrand factor antigen (vWF antigen, previously known as factor VIII-related antigen), abnormal ristocetin cofactor activity, and low factor VIII activity (usually < 10%). Quantitative deficiency of von Willebrand factor can be differentiated from qualitative defects by electrophoretic analysis of von Willebrand factor multimers. Determining the subtype of von Willebrand's disease by multimer analysis is important for proper management of bleeding episodes.

Differential Diagnosis

Bleeding associated with abnormal coagulation tests may also result from acquired coagulation disturbances, including liver disease, vitamin K deficiency, disseminated intravascular coagulation, inhibitors of specific factors, or therapeutic anticoagulation. Abnormal coagulation tests may result from contact factor deficiencies or from antiphospholipid antibodies ("lupus anticoagulant"), neither of which cause bleeding and may be associated with thrombosis. Mild coagulation factor deficiencies may be associated with normal or minimally prolonged clotting times and may result in bleeding only if major vascular injury occurs. Bleeding in the presence of normal coagulation times suggests the presence of an underlying vascular defect, abnormal supporting connective tissue, thrombocytopenia or platelet dysfunction, excessive fibrinolysis, or factor XIII deficiency. Inhibitors to coagulation factors may be found in patients with inherited factor deficiencies as a consequence of replacement therapy and may be suspected in those who do not respond adequately to factor replacement. An inhibitor of coagulation can be confirmed by performing a 1:1 dilution test.

Treatment

Factor replacement is appropriate for patients with inherited coagulation disorders who have active bleeding or who require surgical or dental procedures. The activity level necessary for adequate hemostasis varies for each factor and with the type of bleeding or planned procedure. General guidelines for factor replacement are outlined in Table 17–4. Aspirin use and intramuscular injections should be avoided. Surgical procedures should be performed only in centers with adequate blood bank, coagulation laboratory, and hematology consultation services. Treatment strategies for patients with inhibitors complicating factor deficiencies include desmopressin (for minor bleeding), high-dose factor replacement, use of products that bypass the factor inhibitor (eg, activated prothrombin complex concentrate with factor VIII inhibitor bypassing activity, recombinant factor VIIa, porcine factor VIII), and techniques to lower the titer of the inhibitor (eg, plasmapheresis, intravenous immune globulin, immunosuppression, induction of immune tolerance).

Adjuncts to factor replacement include desmopressin acetate, antifibrinolytic agents such as aminocaproic acid and tranexamic acid, and topical hemostatic agents such

Table 17–4. General principles of factor replacement for inherited coagulation disorders.

Factor Deficiency	T½	Hemostatic Level[1]	Preferred Sources[2]	Dose	Interval Between Doses
vWF	12 hours	25–50%	a. Desmopressin[3] b. Humate-P c. Cryoprecipitate[4]	a. 0.3 μg/kg IV/30 minutes or 1.5 mg/mL nasal spray b. 30 units/kg	a. 24–48 hours b. 12 hours for 2 days, then 24 hours
VIII	9–18 hours	25–30%	a. Purified factor VIII b. Recombinant factor VIII	a. 10–15 units/kg (minor), 30–40 units/kg (major) b. 10 units/kg (minor); 15–25 units/kg (moderate); 40–50 units/kg, then 20–25 units/kg (major); 50 units/kg (surgery)	12 hours (6–12 hours following major surgery)
IX	20–25 hours	15–30%	a. Purified factor IX b. Recombinant factor c. Purified PCC	a. 10–20 units/kg b. 100 units/kg, then 7.5 units/kg/h c. 20–30 units/kg, then 15 units/kg (minor); 40–60 units/kg, then 20–25 units/kg (major bleeding or surgery)	24 hours
II	3 days	20–40%	a. FFP b. Purified PCC	a. 15 mL/kg, then 5–10 mL/kg b. 20 units/kg, then 10 units/kg	24 hours
V	36 hours	15–25%	FFP	20 mL/kg, then 10 mL/kg	12–24 hours
VII	4–7	10–20%	a. FFP b. Purified PCC c. Recombinant factor VII	a. 20 mL/kg, then 5 mL/kg b. 30 units/kg, then 10–20 units/kg c. 60–120 μg/kg	4–6 hours
X	40 hours	10–20%	a. FFP b. Purified PCC	a. 15–20 mL/kg, then 10 mL/kg b. 10 units/kg	24 hours
XI	80 hours	10–20%	FFP	15–20 mL/kg, then 5 mg/kg	12–24 hours
XIII	9–12 days	3–5%	a. FFp b. Factor XIII concentrate	a. 5 mL/kg	a. 1–2 weeks
Fibrinogen	3–4 days		Cryoprecipitate	1–2 bags/10 kg	48 hours

[1]Estimated level required for normal hemostasis. Higher levels required for major bleeding or surgery (factors VIII and IX: 100%, factor XIII: 25–50%).
[2]FFP: Fresh-frozen plasma; PCC: Prothrombin complex concentrate (thrombogenic; do not use in combination with antifibrinolytic agents).
[3]Desmopressin is thrombogenic; use with caution in older patients with vascular disease; may induce fibrinolysis, often used in combination with antifibrinolytic agents.
[4]Use only if factor concentrate is unavailable.

as fibrin glue and fibrillar collagen preparations applied directly to local areas of mucosal bleeding, such as epistaxis. Desmopressin by intravenous (0.3 μg/kg over 15–30 minutes) or intranasal (1.5 mg/mL in each nostril) administration increases circulating levels of von Willebrand factor and factor VIII by two to five times baseline within 15–30 minutes by releasing these factors from endothelial storage sites. Desmopressin is useful for most patients with von Willebrand's disease and in patients with mild to moderate hemophilia A. Repeated infusions within 1–2 days may be less effective, however, limiting the usefulness of desmopressin in patients requiring sustained increases in von Willebrand factor, factor VIII, or both. On the other hand, use of desmopressin may completely eliminate the need for blood products in mild bleeding episodes or during minor dental or surgical procedures and may decrease the amount of blood products required for major bleeds or surgical procedures. A test dose of desmopressin should be administered about 1 week before a planned surgical procedure to determine if a patient with von Willebrand's disease or hemophilia A is responsive. Severe hemophiliacs and those with qualitative abnormalities of von Willebrand factor are rarely responsive to desmopressin. Some subtypes of von Willebrand's disease (eg, type 2B) have been associated with thrombocytopenia following desmopressin therapy because of increased binding of aberrant von Willebrand factor to platelets. If the response to desmopressin is unknown and a patient is actively bleeding, factor replacement with blood products is preferable. Desmopressin also stimulates release of tissue plasminogen activator, so antifibrinolytic therapy is often administered simultaneously.

Aminocaproic acid and tranexamic acid are two commercially available antifibrinolytic agents that may be useful for managing bleeding in patients with a wide variety of bleeding disorders. The use of antifibrinolytics in combination with desmopressin often eliminates the need for any blood product administration for patients with von Willebrand's disease or mild hemophilia A with minor bleeding or after dental procedures. Antifibrinolytic therapy may also be useful as an adjunct to factor replacement in any inherited coagulation disorder unless there are contraindications such as hematuria, uncontrolled disseminated intravascular coagulation, or use of prothrombin complex concentrates. For acute bleeding, aminocaproic acid is usually given as an intravenous infusion at a rate of 1 g/h until bleeding is controlled (maximum 24 g in 24 hours), followed by a maintenance dose of 6 g intravenously or orally every 6 hours for 7–10 days. The suggested dose of tranexamic acid is 10 mg/kg intravenously or 25 mg/kg orally three or four times a day beginning 1 day before surgery or at the onset of acute bleeding, to be continued for 2–8 days.

Current Controversies & Unresolved Issues

Current recommendations regarding factor replacement for inherited coagulation disorders stem primarily from anecdotal experience rather than from carefully designed clinical trials comparing one regimen with another. The optimal level of factor activity, the precise interval between doses, and the duration of therapy are somewhat arbitrary, and for most of the rare disorders reflect a lack of clinical experience. Genetic heterogeneity contributes further to the lack of firm data to support current recommendations.

Because of the risks of bleeding, infections, and other transfusion-related complications, elective surgery should be avoided when possible. There is a body of literature demonstrating the success of surgery in hemophiliacs and others with inherited coagulation defects, but clearly, surgery in such patients poses significant risks and increases the demand for scarce resources, including blood products.

Current screening for infectious diseases and processing of factor concentrates to eliminate many (but not all) infectious agents has significantly decreased the risk of transmission of infectious diseases from plasma-derived products. All patients with hemophilia and related coagulation disorders should be vaccinated against hepatitis B. The development of recombinant factors VIII and IX has contributed to a marked decrease in virus-associated illnesses in these patients. However, recombinant factors are two to three times more expensive than plasma-derived factors and are not always available due to limited production capacity. Hemophilia patients who acquired HIV infection prior to widespread availability of screening and purified factors have been successfully treated with protease inhibitors; however, there appears to be an increased risk of spontaneous bleeding in these patients.

The development of inhibitors to factors continues to be a problem for patients with severe hemophilia; recombinant factors do not eliminate this risk (estimated at 10–15%). Recently, recombinant factor VIIa has been licensed as a method for treating patients with hemophilia A with high-titer inhibitors; however, its estimated cost is $50,000 for treatment of a single bleeding episode. Protein A sepharose immunoadsorption may transiently lower factor VIII inhibitors, allowing time for other immunosuppressive therapies to work. Optimal management of inhibitors remains a challenge in management of severe hemophilia.

Factor IX replacement (recombinant or purified plasma-derived) can cause anaphylaxis in 5% of patients with severe hemophilia B. Further replacement therapy in these patients is risky. Recombinant factor VIIa is the only available therapeutic option for these patients and those with factor IX inhibitors.

Gene therapy has been attempted in patients with severe hemophilia A and B, and, while the reported results are promising, long-term safety and efficacy have yet to be demonstrated. Results from preliminary trials suggest a transient benefit. Gene therapy may not prevent inhibitor development, however, and patients who are undergoing treatment for HIV infection or who have hepatitis may not respond to this approach.

ACQUIRED COAGULATION DISORDERS

ESSENTIALS OF DIAGNOSIS

- *Absence of a personal (if newly acquired) or family history of bleeding disorder.*
- *Abnormal screening coagulation tests.*

- *Clinical situation leading to decreased production or increased destruction of coagulation factors or presence of an anticoagulant.*

General Considerations

Acquired coagulation disorders result from four basic mechanisms: vitamin K deficiency, liver disease, consumption of factors, or inhibition of factor activity or fibrin polymerization. Unlike inherited disorders, acquired coagulation disorders are often characterized by multiple factor deficiencies as well as platelet defects (quantitative and qualitative). In addition, many of the clinical symptoms and signs result from the underlying disease process; the coagulopathy is just one of many processes contributing to the overall clinical picture.

A. Vitamin K Deficiency

Vitamin K is a cofactor necessary for synthesis of functional factors II (prothrombin), VII, IX, X, and proteins C and S. Vitamin K is found in dietary sources (green vegetables) and is synthesized by bacteria in the intestinal lumen. It is fat-soluble, requiring bile salts for absorption in the intestine. Vitamin K deficiency is most likely to occur in patients who have disruption of both dietary and bacterial sources of vitamin K (eg, patients who are receiving broad-spectrum antibiotics who are not eating), who have biliary obstruction or fat malabsorption, or who are taking warfarin derivatives that inhibit metabolism of vitamin K in the liver and induce a vitamin K-depleted state. By unclear mechanisms, certain antibiotics—particularly certain cephalosporins—and high doses of aspirin are known to induce a deficiency of vitamin K-dependent coagulation factors that is reversible with administration of vitamin K. Cholestyramine, mineral oil, and other cathartics may interfere with vitamin K absorption when taken for a prolonged period. Normal newborns have low levels of vitamin K-dependent factors, which fall further during the first few days of life. Deficiency of vitamin K results in progressive depletion of all the vitamin K-dependent factors as they are metabolized. Factor VII has the shortest biologic half-life and is depleted first, followed by proteins C and S and then factors IX, X, and II. Bleeding due to vitamin K deficiency is uncommon unless the deficiency is severe (prothrombin time greater than 25–30 seconds) or vascular injury is present.

B. Liver Disease

Coagulation disorders associated with liver disease are complex. With the exception of von Willebrand factor and factor VIII, all of the coagulation factors and other regulatory proteins (α_2-antiplasmin, protein C and protein S, antithrombin III) are synthesized in hepatocytes. The liver is also the site of clearance of activated coagulation factors and degradation products of fibrin and fibrinogen and is responsible for regeneration of vitamin K after it participates in synthesis of the vitamin K-dependent coagulation factors. Liver disease from any cause may result in multiple abnormalities, including decreased synthesis of all the coagulation factors (with the exception of factor VIII), abnormal synthesis of factors and proteins (eg, dysfibrinogenemia), abnormal vitamin K metabolism resulting in functional vitamin K deficiency, impaired fibrin polymerization due to increased fibrin degradation products, and accelerated fibrinolysis. In addition, thrombocytopenia, defective platelet function, or both may complicate severe liver disease. Advanced cirrhosis is often associated with abnormalities of blood vessels (eg, esophageal and gastric varices) and other defects (eg, gastritis, ulcer disease, esophageal tears), which are the major sites of bleeding in patients with liver disease. Hemostatic abnormalities exacerbate bleeding from these sites and contribute to epistaxis, ecchymoses, and increased bleeding with invasive procedures. In general, the presence of a coagulopathy is a sign of advanced liver disease, though passive congestion of the liver due to right heart failure may be associated with coagulation disturbances without irreversible liver dysfunction.

C. Consumption of Coagulation Factors

Consumption of coagulation factors may result from massive internal or external blood loss or from disseminated intravascular coagulation (DIC). Occasional patients who have massive blood loss will develop a clinically significant deficiency of multiple hemostatic factors, but DIC is the most typical condition associated with consumption of coagulation factors. DIC occurs as a result of abnormal activation of coagulation because of vascular injury, direct release of procoagulant materials into the circulation, or both. There may also be decreased function of naturally occurring anticoagulants (the thrombomodulin-protein C pathway) in patients with sepsis-associated DIC.

Consumption of coagulation factors and platelets is accompanied by secondarily accelerated fibrinolysis and results in a generalized bleeding tendency associated with mucosal bleeding, ecchymoses, and oozing from sites of vascular trauma, including venipuncture and surgical sites. Fibrin deposition in the microcirculation may contribute to some of the clinical sequelae of DIC, such as tissue hypoxia. Rarely, purpura fulminans complicates DIC. As a result of widespread arterial and venous thrombosis, patients with purpura fulminans may have skin necrosis and gangrene of the distal extremities and digits. The conditions in which DIC occurs are complex (Table 17–5), with multiple pathophysiologic mechanisms contributing to the overall outcome of pa-

Table 17–5. Causes of disseminated intravascular coagulation (DIC).

Cause	Examples
Infections	Bacterial sepsis (gram-negative and gram-positive), viremia, rickettsiae, malaria, tuberculosis
Trauma	Massive tissue injury, head trauma, fat embolism
Malignancy	Adenocarcinomas, acute leukemia
Obstetrical complications	Abruptio placentae, amniotic fluid embolism, retained dead fetus, septic abortion
Vascular disorders and prosthetic devices	Giant hemangioma (Kasabach-Merritt syndrome), aortic aneurysm
Toxins	Snake venoms, drugs
Immunologic disorders	Severe allergic reaction, hemolytic transfusion reaction, transplant rejection
Metabolic disorders	Hypotension, hypoxia, hyperthermia, hypothermia

tients, but DIC itself contributes to multiple organ failure and death in patients with severe systemic disorders, particularly sepsis.

Localized consumption of coagulation factors and platelets due to massive internal bleeding may mimic DIC but is not associated with intravascular fibrin generation or generalized fibrinolysis. In this situation, depletion of coagulation factors and platelets may be accompanied by elevated circulating fibrin degradation products and may result in a serious bleeding tendency, but it is not associated with microvascular thrombus formation. Primary systemic fibrinolysis is extremely rare and results in rapid destruction of fibrin clots, destruction of circulating fibrinogen, and consumption of plasminogen and its inactivators. Systemic fibrinolysis accompanies DIC and may contribute significantly to clinical bleeding. Primary fibrinolysis can be confused with DIC but usually is not associated with thrombocytopenia and generalized consumption of coagulation factors.

D. Inhibitors of Coagulation

Infrequently, inhibitors of coagulation develop and may result in a serious bleeding diathesis. Inhibitors directed against factor VIII are most frequently encountered and occur with pregnancy as a complication of treatment for severe hemophilia A or as an isolated condition. The abrupt development of factor VIII inhibitors following surgical procedures has recently been reported and may cause unexpected postoperative bleeding. The use of topical bovine thrombin intraoperatively may result in factor V inhibitors. Inhibitors to other coagulation factors, including von Willebrand factor, have been described. These inhibitors are immunoglobulins with neutralizing activity directed against specific factors and result in a clinical picture consistent with a factor deficiency state. Other types of inhibitors include substances that inhibit fibrin polymerization without immunologic specificity for the fibrin molecule (eg, fibrin degradation products or myeloma proteins). The so-called lupus anticoagulant typically prolongs the partial thromboplastin time and therefore may be confused with factor deficiencies or other inhibitors, but it is not associated with bleeding. Heparin is a therapeutic inhibitor of coagulation, accelerating the rate of antithrombin III-mediated inactivation of thrombin and other coagulation factors that act as serine proteases (factors VII, IX, X).

Clinical Features

The clinical history, physical examination, and screening laboratory abnormalities are usually sufficient to determine the nature of the coagulation defect.

A. Symptoms and Signs

Patients with acquired coagulation disorders may occasionally have spontaneous bleeding but more commonly have excessive bleeding from surgical procedures or exacerbations of bleeding from gastrointestinal or other sites. Other clinical features reflect the underlying disorder. Patients with liver disease may have bleeding from esophageal varices as well as signs of hepatic dysfunction. In DIC, bleeding is a common finding, but ongoing coagulation may be manifested as intravascular thrombosis with skin necrosis and gangrene (purpura fulminans). Features of the disease causing DIC—particularly sepsis—may predominate.

B. Laboratory Findings (Table 17–6)

The prothrombin time and partial thromboplastin time are prolonged in all the acquired coagulation defects as a result of multiple factor deficiencies. A 1:1 dilution test that fails to correct the abnormal prothrombin time or partial thromboplastin time indicates the presence of an inhibitor (including heparin and lupus anticoagulant). Complete correction of the prolonged prothrombin time and partial thromboplastin time within 24 hours after administration of intravenous vitamin K confirms the presence of vitamin K deficiency. The diagnosis of DIC is based on the presence of prolonged prothrombin time and partial thromboplastin time, thrombocytopenia, and elevated fibrin degradation products or D-dimer in the presence of an appropriate underlying condition.

Table 17–6. Laboratory diagnosis of acquired coagulopathies.

Laboratory Abnormality	Vitamin K Deficiency	Liver Disease	DIC	Specific Factor Inhibitors	Lupus Inhibitors	Primary Fibrinolysis
PT prolonged	+	+	+	+[1]	(+)	
aPTT prolonged	+	+	+	+[1]	+	
1:1 dilution does not correct				+	+	
Thrombin time prolonged		+	+			+
Thrombocytopenia		+	+		(+)	
FDP elevated		+	+	+		+
D-dimers present		(+)	+			
Protein C/S decreased	+	+	(+)			
Antithrombin III decreased		+	+			
Red blood cells		Targets, macrocytes	Schistocytes, microspherocytes			
Hypofibrinogenemia			(+)			(+)

[1]Pattern of clotting time prolongation depends on specific factor to which inhibitor is directed.
Key: + common; (+) occasional

Hypofibrinogenemia may be present in very severe cases, but—because fibrinogen is an acute phase reactant—fibrinogen levels are often normal. None of these tests are sensitive or specific enough to determine conclusively whether DIC is present. The presence of circulating fibrin monomers (protamine sulfate test) or degradation products of cross-linked fibrin (D-dimer test) confirms the presence of increased thrombin or plasmin generation and are usually present in DIC; they may also be positive occasionally in patients with liver disease.

Coagulation defects due to liver disease may be confused with DIC because of the presence of accelerated fibrinolysis, decreased clearance of fibrin and fibrinogen degradation products, thrombocytopenia, and prolongation of both the prothrombin time and partial thromboplastin time. Therefore, differentiating DIC from the coagulopathy of severe liver disease may be difficult, and clinical experience is required to interpret the often complex laboratory abnormalities. Schistocytes may be found on peripheral blood smear; when present, DIC must be distinguished from microangiopathic hemolytic anemia; this disorder, which can be due to thrombotic thrombocytopenic purpura-hemolytic uremic syndrome, chemotherapy, malignant hypertension, and the HELLP syndrome (hemolysis, elevated liver enzymes, low platelets), results from endothelial injury with subsequent platelet activation, thrombin generation, and fibrinolysis. Thrombocytopenia, hemolytic anemia, and fragmented red blood cells are the hallmarks of microangiopathic hemolytic anemia, without prolongation of coagulation times in most cases.

Differential Diagnosis

Inherited coagulation defects, thrombocytopenia, platelet dysfunction, and accelerated fibrinolysis may all result in bleeding at sites of vascular injury. Prolonged screening coagulation tests may be abnormal owing to technical error (including obtaining blood samples through heparinized lines or inadequate quantity of blood in the tube), because of inhibitors that do not cause bleeding (eg, lupus anticoagulant), and deficiencies of factors that are not important for in vivo hemostasis (eg, factor XII). Finally, impaired surgical hemostasis, mucosal abnormalities, and primary vascular abnormalities may result in clinical bleeding regardless of coagulation status.

Treatment

Treatment of the underlying disease state, avoidance of invasive procedures, and replacement of deficient factors during acute bleeding episodes are the mainstays of treatment. Vitamin K_1 (phytonadione), 1–10 mg subcutaneously (*not* intramuscularly), should be administered to patients at risk for vitamin K deficiency. Intravenous administration should be reserved for patients with impaired circulation to the skin (massive edema, shock) because it may rarely cause severe allergic reactions. Larger doses may be required to reverse massive overdoses of warfarin. Vitamin K_1, 5 mg orally or subcutaneously, should be given twice a week to patients on broad spectrum antibiotics with poor nutritional status. Fresh-frozen plasma administration is necessary to correct multiple factor deficiencies, but this treatment may be complicated by the large volume required to achieve adequate hemostatic levels, especially if factors are being rapidly consumed. The quantity of fresh-frozen plasma administered must be individualized, but in general, 30–40% of plasma volume (eg, 1000–1200 mL) is required to achieve adequate levels of all the deficient factors; this amount must be readministered every 6-8 hours to maintain adequate levels of factor VII. Many patients will not tolerate such a high volume of fresh-frozen plasma replacement, so only partial correction may be possible–yet if increased consumption of factors is present, even more frequent administration may be needed.

A. Liver Disease

Management of liver disease complicated by bleeding is difficult owing to the presence of multiple pathologic processes. Factor replacement with fresh frozen plasma, platelet concentrates for thrombocytopenia, and cryoprecipitate for severe hypofibrinogenemia are reasonable interventions for serious bleeding but must be accompanied by attempts to correct vascular and mucosal defects which are often the main reasons for bleeding. Prothrombin complex concentrate provides essential coagulation factors in a much smaller volume, but because it is associated with increased thromboembolic complications and DIC (particularly with severe liver disease due to decreased clearance of activated clotting factors present in the complex), it should be used only in life-threatening bleeding. Vitamin K_1 administration (10–20 mg) may improve the prothrombin time and partial thromboplastin time in some patients and should be tried. Desmopressin may shorten the bleeding time in some patients with platelet dysfunction complicating cirrhosis, but its efficacy has not been determined for control of bleeding in liver disease. Antifibrinolytic agents have been advocated for patients with evidence of accelerated fibrinolysis, but their safety and efficacy in patients with advanced liver disease have not been proved.

B. Disseminated Intravascular Coagulation

Patients with DIC have diverse underlying conditions (Table 17–5) and heterogeneous complications (both hemorrhagic and thrombotic). Management should be directed primarily at the underlying disorder. If serious bleeding is present or if an invasive procedure is required, factor replacement with fresh frozen plasma to shorten the prothrombin time to within 2–3 seconds of normal, cryoprecipitate to maintain fibrinogen levels greater than 100 mg/dL, and platelet concentrates to raise the platelets to greater than 50,000/μL should be attempted, but these efforts may be compromised by short survival of the hemostatic factors. Prophylactic administration of factors and platelets in the absence of bleeding is not effective, and coagulation factor concentrates should be avoided because activated factors present in the concentrate may increase intravascular coagulation.

Interruption of the primary pathologic coagulation of DIC with heparin may be helpful in selected circumstances. DIC complicating acute leukemia may be associated with marked bleeding due to impaired platelet production and may necessitate the use of low-dose heparin (eg, 5–10 units/kg/h) in order to achieve adequate platelet counts with platelet concentrates, though controlled studies have demonstrated that heparin administration increases platelet transfusion requirements without decreasing complications associated with DIC. Patients with solid tumors and DIC are more likely to experience thrombotic complications and may benefit from long-term administration of heparin. Patients with overt thromboembolism or purpura fulminans should be treated with heparin, but because of an increased risk of adrenal hemorrhage, the initial dose should be relatively low and adjusted based on clinical response. Although secondary fibrinolysis often contributes to the bleeding diathesis, antifibrinolytic agents are generally contraindicated in the presence of DIC because of the potential for unopposed intravascular coagulation, which may result in significant thrombotic complications. If marked symptomatic fibrinolysis is present and there is no evidence of thrombotic complications, however, antifibrinolytic therapy may be attempted in combination with low-dose heparin to control bleeding.

C. Circulating Inhibitors

Circulating inhibitors pose substantial difficulties in management of the bleeding patient. As in patients with hemophilia A with factor VIII inhibitors, strategies include high-dose factor replacement, decreasing the titer of the inhibitor by immunosuppression or plasmapheresis, or using factors that bypass the need for the factor being inhibited (eg, use of activated prothrombin complex concentrates, recombinant factor VIIa). When high concentrations of fibrin and fibrinogen degradation products are present, treatment of the underlying process (eg, sepsis-induced DIC) is more useful than specific hemostatic therapy. Myeloma proteins that inhibit fibrin polymerization should be definitively treated with chemotherapy, but plasmapheresis may be used as a temporizing measure.

Current Controversies & Unresolved Issues

DIC is a syndrome that occurs in diverse clinical conditions and is usually diagnosed on the basis of a combination of laboratory abnormalities in the appropriate situation. Several confirmatory laboratory tests have been proposed as essential for the diagnosis, but the lack of a "gold standard" combined with lack of standardization for the newer tests has resulted in conflicting data on their usefulness. Management of DIC is directed primarily against the underlying condition, but interventions to interrupt the state of pathologic coagulation and fibrinolysis seem to be logical, since these processes may contribute significantly to the pathologic state. Nevertheless, it has been difficult to demonstrate a clear benefit of anticoagulation or antifibrinolytic therapy in any situation complicated by DIC above and beyond that of aggressive supportive care and treatment of the underlying disease, with the possible exceptions of purpura fulminans and thromboses associated with solid tumors. The use of coagulation inhibitor concentrates, such as antithrombin III or activated protein C, may be beneficial in patients with sepsis-associated DIC, but the extremely high costs of these new products must be balanced against the modest gains demonstrated thus far in clinical trials. Recombinant activated factor VII has been successful at controlling severe bleeding in some patients with DIC refractory to treatment with blood product support, but it has not been extensively tested. Attempts to block activation of coagulation with inhibitors of tissue factor are currently being investigated.

Antifibrinolytic therapy has proved to be useful in the management of some of the inherited coagulation disorders as an adjunct to factor replacement. Because the acquired coagulation disorders are often more complex, disruption of fibrinolysis has been attempted infrequently. Potential complications of such therapy, such as unmasking an underlying thrombotic diathesis, have limited its role in the management of acquired coagulation disorders. There is some evidence, however, that patients with severe liver disease may have excessive fibrinolysis as a major contributor to bleeding. Future studies to determine the efficacy and safety of antifibrinolytic therapy are necessary before it can be recommended.

INHERITED PLATELET DYSFUNCTION

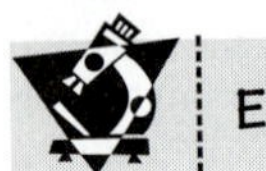

ESSENTIALS OF DIAGNOSIS

- *Lifelong history of easy bleeding.*
- *Prolonged bleeding time out of proportion to platelet count.*
- *Normal platelet count or mild thrombocytopenia.*
- *Normal coagulation times.*

General Considerations

Platelets are involved in multiple aspects of normal hemostasis. Defects in platelet membrane constituents, granules, metabolism, or coagulant function give rise to defective adhesion, aggregation, secretion, or procoagulant activity (Table 17–7). These disorders are generally rare, usually follow autosomal recessive inheritance patterns, and result in varying degrees of bleeding associated with prolongation of the bleeding time or defective or absent platelet aggregation in response to platelet agonists. The most severe defects have onset in the neonatal period or in early childhood with ecchymoses, epistaxis, and other mucosal bleeding, but milder defects may be manifest only after surgery or trauma. Thrombocytopenia is present in some platelet disorders and may contribute to the bleeding tendency. Other congenital abnormalities (eg, albinism) may also be present.

Clinical Features

A clinical history of lifelong bleeding, accompanied by a prolonged bleeding time in the presence of normal platelet count (or mild thrombocytopenia), prothrombin time, and partial thromboplastin time, should sug-

Table 17–7. Inherited disorders of platelet function.

Function	Disorder
Adhesion	Bernard-Soulier syndrome (GP Ib deficiency) von Willebrand's disease.[1]
Aggregation	Glanzmann's thrombasthenia (GP IIb/IIIa deficiency) Afibrinogenemia[1]
Secretion	Gray platelet syndrome (alpha granule deficiency) Storage pool deficiency (delta granule defects) Arachidonic acid pathway abnormalities Defective calcium mobilization
Procoagulant activity	Decreased platelet factor 3

[1]Defect is extrinsic to platelet but affects platelet function, with exception of platelet-type von Willebrand's disease.

gest the possibility of an inherited platelet disorder. A peripheral smear made from fresh nonanticoagulated blood may uncover morphologic platelet abnormalities or absence of platelet aggregation. Platelet aggregation studies using a wide variety of platelet agonists (including ristocetin) are helpful for identifying the specific defect. Confirmation of the specific diagnosis may require specialized studies available only in research laboratories.

Differential Diagnosis

A prolonged bleeding time in the absence of a history of clinical bleeding is unreliable as an indicator of platelet dysfunction or as a predictor of future bleeding. In the presence of bleeding, a prolonged bleeding time may suggest the diagnosis of von Willebrand's disease or an acquired disorder of platelet function (eg, uremia, drug therapy, cardiopulmonary bypass, myeloproliferative disorders) rather than an inherited defect. Mucosal bleeding, ecchymoses, and posttraumatic bleeding may result from severe coagulation disorders, accelerated fibrinolysis, thrombocytopenia, or vascular injury or from multiple hemostatic defects. Adult onset of a severe bleeding tendency makes the diagnosis of an inherited disorder of platelet function very unlikely.

Treatment

Serious bleeding usually requires transfusion of normal platelets. Alloimmunization to HLA antigens and to platelet specific antigens may result in refractoriness to platelet transfusions, so efforts to decrease alloimmunization are recommended (eg, limiting transfusions to life-threatening situations, use of leukocyte-poor platelet preparations, or administration of HLA-matched platelets). For unclear reasons, some defects respond to therapy with desmopressin. Antifibrinolytic agents (aminocaproic acid or tranexamic acid) may be useful for control of minor mucosal bleeding or as adjuncts to platelet transfusions. Hormonal suppression of menses is indicated for control of menorrhagia. Antiplatelet agents are contraindicated, and surgical procedures should be avoided whenever possible.

Current Controversies & Unresolved Issues

Optimal therapy of inherited platelet disorders is hampered by the infectious risk of platelet concentrates and by the risk of alloimmunization to HLA antigens and platelet-specific antigens that renders further transfusions ineffective. The risk of antibody formation is highest in patients with membrane protein defects because of the presence of these proteins on normal platelets. Alternative therapies that may be promising include bone marrow transplantation, desmopressin, and corticosteroids. Bone marrow transplantation can completely correct the bleeding tendency in patients with inherited platelet disorders but remains experimental because of potential lethal toxicity. Desmopressin releases von Willebrand factor and factor VIII from the endothelium, but it may also shorten the bleeding time in some patients with a wide variety of platelet disorders independent of von Willebrand factor and factor VIII levels; its mechanism of action in these intrinsic platelet disorders has not been established. Corticosteroids may decrease bleeding via an effect on vascular integrity and may be indicated for control of bleeding in patients with inherited platelet disorders who have no contraindications to steroid use.

ACQUIRED PLATELET DYSFUNCTION

ESSENTIALS OF DIAGNOSIS

- *Mucosal bleeding, ecchymoses, or excessive surgical bleeding in the absence of thrombocytopenia.*
- *Abnormal bleeding time.*
- *Normal coagulation times.*
- *Clinical condition or medication associated with platelet dysfunction.*

General Considerations

Acquired platelet dysfunction may result from defects in platelet adhesion, aggregation, secretion, or procoagulant function. Drugs, renal disease, cardiopulmonary bypass, antiplatelet antibodies, dysproteinemias, and myeloproliferative or lymphoproliferative disorders may be associated with impairment of platelet function as measured by the bleeding time or by abnormal tests of platelet aggregation. The clinical importance of the laboratory abnormalities in these diverse clinical conditions is not always clear. Bleeding depends not only on the severity of the defect but also on the presence of vascular injury and other hemostatic defects. Typical manifestations reflect impaired platelet function with mucocutaneous bleeding and excessive posttraumatic bleeding. Petechiae are rare unless thrombocytopenia is also present. Spontaneous soft tissue hematomas and joint bleeding are rare.

Thromboxane A_2 is an important mediator of platelet secretion and aggregation. Aspirin irreversibly acetylates and inactivates cyclooxygenase, thus preventing the production of prostaglandins, including thromboxane A_2. Most individuals who take aspirin will have a slight prolongation of baseline bleeding time that may persist for several days, but marked prolongation or clinical bleeding due to platelet dysfunction is rare at doses used in most clinical situations. Patients with other hemostatic defects, however, may experience marked prolongation of bleeding time and clinical bleeding if they take aspirin. Increased gastrointestinal tract bleeding is common in patients chronically taking high doses of aspirin, but this is due to its irritant effect on the mucosa rather than its effect on platelet function. The effect of aspirin on bleeding following major surgery or invasive procedures is controversial. While other nonsteroidal anti-inflammatory agents reversibly inhibit cyclooxygenase, these rarely prolong the bleeding time or induce clinical bleeding even in patients with severe coagulation defects.

Dextran is occasionally utilized for its antiplatelet effect in preventing postoperative deep vein thrombosis without increasing postoperative blood loss. Ticlopidine and clopidogrel are newer antiplatelet agents that inhibit ADP-induced platelet aggregation and prolong the bleeding time, and these may occasionally cause increased mucosal bleeding or bruising. Both agents appear to have irreversible effects on platelet function, requiring 7 days for normal platelet function to appear after withdrawal of the drugs (see Table 40–2). Platelet glycoprotein IIb/IIIa inhibitors are used for treatment of acute coronary ischemia, usually in combination with anticoagulants or fibrinolytic agents, and work by preventing fibrinogen-mediated platelet aggregation. Many other drugs have been linked to prolongation of the bleeding time but rarely result in clinical bleeding.

Renal failure is frequently associated with abnormal platelet function as measured by the bleeding time and by platelet aggregation tests. Impaired platelet function appears to result from biochemical alteration of intrinsically normal platelets, though the precise mechanisms have not been elucidated. Severe anemia seen with renal failure can contribute to prolongation of the bleeding time. Bleeding manifestations attributed to uremia include purpura, epistaxis, and menorrhagia, but the risk of bleeding does not correlate well with laboratory assessment of platelet function. With adequate dialysis and generally improved care of uremic patients in the past 25 years, bleeding may not be significantly increased compared with those without renal failure.

Cardiopulmonary bypass induces both thrombocytopenia and transient platelet dysfunction. Platelet activation while the platelets circulate through the bypass circuit results in a state of functional "refractoriness" that usually reverses within the first few postoperative hours. Multiple mechanisms appear to be responsible for the observed changes in platelet membranes, granule content, and functional activity following bypass. Modest transient coagulation factor deficiencies—due mainly to hemodilution coupled with heparin and protamine usage—may result in prolongation of coagulation times. Bleeding following cardiopulmonary bypass may therefore result from multiple defects in hemostasis, including inadequate surgical hemostasis.

Acquired hematologic disorders cause platelet dysfunction through production of intrinsically abnormal platelets (eg, myeloproliferative disorders, myelodysplastic syndromes, acute leukemias, or hairy cell leukemia) or through production of abnormal substances, usually immunoglobulins, that interfere with platelet function (eg, myeloma or Waldenström's macroglobulinemia; rarely, immune-mediated thrombocytopenia) or with von Willebrand factor (eg, acquired von Willebrand's disease). Clinical bleeding is more often the result of associated hemostatic defects or other hematologic abnormalities, such as severe anemia, thrombocytopenia, marked leukocytosis, or hyperviscosity. Thrombotic sequelae may also result from abnormal platelet function, particularly in the myeloproliferative disorders.

Clinical Features

A. Symptoms and Signs

Mucosal bleeding, ecchymoses, or excessive posttraumatic or surgical bleeding in the absence of thrombocytopenia or abnormal coagulation times should suggest the possibility of an acquired defect of platelet function.

B. Laboratory Findings

In most cases, the underlying condition of the patient and medication use are obvious, and minimal laboratory evaluation is needed to confirm the presence of platelet dysfunction. The bleeding time is a readily available "in vivo" test of platelet function that will identify most patients with significantly abnormal platelet function. In vitro platelet aggregation studies require significant technical experience for reliable results and should be reserved for patients with bleeding suggestive of platelet dysfunction and an unexplained prolongation of the bleeding time—or a very suggestive history of bleeding without prolongation of the bleeding time. Bleeding time and platelet aggregation studies are influenced by multiple factors, and, while useful for diagnosis in patients with significant bleeding, they are not reliable indicators of the risk of future bleeding.

Differential Diagnosis

Inherited disorders of platelet function are usually readily differentiated from acquired disorders by the presence of a long history of bleeding and the absence of underlying conditions associated with acquired platelet dysfunction. Mucosal bleeding, ecchymoses, or excessive posttraumatic and surgical bleeding may result from severe coagulation disorders, thrombocytopenia, excessive fibrinolysis, vascular injury, or multiple hemostatic defects. Prolongation of the bleeding time may result from severe anemia, thrombocytopenia, improper technique, or insignificant platelet dysfunction, and in the absence of bleeding suggestive of platelet dysfunction it is not a reliable indicator of future risk of bleeding.

Treatment

Impaired platelet function in the absence of clinical bleeding usually requires no specific therapy even when invasive procedures are performed. If bleeding is present or if the nature of an invasive procedure is such that any increased risk of bleeding is unacceptable, a variety of therapeutic options are available depending on the underlying cause of the platelet dysfunction. Withdrawal of aspirin or other suspect drugs is usually adequate for management of drug-induced platelet dysfunction. Desmopressin may be useful for management of bleeding in patients with a wide variety of disorders of platelet function, including uremia, cardiopulmonary bypass, and liver disease. Cryoprecipitate infusions, correction of severe anemia with red cell transfusions or epoetin alfa (erythropoietin), aggressive dialysis, and conjugated estrogens are other strategies for controlling bleeding in uremic patients with platelet dysfunction. Aprotinin is a plasmin inhibitor that reduces significant postoperative bleeding following cardiopulmonary bypass.

Platelet transfusions are indicated in the treatment of severe bleeding when platelet dysfunction is due to drugs, cardiopulmonary bypass, or acquired intrinsic abnormalities of platelets (eg, leukemias, myelodysplasias, myeloproliferative disorders) but are not helpful for management of bleeding in uremia. Avoidance of aspirin and other antiplatelet agents, correction of vascular defects, and treatment of the underlying disease process are the most important strategies for prevention and treatment of bleeding associated with platelet dysfunction.

Current Controversies & Unresolved Issues

The bleeding time has enjoyed widespread use as a screening test for patients requiring surgical procedures and as a diagnostic test in bleeding patients. The bleeding time may be affected by technique, the site and depth of the incision, the presence of anemia, and by characteristics of the supporting connective tissues regardless of the functional status of the platelets. A recent review of hundreds of studies of bleeding time produced no convincing evidence that the bleeding time is a useful predictor of bleeding in any clinical situation. Its main value is in diagnosing conditions associated with impaired platelet function, but even when platelet dysfunction is present, the bleeding time does not correlate well with clinical bleeding.

Desmopressin acetate has proved to be useful in shortening the bleeding time in a wide variety of platelet disorders, and it may decrease clinical bleeding as well. Conflicting reports on its efficacy and a lack of understanding of its mechanism of action in diverse diseases have limited its widespread use. In addition, a few case reports have suggested that desmopressin may contribute to thrombotic complications, particularly in elderly patients with cardiovascular disease. Antifibrinolytic agents may prove to have a role as adjuncts to other therapies for treatment of acquired platelet disorders, but the potential for thrombotic complications must be appreciated when considering their use.

THROMBOCYTOPENIA

ESSENTIALS OF DIAGNOSIS

- *Mucocutaneous bleeding; petechiae in severe cases.*
- *Decreased platelet count.*
- *Absence of other hemostatic defects.*
- *Associated condition leading to thrombocytopenia.*

General Considerations

Thrombocytopenia may result from decreased production, increased destruction or utilization, or sequestration of platelets in the spleen (Table 17–8). Decreased production usually affects all hematopoietic cells and rarely results in isolated thrombocytopenia. Mechanical destruction of platelets is often accompanied by evidence of hemolysis with anemia, reticulocytosis, and red blood cell fragmentation on peripheral blood smear as well as clinical manifestations of the underlying disease process. Immunologic destruction of platelets may occur as an isolated problem (eg, autoimmune thrombocytopenic purpura) or may result from drugs, transfusions, or disease states associated with the production of autoantibodies (eg, chronic lymphocytic leukemia, systemic lupus erythematosus, HIV infection). Splenomegaly from any cause may result in thrombocytopenia and is often accompanied by anemia and leukopenia.

Clinical Features

The history and physical examination with attention to bleeding symptoms, medication usage, splenomegaly,

Table 17–8. Causes of thrombocytopenia.

Decreased Production	Increased Destruction or Utilization
Marrow infiltration or replacement	**Mechanical**
Leukemia, lymphoma, metastatic carcinoma	Abnormal heart valves
Aplastic anemia	Vascular devices
Myelofibrosis	Disseminated intravascular coagulation
Granulomatous disease	Vasculitis
Toxic or environmental exposures	Cardiopulmonary bypass
Alcohol	Thrombotic thrombocytopenic purpura
Radiation	Hemolytic uremic syndrome
Chemotherapy	Renal transplant rejection
Chemicals	**Sequestration (hypersplenism, hypothermia)**
Thiazide diuretics	**Massive transfusion**
Ineffective hematopoiesis	**Immunologic**
Vitamin B_{12} or folate deficiency	Drug-induced antibodies or immune complexes
Myelodysplastic syndromes	Systemic lupus erythematosus
Infections	Antiphospholipid antibody syndrome
Viral: HIV, hepatitis, cytomegalovirus	Neoplastic diseases (chronic lymphocytic leukemia, Hodgkin's disease)
Fungal: histoplasmosis	Posttransfusion purpura
Acid fast organisms: *M tuberculosis, M avium-intracellulare.*	Neonatal alloimmune thrombocytopenia
Bacterial sepsis	Viral-associated (HIV, infectious mononucleosis, cytomegalovirus)
Acquired amegakaryocytic thrombocytopenia	Pregnancy
	HELLP syndrome (hemolysis, elevated liver enzymes, low platelets associated with eclampsia)
	Autoimmune thrombocytopenia
	Probably immune
	Malaria
	Bacterial sepsis

Artifactual thrombocytopenias: Anticoagulant-dependent platelet clumping pseudothrombocytopenia platelet satellitism, giant platelets.

and symptoms and signs of underlying disorders will often reveal clues to the diagnosis.

A. Symptoms and Signs

Mucocutaneous bleeding is the most common bleeding manifestation of thrombocytopenia. Petechiae usually occur only with severe thrombocytopenia and may reflect the platelet's essential role in the maintenance of endothelial tight junctions. Spontaneous soft tissue hematomas and hemarthroses are distinctly unusual. The risk of serious bleeding depends on the cause and severity of the thrombocytopenia, the presence of other hemostatic defects or vascular injury, and the condition of the patient. In general, patients with thrombocytopenia due to consumption, destruction, or splenic sequestration are at less risk for serious bleeding than patients with decreased production of platelets, because decreased platelet survival results in production of a younger, more functional population of platelets. The most feared complication of severe thrombocytopenia is central nervous system hemorrhage, which is rare unless the platelet count is less than 10,000/μL and there are other predisposing factors, such as leukemic infiltration, marked leukocytosis, or other vascular injury. Bleeding manifestations associated with various degrees of thrombocytopenia are shown in Table 17–9.

B. Laboratory Findings

Review of the complete blood count and peripheral blood smear is essential to evaluate associated abnormalities in other blood cell lines and to exclude the possibility of "pseudothrombocytopenia" due to in vitro platelet clumping in the presence of EDTA anticoagulant. Other instances of artifactual thrombocytopenia may be due to platelet satellitism around neutrophils or may occur when many giant platelets are present that may not be counted as platelets by automated cell counters. Isolated thrombocytopenia is most often the result of

Table 17–9. Bleeding manifestations associated with thrombocytopenia.

Platelet count (per μL)	Clinical manifestations
> 100,000	No increase in bleeding.
50,000–100,000	Minimal bleeding even with surgery unless platelet dysfunction is present.
30,000–50,000	Increased bleeding with surgery or trauma.[1]
20,000–30,000	Occasionally associated with easy bruising or other minor spontaneous bleeding.[1]
10,000–20,000	Epistaxis, petechiae, menorrhagia, gum bleeding.
< 10,000	Increased gastrointestinal blood loss, spontaneous life-threatening bleeding[2] (eg, intracranial hemorrhage, hematuria, melena, hematemesis).

[1]Minimal in patients with immune thrombocytopenia or other consumptive disorders.
[2]Life-threatening hemorrhage ususally occurs only with underlying vascular defect or if a second hemostatic defect is present (including aspirin ingestion).

immunologic destruction of platelets but may be found in some patients with mild hypersplenism, acute alcohol intoxication, or early acute leukemia and in the rare patient with isolated amegakaryocytic thrombocytopenia. The presence of fragmented red blood cells suggests the possibility of intravascular mechanical trauma to cells, as seen with DIC, thrombotic thrombocytopenic purpura-hemolytic uremic syndrome, eclampsia (ie, HELLP syndrome), or mechanical prosthetic heart valves. Abnormal white blood cells may indicate the presence of leukemia or lymphoma. The combination of nucleated red blood cells and immature white blood cells in the peripheral smear, a "leukoerythroblastic" picture, suggests the possibility of bone marrow infiltration from myelofibrosis or metastatic carcinoma. Macrocytosis and pancytopenia should suggest the possibility of vitamin B_{12} or folate deficiency.

The prothrombin time and partial thromboplastin time should be ascertained to detect a platelet consumptive process, such as disseminated intravascular coagulation. Bone marrow biopsy and aspiration are useful for evaluation of platelet production and should be performed when the diagnosis is not certain or if confirmation of a specific diagnosis (eg, leukemia, aplastic anemia, metastatic carcinoma) is essential to proper management.

Differential Diagnosis

The finding of a normal platelet count in the presence of palpable or nonpalpable purpuric skin lesions (ecchymoses or petechiae) should suggest the possibility of increased intravascular pressure, abnormalities or injury to blood vessels (eg, vasculitis), thromboembolic events (including septic thromboemboli), decreased integrity of the microcirculation and its supporting structures, or primary cutaneous diseases. Severe coagulation disorders may result in mucocutaneous bleeding but are easily distinguished from thrombocytopenia by the presence of markedly prolonged coagulation times and quantitatively normal platelets. Impaired platelet function and von Willebrand's disease should be considered when easy bruising and mucosal bleeding are present and can be identified in most cases by prolongation of the bleeding time in the absence of thrombocytopenia. Abnormalities of coagulation or platelet function rarely result in petechial skin lesions.

Treatment

The most important aspect of treatment is to reverse the underlying disease process. Platelet transfusions should be given only when the risk of bleeding and the probability of efficacy are sufficient to warrant the potential risks of blood component therapy. Prophylactic platelet transfusions are indicated for patients with decreased production of platelets with counts under 10,000/μL to prevent fatal central nervous system hemorrhage. When life-threatening bleeding is present or invasive procedures are required, platelet transfusions may be useful if the platelet count is less than 50,000/μL and no alternative therapies are available. When decreased platelet survival is present, platelet transfusions are not likely to effect a sustained rise in platelet count. Platelet transfusions may be harmful in patients with TTP-HUS syndrome and heparin-associated thrombocytopenia, and should be avoided unless active, life-threatening hemorrhage is present.

Medications such as aspirin that impair platelet function should be avoided when thrombocytopenia is present—with the exception of thrombotic thrombocytopenic purpura, in which antiplatelet agents may be indicated as part of therapy. Correction of severe anemia may decrease clinical bleeding in thrombocytopenic patients. Antifibrinolytic agents such as aminocaproic acid or tranexamic acid may decrease mucosal bleeding in chronically thrombocytopenic patients but should not be used if there is evidence of thrombosis (eg, in DIC) or hematuria. Alternatives to platelet transfusion for patients with bleeding due to thrombocytopenia are outlined in Table 3–2.

Current Controversies & Unresolved Issues

Intravenous administration of human immunoglobulin (IGIV) may rapidly increase the platelet count in patients with immune-mediated thrombocytopenia. Its effect is postulated to be due to competitive blockade of macrophage receptors for immunoglobulin, though other mechanisms may be important. Although it may rapidly increase the platelet count, its usefulness as therapy for immune thrombocytopenia is limited by only transient efficacy combined with its high cost in the face of a low risk of life-threatening bleeding in patients with autoimmune idiopathic thrombocytopenia. It is appropriate for use in patients with serious bleeding with this disorder as a temporizing measure while other therapies are being administered. Anti-D antibodies (Rh_oD immune globulin) may also be useful in the management of immune-mediated thrombocytopenia in patients who are Rh-positive, presumably by a similar mechanism (antibody-coated red cells block macrophage receptors). IGIV has not proved to be useful in treatment of thrombocytopenia due to platelet alloimmunization.

Alloimmunization to platelet-specific antigen or HLA antigens is a common sequela of repeated platelet transfusions and limits the response to subsequent platelet transfusions. For patients requiring long-term platelet support, prevention of alloimmunization is desirable in order to preserve the efficacy of transfusion therapy. Methods to minimize platelet alloimmunization include reducing the total number of all blood product transfusions, adhering to strict criteria for transfusing platelets, removing the source of the HLA sensitization (white blood cells) before transfusion of any blood product (by filtration or irradiation), and using HLA-identical donors.

The optimal management of several conditions associated with thrombocytopenia is under active study. Treatment of these conditions should be undertaken in consultation with a hematologist to ensure accurate diagnosis and up-to-date treatment.

APPROACH TO THE BLEEDING PATIENT

When approaching a patient with a suspected bleeding disorder, it is important to assess quickly the prior personal and family history of bleeding, the pattern of bleeding, and the pattern of laboratory abnormalities. If the personal or family history is suggestive of an inherited bleeding disorder, the apparent inheritance pattern, bleeding manifestations, and laboratory abnormalities should suggest the most likely diagnoses. If the personal and family histories are negative, defective hemostasis is most likely acquired, though some of the milder inherited disorders of hemostasis may not be manifested until significant trauma or surgery occurs later in life. The pattern of bleeding may suggest the nature of the hemostatic defect (Table 17–10), and the pattern of laboratory abnormalities (Table 17–11) will help localize defects in the hemostatic system.

Table 17–10. Approach to the bleeding patient by pattern of bleeding.

Pattern of Bleeding	Possible Disorders
Ecchymoses and mucosal bleeding; petechiae	Thrombocytopenia or platelet dysfunction von Willebrand's disease Severe coagulopathies
Spontaneous hemarthroses, soft tissue hematomas	Hemophilia A and B, other severe coagulopathies
Posttraumatic or surgical bleeding	Thrombocytopenia or platelet dysfunction Von Willebrand's disease Coagulopathies Impaired vascular integrity Inadequate surgical hemostasis Massive injuries
Generalized oozing from mucosal, venipuncture, surgical sites	Consumptive coagulopathies, DIC Excessive fibrinolyis Severe thrombocytopenia or platelet dysfunction

Table 17–11. Approach to the bleeding patient by pattern of screening laboratory abnormalities.

Abnormal Test	Possible Defects
PT only	Factor VII deficiency (inherited, vitamin K deficiency, warfarin effect) or inhibitor
aPTT only[1]	Factor XII, HMW kininogen, prekallikrein, XI, IX, or VIII deficiency or inhibitors to these factors; lupus anticoagulant
PT and aPTT	Deficiency or inhibitor of Factor X, V, II (prothrombin), fibrinogen Multiple factor deficiencies (liver disease, DIC, consumptive coagulopathies, vitamin K deficiency, high dose warfarin effect)
Bleeding time prolonged	Platelet dysfunction or thrombocytopenia
All screening tests normal	Other coagulation abnormalities: Factor XIII deficiency Excessive fibrinolyis Paraproteinemia Vascular defect (including inadequate surgical hemostasis) Supporting tissue abnormality

[1]Deficiencies of factor XII, HMW kininogen, prekallikrein, and lupus-type inhibitors prolong the aPTT but do not cause bleeding.

CURRENT CONTROVERSIES & UNRESOLVED ISSUES

Gastrointestinal Hemorrhage

For more than a century, critically ill patients have been observed to have a high rate of gastrointestinal hemorrhage. Preventive strategies emerged to decrease this complication, including the use of antacids, histamine receptor-2 (H_2) blockade, proton pump inhibitors, and mucosal protective agents. More recent data suggest that only the most severely ill patients—those requiring prolonged mechanical ventilation or who have impaired hemostasis, head trauma, or a history of previous gastrointestinal hemorrhage—are at significantly increased risk for bleeding, and that treatment with acid-lowering agents could actually increase the risk of hospital-acquired pneumonia. Preventive therapy with mucosal protectant agents (eg, sucralfate) or H_2 blockade is recommended for patients identified to be at high risk for bleeding. Underlying hemostatic defects should be treated according to the general principles discussed above. The use of nonsteroidal anti-inflammatory drugs (NSAIDs) and low-dose aspirin increase the risk of gastrointestinal bleeding independent of their effects on platelet function. When *Helicobacter pylori*-associated ulcer is identified, long-term treatment with omeprazole or eradication with antibiotics can decrease the risk of recurrent bleeding associated with aspirin or NSAIDs.

Gastroesophageal variceal hemorrhage is the most serious form of gastrointestinal hemorrhage, with 30% mortality observed with first episodes. Varices occur in the setting of severe liver disease, so that—in addition to mechanical problems—coagulation abnormalities, quantitative and qualitative platelet defects, and excessive fibrinolysis contribute to bleeding. Management of acute variceal bleeding requires gastrointestinal specialists who can diagnose and treat varices endoscopically (ligation, sclerosis, balloon tamponade) but also includes medical therapy with vasoactive agents such as beta-blockers, nitrates, vasopressin, and somatostatin analogs (octreotide, vapreotide). When these approaches fail, transjugular or surgical shunting may be required to control bleeding.

Perioperative Bleeding

Preoperative evaluation of hemostasis should include medical history with attention to adequacy of hemostasis—spontaneous bleeding or bruising or unexpected bleeding after dental extractions or prior surgical procedures suggest the presence of an underlying hemostatic defect. Medical illnesses such as liver or renal disease, myeloproliferative disorders, and paraproteinemias predispose patients to excessive postoperative bleeding. In the absence of symptoms of a bleeding disorder or such medical illnesses, the value of routine laboratory screen-

Table 17–12. Preoperative laboratory screening.

Bleeding History	Type of Surgery	Recommended Laboratory Tests
No suggestive history	Minor (dental, skin biopsy)	None
No suggestive history	Major	Platelet count, aPTT
Possible bleeding history	Major, bypass pump	PT, aPTT, platelet count, bleeding time; if normal, factor XIII assay, euglobulin clot lysis time
Positive bleeding history	Minor or major	Same as above; if negative: thrombin time, factor assays for VIII, IX, XI, alpha$_2$-antiplasmin assay, post-aspirin bleeding time

ing has been questioned. Whether any laboratory screening should be done depends also on the type of planned procedure (minor versus major, use of cardiopulmonary bypass, neurosurgical procedures, etc.). Table 17–12 outlines suggested laboratory screening prior to surgery. If abnormalities in screening tests are detected, further evaluation should be done to define the precise abnormality.

Intraoperative hemostasis with ligature, cautery, and topical thrombogenic substances (fibrin glue, topical bovine thrombin) is essential to prevent postoperative bleeding. In the postoperative period, excessive bleeding may be due to a hemostatic defect that was not detected by the screening tests. Mild coagulation factor deficiencies may not prolong the aPTT, particularly if other factors are elevated (eg, factor VIII increases in acute inflammatory states and may mask mild deficiency of other factors). Preoperative use of aspirin or other antiplatelet drugs may increase postoperative bleeding; if bleeding is severe and the bleeding time is prolonged, desmopressin or platelet transfusions may be required for control of bleeding. Surgery on the prostate gland or uterus may be associated with localized hyperfibrinolysis with excessive bleeding. Antifibrinolytic therapy with aminocaproic acid can be considered for control of bleeding (5 g loading dose followed by 1 g per hour intravenously or orally until bleeding has stopped), though there is some risk of thrombi developing in the ureters (following prostate surgery) which are resistant to lysis. Acute DIC may occur for many reasons following surgery, or decompensation of previously compensated DIC may develop as a result of tissue factor release during surgery (Table 17–13).

Acute renal failure due to hypotension, massive blood loss, or medications can result in platelet dysfunction, which is exacerbated by anemia. Posttransfusion purpura with thrombocytopenia may occur in previously sensitized individuals. The use of intraoperative bovine thrombin as a hemostatic agent may precipitate the development of antibodies to thrombin and factor V. There does not appear to be any significance to the antithrombin inhibitor; however, factor V inhibitors may cause bleeding. Factor VIII inhibitors may also develop postoperatively; the mechanism for this has not been defined. Hetastarch, a plasma volume expander, may cause persistent coagulation abnormalities, particularly in elderly patients, those with preexisting hemostatic defects, or with prolonged use. If bleeding is severe, plasmapheresis to remove these large molecules may be required to control bleeding.

Table 17–13. Causes of postoperative DIC.

- Sepsis
- Hypotension
  - Acute hepatic necrosis
  - Release of bone marrow thromboplastins
- Liver injury (drugs, hypotension, blunt or penetrating trauma)
- Tissue factor release during surgery
- Peritoneovenous shunting
- Use of cell saver device with excessive suction
- Release of tissue factor from placenta
  - Aruptio placentae
  - Amniotic fluid embolism
  - Septic abortion
  - Placenta previa
  - Retained dead fetus
- Trauma
  - Fat embolism
  - Brain injury
  - Extensive soft tissue injury
  - Burns
- Decompensation of chronic (compensated) DIC
  - Dissecting aortic aneurysm
  - Kasabach-Merritt syndrome
  - Cancer
- Infusion of activated clotting factors
  - Prothrombin complex concentrates
  - Recombinant activated factor VII

When postoperative bleeding is encountered, immediate evaluation with history (to uncover preexisting risks, medication use) and laboratory testing (PT, aPTT, platelet count) should be done. Medical treatment of hemostatic defects will depend on the specific abnormalities identified. If history and screening laboratory tests are unrevealing, consideration should be given to reexploration of the surgical site to identify adequacy of surgical hemostasis.

Posttraumatic Bleeding

In the setting of massive trauma, multiple pathophysiologic processes contribute to severe bleeding, including multiple vascular defects, massive transfusion with dilution of coagulation factors and platelets, DIC with acceleration of fibrinolysis, and hypotension. Severe coagulation disturbances associated with trauma may result in adrenal hemorrhage, which can further exacerbate hypotension. Certain types of injuries are particularly associated with DIC: fat embolism, brain injury, extensive soft tissue injury, and extensive burns. Pelvic ring fractures are associated with massive blood loss, often hidden due to tracking of bleeding up into the retroperitoneal space. Control of bleeding in such circumstances may be difficult, even with aggressive blood product support—with fresh frozen plasma, platelets, red blood cells, and cryoprecipitate. Recombinant activated factor VII has been used to treat massive hemorrhage in trauma patients with some success, and it may also be useful in the treatment of refractory bleeding in other settings of DIC.

REFERENCES

Cook D et al: Risk factors for clinically important upper gastrointestinal bleeding in patients requiring mechanical ventilation. Crit Care Med 1999;27:2812–7.

Faust SN, Heyderman RS, Levin M: Coagulation in severe sepsis: a central role for thrombomodulin and activated protein C. Crit Care Med 2001;29(7 Suppl):S62–8.

Grunewald M et al: Acquired haemophilia: experiences with a standardized approach. Haemophilia 2001;7:164–9.

Levi M, ten Cate H: Disseminated intravascular coagulation. N Engl J Med 1999;341:586–92.

Levi M et al: Novel approaches to the management of disseminated intravascular coagulation. Crit Care Med 2000;28(9 Suppl): S20–4.

Lind SE: The bleeding time does not predict surgical bleeding. Blood 1991;77:2547–52.

Mannucci PM: How I treat patients with von Willebrand disease. Blood 2001;97:1915–9.

Mannucci PM, Tuddenham EG: The hemophilias—from royal genes to gene therapy. N Engl J Med 2001;344:1773–9.

Martinowitz U et al: Recombinant activated factor VII for adjunctive hemorrhage control in trauma. J Trauma 2001;51:431–9.

McKenna R: Abnormal coagulation in the postoperative period contributing to excessive bleeding. Med Clin North Am 2001;85:1277–1310.

Miller DG, Stamatoyannopoulos G: Gene therapy for hemophilia. N Engl J Med 2001;344:1782–4.

Moscardo F et al: Successful treatment of severe intra-abdominal bleeding associated with disseminated intravascular coagulation using recombinant activated factor VII. Br J Haematol 2001;113:174–6.

Rice L: Surreptitious bleeding in surgery: a major challenge in coagulation. Clin Lab Haematol 2000;22(Suppl 1):17–20.

Schuster DP: Wringing blood from a turnip. Crit Care Med 1999;27:2846–7.

Sharara AI, Rockey DC: Gastroesophageal variceal hemorrhage. N Engl J Med 2001;345:669–81.

ten Cate H et al: Microvascular coagulopathy and disseminated intravascular coagulation. Crit Care Med 2001;29:S95–8.

Teitel JM: Clinical approach to the patient with unexpected bleeding. Clin Lab Haematol 2000;22(Suppl 1):9–11.

Teitel JM: Unexpected bleeding disorders: Algorithm for approach to therapy. Clin Lab Haematol 2000;22(Suppl 1):26–9.

Psychiatric Problems

18

Stuart J. Eisendrath, MD, & John R. Chamberlain, MD

Intensive care units provide the most advanced technology available to patients with the most serious medical and surgical illnesses. Perhaps as a consequence, these facilities are often associated with some of the most stressful psychiatric conditions within the hospital. Indeed, some physicians have jokingly referred to the Intensive Care Unit as the Intensive Scare Unit. These conditions in ICUs may affect both patient and staff. This chapter will describe some of the significant problems.

Most patients entering the ICU will attempt to manage the stress of their stay with their characteristic coping mechanisms. Some regression generally occurs, however, as most patients experience stressors such as fear of death, enforced dependency, and potential permanent loss of function. Separation from family and the loss of autonomy that accompanies medical treatment in the ICU frequently lead to further psychologic regression. They may try to cope with stress by suppressing their feelings, using humor to laugh at stressful aspects of their situation, or trying to anticipate a return to good health. If these techniques fail, the individual may turn to more primitive mechanisms such as projection, passive-aggressive maneuvers, acting-out behavior, and gross denial of illness. All of this takes place during the time when the patient must deal with serious and usually multiple medical problems.

A number of clinical syndromes may develop as a result of the stressors inherently associated with occupancy of a bed in the ICU. This discussion will focus on several that may adversely influence recovery. **Delirium,** the so-called **intensive care unit psychosis,** is generally not due to psychologic stress alone but develops in association with altered brain function. **Anxiety** may occur at any time during the patient's stay in the ICU—entry, midpoint, or discharge. **Depression** may also occur at any point during the patient's stay but most often occurs after the immediate threat to life has been dealt with and the patient must contemplate the subacute prognosis and ultimate outcome of the disease. Finally, we will discuss how the ICU environment affects the staff working there.

DELIRIUM

ESSENTIALS OF DIAGNOSIS

- *Waxing and waning of consciousness.*
- *Disorganized thinking.*
- *Perceptual disturbances such as visual hallucinations.*
- *Disorientation.*

General Considerations

Early reports from ICUs gave rise to the diagnosis of an **intensive care unit syndrome** characterized essentially as a delirious state with psychotic features such as hallucinations. It was believed to be due to the stress an ill individual felt in a foreboding environment with little privacy, lack of sleep, and sensory overload. Whether or not this syndrome actually existed as a specific entity, current research indicates that delirium occurring in the ICU is most likely due to factors similar to those patients experience on general medical and surgical wards—with the difference that ICU patients may have more severe reactions because of their more severe illnesses.

Stress may play some role in producing delirium, but it is typically only a contributing one. Other factors that alter brain function are usually the primary etiologic agents. The critical care physician should not automatically attribute delirium to stress. Remembering that delirium is an organic dysfunction of the central nervous system will facilitate the search for likely causes and the provision of appropriate treatment. This aggressive approach is justified given the serious impact of delirium on morbidity and mortality in hospitalized patients. Studies have shown that patients suffering an episode of delirium have an increased risk of death, a longer hospital stay, and a greater need for subsequent nursing home placement.

There are at least three broad hypotheses relating to the production of delirium. Any one or any combination of these factors may cause delirium in a particular patient.

A. Increased Central Noradrenergic Production

Drug or alcohol withdrawal states are the most common condition producing delirium in the hospital and probably also the most common condition responsible for increased noradrenergic discharge. Locus ceruleus-controlled production of brain catecholamines is believed to play a central role in this type of delirium.

B. Dopamine and Cholinergic Systems

Imbalance of brain dopamine and cholinergic systems can be recognized in central anticholinergic syndromes produced by atropinic agents. These may produce a relative excess of dopaminergic activity, giving rise to an agitated delirium. This hypothesis also provides a framework for understanding how dopamine-blocking agents such as haloperidol may act by restoring the relative balance between dopaminergic and cholinergic systems that is disturbed in delirium. Delirium-producing agents such as the amphetamines, which cause a shifting of the balance toward the dopaminergic side, can also be better understood in this framework.

C. Toxic Causes of Delirium

A third framework for understanding delirium involves the environment brain cells operate in. Side effects of medications or endotoxins associated with bacterial infections can affect neuronal functioning. Similarly, conditions such as hyperthermia or hypoxia can disturb functioning throughout the central nervous system. Many of the above abnormalities are believed to affect the midbrain particularly; this may in turn lead to fluctuations in the reticular activating system with alterations in level of consciousness and the ability to attend to stimuli in the environment—a key feature of many cases of delirium.

D. Multifactorial Features

In the ICU there are typically numerous factors that play a role in producing delirium. A patient with asthma and pneumonia provides an example—with fever and hypoxia as well as high levels of circulating corticosteroids and catecholamines. Although single causes should be diligently sought, it is unusual to be able to identify and correct just one causative factor of delirium.

Clinical Features

The clinical criteria for delirium in the ICU setting consists of a number of signs and symptoms. Typically, the patient has a waxing and waning of consciousness—may be somnolent at one moment and highly alert and agitated a short time later. The patient's ability to attend to external stimuli fluctuates over time. Delirious patients usually have disorganized thinking manifested by rambling or incoherent speech. Patients frequently have perceptual disturbances such as misperceptions of real objects (illusions) or frank hallucinations. Patients usually have disorders in normal sleep-wake cycles and altered psychomotor behavior (either agitation or retardation). Patients also typically have disorientation to time, place, and situation. Memory impairment, when present, is generally global for both recent and remote events. Delirium usually develops within hours to days. The presence of delirium signifies primarily organic brain dysfunction and is not a manifestation of psychologic distress alone.

The signs and symptoms listed in the preceding paragraph are useful in making a clear-cut diagnosis. Unfortunately for that purpose, however, many ICU patients present only some of the criteria and may require ongoing vigilance. Indeed, one of the keys to diagnosis in these patients is repeated observations over time. The waxing and waning of consciousness so common in delirious patients requires serial monitoring, since a patient may appear quite lucid at one moment and quite confused a half hour later. Nursing staff often have the best data on mental status because of their continuing contact with the patients.

The physician should examine specifically for the presence of delirium. This involves performing some type of specific cognitive assessment such as the Folstein Mini Mental Status Exam. However, intubated patients can be difficult to assess with this instrument. Newer diagnostic instruments such as the Cognitive Test for Delirium (CTD) can be very useful in this setting. This instrument was developed for use in critical care settings and reliably distinguishes patients with delirium, dementia, and acute psychiatric illness. This type of examination tests the patient's ability to attend to stimuli, concentrate on a task, comply with simple memory requests, demonstrate language capabilities through auditory comprehension, and show orientation to time and situation. More importantly, this type of test allows the examiner to detect cognitive deficits that would otherwise go unrecognized. For example, psychiatric consultation may be sought for a patient who is poorly compliant with the medical regimen. Many of these patients prove to be suffering from delirium and have significant memory deficits that make compliance impossible—they cannot remember instructions for 30 seconds.

The patient may appear quietly confused and in a daze. This type of delirium may be easily missed because the patient presents no behavioral problem. Some delirious patients, on the other hand, present behavioral problems ranging from pulling out catheters and lines to biting or striking members of the staff. These patients appear agitated, fearful, and restless. They may be hallucinating and intensely involved in their psychotic states. One physician described his state of mind during his stay in the ICU as follows: "I saw a vulture flying over me. I worried about any drop of blood spilling onto the sheets because I knew that would bring the vulture down for the attack." This physician had been fearfully watching the ceiling for several days but never told the doctors or nurses because "they couldn't do anything and they'd think I was crazy."

Many delirious patients resort to primitive psychologic coping mechanisms. They may exhibit massive denial of any medical problem or externalize their problem as being the fault of somebody else rather than of their illness. Delirious patients often project anger about their helplessness onto their caregivers. This gives rise to paranoid ideation about caregivers trying to poison or otherwise harm them. Other delirious patients—like the doctor in the above example—experience hallucinations that are often threatening. These hallucinations are usually visual and occur without any external stimulus. Many patients will usually have visual illusions which involve a misperception of actual external stimuli. For example, one patient was convinced that the IV standard in his room was actually a person poised to attack him.

Differential Diagnosis

In the critically ill patient—especially an intubated patient, for whom communication is most difficult—delirium may appear to be similar to other conditions.

A. Anxiety

Anxiety occurs quite frequently in the ICU. In some instances, anxiety may occur in patients who have delirium. Individuals with cognitive processing impairment may be quite difficult to reassure. Thus, many patients may be anxious in the ICU but only some will also have delirium—though the majority of delirious patients will experience anxiety and fear. Patients without delirium do not have the significant cognitive impairment and deficits in reality testing (such as hallucinations) so common in delirium.

B. Underlying Psychosis

ICU patients may have an underlying psychosis (eg, schizophrenia) that can be confused with delirium. Schizophrenic patients rarely have visual hallucinations. Visual hallucinations usually are present due to an organic cause that requires investigation. Schizophrenic patients who have paranoid delusions generally have well-formed ones that are fixed over months and years. Delirious patients, on the other hand, have rapidly developing delusional beliefs that shift over hours to days. Most schizophrenic patients have a history of psychiatric treatment and neuroleptic medications. Delirious patients generally do not have such a history. Furthermore, schizophrenic patients typically have onset of illness by the early to mid-twenties, characterized by a progressive decline in function. In contrast, delirium often affects older patients and causes a precipitous decline in mental status and functioning.

C. Neuroleptic Malignant Syndrome

Schizophrenic patients—or any patient who has received a neuroleptic medication—are at risk for development of **neuroleptic malignant syndrome,** characterized by altered mental status, autonomic instability, and extrapyramidal symptoms that are often severe (eg, "lead pipe rigidity"). This syndrome can develop particularly with high-potency neuroleptic medications when the individual also suffers from complicating conditions such as fever and dehydration. Diagnosis in these patients is often assisted by elevated CPK levels, myoglobinuria, and decreased serum iron levels.

D. Depression

The subdued, quiet delirious patient may be mistaken for a depressed one. The depressed patient, however, usually has the depressive view of the world associated with that disorder along with symptoms such as a sense of worthlessness, guilt, and global pessimism. In some instances, small test doses of dextroamphetamine (eg, 2.5 mg twice daily) may allow the clinician to differentiate depressive and delirious patients. The depressed patient may become less depressed after medication, while the delirious patient usually becomes more agitated. A past psychiatric history of depressive disorder may also help differentiate the disorders.

E. Personality Disorder

It is not unusual for staff to apply the pejorative label **personality disorder** to a patient who fails to comply with their requests. Whenever such a diagnosis is contemplated, one should seek confirmation from family or friends. Personality disorders represent long-standing patterns of maladaptive behavior. They do not develop acutely, though they may be exacerbated by the stress of illness. They may emerge in patients after the immediate threat to life has passed. Psychiatric consultation is often helpful in confirming this diagnosis.

F. Dementia

One way of conceptualizing the difference between dementia and delirium is by applying the analogy of acute and chronic renal failure. Delirium represents acute cerebral insufficiency, while dementia is typically a chronic condition. Dementia syndromes may represent a variety of conditions (multi-infarct dementia, Alzheimer's disease) characterized by generalized diminution of intellectual functioning. Most dementias—except for the subcortical ones, such as in Parkinson's disease—show some evidence of cortical dysfunction such as aphasia or apraxia. Dementia syndromes develop over months or years rather than hours or days. The patient's family should be consulted to clarify baseline mental functioning.

A key finding is that delirious patients typically have a waxing and waning of consciousness and the ability to attend to stimuli; deficits in demented patients are generally fixed throughout the day until nightfall, when "sundowning" may occur. It is quite common to see dementia patients who have preserved remote memory, whereas in delirium all forms of memory may be impaired. It is unusual for dementia patients to suffer hallucinations, while delirious patients frequently have hallucinations.

Electroencephalograms may aid in the differentiation of delirium and dementia. The former often show generalized slowing, whereas the latter do not.

Treatment

A. Establish the Cause

The key to treatment of delirium is identification of its cause or causes whenever possible. Since delirium is usually an acute process, a vigorous investigation of reversible causes should be undertaken, much as one would investigate the cause of acute renal failure and attempt to correct it as rapidly as possible. Delirium should be regarded as an example of acute cerebral failure that is associated with significantly increased morbidity and mortality. There are studies in which patients with delirium had a markedly higher mortality rate than other patients (8% versus 1%; Likelihood Ratio 2.3), a higher rate of admission, and a higher rate of institutionalization. Hospital stays are often prolonged by an average of 7 days in delirious patients.

There are many causes of delirium. The most common causes in the ICU are listed in Table 18–1. **Withdrawal states** are among the most common causes of delirium in the general hospital and should always be considered in assessing the patient. In some instances, the patient may conceal or be unable to provide information about drug or alcohol use. Family and friends will be able to help establish this history. In some instances, considerable probing may be necessary. For example one postoperative vascular surgery patient denied the use of alcohol or drugs; persistent questioning, however, revealed that she had increased her usual daily 0.5 mg alprazolam dosage fourfold in the month prior to surgery because of anxiety. When she entered the hospital, this medication had been discontinued. Two days later, she had a florid delirium that responded rapidly to alprazolam. The benzodiazepines are the prototypical agents for the treatment of alcohol and sedative withdrawal. They are safe in large doses, prevent seizures, and are well tolerated. An important feature for ICU use is that they are available in oral, parenteral, and sublingual formulations.

Table 18–1. Common causes of delirium in the ICU.

Drug or alcohol withdrawal or intoxication
Medication effects (eg, corticosteroids, cimetidine, lidocaine)
Hypoxia
Hypoperfusion
Infections (eg, systemic or central nervous system, HIV)
Structural lesions (eg, subdural hematomas)
Metabolic disorders (eg, electrolyte abnormalities, hypercalcemia, hyperglycemia)
Ictal or postictal states
Postoperative states
Fat emboli
Dehydration
Sleep deprivation
Environmental stress
Pulmonary embolism

Medications given in the ICU can frequently produce significant psychoactive effects. Table 18–2 lists a number of drugs that have been established as having these effects. Switching medications is certainly one of the easiest changes to make in trying to manage a delirious patient.

Other causes such as **hypoxia** and **hypoperfusion** need to be reversed before improvement from delirium can occur. Delirium may be the first sign of an **infectious process** and should suggest that possibility when no other cause is discovered. For example, a postoperative patient who develops delirium without any identifiable cause may be suffering from a wound abscess that only becomes apparent several days later.

B. Nonpharmacologic Management

Once one or more causes are identified, the primary goal of treatment is to reverse the disorder. In a significant number of cases of delirium, no specific cause can be identified; in others, the identified cause cannot be easily reversed (eg, an asthmatic on high-dose corticosteroids). In these instances, symptomatic treatment may be required. Family may be enlisted to spend time at the bedside to provide an orienting stimulus. Other environmental measures may include providing a clock,

Table 18–2. Drugs that may cause delirium in the ICU.[1]

Acyclovir	Fluoroquinolone antibiotics
Amiodarone	Ganciclovir
Amphetamines	Histamine H_2 blockers
Amphotericin B	Interferon alfa
Anticonvulsants	Isoniazid
Antidepressants	Ketamine
Antihistamines	Ketonazole
Atropine and other anticholinergics	Levodopa
	Lidocaine
Barbiturates	Methylphenidate
Benzodiazepines	Metoclopramide
Beta-adrenergic blockers	Metronidazole
Cimetidine	Nonsteroidal anti-inflammatory drugs
Corticosteroids	
Cycloserine	Opioids
Cyclosporine	Procaine derivatives
Digitalis glycosides	Propafenone
Dronabinol	Quinidine
Epoetin alfa (erythropoietin)	Trimethoprim-sulfamethoxazole

[1]Modified from: Drugs that cause psychiatric symptoms. Med Lett Drugs Ther 1988;40:21–24.

calendar, and soft music. Staff should attempt to provide adequate day-night orientation and allow the patient to sleep at night as much as possible. Four-hour periods that allow for all stages of sleep may be the most beneficial.

C. Pharmacologic Management

For many patients with delirium, the aforementioned measures will not be enough. Medications become indicated when behavioral control is necessary or when distress is severe. For example, a quietly delirious patient suffering with frightening hallucinations is a candidate for pharmacotherapy.

1. Management of withdrawal syndromes—A number of principles must be considered in initiating therapy. If a withdrawal state is present, the appropriate agent to cover the withdrawal should be given as soon as possible. Sufficient medication must be given to abort the withdrawal process and keep it from reemerging. Alcohol withdrawal is the most common of these conditions. A frequent mistake is to underdose with a benzodiazepine early in the withdrawal process and then try to catch up with a full-blown delirium later. Early substantial doses of long-acting agents such as diazepam may provide timely control. However, lorazepam may be preferred in patients with liver disease because its metabolism (via glucuronide conjugation) is less affected in such individuals.

2. Management of delirium of unknown cause—

a. Benzodiazepines—When the cause of delirium is not known but withdrawal from sedatives or alcohol is suspected, one might consider a pharmacologic probe by giving a benzodiazepine such as 1–4 mg of lorazepam. If the patient's condition worsens, that essentially rules out alcohol and most benzodiazepine withdrawals. A different course of pharmacotherapy must then be pursued. In addition, these agents are preferred for the agitation present with anticholinergic overdose or when there is a need to raise the seizure threshold. Relatively short-acting agents with no active metabolites, such as lorazepam, are preferred for this application.

b. Haloperidol alone or with lorazepam—Haloperidol is often administered intravenously even though the intravenous form is not approved by the FDA. Before initiating haloperidol, some cardiovascular considerations must be addressed (discussed below). Initial dosage depends on the age and size of the patient. A small elderly woman may benefit from 0.2–0.5 mg of haloperidol every 4 hours. A younger 70-kg man may start with 1–2 mg every 2 hours or even higher doses. A more agitated patient should receive larger doses, and some studies have advocated an initial infusion of 5–10 mg followed by a continuous infusion at a rate of 5–10 mg/h. This medication has a mean distribution time of 11 minutes and a half-life of 14–17 hours. If the first dose fails to produce significant improvement, the dose should be repeated at 30-minute intervals to allow time for distribution to occur. The second dose is usually twice the first dose. If monotherapy fails to produce the desired effect, one may add 0.5–1 mg of lorazepam. This combination has been found to improve symptom control while decreasing the side effects of treatment. If the patient remains agitated 30 minutes following the addition of lorazepam, one may give doses of haloperidol up to 5 mg and lorazepam 0.5–2 mg at 30-minute intervals until control is established. In many instances, control of delirium can be achieved with 5–30 mg of haloperidol and 2–4 mg of lorazepam. Some patients may require amounts substantially above these levels. Doses up to 975 mg of haloperidol in a 24-hour period have been reported.

Once control is established, approximately half of the first 24-hour total dosage can be given on the following day in equally divided doses. Each subsequent day's dosing is reduced by half until further dosing is no longer necessary. The goal, once symptom control is achieved, is to taper the patient to the minimally required dose. Many cases of delirium will clear within a few days, particularly when the cause has been reversed.

When giving intravenous haloperidol, several points need to be considered. Generally speaking, intravenous haloperidol imposes a much lower risk of extrapyramidal side effects than oral or intramuscular forms. The reason is not completely clear. It may be that the intravenous route allows brain receptors to bind with different forms of the drug. It is possible also that most patients who receive intravenous haloperidol have some form of central anticholinergic process by virtue of their delirium which provides a protective effect against extrapyramidal reactions. Nonetheless, when giving haloperidol, the clinician should continue to monitor the patient for adverse reactions, which include dystonias, akathisia, and neuroleptic malignant syndrome.

The incidence of cardiovascular side effects from haloperidol is very low. Haloperidol has been found to prolong the QT interval and has been linked with rare episodes of torsade de pointes, ventricular fibrillation, and sudden death. These effects generally seem to occur with high doses of the medication and have led to recommendations for establishing a baseline ECG and subsequent monitoring of the QT interval. Additional recommendations are to monitor serum magnesium and potassium. Most cases of hypotension with haloperidol have been in association with hypovolemia. Administering the medication in a slow infusion over 5–10 minutes may be helpful in preventing hypotension, so intravenous pushes should be avoided.

c. Newer agents—Newer agents such as the atypical antipsychotics risperidone and olanzapine are receiving increasing attention for the treatment of delirium. They have fewer side effects than the typical antipsychotics (eg, haloperidol) and in small reports have been effective against delirium. The main drawback to their use is that they are currently not available in parenteral formulations.

d. Other pharmacologic interventions—When the combination of haloperidol (or another antipsychotic) and lorazepam fails to achieve control, additional interventions may be necessary, including sedation (with opioids, propofol, barbiturates, or benzodiazepines), pharmacologic paralysis, and mechanical ventilation. These measures, however, do not enhance the patient's sense of control, and if sedation is inadequate they can be quite terrifying to the patient.

D. Social and Psychologic Management

A key consideration in managing delirium involves the psychologic aspects. The patient's family often has major concerns about the prognosis for mental recovery. The physician should reassure both the family and the patient that the condition is usually reversible and that return to baseline mental functioning can be expected. Empathically telling the patient that the physician understands the confusion the patient feels may convey a real sense of hope. Encouraging the patient to report any strange phenomena such as hallucinations may make the patient feel more at ease. Similarly, informing the family that accusations and delusional ideas brought forth during an episode of delirium have no real meaning is obviously useful.

Current Controversies & Unresolved Issues

Delirium is such a heterogeneous entity that many issues remain to be delineated by prospective studies. Molecular mechanisms for delirium and the role of neurotransmitters need to be established. We still do not know what are the optimal medications for controlling delirium, the maximum daily dosage of haloperidol and other agents, and whether patients really benefit from large doses of medications or if the practice helps the staff more than the patient. Other questions relate to possible preventive measures, whether psychologic factors alone can cause delirium in the absence of organic factors, and a possible final common pathway for all cases of delirium.

DEPRESSION

ESSENTIALS OF DIAGNOSIS

- *Depressed mood.*
- *Feelings of worthlessness and inappropriate guilt.*
- *Negative thinking.*
- *Recurrent thoughts or wishes for death or suicide.*

General Considerations

Depression occurs in 20–42% of the medically ill. Any patient with a medical illness severe enough to require admission to the ICU faces a number of psychologic issues, including real and potential losses. For example, the patient with myocardial infarction must deal with the threat to life as well as the potential loss of future health and normal function. These losses are enough to produce depressive symptoms in many patients and sad feelings in most patients. An individual undergoing major surgery must deal with the loss of bodily integrity and the threat of death. These actual and potential losses may produce a sense of helplessness in many patients.

Patients are usually placed in unfamiliar surroundings with little sense of autonomy. These conditions may generate a depressive view of the world. Cognitive distortions can develop so that the individual begins to make mistakes in judgment such as forecasting catastrophe or interpreting innocuous events negatively. Patients may begin to think of themselves as worthless and feel they are a burden to family and friends. Motivation to participate in medical care may be impaired.

This depressive picture is often associated with biologic changes. Neurotransmitter levels and receptor function change significantly. Serotonin and noradrenergic systems have substantial alterations. Endocrine dysfunction in both the pituitary-adrenal and thyroid axis may become disturbed. Even immune function may be altered.

Clinical Features

Patients in the ICU who have clinically significant depression can by assessed by general criteria for depression. These criteria, however, have only limited usefulness in the ICU patient because of the context. For example, neurovegetative symptoms are of limited value; many ICU patients have appetite and sleep disturbances, but that does not mean they are depressed.

Nonetheless, some signs and symptoms of depression in ICU patients can be utilized to make a diagnosis of depression. The presence of a depressed or lowered mood is a hallmark. Irritability, particularly, when out of character for an individual, is another marker of depression. Diminished interest in activities such as interacting with family or viewing television often indicates depression. Pronounced thoughts about death or wishes for it in the form of suicidal ideation also indicates depression.

Additional criteria can be used in assessing a patient for depression. One group of factors involves the depressive view of the world a depressed patient develops. For example, seeing oneself, one's doctor, and one's future in negative terms correlates positively with a diagnosis of depression. Feelings of guilt, worthlessness, and hopelessness are also common in depression. Feeling helpless means the individual feels unable to help himself or herself get better; feeling hopeless means the individual does not believe anyone else can help either. The physician should always ask a depressed patient about any suicidal ideation. As a practical matter, very few ICU patients have the means to commit suicide in the unit, but knowing the patient's feelings about suicide may help the physician gauge the level of depression.

In addition to these cognitive factors, assessing the patient's self-esteem often serves as a clue to depression. The patient who is grieving normally usually feels sad in reaction to losses sustained or anticipated. The grieving individual may appear sad but still maintain a proper sense of self-esteem: "I'm okay, really—I'm still a good person despite my medical problem." The depressed individual, on the other hand, feels worthless and useless: "I'm washed up—a burden to my family."

Another way of identifying the depressed individual engages the physician in using his own feelings as an assessment tool. Depressed patients often generate a feeling of depression in their physicians; they may also produce a sense of aversion, so that the physician is eager to get away from the bedside. An appropriately grieving patient, on the other hand, usually generates a sense of sympathy and sadness in the physician. Thus, the physician who is sensitive to his or her own responses to a patient may be able to confirm a diagnosis of depression quite readily.

Differential Diagnosis

The key differential diagnosis in a patient who is being considered for a diagnosis of depression is appropriate grief or organic mood disturbances. A number of conditions may produce depressive symptoms. It is completely normal for an individual to experience sadness and some emotional withdrawal in response to a loss. Disease often produces a sense of loss for many individuals, and it may be difficult for the physician to differentiate appropriate grieving from a clinical depression. One should consider the degree of dysfunction as an indicator of depression. Thus, when a patient's emotional state is seriously interfering with medical recovery or compliance with medical care, some form of treatment should be offered. Depression becomes a likely diagnosis when the patient makes a decision to terminate treatment for a disease whose prognosis is favorable.

Certain medical conditions frequently produce depressive symptoms. Examples are Cushing's disease, hypothyroidism, and pancreatic carcinoma. Virtually all of the organic causes described in the section on delirium can also produce depressive states. In fact, a smoldering delirium may be mistaken for depression unless cognitive function is assessed. Some hypoxic individuals, for example, will appear lethargic and depressed. Medications such as beta-blockers, corticosteroids, digoxin, cimetidine, levodopa, diazepam, and antihypertensives may produce a depressive picture. Some dopamine antagonists such as prochlorperazine or metoclopramide produce psychomotor retardation or akathisia that may mimic depression.

Treatment

A key point in the treatment of depression is for the physician to recognize that depression is a painful and serious condition that should not be considered "normal." Just because a knifing victim might be expected to exsanguinate and experience a fall in blood pressure, medical treatment is not withheld; similarly, the identification of depression warrants appropriate interventions. In serious cases of depression, there may be a substantial risk of failing to provide treatment. A depressed patient is poorly compliant and poorly motivated to participate in recovery—or may fail to take adequate nutrition and participate in other aspects of recovery such as being weaned from a ventilator.

The initial treatment of depression in the ICU should emphasize psychosocial measures. To the extent possible, the patient should be permitted to feel some control over what is happening. Nurses should offer the patient a choice whenever possible. For example, the patient can be asked whether or not pain medication is needed, whether it is time to be moved, etc. Asking the patient to help plan the day's bath and hygiene schedule is very helpful. Encouraging the family to visit as much as possible may also help counter depression. The physician can help reduce depression by providing realistic encouragement and support.

If these measures fail to reduce the depression, psychiatric consultation is indicated followed by pharmacologic treatment. The consultant will inquire about the patient's psychiatric history, particularly to see if some specific antidepressant medication has been successful in the past. If so, that drug should be used. If the patient has not had a prior trial of antidepressant, a psychostimulant such as dextroamphetamine or methylphenidate should be considered unless there is a medical contraindication such as tachyarrhythmia. In the usual starting dextroamphetamine dosage of 2.5 mg at 7 AM and 1 PM, there is little risk of side effects. In an occasional patient, there may be some increase in blood pressure or pulse, but these are usually minimal and do not require stopping the trial. If the patient fails to respond to the above dosage, on the next day one can double the dose to 5 mg given twice. The maximum dosage is 15 mg twice daily, but this level is rarely necessary. The medication is given early in the day so as not to interfere with sleep. Many people have the misconception that dextroamphetamine may worsen appetite, since it has been used in the past for dieting; in depressed patients, however, it generally improves appetite.

Dextroamphetamine has the advantage of being essentially free of side effects in most patients; some may have slight tremor or anxiety. A rare patient may develop persecutory feelings with this drug, but typically only at much higher doses. The tremendous advantage of dextroamphetamine is the rapidity of response when it is successful. The physician can often observe a beneficial effect 1–2 hours after the first or second dose. Many patients report improved mood, energy, appetite, and will to live. The response rate varies in different studies from 48–80% improvement in depressive symptoms.

A number of other agents are effective and well tolerated for the treatment of depression. An example is fluoxetine, which was the first serotonin reuptake inhibitor released in the United States. Although fluoxetine has essentially no anticholinergic or blood pressure effects, it elevates many other drug plasma levels by displacing them from their plasma protein binding sites. This makes fluoxetine an undesirable medication for most ICU patients. Other newer agents have been developed that appear well suited for use in ICU patients. Citalopram, sertraline, and venlafaxine are effective antidepressants that share fluoxetine's lack of blood pressure and anticholinergic effects but are associated with fewer drug interactions. Bupropion has little blood pressure or anticholinergic effect, but in its immediate-release form it has been associated with a higher incidence of seizures than other antidepressants. All of these agents have the limitations of being available only in oral formulations and taking 1–4 weeks to have an effect.

Tricyclic antidepressants can be considered for ICU patients, but, like the newer agents mentioned briefly above, they take 1–4 weeks to show an effect. Their anticholinergic and quinidine-like side effects can also cause problems. Tricyclic antidepressants also have the disadvantage of producing marked alpha-adrenergic blockade, which can have troublesome effects on blood pressure. If treatment with a tricyclic is elected, nortriptyline is the best choice since it has the least effect on postural hypotension and only modest anticholinergic effects. It also has a clear therapeutic window of maximum effectiveness of 50–150 ng/mL.

Current Controversies & Unresolved Issues

Depression may be hard to differentiate at times from normal grief and sadness, so it would be useful to have a biologic marker for the condition. Several years ago, there was excitement about using the dexamethasone suppression test as a marker for major depression. Although this was of important research significance, it has not been useful clinically since 50% of patients will suppress but still have the disorder. Therefore, the test is of very little significance in trying to decide on a diagnosis. It will be important for further research in depression to develop biologic markers the clinician can use.

Another important area for further research involves the identification of subtypes of depression so that specific pharmacotherapy can be tailored appropriately. There have been attempts to differentiate depression by global measures of neurotransmitter levels. Cerebrospinal fluid and urinary levels of methoxyhydroxyphenylglycol (MHPG) and serotonin have been used to predict response to serotonergic and noradrenergic antidepressants. These efforts have not yet produced clinically useful applications.

ANXIETY & FEAR

ESSENTIALS OF DIAGNOSIS

- *Overt terror and panic.*
- *Hypervigilance.*
- *Fear of being alone.*
- *Autonomic arousal.*

General Considerations

Anxiety is the unpleasant feeling associated with an unknown internal stimulus and is out of proportion to the threat from the environment. Fear, on the other hand, is the same feeling state but derived from a known external stimulus and proportionate to the threat. Obviously in the ICU, these two feelings are hard to distinguish, and they will be discussed here under the term fear, which refers to both entities.

Fear is often prominent when the patient first enters the ICU because of awareness of a substantial threat to his or her continued existence resulting from the medical or surgical problem that necessitated the admission.

The ICU patient may be reacting not only to the fear of death but to other unspoken fears as well. The patient may be anxious about how the family is responding to the illness and may have concerns about ability to return to work, or may harbor unrealistic ideas about the nature of the problem and the treatment required. For example, some patients jump to the conclusion that they will need open heart surgery for any type of cardiac problem. The patient may also associate the illness with a loved one who had a similar problem. For example, one 59-year-old man admitted to the coronary care unit feared he would not survive his heart attack because his father had died of one at the same age. Asking the patient about whom he knows who had the same medical problem or treatment may reveal a significant factor contributing to the patient's fears.

Fear and anxiety may produce significant physiologic changes. Catecholamine and corticosteroid levels may fluctuate along with anxiety levels. It has been demonstrated that the perception of physical or emotional stress results in the activation of several brain regions—serotonergic, catecholaminergic, and perhaps cholinergic nuclei. These pathways are apparently then integrated by unknown mechanisms into the hypothalamus. The end result of this complex response is the secretion of glucocorticoids. Evidence has also accumulated for a variety of links between the serotonergic region and the hypothalamic-pituitary axis that may underlie the connection between stress and mood.

Clinical Features

The physician can observe fear in many guises in the ICU. Patients with a past history of generalized anxiety, panic, or "nervous" disorders should be expected to have increased fearfulness in the ICU. Some patients will demonstrate their terror and panic overtly. Others may appear hypervigilant, constantly scanning the environment. Others will talk excessively or seek the presence of the nurse so as not to be left alone. Some patients will fight going to sleep because of fears of dying while asleep. Blood pressure and heart rate may be elevated as the autonomic accompaniments of fear ensue.

Some patients may exhibit their fear by major denial of illness. These individuals may attempt to demonstrate their good health by exercising in the coronary care unit. Others will try to sign out of the hospital against medical advice. Fear is perhaps recognized most easily in the patient being weaned from the ventilator "before I'm ready." These patients often show stark terror as the ventilator settings are reduced. In such cases, anxiety may grossly interfere with medical treatment.

Furthermore, anxiety related to experiences in the ICU does not dissipate at the door upon departure from the unit. Patients may continue to have nightmares and experience episodes of hypervigilance and panic even after returning to home care, thus suggesting the diagnosis of posttraumatic stress disorder (PTSD). Research is still needed to help predict which individuals are at the greatest risk for development of this syndrome. Some studies have linked its development to adverse experiences in the ICU.

Differential Diagnosis

Anxiety and fear can be confused with the agitation of delirium. The delirious patient will, however, have significant cognitive impairment that is usually not present in the anxious patient. The physician should continuously assess the anxious patient for organic factors that could contribute to anxiety. Medications such as corticosteroids, theophylline, and lidocaine can produce anxiety and fearfulness. Medical conditions such as hypoxia, pulmonary emboli, pheochromocytoma, Cushing's disease, and early drug or alcohol withdrawal may have anxiety as a major symptom (Table 18–3).

Treatment

The best treatment of anxiety is prevention. Psychologically preparing a patient for surgery can have a beneficial effect. These efforts, as well as those offered by the pa-

Table 18–3. Medical disorders commonly associated with anxiety.

Pulmonary disorders
COPD
Pulmonary embolus
Asthma
Hypoxia
Drugs
Drug withdrawal
Drug intoxication (eg, amphetamines, cocaine)
Infections
Tuberculosis
Brucellosis
Cardiac disorders
Mitral valve prolapse
Paroxysmal atrial tachycardia
Subacute infective endocarditis
Angina
Endocrine and metabolic disorders
Insulinomas
Carcinoid tumors
Pheochromocytomas
Hypoglycemia
Thyroid disease
Hypocalcemia
Porphyria
Cushing's disease
Neurologic disorders
Multiple sclerosis
Akathisia
Temporal lobe epilepsy

tient's primary physician, can be very effective in preventing anxiety. Similarly, the physician can intervene postoperatively to minimize patients' anxiety. One study suggests that playing a brief tape-recorded message from the surgeon—explaining that surgery went well, giving an orientation to the ICU, and reassuring the patient about early recovery—markedly reduces anxiety.

Nonetheless, for many patients, fear and anxiety will develop in the ICU. The first step in treating the fearful patient involves exploring precisely what the patient is most fearful about. This information may be obtained directly from the patient who is prepared properly and trusts the physician. The physician can start by saying, "Most people have some worries or fears in this situation. What are yours?" This approach normalizes the presence of fears and makes it easier to talk about them. Whatever the patient brings up as a concern should be explored.

Another valuable technique for helping a patient deal with fears is reframing the patient's view of the situation. For example, one 45-year-old African-American wanted to sign himself out of the coronary care unit, saying he refused to believe he had had a bad heart attack. The doctors repeatedly tried to warn the patient of the risks of not accepting hospital treatment. The patient responded by doing ten one-handed push-ups. Finally, psychiatric consultation was requested. The psychiatrist realized that frightening the patient only escalated his fear and increased his need to deny the fear by signing out against advice. The psychiatrist suggested to the patient that it took a strong man to put up with the bed rest and testing the cardiologists wanted. The consultant suggested that the patient could prove his strength in this way. In essence, the patient no longer had to equate staying in the unit as a loss of strength and self-esteem. With this reframing of his medical care, the patient accepted the remainder of his treatment without difficulty.

In some ICUs, the psychiatric consultant or liaison nurse may teach relaxation with the aid of audio tapes. Some patients may be receptive to learning self-hypnosis. These techniques may help by restoring the patient's sense of control over the environment. These techniques may also be helpful in the patient being weaned from the ventilator.

If psychosocial interventions do not work or are not available, medication can be used. Lorazepam is the anti-anxiety drug of choice. Its intermediate half-life (10–20 hours) is long enough to prevent the withdrawal syndrome that can occur with shorter-acting agents but not so long that the drug tends to accumulate. Lorazepam is metabolized in a one-step conjugation and so can be used with patients with liver disease. For most patients with mild to moderate anxiety, the dosage of lorazepam is 1–2 mg (depending on age and weight) every 4–6 hours. For more severe anxiety, one may double these doses. Antidepressants such as sertraline and citalopram can also be useful against anxiety. As with their use in depression, however, they can take up to 4 weeks to have a significant effect and must be given orally. When anxiety is extreme and interfering grossly with the patient's care, a shift to antipsychotic medications has been advocated. Although haloperidol has been advocated for this purpose, newer agents should also be considered. A recent report described the use of risperidone for patients with irritability and hostility. The authors noted that this agent caused fewer side effects than haloperidol, imposed fewer risks than benzodiazepines, and was effective with a more rapid onset than antidepressants.

Current Controversies & Unresolved Issues

There is a continuing quest for the anxiolytic agent that gives relief without clouding the sensorium or producing troublesome withdrawal states. For example, triazolam is a popular sedative benzodiazepine in some regions because it has a short half-life that makes it unlikely to produce a hangover. The short half-life, however, has a major disadvantage in that it may lead to withdrawal syndromes the next day, leaving the patient anxious until the next dose is given. Until the neurotransmitter systems involving various agents such as gamma-aminobutyric acid are further elucidated, the quest for the ideal agent will have to continue.

STAFF ISSUES

The ICU staff considered as a group has many psychologic features similar to those found in individual health providers. Many doctors and nurses, for example, bring certain psychologic motivations to their work. They may feel a strong need to save and rescue their patients. They also may demand perfection from themselves. In some sense, whether it is consciously realized or not, the ICU staff may make the same demand as a group. This may be manifested in attempts to save the unsalvageable patient and reluctance to let any patient die. On the other hand, many patients have unclear prognoses, and these may be particularly challenging for the staff. Research suggests that the most difficult patients for staff to care for are those with multisystem failure and a poor prognosis.

A useful equation for conceptualizing a staff's self-esteem is the following:

$$\text{Self-esteem} = \frac{\text{Realistic achievement}}{\text{Expectations}}$$

In this equation, how staff feel about themselves is equal to what realistic achievement they can accomplish "divided by" their expectations. The equation represents a shorthand way of viewing how the relationship between expectations and achievements influence self-esteem. In instances where the expectation is one of omnipotence, unless the achievement is perceived as a perfect performance, the staff will end up feeling like a failure. In this equation, we should note that the realistic achievement is relatively fixed within a narrow range accomplished by most competent staff. The variable that can be most easily adjusted is the denominator, expectations. If staff are successful in reducing this value, the staff can feel much more satisfied with their accomplishments. This issue is highlighted when staff have to deal with a dying patient. When the staff are able to shift their expectations away from an unrealistic omnipotent fantasy of saving the patient, they can shift to a more realistic one such as providing a comfortable, dignified death. Such a goal is much more easily accomplished.

Identifying Staff Problems

Staff issues can often be identified in staff attitudes toward patients. For example, following a period in which there had been an unusually high number of deaths in an intensive care unit, an 80-year-old patient was admitted to the unit with pneumonia. She required intubation and ventilation. Although her infection was rapidly controlled, she had difficulty being weaned from the ventilator. Staff nurses began to voice concerns such as, "Why are we putting such effort into an 80-year-old woman? She won't make it anyhow." When those concerns were raised in a staff meeting, other staff members pointed out that the patient had been living independently until her pneumonia developed and that her only current problem was one of pulmonary mechanics that should clear with time. This discussion helped the staff to perceive that their view of the patient had been unfairly pessimistic, probably related to the several recent deaths that had led to a sense of inadequacy, helplessness, and group depression. They left the meeting with a clearer understanding of what they could accomplish with the patient. She eventually was weaned from the ventilator and returned to her home.

Interventions

There are various approaches to helping the ICU staff deal with the stress of working with critically ill patients. Units emphasizing a culture of cooperation and communication have a reduced length of stay, increased staff longevity, and a higher perceived quality of care. These observations reinforce earlier recommendations to schedule regular staff meetings, including in the invitation a psychiatrist or social worker familiar with the unit. Ideally, both physicians and nursing staff should attend this meeting. Staff should raise any feelings they have about patients or ward situations. These feelings can be clarified, shared, and discussed with others. Identification of exaggerated expectations or other problems such as group depression can be investigated and resolved. Junior staff can gain broader perspectives from more experienced staff. These meetings can also facilitate communication and humor, which are important ways for a staff to cope. They can help staff deal with the multisystem patient with a poor prognosis. Staff can become more comfortable realizing they are doing the best job possible with this difficult population and accepting death if it becomes clear that the patient will have to die despite the best critical care that could be offered. Recent studies have found that clinicians perceive conflict in up to 78% of cases requiring decision making for critically ill patients. The conflict was perceived to occur with equal frequency between staff and family members and within the staff. While the presence of conflict was not always felt to be detrimental, it can be disruptive and lead to morale problems. Thus, meetings in which such issues can be identified and discussed will benefit the ICU team.

In addition to staff meetings, there are a host of practical interventions that can help staff deal with the stress of working in an ICU. Nursing and physician staff can be encouraged to take adequate time off for restorative recreation and family life. Some institutions schedule fewer but longer shifts (such as three 18-hour shifts per week) in order to provide longer stretches of time off. House staff might be given the afternoon off on the day following a night on call—which is probably the single most important variable in reducing house staff distress. Providing strong medical and nursing directors is extremely helpful for staff dealing with the ambiguities of complex illnesses. Having the services of an ethicist and a chaplain available on a regular basis can be an invaluable support strategy.

Current Controversies & Unresolved Issues

The difficulty of working in an ICU will undoubtedly persist. As technologic advances allow staff to sustain life in the face of severe, previously untreatable conditions, the ethical and philosophical tensions these situations give rise to are likely to increase. Helping the staff to cope with these stressors will remain an ongoing challenge.

REFERENCES

American Psychiatric Association: *Diagnostic and Statistical Manual of Mental Disorders,* 4th ed. Text Revision. American Psychiatric Association, 2000.

American Psychiatric Association: *Practice Guideline for the Treatment of Patients With Delirium.* American Psychiatric Association, 1999.

Barie PS, Bacchetta MD, Eachempati SR: The Contemporary Surgical Intensive Care Unit: Structure, Staffing, and Issues. Surg Clin North Am 2000;80:791–804.

Breen CM et al: Conflict associated with decisions to limit life-sustaining treatment in intensive care units. J Gen Intern Med 2001;16:283–89.

Carter GL, Dawson AH, Lopert R: Drug induced delirium: Incidence, management and prevention. Drug Saf 1996;15:291–301.

Di Salvo TG, O'Gara PT: Torsade de pointes caused by high-dose intravenous haloperidol in cardiac patients. Clin Cardiol 1995;18:285–90.

Eisendrath SJ, Dunkel J: Psychological issues in intensive care unit staff. Heart Lung 1979;8:751–8.

Eisendrath SJ, Link N, Matthay M: Intensive care unit: How stressful for physicians? Crit Care Med 1986;14:95–8.

Eisendrath SJ: Reframing techniques in the general hospital. Family Systems Medicine 1986;4:91–5.

Flacker JM, Lipsitz LA: Neural mechanisms of delirium: Current hypotheses and evolving concepts. J Gerontol 1999;6:B239–46.

Folstein MF, Folstein SE, McHugh PR: "Mini-Mental State": A practical method for grading the cognitive state of patients for the clinician. J Psychiatr Res 1975;12:189–98.

George J, Bleasdale S, Singleton SJ: Causes and prognosis of delirium in elderly patients admitted to a district general hospital. Age Ageing 1997;26:423–27.

Hart RP et al: Abbreviated cognitive test for delirium. J Psychosom Res 1997;43:417–23.

Hassan E, Fontaine DK, Nearman HS: Therapeutic considerations in the management of agitated or delirious critically ill patients. Pharmacotherapy 1998;18:113–29.

Hwang SL et al: Stress-reducing effect of physician's tape-recorded support on cardiac surgical patients in the intensive care unit. J Formos Med Assoc 1998;97:191–96.

Jones C et al: Memory, delusions, and the development of acute posttraumatic stress disorder-related symptoms after intensive care. Crit Care Med 2001;29:573–80.

Karlsson I: Drugs that induce delirium. Dement Geriatr Cogn Disord 1999;10:412–15.

Lerner DM et al: Low-dose risperidone for the irritable medically ill patient. Psychosomatics 2000;41:69–71.

Lopez JF, Akil H, Watson SJ: Role of biological and psychological factors in early development and their impact on adult life: Neural circuits mediating stress. Biol Psychiatry 1999;46:1461–71.

Masand PS, Tesar GE: Use of stimulants in the medically ill. Psychiatr Clin North Am 1996;19:515–47.

McGuire BE et al: Intensive care unit syndrome: A dangerous misnomer. Arch Intern Med 2000;160:906–9.

Saravay SM, Lavin M: Psychiatric comorbidity and length of stay in the general hospital: A critical review of outcome studies. Psychosomatics 1994;35:233–52.

Schelling G et al: Health-related quality of life and posttraumatic stress disorder in survivors of the acute respiratory distress syndrome. Crit Care Med 1998;26:651–59.

Trzepacz P: Update on the neuropathogenesis of delirium. Dement Geriatr Cogn Disord 1999;10:330–34.

van der Mast RC: Delirium: The underlying pathophysiological mechanisms and the need for clinical research. J Psychosom Res 1996;41:109–13.

Care of the Elderly Patient

19

Shawkat Dhanani, MD, MPH, & Dean C. Norman, MD

The elderly are a highly heterogeneous group, and individuals become more dissimilar as they age. Individuals over 65 years of age—with or without chronic diseases—vary widely in their physical, behavioral, and cognitive functions. Any clinician can relate the "Tale of Two Octogenarians" seen in practice on the same day: the end-stage patient afflicted with Alzheimer's disease seen at the nursing home and the vigorous retiree seen after his golf game for monitoring of his historically well-controlled hypertension.

Physiologic age rather than chronologic age should be the major determinant of the health care requirements of the elderly. An abrupt decline in any organ or function is almost certainly due to disease and not due to "normal aging." Therefore, symptoms in the geriatric population should not be automatically attributed to old age, and it is important to look for potentially reversible causes of symptoms. Moreover, treatable conditions should not be undertreated for fear of side effects of medication.

Improvement or maintenance of functional abilities is the major goal of medical care in the geriatric population. Functional disability occurs faster and takes longer to correct in the elderly, necessitating early preventive measures. Active efforts should be made to maintain functional level even during intensive care. Even small changes in function can make large differences in the quality of life. For example, regaining the ability to oppose the thumb to other fingers may enable a geriatric patient to become independent in feeding. Prevention of iatrogenic diseases is also important. For example, close attention should be paid to prevent the development of decubitus ulcers. A decubitus ulcer can develop in just few hours, and the mortality rate of those who develop the lesions in the first 2 weeks of intensive care has been reported to be as high as 73%. Other iatrogenic problems in the ICU include aspiration pneumonia, drug toxicity and interactions, and renal insufficiency.

Multiple concurrent illnesses, cognitive and sensory impairments, age-related changes in physiology and pharmacodynamics, increased vulnerability to delirium, and complications from immobility make management of acute illness in the elderly a clinical challenge for all physicians and other health care providers who care for patients in this age group.

PHYSIOLOGIC CHANGES WITH AGE

The Aging Heart

Heart disease is the leading cause of death in people over 75 years of age, and the fourth most prevalent chronic disease in the elderly. Nearly 30% of elderly people have some abnormality affecting the heart. Moreover, occult cardiac disease can cause marked functional impairments in otherwise apparently healthy elderly people. Coronary atherosclerosis increases exponentially with age and in the elderly can present as heart failure, pulmonary edema, arrhythmias, or exercise intolerance rather than as angina or obvious myocardial infarction.

In healthy subjects, the resting heart rate does not change with age, but the maximal heart rate with exercise decreases with age (Table 19–1). Age-related changes in collagen and elastin contribute to progressive stiffness and loss of recoil of elastic tissues. In the systemic arteries, this process contributes in part to an increase in systolic blood pressure. Systolic pressure rises approximately 6–7 mm Hg per decade, but diastolic pressure changes little with age and may even fall as the systolic pressure rises. In addition, the systolic pressure is underestimated by the cuff sphygmomanometer with increasing age. Resistance to blood flow leads to increased left ventricular wall tension and compensatory left ventricular hypertrophy. Moderate myocardial hypertrophy has been shown to occur with aging in several studies regardless of how subjects were chosen. The myocardium also is affected by changes in collagen and elastin that cause stiffness of the left ventricle which can result in diastolic dysfunction. The left ventricular filling rate during early diastole declines markedly with age (approximately a 50% reduction between age 20 and age 80). Enhanced active filling in late diastole during atrial contraction compensates for decreased passive diastolic filling, and this explains the vulnerability of older persons to congestive heart failure when atrial fibrillation or flutter occurs. Decreased filling also makes them more vulnerable to small decreases in venous filling with volume loss or when given opioids, diuretics, or positive-pressure ventilation. On the other hand, systolic function is relatively preserved in the healthy elderly.

Table 19–1. Summary of age-related change in cardiac physiology.

Heart rate	At rest: unchanged Maximal heart rate with exercise: decreases
Stroke volume	At rest: unchanged With exercise: increases
Ejection fraction	At rest: unchanged With exercise: fails to increase as much as in younger subjects
Cardiac output	At rest: unchanged Low- and medium-intensity exercise: unchanged High-intensity exercise: fails to increase as much as in younger subjects
Early diastolic left ventricular filling rate	Decreases
Late diastolic left ventricular filling rate (atrial "kick")	Increases
Ventricular compliance	Decreases

Despite these disturbances, cardiac output at rest remains relatively constant across the life span. During low- and medium-intensity exercise, increases in stroke volume compensate for the lower heart rates observed in the elderly. This increase in stroke volume with exercise is the result of an increase in end-diastolic volume by as much as 30% (Frank-Starling law). However, with high-intensity exercise, a decline in cardiac output is observed due largely to the age-related lower ceiling on heart rate. This hemodynamic profile is strikingly similar to that observed in younger patients who exercise in the presence of beta-adrenergic blockade. Since beta-adrenergic modulation of pacemaker cells partly explains the increased heart rate during exercise, this observation led to the hypothesis—later confirmed—that diminished response to beta-adrenergic modulation is one of the most notable age-related changes in the cardiovascular system. Chronotropic and inotropic responses of the aging heart to norepinephrine, isoproterenol, and dobutamine are diminished. Virtually all studies show higher mean circulating blood norepinephrine and epinephrine levels in the elderly compared with younger persons.

Both arterial and venous dilation in response to beta-adrenergic stimulation decrease with age. This deficiency in arterial dilation in addition to any age-related structural changes within the large vessels may contribute to increased vascular impedance in advancing age.

The Aging Lung

Cross-sectional population studies consistently show a progressive age-related decline in pulmonary function. The decrements in flow rates and lung volumes are not uniform throughout life but tend to accelerate with age. Given the large individual differences in the elderly, longitudinal studies would be preferable for observing the change in pulmonary function, which is influenced not only by age but also by environmental factors such as smoking, air pollution, infections, and other comorbid conditions.

Age-related changes in collagen and elastin produce a decrease in lung compliance, but this is not physiologically significant. However, rigidity of the chest wall with aging has measurably negative mechanical implications resulting in significantly increased work of breathing. Starting around age 35 years, there is a decrease in forced vital capacity (FVC) averaging 14–30 mL per year and a decrease in forced expiratory volume in 1 second (FEV_1) averaging 23–32 mL per year for nonsmoking men. Nonsmoking women show slightly lesser rates of decline (FVC 15–24 mL per year and FEV_1 19–26 mL per year). All expiratory flow rates decrease with age and tend to fall faster in men, taller individuals, and those with increased airway reactivity. The decrease in FVC is associated with an elevation in functional residual capacity (FRC) and residual volume (RV). Only minor changes occur in total lung capacity.

Age-related changes in lung structure and chest wall mechanics lead to premature closure of terminal airways. This phenomenon occurs predominantly in the dependent parts of the lungs that are the best perfused, accounting for increasing ventilation-perfusion mismatching that results in a progressive decrease in arterial P_{O_2} and an increased alveolar-arterial oxygen difference—$P(A\text{–}a)_{O_2}$—with age. The following equation predicts arterial oxygen tension—Pa_{O_2}—at sea level in the adult:

$$Pa_{O_2}\ (\text{mm Hg}) = 100.1 - 0.325 \times \text{Age (years)}$$

The normal highest value for the $P(A\text{–}a)_{O_2}$ at rest for a given age can be calculated as follows:

$$P(A-a)_{O_2}\ (\text{mm Hg}) = 1.4 + 0.3 \times \text{Age (years)}$$

Based on this formula, a 90-year-old subject will have a predicted Pa_{O_2} of 71 mm Hg and a maximum normal $P(A\text{–}a)_{O_2}$ of 40 mm Hg at sea level.

Changes in position also influence the arterial P_{O_2}. Arterial P_{O_2} is 6–10 mm Hg lower in the supine position compared with the upright position in the elderly. Postoperative hypoxemia is especially common in the elderly, in whom it may persist for several days. There is no significant change in arterial pH or P_{CO_2} with age.

Ventilatory control is also affected by age and is more striking compared with the changes in lung volumes and flow rates. The ventilatory response to hypoxemia is reduced by half in healthy elderly men 64–73 years of age, while the response to hypercapnia is reduced by 40%. Reasons for these decreased responses are unclear. Suggested explanations include altered central or peripheral chemoreceptor function as well as reduction in neuromuscular inspiratory output.

Right atrial, pulmonary artery, and pulmonary capillary wedge pressures are unchanged in the healthy elderly at rest. In contrast, the older person's increased pulmonary artery and pulmonary capillary wedge pressures with exercise are significant, and increases of pulmonary artery resistance are highly significant with age.

With age also comes a reduction in the effectiveness of cough and mucociliary clearance and a decline in the cellular and humoral components of pulmonary immunity. These predispose this population to pulmonary infections. Similarly, a diminished gag reflex, dyscoordination of swallowing, prolonged periods in the supine position, and sedation contribute to an increased risk of aspiration. Table 19–2 summarizes these findings.

The Aging Kidney

Many cross-sectional and longitudinal studies of large human populations have shown a steady decline in creatinine clearance with age. As in any other area, the decline of renal function with age is highly variable among individuals. In general, changes due to disease and to aging are in the same direction and are additive. With aging, there is a loss of nephrons at a rate of 0.5–1% a year. By the seventh decade of life, there is a 30–50% loss of functioning glomeruli due to age alone. This loss occurs primarily in the renal cortex, with relative sparing of the medulla. A progressive reduction in renal plasma flow has also been demonstrated with age. A 50% reduction has been shown between young adulthood and the eighth decade, averaging 10% per decade.

The major clinically relevant renal functional defect arising from these histologic and physiologic changes is a progressive decline, after maturity, in the glomerular filtration rate (GFR). Age-adjusted normative standards for creatinine clearance have been established. The rate of decline has been estimated as 8 mL/min/1.73 m^2 per decade after the fourth decade (or 0.8 mL/min per year). This rather drastic age-related loss of renal function is not completely reflected in the serum creatinine because of the proportionate decline in skeletal muscle mass. Therefore, in order to make an estimation of the glomerular filtration rate in the elderly, the serum creatinine value should be incorporated in the Cockcroft and Gault formula that takes into account the age, sex, and weight of the patient:

$$\text{Estimated creatinine clearance} = \frac{(140 - \text{Age [years]}) \times (\text{Body Weight [kg]})}{(72) \times (\text{Serum creatinine [mg/dL]})}$$

In women, the result should be multiplied by 0.85. Actual body weight is used in this equation, but for obese individuals (BMI ≥ 30), ideal body weight should be used.

For the above reasons, dosage adjustments of medications excreted primarily by the kidneys should not be based on serum creatinine values but rather on measured or at least estimated creatinine clearance. Drugs that are predominantly excreted through kidneys and have low therapeutic indices (eg, digoxin, procainamide, vancomycin) require close monitoring of serum levels.

Since medullary nephrons, which are relatively spared compared with cortical nephrons, have reduced concentrating ability, the elderly tend to excrete more free water. They release more antidiuretic hormone in response to hypertonicity, yet water retention is less than in younger individuals because of reduced end-organ response in older persons. Older individuals tend to have diminished thirst perception and diminished awareness of volume contraction. The response to aldosterone is impaired, and the ability to conserve sodium limited.

Table 19–2. Summary of age-related changes in pulmonary physiology.

Forced vital capacity (FVC)	Decreases
Forced expiratory volume in 1 second (FEV_1)	Decreases
Residual volume	Decreases
Arterial P_{O_2}	Decreases
Alveolar-arterial oxygen difference	Increases
Arterial P_{CO_2}	Unchanged
Regulatory response to hypoxia or hypercapnia	Decreases
Mucociliary clearance	Decreases

The age-related decline in other renal functions such as urine concentration and dilution, tubular secretion and reabsorption, and hydrogen ion secretion render the elderly susceptible to disorders of fluid, electrolyte, and acid-base imbalance. Low renin and aldosterone can contribute to hyperkalemia and hyponatremia.

MANAGEMENT OF THE ELDERLY PATIENT IN THE ICU

Clinical Presentation of Disease in the Elderly

Elderly patients may present with multiple pathologic processes in different organ systems. Various studies have found an average of three or four medical conditions in ambulatory aged patients and five to nine medical diagnoses among elderly patients in chronic care facilities.

Owing in part to the progressive decrease in physiologic reserve with age and comorbidity, the elderly may have unusual presentations of diseases. The onset of a disease in the elderly generally affects the most vulnerable organ system first. This explains the frequent apparent lack of relation between the presenting symptom and the underlying disease. Thus, delirium, functional impairment, frequent falls, incontinence, or syncope could be the presenting manifestations of a variety of illnesses such as congestive heart failure, pneumonia, myocardial infarction, urinary tract infection, or gastrointestinal bleeding. Moreover, painless myocardial infarction may occur in up to 30% of cases. This emphasizes the need for a thorough evaluation when searching for the cause of nonspecific symptoms.

Drug Therapy

Iatrogenic illness is common and often preventable in the elderly. The incidence of iatrogenic problems among acutely hospitalized geriatric patients is close to one in three. By far the most common iatrogenic disorders in the elderly are adverse drug reactions. Changes in pharmacokinetics and pharmacodynamics and polypharmacy predispose geriatric patients to adverse reactions and drug interactions.

Pharmacokinetics is the study of the time course of absorption, distribution, metabolism, and excretion of drugs and their metabolites from the body. Absorption and metabolism are minimally affected by aging. Distribution is affected by changes in body composition. For example, aging is associated with an increased percentage of fat (50% increase in men and 25% increase in women from age 40 to age 80) and a concomitant decrease of total body water. Thus, medications that distribute in the water space (hydrophilic drugs such as digoxin and theophylline) have a lower volume of distribution and tend to reach higher levels in a shorter time in an older patient. On the other hand, drugs that are lipid-soluble (lipophilic drugs such as the psychotropics) will have a larger volume of distribution, resulting in progressive accumulation of these drugs. The net effect of this will be to increase the half-life of these drugs and prolong the duration of action. This effect is further compounded by impaired drug excretion, since both renal and, to a lesser extent, hepatic function tend to decrease with aging.

In addition, some plasma protein levels may alter with age. For example, serum albumin often falls with chronic comorbid conditions, resulting in higher free drug levels and a potential for greater pharmacologic effect at the same dosage or total serum level.

As discussed above, renal function tends to decrease with age, but concurrent changes in muscle mass keep the serum creatinine constant at approximately 1 mg/dL, masking the declining renal function. Thus, measurement of creatinine clearance or estimation with the Cockcroft and Gault formula should be used to assess the glomerular filtration rate and make the necessary adjustment of doses of drugs excreted by the kidneys (see Chapter 4).

Cytochrome P450 enzymatic activity tends to decrease with age. Warfarin and theophylline are examples of drugs eliminated by this system. Hepatic blood flow also decreases. On the other hand, normal aging does not significantly impair the conjugation capacity of the liver. Compared with renal function, hepatic function is extremely difficult to quantitate. Only sparse data are available on hepatic drug metabolism in aging human subjects, and evidence for altered hepatic metabolism in humans is largely indirect and frequently inconsistent. For example, in studies with antipyrine (a useful model compound for the study of drug metabolism), large individual variation frequently exceeds the effect of age, such that only 3% of the variance in metabolic clearance is explained by age alone.

Pharmacodynamics is the study of the physiologic response to a drug or combination of drugs and is based on drug-receptor interactions. For reasons that are not well understood, the aging process appears to be associated with an altered sensitivity of receptors for many commonly used medications. In general, elderly subjects are more sensitive to some medications, including warfarin, narcotics, sedatives, and anticholinergic medications, and less sensitive to others, such as beta-adrenergic agonists and antagonists. Once more, given the marked heterogeneity of the elderly as a group, careful individualization should be the general rule when drawing conclusions about such matters.

Because of multiple disease states and extensive prescription of medications in the elderly, the clinician should always check for possible drug-drug and drug-disease interactions before prescribing any new medication. The probability of a significant drug-drug interaction is nearly 7% for patients using more than five drugs and 24% for those using more than ten medications. Special attention should be paid when prescribing medications with long half-lives, or with anticholinergic or potential central nervous system side effects.

Adverse drug effects can mimic almost any clinical syndrome in geriatrics and should be considered in the differential diagnosis of vague symptoms or deterioration of function. For example, timolol eye drops—a beta-blocker used for glaucoma treatment—may be absorbed systemically and can cause cardiac decompensation in a patient with poor cardiac function.

Hydration & Nutrition

Hydration status is a major concern in the hospitalized elderly. One of the most common reasons for electrolyte abnormalities or fluid disturbances in this population is dehydration. Contributing factors may include laxative or diuretic use, the presence of fever or infection, decreased ability to recognize or express thirst, and limited access to water. There is also an age-related decline in urine concentrating ability, which can lead to frequent urination and fluid loss. Accurate fluid balance assessment is essential in nutritional screening, as alterations in hydration state may contribute to inaccurate anthropometric and biochemical markers. Because of the high prevalence of congestive heart failure in this population, intravenous fluid administration must be individualized and approached cautiously.

As stated earlier, aging is associated with a change in body composition with increase in fat content and a concurrent decrease in muscle mass and total body water. Decrease in muscle mass and a reduction in physical activity result in a fall in total energy expenditure with increasing age. Energy requirements may decrease by about a third between the ages of 30 and 80 years. However, during periods of stress such as trauma, surgery, or infection, daily energy requirements may be more than doubled. In addition to the total energy intake, attention should be paid to macronutrient and micronutrient requirements.

The elderly are particularly vulnerable to malnutrition. The reported incidence of malnutrition in elderly hospitalized patients varies from 17% to 65%. As the duration of hospital stay increases, the likelihood of malnutrition rises. In the elderly, a functional nutritional assessment should include evaluation of sight, taste, smell, dentition, degree of cognitive impairment, presence of depression, swallowing abnormalities, respiratory dysfunction, hand-to-mouth coordination, level of assistance required at meals, and perhaps drug-appetite and drug-nutrient interactions.

Whenever possible, feeding should be started as soon as possible in hospitalized or postoperative elderly patients. The enteral route is greatly preferred, but parenteral nutritional support can be used, if needed. Increased mortality occurs in underweight people, but mortality is not clearly increased in overweight elderly patients.

SPECIAL CONSIDERATIONS

The current disease-oriented model of acute medical care promotes a sequential approach to diagnosis and treatment that generally ignores the practice of restorative care until after the patient is discharged from the hospital. In the frail elderly, this approach may lead to a decline in functional abilities despite effective treatment of acute medical illnesses.

The high rate of delirium and psychologic decompensation in the acutely hospitalized elderly may lead to excessive bed rest with accompanying loss of mobility, muscle atrophy, contractures, pressure sores, greater tendency to fall, thromboembolism, incontinence, anorexia, constipation, and lack of motivation. This has been called the "cascade of illness and functional decline."

Since the physiologic characteristics of the aging population include both a decreased functional reserve and large individual variation, medical management should center on individualized treatment plans that incorporate maintenance of functional status, protection from the hazards of immobility, and low risk of complications from treatment.

Delirium

Approximately one-third to one-half of elderly patients will have a delirious episode during the course of hospitalization for medical or surgical care. The presence of altered level of consciousness, easy distractibility, rambling conversation, illogical flow of ideas, unpredictable switching from subject to subject, perceptual disturbances, and psychomotor agitation or retardation should clue the clinician to the diagnosis of delirium. Risk factors are listed in Table 19–3. Delirium could be the presenting symptom of a variety of illnesses (Table 19–4). Early diagnosis is important because most patients can recover if the underlying cause is recognized and treated. Failure to identify delirium can lead to treatment of the effect instead of the cause. Moreover, the use of sedatives, psychotropic drugs, or physical restraints to treat delirium could worsen the existing situation, placing the patient at higher risk for aspiration pneumonia, pressure ulcers, and other immobility-related complications ("cascade effect").

The *DSM-IV* criteria for diagnosis of delirium include the following: (1) disturbances of consciousness

Table 19–3. Risk factors for delirium.

Prior cognitive impairment
Fracture on admission
Age over 80 years
Neuroleptic use
Infection
Opioid use
Male sex

(ie, reduced clarity of awareness of the environment) in conjunction with reduced ability to focus, sustain, or shift attention; (2) a change in cognition (such as memory deficit, disorientation, or language disturbance) or the development of a perceptual disturbance that is not better accounted for by a preexisting, established, or evolving dementia; (3) development of the disturbance during a brief period (usually hours to days) and a tendency for fluctuation during the course of the day; and (4) evidence from the history, physical examination, or laboratory findings that the disturbance is caused by a general medical condition. Recently, a specific instrument for diagnosis of delirium (the Confusion Assessment Method; CAM) has been validated. In contrast with dementia, delirium generally has an abrupt onset, disturbance of consciousness, fluctuations during the course of the day, and frequently an identifiable and potentially reversible cause.

Several tests can be used to assess decreased attention span as seen in delirium. A simple test is the "A" test, in which the interviewer vocalizes letters at a rate of one per second and the patient is instructed to raise his or her finger at each occurrence of the letter "A." In the "one tap, two taps" test, the patient is instructed to tap twice each time the interviewer taps once and vice versa. More complex tests include spelling the word "world" backward or counting backward from 100, subtracting 7 each time until 72 is reached (100, 93, 86, 79, 72). These tests are often abnormal in patients with delirium.

As mentioned before, diseases in the elderly generally affect the most vulnerable organ system first. Prior cognitive impairment is the most frequent independent factor for delirium. Other factors that predispose to the development of delirium include the presence of fracture on admission, age over 80 years, infections, use of multiple medications (specifically neuroleptics or opioids), unfamiliar surroundings, social isolation, visual or hearing impairment, structural brain disease, concurrent chronic illness, sleep deprivation, and alcohol or drug abuse.

Delirium is indicative of diffuse brain dysfunction and has been associated with four classes of diseases: (1) primary cerebral diseases, such as central nervous system infections, brain tumors, and stroke; (2) systemic illnesses that secondarily affect brain function, including cardiac disease, pulmonary failure, hepatic dysfunction, uremia, deficiency states, anemia, endocrine disturbances, systemic infections, and inflammatory diseases; (3) intoxication with exogenous substances (alcohol, illicit drugs, prescribed medications, industrial toxins); and (4) withdrawal from dependency-producing agents (alcohol, barbiturates, benzodiazepines).

The approach to patients with delirium includes a focused history and physical examination, review of medications, and basic laboratory studies such as complete blood count, serum electrolytes, serum urea nitrogen, glucose, and urinalysis. Further specialized tests can be done in individual cases. These include chest radiography, electrocardiography, pulse oximetry, selected drug levels, selected cultures, vitamin B_{12} level, thyroid function tests, brain imaging, lumbar puncture, and electroencephalography.

Treatment of delirium should include identification and treatment of the underlying cause and review of the medication regimen. Neuroleptics, opioids, or any medication with high anticholinergic or sedative side effects should be discontinued or reduced in dosage whenever possible. When available, constant observation is preferable to restraints. A well-lighted and predictable environment, eyeglasses and hearing aids in place, frequent reorientation by family and nurses, simple explanations of any procedure or confusing stimuli, encouragement to stay awake during the daytime, and nursing routines that permit uninterrupted nighttime sleep are all valuable in the management of delirium. Finally, it may be necessary to treat agitated behavior with medication. Generally, the lowest effective doses of one of the atypical antipsychotics (risperidone, olanzapine) should be used because of the low incidence of extrapyramidal side effects. Total resolution of all symptoms can take days to months.

Table 19–4. Common causes of delirium.

Decreased cardiac output	Hypothermia and hyperthermia
Congestive heart failure	Metabolic disorders
Acute myocardial infarction	Electrolyte abnormalities
Acute blood loss	Acid-based disturbances
Dehydration	Hypoxia
Infections	Hypercapnia
Fractures	Hypoglycemia and hyperglycemia
Stroke	Azotemia
Poorly controlled pain	Transfer to unfamiliar surroundings
Drugs	
Urinary retention	
Fecal impaction	

Communicating With the Elderly Patient

Many elderly patients have hearing and vision problems that interfere with communication and cause difficulty in orientation and adaptation to a new environment. Being able to see and hear properly becomes critical when one must cope with new experiences such as ventilatory support devices and other invasive interventions.

Communication problems generate great anxiety in the patient and frustration in the caregiver. There is a risk of mislabeling the patient as "confused" and disregarding the patient's role as a participant in health care decisions. The elderly patient who reacts to an unfamiliar situation by becoming "agitated" is thus at risk for physical restraint or psychotropic medication. This may lead to worsening of the clinical status and may lead to the "cascade effect" described above. The importance of efforts to maximize communication with the elderly individual is thus emphasized, especially in the ICU setting.

Adequate vision makes communication easier, especially for those who have impaired hearing or comprehension. Eye contact helps the caregiver assess the extent to which the older person hears and understands what is being said. If the patient wears glasses, they should be clean and in place. The head of the bed should be elevated so the patient can see the speaker's lips and eyes. A glare-free light source coming from behind the patient helps the patient see the face and lips of the speaker. If the patient has a hearing impairment, background noise should be reduced by turning the television or radio off, by closing the door, and by asking others in the area to be quiet. The speaker should lean forward so the lips can be seen, but shouting is not helpful. Most elderly people suffer from a selective high-frequency hearing loss with decreased ability to identify high-frequency tones and pitches in the consonants *s, f, t,* hard *g,* and *j.* Increasing the volume of sound is of little help, and shouting may be misinterpreted as hostility or anger. The manner of speaking should be natural and not distorted by exaggerated lip movements. When it is necessary to repeat a comment or question, it is better to rephrase than to say the same thing in a louder voice. If the patient has a hearing aid, it should be properly in place and in good working condition. Older people are often not aware of their hearing inadequacies, and their perceptions of what they have heard may not be accurate. Therefore, an attempt should be made to determine whether the patient has properly interpreted what has been said.

Health care personnel and family members should not whisper or speak together in low tones near a hearing-impaired older adult. A few words may be heard that will result in misinterpretation, increasing the possibility of unwarranted fears, paranoid behavior, or hostility. Glasses and hearing aids should be worn consistently during the day. If the patient is able to talk, dentures should be in place to facilitate clear speech.

Immobility

Elderly patients are particularly vulnerable to the untoward effects of immobility. Contractures, pressure ulcers, and deconditioning can develop rapidly. Some of the other consequences of immobility include muscle atrophy, deep venous thrombosis, increased calcium mobilization from bone, atelectasis, hypostatic pneumonia, constipation, functional fecal and urinary incontinence, and loss of motivation.

Pressure ulcers are a common and frequent complication of immobility. Any disease process leading to immobility (eg, severe congestive heart failure, respiratory failure, delirium, complicated postoperative course, or spinal cord injury) places the elderly patient at high risk for development of a pressure ulcer. Sites commonly involved are the sacrum, ischial tuberosities, hip, heel, elbow, knee, ankle, and occiput. More than 50% of pressure ulcers occur in persons over age 70. Their prevalence among patients expected to be confined to a bed or in a chair for at least 1 week is as high as 28%. Pressure ulcers generally occur within the first 2 weeks of hospitalization. Moreover, the development of pressure sores has prognostic implications; the mortality rate among those who develop them in the first 2 weeks has been observed to be as high as 73%. Sepsis is the most serious complication of pressure ulcers. Among bacteremic patients with a pressure ulcer as the probable source of infection, the in-hospital mortality rate can be as high as 60%.

Frequent repositioning (whether supine or in the sitting position) has been the primary method of preventing pressure ulcers. The evidence of structural changes in experimental animal model tissues after 2 hours of pressure bearing has set the standard, leading to the recommendation for repositioning every 2 hours. Repositioning should be performed so that a person at risk is positioned without pressure on vulnerable bony prominences. This is accomplished in practice by positioning patients horizontally with the back resting partially over pillows that maintain the body at a 30-degree angle to the support surface. Additional pillows between the legs and supporting the arms will aid in maintaining optimal positioning. A person with limited ability to change position who must sit in a chair or have the head of the bed elevated should not remain in this position for more than 2 hours at a time. To diminish the shearing forces over the sacral area, the head of the bed should not be elevated more than 30 degrees. Particulate matter (eg, food crumbs) should be removed from the bed. Sheets should be loose, and tucking of the sheet at the foot of the bed should be avoided so that movement is not restricted and the feet can assume their natural position. Heel and elbow pads can be used as adjunctive measures. Patients should be lifted, not dragged. The skin should be patted dry, not rubbed. Moisture control depends on timely skin care. The evaluation and management of urinary and fecal incontinence are of crucial importance in these patients.

With good nursing care, it is possible to prevent most pressure sores without the use of special equipment. However, in the high-risk patient, pressure-relieving supports such as constant low-pressure supports, alternating-pressure supports or pressure-relieving cushions may be needed. Attention should also be directed toward proper nutrition, hydration, and pain control.

Educational programs aimed at physicians, nurses, and other caregivers, family members, and the patients themselves have beneficial results. One study found that when physicians ordered preventive measures for high-risk patients, the incidence of pressure ulcers was half that observed among patients for whom such orders were not written.

Bed rest also results in immobility and loss of weight-bearing forces on joints. These effects cause changes in periarticular and articular structures that result in joint contractures and changes similar to those of osteoarthritis. Changes in periarticular tissues occur within days. Muscles that bridge the immobilized joint shorten. These changes produce decreased range of motion that can be permanent, depending on the length of immobilization.

Bed rest is accompanied by progressive cardiovascular deconditioning with exaggeration of the hemodynamic changes normally seen with standing, as manifested by orthostatic intolerance and decreased exercise tolerance. Although orthostatic hypotension is not always documented, signs and symptoms of orthostatic intolerance such as tachycardia, nausea, diaphoresis, and syncope are common after prolonged bed rest. A decrease in coordination as measured by pattern tracing and a marked increase in body sway in a standing position has been documented after several weeks of bed rest.

The rate of decrease in muscular strength may be as high as 5% per day and varies with the degree of immobility. Leg muscles tend to lose strength about twice as fast as arm muscles. For some elderly patients who normally use 100% of their quadriceps muscle strength just to stand up, a loss of 5% per day results in significant loss of function in a short time.

Given the numerous complications resulting from immobility, early mobilization of the elderly patient in the intensive care setting should be a high-priority. The rate of loss of muscle strength will slow when active contraction of muscles is encouraged, particularly if resistance is added. Simple devices such as elastic fabrics (Theraband) make exercise against resistance available for patients in beds or in chairs. Active movement in bed and full range of motion exercises should be encouraged in alert patients. For other patients, passive full range of motion should be done on every nursing shift.

Intermittent sitting—and standing when possible—will reduce the frequency of orthostatic hypotension. The sitting position also improves oxygenation (PaO_2 increases by 6–10 mm Hg in the sitting position in the elderly) and diminishes cardiac work, since cardiac output and stroke volume decrease in the sitting position. Finally, rehabilitation service consultation may be useful in the management of elderly patients in the intensive care unit.

REFERENCES

Corcoran PJ: Use it or lose it: the hazards of bedrest and inactivity. West J Med 1991;154:536–8.

Ely EW et al: Evaluation of delirium in critically ill patients: validation of the Confusion Assessment Method for the Intensive Care Unit (CAM-ICU). Crit Care Med 2001;29:1370–9.

Geokas MC et al: The aging process. Ann Intern Med 1990;113:455–66.

Giraud T et al: Iatrogenic complications in adult intensive care units: a prospective two-center study. Crit Care Med 1993;21:40–51.

Harper CM, Lyles YM: Physiology and complications of bed rest. J Am Geriatr Soc 1988;36:1047–54.

Hazzard WR et al (editors): *Principles of Geriatric Medicine and Gerontology,* 4th ed. McGraw-Hill, 1998.

Inouye SK et al: Clarifying confusion: the confusion assessment method. A new method for detection of delirium. Ann Intern Med 1990;113:941–8.

Intensive care for the elderly. (Editorial.) Lancet 1991;337:209–10.

Kitzman DW, Edwards WD: Age-related changes in the anatomy of the normal human heart. J Gerontol 1990;45:M33–9.

Kyriakides ZS et al: Systolic functional responses of normal older and younger adult left ventricles to dobutamine. Am J Cardiol 1986;58:816–9.

Lefevre F et al: Iatrogenic complications in high-risk, elderly patients. Arch Intern Med 1992;152:2074–80.

Levkoff SE et al: Delirium: The occurrence and persistence of symptoms among elderly hospitalized patients. Arch Intern Med 1992;152:334–40.

McGee M, Jensen GL: Nutrition in the elderly. J Clin Gastroenterol 2000;30:372–80.

Mahler DA, Rosiello RA, Loke J: The aging lung. Clin Geriatr Med 1986;28:215–30.

Meyer BR: Renal function in aging. J Am Geriatr Soc 1989;37:791–800.

Oskvig RM: Special problems in the elderly. Chest 1999;115 (Suppl):158S–164S.

Roca R: Psychosocial aspects of surgical care in the elderly patient. Surg Clin North Am 1994;74:223–43.

Rowe JW et al: The effect of age on creatinine clearance in men: A cross-sectional and longitudinal study. J Gerontol 1976; 31:155–63.

Schor JD et al: Risk factors for delirium in hospitalized elderly. JAMA 1992;267:827–31.

Steel K et al: Iatrogenic illness on a general medical service at a university hospital. N Engl J Med 1981;304:638–42.

Warshaw GA et al: Functional disability in the hospitalized elderly. JAMA 1982;248:847–50.

Woodhouse K: The pharmacology of aging. In *Brocklehurst's Textbook of Geriatric Medicine and Gerontology,* 5th ed. Tallis RC et al (editors). Churchill Livingstone, 1998.

Wu AW, Rubin HR, Rosen MJ: Are elderly people less responsive to intensive care? J Am Geriatr Soc 1990;38:621–7.

Critical Care of the Oncology Patient

20

Darrell W. Harrington, MD, & Hassan J. Tabbarah, MD

Complications of cancer that may require critical care include (1) central nervous system disorders (spinal cord compression and increased intracranial pressure); (2) metabolic disorders (hypercalcemia, hypocalcemia, tumor lysis syndrome, hyponatremia, hyperglycemia, hypoglycemia, and hypokalemia with ectopic ACTH production); (3) orthopedic disorders, such as pathologic fracture; (4) urologic disorders (hematuria, hemorrhagic cystitis, acute obstructive uropathy); (5) general surgical disorders (gastrointestinal bleeding, bowel perforation, bowel obstruction, extrahepatic biliary obstruction, and intra-abdominal abscess formation); (6) malignant effusions (pericardial effusion with cardiac tamponade and pleural effusion with lung compression); and, rarely, (7) superior vena cava syndrome. Central nervous system disorders, metabolic disorders, and superior vena cava syndrome will be addressed in this chapter.

CENTRAL NERVOUS SYSTEM DISORDERS

SPINAL CORD COMPRESSION

ESSENTIALS OF DIAGNOSIS

- *Axial (back) pain that may radiate to arms or legs, or band-like discomfort around the chest.*
- *History of malignancy usually but not always present.*
- *Neurologic deficits.*
- *Abnormal images of spine: plain x-rays, CT scan, myelography, MRI.*

General Considerations

Spinal cord compression from epidural metastases is a potentially devastating complication in cancer patients. It occurs in about 5% of cancer deaths and therefore will develop in about 25,000 of the annual 500,000 cancer deaths. The most common primary tumors that cause spinal cord compression are cancers of the lung, breast, and prostate, lymphomas, and multiple myeloma. Cord compression is also seen in patients with leukemia and a wide range of other solid tumors. It may present as the first and only manifestation of cancer.

Epidural spinal cord compression develops via two mechanisms: (1) by metastatic spread to the vertebral bodies, where tumor expands and erodes into the epidural space; and (2) by cancerous involvement of the paravertebral region with extension into the epidural space through the intervertebral foramina. Bone scans and spine x-rays may be normal in the latter cases but usually abnormal in the former. Vertebral body metastases account for epidural spinal cord compression in approximately 85% of patients with solid tumors and 25% of patients with lymphomas. Epidural metastases extend from the paravertebral region in the remainder. In addition to spinal cord compression, sudden irreversible spinal dysfunction may occur from vascular compromise, resulting in spinal cord infarction.

The thoracic spine occupies 47% of the total length of the spine but is the affected area in approximately 70% of patients; the lumbar spine occupies 30% and is affected in 20%; and the cervical region occupies 22% and is affected in 10% of patients. Spinal cord involvement may occur at multiple levels in 10–38% of cases. The greater chance of thoracic spine involvement may be related to the presence of physiologic kyphosis and the narrower spinal canal in this region. Metastases never traverse the intervertebral disks and rarely traverse the dura.

Clinical Features

A. Symptoms and Signs

The clinical presentation of epidural spinal cord compression is well known and depends on the level of spinal involvement. Axial pain is the most common presenting symptom (prodromal phase), occurring in 95% of adults and 80% of children with epidural spinal cord compression. Therefore, spinal cord compression should be considered in any patient with cancer and axial pain.

The local pain corresponds to the site of the lesions and is described as dull and aching. Tenderness over the affected spinal element is usually readily elicited. Approximately 15% of patients will develop paraplegia despite a long duration of painful symptoms (compressive phase), because spinal cord compression is not anticipated. Pain may persist for several weeks or months before symptoms of radiculopathy are manifested. Cervical or lumbar disease usually but not always presents as unilateral radiculopathy, whereas thoracic disease produces bilateral symptoms resulting in a band-like distribution of pain. Radicular pain may be accompanied by sensory or motor loss as determined by the involved nerve root and may easily be confused with disk herniation. Pain is usually worse at night and is aggravated by movement, coughing, or the Valsalva maneuver.

Neurologic deficits usually begin with motor impairment, more commonly in the distal part of the body or the lower extremities, owing to the greater frequency of thoracic and lumbar spine involvement. Anterior spinal cord compression is more common than posterior involvement. Accordingly, patients usually have more motor than sensory disability, at least in the early stages. Sensory impairment follows, parallels the development of motor deficit, and is present in half of patients at the time of diagnosis of spinal cord compression. Autonomic dysfunction occurs later and is present in half of cases.

The neurologic deficit is caused either by mechanical compression by the tumor on the spinal cord or cauda equina or by destruction of a vertebral body sufficient to make it collapse and compress the spinal cord. Once spinal cord compression occurs, progression may be very rapid. The presence of myelopathy is a neurologic emergency. Disease presentation and progression depends on the level of spinal involvement. For example, high cervical cord lesions (C3–5) may be life-threatening, as both quadriplegia and respiratory muscle impairment are common features. Involvement of the thoracic cord is typically characterized by identification of a sensory level on the trunk. In addition, lower extremity weakness and autonomic dysfunction may accompany thoracic cord compression. The specific site of lumbosacral spinal cord compression is less easily determined by physical examination. Patients may present with radiculopathy and loss of associated reflexes or with isolated autonomic dysfunction as seen in the conus syndrome. It is important that each patient have a complete neurologic examination, paying close attention to subtle asymmetries in muscle strength and reflexes. It is important to note that patellar and ankle reflexes provide information only about L4 and S1 nerve roots, respectively. Therefore, normal reflexes of the lower extremity should not be used to exclude the presence of significant myelopathy.

B. Laboratory Findings

In the presence of complete blockage of the spinal canal and to avoid worsening of neurologic status, only a few drops of cerebrospinal fluid should be removed and sent for cytologic examination and protein determination. Lumbar puncture should otherwise be reserved for patients suspected of concomitant leptomeningeal dissemination of tumor. Cerebrospinal fluid findings consist of elevated protein levels, normal or low glucose, and a lymphocytic pleocytosis. A tissue diagnosis of malignancy is usually unnecessary in a patient with a known preexisting malignancy. However, it is prudent to specifically identify malignancy causing spinal cord compression in an individual without an underlying history of cancer. This is because localized infection causing spinal cord compression may mimic malignancy.

C. Imaging Studies

Plain x-rays of the involved area, radionuclide bone scans, examination of the spinal fluid, myelography, CT scan, and MRI are potentially useful in the diagnosis of epidural spinal cord compression. Imaging should be acquired as early as possible and should not be delayed more than a few hours in patients with neurologic symptoms and signs. Plain x-rays may be very helpful in localizing the anatomic origin of compression symptoms. Hematologic malignancies less often are manifested by abnormal plain spine x-rays than solid tumors. The most common findings include loss of pedicles, destruction of the vertebral body, and vertebral body collapse. Plain x-rays will, however, be unsuccessful in identifying up to 20% of vertebral body lesions and will also fail to demonstrate paravertebral masses that spare vertebral body destruction but encroach upon the epidural space via the intervertebral foramina. The overall diagnostic value of plain spine films is about 83%.

The role of radionuclide bone scans is unclear in the setting of suspected epidural spinal cord compression. Bone scans are less accurate than plain spine x-rays in predicting epidural involvement. Moreover, bone scans often will suggest multiple areas of abnormality without identifying the level associated with pain or neurologic deficit. Bone scans may not reflect the extent of vertebral involvement. These studies are reserved for patients with skeletal pain, negative plain x-rays, and a low suspicion for spinal cord compression.

CT scans cannot investigate multiple levels of involvement without extensive scanning and may miss the area of maximal impingement because CT scan "cuts" are too widely spaced. However, CT scans can assess the extent of a paravertebral mass, detect small areas of bone destruction, quantify the extent and characterize the direction of spinal cord impingement, and assess response to treatment.

Myelography remains an important diagnostic method for epidural spinal cord compression, especially when MRI is unavailable. Water-soluble contrast media are preferred. Once a complete block of the spinal canal is demonstrated by a lumbar myelogram, a C1–2 or suboccipital myelogram should be done to define the upper level of block. Myelography may disclose silent epidural metastasis. Lumbar myelography may cause further deterioration of neurologic findings in approximately 14% of patients even with the removal of only a small amount of cerebrospinal fluid. Myelography has been associated with complications such as headaches, seizures, allergic reactions, and deterioration of neurologic status.

MRI has become the diagnostic method of choice for suspected spinal cord compression. It is no more sensitive than bone scanning for detecting bony metastases but is more specific. Vertebral metastases can be seen on unenhanced T1-weighted images as a focus of low signal intensity (dark) that contrasts with the adjacent high signal intensity (bright) of normal adult marrow. The administration of contrast results in normalization of the tumor, making its appearance similar to that of the marrow. Vertebral metastases rarely cross the disk space, as often seen in infection. However, it may be difficult to distinguish between malignancy and infection with MRI. Diffuse bone marrow involvement may make interpretation by MRI difficult. This is also true in younger patients with relatively little fatty marrow. MRI is superior to CT scan without intrathecal contrast and often is superior to CT scan with myelography.

The most important attribute of spinal MRI is the ability to evaluate directly the full length of the cord, thus making it possible for multiple levels of compression to be identified and to determine whether these lesions are related or unrelated to bony erosion or bone destruction by tumor. At least 35% of patients who present with focal symptoms have evidence of subclinical epidural compression at other sites along the spine. MRI also can determine the number of segments and vertebrae involved, the location of a compressive mass, if present (anterior, posterior, or encircling), and perhaps the percentage loss of bone mass. Imaging of the entire spine is usually not done because of the length of time needed (as much as 3 hours), but not taking the time may miss lesions that cause later neurologic compromise. MRI is comparable to myelography and CT with contrast in detecting leptomeningeal metastasis. However, MRI may be inadequate in patients who may have had previous spinal surgery because metal-induced artifacts may be seen and the patient's movements cannot be controlled.

Differential Diagnosis

The differential diagnosis of spinal cord compression includes intervertebral disk herniation, vascular disease (hemorrhage or infarction), infectious processes such as epidural abscess, benign neoplasms (meningioma, neurilemoma, chordoma), neurologic disorders (multiple sclerosis, amyotrophic lateral sclerosis), transverse myelitis, leptomeningeal carcinomatosis, and paraneoplastic syndromes (eg, necrotizing myelopathy, carcinomatous neuropathy).

Treatment

Early recognition, diagnosis, and treatment of epidural spinal cord compression are of utmost importance. Either the presence of neurologic symptoms or radiographic evidence of epidural compression is sufficient to justify beginning treatment. Cord compression diagnosed after the onset of myelopathy has the most profound impact on the patient's quality of life. The drastic difference is between 2 and 6 months of ambulatory survival versus 2–6 months of bed or wheelchair confinement with a urinary catheter, potential urosepsis, pneumonia, and decubiti—and dependence on professional care or family members.

Two factors appear to predict a good prognosis: a normal pretreatment neurologic examination and urgent appropriate treatment. Other prognostic factors include the rate and onset of progression of neurologic dysfunction, histologic features of the primary tumor (myeloma, lymphoma, breast, and prostate have a better prognosis), the presence of vertebral collapse, and the location of the compressing lesion (anterior or posterior). In general, if patients are ambulatory before the start of treatment, two-thirds will remain ambulatory after treatment. If patients are paraparetic before treatment, one-third will be ambulatory after treatment; but if patients are paraplegic (especially if unresponsive to dexamethasone therapy), only a few—if any—will become ambulatory after treatment. The most commonly used treatment regimen consists of high-dose corticosteroid therapy plus external beam radiation. Surgery is used selectively either as initial treatment or when specifically indicated.

A. Corticosteroids

To reduce edema of the cord adjacent to the tumor, corticosteroids are frequently used in the treatment of spinal cord compression. These should be started as soon as the diagnosis is suspected. Delaying therapy while awaiting formal studies is unnecessary and may lead to further progression of the neurologic deficit. These drugs clearly improve the initial rate of neurologic recovery and often lead to stabilization of the neurologic deficit. The optimal dose of corticosteroids is not known and varies with the degree of neurologic impairment. In the presence of pain or radiculopathy alone, dexamethasone, 16 mg intravenously, followed by 4–6 mg intravenously or orally every 6 hours, is adequate. Patients with rapidly progressive symptoms or significant myelopathy should be treated with dexamethasone, 100 mg intravenously, followed by 24 mg intravenously every 6 hours. Therapy should be continued until benefit is demonstrated from definitive therapy (radiation or surgery) or neurologic deficits are considered irreversible. Tapering of corticosteroids is accomplished by reducing the dose by about one-third every 3–4 days over a period of 2–3 weeks. Corticosteroids should be reinstituted if neurologic deficits recur. Patients failing to improve after a 7-day trial at 100 mg/d should be rapidly tapered to the lowest dose that will maintain stable neurologic function. Such steroid regimens do not appear to be toxic, though vaginal burning may occur with rapid intravenous administration of dexamethasone. Conversely, corticosteroids may result in serious and fatal complications when used in high doses for more than 40 days or when given to patients with serum albumin < 2.5 g/dL.

B. Radiation Therapy

Radiation therapy alone produces neurologic improvement in 30–50% of patients with epidural spinal cord compression. Pain relief is obtained in the majority of patients with radiation therapy. Radiation-sensitive tumors such as hematologic malignancies and seminomas have the best outcome; breast and prostate cancer have moderately good outcomes; and lung and renal cancer, sarcomas, and melanoma are radioresistant and have the worst outcomes. Radiation therapy and surgical therapy appear to be of equal effectiveness in the treatment of radiosensitive tumors. The usual dose of radiation is 3000-4000 cGy over a period of 3–4 weeks. Complications of radiation therapy include radiation myelopathy and impaired wound healing in patients who undergo subsequent surgery.

C. Surgery

The surgical approach selected—laminectomy, anterior surgical decompression, or posterolateral surgical decompression—depends on several variables, including the specific element of vertebral involvement, cord level, and stability of the spine. The concept that surgery is not indicated in the treatment of spinal cord compression is based on retrospective analysis of several surgical series that compared decompressive laminectomy followed by radiation therapy with radiation therapy alone. No difference in neurologic outcome was initially reported. Better understanding of the pathogenesis of cord compression combined with advances in operative technique and materials have resulted in improved outcomes after surgical decompression. For example, results were reported in 54 patients with cord compression. Laminectomy was performed for posterior or lateral tumors and vertebral body resection for anterior ones. Occasionally, a combination of both was needed. Spine "stabilization" was performed when indicated, and radiation therapy was given to patients with radiosensitive tumors. All 54 patients improved, and 23 out of 25 patients surviving for 2 years remained ambulatory. The 30-day mortality rate in this series was 6% and the morbidity rate was 15%. The results of this study appear to be superior to those previously reported. It is important to note, however, that surgery is a major procedure associated with a significant rate of complications. Therefore, surgery should be used only in patients who have less extensive disease and longer life expectancy.

Laminectomy allows for direct access to posterior tumors and posterior lateral tumors involving the dorsal elements, laminae, and pedicles but is associated with increased instability of the spine. In addition, laminectomy may not reduce symptoms, as most tumors involve the anterior cord. Anterior surgical decompression provides immediate mechanical stability and the best opportunity for neurologic stabilization and recovery. Compared with laminectomy, there is less blood loss and a superior success rate, usually over 80%. The vertebral body is completely removed in the anterior approach and the spine is reconstructed with methyl methacrylate combined with metal plates or bone grafts when prolonged survival is anticipated. Posterolateral surgical decompression is usually reserved for lesions above the sixth thoracic vertebra and has the advantage of avoiding thoracotomy. However, access to the tumor is usually limited. Patient recovery is often rapid, though neurologic recovery from cord compression is variable and not as predictable as seen in the anterior approach. Newer and less invasive procedures are promising and include vertebroplasty, which utilizes a percutaneous fluoroscope-guided technique to inject methyl methacrylate into the diseased vertebra.

There is general agreement that in the absence of medical contraindications, surgery may be considered (1) when the diagnosis is not known or is in doubt; (2) when there is spinal instability or bone deformity; (3) when there is failure to respond to radiation therapy; (4) when there is a history of previous radiation therapy up to cord tolerance; (5) when there is high cervical spinal cord compression (because of the danger of respiratory failure); (6) in the presence of a radioresistant tumor, especially when the onset of signs is rapid and complete block is present; (7) when atlantoaxial compression is present; (8) when a solitary spinal cord metastasis is present; and (9) as a form of primary treatment before radiation therapy. When possible, it is recommended that adjuvant chemotherapy be delayed for 3–6 weeks after surgical therapy to minimize wound complications.

Table 20–1 offers an approach to the patient with known or suspected malignancy that presents with back pain and possible spinal cord compression.

Byrne TN: Spinal cord compression. N Engl J Med 1992;327: 614–9.

Daw HA, Markman M: Epidural spinal cord compression in cancer patients: diagnosis and management. Cleve Clin J Med 2000;67:497, 501–4.

Ingham J, Beveridge A, Cooney NJ: The management of spinal cord compression in patients with advanced malignancy. J Pain Symptom Manage 1993;8:1–6.

Janjan N: Bone metastases: approaches to management. Semin Oncol 2001;4(Suppl 11):28–34.

Loblaw DA, Laperriere NJ: Emergency treatment of malignant extradural spinal cord compression: an evidence-based guideline. J Clin Oncol 1998;16:1613-24.

INCREASED INTRACRANIAL PRESSURE

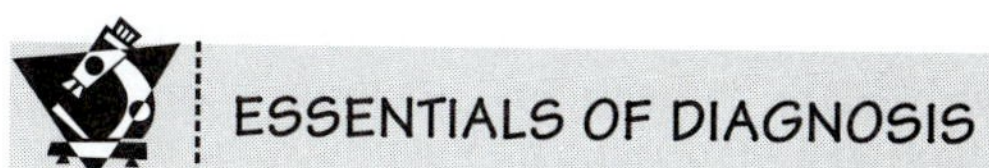
ESSENTIALS OF DIAGNOSIS

- *Mental deterioration, lethargy, somnolence, or confusion.*
- *Changes in heart rate and blood pressure.*
- *Pupillary changes.*
- *Neurologic deficits, focal or nonfocal.*
- *Abnormal brain CT or MRI diagnostic or suspicious of intracranial tumor or metastases.*

General Considerations

Increased intracranial pressure can cause neurologic damage either directly or indirectly by way of herniation of the cerebellar tonsil or uncus or by secondary vascular compromise. It is essential that prompt management be instituted in order to prevent loss of cerebral function.

Increased intracranial pressure can be caused by primary or metastatic tumors. At least one-fourth of patients dying from malignancy will have brain metastases discovered at autopsy. Hematogenous spread is the most common route of dissemination. Thus, most lesions (approximately 80%) are supratentorial. The most common tumors responsible include lung cancer, renal cancer, breast cancer, and melanoma. Hemorrhagic transformation is commonly seen in brain metastases from choriocarcinoma, melanoma, and breast cancer. The tumors may be single or multiple and should be distinguished from diffuse infiltrative processes that also may cause in-

Table 20–1. Management of patients with back pain and suspected malignancy.

Other Clinical Findings	Diagnostic Studies	Treatment
Normal or neurologic examination Normal plain spine x-rays	MRI for high-risk tumors or in the presence of other metastatic disease. If MRI is not available, then CT, CT with myelography, or myelography. Observe closely for low-risk primary tumors.	Treatment depends on MRI or CT findings.
Normal neurologic examination Abnormal plain spine films	None	Radiation therapy to symptomatic vertebral metastases without further imaging. **Advantages:** No delay in treatment, no further expense. **Disadvantages:** May miss other sites of disease that may become symptomatic later and compromise further radiotherapy because of overlapping radiation therapy ports. Disadvantages reduced if x-ray of entire spine is obtained, radiation port includes two segments above and below lesions, or bone scan is performed to document that disease is limited to one area of the spine.
	MRI, or CT with myelography.	Treatment depends on MRI or CT findings.
Abnormal neurologic examination Abnormal or normal plain spine x-rays	MRI of symptomatic area to identify adjacent levels of involvement. If MRI is unavailable, consider CT with myelography.	Treatment (radiation therapy) depends on MRI or CT findings. Consider selective surgery.

creased intracranial pressure. Leukemic meningitis and diffuse leukemic infiltration can also cause increased intracranial pressure without the focal neurologic or radiographic findings usually seen in primary or metastatic brain tumors. In the diffuse process, intracranial pressure increases without evidence of other concomitant findings, eg, localizing findings from a mass lesion.

Studies on the formation, speed, and resolution of brain edema have concluded that increased capillary permeability occurs within the brain tumor itself and not in the surrounding brain tissue. This increased capillary permeability varies depending on the histology of the tumor and its size. Brain edema occurs preferentially in the cerebral white matter. It is not clear how brain edema results in neurologic dysfunction, but it is thought to be related to ischemia from a mass effect or from metabolic abnormalities in the surrounding extravascular fluid.

Untreated, metastatic brain tumors ultimately lead to progressive neurologic function and death. The median survival in this setting is 4–6 weeks.

Clinical Features

A. Symptoms and Signs

Headache, nausea, vomiting, mental deterioration, lethargy, somnolence, and confusion are the key findings in patients with increased intracranial pressure. In addition, decrease in heart rate and increase in blood pressure are often present but are late findings. Cerebellar masses may, however, have a reversed clinical picture. Dilation of one or both pupils suggests rapid and significant increases in intracranial pressure. Focal neurologic deficits and abnormal reflexes may be found. Early diagnosis is usually based on the timely observation of subtle alterations in the mental status or state of consciousness of the patient.

B. Laboratory Findings

Lumbar puncture for diagnosis is to be discouraged, as removal of fluid from the intrathecal sac may result in an acute drop in intracranial pressure, thereby precipitating or worsening herniation.

C. Imaging Studies

Head CT scan and MRI are the safest diagnostic tests. The size and location of a tumor mass or masses, the amount of peritumoral edema, shifts in intracranial structures, and ventricular size can be easily determined. MRI is more sensitive than CT, especially when evaluating lesions of the posterior fossa. However, CT may better detect bony involvement of the skull. Both noncontrast and contrast studies are recommended, as the combination may not only detect hemorrhagic lesions but will allow for the detection of small lesions.

Differential Diagnosis

The differential diagnosis of increased intracranial pressure should include metabolic encephalopathy (hypo- and hypernatremia, hypercalcemia, uremia, hypoxemia, hypoglycemia, and thyroid dysfunction), central nervous system infection, cerebrovascular disease, drug-induced encephalopathy (especially from sedatives and analgesics), and nutritional deficiencies.

Treatment

A. Medical Treatment

If signs of cerebral herniation are evident, emergent reduction of intracranial pressure is warranted. Emergent maneuvers include elective intubation and hyperventilation to maintain $Pa{CO_2}$ between 25–30 mm Hg, followed by administration of mannitol, 1–1.5 g/kg intravenously every 6 hours. Use of mannitol should be avoided when definitive therapy (surgery or radiation) is delayed. Early corticosteroid (dexamethasone) administration and fluid restriction appear to be the best means of achieving a decrease of intracranial pressure and brain edema. The specific mechanism of action of corticosteroids on brain edema is not known. These agents may either decrease edema production or increase edema resorption. Corticosteroids appear to decrease tumor capillary permeability and alter the exchange of sodium and water across the endothelial cells and decrease cerebrospinal fluid production at the choroid plexus. Corticosteroid administration may result in symptomatic improvement within 4–5 hours, but more commonly such improvement occurs gradually over several days, with 70% of patients showing late significant clinical improvement. Dexamethasone is administered at a dosage of 16 mg/d in four divided doses, and the dosage may be increased to 100 mg/d. Some patients must remain on steroids for long periods and whenever they undergo definitive treatment such as surgery or radiation.

B. Surgical and Radiation Treatment

Surgery and radiation therapy are important methods of treatment of primary and metastatic brain tumors, either as initial or as adjunctive therapy. Candidates for surgical resection should be patients with solitary lesions and limited systemic disease. Radiation therapy usually involves the whole brain and requires an average of 3000 cGy. Most recently, radiosurgery has evolved as a new technique to deliver a single large dose of radiation to a specific target. Local control rates appear to be equal to those achieved with surgery. Radiosurgery is especially useful in patients with multiple or poorly accessible lesions.

Alexander E et al: Stereotactic radiosurgery for the definitive, noninvasive treatment of brain metastases. J Natl Cancer Inst 1995;87:34–40.

Boyd TS, Mehta MP: Stereotactic radiosurgery for brain metastases. Oncology 1999;13:1397–409.

Flickinger JC: Radiotherapy and radiosurgical management of brain metastases. Curr Oncol Rep 2001;3:484–9.

Sawaya R: Considerations in the diagnosis and management of brain metastases. Oncology 2001;15:1144–58.

METABOLIC DISORDERS

HYPERCALCEMIA OF MALIGNANCY

ESSENTIALS OF DIAGNOSIS

- *Mental status changes, lethargy, confusion, weakness.*
- *Decreased deep tendon reflexes without localized neurologic signs.*
- *History of malignancy, usually far-advanced.*
- *Elevated serum calcium, chloride:phosphate ratio, and parathyroid hormone-related polypeptide (PTHrP).*

General Considerations

Hypercalcemia is the most serious metabolic disorder associated with cancer. Ten to 20% of patients with cancer will develop hypercalcemia at some point during their course, and life expectancy is poor in these patients even when they are actively treated. Treatment of hypercalcemia of malignancy is usually palliative, as most of these patients have advanced disease. However, symptoms are usually improved with treatment, and many patients may be made well enough to go home from the hospital. While treatment of hypercalcemia may not prolong survival, it clearly improves quality of life.

Pathogenesis

Serum calcium is regulated by hormones and locally acting cytokines at three main sites: the gut, the skeletal system, and the kidneys. Parathyroid hormone (PTH) increases the number and function of osteoclasts, inhibits osteoblasts, and increases renal tubular reabsorption of calcium, all of which increases extracellular calcium levels. The hormone also increases production of active vitamin D, which increases the absorption of calcium from the gut.

In all cases of cancer-related hypercalcemia, there is increased calcium resorption from bones relative to bone formation (Figure 20–1). Increased bone resorption is maintained through the destructive action of tumor cells that spread to the bone by increased osteoclast activation mediated through the action of PTH-related polypeptide (PTHrP) and by locally acting cytokines. Squamous cell carcinomas originating in the lung, head and neck, esophagus, uterine cervix, vagina, and penis—as well as cancers of the breast, lung, and kidney—produce PTHrP. This hormone shares homology with the amino terminal portion of parathyroid-produced PTH only in eight of the first thirteen amino acids. It has predicted isoforms of 139, 141, and 173 amino acids, as compared with 84 amino acids in PTH. PTHrP, like PTH, can mediate bone resorption of calcium and renal tubular absorption of calcium, but unlike PTH, serum calcium levels do not regulate its secretion. PTH and PTHrP are distinguishable by radioassay, and for that reason it is possible to distinguish humoral hypercalcemia of malignancy from coexisting primary hyperparathyroidism. Despite a high frequency of bony metastases, prostate, small cell lung cancer, and colorectal carcinoma are rarely associated with hypercalcemia.

In addition to PTHrP, a variety of locally active **cytokines** augment resorption of calcium from bone, including interleukin-1 (IL-1), IL-3, and IL-6, tumor necrosis factors (TNF-α and TNF-β), and lymphotoxins—all of which are components of what was formerly called osteoclast-activating factor. Furthermore, transforming growth factor (TGF-α), platelet-derived growth factor, and certain hematopoietic colony-stimulating factors such as GM-CSF can also augment bone resorption. In patients with myeloma, increased bone resorption from cytokines is the primary mechanism for hypercalcemia. Finally, prostaglandin E_2 also can increase bone resorption. However, there are two locally acting cytokines that decrease the amount of calcium from bone: interferon-γ and transforming growth factor-beta (TGF-β). Both cytokines inhibit osteoclasts and bone resorption, and TGF-β promotes osteoblast activity.

Some lymphomas can convert sufficient amount of vitamin D to increase gut absorption of calcium and, together with the calcium resorption from cytokines acting locally in bone, may produce hypercalcemia. Hypercalcemia is a prominent feature of adult T cell lymphomas (45% of cases) and of lymphomas and leukemias associated with HTLV-1 (90%).

Clinical Features

When hypercalcemia results from malignancy, the cancer is rarely occult. Patients with severe hypercalcemia (serum calcium > 14 mg/dL) are usually symptomatic. These symptoms are often related to the rapidity of onset

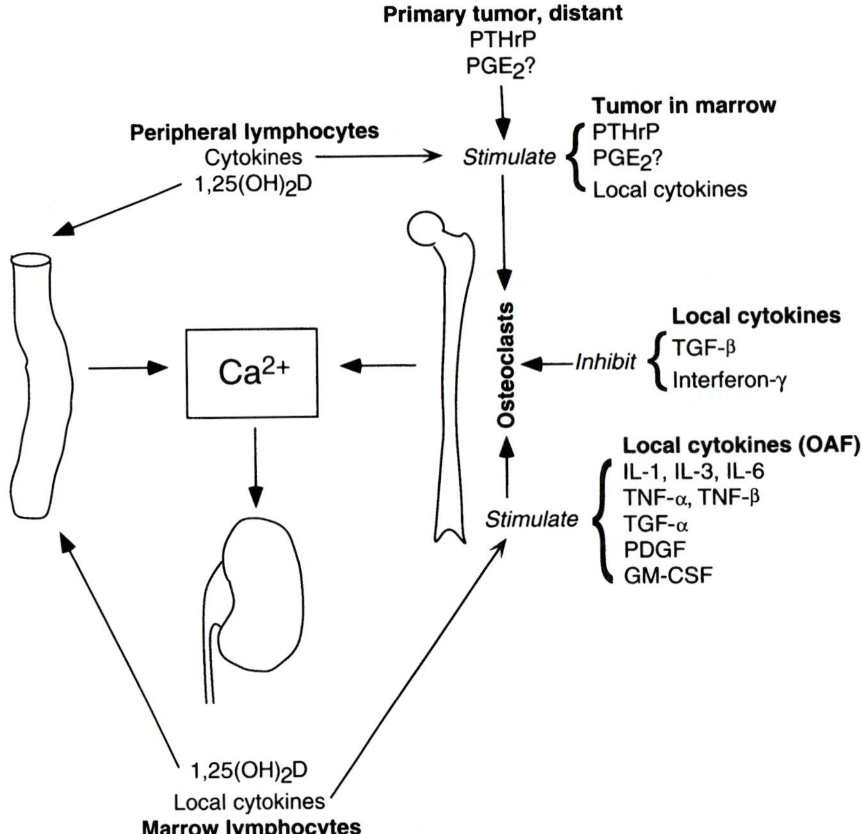

Figure 20–1 Mechanisms of hypercalcemia of malignancy. Osteoclast activity can be stimulated by hormones, cytokines, and other substances from certain primary tumors distant from bone or by tumor in the bone marrow. In other patients, local production of cytokines previously known as osteoclast-activating factors are the primary mediators of increased calcium mobilization. Both peripheral blood and marrow lymphocytes produce cytokines that affect osteoclasts. $1,25(OH)_2$ vitamin D increases calcium absorption from the small intestine. Other local cytokines have an inhibitory effect on osteoclast activity ($1,25[OH]_2D$, vitamin D; PTHrP, parathyroid hormone-related polypeptide; IL, interleukin; TGF-α and TGF-β, transforming growth factors alpha and beta; TNF-α and TNF-β, tumor necrosis factors alpha and beta; PDGF, platelet-derived growth factor; GM-CSF, granulocyte-macrophage colony-stimulating factor.)

of hypercalcemia. The clinical features of hypercalcemia and, in particular, its neuromuscular manifestations tend to be much more prominent in the elderly. Other factors such as the patient's performance status, the use of chemotherapy, sites of metastasis, and the presence of hepatic or renal dysfunction may increase the severity of symptoms. As calcium is a critical regulator of cellular function, patients with hypercalcemia may have a wide range of symptoms affecting different organ systems. Conversely, the most common symptoms of hypercalcemia may be nonspecific and are similar to those seen in patients with chronic or terminal illnesses, such as nausea, anorexia, weakness, fatigue, lethargy, and confusion. In late stages, patients may be stuporous or comatose, and their symptoms may mimic a neurologic emergency.

A. Neurologic

The major neurologic manifestations include weakness, altered mental status, and decreased deep tendon reflexes. Initial manifestations may include personality changes, impaired concentration and apathy, mild confusion and irritability, lethargy, hallucinations, and psychosis, with progression to stupor and coma. Localized neurologic signs are usually absent.

B. Gastrointestinal

Because of the depressive action of hypercalcemia on autonomic nervous tissue, nonspecific symptoms such as anorexia, nausea, and vomiting may occur. These often progress to include abdominal pain, constipation, frank obstipation, increased gastric acid secretion, and acute pancreatitis.

C. Renal

Hypercalcemia causes a reversible tubular defect in the kidney that results in loss of urinary concentrating ability and promotion of dehydration or hypovolemia. If able, patients will admit to polyuria, nocturia, and polydipsia. Metabolic alkalosis is common, and acidosis occurs only when azotemia supervenes. This contrasts with the effects of parathyroid hormone, in which a mild hyperchloremic acidosis is seen. Hypercalcemia can also lead to precipitation of calcium phosphate crystals in the kidneys and ureters and the formation of renal calculi. Such complications, however, are not commonly associated with hypercalcemia of malignancy, and when it occurs the possibility of coexisting primary hyperparathyroidism should be considered.

D. Cardiovascular

Hypercalcemia is associated with electrocardiographic disturbances such as prolongation of the PR and QRS intervals and shortening of the QT interval. With severe hypercalcemia (> 16 mg/dL), the T wave widens, increasing the QT interval. At higher serum calcium concentrations, bradyarrhythmias and bundle branch block may develop, followed by complete heart block and cardiac arrest in systole.

E. Bone and Extraskeletal Tissues

Hypercalcemia can result either from humorally mediated bone resorption or from osteolytic metastasis. Pain, fractures, and skeletal deformities can occur. Metastatic calcification occurs in long-standing and very severe hypercalcemia. Extraskeletal deposition of calcium has been observed with hypercalcemia in several organs, including the heart, lungs, kidneys, skin, joints, and conjunctiva.

F. Laboratory Findings

Serum calcium, phosphate, and albumin levels should be determined in all patients. Ionized calcium accounts for almost half of the serum calcium and is in equilibrium with protein-bound calcium circulating in sera. The corrected serum calcium (mg/dL) is equal to the measured calcium plus $0.8 \times (4 - \text{measured albumin})$. This calculation is especially helpful when malnutrition coexists with hypercalcemia. Hypophosphatemia in the presence of hypercalcemia strongly suggests primary hyperparathyroidism. Elevated alkaline phosphatase is usually not helpful, as this is seen in both primary hyperparathyroidism and hypercalcemia of malignancy. Direct measurement of PTH and PTHrP may be necessary in some cases.

G. Radiographs

Nephrocalcinosis and nephrolithiasis may be present in long-standing hypercalcemia and suggest hyperparathyroidism.

Differential Diagnosis

The differential diagnosis of hypercalcemia of malignancy includes a wide variety of conditions (Table 20–2). Among all patients, the two most common causes of hypercalcemia are malignancy (35%) and primary hyperparathyroidism (54%). Among hospitalized patients with hypercalcemia, 77% have malignancies, 4% have

Table 20–2. Causes of hypercalcemia.

- **I. Primary hyperparathyroidism (54%)**
- **II. Cancer (35%)**
  - A. Caused by hormones (HHM) (80%)
    - 1. Most common: Lung cancer (especially epidermoid) and renal cell carcinoma.
    - 2. Less common: Head and neck cancer, ovarian cancer, hepatoma, pancreatic cancer, bladder cancer, endometrial cancer, lymphomas, leukemia, multiple myeloma.
    - 3. Isolated case reports: Esophageal cancer, colon cancer, rectal cancer, cervical cancer, uterine leiomyosarcoma, vulvar cancer, cancer of the penis, prostate cancer, adrenal cancer, melanoma, hemangiopericytoma, branchial rest cancer, parotid cancer, breast cancer, mammary dysplasia.
  - B. Caused by metastatic destruction of bone (20%). Breast cancer (most common), multiple myeloma, lymphoma, and leukemia.
- **III. Others (11%)**
  - A. Nonparathyroid endocrine disorders: Thyrotoxicosis, pheochromocytoma, adrenal insufficiency, vasoactive intestinal polypeptide hormone-producing tumor.
  - B. Granulomatous diseases: 1,25 $(OH)_2$ vitamin D excess, sarcoidosis, tuberculosis, histoplasmosis, coccidioidomycosis, leprosy.
  - C. Medications: Thiazide diuretics, lithium, estrogens, and antiestrogens.
  - D. Milk-alkali syndrome.
  - E. Vitamin A or vitamin D intoxication.
  - F. Familial hypocalciuric hypercalcemia.
  - G. Immobilization.
  - H. Parenteral nutrition.

HHM = humoral hyperglycemia of malignancy.

coexistent hyperparathyroidism, 2% have vitamin D intoxication, 2% have tamoxifen-induced hypercalcemia, and 16% are due to other causes. Table 20–3 lists features that may be used to differentiate primary hyperparathyroidism from hypercalcemia of malignancy.

Treatment

There is no one regimen that should be applied to the acute management of all cases of hypercalcemia. Moderate hypercalcemia with minimal symptoms may be managed with administration of intravenous normal saline. If the hypercalcemia is more severe and is symptomatic, furosemide and calcitonin may be added. As the effects of calcitonin are not long-lasting, the use of bisphosphonates early in treatment is probably indicated. In patients with lymphoma or myeloma and hypercalcemia, corticosteroids are useful because of the significant role of cytokines to the hypercalcemia. Intravenous administration of sodium phosphate can lower serum calcium rapidly, but its use is dangerous because calcium phosphate complexes will deposit in blood vessels, lungs, and kidneys with resulting severe organ damage and even fatal hypotension. Therefore, intravenous phosphates are not recommended. Oral phosphates are of limited value because diarrhea often develops with an intake of more than 2 g/d. Azotemia and hyperphosphatemia are contraindications to phosphate therapy.

Therapy for hypercalcemia in cancer patients centers on four main mechanisms: (1) correction of volume depletion; (2) inhibition of bone resorption of calcium; (3) enhancement of renal calcium excretion; and (4) treatment of the underlying malignancy. Table 20–4 summarizes the available drugs and their dosages.

A. Fluid and Electrolytes

Volume and electrolyte repletion are the first priorities. Normal saline (0.9% NaCl), usually containing potassium chloride (10–20 meq/L), is given at a rate of 2–3 L/d. Loop diuretics such as furosemide (40–80 mg intravenously) are used to induce calciuresis once fluid deficits are corrected. Judicious fluid administration or central venous pressure monitoring may be appropriate in patients with poor urine output or congestive heart failure. As a result of calcium-related renal tubular impairment and the resulting polyuria, urine output may not be a reliable measure of intravascular volume repletion.

B. Calcitonin

Calcitonin is a useful adjunct in the initial phase of therapy. It is nontoxic and acts within 4–24 hours. Calcitonin promotes renal excretion of calcium, inhibits bone resorption, and inhibits gut absorption of calcium. The effects of calcitonin, however, are minor and of short duration. Calcitonin is usually administered over 24 hours as an intravenous infusion in a dose of 3 units/kg or 100–400 units subcutaneously every 8–12 hours.

C. Corticosteroids

Corticosteroids decrease intestinal calcium absorption and inhibit bone resorption and in that way act as vitamin D antagonists. They also inhibit the action of some of the locally acting cytokines that mediate calcium mobilization from bone. They are effective primarily in hematologic malignancies and breast cancer, primarily to control chronic hypercalcemia.

Table 20–3. Features used to differentiate primary hyperparathyroidism from malignancy-related hypercalcemia.

	Primary Hyperparathroidism	Hypercalcemia of Malignancy
Symptoms	Mild or absent	Symptomatic
Serum calcium	Mildly increased (< 14 mg/dL)	Significantly increased (> 14 mg/dL)
Serum phosphorus	Decreased	Variable
Serum potassium	Normal	Usually decreased
Serum chloride	Increased[1]	Low or normal
Serum bicarbonate	Decreased (hyperchloremic acidosis)	Normal or increased (hypochloremic alkalosis)
Urinary calcium	Increased	Markedly increased
Urinary cAMP	Increased	Variable
1,25 $(OH)_2$ vitamin D	Increased	Usually decreased

[1]Serum chloride:phosphate ratio is increased.

Table 20–4. Drugs used in the treatment of hypercalcemia of malignancy.

1. IV hydration with 3–6 L of 0.9% NaCl with 40–80 mg of potassium chloride per liter over 24 hours.
2. Furosemide, 40–160 mg IV over 24 hours.
3. Bisphosphonates:
   Pamidronate, 60–90 mg in 1 L 0.9% NaCl over 4–24 hours.
   Etidronate, 7.5 mg/kg in 300 mL 0.9% NaCl over 3 hours for 3–5 days.
4. Calcitonin: Extremely useful in patients with life-threatening hypercalcemia. It has the most rapid action: 2–4 hours.
   600 IU in 1 L 0.9% NaCl over 6 hours.
   6–8 IU/kg IM every 6–8 hours for 2–3 days.
5. Corticosteroids: 200–300 mg of hydrocortisone per day or equivalent.
6. Gallium nitrate: 200 mg/m^2 in 1 L 5% dextrose over 24 hours for 5 days.
7. Plicamycin: 25 μg/kg for total dose of 1.5–2 mg IV administered in brief infusion or over 12 hours. No benefit from prolonged infusion.
8. Phosphates: Oral phosphates, 0.5–3 g/d diluted in water. IV phosphates should not be given.

Formula to correct serum calcium for changes in serum albumin concentration: Corrected serum calcium = Measured total calcium value (mg/dL) – serum albumin valve (g/dL) + 4.

D. Bisphosphonates

Bisphosphonates are routinely used because of their efficacy and low toxicity. They are potent inhibitors of osteoclasts and bind to hydroxyapatite in bone to inhibit dissolution of crystals. Two preparations of bisphosphonates are available in the United States for treatment of hypercalcemia of malignancy: pamidronate disodium and etidronate disodium. A single dose of pamidronate (60–90 mg in 1 L of normal saline over 4–24 hours) by intravenous infusion is safe and is more effective than intravenous etidronate (7.5 mg/kg in 500 mL of normal saline over 3 hours daily for 3–5 days). Significant reductions in serum calcium usually occur in 1–2 days and persist for several weeks. Oral etidronate (20 mg/kg per day) may be used for maintenance in patients with prolonged hypercalcemia.

E. Dialysis

Peritoneal dialysis or hemodialysis is very effective in treatment of hypercalcemia but is usually reserved for management in the setting of renal failure or life-threatening manifestations.

F. Other Therapies

Plicamycin and gallium nitrate decrease bone resorption. Prostaglandin synthetase inhibitors and other investigational drugs such as amifostine (WR-2721) have been used. Amifostine inhibits parathyroid hormone secretion and bone resorption and facilitates urinary excretion of calcium.

All patients should be encouraged to avoid immobilization and ambulate. In addition, liberal fluid intake and avoidance of large amounts of foods rich in calcium is also suggested.

Bajournas DR: Manifestations of cancer related hypercalcemia. Semin Oncol 1990;17:16–25.

Bilezikian JP: Management of acute hypercalcemia. N Engl J Med 1992;326:1196–203.

Bushinsky DA, Monk RD: Calcium. Lancet 1998;352:305–11.

Flombaum CD: Metabolic emergencies in the cancer patient. Semin Oncol 2000;27:322–34.

Heys SD, Smith IC, Eremin O: Hypercalcaemia in patients with cancer: aetiology and treatment. Eur J Surg Oncol 1998; 24:139–42.

Leyvraz S et al: Pharmacokinetics of pamidronate in patients with bone metastases. J Natl Cancer Inst 1992;84:788–92.

Mundy GR, Guise TA: Hypercalcemia of malignancy. Am J Med 1997;103:134–45.

Odell WD: Endocrine/metabolic syndromes of cancer. Semin Oncol 1997;24:299–317.

Orloff JJ, Stewart AF: Disorders of serum minerals caused by cancer. In: *Disorders of Bone and Mineral Metabolism.* Coe FL, Favus MJ (editors). Raven Press, 1992.

HYPOCALCEMIA IN MALIGNANT DISEASE

ESSENTIALS OF DIAGNOSIS

- *Tetany; paresthesias of the face, hands, and feet.*
- *Positive Chvostek and Trousseau signs.*
- *Muscle cramps, laryngeal spasm, headache, lethargy.*
- *Low serum calcium.*
- *Osteoblastic metastases (breast or prostate cancer) or tumor lysis syndrome with elevated serum phosphorus.*

General Considerations

Hypocalcemia is a rare complication of cancer, resulting from osteoblastic metastasis secondary either to rapid bone healing in patients with prostate or breast cancer receiving hormonal therapy or to hyperphosphatemia in patients with tumor lysis syndrome. The most common neoplasm associated with hypocalcemia is prostate cancer, and 31% of patients with prostate cancer and extensive osteoblastic bone metastasis develop hypocalcemia. The skeleton in these cases has been described as a "calcium sink." Hypocalcemia secondary to tumor lysis syndrome may be severe and appears to result from a rise in the serum calcium × phosphorus product, leading to precipitation of calcium in soft tissues, including the kidneys, and the development of secondary hyperparathyroidism.

Hypocalcemia may also occur secondarily in patients with low circulating 1,25$(OH)_2$ vitamin D and calcifying chondrosarcoma. Magnesium deficiency results in hypocalcemia in patients with prolonged nasogastric drainage, parenteral hyperalimentation without magnesium supplementation, cisplatin therapy, long-term diuretic therapy, chronic diarrhea, and chronic alcoholism and does not respond to calcium replacement alone. Treatment with plicamycin or intravenous phosphate may also cause hypocalcemia.

Clinical Features

The diagnosis of hypocalcemia is made with ease in patients who develop tetany. Paresthesias of the face, hands, and feet associated with muscle cramps, laryngeal spasm, diarrhea, headache, lethargy, irritability, or seizures are the common clinical manifestations. Chvostek's and Trousseau's signs are usually present. The ECG usually shows a prolonged QT interval. In long-standing cases dry skin, papilledema, and cataracts may develop.

Differential Diagnosis

The differential diagnosis of hypocalcemia should include severe alkalosis secondary to vomiting, nasogastric suction, or hyperventilation and severe muscle cramps resulting from vincristine or procarbazine therapy.

Treatment

Treatment of acute severe hypocalcemia (serum calcium < 6 mg/dL) consists of intravenous administration of calcium gluconate or calcium chloride, 1 g every 15–20 minutes until tetany disappears, and magnesium sulfate, 1 g intravenously or intramuscularly every 8–12 hours if the serum magnesium level is less than 1.5 mg/dL or is unknown. In patients with moderate hypocalcemia (serum calcium > 7 mg/dL), calcium and magnesium may be replaced more slowly.

Tohme JF, Bilezikan JP: Hypocalcemic emergencies. Endocrinol Metab Clin North Am 1993;22:363–75.

TUMOR LYSIS SYNDROME

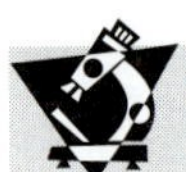

ESSENTIALS OF DIAGNOSIS

- *Lethargy, tetany, muscle cramps, convulsions.*
- *History of administration of chemotherapy to patient with rapidly proliferating malignancy.*
- *Elevated serum uric acid, potassium, phosphate, and urea nitrogen.*

General Considerations

Chemotherapy may release massive amounts of potassium, phosphate, uric acid, and other breakdown products of dying tumor cells into the bloodstream. Hypocalcemia due to hyperphosphatemia may occur. This syndrome occurs most commonly in patients with rapidly proliferating and chemotherapy-sensitive malignancies such as acute leukemia and Burkitt's lymphoma and, on rare occasions, following treatment of solid tumors and chronic lymphocytic leukemia (CLL). Life-threatening complications may occur, including renal failure from hyperuricemia and cardiac arrhythmias induced by hyperkalemia or hypocalcemia.

Diagnosis of tumor lysis syndrome is made because of lethargy, tetany, muscle cramps, and convulsions occurring in a patient with an appropriate tumor who has just received chemotherapy. Hyperkalemia, hyperphosphatemia, azotemia, and oliguria are usually present.

Treatment

Early recognition of risk is the key to prevention and treatment of this complication of cancer therapy. In spite of appropriate treatment, renal insufficiency may still occur. However, prognosis is good and recovery to baseline renal function is expected.

A. Hyperkalemia

Immediate treatment of hyperkalemia consists of administration of 50–100 mL of 50% dextrose in water and 10 units of regular insulin. Removal of potassium can be achieved with oral sodium polystyrene sulfonate, 20–30 g every 6 hours. Hyperkalemia due to adrenal insufficiency may be corrected with mineralocorticoid replacement (ie, with fludrocortisone) 0.05–0.2 mg daily. Hemodialysis may be necessary for the management of chronic or refractory hyperkalemia.

B. Hyperphosphatemia

Hyperphosphatemia is typically severe, with serum levels ranging from 6 mg to 35 mg/dL resulting from tumor cell lysis and renal failure. Patients should be given 20% dextrose in water and insulin until the serum phosphate level falls below 7 mg/dL. Aluminum hydroxide, 30–60 mL orally every 2–6 hours, is used to bind phosphate in the intestines. Oral fluids are given at the rate of 2–4 L every 24 hours. Dialysis may be necessary for patients with renal failure.

C. Hyperuricemia and Hyperuricosuria

Increase in urinary uric acid excretion may occur in untreated patients with rapidly growing malignancies or during their treatment with chemotherapy or radiation therapy. Excessive production of uric acid may result in uric acid nephropathy secondary to the precipitation of uric acid crystals in the kidneys. Hyperuricemic nephropathy, uric acid nephrolithiasis, or interstitial nephritis may also result. When massive doses of allopurinol are used to prevent uric acid production, renal oxypurinol stones may form.

Prevention of hyperuricemia is the cornerstone of management. Allopurinol should be given to patients with myeloproliferative disorders and hematologic malignancies at least 12 hours before starting chemotherapy. Vigorous hydration and alkalinization of the urine are essential to decrease risks of urinary tract precipitation of uric acid. Urine flow should be maintained at a rate of more than 100 mL/h, and urine pH should be between 7.0 and 7.5. Sodium bicarbonate or acetazolamide may be given to alkalinize the urine.

Altman A: Acute tumor lysis syndrome. Semin Oncol 2001;28(2 Suppl 5):3–12.

Lorigan PC et al: Tumour lysis syndrome: case report and review of the literature. Ann Oncol 1996;7:631–9.

HYPONATREMIA IN MALIGNANCY

ESSENTIALS OF DIAGNOSIS

- *Nausea, anorexia, lethargy, confusion, weakness, convulsions, coma.*
- *Low serum sodium with persistent excretion of urinary sodium.*
- *Normal renal function with low serum urea nitrogen, absence of fluid retention, and absence of intravascular volume contraction.*
- *History of malignancy, most frequently small cell carcinoma of the lung.*

General Considerations

Hyponatremia is most often associated in malignant disease with the syndrome of inappropriate antidiuretic hormone secretion (SIADH), resulting from secretion of ADH by the tumor. SIADH causes an increase in total body water with moderate expansion of plasma volume, hyponatremia, plasma hypo-osmolality, and inability to excrete maximally diluted urine. It may occur with any malignancy but is most frequently associated with small cell carcinoma of the lung and mesothelioma. Other causes of SIADH are the administration of thiazide diuretics, vincristine, cyclophosphamide, chlorpropamide, tolbutamide, carbamazepine, intravenous opioids, and psychotropic drugs (amitriptyline and thioridazine) in the setting of treatment of the cancer patient.

Clinical Features

A. Symptoms and Signs

Lethargy, nausea, anorexia, and generalized weakness are the most common symptoms. Such symptoms, however, are nonspecific and may be caused by the primary cancer rather than hyponatremia. Confusion, convulsions, coma, and death may occur if hyponatremia is severe or of rapid onset.

B. Laboratory Findings

Serum sodium is less than 135 meq/L, and there is persistent excretion of urinary sodium. Renal function tests are normal, and edema and intravascular volume contraction do not occur. BUN is characteristically low.

Diagnostic criteria for SIADH include: hyponatremia with low serum urea nitrogen (< 10 mg/dL), absence of intravascular volume contraction, persistent urinary excretion of sodium (> 30 meq/L), absence of fluid retention such as peripheral edema or ascites, normal renal function, and serum hypotonicity in the presence of urine that is not maximally dilute (urine osmolarity > 100–150 mosm/L with plasma osmolarity < 260 mosm/L).

Differential Diagnosis

The differential diagnosis in patients with low serum sodium comprises a long list that includes edematous states (heart failure, nephrotic syndrome, cirrhosis), myxedema, salt-wasting states (mineralocorticoid deficiency, glucocorticoid deficiency, chronic renal failure), gastrointestinal electrolyte losses with hypotonic fluid replacement, compulsive water drinking, and hypothalamic disorders. Pseudohyponatremia secondary to hyperglycemia, mannitol administration, marked hyperlipidemia, and paraproteinemia should be excluded.

Treatment

Treatment of hyponatremia is discussed in Chapter 2. The management of severe hyponatremia (serum sodium < 110 meq/L) should be aggressive in a patient who is comatose or convulsing, with the goal of raising serum sodium above 120 meq/L but no higher than 130 meq/L. In other patients, a maximum increase of serum sodium of 8 meq/L in 24 hours should be the target because of the complication of osmotic demyelination syndrome.

Patients with serum sodium ≤ 125 meq/L should be restricted to 500–700 mL of fluid a day. Patients with higher serum sodium concentrations are restricted to 1000 mL/d. Severe hyponatremia or symptomatic hyponatremia of any severity may require other treatment. Administration of normal saline solution (0.9% NaCl) does not correct the hyponatremia in patients with SIADH. In these patients, hypertonic saline (3% NaCl, 1000 mL over 6–8 hours) and furosemide, 40–80 mg every 6–8 hours as needed, may be necessary. Central venous pressure monitoring can reduce the risk of the precipitous development of pulmonary edema. Serum sodium and potassium concentrations should be monitored hourly. Furosemide and hypertonic saline are discontinued when serum sodium exceeds 110 meq/L and fluid restriction is started.

For chronic hyponatremia, demeclocycline, 150–300 mg orally four times daily, may be given to patients who cannot tolerate chronic fluid restriction or do not improve with fluid restriction. Demeclocycline induces nephrotoxic diabetes insipidus and may cause azotemia. Lithium salts may also be used but are not reliable.

Adrogue HJ, Madias NE: Hyponatremia. N Engl J Med 2000;342:1581–9.

Gross P et al: Treatment of severe hyponatremia: conventional and novel aspects. J Am Soc Nephrol 2001;12(Suppl 17):10–4.

Kovacs L, Robertson GL: Syndrome of inappropriate antidiuresis. Endocrinol Metab Clin North Am 1992;21:859–75.

Odell WD: Endocrine/metabolic syndromes of cancer. Semin Oncol 1997;24:299–317.

HYPOKALEMIA & ECTOPIC ACTH SECRETION

A variety of tumors secrete ACTH, stimulate adrenal production of corticosteroids, and result in Cushing's syndrome. The tumors include small cell lung cancer; carcinoid tumors of the bronchi, pancreas, thymus, and ovary; islet cell tumors; and cancers of the ovary, thyroid, and prostate as well as pheochromocytoma, hematologic malignancies, and sarcomas. Unfortunately, most malignant causes of ectopic ACTH production are rapidly fatal. Patients typically present with weakness, cachexia, and hypertension. Typical features of nonmalignant chronic Cushing's syndrome are often absent.

The differential diagnosis of hypokalemia includes gastrointestinal losses associated with alkalosis, vomiting, prolonged nasogastric suction, villous adenoma of the colon, Zollinger-Ellison syndrome, and chronic laxative abuse. Hyperaldosteronism, hypercortisolism, hypercalcemia, and licorice ingestion may also cause hypokalemia.

The most effective treatment of hypokalemia is control of the underlying tumor. Carcinoid, thyroid tumors, pheochromocytoma, and islet cell tumors are treated surgically if they are resectable. If the tumors are nonresectable, chemotherapy may be used (mitotane, metyrapone, ketoconazole, and aminoglutethimide). Potassium replacement should be accomplished as early as possible. Spironolactone, 100–400 mg daily, is helpful.

HYPOPHOSPHATEMIA IN MALIGNANCY

Hypophosphatemia (serum phosphorus < 3 mg/dL) is occasionally associated with rapidly growing tumors (acute leukemia) and marked nutritional deprivation and cachexia. Symptoms may include generalized weakness, respiratory muscle weakness causing respiratory failure, decreased myocardial function, platelet dysfunction, and leukocyte dysfunction. Hemolysis and rhabdomyolysis may occur with serum phosphorus < 1 mg/dL. The management of severe hypophosphatemia (serum phosphorus < 1 mg/dL) consists of intravenous administration of a solution of 30–40 mmol/L of neutral sodium phosphate or potassium phosphate at the rate of 50–100 mL/h. Intravenous administration of phosphates should be monitored very carefully. Patients with mild hypophosphatemia (serum phosphorus 1–2 mg/dL) can be given inorganic phosphate supplements orally unless severely symptomatic.

HYPERGLYCEMIA IN MALIGNANCY

Hyperglycemia not due to insulin deficiency is present in many patients with cancer. It occurs in patients with glucagonoma, somatostatinoma, pheochromocytoma, and ACTH-secreting tumors. Nonketotic hyperglycemia with hyperosmolar coma may occur as a complication of treatment with cyclophosphamide, vincristine, or prednisone in patients with mild diabetes mellitus and in patients who are receiving hyperalimentation.

Hyperglycemia caused by a tumor may respond to treatment of the primary tumor with surgical resection, radiation therapy, or chemotherapy. Hyperosmolar coma is treated with replacement of fluid losses (intravenous NaCl solutions) and insulin administration.

HYPOGLYCEMIA IN MALIGNANCY

Hypoglycemia may be secondary to inappropriate secretion of insulin (insulinoma) or to nonsuppressible insulin-like substances that are produced by some tumors. Large retroperitoneal fibrosarcomas, mesotheliomas, and renal, adrenal, and primary hepatocellular carcinomas are the most common tumors associated with hypoglycemia. Patients with extensive hepatic metastases may develop severe hypoglycemia secondary to depletion of glycogen and impaired gluconeogenesis. Other causes of hypoglycemia include administration of drugs such as insulin, oral hypoglycemic agents, alcohol, and salicylates. Starvation, chronic liver disease, hypoadrenalism, hypopituitarism, and myxedema may also cause hypoglycemia. Pseudohypoglycemia may occur in patients with marked granulocytosis, especially in the setting of myeloproliferative disorders.

Tumor-associated hypoglycemia produces changes that are characteristic of hypoglycemia in the fasting state such as fatigue, convulsions, or coma. On the other hand, tremors, sweating, tachycardia, and hunger are symptoms more characteristic of reactive hypoglycemia in the fed state.

Intravenous glucose is the treatment of choice and should be given to all patients with blood glucose < 40 mg/dL and symptomatic patients with glucose < 60 mg/dL. Continuous infusion of 20% dextrose in water should be given at a rate to maintain a blood glucose > 60 mg/dL. If blood glucose levels cannot be increased to a safe level, prednisone, diazoxide, or glucagon may be administered.

Service FJ: Hypoglycemic disorders. N Engl J Med 1995;332: 1144–52.

SUPERIOR VENA CAVA SYNDROME

ESSENTIALS OF DIAGNOSIS

- *Distention of neck and anterior chest wall veins.*
- *Edema of the face; cyanosis and edema of upper extremities.*
- *Clinical evidence of intrathoracic malignancy.*

General Considerations

Contrary to common belief, there are no clinical or experimental data to support the concept that superior vena cava obstruction is an oncologic emergency except perhaps on very rare occasions when the patient presents with symptoms caused by tracheal obstruction or severe cerebral edema.

Superior vena cava syndrome was first described in 1751. Malignant tumors are the most common cause (nearly 90% of cases). Because of the significant increase in the incidence of bronchogenic carcinoma over the last several decades, bronchogenic carcinoma is presently the leading cause of superior vena cava syndrome and is responsible for nearly 80% of all malignant causes. Approximately 5% of all patients with bronchogenic carcinoma develop superior vena cava syndrome during their lifetime. Malignant lymphomas are responsible for approximately 15% of malignant cases. Other causes (< 5%) include metastatic disease to the mediastinal lymph nodes (from primary breast and testicular cancer and, rarely, sarcomas) and benign conditions such as aortic aneurysm, mediastinal fibrosis secondary to histoplasmosis, tuberculosis, pyogenic infection, and radiation therapy to the mediastinum. Thrombosis of the superior vena cava is reported to occur secondary to long-term central venous catheters, pulmonary artery catheters, transvenous pacemakers, or peritoneovenous shunts. Very rarely, superior vena cava syndrome may be caused by benign mediastinal tumors such as dermoids, teratomas, thymomas, retrosternal goiters, sarcoidosis, and aneurysms of the ascending thoracic aorta.

Obstruction of the superior vena cava may be caused by the tumor compressing its thin wall or invading it. Thrombosis with clot formation is usually present. Collateral circulation gradually develops. The collateral circulation involves the internal mammary, intercostal, azygos, hemiazygos, superior epigastric, and inferior epigastric veins. It should be noted that in rapidly growing tumors, engorgement of the venous collateral circulation may be absent. Incompetence of the valves of internal jugular veins may result only rarely in severe cerebral edema. Obstruction of the trachea by mediastinal tumors is a serious associated complication.

Clinical Features

The most common physical findings in superior vena cava syndrome are neck and anterior chest wall vein distention (60%), tachypnea (50%), edema of the face (50%), and cyanosis and edema of the upper extremities (15%).

The diagnosis of superior vena cava syndrome is made on clinical grounds in almost all cases. Superior vena cavography may be used to verify the diagnosis and localize the site of obstruction. Chest x-ray, chest tomography, and axial chest CT are used in order to demonstrate, evaluate, and define the extent of the mediastinal lesion. Chest radiographs readily demonstrate a mass in more than 90% of cases. MRI has no advantage over CT in this disorder.

Although the symptoms of superior vena cava syndrome are quite distressing to the patient, attempts to obtain a definite histopathologic diagnosis should be vigorously pursued at the earliest opportunity. More than 60% of these patients have small cell lung cancer or lymphomas that are appropriately treated with chemotherapy, and early treatment with radiation therapy or corticosteroids before making a definite histopathologic diagnosis may make subsequent diagnosis difficult or impossible. The diagnosis may be established by sputum cytology, bone marrow biopsy, bronchoscopy, lymph node biopsy, mediastinotomy, and anterior thoracotomy. Mediastinoscopy with biopsy is not recommended due to the high incidence of severe hemorrhage, increasing neck edema, and failure of wound healing. Adequate tissue biopsy and a touch-preparation for pathologic examination should be done when the diagnosis of lymphoma is suspected. Ample data support the safety of invasive diagnostic procedures in patients with superior vena cava syndrome except those with tracheal obstruction or laryngeal edema.

Treatment

Supportive therapy should be instituted as soon as the patient is admitted to the hospital. Upper airway obstruction from tracheal compression with resulting hypoxia should be promptly addressed. Initiation of oxygen therapy is critical. Corticosteroids should be administered to reduce brain and possibly tracheal edema and to lessen secondary inflammatory reaction. Endotracheal intubation should be avoided if possible in patients with tracheal obstruction to prevent further edema. Frequently, the tracheal obstruction is present in the more distal part of the trachea and cannot be bypassed with endotracheal intubation. Tracheostomy is rarely indicated for the same reasons. Stenting with a self-expanding metal endoprosthesis provides rapid relief and is successful in over 90% of patients.

Chemotherapy is the treatment of choice for patients with small cell lung cancer, lymphomas, and germ cell tumors—more than 60% of patients with superior vena cava syndrome. Radiation therapy is the only treatment available for other cancers. Spiral saphenous vein bypass grafting may also be useful in selected patients. Anticoagulants and antifibrinolytic agents are of no value and may be harmful. Diuretics are of little help.

Overall, it has been observed that improvement in symptoms occurs in 50–70% of patients over a period of 1–2 weeks of treatment rather than within the first few days. It is suggested that such improvement may be due to the development of collateral circulation rather than to relief of the vena caval obstruction. Studies have shown that in patients with complete clinical symptomatic relief, the superior vena cava lumen remained completely obstructed in 46% of cases on venography and in 76% at autopsy. Individual mortality is related to the underlying malignancy rather than the presence of superior vena caval obstruction.

Doty JR, Flores JH, Doty DB: Superior vena cava obstruction: bypass using spiral vein graft. Ann Thorac Surg 1999;67:1111–6.

Hochrein J: Percutaneous stenting of superior vena cava syndrome: a case report and review of the literature. Am J Med 1998;104:78–84.

Walker DL, Casciato DA: Thoracic complications. In: *Manual of Clinical Oncology*, 4th ed. Casciato DA, Lowitz BB (editors). Lippincott Williams & Wilkins, 2000.

Cardiac Problems in Critical Care 21

Shelley Shapiro, MD, PhD

Critically ill patients can present challenging cardiac problems for both diagnosis and management. Many ICU patients develop cardiac problems secondary to the metabolic and hemodynamic consequences of their underlying illness. Others have preexisting cardiac conditions that are either well compensated or asymptomatic prior to presentation to the ICU and become clinically relevant while in the ICU. A final group of patients are treated in the ICU for known cardiac conditions or have their heart condition diagnosed in the ICU. In all of these patients, the interplay of the cardiac illness with other medical problems critically influences the outcome. Therefore, defining the type and severity of the underlying cardiac problem, considering their relationship to other medical problems, and treatment of the heart disease are important considerations. As always, the key factor in the management of cardiac problems is a high degree of suspicion and early diagnosis. Methods for identifying and diagnosing cardiac disease in critically ill ICU patients will be emphasized throughout this chapter.

CONGESTIVE HEART FAILURE

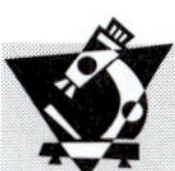

ESSENTIALS OF DIAGNOSIS

- *Acute pulmonary edema: Dyspnea, orthopnea, rales, and wheezing. Abnormal chest x-ray showing perihilar congestion. Hypoxemia.*
- *Cardiogenic shock: Hypotension; abnormal renal, hepatic, and central nervous system function due to decreased perfusion; lactic acidosis.*
- *Cardiomegaly, decreased ventricular ejection fraction or abnormal ventricular wall motion, elevated pulmonary artery wedge pressure, low cardiac output.*
- *May have a previously known cause such as valvular heart disease or cardiomyopathy but may present also as a result of ischemia or secondary to severe systemic hypertension.*

General Considerations

Congestive heart failure is a major therapeutic and diagnostic challenge because of the number of its possible causes, the number of patients who have heart failure, and the associated disability. Congestive heart failure is the most frequent diagnostic category coded in Medicare patients. Determining the cause and severity of congestive heart failure is extremely important for effective treatment. Although coronary artery disease is a frequent cause of congestive heart failure, particularly in the elderly, there are many other causes.

For example, congestive heart failure with pulmonary edema secondary to mitral stenosis is managed quite differently from that due to dilated cardiomyopathy. Therapy effective in treating congestive heart failure in a patient with severe mitral regurgitation could be lethal in a patient with critical aortic stenosis. With the ability to perform valve replacement and repair, coronary bypass grafting and angioplasty, and the possibility of cardiac transplantation, a specific cardiac diagnosis has implications for interventional management as well as drug therapy.

The causes of chronic congestive heart failure may be very different from the causes of acute failure. Acute congestive heart failure in critically ill patients is due to acute myocarditis, myocardial ischemia or infarction, acute valvular insufficiency (mitral or aortic regurgitation), worsening aortic stenosis or mitral stenosis, cardiotoxic drugs, alcohol, and sepsis. Chronic congestive heart failure is often idiopathic, though in many cases it is associated with ischemic heart disease, chronic valvular heart disease, and hypertension.

A high degree of suspicion of congestive heart failure is required to identify subtle cases or patients with coexisting heart failure. Patients in the ICU with dyspnea and hypoxia often have combined heart and pulmonary disease, and patients with known pulmonary disease can develop cardiac disease as a result of the increased stress of sepsis, hypoxia, or deterioration of pulmonary function. Any patient with unexplained hypoxemia, hypotension, or a worsening clinical state requires assessment of cardiac function.

A. Cardiac Function in the Normal Heart

Cardiac output is the product of stroke volume and heart rate. Stroke volume is determined by three factors: preload, afterload, and contractility. In the intact heart, preload is the end-diastolic tension or wall stress and is ultimately determined by the resting length of the muscle or the degree of stretch of the muscle fibers. Preload is directly related to the compliance of the ventricle and the end-diastolic pressure. Although preload is a measure of force, in conceptual terms it can be thought of as being most closely related to the end-diastolic volume of the ventricle. As the ventricular volume and pressure increase, so does the preload. Pulmonary capillary wedge pressure is often used when clinically describing a patient's preload.

Afterload is the resistance against which the ventricle ejects blood. Afterload or tension on the left ventricle can be described by the formula $\Delta P \times r/h$, where ΔP is the transmural pressure during ejection, r is the radius of the left ventricular chamber, and h is the thickness of the ventricular wall. Stroke volume is inversely proportionate to afterload.

Contractility is the inherent ability of the muscle to contract and is independent of the loading conditions on the heart (preload and afterload). Circulating catecholamines and increased sympathetic efferent activity increase contractility. Cardiac performance can be improved for a given level of myocardial contractility by changing the loading conditions.

B. Cardiac Function in Congestive Heart Failure

Congestive heart failure develops when cardiac function is inadequate to maintain sufficient cardiac output to supply the metabolic needs of the body at normal filling pressures and heart rate. In mild heart failure, cardiac function may be adequate at rest. However, exercise or illness can increase metabolic demands that may not be met when cardiac reserve is inadequate. Thus, congestive heart failure may be precipitated by critical illness with attendant fever, anemia, and vasodilation. In heart failure due to decreased left ventricular function with reduced stroke volume, cardiac output may be transiently maintained by increased heart rate or by increased preload with ventricular dilation and increased volume. Acutely, however, cardiac output may be insufficient, and signs and symptoms of hypoperfusion, including hypotension, cyanosis, and peripheral vasoconstriction, may be present ("forward failure"). Inadequate ventricular emptying (low forward flow) results in elevated left atrial and left ventricular end-diastolic volume and pressure that is transmitted back into the lungs and the pulmonary venous system with transudation of fluid. Clinically, this is manifested by rales, hypoxemia, and dyspnea ("backward failure").

A variety of neurally and hormonally mediated responses develop in an attempt to compensate for inadequate cardiac performance. These compensatory responses include renal-mediated fluid retention and peripheral vasoconstriction, tachycardia, and ventricular dilation, which attempt to maintain systemic blood pressure and cardiac output. However, these compensations are frequently counterproductive and worsen hemodynamic status. For example, vasoconstriction, while maintaining systemic blood pressure, increases ventricular afterload, ultimately decreasing stroke volume and cardiac output; fluid retention increases preload (improving stroke volume), but it also raises pulmonary venous pressure and is detrimental to lung gas exchange. Tachycardia increases cardiac output but also increases myocardial oxygen demand—particularly devastating in the setting of myocardial ischemia—and decreases diastolic time needed for optimal ventricular filling.

It is now well recognized that vasoconstriction and tachycardia, previously considered compensatory and useful to the patient, play important roles in the progression of congestive heart failure. This is why afterload reduction therapy with ACE inhibitors or other agents, beta-adrenergic blockade, and aggressive diuretic therapy have greatly improved survival in this disorder.

Clinical Features

A. Symptoms and Signs

Patients with congestive heart failure may develop symptoms slowly or acutely. They may complain of peripheral edema or of congestive symptoms such as dyspnea, orthopnea, or paroxysmal nocturnal dyspnea. Symptoms consistent with decreased cardiac output include fatigue and exercise intolerance. Chest pain may be a feature of acute-onset congestive heart failure associated with myocardial ischemia, infarction, or severe hypertension. Because of sedation or decreased activity, ICU patients may not complain of symptoms. An increasing heart rate, decreasing oxygen saturation, or increasing oxygen requirement may be the only clue.

Patients who present with acute pulmonary edema may have pink frothy sputum, rales, expiratory wheezes, and central and peripheral cyanosis. Tachycardia and hypotension are manifestations of decreased cardiac output; in these patients, low output may be accompanied by peripheral vasoconstriction, with peripheral cyanosis, cold extremities, and diaphoresis. In patients in whom severe systemic hypertension is causally related to congestive heart failure, blood pressure may be high despite low cardiac output. In patients with cardiogenic shock, hypotension is accompanied by evidence of very poor peripheral perfusion. On examination, patients with dilated cardiomyopathy may have an S_3 gallop, a murmur consistent with mitral regurgitation, and elevated jugular venous pressure. Other findings depend on the specific cause and may include murmurs consistent with valvular heart disease and an S_4 gallop.

B. Laboratory Findings

Patients may present with hypoxemia, metabolic acidosis from lactic acidosis, and hyponatremia. In patients with hypotension or shock, renal and hepatic function tests may be abnormal.

C. Electrocardiography

The ECG should be examined for evidence of myocardial ischemia or infarction, atrial hypertrophy, and ventricular hypertrophy. Rhythm disturbances (eg, atrial fibrillation or flutter) may be a cause or an effect of congestive heart failure. Patients with dilated cardiomyopathy or severe left ventricular hypertrophy due to hypertension or hypertrophic processes may have conduction or voltage abnormalities consistent with left ventricular hypertrophy. Tachycardia may indicate poor hemodynamic performance.

D. Imaging Studies

1. Chest x-ray—Chest x-ray may show cardiomegaly in patients with dilated or hypertrophic cardiomyopathy. However, patients with valvular heart disease may have only mild increase in heart size or isolated chamber enlargement. Cardiogenic pulmonary edema is usually marked by central or perihilar infiltrates, increased size of vessels serving the upper portions of the lungs in the upright position, and increased prominence of interlobular septa—usually bilateral and symmetric. Pleural effusions are common. Chest x-rays are very important to exclude pulmonary disease that may mimic heart failure, in particular ARDS and severe pneumonia.

2. Echocardiography—Noninvasive testing, particularly in a critically ill patient, may be difficult but gratifying if successful in identifying a treatable cause of congestive heart failure. Echocardiography, because of its portability, repeatability, and ability to evaluate myocardial and valvular function, is a valuable tool in the assessment of ICU patients. Hemodynamic data, including an estimate of right ventricular pressure, estimates of left atrial pressure, valve areas, left ventricular ejection fraction, and ventricular volumes, can be obtained at the bedside if image quality is adequate. Myocardial ischemia can be inferred by identification of segmental wall motion abnormalities at rest or during special interventions designed to bring out abnormalities in ischemic regions. Pericardial effusions can be diagnosed and measured and their hemodynamic impact evaluated. Echocardiography is a sensitive technique for diagnosing cardiac tamponade. Assessment of valvular regurgitation and monitoring the response to therapy are other uses for echocardiography.

Echocardiography is technically difficult in about 10% of patients overall. ICU patients, because they are often mechanically ventilated and have multiple intravenous or central lines, are difficult to position ideally and are often more difficult to image with echocardiography. Transesophageal technology has increased the value of echocardiography by providing images of good quality in patients who have had inadequate transthoracic studies. With transesophageal echocardiography, the heart is imaged via a transducer inserted into the esophagus through the mouth. The close proximity of the esophagus to the left atrium provides an excellent acoustic window resulting in better images. Views unobtainable with conventional transthoracic echocardiography are possible with this technique. The pulmonary veins, both atrial appendages, and the ascending and descending aorta can be well imaged in addition to the ventricles and valves.

3. Radionuclide angiography—Radionuclide angiography can measure right and left ventricular ejection fractions and evaluate wall motion. Myocardial uptake of technetium pyrophosphate can at times be useful to identify myocardial infarction or cardiac contusions. A variety of radionuclide techniques are used to assess coronary artery disease.

4. CT—In patients who can be moved to the scanner, ultrafast CT provides high-resolution tomographic imaging of the heart and great vessels and can assess right and left ventricular size. CT scans can also assess lung parenchyma to rule out a primary lung process and differentiate congestive heart failure from other lung disease. With the use of contrast, pulmonary thromboemboli or proximal pulmonary artery thrombosis can be seen with ultrafast CT (CT angiogram).

5. Cardiac catheterization—When noninvasive studies cannot fully answer questions about cardiac function, bedside balloon-tipped flow-directed (Swan-Ganz catheter) cardiac catheterization is performed. The catheter is used to measure a variety of hemodynamic parameters, including left ventricular end-diastolic pressure (pulmonary artery wedge pressure) and thermodilution cardiac output. It is placed transvenously into the pulmonary artery by way of the right atrium and right ventricle, usually without fluoroscopic guidance. The catheter is often of critical importance in defining cardiac function and differentiating cardiac from pulmonary disease in patients with pulmonary infiltrates and dyspnea. The pulmonary artery catheter is particularly useful for monitoring the effect of intravenous drugs on hemodynamics when cardiac output is low. In patients with acute severe congestive heart failure, the goal is to maximize cardiac output while lowering wedge pressure in order to relieve pulmonary edema.

In selected patients, left heart catheterization allows direct measurement of left ventricular pressures and function, imaging of the coronary arteries to rule out critical obstruction, and angiographic measurement of cardiac output and left ventricular ejection fraction. Left heart catheterization requires fluoroscopy and cannot be done in the ICU.

Differential Diagnosis

Patients with clinical features of congestive heart failure presenting with dyspnea, orthopnea, rales, and wheezing may instead have pneumonia, ARDS, fluid overload, or exacerbation of COPD or asthma. Cardiomegaly may be due to pericardial effusion rather than an enlarged heart itself. In patients who present with symptoms and signs of primarily right heart failure—such as elevated jugular venous pressure, ascites, edema, and evidence of right ventricular hypertrophy—lung disease resulting in cor pulmonale, or pulmonary arterial hypertension (pulmonary arteriopathy, primary or secondary pulmonary hypertension, or pulmonary emboli) should be considered. Patients with hypotension from cardiac failure should be distinguished from those with volume depletion, sepsis, and pulmonary embolism.

Treatment

A. General Measures

After determining the underlying cause of congestive heart failure, treatment in the ICU consists of quickly reversing the hemodynamic problem without adding further ones.

In very ill patients, initial management of congestive heart failure should utilize intravenous medications. These can be titrated rapidly and stopped quickly if necessary. Intravenous administration of drugs guarantees absorption, particularly in patients with bowel edema and decreased bowel motility. Although some intravenous agents have long half-lives and slow onsets of action, nitroprusside, nitroglycerin, dopamine, dobutamine, and milrinone act quickly and are easily reversed.

Cardiogenic shock may require the initial or concomitant use of vasopressor drugs such as dopamine and inotropic drugs such as dobutamine or milrinone to allow the institution of afterload reduction therapy. Nitroprusside is a potent reducer of left ventricular afterload and is particularly valuable in treating severe congestive heart failure. Disadvantages include toxicity in patients with renal insufficiency who are given nitroprusside over a prolonged period. Intravenous preparations of ACE inhibitors are effective and have longer durations of action. Digoxin and diuretics are still important despite development of newer classes of drugs. Because of negative inotropic effects, calcium channel blockers and beta-blockers are used with extreme caution if at all in patients with acute congestive heart failure. Occasionally, however, congestive heart failure may be secondary to tachyarrhythmias, left ventricular diastolic dysfunction, or severe transient ischemia, and these drugs then play an important role. Close hemodynamic monitoring, usually with a pulmonary artery catheter, allows the physician to titrate multiple drugs optimally.

General treatment of congestive heart failure in critically ill patients includes oxygen, bed rest, and reduction of metabolic derangements that increase myocardial oxygen demand, eg, fever and anemia. Endotracheal intubation and mechanical ventilation are usually not necessary except in severe cardiogenic pulmonary edema.

B. Specific Treatment of CHF

Patients with congestive heart failure can be subdivided into several groups for which specific treatments can be described, as follows.

1. Systolic dysfunction without hypotension— These patients have low stroke volumes and ejection fractions and usually have tachycardia. Pulmonary edema may accompany systolic dysfunction. Digoxin, diuretics, and ACE inhibitors are the mainstays of therapy. Several studies have shown that ACE inhibitors prolong life in patients with chronic congestive heart failure due to left ventricular dysfunction and in patients with myocardial infarction associated with reduced left ventricular function. If the patient is felt to be stable enough to tolerate oral therapy, small doses of an ACE inhibitor and digoxin can be initiated. Hypotension may accompany ACE inhibitor therapy if cardiac output fails to increase after vasodilation, and inotropic drug support of blood pressure may be required. Withholding or reducing the dosage of diuretics when ACE inhibitors are added often can prevent the development of hypotension. Serum creatinine and potassium must be observed carefully because of the effect of ACE inhibitors on renal function (particularly in patients with renal artery stenosis) and on the renin-aldosterone system.

Diuretics are useful in reducing volume overload, particularly when signs of right-sided failure such as peripheral edema, elevated jugular venous pressure, and liver engorgement are present. Intravenous furosemide can be given in a dose of 10–40 mg (more in patients with poor response) and repeated as needed. Continuous infusion of furosemide at a rate of 5–10 mg/h is also effective. Metolazone or hydrochlorothiazide can augment the effectiveness of furosemide by further inhibiting reabsorption of sodium. Sustained diuresis with any of these agents is associated with significant loss of potassium. Nesiritide is a recombinant human B-type natriuretic peptide that is indicated for intravenous treatment of acutely decompensated congestive heart failure. It is given as an initial bolus of 2 μg/kg followed by continuous infusion of 0.01 μg/kg/min for less than 48 hours. Hypotension is a known side effect. Spironolactone has been shown to decrease mortality in chronic congestive heart failure and can be added to help spare potassium loss in the acute situation. Finally, patients in severe congestive heart failure with renal dysfunction may be unable to excrete large amounts of sodium and water, so ultrafiltration may be needed to correct volume overload.

Noninvasive positive-pressure ventilation using tight-fitting masks has proved very useful in acute pulmonary edema. Positive-pressure breathing lowers preload and left ventricular afterload, improves oxygenation, and provides time for pharmacologic therapy to work. (See Chapter 12.)

The effect of various drugs on filling pressures and cardiac output can be demonstrated on the Frank-Starling curve (Figure 21–1). Both digoxin and afterload reducing agents improve the patient's cardiac output or stroke volume for a given filling pressure (move the patient to a more effective curve). In contrast, diuretics lower the left ventricular filling pressure, relieving symptoms of dyspnea, but they may also reduce cardiac output. The patient moves down along the same function curve. Optimal treatment, therefore, should utilize agents that move the patient to a better function curve, and diuretics are employed to help lower filling pressures—if they remain elevated—and expedite symptomatic improvement. In some patients with mild to moderate congestive heart failure, bed rest alone will result in significant diuresis. In addition, improvement of cardiac output with afterload reducing agents and digoxin will ultimately result in diuresis. On the other hand, both preload and afterload reducing agents can result in venodilation and thus fluid retention, so that diuretics may be needed to counteract this unwanted side effect.

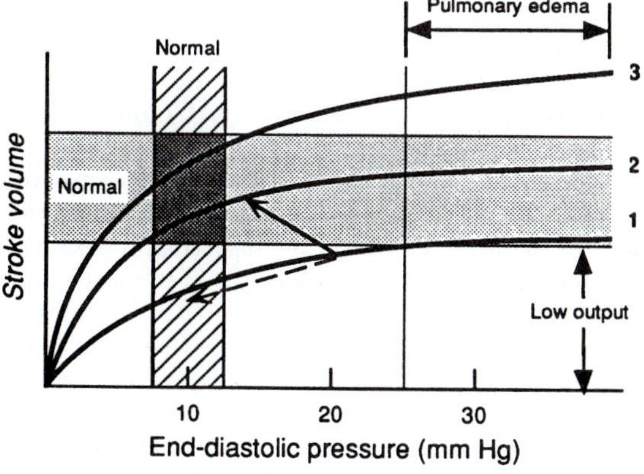

Figure 21–1. Curves demonstrating the relationship between stroke volume and left ventricular end-diastolic pressure (preload), showing the normal range for each variable. End-diastolic pressures > 25 mm Hg are associated with pulmonary edema. **Curve 1** represents severely depressed left ventricular function, with normal stroke volume being achieved only at substantially elevated preload (high left ventricular end-diastolic pressure). **Curve 2** demonstrates a normal relationship between stroke volume and preload. **Curve 3** represents a condition of increased inotropy. Treatment with afterload-reducing agents or inotropic drugs can improve stroke volume by moving an individual from curve 1 to curve 2 (solid arrow). Diuretics can lower filling pressure by moving a patient along his or her own curve (dashed arrow).

Although major emphasis has been placed on ACE inhibitors in the treatment of chronic congestive heart failure, other drugs are effective, including preload-lowering drugs such as nitrates and afterload-reducing drugs such as hydralazine. For example, the combination of hydralazine and nitrates has been shown to prolong life in patients with chronic congestive heart failure.

2. Severe congestive heart failure with hypotension (cardiogenic shock)—Patients with severe congestive heart failure associated with hypotension, pulmonary edema, and metabolic acidosis require aggressive and immediate intervention. These patients often have some reason for acute deterioration such as ischemia, myocardial infarction, new or worsening valvular insufficiency, poor adherence to medical therapy, volume overload, or concomitant medical problems. Even before invasive hemodynamic monitoring is instituted, hemodynamic support can be started using intravenous agents. With severe hypotension, blood pressure support is required—intravenous dopamine should be administered in dosages titrated to achieve a systolic blood pressure of approximately 90 mm Hg or greater. An exception to this precept would be a patient with cardiomyopathy whose known systolic blood pressure is chronically 80 mm Hg. In such cases, clinical markers of hypoperfusion such as decreased mental status or acidosis should help determine the appropriate blood pressure goal. The inotropic drugs dobutamine and milrinone can be used in conjunction with or as an alternative to dopamine to increase cardiac output. Dobutamine has the further advantage of peripheral vasodilation with reduction in left ventricular afterload.

In patients with either adequate blood pressure (systolic blood pressure > 100 mm Hg) or even marginal pressure (systolic pressure 90–100 mm Hg), nitroprusside can be started at small dosages (0.05–0.1 μg/kg/min) and titrated upward every 3–5 minutes while blood pressure is closely observed. Although these are low starting doses, they may avoid the significant and rapid hypotension that sometimes occurs with larger doses, and rapid dose adjustments make it possible to reach the effective dose in a relatively short time. The goal of reducing left ventricular afterload with nitroprusside is to increase cardiac output. However, if peripheral resistance drops in response to nitroprusside without an increase in cardiac output, hypotension will occur. The drop in blood pressure following nitroprusside administration can be dealt with by immediately discontinuing the drug and providing inotropic support if needed. The extremely short half-life of intravenous nitroprusside makes this a safe and valuable agent to try even before invasive hemodynamic monitoring can be started.

Loop diuretics are also extremely valuable in this setting if marked volume overload (pulmonary edema) is evident, and furosemide causes a lowering of preload even before diuresis occurs. Intravenous furosemide can be given in a dose of 10–40 mg (more in patients with poor response) and repeated as needed. Continuous infusion of furosemide at a rate of 5–10 mg/h is also very effective. Intravenous nitroglycerin has preload-reducing as well as some afterload-reducing properties and can be used alone or in conjunction with intravenous nitroprusside to improve cardiac output and reduce left-sided pressures. Nesiritide must be used with caution in cardiogenic shock to avoid worsening of hypotension.

Intraaortic balloon pumps and left ventricular assist devices have been used to treat patients with extreme cardiogenic shock. They are used acutely to allow time to explore opportunities for additional interventions, eg, angioplasty, heart transplantation, or cardiac surgery. This level of tertiary management is undertaken in referral centers with appropriate equipment and in selected patients with potential for good outcomes.

Echocardiography assists in the management of patients with cardiogenic shock in several ways: (1) by identifying surgically correctable valvular abnormalities such as severe aortic or mitral valvular disease that may be contributing to failure; (2) by identifying segmental wall motion abnormalities suggestive of ischemia; and (3) by establishing baseline left ventricular function in patients with new onset of congestive heart failure.

A pulmonary artery catheter will enable the physician to adjust drugs more carefully, with the goal of maximizing cardiac output at acceptably high end-diastolic filling pressure. The pulmonary artery catheter is strongly recommended for treatment of congestive heart failure patients who have hypotension and congestive symptoms. Using a pulmonary artery catheter, a cardiac index (cardiac output divided by body surface area) < 2 L/min/m^2 is considered cardiogenic shock and incompatible with prolonged survival. Heart rate and cardiac output need to be considered in optimizing hemodynamics, particularly in patients with congestive heart failure and myocardial ischemia. If an adequate cardiac index is maintained by an increased heart rate rather than improved stroke volume, ultimate outcome will be poor. Conversely, patients with bradycardia in the setting of congestive heart failure may have dramatically improved cardiac output with a pacemaker or the use of pharmacologic agents to increase the heart rate.

Calculation of stroke volume to assess therapy is very useful. The mixed venous O_2 saturation ($S\bar{v}O_2$) is another way of assessing severity and response to therapy. It reflects delivery and utilization of O_2 and the effectiveness of cardiac output. Some pulmonary artery catheters have an oximeter probe at their tips to continuously monitor $S\bar{v}O_2$ in addition to pulmonary artery pressures. A decrease in $S\bar{v}O_2$ can be an early marker of decreased cardiac output and function. A desirable goal of therapy in treating cardiogenic shock is to attain a mixed venous O_2 saturation > 65%.

After optimizing hemodynamic variables with intravenous medications and attaining a period of stability, a gradual change to oral medication is appropriate. Oral afterload-reducing agents (ACE inhibitors, angiotensin receptor blockers, or hydralazine) should be added while reducing the dosages of intravenous agents. An intravenous ACE inhibitor such as enalaprilat given every 6 hours is an alternative to oral ACE inhibitors.

3. Congestive heart failure with severe systemic hypertension—Treatment is directed at the pathophysiologic mechanisms of congestive heart failure in severe hypertension, ie, reduction of systemic blood pressure and intravascular volume. In these patients, left ventricular systolic function may be normal whereas left ventricular diastolic dysfunction is a major feature, resulting in congestion and pulmonary edema. Systolic dysfunction, if present, may improve significantly following afterload reduction.

Control of blood pressure with reduction of left ventricular afterload is the major focus of initial therapy. Particularly if systolic function is unknown, an intravenous agent such as nitroprusside or nitroglycerin is recommended to lower systemic pressures and improve filling pressures acutely. Intravenous enalaprilat can also be considered. (See section on Hypertensive Crisis.)

For continued treatment of hypertension, beta-adrenergic blockers or calcium channel blockers can be added after congestive heart failure has improved and acceptable left ventricular systolic function has been documented. However, these agents should be used with caution in patients with high filling pressures and severe hypertension because they may depress myocardial function without adequately reducing the afterload. The net result may be worsening congestive heart failure or hemodynamic collapse. Pulmonary artery catheterization may be helpful when considering the use of beta-adrenergic blockers or calcium channel blockers in these patients, but catheterization is not needed to initiate therapy with nitroprusside unless hypotension develops early in treatment, raising the possibility of complicating cardiac or pulmonary problems.

4. High-output or volume-overload CHF—These patients present with congestive symptoms and signs (pulmonary edema, peripheral edema), but systolic cardiac function is normal and cardiac output may be elevated. Treatment should be directed at the cause of the high cardiac output (eg, anemia, thiamin deficiency, sepsis, hyperthyroidism) or volume overload state (renal failure, excessive sodium intake). Rapid lowering of intravascular volume by ultrafiltration may improve blood pressure, hypoxemia, and edema, especially in patients who do not respond well to diuretic therapy. In the ICU patient, volume overload may be due to obligate fluid intake from hyperalimentation, blood product replacement, or antibiotic therapy.

5. Congestive heart failure with diastolic dysfunction—Diastolic dysfunction is seen commonly in patients who have hypertension with left ventricular hypertrophy and ischemia. Patients with amyloidosis also have low ventricular compliance. Diastolic dysfunction means that ventricular filling is impaired, and left ventricular end-diastolic pressures may be elevated. Patients have congestive symptoms (shortness of breath, pulmonary edema) despite normal ejection fraction and normal systolic wall motion. Treatment includes beta-adrenergic blockade to slow the heart rate, allowing more time for diastolic filling. On occasion, aggressive diuretic therapy is counterproductive in patients with diastolic dysfunction. This is because the noncompliant left ventricle requires higher pressure (volume) to generate a certain degree of preloading and subsequent stroke volume. Excessive diuresis may cause stroke volume, systemic blood pressure, and cardiac output to fall.

6. Isolated right heart failure with pulmonary hypertension—Patients may have isolated right heart failure secondary to pulmonary hypertension. Pulmonary hypertension may be related to congenital heart disease, lung disease (most common), medications, HIV infection, and collagen-vascular diseases (scleroderma, mixed connective tissue disease) or may be idiopathic (primary pulmonary hypertension). In primary pulmonary hypertension, the pathophysiologic mechanism of the dyspnea and orthopnea is not entirely clear, though gas exchange in the lungs is inefficient because of maldistribution of perfusion. Compression of the left ventricle with abnormal septal motion and relative left ventricular filling difficulties because of right ventricular encroachment into the pericardial space is another possible mechanism.

Diuretics are used to reduce right atrial pressure and right ventricular and right atrial volume. Oxygen may reduce pulmonary hypertension in patients with primary pulmonary hypertension or lung diseases. As oxygenation improves, liver engorgement, abdominal distention, and lung mechanics improve. One goal is to reduce right atrial pressure to < 10 mm Hg. Finally, digoxin may be helpful by increasing right ventricular inotropy. Reduction of pulmonary artery pressures and right ventricular afterload with nitric oxide or intravenous prostacyclin should be considered when a clear diagnosis of primary pulmonary hypertension is made (in the absence of left heart failure). This is in the realm of tertiary care at institutions able to administer such therapy.

Bertini G et al: Intravenous nitrates in the prehospital management of acute pulmonary edema. Ann Emerg Med 1997;30:493–9.

Colucci WS: Intravenous nesiritide, a natriuretic peptide, in the treatment of decompensated congestive heart failure. Nesiritide Study Group. N Engl J Med 2000;343:246–53.

Elesber AA, Redfield MM: Approach to patients with heart failure and normal ejection fraction. Mayo Clin Proc 2001; 76:1047–52.

Gandhi SK et al: The pathogenesis of acute pulmonary edema associated with hypertension. N Engl J Med. 2001;344:17–22.

Loh E: Maximizing management of patients with decompensated heart failure. Clin Cardiol 2000;23(3 Suppl):III1–5.

Pang D et al: The effect of positive pressure airway support on mortality and the need for intubation in cardiogenic pulmonary edema: a systematic review. Chest 1998;114:1185–92.

Stevenson LW, Perloff JK: The limited reliability of physical signs for estimating hemodynamics in chronic heart failure. JAMA 1989;261:884–8.

Vasan RS, Benjamin EJ: Diastolic heart failure—no time to relax. N Engl J Med 2001;344:56–9.

Vitarelli A, Gheorghiade M: Transthoracic and transesophageal echocardiography in the hemodynamic assessment of patients with congestive heart failure. Am J Cardiol 2000; 86(4A):36G–40G.

VALVULAR HEART DISEASE

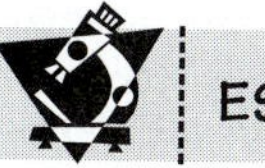

ESSENTIALS OF DIAGNOSIS

Valvular insufficiency:

- *Dyspnea, pulmonary edema, new murmur.*
- *Echocardiogram with Doppler demonstrating regurgitation.*

Valvular stenosis:

- *Dyspnea, pulmonary edema, murmur, syncope, hypotension. Decreased carotid pulses (aortic stenosis).*

- *Atrial fibrillation (mitral stenosis), left ventricular hypertrophy (aortic stenosis).*
- *Echocardiogram documenting decreased valve area.*

Prosthetic valve dysfunction:

- *New onset of symptoms of congestive heart failure, syncope. Change in examination (new murmur, change in intensity of valve sounds).*
- *Echocardiographic evidence of increased valve pressure gradient, thrombosis, or other dysfunction.*

Infective endocarditis:

- *May or may not have history of valvular heart disease or prosthetic valve.*
- *New onset of heart failure with valvular insufficiency or unexplained fever and pathologic heart murmur.*
- *Echocardiographic evidence of valvular disease, positive blood cultures.*

General Considerations

As with congestive heart failure, treating valvular heart disease in the ICU setting involves considering the possibility and proceeding to assess its severity. Few ICUs can afford the luxury of a quiet place to auscultate the heart, but with patience and perseverance the experienced clinician can detect important murmurs. The acoustic qualities of the murmurs are affected by cardiac output. Patients in shock with low-output states and febrile or anemic patients with high-output states may present with misleading physical findings that under- or overestimate the severity of valvular heart disease. At the bedside, echocardiography affords the physician a convenient window on the heart and a way to quantitate valve dysfunction and clarify the relationship between valve function and myocardial function.

Acute valvular insufficiency with regurgitation may be due to endocarditis, trauma, papillary muscle dysfunction (mitral valve), or ischemia. But patients may present with worsening of chronic valvular disease from myxomatous degeneration or prolapse with and without connective tissue disorders or rheumatic heart disease. Isolated aortic valve insufficiency may be due to aortic diseases such as aortic dissection, cystic medial necrosis, and syphilitic aortitis. Most commonly, however, chronic aortic regurgitation results from a congenital bicuspid aortic valve. Mitral stenosis is most often due to rheumatic heart disease. Aortic stenosis is occasionally due to rheumatic heart disease but more often to progressive valvular calcification either of a normal valve or of a congenital bicuspid valve.

Patients with previous valve surgery with prosthetic or bioprosthetic valves represent a special circumstance. These valves are subject to a variety of chronic and acute complications, including infective endocarditis, calcification with simultaneous stenosis and incompetence, thrombosis with valve dysfunction, and peripheral embolic events such as strokes, valve dehiscence, and paravalvular leaks.

Clinical Features

A. Symptoms and Signs

Specific findings depend on which valve is abnormal. Patients with aortic or mitral valvular stenosis or insufficiency may present with congestive heart failure, including pulmonary edema and evidence of decreased cardiac output. Physical findings include rales, S_3 gallop, wheezing, peripheral vasoconstriction, tachycardia, and murmurs. Other important findings to be sought include the character of arterial pulses, intensity of the heart sounds, and changes in the quality of murmurs with different maneuvers, such as Valsalva. Chest pain is a frequent accompanying symptom in patients with significant aortic stenosis or aortic regurgitation. Atrial arrhythmias frequently accompany mitral valve disease with left atrial enlargement.

B. Electrocardiography

The ECG may suggest features of specific valvular heart diseases—eg, left ventricular hypertrophy, seen in aortic stenosis and regurgitation; and left atrial enlargement and right ventricular hypertrophy, seen in mitral stenosis.

C. Imaging Studies

The chest x-ray may show cardiomegaly with specific chamber enlargement. Echocardiography is extremely useful in assessing valvular heart disease. It can provide evidence of leaflet abnormalities, including vegetations and decreased motion of valve leaflets, as well as estimates of valve cross-sectional area in valvular stenosis. The size of the atria and ventricles can be determined and wall motion and ejection fraction estimated. With Doppler techniques, one can quantitatively estimate regurgitant blood flow across an abnormal valve, measure valve pressure gradients, and calculate valve areas.

Pulmonary artery catheters directly measure pulmonary artery pressures, cardiac output, and an estimate of left atrial pressure (pulmonary artery wedge pressure). Cardiac catheterization is usually required to assess valve function prior to surgery and to identify coexistent coronary artery disease. Echocardiography utilizing Doppler techniques may preclude the need for cardiac catheterization in some patients.

Treatment: Native Valves

A. Valvular Regurgitation

The management of left-sided valvular regurgitation is determined by the severity of the regurgitation, the specific cause, and the degree of left ventricular dysfunction. The severity of regurgitation can be estimated echocardiographically using colorflow and continuous wave Doppler and calculating left ventricular and left atrial pressures noninvasively. Echocardiography will also help define operability and determine the cause of the valve dysfunction. Mild to moderate aortic or mitral regurgitation without symptoms requires no treatment. Infective endocarditis prophylaxis should be given when indicated.

In patients with more severe left-sided valvular regurgitation, associated congestive heart failure (pulmonary edema) can be treated with diuretics and digoxin. However, the most important therapy is the use of unloading agents such as ACE inhibitors, hydralazine, and, if needed, nitroglycerin and nitroprusside. These drugs work by decreasing downstream resistance and increasing downstream compliance. Forward blood flow increases while regurgitant flow decreases, so that ventricular filling pressures decline while cardiac output improves. The management of congestive heart failure due to aortic or mitral regurgitation is quite similar to the management of congestive heart failure secondary to systolic ventricular dysfunction.

In patients with such severe valvular regurgitation that cardiac output is very low and there is hypotension (cardiogenic shock), emergent valve surgery may be necessary. Invasive hemodynamic monitoring with a pulmonary artery catheter is essential, and maximum unloading of the left ventricle with intravenous nitroprusside should be started immediately. Inotropic drugs such as dopamine may be required to maintain adequate systemic blood pressure even though—by increasing afterload—valvular regurgitation may be transiently worsened. Mitral regurgitation associated with cardiogenic shock may benefit from intraaortic balloon pumps, but this therapy is contraindicated in those with aortic valve regurgitation.

B. Valvular Stenosis

Aortic stenosis is treated with surgery when it results in congestive heart failure. Resources for medical management are limited, but possible pharmacologic interventions include mild diuresis and the use of digoxin. Systemic vasodilators, useful in other forms of heart failure, may cause severe hypotension in patients with aortic stenosis. Dopamine can be tried if shock develops, but by this time surgery is essential. A rapid and limited search for confounding problems can be undertaken to try to find ways to improve the patient acutely. Atrial fibrillation, for example, because it results in a decrease in left ventricular filling in the patient with severe aortic stenosis, should be treated aggressively with the goal of returning the patient to sinus rhythm. Successful cardioversion of atrial fibrillation may result in acute improvement in cardiac output.

Severe mitral stenosis is also a surgical problem, though it is somewhat more amenable to pharmacologic therapy. The most important goal is to decrease the heart rate, thereby prolonging diastolic filling time. Left atrial pressure and, therefore, pulmonary venous pressure are determined by the degree of left atrial emptying. In patients with mitral stenosis, left atrial emptying is limited by decreased mitral orifice size; and the smaller the valve area, the longer it takes for the atrium to empty. Inadequate time for emptying leads to increased left atrial pressure and volume and worsening pulmonary congestion. Thus, by slowing the heart rate and lengthening diastole, the left atrium has more time in which to empty. Therefore, if left ventricular function is preserved and there is only mild to moderate mitral regurgitation, heart rate control using beta-blockers or calcium channel blockers (or digoxin, if the patient has atrial fibrillation) will often greatly improve symptoms.

Treatment: Prosthetic Valves

A. Dysfunction of Prosthetic Valves

This entity can be a true medical emergency resulting in rapid deterioration of a stable patient and can frequently lead to death if not promptly recognized and treated. Bioprosthetic valves tend to calcify and become both stenotic and incompetent over time. Once the valve becomes dysfunctional, further progression can be rapid, with a rigid leaflet suddenly becoming severely incompetent and producing fulminant congestive heart failure. Mechanical prosthetic valves are more durable, with, for example, Starr-Edwards valves (ball-cage valves) functioning for more than 30 years. However, ingrowth of tissue (pannus formation) or thrombosis secondary to inadequate anticoagulation can result in the development of valve dysfunction with either obstruction, regurgitation, or both (depending on where the tissue ingrowth or clot develops). Progressive thrombosis, particularly on a single-leaflet mechanical valve, can result in death, as the valve may stick in closed position. The St. Jude valve, because it is a bileaflet device, usually develops both insufficiency and stenosis. Other less frequent problems have resulted from mechanical damage of the valve, such as strut fracture with Bjork-Shiley type valves and loss of poppets due to ball variance and fractures in older Starr-Edwards valves.

In evaluating patients with suspected prosthetic valve dysfunction, physical examination may show evidence of congestive heart failure. The murmurs that accompany the prosthetic valve may be fainter than usual because of low cardiac output or high filling pressures. The key to the diagnosis of prosthetic valve dysfunction is a high degree of clinical suspicion and noninvasive assessment of valvular function. Patients with prosthetic valves who present with worsening heart failure should undergo Doppler evaluation of the valves to assess transprosthetic valve gradients and to estimate valve area. Transesophageal echocardiography is extremely useful in this setting and can confirm valve obstruction by demonstrating the presence of a clot and reduced prosthetic leaflet motion. A large pressure gradient across the valve or the presence of substantial transvalvular regurgitation is suggestive of valve thrombosis. Cinefluoroscopy can be used to assess opening angles of the mechanical prosthetic valves by measuring the angle on still frames. The angle of opening for specific valve models is known. If the valve does not open to the expected amount, valve dysfunction and thrombosis can be suspected.

Treatment includes immediate heparinization if thrombosis is suspected, hemodynamic monitoring, and surgical evaluation for urgent valve replacement. Valve replacement is critical and can be lifesaving. Patients who present with severe heart failure in this setting can sometimes be dramatically helped by use of thrombolytic agents, including alteplase or streptokinase. Risks of thrombolytic therapy include embolization of lysed clots and central nervous system hemorrhage, but the risks may have to be accepted when cardiogenic shock occurs secondary to valve thrombosis and operation is considered too hazardous. Results with alteplase can be seen within 90 minutes. Heparinization must be continued after thrombolytic therapy to prevent immediate reclotting.

B. Emboli

Thrombi forming on prosthetic valves are a source of thromboemboli, which can cause complications based on where the emboli lodge, including strokes, renal infarction, ischemic limbs, pulmonary emboli, and coronary artery occlusion. Emboli occur uncommonly in anticoagulated patients; however, inadequate anticoagulation or discontinuation of anticoagulation—particularly with mechanical valves—can result in embolic events. Treatment is supportive, with use of intravenous anticoagulation for treatment of peripheral embolization and prevention of further emboli. Surgical removal of emboli can be performed if they are in accessible locations, such as in limb vessels. In patients who are already adequately anticoagulated with warfarin, the addition of aspirin or dipyridamole has been shown to decrease the frequency of recurrent embolization.

In patients with cerebral emboli, the decision to anticoagulate may be difficult because of the risk of conversion of a bland embolic stroke to a hemorrhagic one. Most neurologists recommend waiting 48–72 hours before anticoagulating such patients unless the concern for recurrent emboli is felt to outweigh these risks. Finally, surgical replacement of a partially thrombosed valve in the patient with stroke is associated with a very high risk of perioperative intracerebral hemorrhage due the combination of low cerebral perfusion and the need for heparin during the procedure.

C. Paravalvular Leaks and Valve Dehiscence

Valve dehiscence is another form of valve dysfunction seen with both bioprosthetic and mechanical valves. The artificial valve is attached to the myocardium or to the annulus where the native valve previously resided. Paravalvular leaks can be a result of technical problems occurring at the time of surgery or may develop years later as a result of prosthesis infection (endocarditis). Paravalvular leaks are a result of space developing between the sewing ring of the valve and the annulus or cardiac tissue. Small, hemodynamically insignificant leaks are often seen as a result of minor surgical imperfections and can remain stable for years. Paravalvular leaks secondary to infective endocarditis are often associated with valve dehiscence, and these paravalvular leaks tend to progress, often rapidly. This results in severe hemodynamic dysfunction, further dehiscence of the valve, instability of the valve, and, frequently, hemolysis due to mechanical destruction of red cells as they pass through the disordered valve.

Development of a paravalvular leak in the setting of endocarditis is a surgical emergency. Complications include progressive uncontrollable congestive heart failure, sepsis, or complete dehiscence of the valve resulting in death. Echocardiography—particularly transesophageal—or cardiac catheterization is required to define the severity of the valve lesions, assess overall cardiac function, and guide valve replacement.

Treatment: Infective Endocarditis (Prosthetic or Native Valve)

Infective endocarditis is a pleomorphic disease that can be rapidly progressive when caused by invasive organisms or can be slowly progressive and debilitating, resulting in chronic congestive heart failure and wasting. Diagnosis and identification of the organism are essential for proper management. Clinical features of endocarditis, including fever, heart murmur, unexplained anemia, and peripheral or immunologic stigmas, should alert the physician. In particular, endocarditis needs to be considered in any febrile patient with a known history of valvular heart disease, a pathologic murmur, or a prosthetic valve. Patients with community-acquired *Staphylococcus aureus* or viridans streptococcal bacteremia have a high incidence of endocarditis (20% and 80%, respectively) and should be considered to have endocarditis unless proved otherwise.

The diagnosis of endocarditis is made on clinical grounds (see Chapter 15). Positive blood cultures are found in as many as 90% of patients, but the frequency of this finding depends on the type of organism and the number of blood cultures obtained. Therefore, one should obtain an adequate number of samples of blood for culture before starting antibiotic therapy or specify laboratory techniques to minimize the effect of antibiotics on the culture results. Obtaining cultures for fungi, anaerobic bacteria, and fastidious or slow-growing organisms may increase the likelihood of an etiologic diagnosis in susceptible patients. Echocardiography, especially using the transesophageal approach, is extremely useful in detecting valvular vegetations in endocarditis and for assessing the degree of valvular incompetence, if any (Figure 21–2).

Effective antibiotic therapy requires selection of bactericidal or fungicidal drugs to which the organism is sensitive and then delivering intravenous antibiotics in adequate quantities for a prolonged period. Fungal endocarditis is almost never eradicated using pharmacotherapy. The duration of therapy is in part dependent on the organism. Prosthetic valve endocarditis often necessitates valve replacement because antibiotics fail to eliminate the infection or because of valve dysfunction, valve dehiscence, or ring abscess.

The outcome of both native and prosthetic valve endocarditis is dependent on cardiac function. Patients developing congestive heart failure do quite poorly without valve replacement. Valve replacement, even while the patient is still infected or septic, can be lifesaving after con-

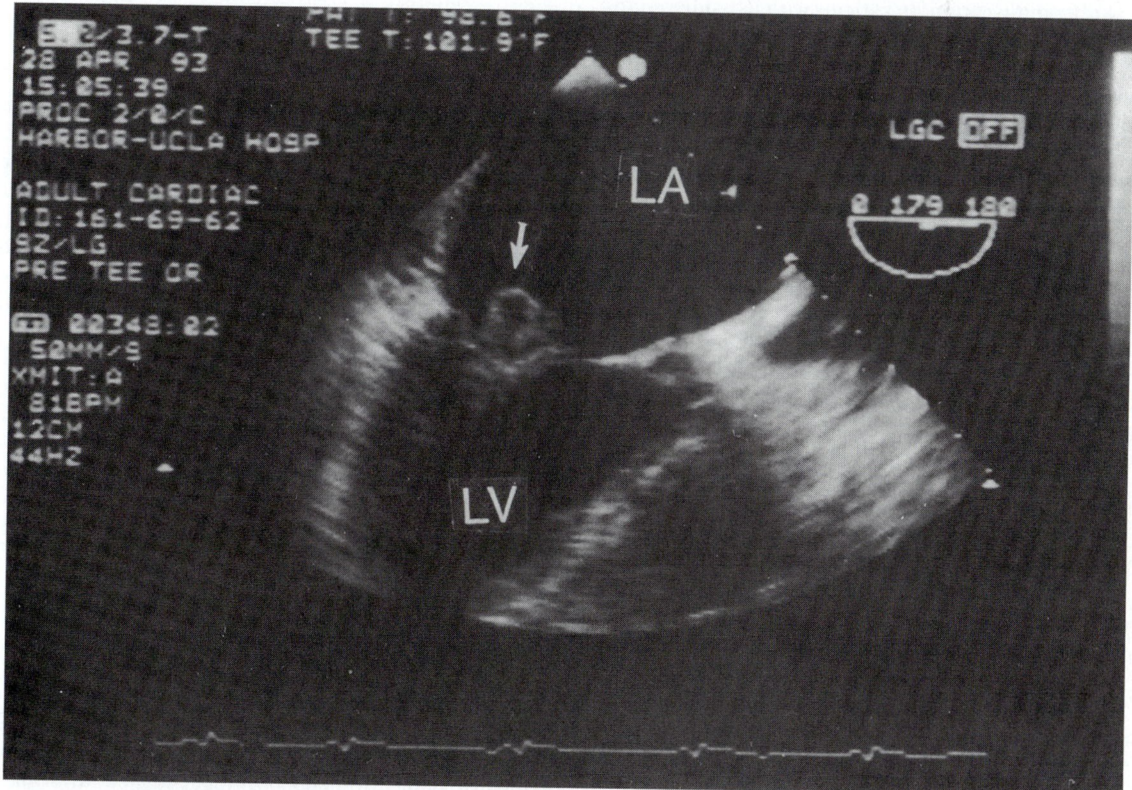

Figure 21–2. Transesophageal echocardiogram demonstrating mitral valve endocarditis with a prolapsing and partial flail mitral valve leaflet ***(arrow).*** A vegetation can be seen as well. The left ventricle and left atrium are indicated by "LV" and "LA," respectively. At surgery, the valve was found to be necrotic. The mitral valve was incompetent, with severe mitral regurgitation, as seen on colorflow Doppler, but this is not shown in this still frame image.

gestive heart failure has developed. When to operate in cases of native valve endocarditis depends in part on the hemodynamic consequences of the infection (eg, severe valvular regurgitation, intracardiac shunts, or congestive heart failure). Surgery is required if antibiotic therapy fails to clear the infection, if there are persistent fevers or a valve ring abscess, or if cultures have identified a fastidious organism known to be difficult to eradicate medically. Patients who have more than one major embolic episode with left-sided endocarditis almost always undergo valve replacement. Larger vegetations, particularly on the left side of the heart, are associated with higher complication rates and poorer outcomes.

In patients suspected of having infective endocarditis, echocardiography should be performed to identify valvular vegetations or valve destruction and qualitatively assess the degree of valvular regurgitation present. Echocardiography can then be used to monitor therapy. Increase in vegetation size, worsening of regurgitation, or the development of mycotic aneurysms, intramyocardial abscesses, or fistula suggests treatment failure and the need for further intervention. In patients with left-sided endocarditis, aortic valve ring abscess, left-to-right shunts, valvular incompetence, and large vegetations have important implications for outcome and the need for valve surgery. Transesophageal echocardiography has superior sensitivity for identifying valvular vegetations, valve ring abscesses, and intracardiac shunts. It is particularly valuable for visualizing lesions in patients with prosthetic valve endocarditis. For these reasons, transesophageal echocardiography is recommended for all patients suspected of having left-sided endocarditis, aortic valve endocarditis, or suspected prosthetic valve endocarditis and for patients with endocarditis who are hemodynamically unstable or deteriorating. The transesophageal echocardiogram should also be used in the preoperative and intraoperative management of these patients to identify unsuspected pathologic findings, including aortic-to-atrial fistulas and valve ring infection, and to verify the adequacy of surgical repair.

ACC/AHA guidelines for the management of patients with valvular heart disease. A report of the American College of Cardiology/American Heart Association. Task Force on Practice Guidelines (Committee on Management of Patients with Valvular Heart Disease). J Am Coll Cardiol 1998;32:1486–588.

Bayer AS et al: Diagnosis and management of infective endocarditis and its complications. Circulation 1998;98:2936–48.

Becker RC, Eisenberg P, Turpie AG: Pathobiologic features and prevention of thrombotic complications associated with prosthetic heart valves: fundamental principles and the contribution of platelets and thrombin. Am Heart J 2001;141:1025–37.

Carabello BA, Crawford FA Jr: Valvular heart disease. N Engl J Med 1997;337:32–41.

Hayek E, Griffin BP: Current medical management of valvular heart disease. Cleve Clin J Med 2001;68:881–7.

Vongpatanasin W, Hillis LD, Lange RA: Prosthetic heart valves. N Engl J Med 1996;335:407–16.

CARDIAC TAMPONADE

ESSENTIALS OF DIAGNOSIS

- *Evidence of elevated pericardial pressure manifested as elevated systemic venous pressure. Decreased cardiac output and hypotension; evidence of decreased peripheral perfusion.*
- *Echocardiography: Diastolic collapse of right ventricle, systolic collapse of right atrium, large pericardial effusion.*
- *Equalization of right atrial, left atrial, and ventricular end-diastolic pressures.*

General Considerations

Pericardial effusions occur in a variety of patients seen in the ICU, including those with malignancy, tuberculosis, fungal infections, myocardial infarction, trauma, acute and chronic renal failure, thyroid disease, autoimmune conditions, and, more rarely, in patients with endocarditis or aortic dissection. Patients after cardiac surgery can develop pericarditis and pericardial effusions for several reasons. The size of the effusion and the rapidity with which it develops are the major determinants of its hemodynamic effects. Cardiac tamponade ensues when adequate ventricular and atrial filling are prevented by increased intrapericardial pressure due to pericardial effusion. Left atrial, right atrial, left ventricular end-diastolic, and right ventricular end-diastolic pressures increase and equalize. Stroke volume, cardiac output, and systemic blood pressure fall greatly, and patients may develop shock with evidence of underperfusion of organs.

Clinical Features

A. Symptoms and Signs

Symptoms and signs may reflect the underlying cause of pericardial effusion, especially if there is inflammation of the pericardium with acute pericarditis. Chest pain that is pleuritic and positional suggests this diagnosis. However, patients with tamponade need not have chest pain, especially if tamponade is due to other causes such as malignancy or uremia. When cardiac tamponade develops, patients may have associated dyspnea and orthopnea.

Physical findings in cardiac tamponade include distended neck veins, tachycardia, hypotension, and pulsus paradoxus. Elevated pericardial pressure will cause distended neck veins (which should be looked for in the upright position since the meniscus may not be visible in a semisupine patient when the pressures are markedly elevated), pulsus paradoxus (augmented respiratory variation in the pulse pressure, usually > 10 mm Hg), and, usually, hypotension. Although in general the blood pressure is reduced, normal or elevated blood pressure can be seen with tamponade in patients with previous hypertension. Tachycardia, tachypnea, and orthopnea are important supporting signs suggesting elevated pressures affecting the left heart. Heart sounds as well as the left ventricular impulse may be muted because the heart is surrounded by fluid and farther away from the chest wall. Hepatomegaly and peripheral edema may be present.

B. Laboratory Findings

Laboratory abnormalities may identify a specific cause of pericardial effusion. If diagnostic pericardiocentesis is performed, a specific diagnosis may be made from bacterial, fungal, or mycobacterial cultures, cytologic examination, and other studies.

C. Electrocardiography

Electrocardiography may show decreased voltage. Acute pericarditis may present with diffusely elevated ST segments on ECG. Electrical alternans is an important clue supporting the diagnosis of cardiac tamponade but is neither sensitive nor specific.

D. Imaging Studies

The chest x-ray may show cardiomegaly with a characteristic "water bottle" shape, but, if the development of pericardial effusion and tamponade is rapid, heart size may be only slightly increased. At the bedside, echocardiography can rapidly and accurately determine if pericardial fluid is present and estimate ventricular function (Figure 21–3). In addition, there are several echocardiographic criteria for diagnosis of tamponade in patients with pericardial effusions. These findings include the "swinging heart," right ventricular diastolic or right atrial systolic collapse, respiratory variation in left ventricular and right ventricular chamber sizes, and right atrial indentation. Although helpful, these signs are neither sensitive nor specific. Therefore, after identifying a moderate to large pericardial effusion by echocardiography in a symptomatic patient, a bedside pulmonary artery catheter should be placed to confirm the hemodynamic findings of tamponade.

Treatment

Initial treatment of cardiac tamponade consists of rapid intravenous fluid loading and dopamine. The goal is to increase intravascular pressures enough to overcome the increased pericardial pressure as well as maintain adequate systemic blood pressure. Although these agents may improve the hemodynamic status for a short time, pericardiocentesis when tamponade is present is essential to avoid hemodynamic collapse and death. This procedure should be performed rapidly to relieve the hemodynamic compromise and to determine the cause of the effusion.

An intrapericardial catheter can be placed through a subxiphoid approach using a wire placed through a thin-walled needle (Seldinger technique). Positioning is done using electrocardiographic guidance, echocardiographic guidance, or fluoroscopy. The catheter should remain in place to permit repeated aspirations of fluid. Fluid should be sent for culture, cytologic examination, and serologic testing. Patients with moderate to large effusions and elevated filling pressures but not satisfying the criteria for cardiac tamponade should have hemodynamic measurements made before and after pericardiocentesis to verify hemodynamic benefit as well as to obtain fluid for diagnosis. Cardiac tamponade secondary to renal failure may benefit from injection of a nonabsorbable corticosteroid into the pericardial space after drainage of the fluid.

In patients with malignant pericardial effusion and cardiac tamponade, drainage followed by sclerotherapy using bleomycin or fluorouracil may decrease the recurrence of tamponade. Alternatively, balloon pericardiotomy may allow drainage of fluid into the pleural or mediastinal space—thus preventing reaccumulation of fluid, which would result in tamponade. However, in patients whose life expectancy is greater than 6 months (a small number of patients with malignant pericardial effusions and tamponade) and in those whose effusion cannot be controlled with sclerosis of the pericardial space, pericardiectomy should be considered.

Soler-Soler J, Sagrista-Sauleda J, Permanyer-Miralda G: Management of pericardial effusion. Heart 2001;86:235–40.

HYPERTENSIVE CRISIS & MALIGNANT HYPERTENSION

ESSENTIALS OF DIAGNOSIS

- *Hypertensive crisis: Systemic blood pressure > 240/130 mm Hg without symptoms, or elevated blood pressure with chest pain, headache, or heart failure. May have intracranial hemorrhage, aortic dissection, pulmonary edema, myocardial infarction, or unstable angina.*

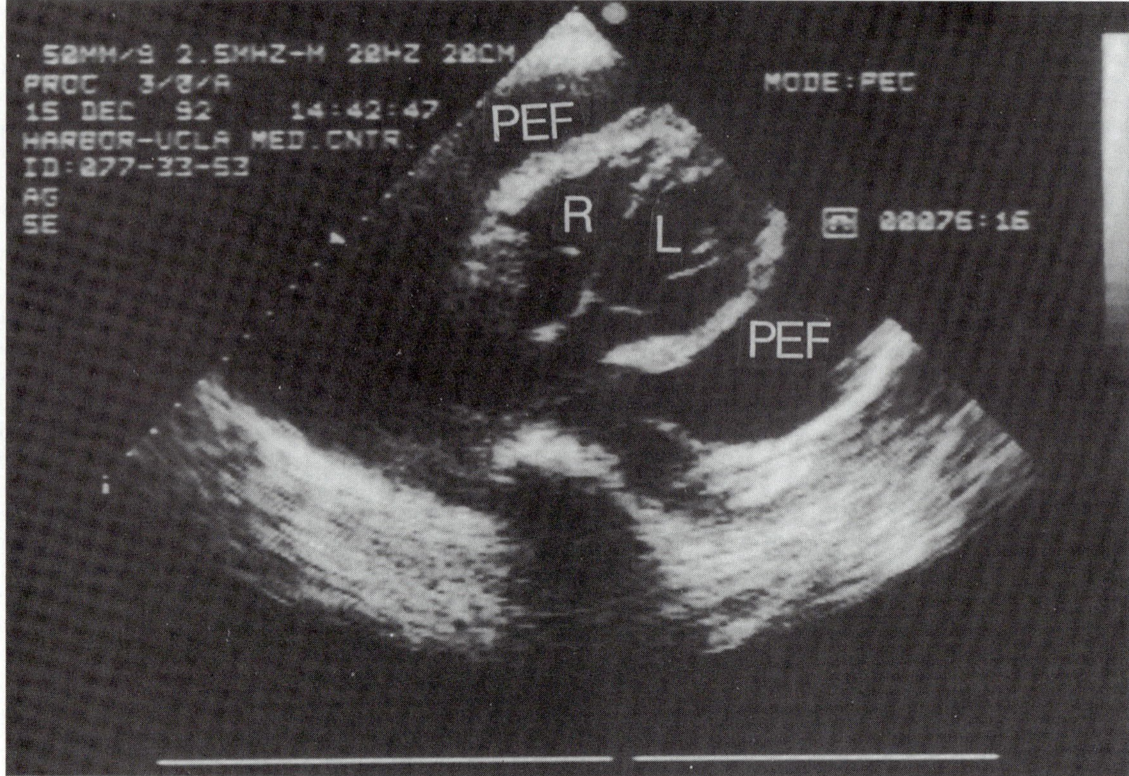

Figure 21–3. Two-dimensional echocardiogram taken from the subcostal window demonstrating a large pericardial effusion with cardiac tamponade. "PEF" locates the pericardial effusion surrounding the heart. "R" and "L" indicate the right and left ventricles, respectively. Note that the chambers are quite small because of the massive pericardial effusion.

- *Malignant hypertension: Severe hypertension associated with encephalopathy, renal failure, or papilledema.*

General Considerations

Hypertension in adults is usually a chronic condition which if untreated is a significant risk factor for the long-term development of coronary, cerebral, and peripheral vascular disease. Mild to moderate hypertension usually poses no immediate danger to the patient if the pressure is below 170/110 mm Hg. Patients with mild to moderate hypertension are often asymptomatic, and control of their blood pressure can be achieved using oral medications and modification of diet. Antihypertensive treatment is usually begun on an outpatient basis after documentation of persistent hypertension and evaluation for potentially reversible causes.

A subset of patients present with or develop severe life-threatening hypertension or have other coexisting medical problems requiring urgent control of blood pressure; these patients are defined as having a hypertensive crisis (sometimes called a hypertensive emergency). For example, patients with acute myocardial infarction or unstable angina benefit greatly from reduction of elevated blood pressure and lowering of left ventricular afterload. Blood pressure represents a major factor in myocardial oxygen demand. When congestive heart failure due to left ventricular dysfunction or aortic or mitral regurgitation is associated with severe hypertension, rapid lowering of blood pressure will accelerate treatment of the hemodynamic dysfunction. Patients with acute aortic dissection and elevated blood pressure have greatly increased stress on the aorta, and urgent control of blood pressure is mandatory. Patients with intracranial hemorrhage—intracerebral or subarachnoid—also require control of blood pressure and may become acutely hypertensive as a result of the central nervous system event. Severe hypertension results in local and systemic effects that start a cascade of events which further elevate blood pressure. Dilation of cerebral blood vessels results in hypertensive encephalopathy, and damage to the blood vessel wall can increase permeability, resulting in edema or bleeding.

Malignant hypertension is defined by some as severe hypertension associated with specific end-organ damage, namely, encephalopathy or nephropathy with papilledema. Treatment of malignant hypertension is important because rapid and effective lowering of blood pressure is essential for reversal of complications.

Any of the causes of hypertension can be associated with hypertensive crisis, including renovascular, primary, or endocrine hypertension (eg, pheochromocytoma). Most patients who present with hypertensive crises have preexisting hypertension.

Clinical Features

A. Symptoms and Signs

Patients with severely elevated blood pressure are frequently asymptomatic, but most will present with headache, confusion, stupor, seizure, or coma depending on the severity of hypertension and the degree of end-organ involvement. Chest pain may be due to angina pectoris, unstable angina, or myocardial infarction associated with hypertension, but chest pain should also raise the possibility of aortic dissection. In malignant hypertension, encephalopathy with papilledema is present. Acute oliguric renal failure as well as signs and symptoms of congestive heart failure may be seen. The blood pressure is usually quite elevated, with diastolic blood pressure exceeding 130 mm Hg. Ophthalmoscopic examination may demonstrate retinal hemorrhages and exudates as well as papilledema. Patients may have evidence of congestive heart failure. Neurologic findings due to severe hypertension may include focal motor or sensory abnormalities as well as altered mental status. However, other causes of acute neurologic impairment with hypertension must be excluded, including primary central nervous system events such as strokes, tumors, head injury, encephalitis, and collagen-vascular disease.

B. Laboratory Findings

Serum creatinine and urea nitrogen may be elevated. In those with acute hypertensive nephropathy, urinalysis shows red blood cells and red blood cell casts and proteinuria.

C. Electrocardiography

Electrocardiography may show left ventricular hypertrophy, particularly with chronic hypertension. Acute ST and T wave changes may be secondary to hypertension but may also represent acute ischemia.

D. Imaging Studies

The chest x-ray may show cardiomegaly and pulmonary edema. Aortic dissection should be considered when reviewing the film. Imaging of specific organs depends on symptoms and signs and may include head CT (strokes, focal neurologic findings), renal ultrasound (acute renal insufficiency), and echocardiography (aortic dissection).

Treatment

The most important consideration in patients with hypertensive crisis is rapid reduction of blood pressure with a short-acting, easily titratable agent. The goal is to prevent permanent vascular and neurologic damage and to avoid worsening heart failure or causing uncontrollable hypotension. Blood pressure should be controlled aggressively in these patients, and therapy should be instituted even while etiologic investigation is still under way. Of particular concern, patients with strokes or other types of neurologic dysfunction may sustain further neurologic damage if blood pressure is lowered too abruptly or is lowered excessively. Therefore, the initial goal of antihypertensive therapy is to lower blood pressure to not less than 150/110 mm Hg. Further lowering should take place more gradually.

A. Nitroprusside

Intravenous nitroprusside, which acts as a peripheral arteriolodilator, is the drug of choice in hypertensive crises because it can be titrated rapidly and safely. Excessive hypotension can be avoided by careful blood pressure monitoring, usually with an arterial catheter, but a noninvasive automated cuff manometer is usually satisfactory. If hypotension occurs with nitroprusside therapy, discontinuation of the drug results in rapid restoration of blood pressure. Nitroprusside is given intravenously at a rate of 0.25–10 μg/kg/min. Usually one begins at a low infusion rate and adjusts the rate as needed every 5 minutes over a period of 1–2 hours. Thiocyanate toxicity can occur, particularly in patients with renal failure. However, over the first 24 hours, when control of blood pressure is essential, this is not a concern. After blood pressure is lowered to a satisfactory level, institution of oral antihypertensive drugs is begun with the goal of discontinuing nitroprusside within 24–48 hours.

B. Fenoldopam

Fenoldopam is an intravenous dopamine DA_1 receptor agonist that lacks DA_2 or adrenergic agonist effects. Theoretically, fenoldopam may have beneficial effects on renal perfusion. It is indicated for treatment for severe hypertension for up to 48 hours of and appears to be as effective as nitroprusside. The initial infusion of fenoldopam is 0.1 μg/kg/min, titrated slowly (0.05–0.1 μg/kg/min) every 15–20 minutes to a maximum of 1.6 μg/kg/min. Oral antihypertensive drugs should be started to maintain blood pressure control as the fenoldopam infusion is gradually withdrawn. Side effects include hypotension, tachycardia, headache, flushing, and nausea.

C. Other Antihypertensive Agents

Other parenteral agents that can be used in patients with severe hypertension include esmolol, hydralazine, labetalol, nitroglycerin (usually a mild blood pressure-lowering agent), and enalaprilat, an ACE inhibitor.

Esmolol is a short-acting beta-adrenergic blocker indicated for short-term use. It should be avoided in patients with bronchospasm, severe heart failure, heart block, or bradycardia. Hydralazine is a peripheral vasodilator that can be given orally or intravenously. Reflex tachycardia is common, and beta-adrenergic blockers are almost always given simultaneously. Labetalol has both alpha- and beta-adrenergic blocking effects. Nitroglycerin has primarily venodilator effects. The degree of lowering of blood pressure with intravenous nitroglycerin varies from patient to patient, and there is some risk of lowering cardiac output excessively with this drug. On the other hand, nitroglycerin has the advantage of being a coronary artery vasodilator and therefore is useful in patients with hypertension and myocardial ischemia. Enalaprilat is the only intravenous ACE inhibitor available. It is converted to the active drug enalapril after infusion. It has modest antihypertensive effects at the dosages recommended (starting dose: 0.625 mg). Side effects include worsening of renal failure and hyperkalemia.

Oral calcium channel blockers, including amlodipine and diltiazem, are useful in less severe hypertension. In patients with severe hypertension and heart failure, calcium channel blockers and beta-blockers may result in unacceptable depression of ventricular function, in some cases worsening congestive heart failure. However, beta-adrenergic blockers must be used in patients with dissecting aortic aneurysms before systemic vasodilators (hydralazine, nitroprusside) are given to prevent an increase in shear stress on the aortic wall. Diuretics may be needed in addition to the antihypertensive medication to help relieve the volume overload associated with treatment with many of the vasodilator drugs.

Stable patients with severe hypertension without encephalopathy may be managed with oral agents, including beta-blockers, calcium channel blockers, clonidine, hydralazine, minoxidil, and ACE inhibitors. Combinations of drugs are often necessary to maximize effects and minimize side effects and toxicities.

Elliott WJ: Hypertensive emergencies. Crit Care Clin 2001;17:435–51.

Ferguson RK, Vlasses PH: Hypertensive emergencies and urgencies. JAMA 1986;255:1607–13.

Houston MC: Pathophysiology, clinical aspects, and treatment of hypertensive crises. Prog Cardiovasc Dis 1989;32:99–148.

Murphy MB, Murray C, Shorten GD: Fenoldopam—a selective peripheral dopamine receptor agonist for the treatment of severe hypertension. N Engl J Med 2001;345:1548–57.

Varon J, Marik PE: The diagnosis and management of hypertensive crises. Chest 2000;118:214–27.

COMPLICATIONS OF CARDIAC CATHETERIZATION

ESSENTIALS OF DIAGNOSIS

- *Bleeding or thrombosis at vascular access site.*
- *Peripheral arterial emboli from clot at access site.*
- *Central nervous system complications from cerebrovascular emboli.*
- *Arrhythmias, myocardial infarction, cardiac tamponade from myocardial perforation, aortic dissection.*

General Considerations

Patients may be admitted to the ICU after cardiac catheterization for monitoring or because of complications. Complications may result from the underlying cardiac problem, but complications from the cardiac catheterization procedure itself should be anticipated. Complications can be grouped into problems related to the vascular access site, the aorta, and the heart.

A. Vascular Access Complications

Vascular access, particularly in an atherosclerotic vessel, can result in the development of dissection or occlusion at the vascular site or may provide a nidus for thrombus with or without peripheral embolization. In addition, large hematomas may develop at the entry site if adequate hemostasis is not achieved or if vascular damage with a pseudoaneurysm or intimal tear has occurred. The use of heparin, aspirin, and glycoprotein IIb/IIIa receptor inhibitors for treatment of unstable angina, and prolonged catheter placement after catheterization have increased the risk of bleeding and the need to pay attention to local hemostasis. Several kinds of devices have been developed to close arterial catheter puncture sites when catheterization is completed, including those with arterial sutures and devices that provide internal compression with a collagen plug. These devices have significantly reduced the risk of bleeding.

In patients with bleeding at the access site, the hematoma should be measured, outlined with a marker, and then observed for any increase in size. An enlarging hematoma or swelling at the access site indicates a need for rapid evaluation to exclude or control significant bleeding. Distal peripheral pulses, leg temperature, and the arterial site should be checked and findings recorded frequently. Doppler studies are indicated if changes occur or pain develops in the distal portion of the extremity or if a pseudoaneurysm or dissection is suspected. Patients undergoing percutaneous transluminal coronary angioplasty (PTCA) and stent placement usually have the arterial sheath left in place for 12–24 hours or may undergo repeat catheterizations to treat multiple lesions. These repeat and prolonged interventions may increase the risk of complications and require diligent anticoagulation to avoid arterial thrombosis.

B. Central Nervous System Complications

Strokes can occur during and after cardiac catheterization because of embolization of intracardiac thrombi, aortic intimal plaque disruption, catheter thrombosis and embolization, or, more rarely, from dissection of carotid arteries or air inadvertently injected during catheterization. Strokes due to catheterization are not infrequent occurrences. A careful neurologic evaluation prior to cardiac catheterization makes evaluation after catheterization more useful. Interpretation of neurologic findings can be complicated by the use of sedation for catheterization; however, a localizing finding such as hemiplegia or aphasia is highly suggestive of postcatheterization emboli. CT scan or MRI of the head should be performed to help determine whether the event is associated with hemorrhage. Whether acute thrombolysis will have a place in management of postcatheterization strokes is unclear.

C. Other Complications

Cardiac complications related to catheterization include myocardial infarction, arrhythmias, cardiac tamponade, and aortic dissection. Echocardiography should be performed with little hesitation in patients complaining of dyspnea or chest pain after catheterization, and this technique can be useful to look for new cardiac wall motion abnormalities, aortic dissection, or the development of a pericardial effusion.

Pericardial effusions developing after catheterization are relatively rare but require close observation for development of tamponade, particularly in patients who have had interventions (eg, angioplasty) or are receiving platelet inhibitors or anticoagulation. Tamponade with hemodynamic collapse can develop rapidly in these situations. Acute shortness of breath with chest pain may be due to acute ischemia, and this must be differentiated from acute cardiac tamponade.

Radiologic contrast media-related problems include histamine-mediated reactions (urticaria, angioedema, hypotension), volume depletion and hypotension secondary to the osmotic diuresis, and acute renal failure. Close monitoring of patients after cardiac catheterization requires attention to electrolyte and fluid balance. Patients with diabetes and preexisting renal disease are at increased risk for acute renal failure.

Urticaria and other histamine reactions can be reduced by pretreatment with antihistamines and H_2 blockers 1 hour before the procedure. Patients with known allergic reactions to contrast should also be pretreated with corticosteroids 8–12 hours before the procedure. Hydration before and after contrast administration is the best way to prevent renal failure. Patients with renal insufficiency may have a reduced risk of further deterioration if given acetylcysteine prior to the administration of contrast.

Chandrasekar B et al: Complications of cardiac catheterization in the current era: a single-center experience. Catheter Cardiovasc Interv 2001;52:289–95.

Tepel M et al: Prevention of radiographic-contrast-agent-induced reductions in renal function by acetylcysteine. N Engl J Med 2000;343:180–4.

AORTIC DISSECTION

ESSENTIALS OF DIAGNOSIS

- *Severe chest pain without features of ischemic heart disease in the presence of hypertension.*
- *Widened mediastinum on chest x-ray. Aortic dissection identified by echocardiogram, CT, or MRI. May be associated with hypertensive heart disease.*

General Considerations

Acute aortic dissection is seen in patients with underlying atherosclerotic vascular disease, hypertension, and connective tissue abnormalities such as Marfan's syndrome. Aortic dissection is the acute development of a tear in the intima of the aorta. Arterial blood under high pressure enters the intima, extending the tear and causing progressive destruction of the aortic media. This process is potentially catastrophic. The path the dissection takes is quite variable, spiraling superiorly and retrograde to the aortic valve and the coronary arteries, antegrade to the abdominal aorta, or both. The hemodynamic manifestations and clinical findings will depend on the path the dissection takes.

Dissections occur most frequently in the ascending aorta near the aortic valve or in the proximal descending aorta beyond the takeoff of the left subclavian artery. There are several classification systems for describing the location of aortic dissection. The easiest to understand and most relevant in terms of clinical decision making divides aortic dissections into two types. The proximal or ascending (type A) dissection involves the proximal aorta but may extend beyond the aortic arch. This type is analogous to the DeBakey type I and type II classification of aortic dissections. Descending or distal (type B) dissection involves only the descending portion of the aorta, similar to DeBakey type III. Type A dissections are often lethal, causing acute aortic insufficiency, congestive heart failure, pericardial effusions often with tamponade, and acute myocardial infarctions. Treatment is almost always surgical. Type B dissections are initially treated medically but may require surgery after stabilization.

Clinical Features

A. Symptoms and Signs

The most common clinical presentation of patients with aortic dissections is the abrupt onset of severe chest pain or back pain. The pain is at maximum intensity at onset. The pain often tracks the progression or pathway of the dissection and is often described as tearing or ripping in quality. The severity of the pain may precipitate vagal reflexes, including hypotension and bradycardia. If the aortic valve or coronary arteries are involved, congestive heart failure can develop acutely. Cardiac tamponade may occur if the tear extends into the proximal aortic root, allowing blood to enter the pericardial space. Physical findings include diminished or unequal peripheral pulses and blood pressures. A murmur of aortic regurgitation may be heard along with findings consistent with acute pulmonary edema or tamponade.

In this age of thrombolytic therapy and anticoagulation for acute myocardial infarction, it is critically important to distinguish aortic dissection from myocardial ischemia. Although both present with chest pain, the pattern of pain—quality, location, duration, and onset—should help distinguish the two. Pain from aortic dissection is more abrupt in onset, more often reaches maximum intensity immediately, and is often described as tearing in quality. Location is more often in the back rather than substernal. Unlike myocardial pain, the pain of aortic dissection usually does not respond to nitrates or beta-blockers acutely but may do so if a reduction of blood pressure decreases the stress on the aorta. Also unlike myocardial ischemia, aortic dissection pain is usually unrelated to activity. In contrast, ischemic pain usually begins slowly and increases in intensity. It radiates to the neck, jaw, and arm but never below the umbilicus. Beta-adrenergic blockers and nitrates usually relieve ischemic pain, though not necessarily the pain of myocardial infarction. Ischemia and infarction often have electrocardiographic findings of ST and T wave changes. On examination, the presence of a new aortic diastolic murmur, unequal peripheral pulses, and absence of rales in a patient with chest pain should raise the question of aortic dissection.

If aortic dissection is a consideration, diagnostic tests should be undertaken expeditiously since the treatment—surgical repair, lowering of blood pressure, and decreasing myocardial contractility with beta-blockers—must be administered urgently. Anticoagulation and thrombolytic therapy are clearly contraindicated. Unfortunately, because aortic dissection can cause acute myocardial infarction by involving coronary arteries in the dissection, the distinction between aortic dissection and myocardial ischemia is not always clear.

B. Imaging Studies

Initial evaluation with chest x-ray may identify a widened mediastinum, but more definitive information can be obtained using transthoracic echocardiography. Although the sensitivity for identifying aortic dissection is relatively low with transthoracic echocardiography, this test provides other useful additional information on cardiac function, ventricular wall motion, and valvular abnormalities and can identify the presence of pericardial effusion. In addition, the echocardiogram can be used to measure the aortic root size, and Doppler echocardiography can determine the degree of valvular regurgitation (Figure 21–4).

Transesophageal echocardiography, MRI, and CT scan are 80–100% sensitive and specific for the diagnosis of aortic dissection. MRI is probably the most sensitive and specific procedure, but the availability of transesophageal echocardiography and the ability to monitor the patient more closely during echocardiography than during MRI or CT scanning are important considerations. Monitoring patients during MRI scanning can be difficult, and unstable or hypotensive patients should instead undergo transesophageal echocardiography at the bedside. One of these tests should make the diagnosis rapidly (Figure 21–5). If the imaging technique identifies aortic dissection, therapy is based on the location of the dissection and the extent of aortic involvement. Further studies may be indicated to assess coronary anatomy and aortic valve function. Cardiac catheterization may be needed to help guide operation.

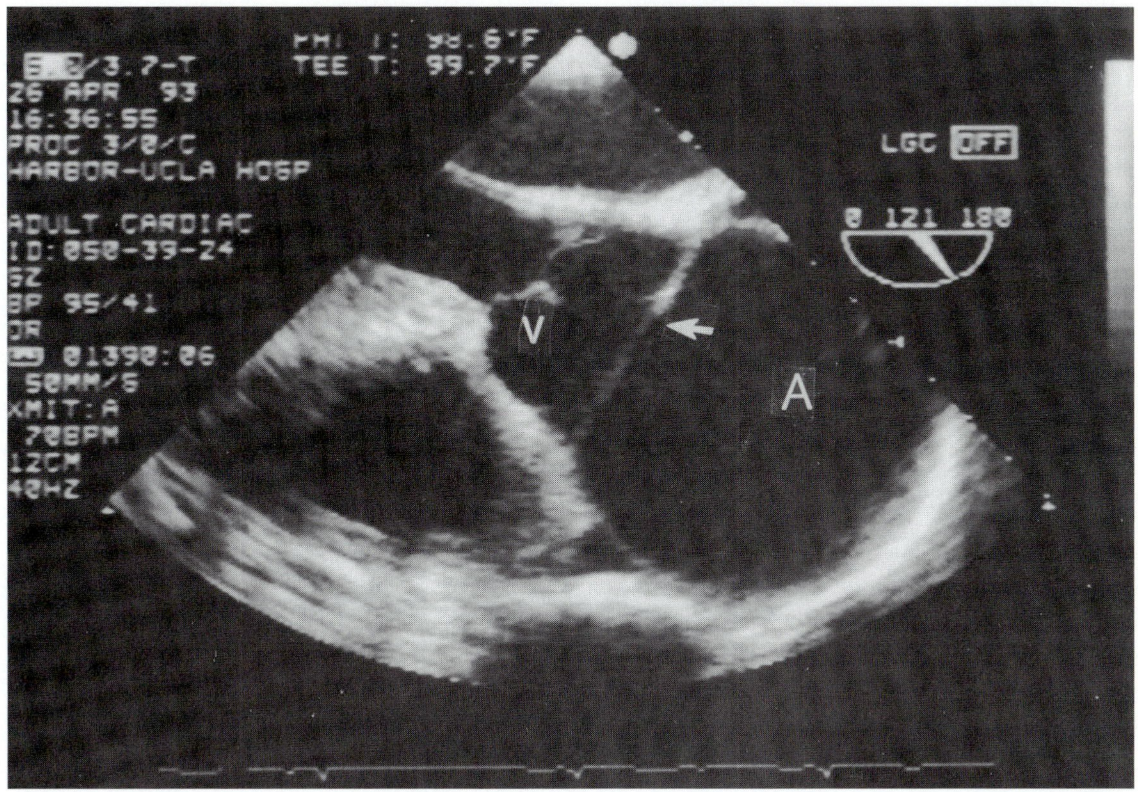

Figure 21–4. Aortic dissection and aneurysm with an intimal flap demonstrated by transesophageal echocardiography. The aneurysm of the ascending aorta is at "A." The aortic valve is at "V." The arrow points to the intimal flap approximately 2 cm above the aortic valve in the proximal ascending aorta.

Treatment

In general, type A aortic dissections require surgery because medical management alone for proximal ascending aortic dissection has a high short-term and 1-year mortality rate. Type B aortic dissections that involve the descending portion of the thoracic aorta only are managed medically unless there is compromise of the renal or mesenteric circulations. Complicated dissections involving the arch and arch vessels have high surgical and medical mortality rates, making therapeutic decisions more difficult.

Immediate management of all aortic dissections requires aggressive medical and pharmacologic therapy to reduce systolic blood pressure and to decrease the peak systolic velocity of aortic blood flow and, thereby, reduce sheer forces on the aortic wall. The goals of therapy include control of pain, reduction of systolic blood pressure to 100–120 mm Hg (as long as renal, myocardial, and cerebral perfusion are maintained), and stabilization of the patient's hemodynamic variables to permit a thorough diagnostic evaluation. Beta-adrenergic blockers are used aggressively to decrease the force of ventricular contraction. Heart rate is used as a guide to the degree of beta blockade, and enough beta-adrenergic blockade should be given to lower the heart rate to 55–65 per minute. Nitroprusside is used to control blood pressure initially and is adjusted as required when beta blockade is achieved. Calcium channel blockers, because of their negative inotropic and antihypertensive properties, are ideal alternatives in patients who are unable to tolerate beta-blockers. Hydralazine and other direct vasodilators should not be given to control blood pressure in the absence of beta-adrenergic blockade. Although blood pressure will fall, the force of aortic blood flow may increase, further increasing stress on the damaged aortic wall.

Survival rates approach 80–90% when appropriate therapy is rapidly instituted in both type A and type B aortic dissections. Outcome is in part determined by

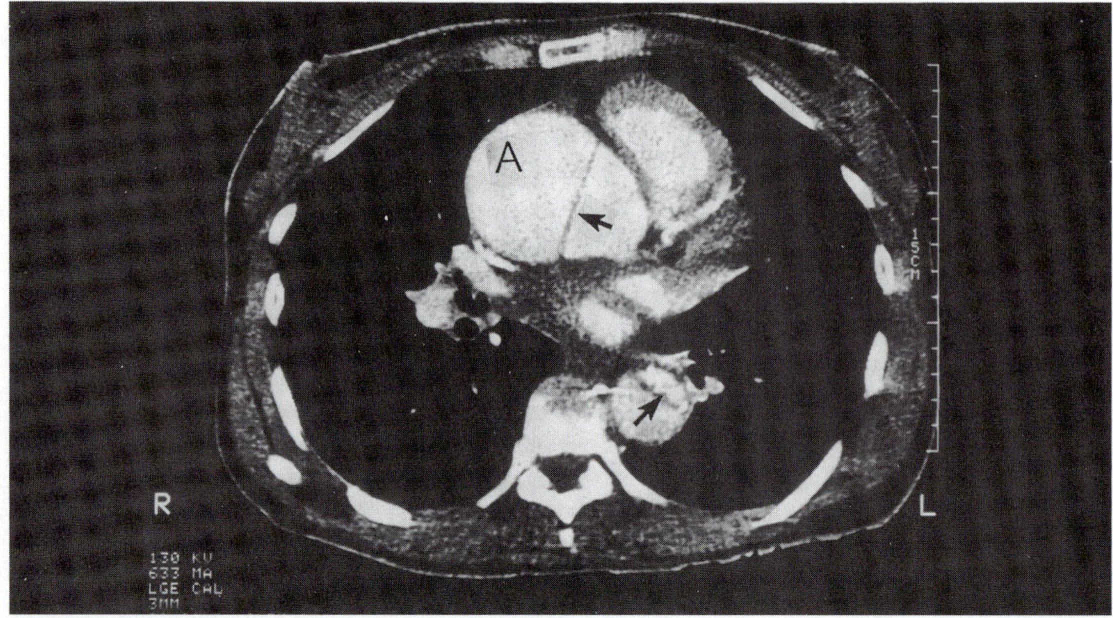

Figure 21–5. Aortic dissection and aneurysm with an intimal flap as demonstrated by ultrafast CT scan in the same patient as shown by transesophageal echocardiography in Figure 21–4. The arrows point to the intimal flap. The aneurysm is marked by an "A."

the degree of damage to vital organs (kidneys, brain, heart, and bowel), the underlying condition of the aorta, and the extent of the repair needed.

Cigarroa JE et al: Diagnostic imaging in the evaluation of suspected aortic dissection. Old standards and new directions. N Engl J Med 1993;328:35–43.

DeSanctis RW et al: Aortic dissection. N Engl J Med 1987; 317:1060–6.

Erbel R et al: Diagnosis and management of aortic dissection. Eur Heart J 2001;22:1642–81.

Hagan PG et al: The International Registry of Acute Aortic Dissection (IRAD): new insights into an old disease. JAMA 2000;283:897–903.

ATRIAL ARRHYTHMIAS

Critically ill patients—particularly those with pulmonary disease and respiratory failure—are at high risk for development of atrial arrhythmias. Atrial distention, electrolyte imbalances, hypoxia, and high catecholamine levels all contribute to electrical instability and increased atrial automaticity. Identifying the type of supraventricular arrhythmia is essential in choosing the correct treatment. A 12-lead ECG permits more careful evaluation of P wave morphology and axis than a single-lead ECG from the bedside monitor or "rhythm strip." The morphology of the ST segments and T waves should be examined for evidence of ischemia. The PR interval and initial activation of the QRS segment can identify the presence of an AV nodal bypass tract and show evidence of preexcitation.

Treatment is directed primarily toward eliminating or reversing the precipitating or exacerbating causes. Correction of alkalosis, hypokalemia, hypomagnesemia, or hypoxemia will increase the likelihood of rate control and eventual conversion to sinus rhythm. The major goal of acute treatment is to slow the ventricular rate so as to improve cardiac output and blood pressure. In the setting of hemodynamic compromise (hypotension, syncope, chest pain, or electrocardiographic evidence of ischemia), rapid treatment using electrical cardioversion may be indicated. This treatment should also be performed immediately if the ventricular rate is extremely rapid or the patient will not tolerate prolonged tachycardia because of other conditions such as aortic or mitral stenosis, hypertrophic cardiomyopathy, or unstable angina. The high likelihood of recurrence of these arrhythmias makes rhythm identification and appropriate pharmacologic treatment important even if initially corrected by electrical cardioversion.

ATRIOVENTRICULAR NODAL OR REENTRANT TACHYCARDIA

Atrioventricular nodal reentrant (circus movement) tachycardias are rhythm disturbances that depend on the properties of the atrioventricular node and the conducting tissue around it for propagation. The arrhythmia results from an endless circle of electrical impulses conducted down one pathway and up another, with slow and fast pathways cooperating to facilitate and maintain the circuit. Alteration of refractoriness or conduction velocities in the atrioventricular node or atrial tissue can immediately stop the arrhythmia. The arrhythmia can be prevented by altering the electrical properties of the involved pathways or by decreasing the frequency of the premature atrial contractions that often initiate the cycle.

Atrioventricular nodal reentrant tachycardias usually have ventricular rates of 140–220 beats/min, and AV conduction is usually 1:1 but occasionally 2:1. The P wave may not be obvious if atrial and ventricular depolarization occur simultaneously, though a retrograde P wave may be seen. Differential diagnosis includes sinus tachycardia, atrial flutter, and atrial fibrillation. If the diagnosis is unclear, adenosine (6–12 mg intravenously) will usually cause the ventricular rate to fall all at once to the underlying sinus rate and rhythm. Sinus tachycardia will slow gradually in response to adenosine, then resume the pretreatment rate.

Atrioventricular nodal reentrant tachycardias are treated effectively with adenosine (6–12 mg intravenous bolus), verapamil (5–10 mg intravenous bolus), diltiazem (continuous infusion), or beta-adrenergic blockers (eg, metoprolol, 5–15 mg intravenously). These drugs alter conduction velocity through the atrioventricular node. Because of adenosine's extremely short half-life (measured in seconds), it is the drug of choice for acute treatment but is not useful in preventing recurrences. Therefore, if the risk of recurrence is great in patients with an underlying predisposing medical condition, one of the other drugs can be administered to decrease the likelihood of recurrence and can be tried if adenosine fails to convert the patient to sinus rhythm. In patients with compromised ventricular function, digoxin may be a more appropriate long-term drug than either calcium channel blockers or beta-adrenergic blockers, both of which are myocardial depressants.

Procainamide is effective in treating atrial arrhythmias by preventing premature atrial beats and decreasing atrial automaticity. When the atrioventricular nodal reentry tachycardia utilizes concealed retrograde conduction through a bypass tract, procainamide may also help by slowing conduction through the bypass tract. A bypass tract may be suspected when the ventricular rate exceeds 200 beats/min in an adult or when a baseline ECG demonstrates a short PR interval and evidence of preexcitation. Digoxin, beta-adrenergic blockers, and calcium channel blockers can be dangerous in patients with concealed bypass tracts who have atrial fibrillation because these drugs block atrioventricular nodal conduction and thereby facilitate conduction through the bypass tract. The ventricle is bombarded by an increased number of impulses from the atria, resulting in a very rapid ventricular rate. Ventricular fibrillation may follow. Class Ic and class III antiarrhythmic agents such as flecainide and amiodarone can also be helpful for medical management of patients with bypass tracts. The development of transvenous catheters for radiofrequency ablation of bypass tracts obviates the need for long-term pharmacologic therapy for most patients and have largely replaced operation. Atrioventricular nodal reentry arrhythmias without bypass tracts and atrial flutter are also effectively treated with ablation.

ATRIAL TACHYCARDIA

Atrial tachycardia is an automatic rhythm (repetitive single focus) and does not depend on the atrioventricular node and reentry to continue. Atrial tachycardia is less common than AV nodal reentrant rhythms and usually has a regular ventricular rate of 140–220 beats/min, though AV block may cause the ventricular rate to be considerably slower. P waves have uniform morphology and relationship to the QRS.

Although calcium channel blockers, beta-blockers, and digoxin will usually not terminate these atrial arrhythmias, they will decrease the ventricular response rate by slowing atrioventricular nodal conduction and therefore can effectively improve hemodynamics. Slowing of the ventricular rate may be helpful in identifying underlying atrial activity on the ECG, so that a distinction can be made between atrial tachycardia, AV nodal reentry, atrial flutter, or atrial fibrillation. After the ventricular rate is controlled, conversion to sinus rhythm can be attempted with class Ia, Ic, or III antiarrhythmic agents or electrical cardioversion. Radiofrequency ablation can be considered in selected cases when the focus of the arrhythmia can be localized and the arrhythmia occurs frequently

ATRIAL FLUTTER

Atrial flutter is a microreentrant arrhythmia and in many ways behaves like atrial tachycardia. Atrial flutter should always be considered when a patient presents with supraventricular tachycardia with a rate of approximately 150 beats/min. The atrial flutter rate is usually approximately 300 beats/min, but, because of normal delays in conduction through the atrioventricular node, the ventricular response rate is slower than the atrial rate, with only every other (2:1 AV block) or every third beat (3:1 AV block) effectively conducted to the ventricle. Increasing the degree of atrioventricular nodal block with drugs (adenosine) or by carotid massage brings out the underlying flutter waves on the ECG and establishes the diagnosis.

Drugs that increase atrioventricular nodal block can usually—though not always—control the ventricular rate at rest, but conversion to sinus rhythm usually requires either antiarrhythmic drugs or, more commonly, electrical cardioversion. Ibutilide, sotalol, or amiodarone can be tried. In general atrial flutter is more resistant to pharmacologic conversion than AV nodal reentrant tachycardia. However, unlike atrial fibrillation and atrial tachycardia, atrial flutter can be converted using fairly small amounts of electrical energy, usually less than 50 J. Atrial flutter can also be converted to sinus rhythm with overdrive pacing using a transvenous right atrial pacemaker electrode or an esophageal pacemaker electrode. Atrial flutter has become a rhythm which is amenable to radiofrequency ablation, with success rates that are approaching those for other supraventricular tachycardias. Given the difficulty of treating atrial flutter and converting it with medical therapy, ablation provides effective long-term treatment.

A subset of patients with atrial tachyarrhythmia may develop bradycardia after electrical cardioversion or drug therapy. Patients with tachy-brady syndrome pose a particular problem in designing therapy and may require temporary pacing if cardioversion is attempted. They may also require a permanent pacemaker to generate an adequate ventricular rate when receiving necessary drug therapy to control the tachyarrhythmias.

ATRIAL FIBRILLATION

Atrial fibrillation is a chaotic arrhythmia probably due to multiple reentry circuits within the atria that results in loss of atrial contraction and an irregular, often rapid ventricular rate. Because of the rapid but unpredictable bombardment of the atrioventricular node by the atrial fibrillatory impulses and variable penetration of the impulses through the atrioventricular node to the ventricle, the ventricular rate is highly variable. An irregularly irregular ventricular rate with the absence of P waves is the hallmark of atrial fibrillation and makes it easily distinguishable from the other more organized and regular atrial arrhythmias. Patients with acute atrial fibrillation may develop hypotension, myocardial ischemia, decreased perfusion of vital organs, and acute congestive heart failure. Those with chronic atrial fibrillation have an increased risk of atrial mural thrombus formation, with subsequent systemic embolization. Atrial fibrillation is very common in patients with mitral stenosis, lung disease, sepsis, and hyperthyroidism as well as in any form of heart disease or after cardiac surgery.

Therapy is directed at slowing the ventricular rate initially, followed—in appropriate patients—by conversion of atrial fibrillation to sinus rhythm. Slowing of the ventricular rate can be achieved with beta-adrenergic blockers, calcium channel blockers, or digoxin, any of which enhance the atrioventricular nodal refractory period. Control of the ventricular rate is particularly important in patients with ischemia and chest pain, congestive heart failure, mitral stenosis, and hypotension. Intravenous verapamil can be given at a dose of 5–10 mg. Alternatively, intravenous digoxin is effective when given at a dosage of 0.125–0.25 mg every 4–6 hours until the desired rate is achieved, or until 1–1.5 mg has been given. In some patients, combinations of these drugs are necessary, but excessive AV nodal blockade should be avoided. The goal of rate control is to lower the ventricular rate to about 80–100 beats/min.

Ibutilide, an intravenous short acting class III antiarrhythmic agent, can be used to convert atrial fibrillation to normal sinus rhythm. When given before DC cardioversion, it increases the likelihood of success. It has proarrhythmic effects, including torsade de pointes, that necessitate close monitoring during its infusion and for several hours after. Combined use with amiodarone may increase heart block or arrhythmias. Sotalol, a class III antiarrhythmic with beta-adrenergic blocking properties, or amiodarone can also be used. These agents can be continued to help maintain normal sinus rhythm. Long-term use of sotalol and amiodarone, however, may result in bradycardia, which may be prolonged because of the 32-day half-life for amiodarone.

Conversion to sinus rhythm may be attempted using class Ia antiarrhythmic drugs such as quinidine or procainamide or by electrical cardioversion. Before administering class Ia drugs, the ventricular response rate must be well controlled because—and this is also seen with atrial flutter and atrial tachycardia—acceleration of the ventricular rate may occur when these drugs are given. It should also be noted that the administration of quinidine may result in nearly a doubling of the serum digoxin level. Thus, a patient with atrial fibrillation whose ventricular rate is controlled with digoxin and who has no evidence of digoxin toxicity may develop digoxin toxicity when quinidine is given. Procainamide may therefore be a better short-term choice in the critically ill patient receiving digoxin. Neither quinidine nor procainamide is well tolerated as a long term oral medication, and both also have significant proarrhythmic effects. They are being replaced by newer type III agents. Electrical cardioversion of atrial fibrillation to sinus rhythm generally requires higher amounts of electrical energy compared with other atrial arrhythmias, often > 100 J.

Atrial fibrillation poses a risk of embolization because the noncontracting atria are potential sites for thrombus formation, and the risk of embolization increases with cardioversion. The greatest risk of embolization is associated with atrial enlargement and atrial fibrillation of long duration. Therefore, patients who have had atrial fibrillation for more than 1 week should be anticoagulated for 3–4 weeks before conversion is attempted. Alternatively, it has been shown to be safe to undertake cardioversion if a transesophageal echocardiogram performed while on anticoagulation demonstrates no atrial thrombi and anticoagulation is continued for 4 weeks after cardioversion. This approach allows fairly immediate cardioversion of patients in whom the duration of atrial fibrillation is unknown and avoids leaving the patient in atrial fibrillation for several additional weeks. Patients without mitral stenosis who develop acute atrial fibrillation can be cardioverted within the first several days without anticoagulation.

Patients with atrial fibrillation who cannot be converted to sinus rhythm are managed by controlling their ventricular rates. Anticoagulation with warfarin should be considered in patients with chronic atrial fibrillation because of the increased frequency of embolic strokes even in the absence of intrinsic heart disease. Aspirin may be an adequate alternative in healthy patients or those with contraindications to anticoagulation with warfarin.

MULTIFOCAL ATRIAL TACHYCARDIA

Multifocal atrial tachycardia is an atrial arrhythmia that can be confused with atrial fibrillation, but it is managed quite differently. This arrhythmia is generally seen in patients with severe lung disease and respiratory failure. The hallmark of this atrial tachycardia is an irregular ventricular rate but with multiple atrial foci (P waves with different morphologic appearances). Atrial fibrillation also has an irregular ventricular response, but P waves are absent.

Treatment of the underlying lung disease and respiratory failure usually corrects the arrhythmia. Once the precipitating pulmonary process resolves, sinus rhythm often returns. Multifocal atrial tachycardia responds poorly to digoxin, with neither slowing of the ventricular rate nor conversion to sinus rhythm. Verapamil may be effective sometimes in slowing ventricular rate and decreasing the frequency of ectopic atrial beats.

VENTRICULAR ARRHYTHMIAS

Management of ventricular arrhythmias in the ICU is often more complicated than management of atrial arrhythmias because the treatment is sometimes worse than the disease, and because these arrhythmias may be poorly tolerated by critically ill patients. Rapid ventricular arrhythmias (eg, ventricular tachycardia) require immediate treatment, particularly in patients who have severe underlying cardiac disease. Almost all antiarrhythmic agents used for the treatment of ventricular arrhythmias may facilitate arrhythmias ("proarrhythmic" effect) and have a variety of other unpleasant or life-threatening side effects. Therefore, treatment of ventricular arrhythmias should be limited to those known to cause hemodynamic compromise or those that occur in the setting of underlying myocardial disease. In general, the more malignant the arrhythmia appears—ie, the more rapid the rate, the longer the duration of the arrhythmia, the more frequent the occurrence, and the greater the hemodynamic compromise (hypotension, syncope)—the more important it is to treat. In addition, the presence of ventricular tachycardia should always raise the question of ischemia with underlying coronary artery disease.

The nuances of evaluation and management of sudden cardiac death and nonsustained and sustained ventricular tachycardia in the presence or absence of ventricular dysfunction are beyond the scope of this text. However, development of significant ventricular arrhythmia justifies and necessitates consultation with an electrophysiologist to determine whether medical therapy is indicated, to assess drug efficacy, and to consider more definitive treatment, including implantable defibrillators and transvenous ablation. The development of sudden cardiac death and sustained ventricular tachycardia in patients without known cardiac disease should result in a careful search for cardiac disease, particularly ischemia. Cardiac catheterization with coronary arteriography may be indicated.

VENTRICULAR ECTOPY (PREMATURE VENTRICULAR CONTRACTIONS)

Treatment of asymptomatic ventricular ectopy (premature ventricular contractions, PVCs) is usually not indicated, particularly in light of many studies demonstrating both the lack of efficacy and potential catastrophic side effects resulting from treatment of non-life-threatening ventricular arrhythmias in certain populations.

Ventricular ectopy is often benign and requires no treatment. However, development of PVCs may be a clue to the presence of digoxin toxicity or electrolyte or other metabolic imbalance—particularly hypokalemia but also hypomagnesemia, alkalosis, hyperkalemia, hypoxemia, and ischemia. Correcting these abnormalities often eliminates the PVCs.

Unifocal PVCs, bigeminy, and couplets (paired PVCs) do not usually require treatment even in a patient with myocardial ischemia. Antiarrhythmic therapy should be reserved for patients with sustained or nonsustained ventricular tachycardia accompanied by hemodynamic compromise. However, the indications for short-term therapy of premature ventricular contractions are less rigorous than the indications for long-term antiarrhythmic treatment, and short-term therapy to suppress PVCs may be appropriate while a patient is medically unstable in the ICU. In patients with congestive heart failure and ventricular ectopy, PVCs may not generate an adequate stroke volume, and frequent PVCs therefore may result in a reduced cardiac output. Suppression of the ectopy may therefore be indicated to increase cardiac output. This goal can usually be achieved with administration of intravenous lidocaine. Procainamide and quinidine are alternatives.

Lidocaine toxicity is most often seen in elderly patients and those with decreased liver function, and the proarrhythmic effects of lidocaine are quite minimal. Both quinidine and procainamide can cause torsade de pointes and worsening of ventricular arrhythmias; use of these agents calls for close monitoring and careful consideration of indications for therapy. The use of beta-blockers, particularly in a patient who has evidence of a high-catecholamine state (tachycardia, agitation, hypertension) may result in a reduction in PVCs, heart rate, and blood pressure.

VENTRICULAR TACHYCARDIA

Ventricular tachycardia is defined as more than three consecutive ventricular beats and is generally considered to be a reentrant type of tachycardia. Nonsustained ventricular tachycardia lasts for less than 30 seconds and spontaneously terminates, in contrast to sustained ventricular tachycardia. Myocardial ischemia is the most common situation in which ventricular tachycardia is seen, but valvular heart disease, myocarditis, and other forms of heart disease also predispose to this arrhythmia. Patients with prolonged QT intervals with or without administration of quinidine or another drug that prolongs the QT interval (such as a tricyclic antidepressant) may have a form of ventricular tachycardia known as torsade de pointes. This arrhythmia presents as ventricular tachycardia marked by a pattern of multiform ventricular beats with the axis shifting with each beat, yielding an undulating QRS pattern (Figure 21–6). Rapid ventricular tachycardia almost always deteriorates into ventricular fibrillation.

In the presence of underlying cardiac disease, ventricular tachycardia often deserves therapy. Nonsustained ventricular tachycardia in the setting of acute ischemia or infarction justifies antiarrhythmic suppression at least over the first 24–48 hours; a similar arrhythmia in a healthy 20-year-old postoperative patient might be observed without therapy, or the patient might be given a beta-adrenergic blocker to decrease the effects of excess catecholamines. Electrolyte imbalances (particularly hypokalemia, hypomagnesemia, and alkalosis) and hypoxia increase ventricular irritability and therefore may predispose to ventricular arrhythmias. In addition, there is evidence that magnesium administration may decrease or prevent ventricular arrhythmias even in the absence of hypomagnesemia. Digoxin toxicity, alcohol withdrawal, and ischemia must also be considered in ICU patients who develop ventricular arrhythmias.

As a general rule, patients with sustained ventricular tachycardia that produces hemodynamic instability with hypotension, congestive heart failure, or chest pain should be immediately electrically cardioverted using 100–400 J. Persistent myocardial ischemia or hypotension that occurs while trying various pharmacologic agents puts the patient at risk of further deterioration and ventricular fibrillation. As the ventricle becomes more ischemic, stabilization becomes more difficult, and intractable ventricular fibrillation and death may ensue.

Pharmacologic conversion of ventricular tachycardia can be used in patients with ventricular tachycardia who are tolerating this rhythm without chest pain, hypotension, or congestive heart failure. Initial therapy is lidocaine administered by an intravenous bolus of 1–2 mg/kg, followed by an intravenous infusion of 1–4 mg/min. Procainamide can be given intravenously as a loading dose (500–1000 mg given at a rate of 50 mg/min), followed by an intravenous infusion (2–4 mg/min) as an alternative if lidocaine fails. Intravenous amiodarone is an effective alternative and is being used more frequently, particularly in patients with recurrent ventricular tachycardia. Amiodarone has a fairly complicated loading schedule: 150 mg is given over 10 minutes followed by 1 mg/min for 6 hours and then 0.5 mg/min for 18 hours. Loading of amiodarone can be repeated if ventricular tachycardia recurs. Bretylium can be used to increase the fibrillation threshold and to convert ventricular tachycardia, but use of this drug is associated with nausea, vomiting, and hypotension. It is now infrequently used. Overdrive pacing to suppress ventricular arrhythmias is helpful in occasional patients.

Patients with torsade de pointes or polymorphic ventricular tachycardia with long QT interval are treated differently. Antiarrhythmic drugs that prolong the QT interval should not be given, including class Ia (quinidine, procainamide), class Ic (flecainide, propafenone), and some class III agents (bretylium, sotalol). These drugs should be stopped if the arrhythmia occurs during their use. Isoproterenol or ventricular overdrive pacing may be helpful in suppressing the initiating ectopic

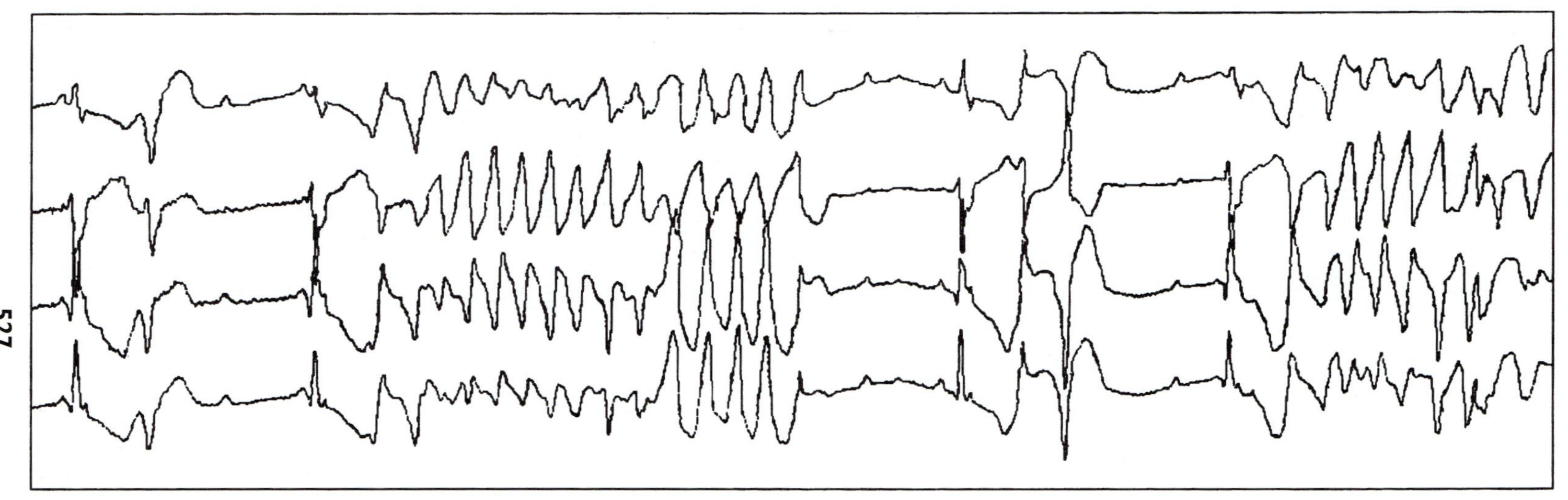

Figure 21–6. Four-channel ECG demonstrating torsade de pointes. This multiform ventricular tachycardia changes its axis with changing height and direction of the QRS complex shifting over the episode. The arrhythmia was initiated by a premature ventricular contraction during a period of high-degree heart block. Note that not all of the P waves are conducted to the ventricle and that the ventricular rate is quite slow.

beats and shortening the QT interval; this is unlike other ventricular arrhythmias, in which beta-adrenergic agonists may exacerbate the arrhythmia.

HEART BLOCK

Heart block occurs when one or more segments of the cardiac conduction system generate or transmit impulses at an inadequate rate. Heart block can be divided into (1) sinus node problems, including sinus arrest, sinus node Wenckebach, and sinus bradycardia; (2) atrioventricular nodal block, including Mobitz type I (Wenckebach); and (3) infranodal block, including bundle branch block, Mobitz type II atrioventricular nodal block, and third-degree heart block. In addition to degeneration caused by aging of the conduction system, heart block can be iatrogenically induced with medications or may be due to myocardial ischemia or infarction; metabolic abnormalities; enhanced vagal tone from tracheal irritation, suction, or intubation; abdominal distention; or severe vomiting. Heart block can sometimes be confused with other cardiac dysrhythmias.

It is important to determine whether the arrhythmia is due to an inadequate impulse formation or poor conduction from the atrium to the ventricles (default) or to a fast nodal or ventricular rate relative to the atrial rate (usurpation). Accelerated idioventricular rhythms, junctional tachycardia, and isorhythmic dissociation are not due to heart block but rather result from an acceleration of infranodal pacemakers. As there is no heart block, speeding of the atrial rate will entrain the ventricles normally.

Heart block is managed differently depending on whether the ventricular rate is adequate or there is clinically significant bradycardia. Treatment of heart block should focus on several issues: (1) identification of reversible causes; (2) the hemodynamic consequences of the arrhythmia; (3) the potential to progress or recur; and (4) the patient's underlying medical condition. For example, the management of patients with second-degree heart block secondary to the combined use of a calcium blocker and a beta-adrenergic blocker for hypertension is different from management of a similar degree of heart block due to intrinsic conduction system disease. Time, calcium, and perhaps isoproterenol might obviate the need for even temporary pacing support in the former, but permanent pacing will probably be required for the latter.

External cardiac pacing may be used for short periods, permitting stabilization with adequate ventricular rates and decreasing the urgency of the need for temporary transvenous pacing. Temporary transvenous pacing should be used in patients who are hemodynamically compromised by heart block. Indications for both temporary and permanent pacing in coronary artery disease are discussed in Chapter 22.

HEART BLOCK & CONDUCTION DISTURBANCES

Sinus Bradyarrhythmias

The name "sick sinus syndrome" has been given to a variety of bradyarrhythmias arising in the sinus node. These include sinus arrest and symptomatic sinus bradycardia. When seen in association with alternating bradycardia and supraventricular tachycardia, the term tachy-brady syndrome is sometimes used. Many patients with sinus bradyarrhythmias have intrinsic heart disease, but digoxin, beta-blockers, calcium channel blockers, and other drugs may precipitate bradycardia with syncope, hypotension, and heart failure. In patients with drug-related bradyarrhythmias, discontinuation of the drug is necessary; in others with symptomatic bradycardia, a pacemaker may be necessary. As described above, treatment of supraventricular tachycardia associated with alternating bradycardia may require drug treatment of the tachycardia (digoxin, beta-blockers) and a pacemaker (because of drug-induced bradycardia).

Atrioventricular Block

Temporary or permanent alteration of conduction through the atrioventricular node or bundle of His is classified as atrioventricular block. Patients with prolonged PR intervals (> 210 ms) have first-degree atrioventricular block; this can be due to intrinsic conduction system disease, increased vagal tone, or, more commonly, cardiac medications or ischemia. First-degree atrioventricular block is usually benign. Second-degree atrioventricular block is diagnosed when atrial impulses are intermittently conducted through to the ventricles. In Mobitz type I second-degree atrioventricular block (Wenckebach block), the PR interval lengthens on successive beats prior to a nonconducted atrial beat (P wave without a following QRS). The electrocardiographic pattern that emerges is grouped beating in which the number of ventricular complexes is equal to the number of P waves minus 1. This rhythm is usually due to increased vagal tone and is often seen in conjunction with reversible ischemia of the atrioventricular node. Treatment of symptomatic or severe bradycardia with Mobitz type I block is begun with atropine. Isoproterenol and dopamine may be tried; a temporary pacemaker is occasionally necessary if the ventricular response is inadequate and prolonged.

Mobitz type II second-degree atrioventricular block is due to disease in the infranodal conduction system. The PR interval is constant in conducted beats. The QRS is usually mildly prolonged secondary to the infranodal conducting system disease. In the nonconducted or blocked beats, a P wave is seen without a QRS. This form of block may occur in a pattern or may occur randomly. Several P waves without accompanying ventricular beats may be seen (3:1 or 4:1 block). A temporary pacemaker is often necessary with this type of block because of the higher likelihood of progression to complete atrioventricular block, and the escape pacemaker with type II block originates in the ventricle and may not generate an adequate ventricular rate.

During complete heart block (third-degree atrioventricular block), no atrial impulses are conducted to the ventricles because of usually infranodal or severe atrioventricular nodal conduction system disease. There is no relationship between P waves and the QRS (AV dissociation). The prolonged QRS interval indicates that ventricular activation is initiated by a ventricular pacemaker (automatic focus). Ventricular rates of 35–40 beats/min are seen with these ventricular escape rhythms and are usually inadequate to maintain acceptable cardiac output and blood pressure. Temporary and often permanent pacing is required in adults with type II second-degree heart block and third-degree heart block.

MALFUNCTION OF PERMANENT ARTIFICIAL PACEMAKERS

Permanent pacemakers are used to support cardiac electrical activity and maintain adequate heart rate by providing electrical stimulation to the cardiac chambers. Pacemaker leads are placed transvenously, though occasionally they may be placed epicardially in association with other cardiac surgery. Pacemakers have become increasingly more complex and sophisticated in the last 5–10 years. In addition to the familiar single-lead pacemakers, which sense and pace in the ventricular chamber, pacemakers now are often dual-chamber, sensing and pacing in both the atrium and the ventricle. Pacemakers can be programmed to interrupt arrhythmias by overdrive pacing or by administering ectopic beats. Pacemakers can have rate-responsive features that allow the heart rate to increase in response to increased physiologic demand.

Because of these added features, assessing pacemaker function has become extremely complex and requires knowledge of the type of pacemaker, understanding of the algorithms the pacemaker uses, and information about the mode in which the pacemaker is functioning. For example, for a rate-responsive pacemaker, knowing the rate at which the pacemaker should be inhibited involves not only knowing its backup settings but the ramp used to adjust the pacing rate and the stimulus to which it is responding.

In a critically ill patient, the major concerns about permanent pacemaker function are (1) that the electrical impulse from the pacemaker results in stimulation and electrical activation in the heart; (2) that the pacemaker is providing an adequate heart rate to meet the patient's needs; and (3) that the pacemaker is sensing the intrinsic cardiac activity and not competing with it. A properly functioning pacemaker is able to sense the intrinsic electrical activity of the heart, so that the pacemaker-generated rhythm and intrinsic rhythm are not competing with each other. Failure to sense the intrinsic rhythm raises the possibility of pacemaker-induced arrhythmia; for example, ventricular tachycardia may result from a pacemaker-triggered QRS occurring on a T wave from the intrinsic rhythm.

In general, in the absence of battery failure, pacemaker failure is almost always due either to lead malfunction from wire fracture, loss of insulation, or fibrosis at the endocardial contact site or to dislodgment in the cardiac chamber or at the junction between the pacemaker and the pacemaker lead. Lead malfunctions produce problems with both the sensing mode and the capturing mode, but often the malfunction is intermittent (occurring when the lead is moved in a particular way), making detection difficult. Interrogation of the pacemaker using the programming device provided by the manufacturer will produce information about the pacemaker's settings as well as lead impedance, thresholds, amplitude of sensed electrical activity, and strength and remaining life of the pacemaker. This information can often differentiate lead malfunction from component malfunction. Unfortunately, the older the pacemaker, the less information can be derived from the programmer; and the older the pacemaker, the more likely it is that malfunction will occur.

Programmability of the pacemaker—ie, the ability to change the rate of pacing or the relationship of ventricular to atrial activation—allows manipulation of the patient's hemodynamics. For example, in a febrile or septic patient or one with heart failure, increasing the ventricular rate may be needed to increase cardiac output. In patients who develop atrial tachyarrhythmias, changing the pacemaker function to ignore the atrial activity can sometimes allow much better rate control.

Desai AD, Chun S, Sung RJ: The role of intravenous amiodarone in the management of cardiac arrhythmias. Ann Intern Med 1997;127:294–303.

Falk RH: Atrial fibrillation. N Engl J Med 2001;344:1067–78.

Fuster V et al: ACC/AHA/ESC guidelines for the management of patients with atrial fibrillation: executive summary. A Report of the American College of Cardiology/American Heart Association Task Force on Practice Guidelines and the European Society of Cardiology Committee for Practice Guidelines and Policy Conferences (Committee to Develop Guidelines for the Management of Patients With Atrial Fibrillation): developed in Collaboration With the North American Society of Pacing and Electrophysiology. J Am Coll Cardiol 2001;38:1231–66.

Ganz LI, Friedman PL: Supraventricular tachycardia. N Engl J Med 1995;19;332:162–73.

Gregoratos G et al: ACC/AHA guidelines for implantation of cardiac pacemakers and antiarrhythmia devices: a report of the American College of Cardiology/American Heart Association Task Force on Practice Guidelines (Committee on Pacemaker Implantation). J Am Coll Cardiol 1998;31:1175–209.

Kaushik V et al: Bradyarrhythmias, temporary and permanent pacing. Crit Care Med 2000;28(10 Suppl):N121–8.

Kowey PR et al: Intravenous antiarrhythmic therapy in the acute control of in-hospital destabilizing ventricular tachycardia and fibrillation. Am J Cardiol 1999;84:46R–51R.

McCord J, Borzak S: Multifocal atrial tachycardia. Chest 1998;113:203–9.

Naccarelli GV et al: Cost-effective management of acute atrial fibrillation: role of rate control, spontaneous conversion, medical and direct current cardioversion, transesophageal echocardiography, and antiembolic therapy. Am J Cardiol 2000;85:36D–45D.

Ommen SR, Odell JA, Stanton MS: Atrial arrhythmias after cardiothoracic surgery. N Engl J Med 1997;336:1429–34.

Trohman RG: Supraventricular tachycardia: implications for the intensivist. Crit Care Med 2000;28(10 Suppl):N129–35.

Van Gelder IC et al: Pharmacologic versus direct-current electrical cardioversion of atrial flutter and fibrillation. Am J Cardiol 1999;84:147R–51R.

CARDIAC PROBLEMS DURING PREGNANCY

Pregnant patients with cardiac disorders may pose difficult management problems. One must always consider the impact of therapy on both the patient and the fetus. It is often possible to pick a medication that will achieve the desired clinical effect without injuring the fetus. However, when the issue of fetal injury secondary to medication arises, the risks need to be defined and the patient advised. Knowledge of which medications cross the placenta and have known teratogenic effects is mandatory. Ultimately, it is the patient and physician who need to make the decision about fetal risks to be accepted or avoided.

Common cardiac problems that occur in pregnant women and may lead to admission to the ICU include arrhythmias, congestive heart failure, pulmonary hypertension, and valvular heart disease.

VALVULAR HEART DISEASE DURING PREGNANCY

Valvular heart disease may be unsuspected in a woman of childbearing age who has been previously healthy. Rheumatic heart disease resulting in mitral stenosis is seen with increased frequency in regions that have large Hispanic and Asian populations.

Clinical Features

Women with mitral stenosis are often asymptomatic until the normal increase in blood volume and cardiac output occurring during pregnancy leads to elevated left atrial pressures and pulmonary venous hypertension. Tachycardia or atrial fibrillation is often seen in the acute presentation. These patients present with signs and symptoms mimicking asthma and, if heart disease is unsuspected, become progressively worse due to drug-induced tachycardia from treatment with beta-adrenergic agonists. Atrial fibrillation may also result in atrial thrombus formation, so that the initial presentation is a stroke.

The rapid heart rate does not allow time for atrial emptying, and left atrial pressures therefore rise, resulting in pulmonary edema. The presence of a diastolic murmur and opening snap consistent with mitral stenosis and an echocardiogram showing decreased mitral valve area and increased right ventricular pressure should lead to appropriate management.

Treatment

When mitral stenosis is the dominant cardiac lesion, beta-adrenergic blockers should be used to slow the heart rate and allow more time for ventricular filling. In general, cardioselective beta-adrenergic blockers such as atenolol are preferred because they cross the placental barrier less effectively than propranolol. If atrial fibrillation rather than sinus tachycardia is present, digoxin can also be used to slow the ventricular rate. Although calcium channel blockers such as diltiazem and verapamil will also slow heart rate, their effects on the fetus need to be considered. In pregnant patients with tight mitral stenosis and especially those with atrial fibrillation, anticoagulation is important to reduce the risk of a stroke. Depending on the stage of pregnancy, unfractionated heparin or low-molecular-weight heparin may be most appropriate.

Returning the patient to normal sinus rhythm may improve cardiac function by allowing better rate control, and restored atrial contraction will aid in left ventricular filling. Cardioversion must be done with the patient fully anticoagulated—with plans to continue anticoagulation—and it is necessary to demonstrate that atrial thrombi are not present by transesophageal echocardiography. Finally, in patients with severe mitral stenosis who continue to have severe congestive heart failure symptoms despite medical therapy, percutaneous valvuloplasty can be considered. Patients should be chosen based on appropriate valve morphology and the absence of significant mitral regurgitation. Fetal age and viability should be considered in the timing of the intervention, and neonatologists and obstetricians should be involved in weighing the risk and benefit to the fetus.

In patients with other types of valvular heart disease, management is directed toward maximizing the patient's cardiac output. However, some of the unloading agents used to treat left ventricular dysfunction and left-sided valvular regurgitation may decrease blood supply to the placenta and therefore to the fetus. Thus, the risks of treatment must be carefully weighed. Fetal monitoring can be used to help assess the impact of therapy.

ARRHYTHMIAS DURING PREGNANCY

Atrial and ventricular arrhythmias are often benign. However, sustained rapid atrial or ventricular tachycardia has the potential to impair uterine blood flow, resulting in compromised fetal oxygenation. Late in pregnancy, when systemic venous return is limited by compression of the inferior vena cava by the enlarged uterus, a tachyarrhythmia may result in profound hypotension and syncope. Therefore, pregnant women who complain of dizziness or syncope must be carefully evaluated and monitored. Because of toxic side effects and potential effects on the fetus, antiarrhythmic drugs should be used only for documented sustained arrhythmias, with drugs and dosages chosen to minimize effects on the fetus.

CONGENITAL HEART DISEASE DURING PREGNANCY

Pregnancy in patients with cyanotic congenital heart disease is associated with a high incidence of fetal wastage as well as maternal death. Pulmonary hypertension, atrial tachyarrhythmias, inability to increase cardiac output with increased demand, and hypoxemia all result in inadequate cardiac output to the mother and fetus. Postpartum, acute exacerbation of pulmonary hypertension and sudden death occur frequently. Treatment during the pregnancy is supportive, including restricting activity, avoiding volume overload, and treating polycythemia. A controlled elective delivery using an epidural block or cesarean section to minimize myocardial demand should be considered. Inhaled nitric oxide or intravenous prostacyclin can be used to help manage the worsening pulmonary hypertension seen after delivery in patients with Eisenmenger's syndrome with cyanosis.

Elkayam U, Gleicher N (editors): *Cardiac Problems in Pregnancy: Diagnosis and Management of Maternal and Fetal Disease,* 3rd ed. Wiley, 1998.

Hameed A et al: The effect of valvular heart disease on maternal and fetal outcome of pregnancy. J Am Coll Cardiol 2001;37:893–9.

Siu SC et al: Risk and predictors for pregnancy-related complications in women with heart disease. Circulation 1997; 96:2789–94.

TOXIC EFFECTS OF CARDIAC DRUGS

Cardiac medications have dramatically changed the treatment of patients with heart disease, improving the quality and duration of life, but these drugs have side effects both major and minor. Some of the toxic effects are extensions of a drug's therapeutic effects, while others are idiopathic or autoimmune in nature. In some patients, toxicity may develop only when metabolic changes occur that result in decreased clearance of the drug, but reactions may occur unpredictably even when drugs levels are in the therapeutic range. Thus, drug levels that produce a desirable drug effect in one patient may produce a life-threatening side effect in another. Toxicity may also develop when several drugs interact. Both the toxic and the therapeutic effects of drugs, their interaction with other drugs, and drug metabolism should be understood and considered in making treatment decisions and in evaluating patients receiving cardiac medications.

Discussed below are some of the more common and important side effects of frequently used cardiac medications. The key to treating critically ill patients with cardiac drugs is always to consider the possible or likely side effects and interactions of the drugs, especially when the patient has unexplained problems.

DIGOXIN

Pharmacology

Digoxin is a glycoside that inhibits Na^+-K^+ ATPase and thereby changes the intracellular Na^+ concentration. By altering the amount of Na^+ available for the Na^+-Ca^{2+} exchanger, the net effect of digoxin is to increase the intracellular calcium. Similarly, the effect of digoxin on Na^+-K^+ ATPase also alters the transmembrane potential of other cells and therefore affects cell excitability, conduction velocity, and refractory periods. Various cell types are affected differently; this accounts for the differing effects of digoxin on atrial, atrioventricular nodal, and ventricular tissue. Digoxin, like other cardiac glycosides, also has neurally mediated effects that alter autonomic balance and sympathetic output.

In appropriate doses, digoxin functions as an inotropic agent, increasing contractility. Its clinically important electrophysiologic effect is to block the atrioventricular node, thereby decreasing the ventricular response rate in atrial fibrillation and inhibiting reentrant supraventricular tachycardia. Digoxin has a fairly long half-life of 36–48 hours. It also has a relatively narrow therapeutic ratio. Digoxin is primarily cleared by the kidneys with perhaps some clearance through the gastrointestinal tract.

In critically ill patients, rapidly changing renal function and the requirement for multiple other drugs make the development of digoxin toxicity more frequent. Electrolyte abnormalities such as hypokalemia, hypomagnesemia, and hypercalcemia enhance digoxin toxicity. Serum levels of digoxin are affected by a variety of drugs. Quinidine alters the renal clearance and volume of distribution of digoxin. Therapeutic levels of quinidine double digoxin serum concentrations. Therefore, the dose of digoxin should be reduced by half when instituting quinidine therapy. Amiodarone, verapamil, and propafenone have similar effects on renal clearance of digoxin and digoxin serum level, though the magnitude of the effect is smaller. Periodic determination of drug levels with appropriate dose reduction or cessation can avoid the worse complications.

Toxicity

Digoxin serum levels are generally considered therapeutic in the range of 0.8–2 ng/mL, which unfortunately overlaps with the range in which toxicity may be seen. Toxicity is rare in patients with serum levels under 1.4 ng/mL but is seen with increased frequency when serum levels exceed 2 ng/mL. The positive inotropic effect of digoxin increases in a dose-related manner, and this effect persists even in the face of high drug levels. The toxic effects of digoxin can be broken down into systemic and electrolyte effects and mild and severe arrhythmias. With mild toxicity, the patient may develop nausea, visual disturbances, and decreased appetite. At higher serum levels of digoxin, as the Na^+-K^+ ATPase is poisoned, hyperkalemia develops that may lead to cardiac arrest. Arrhythmias seen at low levels of toxicity reflect the effect of digoxin on automaticity, resulting in paroxysmal atrial tachycardia, junctional tachycardia, and ventricular ectopy (particularly bigeminy). Because digoxin increases atrioventricular nodal block, the atrial tachycardias are associated with heart block.

Treatment

Treatment depends on the severity of toxic manifestations. Withholding digoxin and correcting hypoxia, hypokalemia, and the acid-base disturbances that exacerbate digoxin toxicity usually correct arrhythmias over time. Marked bradycardia in the setting of atrial fibrillation can be treated with atropine in mild cases and temporary pacing for more severe ones. Lidocaine or phenytoin can often control the less serious ventricular arrhythmias. Electrical cardioversion may be necessary acutely to treat sustained ventricular tachycardia from digoxin toxicity when drugs and other measures have failed, but there is an increased risk of arrhythmic complications because of increased ventricular automaticity caused by digoxin. Using less electrical energy (fewer joules) may decrease the risk.

In cases of severe digoxin toxicity that include the development of hyperkalemia, severe bradyarrhythmia, recurrent ventricular tachycardia, or ventricular fibrillation, digoxin immune Fab (ovine) can be lifesaving. This preparation is a sheep antibody fragment that has a high affinity for digoxin, rapidly binding to the drug and reversing its effect. The Fab fragments have a lower molecular weight than complete antibodies and thus have a greater rate and volume of distribution. The Fab-digoxin complexes are excreted in the urine, thus enhancing renal clearance of the drug. Digoxin antibody is indicated in the setting of life-threatening digoxin toxicity or when the ingestion of large amounts of digoxin makes the development of toxic side effects likely. The dosage of digoxin immune Fab is dependent of the digoxin level and the estimated volume of distribution. However, if the desired effect is not achieved with the calculated dose, treatment with the maximum dose is indicated in life-threatening situations. Side effects from digoxin immune Fab are minimal. The drug is expensive, and its use is therefore reserved for patients with severe life-threatening digoxin toxicity. In most patients, prevention of digoxin toxicity is preferable and achievable with forethought. For example, for elderly patients or critically ill patients in the ICU with acute renal failure or cardiogenic shock, digoxin should not be given as a standing order for more than 1 day without careful review and adjustment if necessary.

ANTIARRHYTHMIC DRUGS

Lidocaine

Because lidocaine is metabolized by the liver, hypotension, right heart failure, and liver failure may result in decreased clearance of this drug. Lidocaine has minimal proarrhythmic and myocardial depressant effects. Its side effects are primarily neurologic, consisting of acute onset of agitation, tremulousness, psychosis, and seizures. Withdrawal of the drug and time are the treatments. If indicated, another antiarrhythmic agent can be used when lidocaine is discontinued.

Quinidine & Procainamide

Procainamide, used for treatment of both atrial and ventricular arrhythmias, is cleared by the kidneys. Both the drug and its by-product, *N*-acetylprocainamide, accumulate in patients with renal failure. Procainamide is a myocardial depressant and can cause hypotension. It can also cause QT prolongation, with the development of polymorphic ventricular tachycardia similar to the effects of quinidine. Unlike quinidine, procainamide does not alter serum digoxin levels. A variety of noncardiac side effects are caused by procainamide, the most important being agranulocytosis and the development of a lupus-like syndrome. Agranulocytosis is reversible, but the patient may present with sepsis. The lupus-like syndrome is generally a late development in the course of prolonged administration, with manifestations such as fever, pleuropericarditis, and arthralgias; there are serum antinuclear antibodies as well. This syndrome may be seen more frequently in patients who metabolize the drug slowly ("slow acetylators"). The syndrome is reversible with discontinuation of the drug.

Quinidine, a class Ia agent whose indications are similar to those of procainamide, has less myocardial depressant effects but is only available orally. Its proarrhythmic effects are well known, with QT prolongation resulting in ventricular tachycardia and syncope. Gastrointestinal side effects are frequent, and the development of nausea and diarrhea often limits its use. Neurologic side effects include tinnitus, hearing loss, and confusion. Autoimmune thrombocytopenia or hemolytic anemia occasionally develops unexpectedly, resulting in hemorrhage or death. Quinidine-induced thrombocytopenia is treated as autoimmune thrombocytopenia.

If polymorphic ventricular tachycardia (torsade de pointes) develops during treatment with quinidine or procainamide, the drug should be stopped and other class Ia and Ic agents should be avoided. Beta-adrenergic agonists such as isoproterenol can be used to speed up the heart rate and shorten the QT interval. Overdrive pacing with a transvenous pacing wire can also be used in patients with recurrent ventricular tachycardia until the offending drug is cleared or metabolized. When monitoring the QT interval during administration of quinidine or procainamide, the drug should be discontinued if the QT interval exceeds 500 ms.

Flecainide

Flecainide is a class Ic antiarrhythmic agent which is well tolerated, with minimal noncardiac side effects. It is proarrhythmic, however, and can cause significant and sustained ventricular tachycardia that is resistant to other antiarrhythmic agents. Flecainide slows conduction throughout the conducting system, which can result in bradycardia as well as heart block.

Amiodarone

Amiodarone is a powerful antiarrhythmic agent with minimal proarrhythmic effects. However, it has a variety of cardiac and noncardiac side effects that are magnified by its long half-life. Resulting toxicities can last from days to months depending on the duration of therapy and the dose. Amiodarone slows conduction throughout the heart, resulting in bradycardia and heart block, which may require permanent pacing. Gastrointestinal side effects include nausea and decreased appetite, resulting in weight loss and necessitating dose reduction or termination of therapy. Either hypo- or hyperthyroidism can result from amiodarone's effect on iodine metabolism. Deposits in the skin can result in darkening of skin, especially in sun-exposed areas. Intracytoplasmic lamellar deposits can occur in several parts of the eyes, most commonly causing corneal epithelial opacities in more than 70% of patients and lens opacities in 50–60%. Neither impairs visual acuity, and amiodarone treatment can be continued. Pulmonary fibrosis is a frightening and potentially life-threatening complication that can further compromise patients who already have significant cardiac impairment. Baseline and follow-up pulmonary function tests are mandatory to monitor the development of pulmonary involvement. Amiodarone interacts with and changes the metabolism of a myriad of drugs. Its interactions with digoxin, beta-adrenergic blockers, calcium channel blockers, and warfarin should be carefully monitored.

Sotalol

Sotalol is a class II (beta-adrenergic blocker) and III antiarrhythmic drug that is renally excreted and therefore must be monitored carefully in patients with changing renal function. It is an effective agent for atrial and ventricular arrhythmias, but—like most antiarrhythmic agents—it has proarrhythmic effects, occurring particularly while therapy is being initiated. It can cause significant bradycardia and heart block when used in conjunction with digoxin or calcium channel blockers.

CALCIUM CHANNEL BLOCKERS

These drugs can be categorized into three subclasses: verapamil-like drugs, diltiazem-like drugs, and nifedipine-like drugs. Some of the toxic effects are the logical result of their therapeutic mechanisms and may be beneficial in certain settings. For example, slowing of the heart rate in patients with ischemia is a desirable effect of some of the calcium channel blockers. However, verapamil and diltiazem can also slow atrioventricular nodal and sinus node conduction excessively, resulting in bradyarrhythmias and hypotension. Because they are myocardial depressants, these drugs may precipitate or exacerbate congestive heart failure. The bradycardiac effects of diltiazem and verapamil can be augmented by concomitant use of beta-adrenergic blockers or digoxin. In contrast, nifedipine and other drugs in its class have no effect on the atrioventricular node but can cause reflex tachycardia and hypotension from vasodilation. Calcium administered intravenously may reverse some of the toxic effects of the calcium channel blockers, at least temporarily.

BETA-ADRENERGIC BLOCKERS

Beta-adrenergic blockers are extremely useful drugs for controlling hypertension, treating atrial arrhythmias, and alleviating myocardial ischemia. In a patient with myocardial dysfunction, beta-adrenergic blockers can precipitate profound heart failure and block the normal tachycardiac response to hypotension and low cardiac output. Despite this, however, these drugs have been shown to improve long-term survival in patients with chronic congestive heart failure.

These drugs are myocardial depressants, block the atrioventricular node, and, by blocking the action of catecholamines, decrease the sinus nodal rate. In patients with conduction system disease, beta-adrenergic blockers may cause profound bradycardia. The effects of beta-adrenergic blockers and calcium channel blockers on the myocardium, the sinus node, and the atrioventricular node can be additive, resulting in severe hypotension and heart block. Beta-adrenergic agonists may be used to counteract the excessive depressant effects of beta-adrenergic blockers.

ANGIOTENSIN-CONVERTING ENZYME (ACE) INHIBITORS

ACE inhibitors, of which captopril and enalapril are examples, are commonly used vasodilators valuable in the treatment of congestive heart failure and hypertension. These drugs can cause hyperkalemia even in patients without overt renal disease. Therefore, potassium levels must be observed carefully when initiating or maintaining therapy with ACE inhibitors. Rapidly developing renal failure may occur in patients with renal artery stenosis when ACE inhibitors are started. Angioedema and cough are allergic side effects that should result in terminating the drug. The cough may be confused with cough due to heart failure but responds fairly quickly to removal of the drug. Angiotensin receptor blockers have effects similar to those of ACE inhibitors and may be substituted. As with other antihypertensive agents, profound hypotension may develop when starting ACE inhibitors, particularly in patients who are hypovolemic. In critically ill patients, the benefits and side effects of these drugs need to be carefully considered.

Desai AD, Chun S, Sung RJ: The role of intravenous amiodarone in the management of cardiac arrhythmias. Ann Intern Med 1997;127:294–303.

Hauptman PJ, Kelly RA: Digitalis. Circulation 1999;99:1265–70.

Kowey PR et al: Intravenous amiodarone. J Am Coll Cardiol 1997;29:1190–8.

Kowey PR et al: Intravenous antiarrhythmic therapy in the acute control of in-hospital destabilizing ventricular tachycardia and fibrillation. Am J Cardiol 1999;84(9A):46R–51R.

Zipes DP, Jalife J, Zorab R (editors): *Cardiac Electrophysiology From Cell to Bedside,* 3rd ed. Saunders, 2000.

Coronary Heart Disease

22

Kenneth A. Narahara, MD

Atherosclerotic coronary artery disease is the leading cause of death in the United States. Each year approximately 1.5 million patients experience a myocardial infarction. Approximately 20% of these individuals die before they reach the hospital, and an additional 7–15% die during hospitalization. This chapter will consider the three major coronary artery disease syndromes: angina pectoris, unstable angina pectoris, and acute myocardial infarction.

PHYSIOLOGIC CONSIDERATIONS

Coronary Anatomy

The right and left coronary arteries arise from ostia in the right and left sinuses of Valsalva. Their function is to deliver oxygen and nutrients and to remove toxic metabolites. The origin of the left coronary artery is called the left main coronary and divides into the left anterior descending coronary artery, which feeds the anterior wall of the left ventricle and the left ventricular septum; and the left circumflex artery, which supplies the lateral and posterior walls of the left ventricle. The right coronary artery supplies the right ventricular free wall and in 90% of cases gives off the posterior descending artery, which in turn provides the blood supply for the posterior right ventricle as well as the inferior left ventricular wall and septum. The coronary artery that gives rise to the posterior descending artery is referred to as "dominant." Thus, 90% of people have a "right dominant circulation." The remaining 10% have a posterior descending artery that originates from the left circumflex coronary artery. Coronary collateral vessels span the area between the right and left coronary artery territories. These vessels are very small and difficult to demonstrate even during cardiac catheterization. However, as coronary stenoses develop in the major epicardial coronary arteries, collateral vessels may increase in size and number and provide a protective effect by allowing increased blood supply from the opposite coronary circulation.

Coronary Blood Flow

Coronary blood flow at rest is ordinarily 70–100 mL/min per 100 g of heart tissue. Approximately 80% of the coronary flow occurs during diastole. As a consequence, coronary blood flow is highly dependent on diastolic blood pressure and resistance to coronary flow within the coronary circulation.

In the absence of disease and with a constant myocardial oxygen requirement (MVO_2), coronary blood flow is kept constant by autoregulation of the coronary vasculature by both myogenic and metabolic factors. Diastolic perfusion pressure provides the driving pressure for coronary blood flow. Metabolic factors, particularly adenosine, affect regional myocardial blood flow. As tissue oxygen decreases, ADP is converted to AMP and then to adenosine by the enzyme 5′-nucleotidase. Adenosine then diffuses out of the cell and causes relaxation of local vascular smooth muscle. This action of adenosine is terminated by its deamination to inosine.

Myocardial Oxygen Consumption

Over 90% of the heart's energy is derived from aerobic metabolism, primarily from oxidation of fatty acids. The absence of oxygen forces a transition to anaerobic metabolism of glucose and glycogen. Myocardial O_2 requirements are multiple: Twenty percent of the MVO_2 is used to support the basal metabolism of the heart; less than 5% is used to support electrical activity; and approximately 15% is used to move calcium into the sarcoplasmic reticulum. The most important determinant of MVO_2 is myocardial contractility, accounting for 60% of MVO_2.

A. Heart Rate and Systolic Blood Pressure

An important concept about coronary artery disease is the relation of MVO_2 to the heart rate (HR) and systolic blood pressure (SBP). HR × SBP is commonly referred to as the double product. The double product is proportionate to MVO_2 and can be used as a measure of myocardial work and thus myocardial O_2 consumption. The inotropic state of the myocardium is another important determinant of MVO_2 and myocardial work. However, it is somewhat difficult to measure clinically; fortunately, the heart rate and systolic blood pressure usually provide sufficient information for clinical decision making.

B. Balance of Oxygen Demand and Supply

Myocardial ischemia represents an imbalance between myocardial oxygen demand and myocardial blood supply. A fixed coronary artery stenosis will limit coronary blood supply. In this circumstance, demand for coronary blood flow may increase, but the stenosis will limit the available blood flow. Hence, demand will exceed supply, and myocardial ischemia will result. The ability of the coronary artery to respond to sympathetic stimulation and other local factors can also result in an inadequate blood supply through coronary artery spasm. However, coronary artery spasm (variant angina, Prinzmetal's angina) is seldom the sole cause of inadequate coronary blood flow. More often, fixed coronary artery stenoses exist in combination with some degree of coronary spasm or vasoconstriction to cause a myocardial O_2 demand-supply imbalance.

MYOCARDIAL ISCHEMIA (Angina Pectoris)

ESSENTIALS OF DIAGNOSIS

- *Complaint of heavy, pressure-like or vise-like discomfort. Sometimes choking, a constricting feeling in the throat, or a sensation of strangling. Discomfort located diffusely in substernal region, left arm, jaw, or neck—rarely localized to a single point.*
- *Discomfort lasts 30 seconds to 15 minutes.*
- *May be provoked by exertion, emotional distress, eating, cold.*
- *Should decrease with rest and may be relieved in 1–2 minutes after sublingual nitroglycerin.*

General Considerations

Resistance to blood flow in the coronary arteries becomes significant when there is sufficient narrowing of the coronary artery diameter by atherosclerotic plaques (diameter decreased by more than 50%). The physiologic consequence is that coronary artery blood flow becomes fixed at some value rather than increasing to meet increased myocardial demands. Coronary blood flow may be adequate to supply the myocardium at rest but becomes insufficient during exertion when the myocardial oxygen demand increases. This explains why, in patients with stable angina pectoris, symptoms are seen with exercise and disappear with rest.

Clinical Features

The diagnosis of angina pectoris is typically a clinical one. Pain with the qualities described below should be considered the primary diagnostic criterion—ie, the history is the most important diagnostic clue to ischemic heart disease and myocardial ischemia (angina pectoris).

A. Symptoms

There are six major features of the clinical manifestations of myocardial ischemia (angina pectoris): the quality of the discomfort (patients do not always complain of "pain"), the location, the duration, provoking factors, sources of relief, and actions taken by the patient during the episode.

1. Quality of discomfort—Patients with myocardial ischemia frequently describe the discomfort as a heavy, pressure-like, or vise-like sensation. They may describe choking or a constricting feeling in the throat. Indigestion or a sensation of strangling is also frequently described. The patient should be asked about "discomfort," since many patients do not perceive angina or myocardial ischemia as "pain."

2. Location of discomfort—The discomfort of myocardial ischemia is usually located in the substernal region but may also be located in the arms (the left more often than the right), the jaw, the neck, the left interscapular region, or occasionally the epigastrium. It is often useful to ask the patient to define the extent of the pain with one finger. The pain of myocardial ischemia is not likely to be localized to a single point.

3. Duration of discomfort—Angina pectoris usually lasts 30 seconds to 15 minutes. Longer episodes of ischemic pain are associated with unstable angina or myocardial infarction.

4. Provocation of discomfort—Exertion, emotional distress, eating, cold weather, and sexual activity are frequent initiating events.

5. Relief of discomfort—Pain from myocardial ischemia should decrease with rest or a reduction in exertion. Sublingual nitroglycerin should relieve angina within 1–2 minutes, and this feature can be used both for diagnosis and for treatment.

6. Actions taken by the patient—Angina pectoris is not relieved by inspiration or movement of the upper extremities or torso nor by antacids or food. Pain relief achieved in this way should make one think of other disorders.

B. Physical Findings

During an episode of angina, an S_3 gallop, pulmonary rales, or the murmur of mitral regurgitation may appear. However, these findings are more likely to be noted during stress testing, when the patient's chest pain is provoked with a physician present.

C. Electrocardiography

1. Resting ECG—If ST and T wave changes (ST depression, T wave inversion, or both) are present during an episode of pain and return to normal with spontaneous relief of pain or after administration of nitroglycerin, the diagnosis of myocardial ischemia is confirmed.

2. Exercise stress ECG—The resting ECG is frequently normal in patients with myocardial ischemia due to coronary artery disease or coronary artery spasm, as the pain has usually subsided by the time the patient reaches medical attention. For this reason, stress testing during bicycle or treadmill exercise is frequently employed to reproduce the supply and demand imbalance that triggers myocardial ischemia. The patient is asked to walk on a treadmill or pedal on a bicycle as the work load is progressively increased. Continuous electrocardiographic monitoring permits detection of ST segment depression. Exercise causes an increase in heart rate and blood pressure (an increase in double product); thus, patients with a fixed (and inadequate) myocardial blood supply due to coronary artery disease will frequently experience angina with ST segment depression as myocardial work exceeds a fixed O_2 supply.

D. Imaging Studies

1. Stress testing—Specialized forms of exercise stress testing, including thallium scintigraphy and stress ventriculography, have been introduced to diagnose myocardial ischemia in patients who have resting ECGs that would make the diagnosis of myocardial ischemia difficult on the basis of exercise electrocardiography. For example, patients with resting ST and T wave abnormalities due to left ventricular hypertrophy, from administration of digitalis glycosides, or from prior myocardial infarction may have a stress ECG that is difficult or impossible to interpret with precision. In these circumstances, the use of myocardial perfusion scanning with thallium-201 or technetium-99m sestamibi may be useful. These perfusion agents are taken up by viable myocardium in proportion to coronary blood flow. As coronary blood flow requirements increase (as during exercise), myocardium supplied by normal coronary vessels will have a normal uptake of the tracer. Conversely, areas of myocardium served by stenotic coronary arteries will have reduced coronary blood flow during exercise. As a consequence, the reduced uptake of the perfusion agent will appear as a "cold spot."

Exercise ventriculography using echocardiography, cine-CT, or radionuclide angiography can identify the presence of myocardial ischemia by the development of a new or worsened wall motion abnormality during stress. As myocardial O_2 requirements outstrip the available supply, regional wall motion abnormalities will develop as nutrient flow to the myocardium remains fixed in the face of an increasing metabolic demand. Initially, a localized wall motion abnormality will appear or will worsen (if a previous infarction is present). Next, the global left ventricular ejection fraction will fall. Although these tests are substantially more expensive than the standard electrocardiographic stress test, they may provide a definitive noninvasive means of diagnosing myocardial ischemia.

2. Coronary angiography—Anatomic diagnosis of coronary atherosclerosis is made by injection of radiopaque contrast material directly into the coronary arteries. Patients are taken to the catheterization laboratory, where careful hemodynamic monitoring can be performed. Significant atherosclerotic lesions are seen as a reduction in the diameter of the coronary artery, and the anatomic information can be utilized to decide whether medical therapy or interventional procedures such as coronary angioplasty or coronary artery bypass surgery might be useful.

Differential Diagnosis

Other causes of chest pain that may have features suggestive of angina pectoris include pericarditis (pain is often positional and related to respiration), esophageal spasm (related to meals and swallowing), chest wall pain (often reproduced by applying pressure to the chest wall), aortic dissection (classically "tearing" in quality and radiating to the back; pulses in the arms may be unequal), gastrointestinal pain from esophagitis, gastritis, cholecystitis, and cholelithiasis (often associated with meals and, for esophagitis and gastritis, relieved by antacids), and hyperventilation.

Treatment

The treatment of myocardial ischemia is directed at both reducing myocardial O_2 consumption (myocardial O_2 demand and double product) and increasing myocardial blood supply. Initially, medical therapy is utilized in an attempt to reduce myocardial O_2 consumption (eg, use of beta blockade to reduce heart rate and blood pressure) or to increase myocardial O_2 supply by using coronary vasodilators such as calcium channel-blocking agents or either short-acting (sublingual nitroglycerin) or long-acting nitrates (isosorbide dinitrate).

More aggressive therapy such as percutaneous transluminal coronary angioplasty and coronary artery bypass surgery directly increase coronary blood supply. While effective in reaching this goal as well as in relieving angina, these strategies are invasive and cause a variable degree of morbidity. To date, with the exception of patients with left main coronary artery disease or three-vessel coronary artery disease in the presence of left ventricular dysfunction, neither coronary angioplasty nor coronary bypass surgery will reduce the mortality rate from coronary artery disease. The high cost and stress on the health care network of these procedures would suggest that the management of myocardial ischemia with medical therapy is a reasonable first step.

A. Long-Acting Nitrates

Nitrates are the oldest form of anti-ischemic therapy. Their continued use is a testament to their efficacy as well as their safety. Many clinicians consider long-acting nitrates as initial therapy for prevention of myocardial ischemia. Therapy with long-acting nitrates aims to improve coronary blood flow. Twenty milligrams of isosorbide dinitrate three times a day is a typical starting dose. Although lower doses may be used, they usually have little more than a placebo effect in patients with coronary artery disease. After initial dosing with 20 mg three times daily for 3–5 days, the dose can be increased to either 40 mg or 60 mg three times daily. A target dose of at least 40 mg three times daily would be a reasonable therapeutic goal, assuming that the patient does not suffer from headaches or symptoms of hypotension.

"Nitrate headaches" frequently occur during the first few days of therapy with isosorbide dinitrate. The patient should be encouraged to continue the medication (perhaps with administration of acetaminophen), since headaches frequently subside with time though the antianginal efficacy of the long-acting nitrates persists. Doses of isosorbide dinitrate larger than 60 mg three times daily are generally not necessary for therapy of angina pectoris and produce a smaller incremental improvement in symptoms compared with the increase from 20 mg to 40 mg or 60 mg three times daily. However, in the treatment of unstable angina or for patients who have severe angina pectoris which is not amenable to revascularization, such high doses of long-acting nitrates may be useful in providing an asymptomatic or moderately symptomatic state.

B. Beta-Adrenergic Blockade

Beta-adrenergic blockers are particularly effective in the treatment of patients who have coexisting angina and hypertension. Likewise, the combination of beta-blocker therapy with a long-acting nitrate may be hemodynamically desirable since the long-acting nitrates tend to produce a modest reflex tachycardia that can be blunted or eliminated by beta blockade. In the treatment of exertional angina, beta blockade can be particularly advantageous as it will block catecholamine-induced increases (from exercise or emotional stress) in heart rate and blood pressure.

Initial therapy with beta-blockers can commence with metoprolol, 50 mg twice daily (or 100 mg of sustained-release metoprolol); atenolol, 50 mg once daily; or betaxolol, 10 mg once daily. In the elderly patient, these initial doses should be reduced at the initiation of therapy. Titration of the dose upward can commence after four to five half-lives have elapsed, ie, 2–3 days for metoprolol, 3–4 days for atenolol, and 5–7 days for betaxolol. Upward titration of the dose of beta-blocker should be considered if the resting heart rate or blood pressure are not affected by the initial dose of therapy.

As a general rule, patients who may be operating machinery or driving automobiles should be warned of the possibility of drowsiness or lethargy when taking beta-blockers. Frequently, the administration of longer-acting agents such as atenolol or betaxolol at bedtime can be useful in reducing symptoms of fatigue and reduced attentiveness during the daytime.

Concern is frequently raised about the use of beta blockade in patients with diabetes. However, if the patient does not suffer from episodes of hypoglycemia, judicious therapy with beta blockade is often rewarded by substantial reduction in angina pectoris. The major concern regarding the coadministration of beta blockade with hypoglycemic agents is blunting of symptoms of hypoglycemia. However, this effect is primarily related to a reduction of tachycardia; diaphoresis and hunger are not blunted by beta-blocker therapy. Of course, beta-blockers should be avoided in the brittle type 1 diabetic or in diabetics with a history of ketoacidosis.

C. Calcium Channel-Blocking Agents

1. Dihydropyridines—This class of calcium antagonists is characterized by both a systemic and coronary vasodilator effect. The dihydropyridines have no effect on sinoatrial or atrioventricular nodal function. Therefore, coadministration of a dihydropyridine with beta-blockers for the combined therapy of angina and hypertension is frequently highly effective. Both agents tend to lower blood pressure, and the bradycardiac effect of beta blockade will prevent any reflex tachycardia that may be engendered by the dihydropyridines.

Nifedipine, the first-generation dihydropyridine, had a relatively short half-life and frequently caused symptoms of vasodilation, including flushing, headaches, and peripheral edema. Sustained-release nifedipine is still used for refractory hypertension in doses of 30–90 mg/d or more. However, for the treatment of coronary artery disease, nifedipine and the second-generation dihydropyridines have been replaced by amlodipine.

Amlodipine and felodipine are "long-acting" dihydropyridine calcium channel antagonists. Amlodipine has an inherently long half-life of over 30 hours, whereas felodipine gains its once-a-day dosing from an enteric coating that results in the gradual release of the agent. Amlodipine is approved for both angina and hypertension; felodipine is approved for hypertension only.

Amlodipine is the only calcium channel-blocking agent that can be used safely in patients with impaired left ventricular function. Hence, the agent can be used for antianginal treatment in addition to nitrates and beta-blockers, particularly when coexisting hypertension is present. The starting dose for amlodipine is 2.5–5 mg/d with a recommended maximum of 10 mg/d. Higher doses of amlodipine may afford additional antianginal and antihypertensive effects, but side effects such as peripheral edema become more pronounced. Given the long half-life of amlodipine, the dose of this agent should not be increased more than once weekly.

2. Verapamil—Verapamil is a vasodilating calcium channel-blocking agent which, in addition to causing coronary vasodilation, has a negative chronotropic effect. Conduction through both the sinoatrial node and the atrioventricular node can be slowed by this agent. Verapamil has a side effect profile similar to that of nifedipine. In addition, verapamil causes constipation, and the patient's bowel habits should be carefully evaluated. Many clinicians will start patients on stool softeners or prophylactic milk of magnesia when commencing therapy with verapamil.

Verapamil is a fairly potent peripheral vasodilator and is therefore an effective antihypertensive agent. Additionally, with its bradycardiac effect, it may be particularly useful for patients with ischemic heart disease who are intolerant of beta-blockers, such as those with asthma or type 1 diabetes. It should be recalled that on balance, verapamil exerts the greatest negative inotropic effect of the currently available calcium blockers and should be avoided in patients with a history of congestive heart failure or a known reduction in ejection fraction. Short-acting verapamil is typically administered in a dosage of 80–120 mg every 8 hours. However, the long-acting verapamil preparations are generally preferred for the sake of compliance and convenience. Long-acting verapamil should be initiated at a dosage of 180 mg once daily with upward titration to 240 mg/d. Titration can occur at weekly intervals for symptoms of angina or control of hypertension. Patients should be warned to avoid chewing or crushing the long-acting preparations of verapamil as the entire daily dose may be released rapidly. Long-acting verapamil should be initiated at a dosage of 120 mg/d in the elderly or in underweight patients.

3. Diltiazem—Diltiazem has a modest effect on heart rate and blood pressure in normotensive patients. Like all calcium channel-blocking agents, it exerts a coronary vasodilating effect. Diltiazem's antianginal properties are the result of both coronary vasodilation and a reduction in the product of heart rate and systolic blood pressure. Diltiazem has a favorable side effect profile characterized by minor occurrences of dyspepsia, rash, and edema. Because diltiazem depresses sinoatrial and atrioventricular nodal function, concomitant administration of beta-blockers warrants careful attention to the heart rate.

Starting dosages for diltiazem are 60 mg every 8 hours, and this can be increased to 120 mg every 6–8 hours. Long-acting preparations of diltiazem have been introduced. Therapy with these sustained-release preparations can be initiated at a dosage determined by therapy with the short-acting preparation (eg, patients who tolerate 60 mg every 8 hours can be converted directly to 180 mg/d of the long acting preparation). Frequently, clinicians initiate therapy with 180 mg of the sustained-release compound and increase the dose weekly up to 360 mg/d. For the elderly and underweight patient, a starting dose of 120 mg/d may be preferable.

Like all calcium channel-blocking agents currently marketed (with the exception of amlodipine), diltiazem should be avoided in patients with reduced left ventricular function. A large multicenter trial demonstrated that the administration of diltiazem to patients with left ventricular ejection fractions < 0.40 or with pulmonary congestion after acute myocardial infarction is associated with an approximately 1.4-fold increase in cardiovascular death. Similar results have been seen in trials with verapamil.

4. Bepridil—Bepridil is a calcium channel-blocking agent that has virtually no effect on the demand side of the ischemic heart disease equation. Dose-dependent reductions in heart rate of 2–5 beats/min and in blood pressure of 3–5 mm Hg have been noted. Presumably, bepridil exerts its anti-ischemic effect primarily through coronary vasodilation. Currently, this calcium channel-blocking agent should be reserved for patients who have failed therapy with conventional antianginal agents. The reason for this caution is the ability of bepridil to prolong the QT interval and potentially initiate torsade de pointes. This side effect can be avoided by screening patients before placing them on bepridil. Bepridil should not be administered to patients with a corrected QT interval > 0.44 s or to patients who are prone to hypokalemia, such as those receiving diuretic therapy unless accompanied by potassium-sparing agents such as triamterene or ACE inhibitors. About 1 week after initiation of bepridil, an ECG should be obtained. If the corrected QT interval has increased by more than 25%, the dose of bepridil should be reduced or the drug should be discontinued. Conventional doses of bepridil range from 200–400 mg/d. The 42-hour half-life of this agent makes it an inherently long-acting compound and may be responsible for some of its therapeutic benefit by avoiding troughs in serum levels.

Gibbons RJ et al: ACC/AHA/ACP-ASIM guidelines for the management of patients with chronic stable angina: a report of the American College of Cardiology/American Heart Association Task Force on Practice Guidelines (Committee on Management of Patients With Chronic Stable Angina). J Am Coll Cardiol 1999;33:2092–197.

UNSTABLE ANGINA AND NON-ST SEGMENT ELEVATION MYOCARDIAL INFARCTION

ESSENTIALS OF DIAGNOSIS

- *Increase in the frequency, severity, or duration of stable angina, or angina occurring at a lower threshold (unstable angina with low-risk characteristics).*
- *Prolonged (> 20 minutes) angina at rest now resolved, plus diabetes, age over 65, deep T wave inversions in more than five leads, angina on walking one to two blocks on the level or climbing one flight of stairs at a normal pace in the past 2 weeks, nocturnal angina, or pathologic Q waves (unstable angina with intermediate-risk characteristics).*
- *Ongoing (> 20 minutes) chest pain, ST segment depression ≥ 1 mm, angina plus heart failure, or angina plus hypotension (unstable angina with high-risk characteristics).*
- *Any of the above plus cardiac enzyme markers of myocardial necrosis (troponin I, troponin T, or CK-MB) (non-ST-segment elevation myocardial infarction).*

General Considerations

Patients with non-Q wave myocardial infarctions represent one end of the spectrum of the pathology associated with unstable angina. Fissuring or rupture of an atherosclerotic plaque precedes unstable angina. If the plaque disruption can be stabilized spontaneously or through medical intervention, unstable angina has occurred. Otherwise, non-ST elevation myocardial infarction may occur.

The American College of Cardiology/American Heart Association has issued guidelines for the management of unstable angina pectoris and non-ST-segment elevation myocardial infarction (non-STEMI). The intensity of medical therapy and interventional procedures, as well as the urgency of starting treatment, should be guided by both symptoms and objective findings.

Clinical Features

A. Symptoms and Signs

The signs and symptoms of unstable angina and non-STEMI are the same as those of stable angina pectoris. The distinction between stable and unstable angina or non-STEMI is in the longer duration of the pain episodes, the reduced amount of exertion required to produce angina (including pain at rest), and the increased frequency of chest discomfort.

B. Diagnostic Testing

As in stable angina, patients with unstable angina frequently have normal ECGs. However, the presence of new ST depression, T wave inversion, or both, which resolve spontaneously or with the administration of sublingual nitroglycerin, identifies a category of patients at high risk for subsequent cardiac events, including myocardial infarction or death. Chest pain with ST segment depression now can be managed by specific therapy defined by large randomized clinical trials.

A non-ST segment elevation myocardial infarction is diagnosed when markers of myocardial necrosis (elevated levels of troponins or CK-MB) are present in the absence of ST segment elevation on the ECG.

C. Evaluation of the Stabilized Patient

In patients whose symptoms become well controlled on antianginal therapy after an episode of unstable angina pectoris, three approaches may be followed: (1) Perform coronary arteriography with the anticipation of elective coronary artery angioplasty or coronary artery bypass surgery; (2) treat the patient conservatively with increased doses of antianginal medications; or (3) perform a functional test to select those patients most likely to benefit from more invasive therapies. The latter course is advocated by some cardiologists and is favored by the present author.

A "low-level" stress test can identify patients who are at high or low risk for development of subsequent myocardial infarction, further unstable angina, and death after an initial episode of unstable angina. These exercise stress tests, which are limited either by workload (5–7 mets [ie, five to seven times the resting metabolic rate]) or heart rate (< 120 beats/min or less than 65% of predicted maximum heart rate), are used to determine whether ischemia is present at levels of exercise likely to be encountered in ordinary daily activities. Safety is the primary reason for limiting the test to a lower target workload or heart rate than might be the goal for a patient with stable angina. Furthermore, it makes little sense intuitively to challenge with a conventional stress test a patient who has recently had symptoms with minimal exertion.

In any case, a negative low-level stress test is associated with a relatively good outcome, with over 70% of patients with a negative study having no or mild angina pectoris in the ensuing 6 months to 1 year. Conversely, a positive low-level stress test with development of ST segment depression or the development of chest pain is associated with a high (> 80%) incidence of subsequent undesirable outcome (recurrent unstable angina, myocardial infarction, or death). Thus, the low-level stress test can be used to identify patients at high risk and therefore more likely to benefit from early aggressive management of ischemic heart disease.

Treatment

Patients who experience an increase in the frequency or duration of angina pectoris or a marked decline in the amount of exertion required to provoke chest pain are candidates for hospitalization to reduce the work of the heart (by hospitalization itself) as well as to initiate or intensify pharmacologic therapy for ischemic heart disease.

A. Aspirin

Over two decades ago, two major studies attested to the importance of aspirin in the therapy of unstable angina pectoris. Both the Veterans Administration and the Canadian Cooperative trials demonstrated a 50% reduction in deaths and myocardial infarctions in patients with unstable angina who take one to four 325 mg aspirin tablets a day. The observation that patients with unstable angina or non-STEMI have large amounts of thrombus in patent but atherosclerotic coronary arteries at the time of coronary angioscopy or coronary arteriography provides the pathophysiologic basis for this remarkably successful and inexpensive form of therapy. Patients with true allergies to aspirin can substitute clopidogrel, 75 mg/d.

B. Beta-Blockers

The prevention of the ischemia that underlies unstable angina pectoris and non-STEMI is most easily accomplished by reducing the work of the heart. By lowering both the heart rate and blood pressure, beta-blockers perform this task efficiently and inexpensively. In patients with high-risk characteristics of unstable angina or evidence of a non-STEMI, intravenous administration of beta-blocking agents followed by oral beta-blockers is appropriate and desirable. Metoprolol should be administered intravenously in 5 mg increments more than 2 minutes apart to a total dose of 15 mg (or more if better control of the heart rate is desired). Following intravenous loading of beta-blockers, oral metoprolol, 50 mg twice daily, or oral atenolol, 50 mg once daily, should be initiated.

For patients with contraindications to beta blockade (eg, bronchospastic lung disease), calcium channel-blocking agents may be substituted. Calcium channel blockers, ACE inhibitors, or angiotensin II receptor blockers may be added to beta blockade if additional antihypertensive therapy is required.

C. Nitrates

Oral nitrates may be initiated as 20 mg of isosorbide dinitrate three times per day with a target dose of 40–60 mg three times per day. Long-acting isosorbide mononitrate can be initiated at a dosage of 20 mg/d with a target dosage of 60–120 mg/d. These agents are usually administered to low-risk and intermediate-risk patients who need additional anti-ischemic therapy after beta-blockers.

Intravenous nitrate therapy may be particularly useful in the patient with high-risk unstable angina pectoris who has ongoing pain or the non-STEMI patient with hypertension that is difficult to control. Patients receiving intravenous nitroglycerin should be closely monitored, and the rate of infusion should be titrated to relieve pain as well as to meet blood pressure goals while avoiding hypotension.

D. Thrombolytic Therapy

There is no role for thrombolytic therapy in unstable angina or non-STEMI. Trials designed to test the efficacy of thrombolytic therapy in these settings are negative (thrombolytics increased morbidity and mortality).

E. Anticoagulation

The ESSENCE and TIMI 11B trials have provided convincing evidence supporting the use of the low-molecular-weight heparin enoxaparin in high-risk unstable angina pectoris and non-STEMI patients. While also approved for use in intermediate-risk unstable angina, a close look at the data suggests that the greatest benefit from this agent occurs in patients with pain at rest and 1 mm or more of ST depression or who have elevated troponins or CK-MB. The dose of enoxaparin is 1 mg/kg subcutaneously every 12 hours for 48–72 hours.

Intravenous unfractionated heparin can be given for non-STEMI as well as for intermediate-risk and high-risk unstable angina. However, given the advantages of low-molecular-weight heparin, unfractionated heparin seems most useful as an adjunct to the glycoprotein IIb/IIIa inhibitors or in renal failure, where enoxaparin is not desired because it is cleared by the kidneys.

F. Glycoprotein-IIb/IIIa Receptor Inhibitors

This class of drugs blocks the affinity of the glycoprotein IIb/IIIa receptor for fibrinogen on platelets activated by products released from plaque rupture. In this manner, platelet plugging and clot formation in atherosclerotic lesions are retarded or inhibited.

Like enoxaparin, the glycoprotein IIb/IIIa receptor antagonists (eptifibatide and tirofiban) are indicated for the treatment of intermediate-risk and high-risk unstable angina and for non-STEMI patients. Eptifibatide is approved for use in preventing complications of percutaneous revascularization. Both agents are administered with unfractionated heparin at a dose titrated to result in a twofold increase in the partial thromboplastin time. Eptifibatide is initiated with an intravenous bolus of 180 μg/kg followed by an infusion of 2 μg/kg/min for

72–96 hours. Tirofiban is given as an intravenous loading dose of 0.4 mg/kg/min for 30 minutes, followed by an infusion of 0.1 μg/kg/min for 48–96 hours.

Both glycoprotein IIb/IIIa receptor antagonists reduce the combined end point of death or myocardial infarction or the need for urgent revascularization. Like enoxaparin, the greatest benefit from these agents appears to be conferred upon the more ill patients (ie, those with prolonged chest pain, 1 mm or more ST segment depression, or positive cardiac enzymes). The decision to utilize these costly agents may hinge on the likelihood of side effects of bleeding.

G. Coronary Angioplasty and Coronary Artery Bypass Grafting

Debate continues regarding the advantages of conservative compared with aggressive management of these patients. The clinician may elect to initiate or enhance the therapy of patients with low-risk unstable angina and simply follow the patient symptomatically with or without hospitalization. This option is based on the observation that low-risk patients have a risk of serious events (death and myocardial infarction) that is similar to that borne by patients with stable angina. Even intermediate-risk unstable angina pectoris patients who stabilize their symptoms on medical therapy are at risk only for an increased rate of recurrent unstable angina during the ensuing year. Hence, for stabilized patients, watchful waiting appears to carry little risk and may avoid unneeded revascularization procedures.

Recurrent ischemic pain despite adequate medical therapy should prompt urgent coronary angiography in anticipation of coronary bypass grafting or coronary angioplasty. This recommendation also applies to patients with recurrent pain during treatment of non-STEMI.

Data from TACTICS and TIMI 18 suggest that patients with rest pain plus ST segment depression or who have a non-STEMI may benefit from an early (but not emergent) cardiac catheterization in anticipation of expeditious coronary revascularization.

Antman EM et al: Assessment of the treatment effect of enoxaparin for unstable angina/non-Q-wave myocardial infarction: TIMI 11B-ESSENCE meta-analysis. Circulation 1999;100: 1602–8.

Braunwald E et al: ACC/AHA guidelines for the management of patients with unstable angina and non-ST-segment elevation myocardial infarction: a report of the American College of Cardiology/American Heart Association Task Force on Practice Guidelines (Committee on the Management of Patients with Unstable Angina). J Am Coll Cardiol 2000;36:970–1062.

Cannon CP et al for the TACTICS-Thrombolysis in Myocardial Infarction 18 Investigators: Comparison of early invasive and conservative strategies in patients with unstable coronary syndromes treated with the glycoprotein IIb/IIIa inhibitor tirofiban. N Engl J Med 2001;344:1879–87.

Kong DF et al: Clinical outcomes of therapeutic agents that block the platelet glycoprotein IIb/IIIa integrin in ischemic heart disease. Circulation 1998;98:2829–35.

Lewis HD Jr et al: Protective effects of aspirin against acute myocardial infarction and death in men with unstable angina. Results of a Veterans Administration Cooperative Study. N Engl J Med 1983;309:396–403.

ACUTE MYOCARDIAL INFARCTION WITH ST SEGMENT ELEVATION

ESSENTIALS OF DIAGNOSIS

- *Precordial chest pain with or without radiation to the left arm, shoulder, or jaw.*
- *Pain may be identical in quality and description to that of angina pectoris but may last from 10 minutes to several hours.*
- *> 1 mm ST elevation in two contiguous leads with or without Q wave formation*
- *Confirmation by serial changes in ECGs plus elevation of cardiac enzymes (CK-MB, troponin I, or troponin T)*
- *Complications may include arrhythmias, pulmonary edema, hypotension and shock, ventricular rupture, and pericarditis.*

General Considerations

Coronary thrombosis is the immediate cause of acute myocardial infarction in over 90% of patients with this syndrome. Although early autopsy investigations suggested a variety of other causes of acute myocardial infarction—including coronary vasospasm and emboli—over 86% of those with acute myocardial infarction had coronary artery thrombi when coronary angiography was performed within 4 hours after onset of symptoms.

Current concepts of acute myocardial infarction support the view that the nidus for thrombosis is an atherosclerotic plaque in a coronary artery. The plaque itself may or may not result in stenosis of the artery severe enough to cause symptoms, though more severe atherosclerotic stenoses may be associated with exertional angina. The pathophysiologic sequence of events then probably includes plaque rupture with exposure of the subintimal components of the plaque to coronary blood flow. Platelet activation occurs as the contents of the atherosclerotic plaque (including cholesterol and calcium) interact with circulating blood components. Platelet activation releases thromboxane A_2, a vasoconstrictive substance that may lead to localized vasospasm, which further impedes coronary artery blood flow. The net result of these events is interruption of coronary blood flow by thrombus formation followed by myocardial necrosis if therapy is not effective.

New information regarding the treatment of unstable angina and non-ST elevation myocardial information appears almost weekly. The therapies of unstable angina, non-ST elevation myocardial infarction, and ST elevation myocardial infarction are now driven by large clinical trials that defined current pharmacologic and revascularization strategies.

Clinical Features

A. Symptoms

Acute myocardial infarction is classically associated with precordial chest pain with or without radiation to the left arm, shoulder, or jaw. The pain is identical to that described in the section on angina pectoris but often more severe. The only deviation is duration. The chest pain of myocardial infarction lasts from 10–15 minutes to several hours. The pain is poorly responsive to nitroglycerin and may require morphine for relief. Diaphoresis, syncope, and light-headedness may be present. Dyspnea and orthopnea may be associated with acute congestive heart failure and pulmonary edema.

B. Signs

During myocardial infarction, an S_3 gallop, pulmonary rales, or the murmur of mitral regurgitation may appear. Myocardial infarction may be associated with decreased intensity of S_1 and S_2. Patients should be carefully examined for murmurs of mitral regurgitation and for the presence of pericardial friction rubs. Rales and wheezes may indicate acute pulmonary edema from congestive heart failure.

C. Laboratory Findings

Venous blood should be routinely obtained to measure the cardiac-specific CK-MB and troponin I or troponin T upon admission to hospital and every 6–8 hours thereafter for the first 24 hours. Daily CK-MB and troponin levels may be useful during the balance of the patient's hospital stay to detect silent recurrent myocardial necrosis. A partial thromboplastin time should be obtained on admission and repeated if unfractionated heparin therapy is indicated. Arterial blood gases should be measured if hypoxemia is suspected from physical findings, chest x-ray, or pulse oximetry.

D. Electrocardiography

By definition, acute ST elevation myocardial infarction is associated with specific electrocardiographic findings. However, with modern management, the classic electrocardiographic changes of ST elevation followed by T wave inversion with development of Q waves may be retarded or even abolished. A substantial proportion of patients with myocardial infarction will not develop Q waves after initial ST elevation and may demonstrate only T wave changes or no changes in their ECGs. The development of Q waves portends a worse prognosis.

E. Imaging Studies

Imaging studies should not delay prompt management of acute myocardial infarction.

1. Chest x-ray—The chest x-ray should be reviewed for cardiomegaly, pulmonary edema, and pleural effusions. In upright chest x-rays, fullness and congestion of vessels leading to the upper lung fields is sometimes taken as evidence of mild pulmonary edema from heart failure.

2. Echocardiography—Echocardiography is useful in defining coexisting heart disease—especially valvular or congenital disease—identifying pericardial effusion, evaluating unexplained tachycardia, and assessing ventricular function. Patients with acute myocardial infarction should have an echocardiogram if there is hypotension or shock. Other indications for echocardiography include suspicion of ventricular septal rupture or severe mitral regurgitation (both potentially requiring surgery), a large myocardial infarction as judged from CK-MB or troponin elevation, suspected pericardial effusion, or left ventricular dysfunction that may be worsened by beta-adrenergic blockade or calcium antagonists.

An evaluation of left ventricular function by echocardiography or radionuclide ventriculography should be performed in almost all patients after an acute myocardial infarction to help define prognosis and guide appropriate prophylactic therapy. ACE inhibitors given after myocardial infarction will prolong survival, and the greater the degree of reduction in ejection fraction or severity of heart failure as defined by NYHA functional class, the greater the benefit from the routine use of these agents. Similar statements can be made for the beta-blocker carvedilol in patients with NYHA class II and class III symptoms.

3. Pulmonary artery catheterization (right heart catheterization)—Right heart catheterization allows the determination of right atrial, right ventricular, pulmonary artery, and pulmonary capillary wedge pressures. Since the latter value is a rough estimate of the left ventricular end-diastolic pressure, pulmonary capillary wedge pressure can provide valuable information regarding the necessity for volume expansion or diuresis. The right heart catheters are equipped with a temperature-measuring thermistor that allows determination of cardiac output by thermodilution.

Right heart catheterization should be considered at any point during the course of an acute myocardial infarction when a question exists regarding fluid volume status. For example, a patient with acute myocardial infarction and possible pneumonia may have a lung examination that could represent pulmonary edema, pneumonia, or both. On the other hand, treatment of hypotension in the presence of suspected right ventricular infarction can usually commence without right heart catheter guidance. Patients with an acute inferior infarction who experience hypotension and have clear lungs and no S_3 gallop should receive 500–1000 mL of normal saline to see if volume expansion will increase the blood pressure without causing rales. However, should further volume supplementation seem necessary or should incipient left heart failure be present or suspected, right heart catheterization would be invaluable in determining the true volume status of the patient.

For patients in whom hypotension persists for more than an hour despite use of vasopressors, right heart catheterization is strongly advised.

4. Cardiac catheterization—Cardiac catheterization after acute ST elevation myocardial infarction is generally reserved for patients who develop instability. The routine use of cardiac catheterization after acute myocardial infarction for the purpose of elective angioplasty or bypass surgery has not found justification in randomized trials of elective revascularization after acute ST elevation myocardial infarction. Rather, patients who have an uncomplicated myocardial infarction (no recurrent chest pain) can safely undergo stress testing (usually with a low-level exercise protocol) prior to hospital discharge to identify those at high risk for reinfarction or death who should undergo further study.

Cardiac catheterization before hospital discharge is indicated in two classes of patients: (1) patients who develop chest pain after acute myocardial infarction, which is thought to be ischemic in nature; and (2) patients who have chest pain or evidence of ischemia on electrocardiography or myocardial perfusion scintigraphy during low-level exercise stress testing. These patients have "failed" medical therapy by virtue of having chest pain in the hospital (presumably while on adequate medication) and are likely to be best served by undergoing coronary angioplasty or coronary bypass grafting if their anatomy is found to be suitable by angiography.

Differential Diagnosis

The differential diagnosis of myocardial infarction is essentially the same as that of angina pectoris (see above).

Treatment

Treatment may be divided into immediate and later phases. Immediate therapy is empiric and is initiated after obtaining the history, performing a physical examination, and examining the ECG.

A. Initial Outpatient Treatment

Sublingual nitroglycerin tablets or nitroglycerin spray should be self-administered if the patient has either drug. Otherwise, sublingual nitroglycerin should be administered by paramedics or by personnel in the emergency department. A sublingual nitroglycerin tablet (usually 0.3 mg) can be administered every 3–5 minutes (if pain persists) for an initial total of three to five tablets. Repeat doses of nitroglycerin can be administered once blood pressure monitoring is available and the patient has no significant side effects such as dizziness or severe headaches.

B. Immediate Hospital Therapy

Initial therapy of a patient in the hospital suspected of having myocardial infarction consists of nitroglycerin as indicated above. Oxygen therapy, usually 2 L/min by nasal cannula, is frequently begun empirically and adjusted based on pulse oximetry. One aspirin tablet (325 mg) should be chewed and swallowed by the patient to reduce subsequent morbidity and improve chances for survival. For aspirin-allergic patients or patients already taking prophylactic aspirin, oral clopidogrel, 75 mg, may be substituted.

1. Revascularization—

a. Thrombolytic therapy—If the patient has a classic history for acute myocardial infarction and has > 1 mm ST segment elevation in two contiguous leads (eg, in two inferior leads [II, III, aVF]; or in leads I and aVL; or in two contiguous chest or V leads), thrombolytic therapy should be considered if it can be started within 12 hours after the onset of pain. The presence of a left bundle branch block not known to be old is also an indication for thrombolytic therapy.

Tenecteplase, intravenous streptokinase, or anisoylated plasminogen streptokinase activator complex (anistreplase; APSAC) can be administered if the patient does not have one or more of the following contraindications: active internal bleeding; history of stroke; intracranial or intraspinal surgery or trauma within 2 months; intracranial neoplasm, arteriovenous malformation, or aneurysm; known bleeding diathesis; or severe uncontrolled hypertension. Age over 75 has been used as a contraindication to thrombolytic therapy, but this remains controversial.

Systemic anticoagulation with unfractionated heparin has been routinely utilized to increase the partial thromboplastin time to two times control values in the 48 hours subsequent to thrombolytic therapy. However, recent data suggest that low-molecular-weight heparin in the form of enoxaparin, 1 mg/kg subcutaneously twice daily, may be equally efficacious as an adjunct to thrombolytic therapy with tenecteplase. Low-molecular-weight heparin has the advantage over intravenous unfractionated heparin of subcutaneous administration as well as of obviating the need for frequent determinations of the partial thromboplastin time.

b. Primary angioplasty—Facilities with an active catheterization laboratory may consider urgent coronary angiography and percutaneous angioplasty (with or without stenting) as an alternative to thrombolytic therapy. If the patient can be brought to the angiographic laboratory in an expeditious manner, the angiographer may initiate abciximab, which binds to the platelet glycoprotein IIb/IIIa receptor and inhibits platelet aggregation, to reduce the incidence of subsequent myocardial infarction and death.

Whether angioplasty or thrombolytic treatment is chosen as the therapy for acute ST elevation myocardial infarction, the administration of aspirin and intravenous beta blockade should not be delayed.

2. Beta-adrenergic blockade—Beta-adrenergic blockade with intravenous metoprolol should be accomplished as soon as possible after the diagnosis of acute myocardial infarction has been established by history and electrocardiography. Intravenous beta blockade can be initiated provided the patient has an initial heart rate over 50/min, a systolic blood pressure over 90 mm Hg, has rales less than one-third of the way up the back, has a PR interval less than 0.28 s, and has no other contraindications (eg, asthma). Metoprolol should be administered intravenously in 5 mg increments more than 2 minutes apart to a total dose of 15 mg (or more if greater control of the heart rate is desired). Following intravenous loading of beta-blockers, oral metoprolol, 50 mg twice daily, or oral atenolol, 50 mg once daily, should be initiated.

3. Intravenous nitroglycerin—Intravenous nitroglycerin was frequently administered to all patients with known or suspected myocardial infarction in the hope of reducing morbidity and mortality. Large trials of patients with ST elevation myocardial infarction have failed to justify the enthusiasm for the routine use of this agent in asymptomatic patients with acute myocardial infarction. Current recommendations for intravenous nitroglycerin include relief of ischemic pain and reduction of systolic blood pressure. A dose of 0.5 μg/kg/min (35 μg/min for an average-sized patient) can be initiated and the rate of administration increased until pain relief or a reduction in systolic blood pressure to less than 90–100 mm Hg. The rate of administration should not be further increased if the patient develops dizziness or other evidence of decreased organ perfusion. If long-term nitrate therapy is desired, long-acting nitrates such as isosorbide dinitrate or isosorbide mononitrate should be started within 24 hours. The continuous administration of intravenous nitroglycerin can rapidly lead to "nitrate tolerance" and loss of anti-ischemic effect.

4. Morphine sulfate—Morphine beginning with 2 mg intravenously should be administered if nitroglycerin does not provide prompt relief of pain. Incremental doses of morphine can be administered to a total that is usually less than 20 mg. Much lower doses may be effective. As morphine doses exceed 10–15 mg, the possibility of respiratory depression must be considered.

5. Antiarrhythmic therapy—Patients with acute myocardial infarction who have hemodynamically unstable ventricular arrhythmias (ventricular fibrillation or ventricular tachycardia) lasting for more than 30 seconds or causing hemodynamic collapse or hypotension should be electrically cardioverted.

Sustained monomorphic ventricular tachycardia not associated with symptoms or hypotension (blood pressure < 90 mm Hg) should be treated with one of the following:

a. Lidocaine—An intravenous bolus of lidocaine (1–1.5 mg/kg) is given, followed by supplemental boluses of 0.5–0.75 mg/kg every 5–10 minutes to a maximum loading dose of 3 mg/kg. Loading is followed by an intravenous infusion of lidocaine at a rate of 2–4 mg/min. Nursing staff must be alert to changes in the patient's mental status (somnolence, disorientation, dysesthesias) that may signal lidocaine toxicity. The elderly are particularly susceptible.

b. Amiodarone—Give 150 mg intravenously over 10 minutes followed by an infusion of 1 mg/min for 6 hours, then a maintenance infusion of 0.5 mg/min.

c. Procainamide—Give a loading dose by intravenous infusion of 12–17 mg/kg at a rate of 20–30 mg/min, followed by an infusion of 1–4 mg/min.

The acute administration of antiarrhythmics allows time to diagnose and correct electrolyte abnormalities such as hypokalemia and hypomagnesemia, correct hypoxemia, and allow anti-ischemic therapy (beta blockade) to be intensified.

6. Sedation—Sedatives such as intravenous or oral benzodiazepines may be useful in reducing the level of anxiety engendered by the ICU setting.

C. Additional Care in the ICU

1. General measures—The patient should be placed at complete bed rest during the first 24 hours. Thereafter, in stable uncomplicated patients, the patient should be encouraged to sit up in bed, dangling the legs over the side several times a day, and then spend increasing amounts of time sitting in a chair or ambulating with assistance. The patient should be provided with a clear-liquid diet for the first 12–24 hours after hospitalization for acute myocardial infarction. Stool softeners are often useful to prevent straining during defecation.

Subcutaneous heparin, 5000 units twice daily, should be considered—if no contraindication exists—to prevent deep venous thrombosis and pulmonary embolism. Additional supportive measures for patients in the coronary care unit include daily monitoring of serum electrolytes (including serum Mg^{2+}) for at least 72 hours. In patients with normal renal function, potassium supplements should be administered to keep the serum $K^+ > 4.5$ meq/L, and magnesium should be given intravenously to maintain serum Mg^{2+} levels > 2.0 mg/dL. These maneuvers will reduce the incidence of ventricular arrhythmias in a safe and physiologic manner. While prophylactic Mg^{2+} administration does not reduce mortality overall, there is some suggestion that high-risk groups (nonreperfused patients) may benefit. Magnesium sulfate (10 g [40 mmol] in 100–200 mL of D_5W administered over 2–3 hours) will usually increase the steady state serum levels of Mg^{2+} about 0.3–0.4 mg/dL in patients with normal renal function.

2. Aspirin—One aspirin tablet per day (eg, enteric-coated aspirin, 160–325 mg) should be administered to all patients after myocardial infarction unless there are contraindications. Regardless of whether thrombolytic therapy has been given or not, prophylactic aspirin therapy has reduced the post-myocardial infarction mortality rate by 23%. For aspirin-allergic patients, clopidogrel, 75 mg/d, can be substituted.

3. Beta-adrenergic blockade—Any of the following—propranolol, 180 mg daily in divided doses; timolol, 10 mg twice daily; metoprolol, 100 mg twice daily; or atenolol, 100 mg once daily—should be administered after acute myocardial infarction to prevent sudden death in patients who can tolerate this class of drugs. The criteria used to define patients eligible for prophylactic beta-adrenergic blockade are similar to those applicable in the immediate post-myocardial infarction period: systolic blood pressure > 90–100 mm Hg, heart rate > 50 beats/min, no rales, PR interval < 0.28 s, and no contraindications (eg, asthma, "brittle" diabetes).

Randomized trials of over 50,000 patients in the United States and Europe have consistently demonstrated a 25–35% decrease in post-myocardial infarction sudden death with the prophylactic use of beta blockade. Of particular interest is the observation that if a patient can tolerate beta blockade after acute myocardial infarction, the greatest benefit accrues to those in whom some of the most serious concerns against beta blockade are raised. Specifically, a patient who has had heart block, sudden death (ventricular fibrillation, ventricular tachycardia), or heart failure post-myocardial infarction and can subsequently tolerate beta blockade (ie, if heart failure clears with one or two doses of diuretics) gains the greatest cardioprotective effect from beta blockade. For example, assuming a pool of patients with prior congestive heart failure who subsequently stabilize, it is estimated that prophylactic treatment with beta-blockers of only 26 patients is required to save one life.

4. Antihypertensive agents—Patients with hypertension have an obvious need for lowering systolic blood pressure. A goal for systolic blood pressure of approximately 120 mm Hg or less would be desirable, though any evidence of cerebral hypoperfusion may frustrate this goal in some patients.

While most antihypertensive drugs are potentially suitable for treatment of hypertension in patients with acute myocardial infarction, preference should be given to agents likely to treat both hypertension and the underlying coronary artery disease. For example, beta-blockers would seem an ideal antihypertensive choice, since they reduce the work of the heart (by lowering both heart rate and blood pressure) as well as providing a cardioprotective effect that reduces the incidence of sudden death following acute myocardial infarction.

Angiotensin-converting enzyme (ACE) inhibitors may be useful for the treatment of hypertension and should be strongly considered if the patient has any element of congestive heart failure (rales, cardiomegaly, or known reduction of ejection fraction) in conjunction with an acute myocardial infarction. Survival benefit in the post-myocardial infarction setting has been demonstrated for a host of ACE inhibitors, with greater improvement in survival being observed in the patients with the greatest reductions in ejection fraction. For patients intolerant of ACE inhibitors, the angiotensin II receptor blocking agents (eg, losartan, valsartan) are suitable alternatives.

The calcium channel blockers diltiazem and verapamil are reasonable alternatives to beta-adrenergic blockade in patients with brittle diabetes or bronchospastic lung disease. Both agents have a modest bradycardiac effect in addition to their antihypertensive effects. It should be remembered that these agents should be reserved for patients with preserved left ventricular function, as these drugs increase mortality substantially in patients with ejection fractions under 0.40.

5. Diltiazem—In patients with acute myocardial infarction who do not develop Q waves on the ECG (acute non-Q wave myocardial infarction or subendocardial myocardial infarction), strong consideration should be given to administering diltiazem in a dose of 60 mg four times daily or 90 mg every 8 hours. At these doses, this agent has been shown to prevent reinfarction in the month following an acute non-Q wave myocardial infarction.

Complications

A. Arrhythmias

1. Atrial fibrillation—This disorder, characterized by a narrow QRS complex and an irregular rhythm, is frequently associated with extensive damage to the myocardium.

If rapid atrial fibrillation is associated with symptomatic hypotension or with chest pain, conservative measures should be abandoned and synchronized electrical cardioversion should be performed immediately.

Typically, initial therapy would consist of digoxin given intravenously in a dose of 0.25–0.5 mg to slow the ventricular response and improve left ventricular function. Subsequent doses of 0.125–0.25 mg of intravenous digoxin can be given up to a total of 1–1.5 mg over the initial 24 hours post-myocardial infarction. Oral digoxin, usually 0.125–0.25 mg/d, is administered for maintenance therapy. The goal of digoxin therapy is to reduce the ventricular rate to < 90–100 beats/min.

Concomitant therapy with either beta-adrenergic blockers or the calcium channel-blocking agent diltiazem will achieve acceptable heart rate control in a shorter period of time than with digoxin alone. For example, 5 mg of intravenous propranolol can be administered every 5 minutes to achieve prompt control of rapid atrial fibrillation while digoxin therapy is being initiated. An oral maintenance dose of metoprolol, 50 mg twice daily, can be initiated once the resting heart rate is controlled with the intravenous preparation. Intravenous diltiazem, a loading dose of 20 mg (or 0.25 mg/kg) over 2 minutes, can be given and repeated in 15 minutes. A maintenance infusion of 10–15 mg/h can be prescribed for 24 hours if necessary.

Heparin should be given in the absence of contraindications.

2. Ventricular premature beats—Prophylactic abolition of *asymptomatic* ventricular ectopy after myocardial infarction results in a marked increase in mortality rate. The results of the CAST study (Cardiac Arrhythmia Suppression Trial) have conclusively documented that routine use of antiarrhythmic therapy for asymptomatic ventricular ectopy is contraindicated. It is worth noting, however, that the prophylactic use of beta-adrenergic blockade has been associated with a decrease in the frequency of ventricular ectopy. Since beta-blockers prolong survival after a myocardial infarction, they should be considered the primary form of nonspecific anti-ectopy therapy.

Isolated ventricular premature beats need not be treated, but repetitive forms of ventricular ectopy such as couplets and ventricular tachycardia (more than three ventricular premature beats in a row) are indications for prophylactic lidocaine if they are associated with hypotension (see above). If longer-term antiarrhythmic therapy is believed necessary, intravenous procainamide (2–4 mg/min) or oral sustained-release procainamide (750 mg every 6 hours) would be potentially beneficial. Alternative agents include quinidine sulfate, 200 mg every 6 hours, or sustained-release quinidine gluconate, 324 mg every 8 hours, as well as tocainide, mexiletine, and amiodarone.

HEART FAILURE

Heart failure complicating acute myocardial infarction will increase the mortality rate from 2–3% to as high as 50% per year. A primary goal of therapy for acute myocardial infarction is to prevent the progression of uncomplicated myocardial infarction to reinfarction, with development of heart failure. The administration of intravenous, cutaneous, or oral nitrates as well as beta-adrenergic blockade therapy and thrombolytic therapy are directed toward this goal.

If congestive heart failure develops after myocardial infarction, initial therapy may include the following.

1. Diuretics—Rales and S_3 gallop are sometimes eradicated by a single intravenous dose of furosemide (20–40 mg intravenously in patients who have not previously received this agent). Larger doses of intravenous furosemide may be utilized as the initial diuretic dose if the patient is known to have been receiving diuretic therapy in the past.

2. Vasodilators—ACE inhibitors are first-line therapy for the treatment of congestive heart failure in acute myocardial infarction. In addition to their beneficial hemodynamic effects, these agents improve survival by altering favorably the "remodeling" of the left ventricle that occurs with myocardial infarction. Captopril can be initiated in doses 12.5 mg every 8 hours and then increased to 100 mg every 8 hours. Dose escalation can occur daily (or more frequently), if no orthostatic symptoms are noted. Corresponding doses of enalapril range from 2.5–10 mg twice daily—and for lisinopril, 5 mg once daily initially, titrated upward to 10–20 mg/d. Ramipril is another ACE inhibitor with proof of efficacy and survival benefit in the treatment of congestive heart failure complicating acute myocardial infarction.

Cough and elevation of the serum creatinine can limit the utilization of ACE inhibitors. Some clinicians have substituted angiotensin II receptor antagonists such as losartan and valsartan for ACE inhibitors. Clinical trials in chronic heart failure would support this practice, though the ACE inhibitors remain the vasodilators of choice for prolongation of life with heart failure and depressed left ventricular function. Another alternative therapy for heart failure with proven survival benefits is the combination of the vasodilator hydralazine with isosorbide dinitrate. Hydralazine can be started at 25 mg orally with the dose increased every 3–6 hours to a target of 100 mg every 8 hours. Isosorbide dinitrate can be initiated at 20 mg three times daily and increased with each dose to a target of 60 mg three times daily.

A serum sodium < 135 meq/L developing during the course of acute myocardial infarction or chronic congestive heart failure suggests that the patient's blood pressure is critically dependent upon various compensatory mechanisms designed to support blood pressure, such as production of antidiuretic hormone and angiotensin. In such patients, heart failure therapy with ACE inhibitors may result in substantial or profound hypotension.

3. Digoxin—Digoxin is frequently administered to patients with heart failure who do not respond to one or two doses of intravenous furosemide. Since digoxin may increase myocardial O_2 consumption and may aggravate ventricular arrhythmias, it should be given orally at a dose of 0.125–0.25 mg daily. The administration of a "loading dose" of digoxin is unnecessary unless rapid atrial fibrillation coexists with heart failure and rapid control of ventricular rate is desired.

C. Cardiogenic Shock

The mortality rate for cardiogenic shock complicating acute myocardial infarction still remains over 50%. Treatment may include the following.

1. Increase intravascular fluid volume—Volume expansion with 250–500 mL of normal saline may be utilized as first treatment for cardiogenic shock if no evidence of left ventricular failure is present (no rales, absent S_3 gallop). If no clear response is seen (blood pressure does not increase), more fluid may be administered, but consideration of pressor agents or right heart catheterization (or both) should be high on the list of subsequent priorities.

2. Vasoactive and inotropic agents—Intravenous dopamine in the range of 5–25 μg/kg/min may be given to raise the systolic blood pressure to more than 90 mm Hg or to otherwise maintain organ perfusion. Intravenous dobutamine given in doses of 2.5–25 μg/kg per minute is frequently helpful in cardiogenic shock. This agent is particularly useful because it is both a vasodilator and an inotropic agent. Despite its vasodilator properties, in patients with a markedly reduced cardiac output, dobutamine infusions frequently result in an increase in blood pressure.

If either of these agents is required for more than a few minutes to an hour, placement of a pulmonary artery catheter is warranted so that the dose of each agent can be adjusted to meet hemodynamic goals. The simultaneous administration of dopamine (6–7 mg/kg/min initially) and dobutamine (2–3 μg/kg/min initially) may be useful in increasing both the blood pressure and the cardiac output in patients with acute myocardial infarction and severely compromised hemodynamics. These dosages are an empiric starting point. A right heart catheter is required for rational adjustment of these two pressor agents.

Milrinone has a hemodynamic profile similar to that of dobutamine, but it is much more costly. This phosphodiesterase inhibitor does not demonstrate the rapid tachyphylaxis seen with beta-adrenergic agonists. If long-term high-dose catecholamine support is required to maintain cardiac output, milrinone may be a suitable alternative.

3. Intra-aortic balloon pump—The intra-aortic balloon pump should be considered if acute ischemia is suspected as the primary cause of cardiogenic shock. If a patient has continued chest pain after myocardial infarction and develops cardiogenic shock, intra-aortic balloon pumping may provide a bridge to surgical therapy of shock. The intra-aortic balloon is inflated in the descending aorta during diastole, thereby increasing coronary perfusion pressure. By deflating during systole, it "unloads" the left ventricle.

D. Heart Block

1. Inferior myocardial infarction and heart block—Heart block frequently occurs along with acute inferior wall myocardial infarction during which the blood supply to the atrioventricular node has been compromised either by ischemia or by infarction. However, temporary pacing is not necessarily indicated if the heart block is Mobitz I (Wenckebach) and the patient's blood pressure and clinical status are stable. Atropine is very useful for increasing the heart rate in patients with symptomatic bradycardia. An increase in heart rate and blood pressure is frequently seen after a 1 mg intravenous bolus of atropine sulfate. Atropine can be repeated once or twice if necessary. However, serious side effects (dry mouth, blurred vision, and even psychosis) preclude its continued use. Therefore, the development of heart block with hemodynamic compromise (fall in blood pressure, decrease in mentation, or other evidence of peripheral hypoperfusion) should lead to serious consideration of a transvenous temporary pacemaker.

2. Temporary transcutaneous pacing—Transcutaneous pacing may be very helpful as a temporary expedient. The technique is very painful to the patient and should be replaced by transvenous pacemaker placement in high-risk patients likely to require pacing. Transcutaneous pacing is indicated for symptomatic bradycardia (heart rate < 50 beats/min) or bradycardia with hypotension (systolic blood pressure < 80 mm Hg) unresponsive to drug therapy, Mobitz type II second-degree atrioventricular block, third-degree heart block and bilateral bundle branch block (BBB) (ie, alternating BBB), new BBB or fascicular block, and RBBB or LBBB with first degree AV block.

3. Temporary transvenous pacing—Temporary transvenous pacing in the acute myocardial infarction patient is indicated for the following conditions: asystole, symptomatic bradycardia unresponsive to medications and type I second degree atrioventricular block, bilateral bundle branch block, a new bundle branch block or fascicular block *and* first degree AV block, and Mobitz type II second-degree AV block.

4. Permanent pacing after acute myocardial infarction—Consideration for permanent pacemaker implantation should take place in the presence of persistent Mobitz type II second-degree AV block or complete heart block after myocardial infarction, transient second-degree or third degree AV block plus BBB, and symptomatic atrioventricular block at any level.

E. Right Ventricular Infarction

Right ventricular myocardial infarction complicates roughly one-third of all acute inferior wall myocardial infarctions. The right ventricle is a very thin-walled structure that is poorly adapted to acute changes in either pressure or volume. The diagnosis of this entity can be made through echocardiography, radionuclide ventriculography, cardiac catheterization, or electrocardiography.

1. Diagnosis—ST elevation in the right-sided electrocardiographic chest leads is the most sensitive test for detecting an acute right ventricular infarction. Lead V_4R is the most sensitive and most specific lead. However, all electrocardiographic criteria begin to dissipate within hours after an acute right ventricular infarction, and the hemodynamic consequences may be more apparent than the changes on the ECG. Right ventricular infarction should be suspected in all patients with acute inferior wall myocardial infarction with hypotension, especially if there is evidence that left ventricular function is preserved. The hallmarks of a hemodynamically significant right ventricular infarction include the presence of elevated neck veins, clear lungs, and evidence of poor cardiac output.

2. Treatment—Since right ventricular infarction is a common complication in patients with acute inferior wall myocardial infarction, initial doses of nitroglycerin should be given cautiously to these patients. This is because right ventricular output may decrease markedly in response to systemic venodilation by nitroglycerin. These patients may also be particularly sensitive to diuretics such as furosemide.

To increase blood pressure and cardiac output in the face of a known or suspected acute right ventricular myocardial infarction, initial therapy should consist of intravenous fluids, provided there is no evidence of pulmonary congestion or a left ventricular S_3 gallop. Patients who fail to respond to fluid infusion with an increase in blood pressure and improved systemic perfusion should be treated next with intravenous dobutamine, preferably with a pulmonary artery catheter to help guide therapy.

F. Other Complications

1. Pericarditis—Pericarditis is a common complication of myocardial infarction. If the infarction process involves the epicardium of the left ventricle, irritation of the pericardium may occur. The patient typically complains of chest pain exacerbated by respiration and supine posture; the patient frequently feels more comfortable sitting upright. The appearance of a three-component friction rub representing the left ventricular epicardium rubbing against an inflamed pericardium confirms the diagnosis.

Treatment is generally straightforward. An asymptomatic friction rub heard on routine daily examinations need not be treated. Symptomatic episodes of pericarditis can be treated with either aspirin, 325 mg every 4–6 hours, or with nonsteroidal anti-inflammatory agents. Rarely, corticosteroids are required to control post-myocardial infarction pericarditis pain.

Most episodes of pericarditis are self-limited and require no more than symptomatic therapy. If a question regarding a patient's symptoms arises, an echocardiogram that demonstrates an increase in pericardial fluid may be helpful in establishing the diagnosis of pericarditis.

Thrombolytic therapy and heparin (except for subcutaneous heparin for prevention of deep venous thrombosis) should be terminated if pericarditis is suspected or diagnosed post-myocardial infarction. Rarely, post-myocardial infarction pericarditis leads to a pericardial effusion sizable enough to cause hemodynamic compromise. The hallmarks of a significant pericardial effusion include an increase in heart rate, an increase in the magnitude of paradoxic pulse, a decrease in the systolic pressure, a decrease in the systemic pulse pressure, elevated neck veins, and, in advanced stages, evidence of low cardiac output (cool extremities, decreased mentation, decreased urine output). Should a hemodynamically significant pericardial effusion be suspected, urgent echocardiography should be performed to confirm the diagnosis and to localize the effusion. While the echocardiogram is being performed, cardiac catheterization laboratory personnel should be preparing to perform pericardiocentesis if necessary.

2. Papillary muscle rupture and ventricular septal defect—These are rare but life-threatening complications of acute myocardial infarction. A murmur consistent with acute mitral regurgitation may be heard in up to 50% of patients with acute myocardial infarction during the first 24–48 hours after the event. However, these mitral regurgitant murmurs usually represent transient papillary muscle ischemia and disappear with time or remain hemodynamically unimportant.

Papillary muscle rupture or an acute ventricular septal rupture should be suspected in patients who develop sudden hypotension or evidence of severe heart failure. The hallmark of both lesions is a loud systolic murmur, often with a thrill palpable over the left chest. The diagnosis of these lesions can be confirmed by echocardiography. Alternatively, since these lesions are usually associated with heart failure and a low cardiac output, a pulmonary artery catheter should be placed to help guide subsequent management. The presence of high (near systemic) O_2 saturation in a right atrial blood sample confirms the diagnosis of ventricular septal rupture (with left-to-right shunting of blood). The presence of a large *v* wave in the pulmonary capillary wedge pressure tracing may lend support to the diagnosis of ventricular papillary muscle rupture.

Both of these conditions are acute emergencies. Conservative measures are usually insufficient to allow survival. Consideration should be given to urgent cardiac catheterization with anticipation of emergent open heart surgery.

Dell'Italia LJ et al: Comparative effects of volume loading, dobutamine, and nitroprusside in patients with predominant right ventricular infarction. Circulation 1985;72:1327–35.

Dell'Italia LJ et al: Right ventricular infarction: Identification by hemodynamic measurements before and after volume loading and correlation with noninvasive techniques. J Am Coll Cardiol 1984;4:931–9.

Gottlieb SS, McCarter RJ, Vogel RA: Effect of beta-blockade on mortality among high-risk and low-risk patients after myocardial infarction. N Engl J Med 1998;339:489–97.

Hennekens CH et al: Adjunctive drug therapy of acute myocardial infarction—evidence from clinical trials. N Engl J Med 1996;335:1660–7.

Ryan TJ et al: 1999 update: ACC/AHA guidelines for the management of patients with acute myocardial infarction: a report of the American College of Cardiology/American Heart Association Task Force on Practice Guidelines (Committee on Management of Acute Myocardial Infarction). J Am Coll Cardiol 1999;34:890–911.

Cardiothoracic Surgery

23

Edward D. Verrier, MD, & Craig R. Hampton, MD

Primary cardiovascular disease is the most common single indication for ICU care and monitoring. Many patients with other diseases requiring intensive care develop secondary cardiovascular complications. Moreover, cardiac surgery patients remain the most common group of surgical patients requiring intensive care and monitoring. Many of the ICU concerns relevant to cardiac surgical patients are covered in other sections of this text, but certain aspects are unique to this common subset of patients. The following sections cover these unique problems and include aneurysm and dissection of the great vessels, postoperative arrhythmias, perioperative coagulopathy, complications of artificial circulation, and postoperative low-output states.

ANEURYSMS, DISSECTIONS, & TRANSECTIONS OF THE GREAT VESSELS

ESSENTIALS OF DIAGNOSIS

- *Chest pain.*
- *Differential peripheral pulses.*
- *Aortic insufficiency.*
- *Widened mediastinum on chest x-ray.*
- *Cardiovascular collapse.*
- *End organ ischemic symptoms.*

General Considerations

Disease of the great vessels often presents dramatically and is often lethal if not managed expeditiously. Timely surgical correction or, when appropriate, medical therapy may be lifesaving. However, despite considerable progress in surgical approaches and medical therapies, a minority of patients still face the specter of complications: potential paraplegia, pre- or postoperative mortality, end organ injury, delayed recovery from surgical incisions, or subsequent surgery from disease progression after initial medical or surgical therapy.

Terminology is frequently confusing, in part due to the nature of the pathology, and because of various classification schemes. Aortic dissections, transections, and aneurysms are related but distinct entities. Aortic dissections and transections predispose to false (pseudo) aneurysms, and aneurysms predispose to dissections; but because of therapeutic and prognostic considerations it is desirable, and usually possible, to determine which came first. These three entities frequently present simultaneously as a combined lesion, but the relative contribution of each component of the disease should be considered separately—while appreciating their interrelationships.

Aneurysms of the great vessels (ie, aorta, innominate artery, carotid artery, ductus arteriosus, and subclavian artery) are pathologically either true aneurysms composed of all three layers of the vascular wall or false aneurysms containing only adventitia and periaortic fibrous tissue. True aneurysms result from transmural degeneration of the structural components of the vessel (eg, Marfan's syndrome, residual ductus arteriosus tissue, ectatic vein grafts, and aortic disease associated with obstructive lung disease), or from a localized degeneration of vascular layers (eg, atherosclerosis, vasculitis). False aneurysms are usually due to prior dissection, trauma, prior great vessel surgery, or rarely tumor. Descriptively, both true and false aneurysms are either saccular or fusiform (Figure 23–1). Classification of great vessel aneurysms based on location and extent is helpful for diagnosis, prognosis, and therapy. Aneurysms that involve the arch are more technically complex than those isolated to the ascending or descending aorta. Because they usually require circulatory arrest for repair, they have an increased potential for neurologic injury. Repair of aneurysms that traverse the diaphragm are more prone to cause paraplegia because of their proximity to the arterial supply of the anterior spinal artery. Aneurysms that involve the aortic root are likely to require coronary reimplantation and valve resuspension or replacement. Hence, they have increased risk for myocardial ischemia and the potential complications associated with valvular surgery. Extensive aneurysms of the entire aorta may require a staged approach with initial replacement of the ascending aorta, followed by the arch, and subsequently by the descending thoracic and abdominal portions.

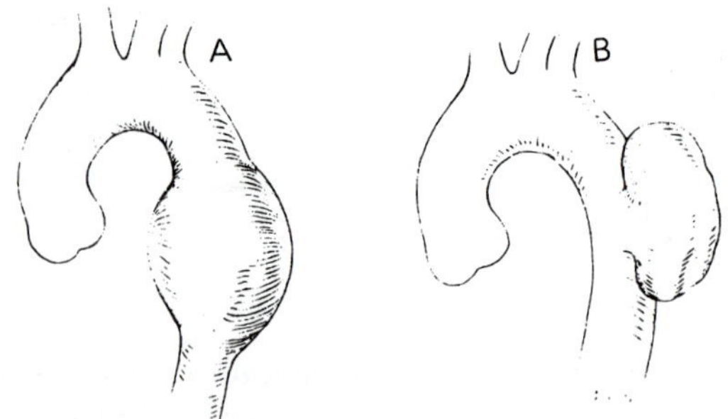

Figure 23–1. Types of thoracic aortic aneurysms. ***A:*** Fusiform. ***B:*** Saccular. (Reproduced, with permission, from Way LW [editor]: *Current Surgical Diagnosis & Treatment,* 10th ed. Originally published by Appleton & Lange. Copyright © 1991 by The McGraw-Hill Companies, Inc.)

Aneurysms presumably cause symptoms by expansion, compression of local structures, distal embolism of contained material, secondary dissection, and either contained or free rupture. The frequency of these complications increases exponentially with aneurysm size.

Etiology

A. Aortic Transection

Aortic transection most commonly occurs after significant blunt trauma and generally occurs at points of relative aortic fixation—in descending order of frequency, near the ligamentum arteriosum, at the diaphragmatic hiatus, the ascending aorta, and the abdominal aorta. Shearing stress from rapid deceleration has been regarded as the primary biomechanism of this injury, but recent evidence suggests that lateral impact collision forces with simultaneous acceleration of the victim and increased hydrostatic pressure within the aorta may also be important mechanisms. In survivable cases, tenuous vascular integrity is maintained by the adventitia. Early symptomatic presentation is usually exsanguinating rupture or distal dissection, while late presentation is in the form of a pseudoaneurysm. Aortic transection is occasionally due to penetrating violent injury or to iatrogenic trauma during cardiac or other surgery.

B. Aortic Dissection

Aortic and other great vessel dissections represent pathologic separation of the vessel layers, thereby creating a true lumen and a false one. Since aortic tissue is intrinsically stable, there is usually associated pathology such as disease of the intima or media (eg, atherosclerosis, cystic medial necrosis, Marfan's syndrome), increased wall tension (preexisting aneurysm, hypertension), or trauma (blunt or sharp). Indeed, the two conditions most frequently associated with aortic dissection are hypertension (about 80%) and Marfan's syndrome. Mechanistically, rupture of the vasa vasorum is probably the most important inciting event. It is not clear whether spontaneous bleeding into the aortic wall (ie, intramural hematoma) may cause aortic dissection. Dissections are usually complex anatomically and dynamic in presentation. Once the intimal tear occurs, there is progressive separation of the adventitia and the intima. This separation typically propagates distally but may occasionally extend proximally. As the separation extends, branch vessels may be themselves dissected, occluded, or completely unaffected depending on the location and extent of the aortic dissection. Ultimately, the dissection reaches an equilibrium between the vessel's intrinsic resistance and shear forces that promote propagation. The dissection then either reenters the true lumen via a second or third tear in the intima or creates a blind pouch. These "neostructures" may then remain permanently patent because of continued flow down the false channel, or they may thrombose due to stasis. These dynamics of aortic dissection are a function of the balance between tissue strength and continued shear forces. Shear forces, in turn, are determined by blood pressure, change in blood pressure with time (dP/dT), size and location of the intimal tear, and blood vessel diameter.

Two classification schemes are commonly used, based on the location and extent of dissection—the Stanford and DeBakey classifications. A Stanford type A dissection begins in the ascending or transverse aorta with variable amounts of aortic involvement. Type B dissections begin distal to the takeoff of the last great vessel, usually the left subclavian artery. By comparison, a type I DeBakey lesion is analogous to an extensive Stanford type A dissection. Both begin in the ascending aorta and extend across the arch and down the descending aorta. A DeBakey type II dissection involves only the ascending aorta, while a type III DeBakey lesion is analogous to a Stanford type B dissection.

These classification schemes are vital to management and prognosis, with particular emphasis on identifying involvement of the ascending aorta. Type A dissections have an 80% mortality within 48 hours without surgical treatment, while selected type B dissections can frequently be managed medically with only a 10% mortality at 30 days. These vastly different outcomes are primarily based on the proximity of type A dissections to vital structures, including the heart, coronary arteries, aortic valve, and carotid vessels. Myocardial infarction, acute aortic insufficiency, intrapericardial rupture causing tamponade, and stroke are all frequent consequences of proximal dissections. In addition, progression of a type A dissection may result in all of the complications normally associated with a type B dissection such as intrathoracic rupture, paraplegia, visceral ischemia, extremity ischemia, and intra-abdominal rupture. Fortunately, many of the structures affected by type B dissections are either paired (eg, renal), tolerate ischemia for long periods of time (eg, extremities), or have collateral pathways (eg, gastrointestinal tract) for blood supply.

Other changes related to the dissection process include (1) lability of the blood pressure to fluid shifts, cardiac decompensation, baroreceptor involvement, and underlying etiology; (2) coagulopathy from massive blood exposure to tissue; (3) metabolic derangements from hypoperfusion; (4) respiratory compromise from systemic inflammation and local airway compression; (5) any variety of neurologic, renal, gastrointestinal, cardiac, and extremity complications; and (6) progression to chronic pseudoaneurysm or, rarely, stenosis or obstruction of the aortic lumen. The surgical risks and adverse effects of therapy multiply with extent and acuity of the disease process.

Clinical Features

A. Symptoms and Signs

Any patient with significant chest pain should be assumed to have an aortic catastrophe until another cause is established. Discrepancies in peripheral pulses and blood pressures occur frequently, particularly in the presence of aortic valve insufficiency. Changes in pulse contour or distribution may help localize the extent of a dissection or transection. Patients with recent or remote trauma, a family history of Marfan's syndrome, hypertension, or prior surgery of the aorta are at increased risk.

Dissections in particular—and sometimes aneurysms—have myriad presentations, making them a diagnostic challenge. By far the most common symptom accompanying aneurysms, transections, and dissections is chest pain, usually sharp and, less frequently, tearing or ripping, with radiation to the back or abdomen.

Aneurysms may present with pressure symptoms related to the recurrent laryngeal nerve, great veins, trachea, esophagus, or chest wall. Significantly, aneurysms may be asymptomatic until they rupture and present with circulatory collapse.

Any number of end organs may become ischemic temporarily or permanently with their own characteristic symptoms. Temporary neurologic findings are particularly common, but any vascular organ can present with initial or subsequent ischemia.

B. Electrocardiography

Because primary coronary artery disease is more common than significant aortic disease, a normal ECG with normal cardiac enzymes should heighten the suspicion of dissection or aneurysm as a cause of chest pain. However, if a type A dissection extends into a coronary (more commonly the right coronary) artery, an ECG cannot make this distinction. Moreover, electrocardiographic findings occur in about 70% of dissection patients, including nonspecific ST–T wave changes, left ventricular hypertrophy, ischemia, myocardial infarction with old Q waves, or myocardial infarction with new Q waves.

C. Imaging Studies

A normal chest x-ray is helpful but does not exclude disease. Overlying structures may compromise aortic visibility. Tortuosity of the aorta may falsely suggest enlargement. Aortic transections and dissections may be present in an aorta of normal caliber. However, the majority of cases will show mediastinal widening that mandates further investigation. To evaluate mediastinal widening, a posteroanterior chest x-ray should be obtained, because anteroposterior views are frequently misleading. If available, prior films should be examined. Other radiographic findings, in decreasing order of frequency, are abnormal aortic or cardiac contour, displacement or calcification of the aorta, and pleural effusion.

Many patients will have more than one special imaging study to determine the presence and extent of disease. All the examinations mentioned below have sensitivities and specificities greater than 90% when performed and interpreted properly. Probably the most important consideration is to establish *in advance* which approach will be used based on resources and expertise, since diagnosis must be rapid.

In the past, angiography was standard for evaluating aortic disease, and it still has many advantages over other techniques. Angiography has sensitivity and specificity similar to those of other examinations, provides an assessment of flow to vessels from both the true and false lumens, permits coronary angiography to be obtained simultaneously in selected cases, allows evaluation of aortic insufficiency, and frequently establishes the etiology of the disease. Disadvantages include its invasive nature, the possibility of iatrogenic catheter injury, peripheral access problems secondary to dissections or underlying obstructive disease, contrast load, occasional inadequate visualization of a nonperfused false channel, and nonvisualization of surrounding structures. Furthermore, angiography is more time-consuming than other diagnostic techniques (see below), and delay in diagnosis may contribute to further morbidity and mortality. With these considerations, echocardiography and CT imaging are the diagnostic tests of choice.

CT and MRI provide similar views. CT is more widely available than MRI and can usually be obtained rapidly, but it requires contrast administration. The sensitivity and specificity of these modalities are excellent, and both provide information about surrounding structures.

Echocardiography—particularly transesophageal echocardiography—has emerged as a valuable technique in the diagnosis of aortic disease and is considered by many to be the preferred diagnostic modality. For adequate visualization, a biplane transesophageal probe is required. Expertise in evaluating the images is crucial. The technique is limited by the presence of intervening structures, particularly those containing air, and distance of the probe from the vessel.

Differential Diagnosis

Pericarditis, myocardial infarction, and primary aortic insufficiency are common cardiac diseases that can have similar presentations. Similarly, pain from esophageal diseases such as spasm, rupture, tumor, achalasia, and reflux can be confused with aortic symptomatology. Tortuosity and atherosclerosis of the aorta may have a similar appearance on chest x-ray. Tumors may widen the mediastinal silhouette, and pulmonary diseases such as pleural effusions and pulmonary emboli can cause densities on radiographs that may be difficult to differentiate from aortic disease. When this occurs, CT or MRI can be of value. Minor ruptures of the aortic vasa vasorum can widen the aortic shadow without actually producing aortic disruption.

Treatment

A. General Measures

The disease extent and, if applicable, the site of intimal injury should be determined based on clinical examination and studies already available. Patients who are exsanguinating may require immediate operation based on chest x-ray findings alone. Others should be rapidly evaluated and, if ascending aortic disease or aortic transection is confirmed, immediately repaired. Many elderly patients with type B dissections or asymptomatic small (< 5 cm) aneurysms may best be managed initially with medical therapy.

Regardless of disease type, patient age, or initial treatment, vigorous continuous medical control of shear forces with antihypertensives and negative inotropes is essential if there is residual abnormal aorta. Patients with aortic transections and localized aneurysms frequently have curative surgery with no remaining diseased aorta. Commonly, when an aortic dissection is present, only a portion of the aorta is repaired, and residual disease requires vigorous treatment and long-term follow-up.

Since diseases of the thoracic aorta can cause morbidity and mortality owing to complex disease, significant comorbidities, and acuteness of presentation, they provide a logical potential application for newer catheter-based therapies that have proliferated in the past decade for the treatment of cardiovascular disorders. Indeed, endovascular stent grafts have been used in both elective and emergent settings for thoracic aortic dissection, aneurysmal disease, and blunt injury to the thoracic aorta. Furthermore, percutaneous fenestration of the intimal flap has been successfully performed to restore perfusion to end organs when ischemia results from dissection. As long-term results of these therapies become available and as new technology develops, the indications for the use of percutaneous-based therapies in diseases of the thoracic aorta will become clearer.

B. Blood Pressure Control

Rapid, continuous control of blood pressure and pulse pressure should be aggressively obtained immediately following diagnosis. Systolic blood pressure should be kept below 110 mm Hg systolic. The force of left ventricular contraction (dP/dt) should be minimized by administering negative inotropes.

An intra-arterial monitoring line is vital during the early phases of treatment because of the potential for rapid alterations in blood pressure. The arterial line should be utilized until documented continuous blood pressure control is accomplished.

Central venous pressures should be monitored and fluid status optimized. Patients with severe blood loss, intrapericardial blood and tamponade, or end organ ischemia may require volume replacement. Cardiovascular function is frequently labile, and inotropes and vasopressors may be required while definitive diagnosis is established.

A single ideal drug applicable to every situation does not exist, but several aspects of the many available antihypertensives are useful. The rapidity of onset, half-life, potency, distribution, metabolism, degradation products, side effects, and physiologic effects should all be considered. Use of a short-acting vasodilator (intravenous nitroprusside) in combination with a negative inotropic agent (intravenous esmolol) effectively reduces both blood pressure and the force of blood ejection.

Vasodilators commonly used include nitroprusside, hydralazine, and nitroglycerin. Nitroprusside is well tolerated, extremely potent, rapid-acting, and has a short half-life. Its disadvantages include: an increase in dP/dT when used alone, elevation of pulmonary shunt, and creation of a toxic metabolite (cyanide) with prolonged high-dose use. Hydralazine is longer-acting and available orally, making it a suitable agent for long-term use. Nitroglycerin decreases cardiac output and blood pressure through direct venodilation but has little effect on arterial relaxation. Thus, its usefulness for disorders of the thoracic aorta is limited, and it should not be regarded as a first-line agent.

Beta-blockers are available in short-acting (esmolol) and long-acting (atenolol) forms. As such, they are usually a part of both short-term and long-term management. Of the many beta-blockers available, esmolol offers the advantage of an extremely short half-life, allowing precise and frequent dosing adjustments toward optimal blood pressure. Labetalol is also an efficacious agent because of its blockade of both alpha-adrenergic and beta-adrenergic receptors. With this said, for acute blood pressure control, beta-blocker therapy combined with sodium nitroprusside, as needed, is regarded as the therapy of choice.

Calcium blockers produce both decreased blood pressure and decreased contractility. They are of greatest benefit in long-term management. Their relatively long half-life limits use acutely during unstable periods.

Central sympatholytics include trimethaphan, clonidine, methyldopa, and reserpine. They are less commonly used but do have a role in acute and chronic care as adjuncts to standard drug regimens.

Chavan A et al: Intravascular Ultrasound-Guided Percutaneous Fenestration of the Intimal Flap in the Dissected Aorta. Circulation 1997;96:2124–7.

Cigarroa JE et al: Diagnostic imaging in the evaluation of suspected aortic dissection: Old standards and new directions. N Engl J Med 1993;328:35–43.

Hagan PG et al: The International Registry of Acute Aortic Dissection (IRAD): New Insights into an Old Disease. JAMA 2000;283:897–903.

Kirklin JW, Barratt-Boyes BG: *Cardiac Surgery: Morphology, Diagnostic Criteria, Natural History, Techniques, Results, and Indications,* 2nd ed. Churchill Livingstone, 1993.

Nienaber CA et al: Nonsurgical reconstruction of thoracic aortic dissection by stent-graft placement. N Engl J Med 1999; 340:1539–45.

Peach SE, Trunkey D: Blunt injury of the thoracic aorta. Eur J Surg 1999;165:1110–5.

Svensson LG, Crawford ES: Aortic dissection and aortic aneurysm surgery: Clinical observations, experimental investigations, and statistical analyses. (Three parts.) Curr Probl Surg 1992; 29:817–911 (Part I); 913–1057 (Part II); 30:1–163 (Part III).

POSTOPERATIVE ARRHYTHMIAS

ESSENTIALS OF DIAGNOSIS

- *Heart rate.*
- *Regular or irregular rhythm.*
- *Electrocardiographic abnormalities.*
- *Altered peripheral perfusion.*

General Considerations

Significant cardiac dysrhythmias occur in up to one-third of postoperative cardiac surgical patients. Age is the most consistently identified predictor of postoperative arrhythmias, though many other risk factors exist, including valvular disease, cardiomyopathy, ischemia, reperfusion, adequacy of myocardial protection, metabolic derangements, adrenergic states, medications, temperature, and mechanical irritants.

Arrhythmias should first be classified by ventricular rate. The rhythm is then subclassified according to its origin—supraventricular or ventricular—by establishing the rate of the atrium and evaluating the status of the atrioventricular conduction system. Bradycardias include sinus bradycardia, heart block, sinus arrest, and slow junctional rhythms. Tachycardias include (1) supraventricular arrhythmias (atrial fibrillation, atrial flutter, premature atrial contractions, paroxysmal atrial tachycardia, and fast junctional rhythms); and (2) ventricular tachycardia, flutter, fibrillation, and premature ventricular contractions. Conduction defects include heart block, bundle branch block, and preexcitation. Sometimes, the origin of a rapid arrhythmia is indeterminate and should be referred to as a nonspecific wide complex tachycardia.

Etiology

The etiology of perioperative arrhythmias is multifactorial. Mechanistically, they can be separated into ectopic foci and reentrant circuits. Both originate either from abnormal cardiac tissue affected by ischemia, hypertrophy, dilation, cardiomyopathy, and scar, or from normal cardiac tissue induced by inotropes, endogenous catecholamines, autonomic stimulation, and metabolic derangements.

A. Intrinsic Factors

Age is associated with supraventricular arrhythmias and heart block in both cardiac and other thoracic surgical patients. The etiology of this association is unclear, but the incidence in patients over 65 years of age is high enough to warrant prophylactic therapy in many cases. To this end, beta-blockers (eg, sotalol) and amiodarone are commonly used agents. Though routine preoperative prophylaxis against postoperative arrhythmias (particularly atrial fibrillation) remains controversial, it is increasingly supported by emerging data. Intrinsic cardiac disease, including cardiomyopathy, acute coronary insufficiency, valvular heart disease, congenital lesions, pulmonary hypertension, ventricular outflow obstruction, or ventricular failure also increases the incidence and severity of arrhythmias in both the preoperative and postoperative periods.

Cardiomyopathy, both ischemic and nonischemic as well as dilated and nondilated, frequently causes both atrial and ventricular rhythm irregularity and is one of the more common presenting complaints. Surgical therapy (excluding aneurysm resection and endocardial ablation) frequently does not eliminate the cause. Atrial arrhythmias can result from primary involvement of atrial muscle or secondary dilation of atrial chambers by ventricular failure. Ectopic foci and reentrant circuits are the primary underlying causes, but the metabolic complications of diuresis and inotropes frequently contribute. Ventricular rhythm disturbances develop by these same mechanisms and are often life-threatening.

Acute coronary arterial insufficiency frequently presents with severe arrhythmias (particularly ventricular) or heart block. They can recur or present postoperatively from residual or recurrent ischemia and reperfusion injury.

Valvular heart disease frequently has residua that predispose to arrhythmias despite correction of the valvular lesion. The conduction system is anatomically close to valvular structures and is easily interrupted.

Endocarditis is particularly likely to be associated with heart block pre- and postoperatively. Aortic disease leads to left ventricular hypertrophy or ventricular dilation, both of which predispose to reentrant circuits or arrhythmic foci. Mitral and tricuspid valve disease most commonly cause atrial arrhythmias, primarily fibrillation. These should be expected to recur with almost 100% certainty in the postoperative period.

Congenital lesions are frequently associated with abnormalities of the location and function of the conduction system and with chamber enlargement or hypertrophy. All of these factors contribute to ectopic foci and reentry. Wolff-Parkinson-White syndrome is a common congenital lesion of the conduction system predisposing to reentrant atrioventricular rhythms. Gross anatomic disease is also occasionally associated with specific rhythm changes. In particular, Ebstein's anomaly may be complicated by Wolff-Parkinson-White syndrome, tetralogy of Fallot is associated with right ventricular arrhythmic foci, and certain types of transposition result in abnormal conduction anatomy and an increased incidence of perioperative heart block. Pulmonary and pulmonary vascular abnormalities are superimposed on all of these lesions and result in right ventricular enlargement and hypertrophy, tricuspid regurgitation, and secondary atrial arrhythmias.

B. Extrinsic Factors

Mechanical irritants (chest tubes, central catheters, blood, tamponade), metabolic derangements (hypo- or hypermagnesemia, -kalemia, -phosphatemia, -calcemia), adrenergic or vagotonic states, and cardiovascular drugs are frequent in the postoperative period and can induce and aggravate arrhythmias.

Clinical Features

The approach to the diagnosis of rhythm disturbances in the postoperative period is similar to that presented elsewhere. However, because of the unique perioperative factors that contribute to arrhythmias, an organized, rapid, and complete evaluation is crucial.

A. Symptoms and Signs

Patients with cardiac arrhythmias in the perioperative period have findings identical to those seen in nonsurgical patients. They may have more profound and acute circulatory compromise due to residual anesthetic agents, cardiopulmonary bypass effects, ongoing hemorrhage, metabolic derangements, volume shifts, hypothermia, and residual cardiac disease.

B. Electrocardiography

Unique to cardiac surgical patients is the frequent presence of ventricular or atrial pacing wires, which can provide valuable information and management options. Twelve-lead surface electrocardiographic tracings should be compared with preoperative and earlier postoperative examinations for evidence of ischemia, rhythmicity, conduction abnormalities, QRS and ST abnormalities, and QT interval prolongation.

If the rhythm cannot be conclusively diagnosed, an atrial ECG should be obtained by attaching one or more of the atrial pacing wires (if not in use for pacing) to the electrocardiographic machine or bedside monitor. A predetermined configuration on the 12-lead machine is usually used, and the tracings based on the atrial wires will emphasize the atrial portion of the rhythm despite its small muscle mass.

Signal-averaged ECGs and programmed electrical stimulation are beyond the scope of this text but should be pursued on an individual basis to establish a diagnosis, stratify risk, and evaluate the effects of treatment.

C. Laboratory Findings

Arterial blood gases and electrolytes should be obtained to exclude acidosis, alkalosis, and electrolyte abnormalities. Serum potassium and calcium levels merit particular attention.

Invasive Hemodynamic Monitoring

Invasive hemodynamic monitoring with arterial lines and flow-directed pulmonary artery catheters is typically performed to assist with management after cardiac surgery. Analysis of these data is invaluable in the diagnosis and management of postoperative arrhythmias. Furthermore, confirmation of appropriate waveforms (pulmonary capillary wedge pressure, pulmonary artery pressure) with the pulmonary artery catheter may decrease the suspicion of mechanical irritation from the catheter, significantly contributing to the arrhythmias.

Differential Diagnosis

Problems peculiar to postoperative cardiac surgical patients which may lead to arrhythmias include hypovolemia, bleeding, pericardial tamponade, tension pneumothorax, thrombosis or dehiscence of a prosthetic valve, coronary ischemia, and hypoxia. Care must be exerted to ensure that the bedside monitor is working correctly and that observed rhythms are not due to electrical interference.

Treatment

A. Antiarrhythmics

Arrhythmias are frequent postoperatively, and prophylaxis with a variety of agents is effective. Beta-blockers in particular reduce the incidence and severity of atrial arrhythmias and probably prevent some ventricular arrhythmias. Magnesium administration has been shown to reduce the incidence of both atrial fibrillation and atrial flutter. It probably decreases the incidence of ventricular arrhythmias as well. Calcium blockers may have similar benefits, but those agents are less well studied in the postoperative context. Further discussion of the medical treatment of arrhythmias is found in detail elsewhere in Chapter 22.

B. Cardioversion

In addition to pharmacologic measures, preparation should be made for rapid cardioversion in patients at high risk for severe ventricular arrhythmias. Patients who have had ventricular fibrillation perioperatively may require immediate cardioversion. Equipment should be ready at the bedside and attached to the patient. Much of the morbidity of severe ventricular arrhythmias can be avoided by immediate cardioversion.

The rhythm type and chamber of origin—atrial, junctional, or ventricular—should be established. If the atrial arrhythmia is fast and poorly tolerated (ie, symptomatic), immediate electrical conversion is warranted. To convert atrial fibrillation or flutter, high-energy shock usually is required and should always be synchronized. Overdrive atrial pacing may be performed at the bedside utilizing the atrial epicardial pacing wires. This is most effective for supraventricular tachyarrhythmias such as atrial flutter and paroxysmal atrial or AV junctional reentrant circuits. Rapid atrial pacing can also interrupt a reentrant circuit such as atrial fibrillation, thereby restoring sinus rhythm, though less effectively. When performing overdrive pacing, great vigilance must be exercised to ensure that the atrial leads—rather than the ventricular leads—are attached to the generator.

Ventricular tachycardia can frequently be terminated with low-energy synchronized cardioversion. Ventricular fibrillation should be immediately treated with high-energy defibrillation, usually unsynchronized. Both defibrillation and cardioversion can worsen the existing rhythm, so one must be prepared to rapidly increase electrical output and defibrillate again. If the rhythm is bradycardiac or becomes so following electrical or chemical conversion, ventricular pacing should be instituted immediately. After an adequate heart rate is obtained with ventricular pacing, the patient can be converted to atrial or atrioventricular sequential pacing if wires are available. If wires are not available or do not function, temporary transvenous pacing (balloon-guided or pacing pulmonary artery catheter wires) can be attempted.

C. Supportive Measures

If prophylaxis has been unsuccessful, the first objective is to maintain adequate oxygen delivery and pH control with optimal ventilation. Circulatory support with CPR may be necessary while preparations are made for electrical cardioversion. Cardiopulmonary resuscitation procedures in cardiac surgery patients are similar to those followed under other circumstances. Closed chest compressions are effective in cardiac surgery patients and should be used when indicated as in any other resuscitation effort. If a pulse is obtained with CPR, continued efforts at external electrical conversion can be pursued, but if perfusion is inadequate or external electrical conversion is unsuccessful, open cardiac massage and internal paddle defibrillation should be considered.

After initial control with electrical conversion in unstable patients—and primarily in stable patients—the rhythm should be evaluated for type and probable causes. Many rhythms are caused by temporary derangements and are best treated by eliminating the primary cause. Almost all antiarrhythmic drugs have adverse side effects even when used appropriately, and many (perhaps all) are proarrhythmic. Careful consideration of the risks and benefits of drug therapy is vital since the complications of therapy are sometimes worse than the underlying arrhythmia. The safest therapies are to optimize electrolytes, decrease sympathetic stimulation, remove mechanical causes, treat ischemia, and allow some temporary arrhythmias (due to reperfusion) to resolve spontaneously with careful monitoring.

Atrial arrhythmias are particularly common and usually cannot be allowed to persist because they are accompanied by symptomatic tachycardia. The rate of conduction of atrial fibrillation and flutter through the atrioventricular node can be blocked with digoxin, beta-blockers, and calcium channel blockers, singly or in combination. After adequate rate control is established, conversion of the arrhythmia can be accomplished with a class Ia antiarrhythmic agent (procainamide or quinidine). The risk of treating relatively benign atrial arrhythmias with class I agents should be appreciated, since there is a chance of inducing ventricular arrhythmias.

Ventricular arrhythmias in the postoperative period require individual evaluation of the circumstances, prior therapy, and risks of drug treatment. Unless a specific cause is found and removed, most arrhythmias will recur, requiring drug or device therapy to block the effects. For that reason, symptomatic ventricular arrhythmias (tachycardia or fibrillation) should almost always be corrected.

Andrews TC et al: Prevention of supraventricular arrhythmias after coronary artery bypass surgery: A meta-analysis of randomized control trials. Circulation 1991;84(5 Suppl):III236–44.

Bojar RM, Warner KG: *Manual of Perioperative Care in Cardiac Surgery,* 3rd ed. Blackwell Science, 1999.

Braunwald E: *Heart Disease: A Textbook of Cardiovascular Medicine,* 4th ed. Braunwald E (editor). Saunders, 1992.

Carlson MD, Biblo LA, Waldo AL: Post open heart surgery ventricular arrhythmias. Cardiovasc Clin 1992;22:241–53.

Frost L et al: Atrial fibrillation and flutter after coronary artery bypass surgery: Epidemiology, risk factors and preventive trials. Int J Cardiol 1992;36:253–61.

Katritsis D, Butrous G, Camm AJ: Three decades of antiarrhythmic therapy. PACE 1992;15:1394–402.

Kolansky DM, Cohen LS: Immediate postoperative management. Cardiovasc Clin 1993;23:277–91.

Rogove HJ, Hughes CM: Defibrillation and cardioversion. Crit Care Clin 1992;8:839–63.

BLEEDING, COAGULOPATHY, & BLOOD PRODUCT UTILIZATION

ESSENTIALS OF DIAGNOSIS

- *Excessive chest tube output.*
- *Hypovolemia.*
- *Bleeding from needle puncture sites.*
- *Gastrointestinal or endotracheal tube bleeding.*
- *Rash, hematuria.*
- *Abdominal or groin distention.*
- *Respiratory compromise.*
- *Neurologic event.*
- *Evidence of tamponade.*

General Considerations

Hypocoagulable and hypercoagulable states are known complications of all major surgery but are particularly common following cardiovascular surgery. Both may adversely affect outcome. Factors contributing to a hypocoagulable state include the underlying pathology and anatomy of the heart or great vessel disease itself and a variety of intrinsic coagulopathies due to hepatic failure, uremia, drugs, and cardiopulmonary bypass. Hypercoagulability results from intravascular stasis, endothelial injury, implanted foreign bodies, and derangement of the normal anticoagulant factors by blood loss, surgical complications, cardiopulmonary bypass, and drugs.

Etiology

A multitude of causes combine to make both bleeding and excessive coagulation two of the most common complications of cardiovascular surgery. Both are reviewed here because of the delicate balance between normal coagulation and pathologic bleeding or clotting. Factors favoring coagulation and decreased bleeding are complicated by the sequelae of excessive thrombosis: myocardial infarction, stroke, or peripheral embolus.

A. Hypocoagulability

The frequency of blood product administration varies widely between institutions, but the incidence of blood and coagulation factor loss in cardiothoracic surgery patients is significant at all centers. The majority of coronary, valvular, congenital, and ascending aortic or arch aortic surgeries performed by current techniques utilize total cardiopulmonary bypass and systemic anticoagulation with heparin, with or without hypothermia. This is true in 2001 even with the recent increased popularity of minimally invasive techniques ("keyhole" surgery) and "beating heart" surgery. Descending thoracic aortic surgery frequently is performed using partial bypass or the "clamp and sew" technique, both of which eliminate or reduce the need for anticoagulation with heparin. Total cardiopulmonary bypass circuits consist of priming solutions, pumps, cannulas, tubing, reservoirs, filters, and oxygenators. Each of these components causes a variety of coagulation changes, including: dilution of all blood components by priming solution, consumption and impairment of clotting factors and platelets by contact with component surfaces, release of cytokines and complement, blood and factor injury by direct air contact in the operative field, and injury by turbulence and mechanical stress. Additionally, many operations utilize hypothermia, which further decreases the activity of existing clotting factors. The length of cardiopulmonary bypass and the degree of hypothermia employed are related to the severity of these changes.

In addition to these deleterious changes are the effects produced by heparin. High-dose heparin (100 units/kg) is necessary in current bypass circuits to prevent disseminated intravascular coagulation. With the use of heparin-bonded bypass circuits, lower-dose heparin may be as efficacious, though this is currently the focus of active investigation. The majority of heparin's effects are counteracted by protamine administration after weaning from cardiopulmonary bypass. Protamine, however, is itself a weak anticoagulant, and the heparin-protamine complex thus formed impairs platelet and factor function until cleared from the bloodstream by the reticuloendothelial system. Occasionally, heparin-induced antibodies or protamine intolerance complicates the perioperative course and requires specific therapy as outlined below. The development of bypass circuits with improved biocompatibility (eg, heparin-bonded circuits) may decrease the heparin—and thus the protamine—requirements. Partial bypass circuits and shunts that do not require an oxygenator (eg, left atrial to femoral or descending aorta) can be accomplished with little or no heparin in many instances. This is particularly important in traumatic aortic injuries, where anticoagulation is usually contraindicated.

Numerous risk factors identify those patients more likely to bleed or require blood products. Perioperative drug therapy can cause a hypocoagulable state. Platelet inhibitors commonly used for treatment and prevention of cardiovascular disorders include newer agents such as the platelet glycoprotein IIb/IIIa receptor inhibitors (eg, abciximab), though aspirin remains the most commonly used medication. Platelet function is dramatically reduced by aspirin for up to 10 days following a single dose. Nonsteroidal anti-inflammatory agents have similar effects but usually are more transient. Heparin therapy preoperatively can result in heparin-antibody-platelet complexes with subsequent thrombocytopenia or occasional thrombotic complications. Warfarin therapy preoperatively is typically reversed by withholding warfarin for several days until measured coagulation tests are normal. Thrombolytics are usually combined with both heparin and antiplatelet therapy and have the additional effect of depleting fibrinogen levels. Antibiotics occasionally result in vitamin K-dependent factor loss. High-dose penicillin-like antibiotics can cause profound platelet dysfunction.

A variety of systemic diseases cause specific defects. Uremia primarily affects platelet function; hepatic failure (primary, or secondary to alcohol or congestive heart failure) results in decreased levels and delayed restoration of clotting factors. Cyanotic disease is believed to cause factor and platelet dysfunction. Thrombocytopenia and factor deficiency frequently occur with septicemia associated with endocarditis. Von Willebrand's disease and other inherited platelet and factor abnormalities can usually be identified by a careful preoperative history. Poor tissues are associated with malnutrition, age, organ failure, advanced endocarditis, and connective tissue disease. Transfusion reactions are sometimes difficult to detect but can cause severe coagulopathies.

Reoperations and procedures requiring multiple suture lines, work on abnormal tissue, and extensive operative dissections increase the risk for bleeding. These include all reoperations, aortic dissections and aneurysms, multiple valves and combined procedures, complex congenital heart disease, and those patients who require ventricular support.

Prolonged cardiopulmonary bypass, hypothermia, circulatory arrest, a history of massive intraoperative blood loss, and perioperative cardiovascular collapse all decrease the level and function of platelets and clotting factors. A history of heparin resistance or a protamine reaction frequently heralds a fibrinolytic state, intravascular coagulation, or severe platelet or factor deficiency.

Recent efforts to modify the bypass circuit with heparin bonding or to improve surgical techniques (eg, by minimally invasive or "beating heart" surgery) appear to meliorate the inflammation and coagulation abnormalities after cardiac surgery. However, as of 2001, these techniques are limited in application and only partially effective; thus, coagulation abnormalities continue to be a major cause of morbidity after cardiac surgery.

B. Hypercoagulable States

Hypercoagulable states are related to Virchow's triad of stasis, endothelial injury, and systemic hypercoagulability. Stasis is present during low-flow states, periods of immobility, during certain arrhythmias, and intraoperatively during vessel or chamber cannulation or clamping. The risk of major arterial thrombosis and deep venous thrombosis appears to be low in patients who have undergone full anticoagulation. In procedures such as descending aortic replacement with heparinless shunts or without bypass, the risk is similar to other thoracotomy and vascular surgery patients. Endothelial injury is common and includes coronary anastomotic sites, vascular clamp sites, tears in aortic dissection patients, conduits, valves, intravascular or cardiac patches, and numerous arterial and venous catheters. Systemic hypercoagulability occurs after all types of major surgery, presumably due to coagulation factor activation and derangements of factor levels. Naturally occurring anticoagulants—including proteins A, C, and S and antithrombin III—are also frequently depleted, particularly in patients receiving heparin, warfarin, or thrombolytics. Inherited hypercoagulable states (eg, activated protein C resistance), which are increasingly being recognized, may also coexist and contribute to a perioperative hypercoagulable state.

Hypercoagulability is less common than hypocoagulability but has dramatic consequences. Heparin, warfarin, and thrombolytics occasionally are complicated by naturally occurring anticoagulant factor depletion (antithrombin III, proteins A and C). Liver disease, either primary or secondary (eg, congestive hepatopathy), may also result in anticoagulant factor depletion. Antifibrinolytics (eg, aprotinin) and desmopressin can result in a hypercoagulable state, and their use should be critically evaluated. Heparin-induced thrombocytopenia can result in thrombi that consist of the platelet-antibody complex. Patients with prior deep venous thrombosis, pulmonary embolism, or thrombophlebitis are especially prone to recurrent thrombosis, and early anticoagulation should be considered. Patients undergoing coronary endarterectomy appear to have an increased risk of graft thrombosis and are usually started on antiplatelet agents immediately after surgery. Areas of stasis are always at risk for thrombosis. These include the deep veins in immobile patients and the left atrium in those with atrial fibrillation or akinetic endocardium after a myocardial infarction. The presence of intravascular foreign bodies may increase the risk of thrombosis. Catheters, patches, valves, conduits, balloon pumps, and ventricular assist devices may cause thrombosis and embolism.

Clinical Features

A. Chest Tube Output

Chest tube output varies widely between patients and over time in individuals. It should be considered in the context of chest x-ray findings, hemodynamics, previous outputs, surgical findings, and the patient's history. Even in the best hands, chest tube output is frequently miscalculated as a result of autotransfusion, multiple tubes and containers, and in unrecorded intervals such as during patient transport. These possible errors should be considered and a reproducible technique of recording and reporting outputs established. Many valid definitions of excessive chest tube output exist; in the descriptions that follow, output > 200 mL/h for 2 hours is considered significant, while > 400 mL/h for 2 hours is considered severe. Chest tube output during the first 2 hours following operation is extremely variable due to retained blood in the pleural space and lack of drainage during transport. Increased drainage can be expected during this period. Greater than 200 mL/h of drainage after the initial period may indicate the need for reexploration. The average chest tube output over 24 hours is approximately 1200 mL in primary low-risk coronary artery bypass graft patients, but it may be significantly higher after more complex procedures.

If chest tubes are clotted or do not communicate with the bleeding site, cardiovascular instability consistent with hypovolemia will frequently be the presenting sign. Inadequate resuscitation of prior or ongoing severe bleeding presents in a similar fashion.

Patients with excessive drainage from chest tubes should be thoroughly examined for diffuse oozing from other sites such as needle punctures, wounds, and nasogastric tubes. A generalized rash and hematuria should alert one to the possibility of hemolysis due to a transfusion reaction. Other findings suggestive of bleeding include abdominal or groin distention, respiratory compromise due to intrapleural blood, low cardiac output due to tamponade, and neurologic changes from hypoperfusion or intracranial hemorrhage.

B. Thrombosis

An uncommon result of a relative hypercoagulable state is prosthetic valve thrombosis. Although most common in patients not adequately anticoagulated chronically, valve thrombosis can occur at any time in the hospital course and requires immediate diagnosis. A new murmur suggesting outflow or inflow obstruction or valvular insufficiency should be immediately investigated with echocardiography. Hemodynamic changes may be severe.

Arterial occlusions due to primary thrombosis or secondary to embolus may be subtle or dramatic and are quite common. The arteries at highest risk for primary thrombosis are recent coronary or peripheral grafts, peripheral cannulation sites, and arteries with preexisting stenoses. An arterial embolus will have a similar presentation, but multiple emboli commonly occur with combined neurologic, coronary, gastrointestinal, and peripheral findings. Subtle neurologic changes are sensitive indicators of arterial thrombi or emboli. Findings associated with arterial occlusion under normal circumstances may be blurred by perioperative low flow states, systemic hypothermia, and preexisting arterial disease.

Venous occlusion is not commonly seen following cardiac surgery, presumably because of systemic anticoagulation during cardiopulmonary bypass. However, patients should be monitored for signs of deep venous thrombosis and pulmonary embolization. Since lower extremity edema following cardiac surgery is common and is further confounded by long venectomy incisions, lower extremity venous duplex ultrasound examination is critical for diagnosis when deep venous thrombosis is suspected. In congenital disease, systemic and pulmonary venous patches and conduits are potential sites for thrombosis.

C. Imaging Studies

The routine postoperative chest x-ray should be reviewed in any patient with suspected bleeding. Changes in mediastinal width (corrected for technique), pleural accumulations, and other lesions causing hemodynamic compromise can be rapidly diagnosed.

D. Laboratory Findings

Activated clotting times (ACTs) are routinely obtained to determine the adequacy of anticoagulation during bypass and to assess its reversal by protamine. A normal ACT is between 100 and 120 seconds. Anticoagulation during bypass increases it to over 400 seconds. Limited anticoagulation usually falls in the range between 150 and 250 seconds.

Thromboelastography gives a rapid assessment of the adequacy of the coagulation cascade and can help predict the subgroup of patients whose bleeding is due to an underlying disorder. Thromboelastography also can identify unsuspected hypercoagulable patients. Five parameters are measured (Figure 23–2). The specific cause of an abnormal thromboelastogram can be further investigated by routine coagulation tests described below.

Platelet counts should be obtained in patients with long or complex bypass runs and those with excessive bleeding. However, platelet dysfunction is common perioperatively despite adequate platelet numbers and is probably the most common cause of excessive bleeding. Unfortunately, no simple reproducible test of in vivo platelet function is currently available. Template bleeding time can provide some information but is not recommended on a routine basis. It should be obtained in patients with a history of bleeding or refractory postoperative blood loss. A very prolonged template bleeding time (> 8 minutes) is suggestive of significant platelet dysfunction.

Routine coagulation tests—international normalized ratio (INR),* partial thromboplastin time (PTT), thrombin time (TT), fibrinogen level, and fibrinogen degradation products (FDPs)—should be obtained in any patient with severe bleeding who will be receiving factor replacement. The INR is frequently mildly elevated early postoperatively in all patients, but an INR > 1.7 in a patient with excessive bleeding should be corrected. Thrombin time is extremely sensitive to the presence of heparin, while PTT accurately reflects the level of heparin activity. Fibrinogen deficiency and elevated FDPs usually indicate excessive fibrinolysis consistent with consumption coagulopathy. Using the above guidelines, the results of routine coagulation tests are used to direct therapy at the specific defects outlined below.

To monitor the proper perioperative anticoagulation in patients with artificial valves and other indications for systemic anticoagulation, the INR is obtained on a daily basis before and after beginning warfarin therapy. The INR is superior to the prothrombin time since it minimizes interlaboratory reagent variation. Appropriate levels for given circumstances are outlined below. In occasional patients at high risk for thrombosis or those who may need further invasive procedures postoperatively, heparin is started when deemed safe, and anticoagulation is maintained at a level appropriate for the relative risks using aPTT assays or the ACT.

* The INR is the equivalent of the prothrombin time (PT) corrected for the wide interlaboratory variation in reagents and PT results.

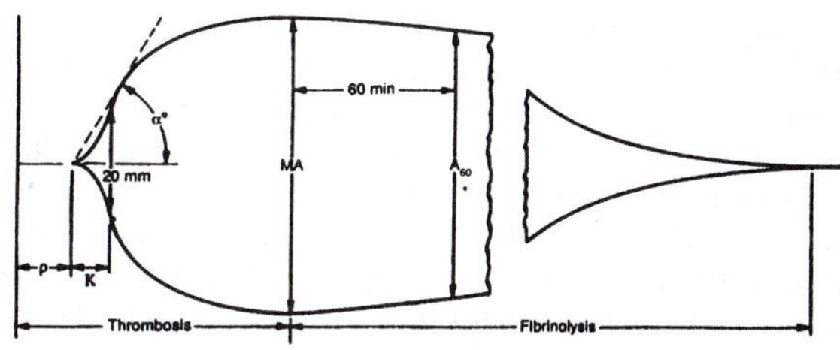

Figure 23–2. Quantification of TEG variables. Analysis of the thrombelastograph. *r* = reaction time (time from sample placement in the curette until TEG tracing amplitude reaches 2 mm [normal range 6–8 min]). This represents the rate of initial fibrin formation and is related functionally to plasma clotting factor and circulating inhibitor activity (intrinsic coagulation). Prolongation of the *r* time may be a result of coagulation factor deficiencies, anticoagulation (heparin) or severe hypofibrinogenemia. A small *r* value may be present in hypercoagulability syndromes. *K* = clot formation time (normal range 3–6 min); measured from *r* time to the point where the amplitude of the tracing reaches 20 mm. The coagulation time represents the time taken for a fixed degree of viscoelasticity to be achieved by the forming clot, as a result of fibrin buildup and cross-linking. It is affected by the activity of the intrinsic clotting factors, fibrinogen and platelets. Alpha angle (α°) (normal range 50–60°) = angle formed by the slope of the TEG tracing from the *r* to the *K* value. It denotes the speed at which solid clot forms. Decreased values may occur with hypofibrinogenemia and thrombocytopenia. Maximum amplitude (MA) (normal range 50–60 mm) = greatest amplitude on the TEG trace and is a reflection of the absolute strength of the fibrin clot. It is a direct function of the maximum dynamic properties of fibrin and platelets. Platelet abnormalities, whether qualitative or quantitative, substantially disturb the MA. A_{80} (normal range = MA – 5 min) = amplitude of the tracing 60 min after MA is achieved. It is a measure of clot lysis or retraction. The clot lysis index (CLI) (normal range > 85%) is derived as $A_{80}/MA \times 100$ (%). It measures the amplitude as a function of time and reflects loss of clot integrity as a result of lysis. (Reprinted, with permission, from Mallett SV, Cox DJA: Thromboelastography. Br J Anaesth 1992;69:307–13.)

Differential Diagnosis

Bleeding is usually easy to diagnose while chest tubes are in place if they are not clotted and if they communicate with the bleeding site. Once chest tubes and monitoring lines are removed, the diagnosis becomes much less obvious but remains equally vital. Vasodilation due to rewarming can require large volumes of fluid and can be mistaken for ongoing bleeding. This rewarming process with attendant hemodynamic changes typically occurs over the first 1–2 hours postoperatively in the ICU. Pleural accumulations of blood or serous fluid are common, and their drainage can be alarming but benign, as can mediastinal collections. Hemolysis is rarely confused with significant bleeding but should be considered. Intrinsic cardiac dysfunction and congestive heart failure may present with hypertension, hemodilution, and congestion similar to hypovolemia or tamponade, as can any other cause of shock and hypotension.

Thrombosis or occlusion of peripheral arteries can be confused with poor perfusion due to low-output states and vasoactive drugs. Findings are typically more localized with thromboemboli. Vascular spasm is particularly common with mammary artery grafts and can mimic occlusion. Spasm of peripheral vessels may be observed. Cholesterol emboli from an atherosclerotic aortic wall are probably much more common than thromboemboli due to disseminated clotting. Cholesterol emboli usually present immediately postoperatively and are frequently multiple.

Treatment

A. Bleeding

If postoperative bleeding is apparent, one must immediately ensure the availability of adequate supplies of packed red blood cells or whole blood. Blood loss and replacement are frequently underestimated because of autotransfusion, loss into the pleural space, and what seems to be large volumes of blood replacement. Bleeding is often more rapid than initially thought. Careful fluid balances are crucial and should be reported in a reproducible fashion at appropriate intervals. Patients should be rapidly stratified according to the level of bleeding. Bleeding less than 200 mL/h frequently stops without additional therapy as the effects of cardiopulmonary bypass and anticoagulation resolve. Bleeding greater than 300 mL/h only rarely resolves spontaneously. Severe bleeding (> 400 mL/h) frequently requires operation. If the patient is hemodynamically stable, evaluation for a nonsurgical cause of bleeding may be undertaken provided that preparation for mediastinal exploration is begun and sufficient blood products are available.

If patients can be stabilized and bleeding is less than massive, a check for residual heparin can be performed with an ACT in a few minutes. Protamine should then be administered if the ACT is elevated above baseline. A platelet count should be checked, though an adequate number does not equate with adequate function. Thromboelastography can provide an overview of the level of coagulation, and if it is normal one should suspect a surgical cause for the bleeding. Routine coagulation tests can be obtained to guide specific factor therapy and to rule out ongoing fibrinolysis.

B. Transfusion

Platelets are the first therapy in most cases since they augment platelet function, supply fresh frozen plasma, and provide a source of fibrinogen with the same number of donor exposures. If platelet concentrate fails to correct the deficit or severe factor deficiencies are documented, an elevated INR is usually treated with fresh frozen plasma, and a diminished fibrinogen is treated with cryoprecipitate.

C. Other Agents

Antifibrinolytics such as aminocaproic acid (4–5 g in 250 mL of diluent over 1 hour intravenously, followed by 1 g/h as a continuous infusion) can be added if fibrinolysis is significant; however, most agents should be given preoperatively for full effect. Patients felt to be at high risk for bleeding should be treated prophylactically. Desmopressin acetate (0.3 μg/kg intravenously over 15–30 minutes) is particularly effective in the treatment of patients with platelet deficiency due to uremia or von Willebrand's disease, but it may cause increased graft thrombosis. Conjugated estrogens and serine protease inhibitors may also be helpful in treatment of uremic bleeding, though consideration must always be given to the risks and benefits of these pharmacologic therapies.

If correction of the clotting mechanism does not stop the hemorrhage, immediate surgical exploration is mandatory irrespective of the patient's hemodynamic status.

D. Thrombosis

Excessive thrombosis is less obvious than active bleeding. Clinical (chest pain, hemodynamic changes) and electrocardiographic (ST changes) evidence for coronary graft thrombosis is not infrequently due to graft spasm, particularly with arterial conduits (mammary arteries). In unresolved cases, echocardiography should be obtained to evaluate wall motion in the suspect arterial territory. Antispasmodics should be instituted (calcium channel blocking agents or nitroglycerin) while diagnostic evaluation continues. Many centers give antispasmodics (calcium channel blockers) prophylactically in an attempt to avoid spasm. If wall motion abnormalities are documented and persist with antispasmodics, angiography may be indicated to confirm graft patency. Reexploration of grafts is then considered on an individual basis.

Peripheral thrombosis is not uncommon in open heart surgery and occurs in the presence of a left ventricular thrombus, preexisting vascular disease, and injuries from prior angiography. Additionally, peripheral emboli and thrombosis are frequent in patients with intravascular prostheses or devices, particularly intra-aortic balloon pumps and prosthetic valves. All unnecessary foreign bodies should be removed as soon as possible. Patients should be stratified according to risk of thrombosis, and those who subsequently have a thromboembolism despite one level of anticoagulation should be increased to the next level of anticoagulation and a thorough evaluation of why they failed should be undertaken. Patients with a high risk of thrombosis, delayed onset of long-acting anticoagulants (warfarin), or evidence of current thromboembolism should be treated with rapid-onset anticoagulants, eg, heparin, with appropriate consideration of the risk of bleeding in the perioperative period.

All patients with unexplained or recurrent thrombotic episodes should be evaluated for inherited thrombophilias, including (at least) resistance to activated protein C (factor V Leiden, HR_2 haplotype), heterozygosity or homozygosity for factor V Leiden or G20210A prothrombin mutation, hyperhomocysteinemia, factor VIII levels, and the presence of lupus anticoagulant. If heparin-induced thrombocytopenia is suspected, platelet counts and antiplatelet antibody studies should be obtained. Heparin-induced thrombocytopenia and the resultant platelet thrombi are treated by eliminating all heparin, adding platelet inhibitors, and beginning warfarin. Antithrombin III deficiency can be treated temporarily with fresh frozen plasma and long term with warfarin. The treatment of protein A, C, or S deficiency is approached on an individual basis. Hyperhomocysteinemia is treated indefinitely with folic acid, supplemented with vitamins B_6 and B_{12} if homocysteine levels do not normalize on folic acid alone. Patients with inherited thrombophilias who have thrombotic episodes should be treated with standard heparin overlapped with warfarin toward the goal of INR 2.0–3.0.

Bidstrup BP et al: Effect of aprotinin (Trasylol) on aorta-coronary bypass graft patency. J Thorac Cardiovasc Surg 1993;105:147–52.

Goodnough LT, Johnston MF, Toy PT: The variability of transfusion practice in coronary artery bypass surgery. Transfusion Medicine Academic Award Group. JAMA 1991;265:86–90.

Khuri SF et al: Hematologic changes during and after cardiopulmonary bypass and their relationship to the bleeding time and nonsurgical blood loss. J Thorac Cardiovasc Surg 1992;104:94–107.

Ratnatunga CP, Rees GM, Kovacs IB: Preoperative hemostatic activity and excessive bleeding after cardiopulmonary bypass. Ann Thorac Surg 1991;52:250–7.

Seligsohn U, Lubetsky A: Genetic susceptibility to venous thrombosis. N Engl J Med 2001;344:1222–31.

Sethi GK et al: Implications of preoperative administration of aspirin in patients undergoing coronary artery bypass grafting. Department of Veterans Affairs Cooperative Study on Antiplatelet Therapy. J Am Coll Cardiol 1990;15:15–20.

Walls JT et al: Heparin-induced thrombocytopenia in patients who undergo open heart surgery. Surgery 1990;108:686–92.

Woodman RC, Harker LA: Bleeding complications associated with cardiopulmonary bypass. Blood 1990;76:1680–97.

CARDIOPULMONARY BYPASS, HYPOTHERMIA, CIRCULATORY ARREST, & VENTRICULAR ASSISTANCE

ESSENTIALS OF DIAGNOSIS

- *Decreased peripheral perfusion.*
- *Altered end-organ function.*
- *Hypothermia.*
- *Coagulopathy.*
- *Hemolysis.*
- *Edema, localized or generalized.*

General Considerations

More than 30 years ago, the introduction of cardiopulmonary bypass—and therefore the ability to interrupt and alter circulation locally and systemically—revolutionized the approach to cardiothoracic and other major surgery of vascular structures. Continued advances in technique have made cardiopulmonary bypass well tolerated. Untoward effects still exist, particularly at the extremes of age. Despite the recent popularity of minimally invasive and off-pump techniques in cardiac surgery, full cardiopulmonary bypass is still utilized for most cardiac surgical procedures. An understanding of the pitfalls of cardiopulmonary bypass are crucial to realizing its benefits.

Both total and partial bypass circuits are utilized on a routine basis and are primed with crystalloid, colloid, or blood if estimated hemodilution will be severe. Total cardiopulmonary bypass begins with drainage of systemic venous blood into a cardiotomy reservoir via a venous cannula. A separate pump-driven cardiotomy suction device is usually added to return blood shed in the operative field to the same reservoir. Blood is then actively pumped through an oxygenator-heat exchanger and back to the systemic circulation via the arterial cannula. A variety of additional specialized circuits deliver cardioplegia, provide pulmonary venous and collateral drainage (vents), or perfuse localized areas. Arterial and venous cannulas are usually placed in the ascending aorta and right atrium, but a variety of locations are utilized on an individual basis (Figure 23–3). Partial bypass circuits include venovenous bypass (usually with oxygenator), left atrioarterial or right atriopulmonary

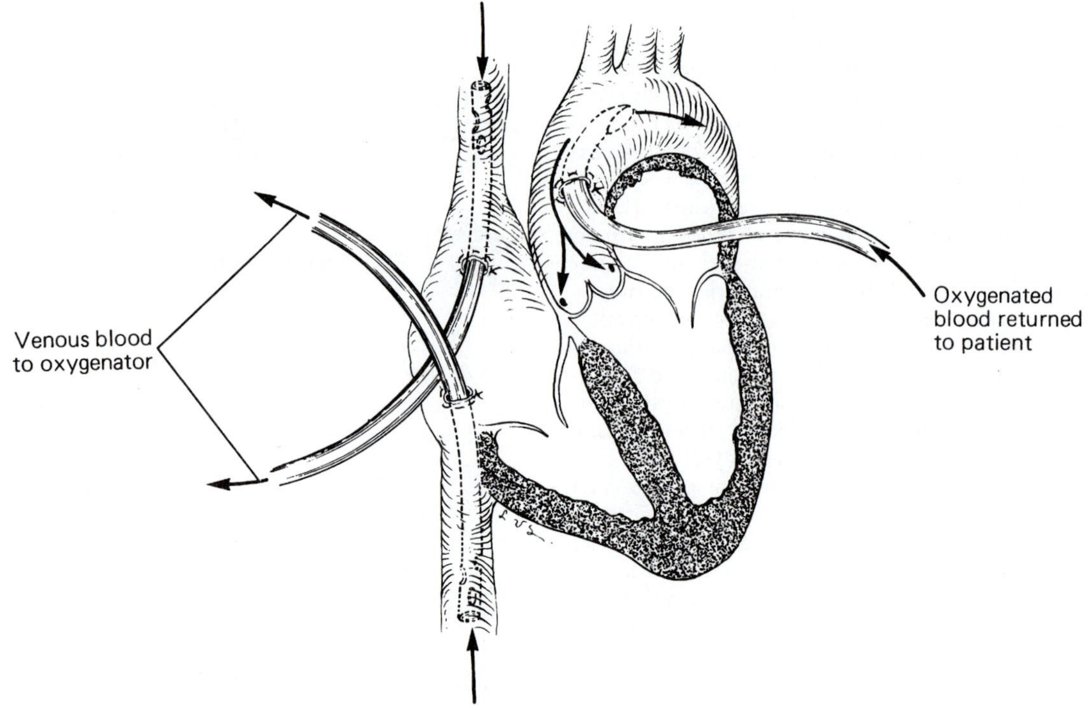

Figure 23–3. Cannulation sites commonly used in connecting the extracorporeal circuit. Venous blood is drained through tubes introduced into both venae cavae. Oxygenated blood is returned to the arterial system through a tube in the aorta. (Reproduced, with permission, from Way LW [editor]: *Current Surgical Diagnosis & Treatment,* 10th ed. Originally published by Appleton & Lange. Copyright © 1991 by The McGraw-Hill Companies, Inc.)

bypass or ventricular assist (usually without oxygenator), and simple arterioarterial and venovenous shunts, with or without pumps or oxygenators. Severe adverse effects of cardiopulmonary bypass strictly due to the circuit itself are rare but include massive air embolism, aortic dissection from cannulas or clamps, general or localized venous congestion from kinked or misplaced return lines, severe hypoxia from oxygenator dysfunction, and a variety of unusual but significant events. One or more lesser effects of the cardiopulmonary bypass circuit are nearly universal. Microscopic air, platelet, and cholesterol emboli, direct blood cell trauma, and endothelial injury may occur secondary to mechanical pump or cannulation injury.

Blood contact with circuit surfaces causes a variety of undesirable effects, including systemic inflammation (elaboration of cytokines, leukocyte activation), complement activation, coagulation abnormalities, and endothelial cell activation. Indeed, these changes contribute to the morbidity and mortality of cardiac surgery. Full anticoagulation with heparin (300 units/kg) is required in all circuits to prevent widespread coagulation, though lower anticoagulation protocols may prove equally efficacious as the biocompatibility of the circuits improves (heparin bonding). Partial-bypass circuits—and some full-bypass circuits with heparin-bonded components—can frequently be maintained with little or no systemic anticoagulation depending on flow, component surfaces, and the effects of the pump, filters, and special devices. Circuit priming solutions and added fluids cause hemodilution, which is frequently helpful in diminishing blood cell loss but may be excessive in patients with low blood volumes. In selected patients with generous prebypass blood cell volumes, whole blood or blood components may be removed prior to bypass for retransfusion postoperatively. This restores coagulation factor activity and reduces homologous blood product utilization.

Perfusion during total cardiopulmonary bypass is almost always nonpulsatile, and flow is maintained at a level to ensure adequate end organ perfusion based on metabolic demands. Perfusion during partial bypass or ventricular support may be pulsatile or nonpulsatile depending on the circuit and device. Flows in these local circuits are determined by arterial resistances in the native perfused and mechanically perfused beds, left- and right-sided pressures during ventricular support, inflow limitations, technical considerations, and device capabilities. Measured pump flows are felt to be more crucial than blood pressure in patients without vascular stenoses. Typical flows at normothermia are 2.4 L/min/m^2, which sustains systemic blood pressure at > 40 mm Hg.

Determinants of tissue metabolic demand include tissue activity (primarily skeletal and cardiac muscle), temperature, tissue mass, and preexisting metabolic debt. Certain organs are intrinsically more susceptible to inadequate flows. Brain and spinal cord, heart, liver, kidneys, gastrointestinal tract, skeletal muscle, and skin tolerate warm ischemia for periods varying between a few minutes to many hours. Metabolic activity of cardiac muscle can be markedly decreased with hyperkalemic or other forms of arrest. Skeletal muscle relaxants vastly decrease the metabolic demands of skeletal muscle. Barbiturates may decrease central nervous system metabolic demands. In addition to minimizing contraction of cardiac and skeletal muscle, hypothermia is often added to extend the period of safe hypoperfusion. Systemic hypothermia further attenuates metabolic demands and may be utilized during certain cardiac surgical procedures (eg, coronary artery bypass grafting) to minimize the sequelae of bypass or circulation arrest. The routine use of systemic hypothermia during cardiac surgery remains controversial. Safe periods of decreased or arrested circulation vary inversely with temperature. Central nervous system protection is the primary limiting factor. At core temperatures near or below 18 °C, circulatory arrest may be well tolerated for periods exceeding 1 hour in extreme circumstances. However, the safety of the central nervous system is not guaranteed owing to temperature variations and undesirable metabolic activity.

Following cardiopulmonary bypass, patients are usually anemic because they have gained significant extracellular and intracellular fluid. The combined effects of anesthesia, surgery, and cardiopulmonary bypass produce hypothermia and coagulopathy. The latter is caused by factor loss and activation, hemodilution, and residual heparin and protamine. Ongoing effects are due to reperfusion of tissues inadequately protected or congested during cardiopulmonary bypass. In addition, a variety of drugs, anesthetics, blood products, and ongoing insults from cardiac instability make the period immediately following cardiopulmonary bypass unique.

All organs are potential sites of dysfunction, and each should be examined as it becomes accessible to evaluation. Cardiovascular and renal complications are almost immediately evident. Neurologic function is frequently slow to return secondary to anesthetics, particularly in the elderly, but is probably the most sensitive measure of the adverse effects of cardiopulmonary bypass. Indeed, much of the impetus for off-pump techniques was directed toward minimizing the neurologic sequelae that occur frequently after bypass. Short-term memory loss, focal defects, choreoathetoid motions, paraplegia, confusion, worsening of previous neurologic deficits, seizures, and visual changes occur frequently and are presumably due to edema, microemboli, hypoperfusion, residual anesthetics, and drugs and the systemic effects of cardiopulmonary bypass. Gastrointestinal function usually returns within 24 hours, and persistent gastrointestinal complaints are rare. The extremities may be hypoperfused individually or in concert and occasionally are sufficiently ischemic to result in tissue (usually muscle) loss.

A. Circuit-Related Complications

Circuit-related complications are infrequent following cardiac surgery but are serious when they occur. Full knowledge of the type, location, and variations of the cannulas used during bypass or ventricular support is essential to evaluate subsequent problems. Complications include aortic dissection from ascending aortic cannulation; arterial occlusion from peripheral cannulation; congestion of the upper body, lower body, or both from venous cannulation mishaps; and obstruction, leakage, and cavitation of indwelling cannulas due to kinking, disrupted connections, or excessive pump flows. Monitoring lines are frequently placed in unusual locations, particularly in congenital disease and with ventricular assist devices. Familiarity with their care and use is essential.

Certain bypass components are related more frequently than others to adverse effects. Oxygenators are either of the membrane or bubble type, with a trend nowadays toward membrane oxygenators because of a perception that they are associated with fewer deleterious effects, since a "membrane" separates blood from air. Roller pumps or centrifugal pumps are used for total cardiopulmonary bypass. Centrifugal pumps are used more commonly because there is less blood component trauma and less chance of massive air embolism. Care providers of patients with ventricular assist devices should familiarize themselves with the anatomy, connections, components, and monitoring associated with individual patient situations. The complications in these patients secondary to circuit failure are characteristically immediate and severe. A familiarity with typical operative circuits also provides excellent background for diagnosis of related problems.

B. Coagulation Parameters

Profound heparin anticoagulation is required for cardiopulmonary bypass. Protamine is used intraoperatively to reverse the heparin effect. Inadequate anticoagulation results in consumption coagulopathy; with inadequate protamine, rebound heparinization may occur. Significant protamine reactions are infrequent but may result in hypotension, coagulopathy, pulmonary hypertension, and massive pulmonary edema.

C. Crossclamp Time and Hypothermia

Crossclamp time primarily applies to cardiac procedures, but any organ that was isolated from systemic cardiopulmonary bypass support should be considered at special risk. With current organ protection techniques, crossclamp time does not always represent ischemia and may in fact be beneficial, but the circumstances and length of altered organ perfusion should be considered.

The degree of hypothermia and the length of decreased or absent systemic perfusion should be established to raise the index of suspicion for complications of these interventions. At the extremes of age, systemic effects are common, as outlined below. The extent of rewarming is variable, and ongoing temperature changes have significant effects.

D. Fluid and Drug Administration

To monitor the course of the operation and to assist with postoperative fluid management, both perfusion and anesthesia records should be evaluated. Intake and output fluids—including blood loss, hemoconcentrators, urine output, cell saver, acute blood donations, cardioplegia, chest tube autotransfusion, rapid infusers, and priming solutions—should be considered carefully.

Inotropes, pressors, vasodilators, inhaled and intravenous anesthetics, paralyzing agents, antiarrhythmics, anticoagulants, and antibiotics are a routine part of cardiopulmonary bypass and have altered effects, kinetics, and distribution volumes in the bypass circuit itself and in cold, artificially perfused organs. As in all critically ill patients, effects of current and past drugs should be considered as the cause of a variety of complications.

E. Surgical Details

The specifics of the operative procedure, particularly in unusual cases, are essential to understanding ongoing problems. Complex aortic procedures, congenital disease, valvular disease, and noncardiac surgery requiring cardiopulmonary bypass frequently have unique complications secondary to old and new anatomy and physiology.

Diagnosis

A. Peripheral Perfusion

Alterations in generalized or local perfusion can result from prior cardiopulmonary bypass or ongoing cardiac support with assist devices. Peripheral pulses should be examined immediately following operation or device placement, so that the severity of subsequent changes can be fully appreciated. Peripheral perfusion is frequently decreased immediately following cardiopulmonary bypass owing to vasoconstriction from hypothermia but should return to normal when normothermia is reached.

A general evaluation of all major tissue beds should be performed early. Examination of the circulation, including peripheral pulses, ankle pressure indices, duplex examinations of vascular beds with abnormal perfusion, ophthalmologic examination, and angiography should be pursued early when localized changes are noted. Cardiovascular parameters, including filling pressures, outputs, vascular resistances, and oxygen saturations, should be reviewed. Pulmonary function may change dramatically with reperfusion, and blood gases—particularly $Pa{CO_2}$ levels—increase rapidly with rewarming and inactivation of muscle relaxants. Renal function is normally quite brisk due to excess fluid and mannitol administration surrounding the period of cardiopulmonary bypass. Low urine output may indicate renal hypoperfusion. Neurologic dysfunction is present in almost all patients to a mild degree when evaluated by psychometric testing. Single and multiple focal central nervous system defects most commonly result from thromboembolism and hemorrhage. Watershed defects are frequently due to inadequate local or generalized flows. More severe psychometric defects, seizures, blindness, and choreoathetoid movements may result from air embolus, microparticulate emboli, hypoxia, profound anemia, or hypoperfusion. Paraplegia from regional hypoperfusion, aortic dissection, or embolism is rarely seen with full cardiopulmonary bypass but may occur in up to 40% of patients with complex thoracoabdominal procedures with or without artificial support. Gastrointestinal and hepatic symptoms, including abdominal pain, ileus, ascites, and gastrointestinal bleeding, may represent prior or ongoing venous congestion or arterial hypoperfusion.

B. Hypothermia

Numerous local temperatures are measured during bypass. Core temperature should be evaluated postoperatively, and other localized temperatures (axillary, rectal) should be correlated.

C. Coagulopathy

Coagulopathy and hemolysis are usually most evident during or immediately after cardiopulmonary bypass, respectively, and both may herald a complicated post-cardiopulmonary bypass course. Examine for diffuse bleeding, blood-tinged urine, evidence of abnormal thrombosis, or abnormal laboratory values.

D. Edema

Differential edema and severe generalized edema should be noted and potential reversible mechanical causes (venous obstruction) evaluated. Accurate pre- and postoperative weights are essential for evaluating fluid accumulations and losses, which may represent 10–20 L in extreme cases.

E. Laboratory Studies

Coagulation studies, free hemoglobin, amylase, liver function tests, and arterial blood gases may delineate secondary adverse effects of cardiopulmonary bypass on tissue beds.

F. Imaging Studies

A chest x-ray should be examined postoperatively for retained foreign bodies, catheter position, ventricular support cannula positions, chest tubes, valves, pulmonary parenchymal and pleural abnormalities, mediastinal contour, aortic calcification and evidence of displacement, endotracheal tube position, and, if applicable, intra-aortic balloon pump placement.

G. Mechanical Problems

In patients with ongoing ventricular support, erratic pump flows or increased tubing motion may herald cannula obstruction or pump failure. Air in the circuit is always an emergency, and, although rare, it should be excluded. Left- and right-sided chamber pressures are vitally interdependent in patients being maintained on ventricular assist devices, since the normal physiologic homeostatic mechanisms do not apply. Filling, arterial, and line pressure require constant vigilance.

Differential Diagnosis

Secondary organ changes due to congenital, valvular, and coronary disease are frequently superimposed on—and magnified by—the effects of cardiopulmonary bypass. An appreciation of the preexisting and subsequent anatomy and physiology is essential. Sepsis, either preexisting or new, mimics almost all the inflammatory, organ failure, and embolic effects of cardiopulmonary bypass, as do many anaphylactic or cardiovascular drug reactions and hemolysis. Superimposed myocardial infarction during cardiopulmonary bypass may have profound systemic effects.

Treatment

A. Minimize Support Period

Decreasing the level and time of artificial circulation is the most direct treatment but is rarely feasible. Changing the type of support device will occasionally be possible, and many available pulsatile support devices are tolerated for long periods of time. As mentioned, improvements in the biocompatibility of the bypass circuit blunt the systemic coagulation and inflammation abnormalities and may improve clinical end points. Despite these "equipment" improvements, they are only partially effective, and optimal therapy in the future will probably combine multiple strategies for optimal outcomes.

B. Restore Perfusion

Organs with documented inadequate flow should have perfusion restored by moving cannulas, administering vasodilators locally, peripheral bypass grafts where appropriate, or thromboembolectomy.

C. Correct Hypothermia

Correction of hypothermia should be ongoing with warmed intravenous fluids, radiant heat, and heated ventilatory gases. However, the efficacy of all these maneuvers is very limited, and in cases of extreme hypothermia consideration should be given to direct blood rewarming with a partial bypass circuit and heat exchanger.

During rewarming, fluid requirements may be substantial secondary to vasodilation and ongoing losses. The significant cellular and extracellular edema that accumulates demands vigorous diuresis as soon as feasible to prevent the increased cardiovascular burden of increasing preload as fluid is mobilized. Robust urine output of 300–500 mL/h may be necessary to keep pace with fluid administration and fluid mobilization.

D. Correct Coagulopathies

Coagulopathies frequently correct spontaneously with rewarming, but the occasional patient with ongoing fibrinolysis, significant factor deficits, or ongoing bleeding needs specific therapy as outlined in the section on coagulation.

E. Organ Dysfunction

Patients who develop myocardial dysfunction, neurologic or ophthalmologic deficits, ARDS, pancreatitis, generalized inflammatory states, renal failure, and extremity ischemia temporally related to cardiopulmonary bypass are treated in fashion similar to what is available for these maladies caused by other insults. Cardiopulmonary bypass should not be assumed to be the cause of these deficits until other primary causes are excluded.

Davis EA et al: Hypothermic circulatory arrest as a surgical adjunct: A 5-year experience with 60 adult patients. Ann Thorac Surg 1992;53:402–6.

Downing SW, Edmunds LH Jr: Release of vasoactive substances during cardiopulmonary bypass. Ann Thorac Surg 1992;54:1236–43.

Golding LA et al: Postcardiotomy centrifugal mechanical ventricular support. Ann Thorac Surg 1992;54:1059–63.

Hammermeister KE et al: Identification of patients at greatest risk for developing major complications at cardiac surgery [published erratum appears in Circulation 1991;84:446.] Circulation 1990;82(5 Suppl):IV380–89.

Huddy SP, Joyce WP, Pepper JR: Gastrointestinal complications in 4473 patients who underwent cardiopulmonary bypass surgery. Br J Surg 1991;78(3):293–96.

Kirklin JW, Barratt-Boyes BG: *Cardiac Surgery: Morphology, Diagnostic Criteria, Natural History, Techniques, Results, and Indications,* 2nd ed. Churchill Livingstone, 1993.

Mills SA, Prough DS: Neuropsychiatric complications following cardiac surgery. Semin Thorac Cardiovasc Surg 1991;3:39–46.

POSTOPERATIVE LOW-OUTPUT STATES

ESSENTIALS OF DIAGNOSIS

- *Diaphoresis.*
- *Cyanosis or pallor.*
- *Poor peripheral perfusion.*
- *Thready pulse; tachycardia or bradycardia.*
- *Tachypnea.*
- *Venous congestion.*
- *Pulmonary rales.*
- *New or increased murmurs.*
- *Mental status changes.*
- *Anxiety.*
- *Low urine output.*

General Considerations

Cardiac insufficiency may complicate the course of postoperative cardiac surgical patients. Intrinsic myocardial dysfunction, valvular disease, and congenital anomalies frequently coexist with extrinsic cardiac factors and complicate the diagnosis and therapy of shock in this group of patients. Rapid diagnosis and reversal of decreased cardiac output are essential to avoid secondary organ damage.

Etiology

A. Intrinsic Factors

The preoperative cardiac and vascular anatomy, rhythm, ventricular function (diastolic and systolic), vascular resistances, valvular gradients and insufficiencies, coronary anatomy, and prior interventions should be reviewed and correlated. This cannot be overemphasized, particularly in patients with cardiomyopathy, acute coronary insufficiency, valvular heart disease, congenital cardiac lesions, pulmonary hypertension, ventricular outflow obstruction, or ventricular failure.

B. Cardiomyopathy

Cardiomyopathy is conveniently classified by etiology as ischemic or nonischemic and by type as dilated or nondilated. Dilated cardiomyopathy is characterized by loss of muscle mass or function which is compensated for by moving residual myocardial function farther along the Starling curve, ie, by increasing myofibril length. Resting cardiac output is preserved, but systolic reserve is limited and compliance is decreased. These cardiomyopathies are frequently associated with ventricular dilation, areas of dyskinesis, mitral incompetence, cardiac rhythm disturbance, pulmonary hypertension, and secondary right ventricular failure. Hypertrophic disease is usually nondilated and causes decreased diastolic function with small chamber size, increased left ventricular mass, functional outflow obstruction, and elevated filling pressures. Many patients with cardiomyopathy undergo revascularization, arrhythmia surgery, valvular replacement, or eventual transplant.

C. Acute Coronary Insufficiency

Preoperative acute coronary insufficiency frequently necessitates emergent revascularization. This may be complicated by reperfusion injury, residual ischemia, and myocardial infarction with secondary mitral regurgitation, ventricular rupture, or ventricular septal defect. Reperfusion injury results in decreased ventricular compliance, decreased systolic and diastolic function, and rhythm disturbances (atrial fibrillation and flutter, premature atrial contractions, ventricular fibrillation, ventricular tachycardia, heart block). Residual ischemia causes similar derangements that may fluctuate with the level of ischemia. Acute papillary muscle rupture with severe mitral regurgitation, ventricular free wall rupture, and ischemic ventricular septal defects can occur pre- or postoperatively. These events are usually associated with large transmural infarcts and usually present acutely with severe compromise.

D. Valvular Heart Disease

Valvular heart diseases frequently leave residua that predispose to poor cardiac function despite correction of the valvular lesion. Aortic stenosis leads to left ventricular hypertrophy and severely reduced ventricular compliance early in its course. Ventricular dilation and reduced systolic function are frequent late consequences. Associated coronary artery disease or left ventricular outflow tract obstruction may also contribute to poor hemodynamics in patients with aortic stenosis. Aortic insufficiency classically evolves into a dilated, hypokinetic left ventricle with decreased compliance. Aortic valve disease of both types is often complicated by pulmonary hypertension and right heart failure. With mitral valve disease, left ventricular dynamics may be near normal (rheumatic mitral stenosis) or severely depressed (ischemic mitral regurgitation). Mitral stenosis frequently coexists with a normally functioning ventricle preoperatively; however, with relief of inflow obstruction, ventricular overload may occur. Mitral regurgitation is often associated with decreased left ventricular function and dilation preoperatively. Function may worsen in the early postoperative period because of an acute increase in afterload and anatomic changes. Left ventricular function is usually less compromised following mitral valve commissurotomy or repair, but prosthetic mitral valve replacement changes ventricular dynamics significantly and in many cases severely impairs left ventricular function. Other confounding factors include left ventricular outflow obstruction following mitral valve repair or replacement, pulmonary hypertension, right ventricular failure, and tricuspid regurgitation.

E. Congenital Lesions

Congenital lesions are beyond the scope of this discussion, but an assessment of preoperative and postoperative anatomy and function is essential to treatment. Specifically, both the systemic status and the pulmonary (if present) ventricle's functional state should be assessed, preoperative and residual shunts quantitated, vascular resistances determined, outflow and inflow obstructions documented, and associated pulmonary and vascular changes considered. Ventricular function may be compromised for a variety of reasons. Patients with a right ventricle as a systemic chamber have minimal reserve function and are a subset of the cardiomyopathies mentioned above. Congenital lesions may be associated with coronary compromise and secondary loss of ventricular function (eg, tricuspid atresia with intact ventricular septum). In patients without a pulmonary ventricle (eg, postoperative Fontan patients), supranormal systemic ventricular function, low systemic-sided filling pressures, and low pulmonary vascular resistance must all be maintained to promote passive pulmonary flow. Patients with left ventricular outflow obstruction (eg, coarctation or aortic stenosis) frequently have significant left ventricular hypertrophy and dysfunction. Shunts at multiple levels are also common. Residual shunts following correction of congenital anomalies may be beneficial by permitting decompression of high filling pressures and maintenance of cardiac output (eg, following Fontan repair) or may cause significant compromise due to ventricular overload or arterial desaturation. In view of these complexities and their interrelationships, a detailed understanding of the function of each ventricle, the volume load presented to each chamber, and the configuration of outflow and inflow is essential to proper management.

F. Arrhythmias

Arrhythmias may complicate the postoperative course and produce low output states. Supraventricular rhythms, including atrial fibrillation and flutter, occur in up to 30% of open heart surgery patients and are particularly detrimental with decreased ventricular compliance or marginal functional reserve. Metabolic derangements, atrial ischemia, atrial dilation, and sympathetic activity all contribute to supraventricular arrhythmias. Similarly, ventricular arrhythmias are common, particularly in dilated cardiomyopathies, hypertrophic disease, and ischemia. Finally, bradycardias and conduction disturbances are common, particularly at the extremes of age.

G. Pulmonary Disease

Pulmonary and pulmonary vascular disease may be superimposed on any of the above lesions. Chronic left ventricular failure compromises lung compliance, air flow, and oxygenation. Pulmonary vascular resistance is frequently elevated and may or may not be reversible. Vascular rings and slings may directly compromise pulmonary blood flow or gas exchange. Additionally, some conditions may be associated with decreased lung parenchyma or vasculature (eg, endocardial cushion defects, tetralogy of Fallot, pulmonary atresia).

H. Extrinsic Factors

Pericardial tamponade, tension pneumothorax, inadequate or excessive resuscitation, and circulating myocardial depressants should all be considered during evaluation of inadequate cardiac output.

Resuscitation is frequently inadequate during the early postoperative course. Patients with ongoing blood loss, decreased ventricular compliance, perioperative infarcts, significant organ damage, or complicated cardiopulmonary bypass courses have particularly high fluid requirements, as also do those who are rewarming following hypothermic bypass or circulatory arrest. Overzealous fluid administration can also result in acute cardiac insufficiency, especially in patients with exceptionally low ejection fractions. This delicate balance between inadequate and excessive fluid administration provides the basis for invasive hemodynamic monitoring in patients with complex problems.

1. Tamponade—Tamponade may result from both early bleeding and late pericardial fluid accumulation. Localized collections can result in atypical but equally dangerous presentations. The causes of tamponade are reviewed in the sections on postoperative hemorrhage and postpericardiotomy syndrome.

2. Tension pneumothorax—Tension pneumothorax should be excluded in any patient with hemodynamic compromise.

Myocardial depressants are frequently active perioperatively. Calcium channel blockers, beta-blockers, antiarrhythmics, and anesthetic agents all contribute to decreased myocardial performance. Endogenous substances such as IL-6 may also play a role in patients with long cardiopulmonary bypass runs or systemic injury from prolonged hypoperfusion.

Clinical Features

A. Symptoms and Signs

Invasive hemodynamic monitoring with pulmonary artery catheters is valuable to assess cardiopulmonary physiology and guide therapy. Confounding problems specific to cardiac surgery patients are due to the frequent presence of endotracheal tubes, residual anesthetic agents, and continued "normal" residual effects of cardiopulmonary bypass. Ongoing hemorrhage, pulmonary insufficiency, metabolic derangements, volume shifts, and temperature changes all contribute to variable cardiac performance.

B. Imaging Studies

Chest radiographs should be obtained early and evaluated for evidence of enlarging cardiac silhouette (tamponade), pulmonary venous congestion (congestive heart failure and tamponade), pleural fluid (ongoing bleeding), mediastinal shift, and extrapulmonary air (tension pneumothorax). Chest radiographs need to be evaluated in comparison with previously obtained films to highlight changes and permit correlation with a changing clinical course.

C. Echocardiography

Surface or transesophageal echocardiography can be invaluable in specific clinical circumstances. Surface echo is usually performed initially. If necessary, transesophageal studies can be added to provide additional information about posterior structures, particularly the mitral valve and thoracic aorta. Echocardiography is useful in the evaluation of tamponade because it can display diffuse or localized fluid collections as well as shift and paradoxical motion of the ventricular septum, which suggest hemodynamic compromise. In addition, echo can confirm poor ventricular function, which occurs with cardiomyopathy or global ischemia. It visualizes localized wall motion abnormalities due to new or recurrent local ischemia. Ventricular filling and insufficient or excess volume resuscitation can also be evaluated. Echo is also helpful in evaluating left ventricular outflow obstruction, frequently present in patients with hypertrophic cardiomyopathies, and after mitral or aortic valve repair or replacement. New or residual valvular disease, dissection of the aorta, and septal defects can also be visualized.

D. Electrocardiography

Electrocardiographic tracings should be compared with preoperative and earlier postoperative examinations for evidence of ischemia, rhythm and rate disturbances, or diffuse changes sometimes seen with pericardial hematoma and pericarditis.

E. Hemodynamic Monitoring

Cardiac output, central venous pressure, and pulmonary artery and pulmonary wedge pressures, as determined with a thermodilution pulmonary artery catheter, are invaluable for assessment of cardiovascular status at the bedside. Indeed, these data are often the earliest and easiest to obtain, further underscoring their importance. A cardiac index of less than 2.0 $L/min/m^2$ always requires prompt evaluation and correction. Even higher indices may be inadequate in specific situations. Inaccurate output measurements can occur if incorrect calibration constants are used or tricuspid regurgitation is present. If measured values appear inappropriate to the clinical situation, their validity should be confirmed by venous O_2 saturation measurement or echocardiography (see below). Central pressures should be evaluated early in the course of low-output states.

F. Oxyhemoglobin Saturation

Venous oxyhemoglobin saturation can be measured intermittently by transcatheter aspiration or continuously by fiberoptic pulmonary artery catheters. Central venous (right atrial) oxygen saturations are typically measured, and resting values are usually 75%. Assuming a 100% arterial saturation, this represents unloading of one-fourth of the available oxygen. Venous desaturation usually indicates inadequate tissue perfusion whether or not the cardiac index is depressed. Oxygen content calculations from specific chambers can also be used to determine intracardiac shunts and flows.

Differential Diagnosis

Intravascular volume changes, including hypovolemia, ongoing bleeding, and overload with impaired right or left ventricular function, can all result in acute cardiovascular insufficiency. Extrinsic factors (pericardial tamponade, tension pneumothorax, or hemothorax) and intrinsic cardiac compromise (ventricular free wall rupture, acute ventricular septal defect, papillary muscle rupture, prosthetic valve dehiscence or thrombosis, coronary ischemia, and arrhythmias) can also be confused with low output syndromes. Systemic hypoxia, hypocalcemia, acidosis, sepsis, and organ ischemia can occasionally present initially as low output states in the postoperative period. Malfunctioning arterial catheters and electronic monitors occasionally prompt a search for the cause of hypotension in a normal patient.

Treatment

A. Supportive Measures

As with any critically ill patient, the first objective is to maintain adequate oxygen delivery and pH control by optimizing ventilation. If the cause of the low-output state is not easily identifiable and remedied, then early reintubation, while the patient is still hemodynamically resuscitatable, is preferable to subsequent emergent intervention. If an endotracheal tube is already in place, its function and position should be rapidly confirmed by assessing breath sounds, ventilatory settings and pressures, and inspired O_2. Pulse oximetry and blood gas analysis should be obtained as quickly as possible, as well as electrolytes and hematocrit. Reversible causes (respiratory disorders, electrolyte imbalance) should be promptly corrected.

During evaluation for specific causes, the circulation should be aggressively supported, and this is best accomplished by a systematic approach to appraisal of the hemodynamic status of the patient. As mentioned, adequate oxygenation and ventilation must be ensured. Preload should then be optimized. The virtues of prompt administration of fluids, when appropriate, cannot be overemphasized. Inadequate volume administration is common in patients who are rewarming following a period of hypothermia, who are being treated with vasodilators, or who have poor left or right ventricular compliance. In these circumstances, prompt fluid administration is all that is required for full restoration of cardiovascular stability. In addition, patients with tamponade frequently respond to fluids while preparations for definitive therapy are being made. Conversely, in the patient who has gradually become volume-overloaded, with subsequent impairment of ventricular performance, it is important to treat with inotropes and afterload reduction instead of with additional volume. Patients with very poor ventricular function are prone to both hyper- and hypovolemia. Occasionally, some of the classic signs of hypovolemia, such as increased creatinine and decreased cardiac output, are the result of excessive fluid administration and subsequent ventricular impairment.

Heart rate and rhythm disturbances should then be assessed and treated as outlined in Chapter 22. Contractility may be enhanced with inotropic agents, with particular attention to right ventricular status. Lastly, afterload may be reduced with vasodilators to further improve cardiac output and systemic perfusion. Though most inotropes are described elsewhere in the text, a few warrant further comment.

There are a variety of inotropic drugs that are commonly used to support the failing heart—including dopamine, dobutamine, and epinephrine. While these agents are all effective for improving the contractile state of the myocardium and have variable effects on heart rate and afterload, their effects are primarily exerted on the left ventricle. More recently, the importance of adequate right ventricular function to cardiovascular success has been appreciated, as well as the sensitivity of the right ventricle to increased afterload, which is manifested as cardiovascular failure. Accordingly, pharmacologic agents that provide physiologic benefit to the right ventricle—in the context of perioperative low cardiac output syndrome—including phosphodiesterase III inhibitors (eg, amrinone, milrinone) and inhaled nitric oxide (NO) have received attention and warrant further comment.

The phosphodiesterase III inhibitors have been termed "inodilators" because of their ability to improve myocardial contractility while simultaneously causing vascular smooth muscle relaxation. As a result, these agents have consistently been shown to improve cardiac index and decrease systemic vascular resistance (SVR) and pulmonary vascular resistance (PVR). Furthermore, they cause little or no increase in myocardial oxygen consumption and have almost no effect on systemic blood pressure and heart rate. Moreover, these agents may act synergistically with β_1-adrenergic agonists (eg, epinephrine). Amrinone and its newer derivative, milrinone, are the most common drugs used in this class. They have similar pharmacodynamic properties, though their pharmacokinetics vary somewhat; milrinone is 20–30 times more potent and has a shorter half-life ($t_{1/2}$ = 2–4 hours) than amrinone. As a result of these beneficial effects on the myocardium and the pulmonary and systemic vasculature, these agents are playing an increasing role in the management of perioperative low cardiac output syndrome.

Nitric oxide (NO), formerly known as endothelium-derived relaxing factor (EDRF), has received much attention in and out of the laboratory since being named molecule of the year in 1992. It has emerged as a critical regulator of vascular tone and reactivity in both normal and pathologic processes. Exogenous (ie, inhaled) NO retains the biologic properties of endogenous NO and is the only known agent that specifically dilates the pulmonary vasculature. Accordingly, it has been used with success when pulmonary hypertension is the primary physiologic disturbance (eg, persistent pulmonary hypertension of the newborn, post-cardiac transplantation, post-pulmonary thromboendarterectomy). When it is used, continuous monitoring of its lethal by-product (nitrogen dioxide) is necessary. Furthermore, therapy with inhaled NO mandates mechanical ventilation and is very expensive—thus, it is infrequently a first-line agent. The role of NO in the treatment of perioperative low cardiac output syndrome is limited at this time, but NO offers specific physiologic benefits that may provide the basis for increased use of NO in this setting.

In patients who continue to have low-output states despite these strategies, intra-aortic balloon counterpulsation should be added. In appropriate patients who fail to respond to intra-aortic balloon counterpulsation, more extensive ventricular support should be considered.

B. Correction of Arrhythmias

Most patients will have continuous electrocardiographic monitoring, and the rate and rhythm should be established and corrected as appropriate. Rate abnormalities may have profound hemodynamic consequences, and a rate of 80–100 should be the goal. Temporary atrial, ventricular, and ground wires are frequently available and can be used to correct bradycardias with atrial, ventricular, or sequential atrioventricular pacing. In emergent settings, simple single-chamber ventricular pacing should be instituted first to restore cardiac function immediately. Then, if atrial wires are available, sequential atrioventricular pacing can be instituted to optimize cardiac function. Electrical cardioversion of hemodynamically significant arrhythmias is preferable to long periods of low cardiac output and is easily performed, particularly in intubated and ventilated patients. In extubated patients, brief intravenous anesthesia is sometimes appropriate for cardioversion of atrial fibrillation, atrial flutter, or sustained slow ventricular tachycardia. This is not indicated in patients who are significantly compromised.

C. Surgical Evaluation of Pericardial Tamponade

Ventilation, rhythm, blood pressure, and fluid status should be established within the first few minutes of evaluation. Classically, cardiac tamponade is suggested by hemodynamic instability in a patient with significant bleeding that recently decreased or stopped. Further evidence includes elevated filling pressures (possibly left-right equilibration), mediastinal widening on serial chest radiographs, and increasing tachycardia (compensatory). If not diagnosed rapidly, pulseless electrical activity may result. Despite full evaluation, tamponade frequently cannot be excluded conclusively, and mediastinal exploration, either in the intensive care unit or in the operating room, is required. If time permits, echocardiography may be performed at the bedside to determine the presence or absence of pericardial tamponade. Any patient with cardiovascular collapse in the early period following cardiac surgery should be considered to have tamponade and should be explored surgically if they are not responding to appropriate therapy—even if other examinations are inconclusive or are negative. Tension pneumothorax can occur in any critically ill patient and should be on the basis of ventilator pressure changes, physical examination, and chest x-ray.

D. Other Modalities

Occasional patients will be incompletely revascularized or may have vein or arterial conduit spasm. If serial ECGs are suggestive of ischemia, vascular antispasmodics (ideally calcium channel blockers) should be administered and consideration given to echocardiography to document localized wall motion abnormalities, angiography to definitively establish localized vascular lesions, or early reoperation to treat acute graft occlusion.

Bojar RM, Warner KG: *Manual of Perioperative Care in Cardiac Surgery,* 3rd ed. Blackwell Science, 1999.

DiSesa VJ: Pharmacologic support for postoperative low cardiac output. Semin Thorac Cardiovasc Surg 1991;3:13–23.

Doyle AR et al: Treatment of perioperative low cardiac output syndrome. Ann Thorac Surg 1995;59:S3–11.

Kirklin JW, Barratt-Boyes BG: *Cardiac Surgery: Morphology, Diagnostic Criteria, Natural History, Techniques, Results, and Indications,* 2nd ed. Churchill Livingstone, 1993.

Sabiston DC, Spencer FC (editors): *Surgery of the Chest,* 6th ed. Saunders, 1995.

Pulmonary Disease 24

Darryl Y. Sue, MD, & Janine R.E. Vintch, MD

STATUS ASTHMATICUS

ESSENTIALS OF DIAGNOSIS

- *Usually unremitting asthma, rapidly increasing in severity, but may present with sudden and severe obstruction.*
- *Poor and decreasing response to beta-adrenergic agonist therapy.*
- *May develop hypercapnic respiratory failure.*
- *Evidence of respiratory (inspiratory) muscle fatigue.*

General Considerations

Status asthmaticus is very severe asthma that is unremitting and poorly responsive to usual anti-asthma therapy. Studies have emphasized the differences between chronic stable asthma and status asthmaticus in terms of pathophysiology, prognosis, management, and response to treatment. Importantly, there has been increased awareness of mortality and morbidity from severe asthma, recognition of the key role of inflammation in the mechanism of severe asthma, changes in the mode of delivery of agents for treating asthma, and revised concepts in management of patients requiring mechanical ventilation.

Many patients with asthma will have episodic attacks that are easily and rapidly treated. These mild exacerbations call for changes in management, but the important feature of such cases is that the patient responds and returns to baseline in a short time. These attacks are to be distinguished from status asthmaticus, characterized by slow and inadequate response to treatment and a poor outlook for resolution of attacks. The recognition of severe acute asthma may in some cases be difficult when the patient is assessed against a background of chronic but stable asthma.

Pathophysiology & Pathogenesis

Asthma prevalence is increasing in the United States, and asthma mortality is a matter of great concern. Airway obstruction is the major feature of this disorder, and asthma is both an acute reversible obstructive disease and a chronic pulmonary disease causing permanent airway obstruction. Failure to control asthma symptoms is associated with a more rapidly progressive decline in lung function and loss of reversibility. This is the basis for several new consensus recommendations for chronic asthma management, which can be summarized as follows: (1) There is a key role for anti-inflammatory therapy (eg, corticosteroids); (2) regular beta-adrenergic agonist use as the sole therapy for asthma should be abandoned; and (3) the goal of asthma treatment is to keep the patient completely symptom-free at all times. Despite widespread dissemination of these recommendations, optimal management of asthma is far from an achieved objective, and many asthmatics have moderate to severe exacerbations requiring hospitalization—with some requiring intensive care management.

Airway obstruction in asthma results from three mechanisms: enhanced bronchial smooth muscle contraction (increased tone and response to stimuli), bronchial mucosal inflammation and edema, and plugging of the bronchi by secretions and inflammatory debris. The response to therapy depends on the relative contributions of each of these mechanisms. For example, bronchodilators relax bronchial smooth muscles but have little or no effect on reducing airway obstruction caused by inflammation or debris. Corticosteroids have no direct effect on bronchial smooth muscle but reduce inflammation in the bronchial walls.

The baseline amount of inflammation and airway narrowing is a major determinant of the severity of exacerbations once an asthma exacerbation is triggered. Exacerbations may be triggered by allergens in susceptible individuals; by cold air or irritants such as dust; by aspirin; or by respiratory infections, especially viral infections. These insults cause release of mast cell products such as histamine, inflammatory mediators (leukotrienes and prostaglandins), and substances that attract and activate leukocytes, especially eosinophils. It often happens that an identifiable precipitating cause for an exacerbation cannot be identified. Bronchial smooth muscle contraction and bronchospasm usually occur first, with mucosal edema, increased mucous gland secretions, and inflammatory cell infiltration rapidly following. The proportion of airway obstruction due to bronchospasm and that due to edema, inflammation, and mucus plugging is highly variable between patients.

There seems to be a key role for eosinophilic infiltration of the bronchial mucosa in asthma, but neutrophils and T-lymphocytes have also been implicated. Eosinophils may be attracted by platelet-activating factor produced by a variety of cells, and there is increased local production of IL-5, an activator of eosinophils.

A number of studies have suggested an association between regular use of short-acting beta-adrenergic agonists and fatal or near-fatal asthma events. Proposed mechanisms are (1) promotion of airway hyperresponsiveness by these drugs, since they are so effective that the patients are more apt to undergo prolonged exposure to allergens or irritants; and (2) heavy use of beta-adrenergic agonists, followed by hypokalemia and cardiac arrhythmias. Other commentators have taken the position that asthma deaths are more strongly associated with undertreatment with beta-adrenergic agonists than with overtreatment, and these workers do not believe the evidence for an association of poor outcome with beta-adrenergic agonist use is compelling. First, they argue that increased beta-adrenergic agonist use in the histories of these patients is the *result* of increased asthma severity and that this is a coincidental and not a causal relationship. Second—increased mortality has been linked to certain beta-adrenergic agonists but much less to others. And finally, heterogeneity of the structure and function of the beta-adrenergic receptor has been documented, and there is evidence that some receptor types are more subject than others to down-regulation by beta-adrenergic agonist exposure. During an exacerbation, asthmatics with down-regulated beta-adrenergic receptors would have poorer responses to beta-adrenergic agonists—and may therefore use excessive amounts of beta-adrenergic agonists and have an increased risk of complications. Thus, the conclusion offered is that certain asthmatic patients are more susceptible than others to problems with beta-adrenergic agonists—not the same as saying that the drugs alone are responsible for increased numbers of deaths from asthma.

Status asthmaticus is characterized by poor responsiveness to bronchodilator therapy, a rapid, unremitting, and often progressive course, and slow recovery to a baseline. Patients who die with status asthmaticus are often found to have severe mucus impaction of airways and marked inflammatory infiltration of the bronchial walls, suggesting a greater role of airway mucosal inflammation over bronchial smooth muscle contraction. In some patients with status asthmaticus, hypoxemia persists much longer than airway narrowing (as measured by peak flow or FEV_1), suggesting that persistent blockage of small airways with mucus prolongs ventilation-perfusion mismatching. It is not known why an asthmatic with exacerbation may sometimes develop a self-terminated bronchoconstrictor response and at other times generate a persistent unremitting response (status asthmaticus) with airway edema and inflammation.

On the other hand, a small number of patients with fatal or near-fatal asthma appear to have rapid onset of symptoms with little airway inflammation. These patients experience very severe bronchospasm that may lead to death within minute or hours. Identification of such patients before they have a fatal or near-fatal episode is difficult, but recent evidence suggests that these patients may have reduced perception of increased airway resistance combined with decreased hypoxic ventilatory drive.

Most patients with asthma exacerbations can be treated successfully before they develop severe respiratory failure. Respiratory failure in asthma comes about from two major mechanisms. First, the diffuse but variable bronchial obstruction causes ventilation-perfusion mismatching with resultant hypoxemia, and if the patient fails to increase alveolar ventilation appropriately there is also hypercapnia. Second is respiratory muscle fatigue, which somewhat paradoxically is more marked for the inspiratory than for the expiratory muscles. Airway obstruction contributes to respiratory muscle fatigue from increased resistance during both inspiration and expiration. Because airway obstruction in asthmatics is intrathoracic, airway narrowing is more marked during the expiratory phase, increasing expiratory work of breathing and lengthening the time needed for adequate exhalation. However, because respiratory drive is increased in asthma as a result of hypoxemia, hypercapnia, and other factors, the respiratory rate increases and expiratory time shortens. This combination of greater expiratory airway obstruction and shorter expiratory time results in hyperinflation (air trapping). Hyperinflation puts an additional burden on the inspiratory muscles because these muscles are shorter than normal prior to contraction and thus are unable to generate as much tension for as long a time. Respiratory failure develops because the patient becomes unable to compensate for the pathophysiologic changes. The result is fatigue of inspiratory muscles, worsening hypercapnia and respiratory acidosis, and, usually, a need for intubation and mechanical ventilation.

Clinical Features

A. Symptoms and Signs

The severity of an asthma exacerbation should be judged in order to make decisions about management. Early response to therapy is the key piece of information on which to base a judgment about the severity of asthma, but other information may be helpful as well. Indicators of severity include prolonged duration of attacks, history of hospitalization for asthma, prior or current use of corticosteroids (especially oral), poor response to bronchodilators, increasingly more frequent or increased dosages of medications, recent or repeated emergency room or office visits for acute asthma, and a history of requiring mechanical ventilation for asthma. Increasing severity of asthma may be manifested by less diurnal variation in asthma severity, diminishing peak flow both before and after bronchodilators, and inability to sleep. A minority of asthmatics present with status asthmaticus after very short duration of symptoms. Some investigators have suggested that these patients presenting with a hyperacute attack may have a variety of asthma marked by sudden severe airway closure, perhaps from a neural mechanism rather than from airway inflammation. Lastly, because pregnancy has a variable effect on women with stable chronic asthma, including causing marked worsening in some individuals, pregnancy in women with child-bearing potential should be considered as a factor for asthma worsening.

The physical examination is helpful for identifying signs of severe airway obstruction (absence of wheezing, use of accessory muscles of respiration, intercostal retractions, pulsus paradoxus) or signs of impending respiratory muscle fatigue (paradoxic abdominal wall movement), but these signs are insensitive or unreliable when used by themselves to assess severity. A number of studies have attempted to assess the value of other signs, such as tachycardia, tachypnea, cyanosis, and hypotension, singly or in combination, but these have not proved to be of discriminating value. The key role of the physical examination is to exclude other acute respiratory problems that may be mistaken for asthma, such as pulmonary edema, anaphylaxis or angioedema, pneumothorax, pneumonia, and upper or central airway obstruction due to tumor, foreign body, or epiglottitis.

B. Laboratory Findings

The majority of patients with acute asthma will have hypoxemia of mild to moderate degree, and hypoxemia is not a particularly discriminating variable for asthma severity. Most asthmatics (80%) presenting with an acute episode have mild respiratory alkalosis. Only a small proportion are reported to have normal or elevated P_{CO_2}, and there is an association between severe airway obstruction and hypercapnia in asthma. Nonetheless, although hypercapnia is of concern in status asthmaticus, hypercapnia is not consistently linked with prolonged severe asthma or the need for mechanical ventilation. There has also been a finding of metabolic acidosis due to increase in blood lactate in patients presenting with acute asthma, especially in association with hypoxemia. Although pulse oximetry gives an estimate of arterial oxygenation, an arterial blood gas determination of pH and P_{CO_2} is mandatory for any asthmatic admitted from the emergency department or being considered for admission to the intensive care unit.

Serum sodium and potassium should be measured because of the association of hyponatremia with pulmonary diseases and respiratory failure and the observation that aggressive beta-adrenergic agonist use can sometimes result in severe hypokalemia. Although magnesium has been used as a bronchodilator and although hypokalemia and hypomagnesemia are closely related, hypomagnesemia has not been associated with asthma exacerbations.

C. Imaging Studies

Chest radiographs during acute asthma almost always show hyperinflation, with low, flat hemidiaphragms and an increased anteroposterior diameter. They are not helpful in assessment of the severity of asthma, precipitating factors, or complications. However, some investigators have claimed that chest radiographs provide important diagnostic information in asthmatics who are admitted to the hospital in that the choice of therapy is altered by the findings on the radiograph. Features to be sought include the presence of pneumothorax, infiltrates suggestive of bacterial or viral pneumonia, findings suggestive of allergic bronchopulmonary aspergillosis (fleeting infiltrates, cylindric bronchiectasis), and lobar or segmental atelectasis suggesting mucous impaction of large airways. Because pulmonary edema may present with acute onset of dyspnea and wheezing, cardiomegaly and features of congestive heart failure should be excluded.

D. Spirometry

Spirometry can be very helpful in the assessment of status asthmaticus, both initially and in following treatment. Although many clinicians have recommended using FEV_1 or peak flow at presentation for initial decision-making, the subjective and objective response to therapy after the first 1–2 hours provides much more meaningful information. It is recommended that FEV_1 or peak flow be measured on initial presentation to the emergency room and then hourly until a decision is made to hospitalize. The frequency of spirometry thereafter depends on clinical assessment, but the response to additional treatment with bronchodilators and, after sufficient time has elapsed, to corticosteroids, may be of additional value in planning treatment and observation. The FEV_1 or peak flow may be compared with predicted values for the patient's age, sex, and size, but improvement in the measured values over time is the most helpful indicator. In one study, good response to treatment at 30 minutes was the single variable most highly correlated with favorable patient outcome.

Differential Diagnosis

Features suggesting status asthmaticus, including acute onset of shortness of breath, cough, wheezing, and progression to respiratory failure, may be seen to varying degrees in congestive heart failure, upper airway obstruction, exacerbation of chronic bronchitis or emphysema, spontaneous pneumothorax, anaphylaxis, acute pulmonary embolism, and foreign body aspiration. Upper airway obstruction is characterized by inspiratory wheezing or stridor, sometimes loudest over the trachea in the neck. Asthmatics who had prior endotracheal intubation—especially for long duration—or tracheostomy should be suspected of having extrathoracic airway obstruction. A small but significant number of patients mistakenly diagnosed as having asthma instead have vocal cord dysfunction syndrome. In this syndrome, the vocal cords adduct inappropriately during exhalation, increasing expiratory resistance and causing expiratory wheezing and hyperinflation. Vocal cord dysfunction may go unidentified for years until direct visualization of the vocal cords during the respiratory cycle makes the diagnosis. On some occasions, patients who are intubated for severe asthma have sudden and complete relief of obstruction and wheezing, and these patients should be suspected of vocal cord dysfunction syndrome.

Treatment

Status asthmaticus is treated with bronchodilators (titrated to patient response), corticosteroids, and oxygen, with endotracheal intubation and mechanical ventilation if necessary. The aim of treatment is to relieve the airway obstruction by relaxing bronchial smooth muscles and reversing inflammation while supporting respiratory function. Support of respiratory function depends on the severity of the asthma and the ability of the patient to sustain inspiratory and expiratory muscle work. An important concept in treatment of status asthmaticus is that the airway obstruction should not be expected to reverse as quickly or completely as in mild asthma exacerbations.

A. Oxygen

Ninety percent of patients presenting with a severe asthmatic attack are hypoxemic to some degree. Severe hypoxemia must be treated with oxygen. Hypoxemia increases respiratory drive and tachypnea, contributing to increased hyperinflation and possible inspiratory muscle fatigue. Oxygen therapy may be helpful in attenuating some respiratory drive and allowing a prolonged expiratory time. Because hypoxemia is usually due to ventilation-perfusion mismatching, hypoxemia in most asthmatics can be treated with low concentrations of supplemental oxygen in sufficient amounts to raise arterial Po_2 to 80–100 mm Hg. In nonintubated patients, oxygen can be given by nasal cannula or Venturi-type masks.

B. Bronchodilators

Bronchodilators of all types have been used in status asthmaticus, including beta-adrenergic agonists (sympathomimetics), methylxanthines (theophylline), anticholinergics, and others. (See Chapter 12.)

Beta-adrenergic agonists are the most effective bronchodilator agents in acute asthma exacerbations. Those that are modified to have more specificity for β_2 receptors, such as albuterol, are most often used because of their decreased effect on heart rate. Aerosolized formulations are much more potent and better tolerated than the same drugs given orally, subcutaneously, or intravenously, having a greater bronchodilator effect and causing less tachycardia and less hypokalemia even in patients who have severe bronchial obstruction. In moderately severe to severe asthma, aerosolized beta-adrenergic agonists can be given with equal effectiveness with either a metered-dose inhaler (MDI) or hand-held nebulizer if a spacer or reservoir device is used with the MDI. Finally, the effective dose of beta-adrenergic agonists is often higher than was formerly recommended; the doses should be titrated in individual patients to tolerance, often using clinical response, tachycardia, tremor, or other observations as guides to dosage. Beta-adrenergic agonists may be given in conventional doses but as often as hourly or even by continuous nebulization. Continuous nebulization has been found to be variably effective. Hypokalemia as a consequence of beta-adrenergic agonist therapy—causing increased transport of potassium into cells—is a known complication when these drugs are given in large doses.

Subcutaneous epinephrine has a long history of effective use in acute asthma, but inhalation of selective beta-adrenergic agonists is more effective. The side effects of epinephrine include tachycardia, increased myocardial oxygen requirement, and hypertension. Salmeterol is a long-acting beta-adrenergic agonist that is structurally similar to albuterol but has a longer side chain that may anchor it near the β_2-receptor site. This drug has no value in acute severe asthma, and salmeterol should be reserved for use only after resolution of the acute attack.

In severe asthma, aerosolized albuterol is recommended. If given by metered-dose inhaler (MDI), a spacer or reservoir is necessary. A starting dosage is 2–4 puffs every 1–2 hours, the number of puffs can be increased to 6–8 or more, if tolerated. Alternatively, a nebulized solution of 0.5 mL of albuterol (0.5%) diluted in 2.5 mL of normal saline can be given by gas-powered nebulizer or intermittent positive-pressure breathing every 2–6 hours, but there is no evidence that this is more effective than administration by MDI. The response to bronchodilators should be objectively measured, preferably by spirometry (FEV_1 or peak flow). Tachycardia, tremors, and changes in blood pressure should be carefully monitored, especially when doses given exceed usual recommendations.

Anticholinergic drugs are generally considered more effective in chronic bronchitis than in asthma. Studies support their use in severe asthma but only in conjunction with optimized beta-adrenergic agonist use. The quaternary anticholinergic drug ipratropium bromide is available for use via metered-dose inhaler or by nebulization. Effective doses of ipratropium bromide may be considerably higher than currently recommended, but its minimal side effects allow it to be well tolerated. Ipratropium should be given to asthmatics with severe exacerbations along with maximal beta-adrenergic agonist therapy. A fixed-dose MDI combination of ipratropium and albuterol is available, but it is not known if this preparation is useful in acute asthma attacks. In severe asthma, ipratropium should be given either by MDI or by nebulization. Ipratropium bromide is available in MDIs or in solution for nebulization. By MDI, the starting dosage should be 2–4 puffs every 4–6 hours. For nebulization, an effective dose is 0.5 mg given every 6–8 hours. Even at the highest doses, side effects of ipratropium are minimal and these doses appear to be safe.

The addition of theophylline to optimized regimens of beta-adrenergic agonist therapy confers little or no additional benefit and increased toxicity and side effects. Some of the side effects of theophylline are identical to those of beta-adrenergic agonists, and this may limit the use of the more beneficial agent. Theophylline should be considered a third-line bronchodilator drug in status asthmaticus, but it might warrant consideration in selected patients who are not responding to other therapy. Theophylline is tolerated only when the serum concentrations are carefully maintained in the therapeutic range, and in some patients toxicity occurs even then.

Intravenous magnesium sulfate has been shown to be an effective bronchodilator in some studies of asthma exacerbation. Doses administered have been in the range of 0.5–1 mmol/min over 20 minutes, corresponding to about 3–5 g of $MgSO_4$. Comparison with beta-adrenergic agonists has not been carried out in the ideal manner for evaluating the precise role of magnesium sulfate in combination with other drugs.

C. Corticosteroids

The importance of corticosteroids in the treatment of status asthmaticus has been documented in several studies, but the ideal dosage remains undetermined. In one study, 15 mg of methylprednisolone given intravenously every 6 hours did not appear to be as effective as larger doses such as 40 mg or 125 mg every 6 hours, and most clinicians agree that a dose of 10–15 mg/kg/24 h of hydrocortisone or equivalent is effective. Larger doses have not resulted in improved outcome or more rapid resolution. These recommendations translate into quite large doses, such as 120–240 mg of prednisone or methylprednisolone per day in divided doses for average-sized adults. Oral administration has been shown to be as effective as intravenous infusion with no difference in time of onset of effect, but intravenous administration is more commonly chosen.

For status asthmaticus, intravenous methylprednisolone, 40–60 mg every 6 hours, or similar dosage of oral prednisone or methylprednisolone is recommended. The dose should be continued, in the absence of acute severe side effects, for several days even if the patient improves. The rate of tapering of systemic corticosteroids depends on clinical response as well as the patient's recent history of asthma severity and previous dosage of corticosteroids.

The beneficial effect of corticosteroids is not clinically apparent until at least 6 hours after administration. Therefore, if corticosteroids are to be optimally effective, they should be given early, and as soon as a diagnosis of status asthmaticus is made. Corticosteroids should be continued initially for at least 24–48 hours, then reduced by approximately 25–50% depending on clinical response. Further reduction can generally take place over about a 2-week period. Most investigators do not believe there is a role for aerosolized corticosteroids in status asthmaticus because of concern about delivery to the airways during acute airway obstruction. However, these agents are quite beneficial as the systemic corticosteroids are tapered, and relatively soon (within a few days) highly potent inhaled corticosteroids (eg., fluticasone) are effective.

The major concern of corticosteroid therapy is the side effects. The usual side effects of high-dose corticosteroids in critically ill patients include hyperglycemia, altered mental status, metabolic alkalosis, and hypokalemia. In asthmatics, however, worsening respiratory failure from acute myopathy has been reported in association with corticosteroids. Three mechanisms have been proposed to explain this phenomenon. First, hypokalemia may develop, especially with high-dose beta-adrenergic agonist use and high-dose corticosteroids. Second, acute steroid myopathy has been reported at the doses used in status asthmaticus. Finally, there is a well-accepted association of prolonged muscle weakness when high-dose corticosteroids are given in combination therapy with nondepolarizing muscle relaxants. In the latter syndrome, temporary pharmacologic denervation of muscles appears to potentiate the acute myopathic effects of corticosteroids. This syndrome, seen in asthmatics and others requiring muscle relaxants to help them accept mechanical ventilation, may prolong the need for mechanical ventilation.

Because of the central role of inflammation in status asthmaticus, other agents that interfere with the inflammatory response have been proposed. Although methotrexate has been used in stable steroid-dependent asthma, there are no studies of this antimetabolite in status asthmaticus. Leukotriene antagonists and inhibitors of leukotriene synthesis are effective in modifying asthma and perhaps reducing exacerbations. They do not appear to have a role in acute asthma exacerbations.

D. Asthma in Pregnancy

Asthma is the most commonly encountered pulmonary problem in pregnant women, and asthma may worsen, improve, or remain unchanged in severity during pregnancy. Fetal outcomes are adversely influenced if the mother's asthma is poorly controlled, and improvement in asthma control is rewarded by a better outcome. Guidelines for treatment developed by the National Asthma Education and Prevention Program emphasize recommendations similar to those for nonpregnant patients. These include close monitoring of lung function, early administration of inhaled corticosteroids or other anti-inflammatory agents, and rapid therapeutic intervention during acute exacerbations to avoid hypoxemia. Clinicians may be reluctant to give medications to pregnant women because of risks to the fetus. Beta-adrenergic agonists are considered safe, as are inhaled corticosteroids, and systemic corticosteroids should not be withheld if needed during acute exacerbations. A more complete discussion of this topic is included in Chapter 39.

E. Mechanical Ventilation

Patients with status asthmaticus who require intubation and mechanical ventilation should be identified either by the extreme severity of the airway obstruction or by anticipating failure of the patient to maintain adequate alveolar ventilation. Although most patients who require intubation and mechanical ventilation develop altered mental status, acute CO_2 retention, or both, a poor response to treatment or evidence of impending inspiratory muscle failure implies a high likelihood of a need for ventilatory support.

1. Dynamic hyperinflation and complications from mechanical ventilation—Mechanical ventilation with positive-pressure ventilation in status asthmaticus was at one time associated with a disproportionate complication rate and increased mortality. Barotrauma (pneumothorax) and other complications of positive-pressure ventilation and endotracheal intubation were much higher in asthmatics than in patients with other forms of respiratory failure requiring mechanical ventilation. Possible reasons for this include failure to recognize the severity and slow reversibility of status asthmaticus, thereby selecting out a more severely afflicted population of patients and delaying intubation and onset of mechanical ventilation; insufficient attention to the high airway pressure and progressive hyperinflation seen during mechanical ventilation of asthmatics; and failure to understand the importance of hyperinflation or air trapping as a cause of gas exchange failure. Identified risk factors for barotrauma in one study included significantly higher minute ventilation and degree of estimated hyperinflation compared with those who escaped complications. Current recommendations for mechanical ventilation have reduced complications and mortality in this disorder to rates comparable to what is reported with other causes of acute respiratory failure.

The most important recommendation is limiting the degree of dynamic hyperinflation, which occurs when end-expiratory lung volume exceeds the end-expiratory volume predicted if there is sufficient time for the patient to completely exhale. Dynamic hyperinflation increases the risk of barotrauma because the lung is highly stretched at end-expiration, and adding the next tidal volume further stretches the lung. It also results in very inefficient gas exchange with a large increase in the ratio of dead space to tidal volume and in hypercapnia. Finally, because of the high air space pressures it engenders during both inspiration and expiration, dynamic hyperinflation may compromise the circulation.

Dynamic hyperinflation results from a combination of factors. First, expiratory resistance is high and the tidal volume requires more time to be exhaled completely. Second, patients with asthma may have high ventilatory drive due to hypoxemia, hypercapnia, or both. High ventilatory drive increases respiratory rate and decreases the time available for exhalation. Third, because of the hypercapnia, clinicians may try to increase minute ventilation by raising tidal volume and increasing respiratory rate during mechanical ventilation. High tidal volume and high respiratory rate during status asthmaticus are predictably associated with high peak airway pressures, high inspiratory plateau pressures, short expiratory times, "auto-PEEP," and hyperinflation. The magnitude of dynamic hyperinflation can be remarkable. In one study, estimates of the volume of "trapped gas" were as much as 12–20 mL/kg above normal end-expiratory volume.

2. Ventilator settings—All asthmatics who are receiving mechanical ventilation potentially have severe dynamic hyperinflation, and a trial of reduced tidal volume, respiratory frequency, or both should be initiated with careful monitoring of arterial pH and P_{CO_2}. Dynamic hyperinflation is especially likely to occur if hypercapnia is worsening in the face of recent increases in tidal volume or respiratory frequency. One key adjustment is to minimize dynamic hyperinflation by maximizing inspiratory flow rate. This adjustment shortens inspiratory time and lengthens expiratory time, providing a greater opportunity to exhale the tidal volume. Inspiratory flow should be at least 80–100 L/min (1.3–1.6 L/s). The resultant I:E ratio should be 1:4 or higher.

A second important strategy is to constrain tidal volume and respiratory rate using volume-cycled positive-pressure ventilation enough to keep inspiratory plateau pressure at 30–40 cm H_2O or less. Tidal volume should be set at 7–10 mL/kg ideal body weight, and respiratory rate should be adjusted to minimize estimated auto-PEEP (< 5 cm H_2O) and inspiratory plateau pressure. Patients may require sedation or muscle relaxants to achieve these goals. Dynamic hyperinflation plays such a dominant role in determining effective gas exchange that reducing hyperinflation may decrease P_{CO_2} despite a seemingly paradoxic lower minute ventilation. However, a more likely result is hypercapnia and respiratory acidosis. The risks and complications of hypercapnia have been reported to be minimal, and the more favorable overall outcome favors allowing some degree of hypercapnia and respiratory acidosis (pH > 7.25). At present, permissive hypercapnia should be allowed as needed to avoid severe dynamic hyperinflation.

The decision to increase minute ventilation and reverse hypercapnia is generally made as peak airway pressure and auto-PEEP decline as the patient's airway resistance improves with treatment. In one study, a 40–60 s apnea period was set for asthmatic patients who were sedated and given muscle relaxants. The total exhaled gas volume was measured; this consisted of the previous tidal volume plus any amount of "trapped gas" that could be exhaled during the prolonged exhalation period. Patients whose total exhaled gas volumes exceeded 20 mL/kg had their respiratory frequency reduced regardless of the measured P_{CO_2}. But the respiratory frequency was increased in the other patients as much as possible without exceeding 20 mL/kg total exhaled volume, and these patients did not have worsening of hypercapnia or evidence of barotrauma. Patients were discontinued from mechanical ventilation when a P_{CO_2} of 40 mm Hg could be obtained and exhaled gas volume was less than 20 mL/kg.

There is limited published experience with administration of intravenous sodium bicarbonate to compensate for the increased P_{CO_2}, and this treatment should be used judiciously in selected patients. In one study, no complications of bicarbonate therapy were identified, but there is concern for development of paradoxic cerebrospinal fluid acidosis, hypernatremia, and intravascular volume overload. The use of other buffers that do not produce additional CO_2 when they react with acids has been proposed.

Current Controversies & Unresolved Issues

A. General Anesthesia for Refractory Asthma

In patients undergoing mechanical ventilation, halothane and ketamine anesthesia has been used in status asthmaticus that is refractory to conventional management, but this management has not been compared with other forms of therapy. Both agents have bronchodilator properties, but this remains an unproved and potentially risky therapy.

B. Mucolytic Administration by Fiberoptic Bronchoscopy

Recognition that severe refractory airway obstruction in status asthmaticus is often due to plugging of small airways with inspissated mucus led to the use of mucolytic agents such as acetylcysteine. However, aerosolization of this agent sometimes led to bronchospasm, and its effectiveness in the dose and manner administered has been questioned. Bronchoalveolar lavage with acetylcysteine and saline has been performed using the fiberoptic bronchoscope. Because of compromise of the airway with the bronchoscope, this must be done only during mechanical ventilation with sedation, muscle relaxants, or general anesthesia. The usefulness of this technique has not been proved, and, because of the high risks to the patient, it should be considered only if other more conventional treatment has failed. Using a strategy to reduce dynamic hyperinflation and waiting for resolution of the underlying asthma in response to corticosteroids is almost always a better option.

C. Helium-Oxygen Inhalation

Helium-oxygen mixtures (21–40% oxygen; balance helium) have less density than nitrogen-oxygen mixtures. Because a less dense gas is more likely to move through airways under conditions resulting in laminar rather than turbulent flow, helium-oxygen mixtures may improve distribution of ventilation and reduce airway pressures needed for effective ventilation. Helium-oxygen has been used in spontaneously breathing asthmatics to unload the work of the inspiratory and expiratory muscles. This may allow enough time for anti-inflammatory therapy to take effect and avoid intubation and mechanical ventilation. Mechanical ventilation with 60% helium and 40% oxygen mixtures has been used with improved arterial blood gases and markedly decreased airway pressures compared with a nitrogen-oxygen mixture. Although there have been no controlled studies of helium-oxygen mixtures in status asthmaticus, it is reasonable to suppose that this form of treatment may be beneficial in some refractory asthmatics. The problems include obtaining the appropriate gas, adapting the ventilator to use the gas mixture, monitoring tidal volume, and ensuring the adequacy of oxygen in the inspired gas mixture.

Corbridge TC, Hall JB: The assessment and management of adults with status asthmaticus. Am J Respir Crit Care Med 1995;151:1296–1316.

Cydulka RK et al: Acute asthma among pregnant women presenting to the emergency department. Am J Respir Crit Care Med 1999;160:887–92.

Fabbri L et al: Similarities and discrepancies between exacerbations of asthma and chronic obstructive pulmonary disease. Thorax 1998;53:803–8.

Guidelines for the diagnosis and management of asthma. Expert Panel Report 2. National Institutes of Health, National Heart, Lung, and Blood Institute, Publication No. 97–4051A, May 1997.

Levy BD, Kitch B, Fanta CH: Medical and ventilatory management of status asthmaticus. Intensive Care Med 1998;24:105–17.

Management of asthma during pregnancy. National Asthma Education Program, 1993. National Institutes of Health, Publication No. 93–3279.

McFadden ER: Dosages of corticosteroids in asthma. Am Rev Respir Dis 1993;147:1306–10.

Turner MO et al: Risk factors for near-fatal asthma. Am J Respir Crit Care Med 1998;157:1804–9.

Tuxen DV et al: Use of a measurement of pulmonary hyperinflation to control the level of mechanical ventilation in patients with acute severe asthma. Am Rev Respir Dis 1992;146:1136–42.

Williams TJ et al: Risk factors for morbidity in mechanically ventilated patients with acute severe asthma. Am Rev Respir Dis 1992;146:607–15.

LIFE-THREATENING HEMOPTYSIS

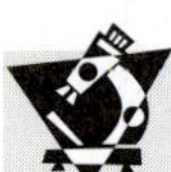

ESSENTIALS OF DIAGNOSIS

- *Expectoration of blood or blood-tinged sputum in sufficient quantity to compromise lung function.*
- *Either a large volume of hemoptysis in a healthy patient or a patient with preexisting lung or heart disease, inability to protect the airway, or altered level of consciousness.*

General Considerations

Hemoptysis can be caused by a wide variety of lung conditions, and hemoptysis sufficient to be acutely life-threatening is not common (5–15% of hemoptysis patients). Acute hemoptysis was formerly classified as massive or nonmassive, and the major decision about whether to perform surgical resection was based on the estimated amount of bleeding. There is now recognition that even large volumes of hemoptysis can be tolerated if the patient is relatively healthy; on the other hand, small amounts of bleeding can cause severe complications in patients who have limited pulmonary reserve from COPD, previous lung resection, tuberculosis, or heart disease. Mortality from severe hemoptysis does correlate with the estimated amount of hemoptysis. However, with additional approaches to diagnosis and management now available, one considers both the severity of bleeding and the patient's ability to tolerate accumulation of blood in the lungs and airways.

Pathophysiology & Pathogenesis

A. Mechanisms of Hemoptysis

Bleeding in the airways and lungs can result from several different mechanisms and two major sources, the bronchial arteries (systemic) and the pulmonary arteries. Disorders associated with hemoptysis are listed in Table 24–1.

1. Inflammation of the bronchi—Inflammation of the tracheobronchial mucosa is the most common cause of hemoptysis but is rarely associated with severe bleeding. Chronic bronchitis stimulates increased blood vessels and engorgement of vessels of the mucosa with blood supplied from hypertrophied bronchial arteries. Chronic bronchitis with acute exacerbation may or may not be associated with bacterial or viral infection.

2. Infection—Worldwide, tuberculosis remains an important cause of hemoptysis, both during active infection and as a consequence of the scarring and cavitation seen

Table 24–1. Common causes of hemoptysis.[1]

Airway
Tracheobronchitis
Chronic bronchitis
Bronchogenic carcinoma
Benign tracheobronchial tumors
Bronchiectasis
Cystic fibrosis
Suctioning or bronchoscopic trauma
Post-transbronchial or endobronchial biopsy
Transthoracic needle aspiration or biopsy
Trauma
Lung parenchyma
Pulmonary infarction (pulmonary embolism)
Invasive pulmonary infection (aspergillus, bacteria)
Necrotizing bacterial or fungal pneumonia
Lung abscess
Tuberculosis with or without cavity
Pulmonary vasculitis
Goodpasture's syndrome
Idiopathic pulmonary hemosiderosis
Trauma
Thrombocytopenia
Cardiovascular
Left-ventricular failure
Mitral stenosis
Pulmonary artery rupture (PA catheter balloon)
Pulmonary artery aneurysm
Aortic aneurysm
Hereditary hemorrhagic telangiectasia

[1]Items in italics are those associated most often with massive hemoptysis.

with chronic disease. Active disease may result in hemoptysis from lung necrosis, often with a cavity visible on chest x-ray. Tuberculous cavities, however, may cause hemoptysis whether or not there are viable mycobacteria present. Bleeding arises from dilated vessels in the wall of the cavity, most often fed by an elaborately developed network of vessels arising from bronchial arteries with interconnections between these and pulmonary arteries. Rarely, aneurysmal dilation of a vessel in the wall has been known to be the cause of severe hemoptysis. An important cause of bleeding from tuberculous cavities is the development of a mycetoma or fungus ball, usually of aspergillus, that seems to further stimulate bronchial artery hypertrophy and blood flow. In tuberculosis patients without cavities, bleeding can be caused by broncholiths (calcified lymph nodes) adjacent to airways that erode through the bronchial wall and chronic bronchiectasis. Patients with other forms of bronchiectasis (previous viral infections, bronchopulmonary aspergillosis syndrome, and idiopathic cases), bacterial lung abscess, and fungal infections with cavitation may present with hemoptysis, and in occasional cases hemoptysis may be severe and life-threatening. Bacterial pneumonia can sometimes present with blood-tinged sputum, but significant bleeding is rare.

3. Noninfectious causes—Infarction of pulmonary parenchyma can result in hemoptysis by causing death of lung tissue, but most patients with pulmonary embolism do not have pulmonary infarction. Inflammation of lung due to involvement by Wegener's granulomatosis may be associated with hemoptysis, occasionally severe. Two autoimmune diseases for which hemoptysis is a characteristic feature, Goodpasture's syndrome and idiopathic pulmonary hemosiderosis, are not associated with inflammation, and bleeding arises from involvement of the alveolar-capillary interface by anti-glomerular basement membrane antibodies. Less frequent causes of hemoptysis include left ventricular failure and mitral stenosis, with bleeding resulting from increased pulmonary venous and capillary pressures. Hemoptysis may be seen with vascular malformations occurring as isolated abnormalities of the pulmonary circulation or in association with hereditary telangiectasia (Osler-Weber-Rendu syndrome).

Bronchogenic carcinoma and benign tumors of the tracheobronchial tree are other important causes of hemoptysis, with bleeding coming from hypertrophied bronchial arteries supplying the tumor. Finally, thoracic trauma may result in hemoptysis due to rupture of pulmonary vessels, resulting in bleeding into the lung parenchyma (lung contusion) or laceration of a major airway.

4. Hemoptysis in ICU patients—In ICU patients who develop hemoptysis unrelated to their primary problems, some unique mechanisms must be considered. The most common source of hemoptysis is upper airway bleeding, which may result from tracheobronchitis due to infection or repeated suctioning. However, other airway problems should be considered, such as trauma from the tip of the endotracheal tube or tracheostomy tube or necrosis of the tracheal mucosa by the tube cuff. Rarely, bleeding can arise from pressure necrosis and erosion of the tube into an innominate or carotid artery or even into the aortic arch. A recognized cause of severe hemoptysis is rupture of a pulmonary artery by a pulmonary artery catheter because of overdistention of the balloon at the tip of a pulmonary artery catheter, perforation by the tip of the catheter, or eccentric balloon placement, causing perforation by the tip during balloon inflation. In these patients, mortality is very high.

Regardless of the cause of hemoptysis, bleeding can be made worse in patients with coagulopathy, qualitative platelet dysfunction from uremia or drugs, or thrombocytopenia. Patients with severe thrombocytopenia may have spontaneous alveolar hemorrhage.

B. Massive Hemoptysis

Large amounts of hemoptysis, often called "massive hemoptysis," usually result from a smaller number of common disorders causing hemoptysis (Table 24–1). The mechanisms are often due to chronic and severe development of enhanced bronchial blood flow (tuberculosis, lung abscess, bronchiectasis, malignancy), necrosis and destruction of lung (abscess, tuberculous cavity, fungal pneumonia in immunocompromised host), or disruption of a pulmonary artery (trauma, rupture by pulmonary artery catheter balloon). In major series of patients with massive hemoptysis, tuberculosis and bronchiectasis are found in a large majority, while bronchogenic carcinoma is quite unusual as a cause of massive hemoptysis.

Clinical Features

A. Symptoms

Patients—especially those with chronic sputum production (chronic bronchitis, bronchiectasis)—may complain of coughing up blood-tinged sputum. Others will note expectoration of bright or dark red material only. The degree of coughing is highly variable, with some patients having intractable coughing and others noting only that the blood wells up into the mouth with little stimulation of cough. The relationship of prior hemoptysis to massive or life-threatening hemoptysis is highly variable. Some patients have prolonged minor hemoptysis; others have no premonitory blood in the sputum prior to severe coughing of blood. The degree of dyspnea is determined by the severity of hemoptysis and the amount of preexisting lung or heart disease. Patients with moderate to severe obstructive lung disease, those with extensive lung destruction from tuberculosis, and those with other heart or lung disorders will be most likely to have respiratory compromise. Fever, night sweats, and weight loss suggest active tuberculosis, but other infections should also be considered. A history of cigarette smoking or other risks for bronchogenic carcinoma should be sought.

An important part of the medical history is to estimate the amount of bleeding. While this cannot always be accurately measured, the patient should be asked to provide an estimate in cups, tablespoons, or other convenient measures and over as precise a time frame as possible.

B. Signs

Physical examination may be unhelpful in evaluating the severity of hemoptysis. However, the upper airway, including the nose, sinuses, pharynx, and upper larynx, should be carefully examined to exclude these sites as the source of bleeding. Localization of a lower respiratory tract site by examination (left or right lung) of hemoptysis is often inaccurate. The presence of blood in the airways may lead to generalized or focal wheezing, crackles, and dullness to percussion if there is sufficient bleeding to fill a portion of the lungs. In patients with chest trauma, rib fractures, superficial injury, and other findings may be helpful in assessing the likelihood of lung contusion, but these indicators are insensitive and nonspecific. Features of heart failure, such as a third heart sound and rales, may be helpful in the differential diagnosis, as well as findings suggesting mitral stenosis. Osler-Weber-Rendu syndrome is suggested by finding single or multiple telangiectases on the skin or mucosal membranes. The physical examination is most useful in determining the severity of respiratory and nonrespiratory disease that contribute to mortality and complications from hemoptysis.

C. Laboratory Findings

Sputum should be examined by acid-fast stain for mycobacteria, Gram stain for bacteria, and for malignant cells. The presence of a large number of red cells often makes these examinations difficult. Cultures should be made from sputum and blood if pneumonia is suspected. Coagulation times, bleeding time, platelet count, and hematocrit should be determined. Blood for transfusion should be arranged for, but blood is not often needed to correct a low hematocrit until operative treatment is indicated. Arterial blood gases are required to determine the extent of bleeding and the tolerance of the patient to further aspiration of blood into the lungs.

The presence of renal insufficiency changes the differential diagnosis of hemoptysis, so it is important to determine renal function. In one study of patients with serum creatinine > 1.5 mg/dL and any hemoptysis, no cause of hemoptysis was determined in 41% of patients, and the yield of fiberoptic bronchoscopy was very low.

D. Imaging Studies

Usual procedures such as chest x-rays and CT scan may show an infiltrate, cavity or cavities, atelectasis, or other features that suggest a lesion from which bleeding is arising. These findings should be interpreted with some caution because another unsuspected source may be present, including the opposite lung. For example, aspirated blood may cause atelectasis and infiltrates remote from the actual bleeding site. Lung cavities are often multiple, bilateral, and involve several lobes, but the cavity whence blood is coming may not be readily identified cavitary lung disease, especially in the upper lung zones, may suggest tuberculosis, but active tuberculosis cannot be diagnosed accurately from imaging studies. Furthermore, cavities are seen in fungal infection, sarcoidosis, necrotizing pneumonia, and other diseases. A mycetoma, however, can sometimes be identified on chest x-rays—especially if taken with the patient in several positions—or by CT scan. High-resolution CT scans may be very helpful in establishing a diagnosis of bronchiectasis in selected patients. Localization of bleeding may require bronchial or, rarely, pulmonary angiography (see below).

Treatment

In life-threatening hemoptysis, maintenance of the airway and removal of blood from the airway take precedence. Diagnostic measures must be deferred until it is established that the patient can maintain adequate gas exchange with or without an artificial airway, oxygen, and other measures to reverse coagulopathies or other bleeding tendencies. After the patient is stabilized, efforts are directed toward determining the site of bleeding as rapidly as possible so that definitive control of bleeding can be achieved.

The outcome of patients with hemoptysis of a large volume of blood is said to be poor, and this has strongly influenced recommended treatment. However, much of these data come from older studies in which tuberculosis caused hemoptysis from severe chronic destruction of the lungs. For example, in a series of patients from the 1950s and 1960s, those who coughed up more than 600 mL of blood within 16 hours had a 75% mortality rate, but those who produced 600 mL over 16–48 hours had a mortality rate of only 5%. About three-fourths of these patients had active or inactive tuberculosis, with the remainder having lung abscess, bronchiectasis, or bronchogenic cancer. Another study of patients who expectorated more than 600 mL of blood within 24 hours reported a 22% overall mortality rate.

The term "life-threatening" hemoptysis is preferred rather than massive hemoptysis, though the volume of expectorated blood does relate to outcome. However, asphyxiation rather than exsanguination is the most common cause of death, and for that reason the most important risk factors for mortality are the *rapidity* of blood loss and the severity of preexisting lung disease. Other prognostic signs are listed in Table 24–2, and most reflect the ability to control blood loss, maintain a patent airway, or provide for adequate gas exchange. Some studies have pointed out that spontaneous cessation of bleeding in those who have had massive hemoptysis does not necessarily predict a good short- or long-term outcome. Rebleeding is very common without definitive treatment and may occur soon after the patient has been judged to be stable or greatly improved.

A. Localization of Bleeding

Severe hemoptysis may occasionally be misidentified as upper gastrointestinal bleeding or bleeding from the nose, nasopharynx, mouth, or upper airway, but the history and examination should confirm or absolve these structures as possible sites of bleeding. The next step is to establish whether bleeding is from the trachea or from the right or left lung. Although it is tempting to conclude that an infiltrate or cavity on chest x-ray or chest CT scan indicates the site of bleeding, bilateral disease in tuberculosis, infection, and inflammatory disorders is common. The infiltrate may also represent a collection of blood brought up from the contralateral side or from a different lobe or segment.

Bronchoscopy is the procedure of choice for identification of a bleeding site in the tracheobronchial tree, and flexible fiberoptic bronchoscopy is generally preferred over rigid bronchoscopy. Bronchoscopy performed early in the course of massive hemoptysis increases the likelihood of localization. The advantages of fiberoptic bronchoscopy are patient comfort and the ability to explore farther generations of bronchi. The fiberoptic bronchoscope may be of limited use in early severe hemoptysis, because the view is easily obscured by small amounts of blood and its suctioning ability is limited by the small-diameter suction channel. Although the fiberoptic bronchoscope can be passed through a large enough endotracheal tube (usually > 8 mm), maintenance of a patent airway may be very difficult if the patient is actively bleeding. The fiberoptic bronchoscope provides very limited treatment options, such as lavage, suctioning, and balloon tamponade. On the other hand, the rigid bronchoscope can be used even during severe hemoptysis because of better ability to suction blood, maintain the airway, and provide adequate ventilation. In general, if hemoptysis subsides and the patient is stable, bronchoscopy can be delayed for several days so that the fiberoptic instrument can be used for careful inspection of the tracheobronchial tree. In more emergent situations, rigid bronchoscopy is the preferred bronchoscopic technique. Isolation of a bleeding lobe or segment by endobronchial balloon tamponade using the fiberoptic or rigid bronchoscope and lavage of the bleeding site with iced saline or vasoconstrictor agents such as epinephrine should be regarded as minor adjuncts to control of hemoptysis, and both may be difficult to perform in the face of severe hemoptysis.

Bronchial arteriography may be useful for localization of bleeding, and bronchial artery embolization (see below) is widely used for control of severe hemoptysis. The angiographic characteristics of potentially involved bronchial arteries include hypervascularity, hypertrophy, aneurysms, and bronchopulmonary anastomoses. Occasionally, no abnormalities are identified. In tuberculosis and other disorders, these changes may be seen in several locations, including bilaterally, suggesting that findings do not establish the site of bleeding with complete confidence. Because extravasation of contrast material injected into a bronchial artery is rarely if ever seen except with rapid blood loss, exact localization of a bleeding site is often not confirmed until after successful embolization. If there is no evidence of potential bronchial artery abnormalities, some investigators suggest that pulmonary arteriography should be performed to examine the pulmonary circulation as a source of bleeding.

Table 24–2. Factors contributing to life-threatening hemoptysis.

Massive hemoptysis (estimated > 600 mL blood over 24 hours)
Decreased pulmonary function (obstructive or restrictive disease)
Altered mental status or level of consciousness
Poor cough due to advanced age, sedation, neuromuscular weakness
Coagulopathy or thrombocytopenia
Mechanism of hemoptysis
Underlying disease

B. Medical Treatment

Supportive care consists of maintaining an adequate airway and introducing measures to control bleeding. Patients should be at bed rest with the suspected or known side of bleeding dependent to protect less involved parts of the lungs from filling with blood. Cough suppressants such as codeine and sedative drugs should be used cautiously, with a balance between decreasing irritation of the airway from coughing and losing the effectiveness of cough in keeping the airways clear. Vitamin K, fresh frozen plasma, and platelet transfusions should be given if indicated. Significant anemia is not usually due to acute hemoptysis, so erythrocyte transfusions are needed only if the patient has underlying anemia or other sources of blood loss. Oxygen is generally administered. Patients are often given antibiotics to decrease any inflammatory component due to acute bacterial bronchitis. If active tuberculosis is suspected, antituberculosis therapy should be started.

The best means of maintaining an adequate airway is the patient's own cough. The decision to place an endotracheal tube implies that the rate and volume of hemoptysis exceed the patient's ability to cough up blood to keep the airway clear. A cuffed endotracheal tube can be introduced into the trachea and the patient suctioned to see if this treatment is adequate to keep the airway clear. A sufficiently large tube—preferably at least 8 mm in diameter—is usually needed. If extensive bleeding continues, selective endobronchial intubation of the *nonbleeding* lung for ventilation can be performed by advancing the endotracheal tube into a main bronchus to protect the nonbleeding lung. For uncontrolled right-sided bleeding, the endotracheal tube should be inserted into the left main bronchus under fluoroscopic or bronchoscopic guidance. The left lung is selectively ventilated, and blood is allowed to come up the trachea around the tube. For left-sided bleeding, however, the endotracheal tube cuff should be placed in the trachea, and a balloon-tipped catheter (such as Fogarty-type 14F balloon) is used to seal the left main bronchus while the right lung is selectively ventilated. This method permits ventilation of the entire right lung, including the right upper lobe. Placement of the balloon-tipped catheter may be difficult while there is active bleeding.

Although the use of double-lumen endobronchial tubes for split lung ventilation during thoracic surgery has been advocated to separate the bleeding lung from the nonbleeding lung, these tubes are not easily placed by inexperienced persons and are subject to displacement even if properly situated. In addition, the two lumens are small, which may limit the amount of blood that can be suctioned. Both Carlens type double-lumen tubes and newer plastic double-lumen tubes with soft low-pressure tracheal and bronchial cuffs have been used to achieve lung separation in hemoptysis, but only experienced personnel familiar with these devices should be asked to insert them.

C. Bronchial Artery Embolization

Bronchial arteriography and selective bronchial artery embolization with artificial material have greatly changed the management of severe hemoptysis. Control of bleeding is achieved with a high degree of success in patients with a variety of causes of hemoptysis. Bronchial artery embolization is performed by identifying bronchial arteries leading to the affected side, the usual patterns consisting of one or two bronchial arteries on each side arising from the aorta between the fifth and sixth thoracic vertebrae. Branches of these arteries may also supply anterior spinal arteries and intercostal arteries. Complications of this procedure include distal arterial embolization if the catheter is not placed far enough into the selected artery and spinal cord damage if embolization is performed into a branch supplying both the bronchial artery and the spinal cord. If performed with proper care, this procedure is highly effective and may lead to long-term resolution of hemoptysis as well as short-term control prior to definitive therapy. Estimates of immediate control of bleeding by bronchial arterial embolization range as high as 90% of patients. Recurrent bleeding after successful embolization may suggest the need for repeat embolization in the same or other areas. In some patients with chronic inflammatory lung disease, identification of collateral arterial vessels may be important. In one study, lasting control of hemoptysis was achieved in 82% of patients during follow-up for as long as 24 months. Recurrent bleeding was seen with significantly greater frequency in patients with residual pulmonary disease and mycetoma.

D. Surgical Treatment

Surgical resection of the bleeding lobe or segment in patients who tolerate the procedure removes the threat of recurrent bleeding. Earlier reports of mortality rates higher than 30% from resectional surgery in massive hemoptysis are now considered to be due to ongoing bleeding, poor pulmonary function, and failure of preoperative localization of the bleeding site. Local control of bleeding by airway management or bronchial artery embolization allows surgery to be performed under controlled conditions, and emergency surgery is now quite rare, with a corresponding decrease in surgical deaths.

On the other hand, many patients with severe hemoptysis will not be surgical candidates because of extensive bilateral lung disease and severe reduction of pulmonary function. Of the remainder, medical management is usually adequate to control bleeding, and early surgical therapy is reserved for those with progressive aspiration of blood or inability to control bleeding.

There is debate about prophylactic surgical resection after severe hemoptysis has resolved. Recurrent bleeding is common after medical management in some series (25–40%), and death from hemoptysis has occurred during the initial bout of hemoptysis without warning or during a recurrent bout after bleeding had apparently ceased. This risk of recurrent life-threatening hemoptysis has prompted some to perform elective resectional surgery in all patients with hemoptysis in whom surgery is deemed tolerable. However, while there is nearly universal agreement that surgery is indicated for recurrent hemoptysis from a tuberculous or other cavity in which a mycetoma is identified, prophylactic surgery is not universally recommended. Potential candidates for resection include those with well-localized disease, adequate pulmonary function, minimal pleuropulmonary adhesions, and a high likelihood of recurrence. Results of surgical resection should be compared with the increasingly long-term experience with arterial embolization (nonsurgical management) for hemoptysis.

Dweik RA, Stoller JK: Role of bronchoscopy in massive hemoptysis. Clin Chest Med 1999;20:89–105.

Hirshberg B et al: Hemoptysis: etiology, evaluation, and outcome in a tertiary referral hospital. Chest 1997;112:440–4.

Jean-Baptiste E: Clinical assessment and management of massive hemoptysis. Crit Care Med 2000;28:1642–7.

Kallay N et al: Hemoptysis in patients with renal insufficiency: the role of fiberoptic bronchoscopy. Chest 2001;119:788–94.

DEEP VENOUS THROMBOSIS & PULMONARY THROMBOEMBOLISM

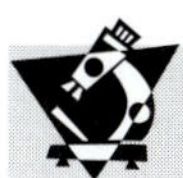

ESSENTIALS OF DIAGNOSIS

Deep venous thrombosis:

- *Risk factors, especially a chronic or acute illness, immobilization, recent surgery or orthopedic injury, hypercoagulable state.*
- *Asymmetric calf or thigh pain, or tenderness, but may be asymptomatic.*
- *Confirmation by contrast venography or duplex ultrasonography.*

Pulmonary thromboembolism:

- *May have evidence of deep venous thrombosis.*
- *Dyspnea, tachycardia, chest pain (especially pleuritic), and tachypnea. If severe, hypotension, syncope, cyanosis, or shock.*
- *Mild to moderate hypoxemia, increased $P(A\text{–}a)O_2$, and mildly reduced $PaCO_2$.*
- *Confirmation by ventilation-perfusion radionuclide scan, pulmonary angiogram, or computed tomographic angiography (helical CT scan).*

General Considerations

Venous thromboembolism is a disease thought to affect approximately 1 in every 1000 hospitalized patients in the United States and Europe. Some studies suggest that this process accounts for or contributes to over 50,000 deaths annually in the United States. Because of the difficulty of recognizing and diagnosing this syndrome, this figure may be an underestimate of its true prevalence. Deep venous thrombosis and pulmonary thromboembolism present three primary problems in the ICU. First, patients with pulmonary thromboembolism may present with severe respiratory failure or hemodynamic instability. Second, critically ill patients with a variety of medical and surgical disorders can develop pulmonary thromboembolism, complicating their underlying conditions. The diagnosis of pulmonary thromboembolism in these intensive care patients is often especially difficult to make or confirm. The usual method of treatment with anticoagulation is hazardous and may be contraindicated in some of these patients. Finally, there is increased emphasis on the prevention of deep venous thrombosis and pulmonary thromboembolism in ICU patients given that they tend to have multiple risk factors for this disease. The causative relationship between the two disorders means that the diagnosis, treatment, and prevention of both must be considered together.

Pathophysiology & Pathogenesis

A. Deep Venous Thrombosis

The pathophysiology of deep venous thrombosis centers around Virchow's triad of stasis of blood flow, intimal vascular injury, and a hypercoagulable state. It is often the failure of mechanisms that prevent the normally circulating blood from clotting in the intravascular space which leads to clot formation. A systemic hypercoagulable state can be either inherited or acquired but is identified in a small fraction of patients with venous thromboembolism. In general, these thrombophilic states do not cause a clinical thrombotic event without the presence of a second acquired risk factor or precipitating circumstance. Factor V Leiden or activated protein C resistance has been identified in up to 5% of the Caucasian population in the United States. Other hypercoagulable states include congenital or acquired deficiency of circulating anticoagulants (deficiency of protein C, protein S, or antithrombin III), prothrombin gene mutation (G20210A), abnormalities in fibrinolysis, the presence of a lupus-associated anticoagulant, and increased procoagulant activity such as occurs in some malignant diseases and severe generalized trauma. More often, patients with deep venous thrombosis have a combination of venous stasis plus local damage to the venous endothelium, exposing subendothelial procoagulant tissue factors to the blood. Obstruction of venous flow leads to edema and pain in the area drained by the affected veins. On occasion, the intravenous clot is palpable on examination as a cord.

Destruction of venous valves by this process eventually may lead to permanent local edema, pain, postphlebitic syndrome, or venous insufficiency.

Risk factors for deep venous thrombosis include immobilization of the extremity, bed rest, trauma to the extremity, severe generalized trauma, preexisting venous insufficiency, peripheral arterial disease, recent surgery, recent termination of pregnancy, pelvic disease, obesity, nephrotic syndrome, congestive heart failure, acute myocardial infarction, malignancy, estrogen therapy, and advanced age. Neurologic disease leading to immobility, especially spinal cord trauma with subsequent paralysis, is a leading risk factor for deep venous thrombosis. Severe acute illness necessitating emergency hospital admission is associated with an increased incidence of deep venous thrombosis. Patients at low but significant risk include those over age 40 who undergo major surgical procedures lasting more than 30 minutes. Lastly, the increasing use of central venous catheters in the ICU setting has led to an increasing incidence of upper extremity deep venous thrombosis.

Deep venous thrombosis develops most frequently in the posterior tibial vein, the popliteal vein just above the knee, and the common femoral vein in the thigh. A smaller number of patients with deep venous thrombosis have thrombi in the pelvic veins. While the calf vein is probably the most common site of deep venous thrombosis, only about 15–20% of these lesions will extend proximally into deep veins above the knee. It has been pointed out, however, that upper extremity deep venous thrombosis may be more frequent than previously speculated. Increased risk for deep venous thrombosis in the upper extremities may be seen in ICU patients who have short- or long-term central venous catheters inserted into internal jugular or subclavian veins. Thrombi may also be found in the right atrium, especially in patients with chronic atrial fibrillation, and in the ventricles of patients with dilated cardiomyopathy or ventricular aneurysms after myocardial infarction. Hypercoagulable states may cause clots to form in the superior and inferior venae cavae, the renal veins (especially in nephrotic syndrome), and the hepatic veins (in Budd-Chiari syndrome).

B. Pulmonary Thromboembolism

As many as 90% of patients with pulmonary thromboembolism have blood clots arising from proximal veins of the lower extremities (deep femoral veins), with the remainder having thrombi coming predominantly from pelvic veins. In a study of patients with deep venous thrombosis, perfusion lung scans were uniformly negative in those with thrombosis limited to calf veins only. This emphasizes the importance of identifying thrombi in popliteal and thigh veins or extension of clot from calf veins to proximal veins in pulmonary thromboembolism. Thrombosis of superficial veins is rarely associated with significant pulmonary embolism. With increasing use of central venous catheters there has been a reported rise in venous thrombosis and subsequent pulmonary thromboembolism from the upper extremity. A 20% risk of embolization has been cited in patients with symptomatic upper extremity thromboses.

The finding of lower extremity proximal vein deep venous thrombosis has become part of several algorithms for the diagnosis of pulmonary embolism because of the association of proximal leg deep venous thrombosis and pulmonary embolism. These data are obtained from the overall population of patients with pulmonary embolism but may not reflect findings in patients already in the ICU. Nevertheless, deep venous thrombosis of the proximal leg veins remains the most frequent source of pulmonary thromboemboli—though the frequency of calf, upper extremity, and pelvic deep venous thrombosis and of clots arising from the inferior vena cava and right atrium and ventricle is unknown in this population of critically ill patients.

The clinical manifestations of pulmonary thromboembolism reflect two pathologic processes: obstruction of the pulmonary circulation resulting in hemodynamic compromise and gas exchange abnormalities. The degree of circulatory compromise depends on the size and number of thromboemboli and the preembolic state of the right heart and pulmonary circulation. The terms massive and submassive pulmonary emboli have been applied to the angiographic occlusion of two or more lobar pulmonary arteries or greater than 50% of the pulmonary circulation as seen by noninvasive radionuclide perfusion scanning. These large or multiple emboli may or may not be associated with circulatory collapse and shock. Patients with a previously normal pulmonary circulation and right ventricular function can generally tolerate occlusion of even a large pulmonary artery with maintenance of sufficient cardiac output to avoid shock. However, acute pulmonary thromboembolism in a patient with preexisting pulmonary hypertension or heart failure may cause acute right heart failure and subsequent circulatory collapse. The same may happen to a previously normal patient in whom a large pulmonary embolus lodges in the main pulmonary artery or who has multiple moderately sized emboli in several major branches.

Occlusion of pulmonary arteries results in decreased regional perfusion of the lungs. If ventilation to these areas is maintained, then high $\dot{V}/\dot{Q}$ areas contribute to increased dead space ventilation. Minute ventilation requirements increase if Pa_{CO_2} is maintained. Arterial hypoxemia is much more common. Although the mechanism of hypoxemia is not completely understood, it probably results from a combination of ventilation-perfusion mismatching from atelectasis, redistribution of pulmonary blood flow, and increased blood transit time.

Occasionally, acute pulmonary hypertension leads to opening of a patent foramen ovale with intra-atrial right-to-left shunt and severe refractory hypoxemia.

The manifestations of pulmonary thromboembolism often appear to be greater than can be explained by the degree of vascular occlusion by thrombi. Although this is often due to lack of cardiopulmonary reserve in patients with chronic illness, it is probable that vasoactive and bronchoactive substances play a role as well as normal compensatory processes in the lung circulation and parenchyma. Among candidates for participation in the response to pulmonary embolism are products released by platelets and endothelial cells. In addition, occlusion of a pulmonary artery is associated with a decreased amount or decreased effectiveness of surfactant in the region of lung supplied by that vessel, contributing to atelectasis.

Pulmonary infarction is another potential manifestation of pulmonary thromboembolism. However, this diagnosis does not seem to alter outcome or management other than by causing different abnormalities on chest x-ray or somewhat different clinical manifestations. Pulmonary infarction is uncommon in pulmonary embolism, probably because of the dual systemic and pulmonary artery blood supplies to the lung. Patients who present with pulmonary infarction are more frequently those with congestive heart failure in whom both pulmonary venous congestion and systemic perfusion may be compromised.

Because the lungs receive the total cardiac output, a variety of other emboli can make their way into the pulmonary arterial circulation. These include pieces of tumors, particularly seen with adenocarcinomas that have eroded into the systemic veins; foreign bodies such as broken intravenous catheters or particulate matter accidentally or deliberately injected into veins; fat and tissue emboli from orthopedic injury, operative procedures, or bone marrow infarction as seen in acute chest syndrome in patients with sickle cell disease; air introduced through intravenous lines, lung rupture, or decompression during ascent from underwater diving; and amniotic fluid introduced into the systemic circulation during a tumultuous obstetric delivery. The pathophysiologic consequences of these emboli depend somewhat on the clinical situation, the size and number of emboli, and concomitant medical problems. In particular, fat emboli may result in a distinct syndrome with systemic manifestations as a result of the breakdown of free fatty acids in the microcirculation and their systemic effects.

Clinical Features

The clinical features of deep venous thrombosis and pulmonary thromboembolism are intertwined, and both can present diagnostic difficulties. Deep venous thrombosis causes nonspecific clinical findings and is sometimes found in patients with pulmonary embolism in whom thrombosis was previously unsuspected. The diagnosis of pulmonary thromboembolism can be difficult because it too presents with nonspecific symptoms, signs, and laboratory tests that suggest other acute lung and heart diseases. In the critically ill patient with preexisting cardiac or respiratory failure, pneumonia, atelectasis, pleural effusion, or infection, diagnosing superimposed pulmonary thromboembolism may be even more difficult. It is often suspected when a critically ill patient undergoes acute deterioration from previous baseline findings, manifested by tachypnea, tachycardia, and impaired gas exchange.

A. Deep Venous Thrombosis

1. Symptoms and signs—Obstruction of the deep venous system of the leg may result in edema of the lower part or the entire leg, pain, tenderness, redness or various other skin changes, and other nonspecific features. Findings are notoriously unreliable and insensitive, with as many as 50% of patients with deep venous thrombosis being asymptomatic or lacking abnormal physical findings. Clinically significant venous thrombi may not completely occlude the vascular lumen, or collateral veins and lymphatics may prevent swelling. Most blood clots do not elicit an inflammatory response unless there is additional vascular injury, so that redness and warmth are most often not present in uncomplicated deep venous thrombosis. Importantly, those patients with proximal deep venous thrombosis may have a somewhat greater tendency to have silent disease compared with those who have calf vein involvement. However, swelling above the knee or below the knee, recent immobility, cancer, and fever were found to have diagnostic value in proximal acute deep venous thrombosis. Only 5% of 95 patients had none of these five findings, while 42% had between two and five of these features.

The differential diagnosis of deep venous thrombosis in symptomatic patients includes cellulitis and other infections, popliteal cysts in those with below-the-knee swelling, septic or inflammatory arthritis, lymphatic obstruction or inflammation, external compression of deep veins, trauma, and hematomas. The finding of unilateral leg swelling does not rule out primary disease in pelvic iliac veins.

2. Diagnostic work-up—Imaging studies for deep venous thrombosis include contrast venography, noninvasive compression ultrasonography, noninvasive impedance plethysmography, radiofibrinogen scans, and magnetic resonance imaging.

Contrast venography uses injection of radiocontrast into peripheral veins of the legs to identify obstructing thrombi in the deep venous system. Twenty to 50 percent of proximal venous thrombi can usually be identified as intraluminal filling defects. Costs and complications make this test less desirable.

Duplex ultrasound uses a combination of real-time ultrasound imaging to demonstrate normal venous collapse with direct compression and Doppler venous flow assessment. Because collapse with compression is the most important feature, a more accurate name for this technique is compression ultrasonography. Failure to collapse or demonstration of intraluminal echoes is indirect evidence of deep venous thrombosis. Compression ultrasonography is practical for the popliteal vein, the common femoral vein, and often the superficial femoral vein and calf veins. It is generally regarded as having as much as 89–98% sensitivity for proximal deep venous thrombosis, and comparable specificity. It is less reliable in imaging the venous plexus in the calf. It cannot detect thrombi limited to iliac or pelvic veins. As discussed below, compression ultrasonography has been incorporated into diagnostic algorithms for diagnosis of pulmonary thromboembolism.

Impedance plethysmography utilizes the change in electrical impedance of the leg when blood flows out of the leg venous system after release of a pressure cuff. Failure to change impedance is presumptive evidence of proximal deep venous thrombosis. This test has been reported to be highly accurate for diagnosing proximal deep venous thrombosis, though other forms of venous obstruction and congestive heart failure can give false-positive results. In addition, the accuracy of the test is likely to be hospital-dependent or operator-dependent. It has been recommended that each facility establish the accuracy of impedance plethysmography compared with contrast venography. Impedance plethysmography must be performed with the leg held immobile and cannot be used if there is a plaster cast on the suspected leg. In a comparison trial of compression ultrasonography and impedance plethysmography, the predictive value of compression ultrasonography was significantly higher in symptomatic outpatients.

Radiofibrinogen leg scans demonstrate the inclusion of radiolabeled fibrinogen into actively forming thrombi. This test is primarily useful for identifying calf and lower thigh deep venous thrombosis. Only clots that are currently forming can be located with this method. It is poor in detecting proximal deep venous thrombosis. This test is rarely used today except in research protocols.

Magnetic resonance imaging and computed tomographic pulmonary angiography accompanied by venography are currently being investigated for their role in the work-up of thromboembolic disease. The advantage of these studies would be evaluation of the pulmonary vascular system for emboli combined with evaluation of the pelvis and lower extremity venous system for the source of the emboli in a single study.

Due to its invasive nature, contrast venography is obviously not appropriate for screening patients at risk for deep venous thrombosis. Both impedance plethysmography and compression ultrasonography can be used effectively for this purpose. In patients at high risk for deep venous thrombosis, such as those with pelvic or hip trauma and those with critical medical illness, compression ultrasonography is probably most sensitive and specific for proximal vein thrombosis even though there has been greater experience with impedance plethysmography. In patients with deep venous thrombosis limited to the calf, serial compression ultrasonography of patients is needed to identify during follow-up the 15–20% of patients who extend their thrombi into the proximal veins. Most clots have been found to extend proximally within the first 7 days. Thus, studies have recommended follow-up examinations within 2–3 days and again in 7–10 days if clinical suspicion for deep venous thrombosis remains high.

B. Pulmonary Embolism

1. Symptoms and signs—The clinical features of pulmonary embolism have been accurately described, and review of these findings demonstrates their nonspecificity. Table 24–3 summarizes data from a series of 500 patients comparing the clinical signs and symptoms in patients with proven pulmonary emboli by pulmonary angiography (202 patients) versus those without pulmonary embolism. Dyspnea and chest pain were the most common complaints; tachycardia, tachypnea, rales, and an increased intensity of the pulmonic component of the second heart sound were the most frequent findings on physical examination. The classic findings of hemoptysis, chest pain, and dyspnea were uncommon as a triad. Less than one-third of the total group had symptoms or signs suggesting deep venous thrombosis. While it is correct that these clinical findings do not distinguish patients with pulmonary embolism from those with other severe heart and lung diseases, patients suspected of pulmonary embolism who have cyanosis, hypotension, shock, syncope, or evidence of coexisting disease deserve particular consideration.

Symptoms and signs, nevertheless, can establish meaningful probabilities for pulmonary embolism. In one study, a clinical model for estimating probability was developed and tested. Patients suspected of this disorder were stratified into low, moderate, and high probability, and these classifications were confirmed by subsequent testing (Table 24–4). A clinical estimate of pulmonary embolism likelihood is the first step in diagnosis, followed by laboratory and imaging studies.

2. Laboratory findings—Arterial blood gases most often show mild to moderate hypoxemia, increased $P(A-a)O_2$, and mildly reduced $PaCO_2$. Almost all patients with pulmonary embolism have a $PaO_2 < 80$ mm Hg, but

Table 24–3. Symptoms and signs in 500 patients with suspected pulmonary embolism (PE).[1]

	PE Present (n = 202)	PE Absent (n = 298)
Symptoms		
Dyspnea		
Sudden onset	78%	29%
Gradual onset	6%	20%
Chest pain		
Pleuritic	44%	30%
Nonpleuritic	16%	10%
Orthopnea	1%	9%
Fainting	26%	13%
Hemoptysis	9%	5%
Cough	11%	15%
Palpitations	18%	15%
Signs		
Tachycardia, HR > 100/min	24%	23%
Cyanosis	16%	15%
Hypotension (SBP < 90 mm Hg)	3%	2%
Neck vein distention	12%	9%
Unilateral leg swelling	17%	9%
Fever > 38 °C	7%	21%
Crackles	18%	26%
Wheezes	4%	13%
Pleural friction rub	4%	4%

[1]Adapted from Miniati M et al: Accuracy of clinical assessment in the diagnosis of pulmonary embolism. Am J Respir Crit Care Med 1999;159:864–71.

no absolute level of PaO_2 can be used to exclude the diagnosis. Diagnostic accuracy may be improved somewhat by using the $P(A–a)O_2$ difference rather than the PaO_2, but again a clear distinction between those with and those without pulmonary embolism cannot always be made. In the Prospective Investigation of Pulmonary Embolism Diagnosis (PIOPED) study, 7% of patients with angiographically documented pulmonary emboli had completely normal arterial blood gas measurements on presentation. Another study found that patients suspected of pulmonary embolism, but without a history of pulmonary embolism or deep venous thrombosis and who had a normal $P(A–a)O_2$ had, only a 1.8% chance of having a pulmonary embolism. Severe hypoxemia refractory to oxygen administration may indicate the opening of a patent foramen ovale. Hypercapnia is unusual and suggests the presence of underlying lung disease.

Sinus tachycardia is the most frequent and nonspecific finding on electrocardiography in acute pulmonary embolism. Arrhythmias are unusual, but supraventricular tachycardia and atrial fibrillation are sometimes present. Features suggesting acute right heart strain on the ECG occur relatively infrequently; these include acute right axis deviation, P pulmonale, right bundle branch block, and inverted T waves and ST segment changes in right-sided leads. In the past, electrocardiographic patterns such as an S wave in lead I, Q wave in lead III, and inverted T in lead III ("S1Q3T3") and S waves in leads I, II, and III ("S1S2S3") were considered highly predictive of pulmonary embolism, but these observations were found in less than 12% of patients with pulmonary emboli in recent studies. In the differential diagnosis of pulmonary embolism, the ECG is particularly useful to assess the presence of myocardial ischemia and infarction.

D-dimer, a fibrin degradation product, is found in the plasma of patients with deep venous thrombosis and pulmonary embolism. D-dimer is the result of plasmin action (thrombolysis) on fibrin monomers that have undergone cross-linking by factor XIII to form fibrin polymers. Various methodologies are available to measure D-dimer levels. Studies have demonstrated that the ELISA assays have a higher sensitivity and negative predictive value (91–100%) when compared with the latex agglutination techniques. However, the ELISA assays are more labor-intensive, require skilled personnel, and take several hours to report a result, making them less useful clinically in an emergent situation while the semiquantitative latex agglutination studies can be performed at the bedside. A measured D-dimer less than 500 μg/L by ELISA is considered the cutoff for excluding venous thromboemboli. Current recommendations are to combine this laboratory finding with the pretest clinical probability as well as some other noninvasive evaluation to guide decision making for diagnosis and management. Thus, a low D-dimer value by itself is not enough to exclude venous thromboembolic disease. D-dimer is also of limited clinical use if the patient has had surgery or trauma in the past 3 months, underlying malignancy, sepsis with or without DIC, or abnormal liver function. Further clinical studies are under way assessing the impact of the use of this test in the diagnosis of pulmonary thromboembolism.

3. Imaging studies—Radiographic studies include nonspecific tests such as chest x-rays, examinations of the pulmonary circulation such as perfusion lung scans, computed tomographic pulmonary angiography (spiral

Table 24–4. Estimating clinical probability of pulmonary embolism (PE).[1]

	Clinical Features Typical for PE[2]						Clinical Features Not Typical for PE[3]		
	No Severe Findings[4]				**Severe Findings[4]**				
Which is more likely, PE or alternative diagnosis?	Alternative diagnosis		PE		Alternative diagnosis	PE	Alternative diagnosis	PE	
Risk factors?[5]	No	Yes	No	Yes	Yes or No	Yes or No	Yes or No	No	Yes
Estimated probability of PE	Low 3%	Mod 28%	Mod 28%	High 80%	Mod 28%	High 80%	Low 3%	Low 3%	Mod 28%

[1]Modified from Wells PS et al: Use of a clinical model for safe management of patients with suspected pulmonary embolism. Ann Intern Med 1998;129:997–1005.
[2]Typical findings for PE: Any two or more of the following: dyspnea, pleuritic chest pain, nonretrosternal nonpleuritic chest pain, arterial O_2 saturation < 92% on room air that corrects with < 40% FIO_2, hemoptysis, pleural rub.
[3]Does not have typical findings for PE listed above.
[4]Severe findings: syncope, SBP < 90 mm Hg and heart rate > 100/min, mechanical ventilation or FIO_2 > 40%, or new-onset RV failure (RBBB, elevated jugular venous pressure).
[5]Risk factors: Surgery < 12 weeks, complete bed rest > 3 days within 4 weeks, prior deep venous thrombosis or pulmonary embolism, lower extremity fracture and immoblization < 12 weeks previously, strong family history of deep venous thrombosis or pulmonary embolism, cancer (palliative treatment or ongoing treatment), postpartum, lower extremity paralysis.

or helical CT scans) and pulmonary angiograms, as well as studies directed at finding deep venous thrombosis.

a. Chest x-ray—The chest x-ray is most useful in identifying coexisting problems such as pneumonia, lung mass, lymphadenopathy, pulmonary edema, atelectasis, or pleural effusion. The most common findings in pulmonary embolism without coexisting disease are nonspecific, including no visible abnormality, plate-like atelectasis, or small pleural effusion. Thus, a normal chest x-ray in a patient with shortness of breath and hypoxemia should prompt a further evaluation for pulmonary embolism. Findings suggestive of pulmonary vascular occlusion, such as an apparent cutoff of a segmental or lobar pulmonary artery, regional hyperlucency of the lung parenchyma or oligemia (Westermark's sign), or a wedge-shaped density consistent with pulmonary infarction, may suggest pulmonary embolism but are insensitive and lack specificity.

b. Radionuclide ventilation-perfusion scan—The ventilation-perfusion lung scan is currently the test most often used to diagnose pulmonary embolism. However, scan results must be considered carefully because these tests do not have perfect diagnostic accuracy. To perform the perfusion lung scan, a small quantity of radionuclide-labeled macroaggregated albumin is injected into a peripheral vein, after which the labeled particles become trapped in the pulmonary capillary bed. Uniform distribution of the radionuclide throughout the lung fields implies the absence of significant localized pulmonary arterial obstruction, whereas a pulmonary embolism occluding a pulmonary artery will result in an area of absent radionuclide (a perfusion defect). Unfortunately, perfusion defects commonly result from other causes, including focal atelectasis, pneumonia, and bronchospasm.

To improve the diagnostic value of the perfusion scan, the uniformity of ventilation is assessed using a ventilation scan, performed by inhalation of either radioactive xenon or an aerosol containing a radiolabeled solute. The perfusion and ventilation scans are then compared. A perfusion defect *without* a corresponding ventilation defect in the same area (mismatched defect) is generally considered supportive of the diagnosis of pulmonary embolism if the perfusion defect is of sufficient size. On the other hand, a perfusion defect with a corresponding ventilation defect (matched defect) is generally considered indeterminate (ie, not helpful in making a diagnosis of pulmonary embolism) or due to other kinds of heart or lung disease such as pneumonia or bronchospasm.

By convention, ventilation-perfusion lung scans are interpreted as normal (no perfusion defects), low or high probability for pulmonary embolism, or intermediate probability (sometimes called indeterminate) for pulmonary embolism. Recent prospective studies have greatly clarified the meaning of these interpretations and have led to the development of currently accepted diagnostic strategies for pulmonary embolism. The PIOPED multicenter study compared lung scan results with pulmonary angiography in patients with suspected pulmonary embolism. Table 24–5 is a modified summary of lung scan categories and criteria used in 931 patients included in this study.

Table 24–5. PIOPED lung scan interpretation criteria (modified).

High probability
- ≥ 2 large (> 75% of the segment), or
- ≥ 2 moderate (25–75% of the segment) plus one large, or
- ≥ 4 moderate mismatched perfusion lung scan defects

Low probability
- Nonsegmental perfusion defects only, or
- One moderate mismatched segmental perfusion defect with normal chest x-ray, or
- Any perfusion defect with a larger chest x-ray abnormality, or
- Limited number of large or moderate perfusion defects with matching ventilation defects (with normal or mildly abnormal chest x-ray)

Intermediate probability
- Not falling into normal, low, or high-probability categories
- Borderline high or borderline low
- Difficult to categorize as high or low

Normal
- No perfusion defects, or
- Perfusion outlines exactly the shape of lungs seen on chest x-ray (chest x-ray or ventilation lung scan may be abnormal)

Of patients with suspected pulmonary embolism enrolled in this study, ventilation-perfusion lung scans were interpreted to indicate a high probability of pulmonary embolism in 13% and were normal or nearly normal in 14% of the scans. Intermediate or low probability was the conclusion in 73%. The sensitivity, specificity, and likelihood ratios of lung scan interpretations for angiographically diagnosed pulmonary emboli are shown in Table 24–6. The likelihood of pulmonary embolism parallels the interpretation of the lung scans, especially when used in conjunction with the pretest clinical likelihood of pulmonary embolism. A reading of *any* probability (low, intermediate, or high) of pulmonary embolism on lung scan resulted in 98% sensitivity but low specificity. This meant that all other readings accounted for only 2% of patients with pulmonary embolism, but the "any probability" group also included an excessively large number without pulmonary embolism. Unfortunately, only 41% of cases of angiographically diagnosed pulmonary embolism were associated with high-probability lung scans, whereas 42% had intermediate-probability scans and 17% had low-probability scans. It is emphasized that patients with low-probability lung scans are found to have pulmonary emboli about 15–30% of the time.

These data, confirmed by results from other well-designed prospective studies, support the idea that ventilation-perfusion lung scans are of greatest utility when they show high probability for pulmonary embolism (87% likelihood of pulmonary embolism in all patients suspected of pulmonary embolism; 96% if clinical suspicion is high) or when they are normal (nil to 4% likelihood of pulmonary embolism during long-term follow-up even if clinical suspicion was high). Thus, high-probability lung scans effectively predict pulmonary embolism, while a normal scan (no perfusion defects) effectively rules out pulmonary embolism. Treatment or withholding of treatment can be guided by this rule with considerable confidence. However, the majority of patients suspected of having pulmonary embolism will fall into the categories of intermediate or low probability, and substantial numbers within each category will or will not actually have the

Table 24–6. Sensitivity, specificity, likelihood ratios, and posttest probabilities of ventilation-perfusion radionuclide lung scanning for pulmonary embolism.

Instructions: For a patient with suspected pulmonary embolism, estimate pretest probability (clinical information or clinical information plus results of prior tests). Find posttest probability at intersection of pretest probability (columns) and scan results (rows).

				Pretest Probability				
				3%	10%	28%	50%	80%
Scan Result	**Sensitivity**	**Specificity**	**Likelihood Ratio**	**Posttest Probability**				
High probability	41%	97%	17.1	35%	66%	87%	94%	99%
Indeterminate	41%	62%	1.1	3%	11%	30%	52%	81%
Low probability	16%	60%	0.4	1%	4%	13%	29%	62%
Near-normal or normal	2%	81%	0–0.1	0%	0–1%	0–4%	0–9%	0–29%

disease. Furthermore, it should be emphasized that these studies have characterized mostly patients who were not critically ill in whom the appropriate studies could be performed and compared. The predictive value of lung scans may not be comparable in patients with multiple medical problems, including severe heart and lung disease.

c. **Combination imaging**—Three approaches for improving diagnostic accuracy when lung ventilation-perfusion scanning is nondiagnostic have evolved (Figure 24–1). The traditionally used strategy is to perform pulmonary angiography for all suspected patients in whom intermediate probability lung scans are found

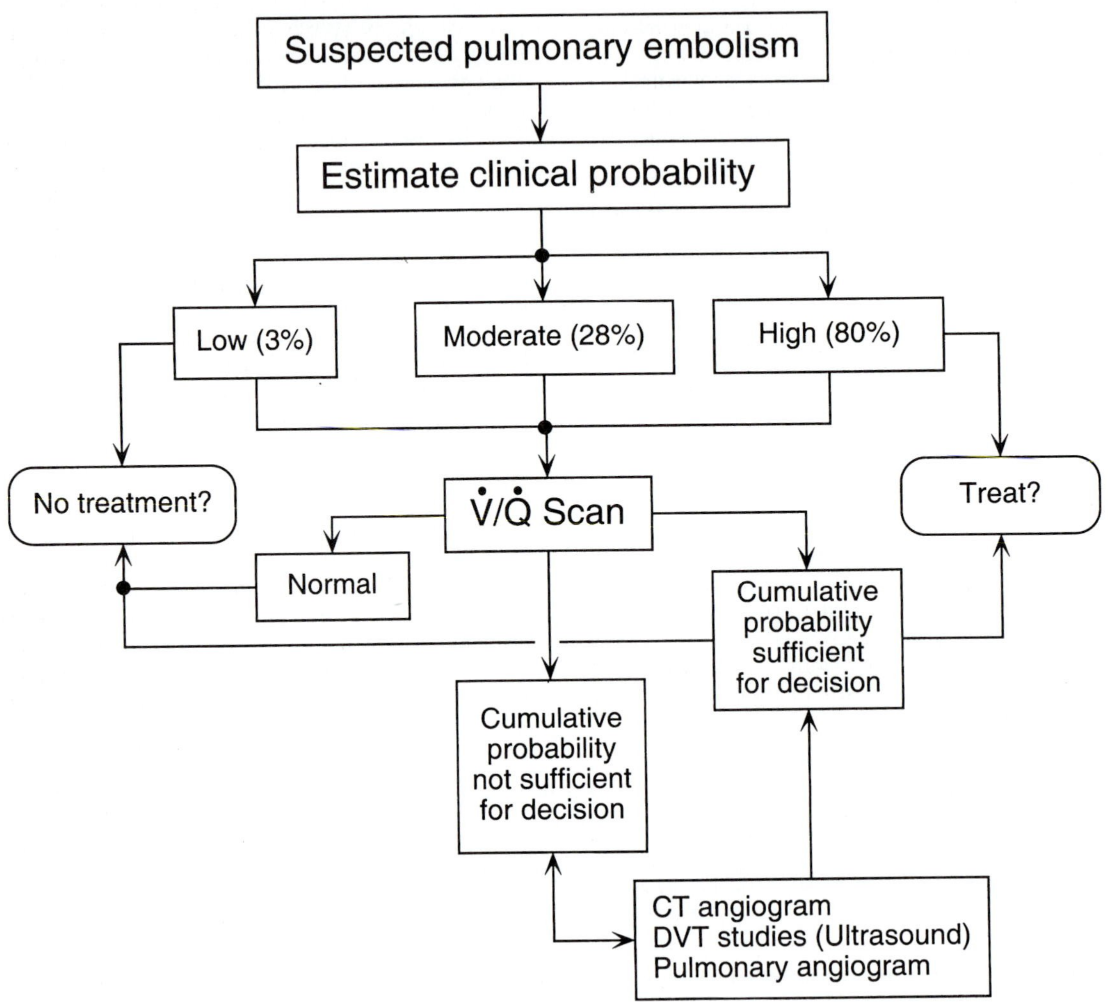

Figure 24–1. One suggested approach to a patient with suspected pulmonary embolism. After estimation of clinical probability (Table 24–4), almost all patients should have ventilation-perfusion scanning. Exceptions include the following: (1) patients with preexisting lung disease likely to result in uninterpretable scans; (2) clinically unstable patients; (3) patients in whom a very strong probability of pulmonary embolism is estimated to be present; and (4) patients with a very low clinical probability of pulmonary embolism in whom the risk of treatment outweighs the potential benefits of treatment. If the cumulative probability of clinical estimation plus ventilation-perfusion scanning is sufficient to begin or withhold treatment, diagnostic studies are completed. If not, further studies are required (CT angiogram, compression ultrasonography, or pulmonary angiography) until a decision can be reached. Any decision to begin or withhold treatment must take into account the risk of treatment compared with the potential benefits of treatment.

(pulmonary embolism present by angiography in 16–66% depending on clinical suspicion), or in whom a low-probability lung scan is associated with high or uncertain clinical suspicion (pulmonary embolism found in 16–40%). A normal pulmonary angiogram is quite accurate in ruling out pulmonary embolism, with fewer than 1% of patients with negative pulmonary angiograms subsequently proving to have pulmonary embolism *without treatment* during long-term follow-up or at autopsy. This approach would be ideal if it were not for problems encountered with obtaining pulmonary angiography, including limited availability, uncertain reliability in all hospitals, and risks of vascular catheterization and radiographic contrast agents. Furthermore, in critically ill patients, the transport to a suitable area for this procedure may be associated with high risk, less-than-optimal monitoring, and fewer therapeutic interventions. Small amounts of contrast material, selective pulmonary angiography, nonionic contrast media, and careful preinjection measurement of pulmonary artery pressure reduce the frequency of complications from pulmonary angiography. Pulmonary hypertension is a relative contraindication because of reported morbidity and mortality from injecting additional volume into a system already under high pressure. Other complications, including death, respiratory distress leading to intubation, renal failure, and hematoma requiring transfusion are reported to occur in up to 4% of critically ill patients undergoing pulmonary angiography.

Using this diagnostic strategy, pulmonary angiography should be performed in patients with indeterminate or low-probability lung scans with high clinical suspicion, especially when treatment is particularly risky or confirmation of diagnosis is particularly important. For example, pulmonary angiography used to be performed in patients being considered for thrombolytic therapy, but this recommendation is being questioned because of the subsequent risk of bleeding. A bleeding risk as high as 20% when thrombolytics are given after an angiogram has been reported. The major disadvantage of this approach is that a large number of patients would require pulmonary angiography because of abnormal but nondiagnostic lung scans. In some studies, patients making up this group comprise 40–60% of the total enrolled.

A second approach recognizes the close relationship between pulmonary thromboembolism and deep venous thrombosis. Proximal vein deep venous thrombosis is found on initial testing in about 50% of patients with pulmonary embolism. In patients with low-probability or intermediate-probability ventilation-perfusion lung scans but with high or uncertain clinical probability of pulmonary embolism, compression ultrasonography or impedance plethysmography may be performed. A combination of high or uncertain clinical suspicion, abnormal (but not high-probability) lung scan, and positive noninvasive test for deep venous thrombosis strongly supports the diagnosis of pulmonary embolism. Treatment should be initiated on the basis of this result. But the absence of evidence of deep venous thrombosis should not rule out pulmonary embolism because the false-negative rate of a single noninvasive test for deep venous thrombosis ranges from as low as 3% to as high as 30%. Therefore, these patients must undergo pulmonary angiography or serial duplex ultrasonography (see below). Nevertheless, the combination of lung scan and noninvasive deep venous thrombosis studies decreases the number of pulmonary angiograms needed in these groups of patients from about 72% to 33%. An outcome analysis of a variety of diagnostic strategies addressing patients in these categories concluded that the most effective strategy was pulmonary angiography if perfusion-ventilation lung scans were nondiagnostic and compression ultrasonography results were negative.

Lastly, a completely noninvasive strategy for selected patients has been proposed. In patients suspected of pulmonary embolism who have abnormal but nondiagnostic lung scans (low or intermediate probability) and adequate cardiopulmonary reserve (lack of respiratory failure, hypotension, severe underlying lung disease, and severe tachycardia), *serial* noninvasive tests for proximal lower extremity deep venous thrombosis are performed (impedance plethysmography or compression ultrasonography). If evidence of deep venous thrombosis is found initially or subsequently, treatment is started. However, if no evidence of deep venous thrombosis is found, anticoagulation is withheld while noninvasive deep venous thrombosis studies are repeated every 2–3 days for about 10 days, then approximately a week later. In a study of 627 untreated patients with suspected pulmonary embolism with nondiagnostic lung scans and negative serial impedance plethysmographic studies over 2 weeks, pulmonary thromboembolism occurred in only 1.9% over the next 3 months. Treatment can therefore be withheld in this group of patients with acceptable results. In fact, this approach clarifies the natural history of pulmonary thromboembolism in that extension of the pulmonary embolus itself rarely occurs without treatment—and treatment is directed solely at prevention of extension of the venous thrombus. This noninvasive approach can be used to avoid pulmonary angiography in some patients with nondiagnostic lung scans. For critically ill patients, however, this strategy may not be feasible because of concomitant heart and lung disease and lack of cardiopulmonary reserve. In addition, patients being considered for therapy other than anticoagulation, such as thrombolytic therapy, cannot be appropriately evaluated using this method. It is likely that further studies using this noninvasive approach will be forthcoming.

d. Helical (spiral) computed tomographic pulmonary angiography—Newer imaging studies are currently being rigorously evaluated for their role in the diagnostic workup of pulmonary thromboembolism. The development of helical (spiral) and electron-beam computed tomographic (CT) pulmonary angiography appears very promising, with reported sensitivities greater than 80% and specificities of greater than 90% for diagnosing pulmonary emboli in the main, lobar, and segmental pulmonary arteries. It has been found to be less accurate in identifying thrombi in subsegmental arteries. The clinical impact of emboli in these subsegmental arteries is unclear and may not pose the same morbidity and mortality risks as emboli in larger segments. However, in patients with a limited cardiopulmonary reserve, emboli in subsegmental arteries could potentially be devastating. Newer CT techniques including thin collimation (2–3 mm instead of 5 mm) and faster acquisition timing may improve the evaluation of these subsegmental vessels. An advantage of these imaging studies is their ability to provide additional information with regard to other disease processes that may be responsible for the patient's clinical presentation such as pneumonic infiltrates, pleural disease, mediastinal lymphadenopathy, or parenchymal masses. CT imaging requires the administration of intravenous contrast and a degree of patient cooperation with the ability to hold the breath for approximately 25 seconds in order to obtain good quality pictures of the vasculature. In a small but important proportion of studies, the results are not acceptable because of movement artifacts or inadequate concentration of contrast boluses in the pulmonary arteries.

The exact role of these CT imaging techniques in the workup of pulmonary thromboembolic disease is still being evaluated, and CT imaging may eventually replace both the ventilation-perfusion scan and the pulmonary angiogram. Because of concern about the overall sensitivity of CT imaging but with acceptable specificity, the helical CT can be used to diagnose pulmonary thromboembolism if a thrombus is seen but may not be able to exclude significant pulmonary artery thrombi if clots are not visualized. A strategy of performing helical CT rather than ventilation-perfusion scanning has been used. A negative study in the face of sufficient clinical suspicion requires a subsequent pulmonary angiogram, while a positive study leads to treatment with anticoagulants. At the present time, this strategy is supported by relatively strong clinical evidence. On the other hand, whether CT imaging is sufficiently sensitive to replace pulmonary angiography remains to be seen; a definitive study would require prospective analysis of suspected pulmonary thromboembolism patients with negative helical CT scans who are not given anticoagulation. If an acceptably low number have recurrent thromboembolism or other complications due to thromboembolism, helical CT may supplant pulmonary angiography.

CT imaging of the pelvis and lower extremities during the same CT study to evaluate the venous system for the source of the embolus is also being investigated. Magnetic resonance imaging (MRI) of both the pulmonary vasculature and the venous system of the pelvis and lower extremity may also have a future role in the workup of this disease. The advantage would be similar to that of the CT scan but without the use of intravenous contrast, which carries its own set of risks including anaphylactic reactions and renal failure.

4. Diagnostic approach to pulmonary thromboembolism—A number of algorithms based on optimizing diagnostic strategies have been proposed. A logical approach is to assess pretest probability (clinical) from symptoms and signs, then apply tests that increase or decrease the probability of disease (posttest probability). In this way, the likelihood of pulmonary embolism can be estimated and the risks of treatment compared. Table 24–4 assigns low, moderate, and high clinical estimates for disease based on clinical findings. Validation of these data using pulmonary angiography or high-probability ventilation-perfusion scans confirmed that these groups had 3%, 28%, and 80% likelihoods of pulmonary embolism.

The clinician must decide whether these probabilities are a sufficient basis for decisions about whether or not to treat a patient. If a more certain diagnosis is warranted—and this is almost always the case with clinical information alone—another diagnostic test is applied. Most often that test is ventilation-perfusion radionuclide scanning. Exceptions include (1) patients with preexisting lung disease likely to result in uninterpretable scans; (2) clinically unstable patients; (3) patients in whom the probability of pulmonary embolism is very high; and (4) patients with a very low clinical probability of pulmonary embolism in whom the risk of treatment outweighs the benefits of treatment. Table 24–6 shows the posttest probability for various scan results for different pretest (clinical) probabilities. If the probability is sufficiently high to justify starting treatment or sufficiently low to justify withholding treatment, further diagnostic tests are not indicated. If more diagnostic certainly is desired, then noninvasive studies—compression ultrasonography, pulmonary angiography, or CT angiography (helical CT)—can be performed. For decision making purposes, the pulmonary angiogram is assumed to have 100% specificity; ie, a negative study excludes pulmonary embolism. The probabilities of pulmonary embolism when assessed by CT angiography, compression ultrasonography, D-dimer, and other diagnostic tests are set forth in Table 24–7. These tests can be applied sequentially to support the diagnosis or to exclude the diagnosis, though, to be sure, these estimates are derived from dif-

Table 24–7. Sensitivity, specificity, likelihood ratios, and posttest probabilities of compression ultrasonography, D-dimer, and helical CT pulmonary angiography for pulmonary embolism.

Instructions: For a patient with suspected pulmonary embolism, estimate pretest probability and find posttest probability at intersection of pretest probability (columns) and test results (rows).

Compression Ultrasonography (for Patient With Symptoms of DVT)

				Pretest Probability				
				3%	10%	28%	50%	80%
Sensitivity	Specificity	Test Result	Likelihood Ratio	Posttest Probability				
95%	95%	Positive	19	37%	68%	88%	95%	99%
		Negative	0.05	0%	1%	2%	5%	17%

Compression Ultrasonography (for Patient Without Symptoms of DVT)

				Pretest Probability				
				3%	10%	28%	50%	80%
Sensitivity	Specificity	Test Result	Likelihood Ratio	Posttest Probability				
62%	97%	Positive	21	39%	70%	89%	95%	99%
		Negative	0.39	1%	4%	13%	28%	61%

D-Dimer (ELISA)

				Pretest Probability				
				3%	10%	28%	50%	80%
Sensitivity	Specificity	Test Result	Likelihood Ratio	Posttest Probability				
31–65%	97–100%	Positive	1.4–2.8	4–8%	14–24%	36–52%	59–65%	92–95%
		Negative	0.0–0.07	0%	0–1%	0–3%	0–6%	0–21%

Helical CT Pulmonary Angiogram

				Pretest Probability				
				3%	10%	28%	50%	80%
Sensitivity	Specificity	Test Result	Likelihood Ratio	Posttest Probability				
78–97%	53–100%	Positive	3.5–32	10–49%	28–78%	58–92%	78–97%	93–99%
		Negative	0.05–0.48	0–1%	1–5%	2–16%	5–33%	17–66%

ferent studies of different populations. While they are not strictly independent estimates, the combined probabilities are still likely to have value. Any decision to begin or withhold treatment must take into account the risk of treatment compared with its potential benefit.

Treatment

A. Anticoagulation

Anticoagulation is the major therapy for deep venous thrombosis involving proximal veins of the leg or pelvic veins and pulmonary embolism. Intravenous heparin is most often given for 4–5 days, overlapping with oral anticoagulant therapy beginning on day 1, and followed by oral anticoagulant agents alone for at least 3 months. There are a variety of other treatment schedules. Heparin therapy can be started immediately before any definitive tests are performed, and a diagnosis of deep venous thrombosis or pulmonary embolism is made if there is a strong clinical suspicion and no contraindications. Heparin should also be started once a diagnosis of deep venous thrombosis or pulmonary embolism is made. Anticoagulants do not directly affect existing thrombi, but if given in sufficient amounts they prevent further clot growth until normal fibrinolysis can act.

In the absence of contraindications, initial treatment should be with heparin in the form of continuous intravenous infusion of unfractionated heparin or subcutaneous low-molecular-weight heparin. To begin therapy with continuous unfractionated heparin, an infusion of heparin is given at a dose that achieves and maintains a stable activated partial thromboplastin time (aPTT) of 1.5–2.5 times control when measured at 6-hour intervals. The partial thromboplastin time can then be measured at approximately daily intervals once this goal range has been achieved. Failure to achieve an aPTT at least in the lower level of this range within the first 24 hours of therapy has been associated with recurrent venous thromboembolism in patients with deep venous thrombosis.

Standard heparin dose adjustment protocols or nomograms for deep venous thrombosis and pulmonary thromboembolism are highly desirable and have been shown to increase therapeutic efficacy and reduce bleeding complications. One weight-based nomogram is shown in Table 24–8. A bolus of 80 units/kg of unfractionated heparin is given, followed by 18 units/kg/h. For a 60 kg adult, this corresponds to 4800 units as a bolus followed by 1080 units/h or about 26,000 units/d. Concern has been expressed that the maintenance dose of heparin is frequently underestimated, resulting in recurrent deep venous thrombosis or pulmonary thromboemboli. The mean heparin requirement in several studies was approximately 1300 units/h (about 31,000 units/24 h) compared with older studies suggesting that 1000 units/h was usually adequate. The dose is adjusted upward or downward as needed based on the aPTT. Although this nomogram should be strictly used only when the same reagent is employed as in the development of the nomogram, it should prove useful as a guide in all hospitals. It is important to remember that a lower therapeutic range for

Table 24–8. Body weight-based dosing of intravenous heparin.[1]

Initial dosing

Loading: 80 units/kg
Maintenance infusion: 18 units/kg/h using 25,000 units in 250 mL D5W (100 units/mL)
Obtain aPTT before and 6 hours after starting heparin

Subsequent dose adjustments based on aPTT measured at 6-hour intervals[2]

aPTT (s)	Rate Change (units/kg/h)	Additional Action	Next aPTT
< 35 (< 1.2 × normal)	+4	Rebolus with 80 units/kg	6 hours
35–45 (1.2–1.5 × normal)	+2	Rebolus with 40 units/kg	6 hours
46–70 (1.5–2.3 × normal)	0	None	6 hours
71–90 (2.3–3.0 × normal)	–2	None	6 hours
> 80 (> 3 × normal)	–3	Stop infusion for 1 hour	6 hours

[1]Modified from Hyers TM: Venous thromboembolism. Am J Respir Crit Care Med 1999;159:1–14.
[2]During the first 24 hours, repeat aPTT every 6 hours. Thereafter, obtain aPTT every morning unless it is outside the therapeutic range.

the aPTT on heparin is recommended for patients with acute myocardial ischemia receiving thrombolytics or glycoprotein IIb/IIIa antagonists. Therefore, heparin dosing schedules cannot be interchanged.

Low-molecular-weight (LMW) heparins differ from standard unfractionated heparin in their pharmacokinetics, bioavailability, and anticoagulant activity and have now found a role in the treatment of deep venous thrombosis and pulmonary embolism. These heparin fractions have greater bioavailability when given subcutaneously, longer duration of action allowing for once or twice daily dosing, and predictable anti-factor Xa activity. The anticoagulation effects of LMW heparin can be correlated with body weight for dosing purposes, and this diminishes the need for following laboratory parameters to ensure adequate anticoagulation. In direct comparisons, LMW heparins have been associated with fewer major bleeding complications, less thrombocytopenia, and a lower incidence of osteoporosis when compared with unfractionated heparins. All LMW heparin formulations cross-react with unfractionated heparins and cannot be used as an alternative form of anticoagulation in patients with heparin-induced thrombocytopenia syndrome. Dosage adjustments may be necessary in patients with morbid obesity and it should not be used in patients with renal dysfunction. Each LMW heparin formulation has its own distinct pharmacokinetic profile, so that data on one form cannot be readily extrapolated to another form in the same class. In the treatment of deep venous thrombosis and pulmonary thromboembolism, the 2001 American College of Chest Physicians (ACCP) Consensus recommendations are as follows: enoxaparin sodium, 1 mg/kg subcutaneously every 12 hours or 1.5 mg/kg subcutaneously daily (single daily dose not to exceed 180 mg/d); or tinzaparin sodium, 175 anti-Xa IU/kg subcutaneously daily.

In addition to heparin, oral warfarin can be started on day 1 unless there are contraindications to its use. Warfarin, an anticoagulant that inhibits synthesis of vitamin K dependent coagulation factors, becomes an effective anticoagulant only after disappearance of previously synthesized circulating coagulation factors. Thus, several days are needed for warfarin to have an antithrombotic effect. In the past, concern has been raised about a potential hypercoagulable state induced by warfarin because synthesis of protein C and protein S, naturally occurring anticoagulants, is also inhibited by this agent. This problem is very rarely encountered.

Almost all patients can be started with a single oral dose of warfarin at 5 mg per day. The goal is to achieve an international normalized ratio (INR) of 2.5 (range 2.0–3.0). This corresponds roughly to a prolongation of the prothrombin time to 1.3–1.5 times normal (using the usual tissue thromboplastin assay employed in laboratories in North America). Nomograms for warfarin dosing suggest that the INR measured at least 15 hours after the first dose is helpful in deciding on subsequent doses. If the first INR > 1.5, a very low maintenance dose (1 mg) is probably sufficient; an INR between 1.2 and 1.3 calls for a dose of 2–3 mg/d. All other patients should receive a second oral dose of 5 mg and should be monitored by continued daily INR measurements. Heparin can be discontinued after 4–5 days if the INR is > 2.0.

The dose of warfarin should be adjusted according to the prothrombin time. Initially, the prothrombin time should be measured daily until a stable INR is achieved. Thereafter, twice-weekly measurements followed by weekly measurements should be adequate. A number of drugs interact with warfarin, both increasing and decreasing its effectiveness. Antibiotics in particular may decrease bacterial flora of the gut that are responsible for a significant amount of vitamin K synthesis. In the ICU, other drugs that may prolong the prothrombin time by potentiating the action of warfarin include aspirin, nonsteroidal anti-inflammatory drugs, omeprazole, and amiodarone as well as antibiotics such as most cephalosporins, erythromycin, fluconazole, and metronidazole. On the other hand, barbiturates, rifampin, and carbamazepine may reduce the effect of warfarin on the prothrombin time. Warfarin and other oral anticoagulant drugs are contraindicated during pregnancy because of the potential for abnormal fetal development.

The optimal duration of anticoagulation therapy for deep venous thrombosis and pulmonary embolism has not been determined for all clinical situations and depends on underlying predisposing risk factors. Studies have shown that heparin followed by 3 months of warfarin results in an acceptably low (< 5%) frequency of recurrent deep venous thrombosis in patients who do not have identifiable risk factors. This applies only to patients with a first event whose predisposing risk factor—such as immobilization from a broken bone, surgery, or trauma—has resolved. For patients with a first episode of idiopathic venous thromboembolism (no identifiable risk factor), at least 6 months of anticoagulation therapy is recommended. On the other hand, patients in whom risk factors are long-term and poorly reversible, such as those with chronic congestive heart failure or hypercoagulable states, should receive a longer period of anticoagulation therapy—on the order of 12 months or even indefinitely. In patients with a hypercoagulable state associated with malignancy, the effectiveness of anticoagulation is highly variable. Patients unable to receive warfarin should be given either subcutaneous heparin at a dosage sufficient to prolong the aPTT more than 1.5 times control (adjusted-dose subcutaneous heparin) or daily LMW heparin.

The major complication of unfractionated heparin therapy is bleeding, occurring in about 5% (about 1% in those with low risk for bleeding, about 10% in those with high risk). Low-molecular-weight heparins have imposed a lower risk of major bleeding events when used in the setting of venous thromboembolism. Bleeding is usually not spontaneous but due to some underlying cause. Heparin-induced thrombocytopenia may contribute to bleeding, as may also simultaneous administration of antiplatelet agents such as aspirin or dextran. Warfarin and other oral anticoagulant agents are also associated with bleeding complications. Bleeding has been demonstrated to be less common when excessively prolonged coagulation times are avoided.

The effect of heparin can be quickly counteracted by protamine and by discontinuing administration. Nonbleeding patients on warfarin with excessively high INR in the range of 4.0–5.0 can safely have warfarin withheld until the INR falls into the therapeutic range. For INR values 5.0–9.0, low-dose vitamin K (1–2.5 mg oral phytonadione) is indicated if there is bleeding or high risk of bleeding. If the INR is greater than 9.0 and associated with bleeding, oral or parenteral vitamin K in larger doses (10 mg) is necessary. Reversal of the effects of warfarin can take several hours to correct the INR. Conversely, restoration of the desired anticoagulated state may be difficult and prolonged if too much vitamin K is given. Fresh frozen plasma contains the vitamin K-dependent factors inhibited by warfarin, and this product can be given to reverse the prothrombin time relatively quickly.

An important complication of heparin use is heparin-induced thrombocytopenia syndrome, an immune-mediated disease that is associated with both bleeding and venous and arterial thrombotic complications. This syndrome should be suspected when the platelet count falls precipitously in a patient receiving any form of heparin. It is seen in approximately 3–4% of patients receiving unfractionated heparin and fewer patients receiving LMW heparin. Treatment for this syndrome includes immediate discontinuation of all heparin administration of any kind, including intravenous flushes. If anticoagulation is still necessary for the patient's primary disease process, heparinoids such as danaparoid or recombinant lepirudin can be used. Warfarin should not be used alone.

B. Thrombolytic Therapy

Thrombolytic agents currently approved for use in venous thromboembolic disease are urokinase, streptokinase, and alteplase (tissue plasminogen activator). Deep venous thrombosis, especially in patients with extensive iliofemoral thrombosis, is now an approved indication for use of thrombolytic agents urokinase or streptokinase for a 48- to 72-hour infusion regimen in the United States. In studies in which thrombolytic therapy was given for pulmonary embolism, deep venous thrombosis resolved more rapidly, and there was evidence that destruction of venous valves was lessened, decreasing the pain, swelling, and potential for postphlebitic venous insufficiency. However, thrombolytic therapy should be individualized, and larger trials are needed to develop recommendations based on the benefits versus the risks of their use in deep venous thrombosis.

In short-term studies of pulmonary embolism, thrombolytic therapy is associated with faster clot lysis compared with heparin, decreased pulmonary hypertension, improved pulmonary perfusion, and subsequent higher pulmonary capillary blood volume as assessed by carbon monoxide diffusing capacity. A trend toward lower death rates in patients with pulmonary embolism treated with urokinase followed by heparin compared with those given heparin alone was seen in one trial; in the first 2 weeks of treatment, 7% died in the urokinase group compared with 9% in the heparin group. Lower numbers of recurrent pulmonary emboli in the urokinase-treated group were also found. Despite these results, many physicians believe that the benefits of thrombolytic therapy compared with anticoagulation alone are not clearly proved for patients with pulmonary embolism. Thus, the vast majority of patients are treated with heparin and oral anticoagulation alone.

Thrombolytic therapy has been considered most often in the setting of "massive pulmonary embolism," described as clot occupying over 50% of the pulmonary vascular bed. If the patient has preexisting cardiopulmonary disease, occlusion of 20% of the pulmonary vascular bed may be considered "massive." Rather than the size of the thromboembolism itself, this syndrome may also be defined by the presence of severe hemodynamic compromise with hypotension, shock, or severe gas exchange abnormalities. Several small clinical trials of patients with severe large pulmonary emboli have shown faster lysis of clot in the pulmonary circulation, reduction of pulmonary artery pressure, and improved cardiac output with the combination of thrombolytic agent and heparin compared with heparin alone.

At present, thrombolytic therapy should be considered in patients with acute massive embolism who are hemodynamically unstable and who appear to be able to tolerate thrombolysis or in patients with "submassive" embolism who show evidence of right ventricular dysfunction. Some physicians reserve thrombolytic therapy for patients who have hypotension and low cardiac output despite initial vigorous treatment with intravenous fluids and vasopressors. Echocardiography has become a key tool used to evaluate right heart function. Evidence of severe right ventricular dysfunction in the face of acute pulmonary embolism may be an indication for thrombolysis.

Most investigators recommend that pulmonary angiography should be used to confirm the diagnosis of pulmonary embolism prior to thrombolytic treatment.

However, one analysis found that the frequency of major bleeding averaged 14% in patients who received tissue plasminogen activator after pulmonary angiography, whereas it was estimated from thrombolytic trials in acute myocardial infarction patients that a noninvasive diagnosis of pulmonary embolism would be associated with only a 4.2% risk of bleeding. The authors suggested that it would be safer to avoid pulmonary angiography for patients chosen to receive thrombolytics who have high-probability lung scans or those with intermediate probability scans plus high clinical suspicion. A comparison of relative risks may prove useful in making decisions about pulmonary angiography and thrombolytic therapy.

Contraindications to thrombolytic therapy include surgery in the past 10 days, recent puncture or invasion of noncompressible vessels, intracerebral hemorrhage or stroke, uncontrolled hypertension, recent trauma, pregnancy, hemorrhagic retinopathy, or other sites of potential bleeding. In addition, streptokinase has been associated with allergic reactions given its antigenic properties and cannot be administered more than once in a 6-month period. Customary invasive vascular procedures such as arterial blood gas measurements and catheterization sites where bleeding cannot be easily controlled should be avoided. Pulmonary angiography, if done, should be approached from the brachial vein rather than from the femoral vein. Heparin should be discontinued before starting thrombolytic agents; antiplatelet agents should not be given simultaneously.

Streptokinase, urokinase, and alteplase have been used in pulmonary embolism. Urokinase and streptokinase are given as a loading dose (streptokinase, 250,000 units over 30 minutes; urokinase, 4400 units/kg over 10 minutes) followed by continuous infusion (streptokinase, 100,000 units/h for 24 hours; urokinase, 4400 units/kg/h for 12–24 hours). Alteplase has usually been administered as a continuous peripheral infusion of 100 mg over 2 hours. Some studies administering a relatively large bolus injection of 0.6 mg/kg (maximum 50 mg bolus) of tissue plasminogen activator over 15 minutes have demonstrated an improvement in resolution of clot and patient safety.

After completion of thrombolytic therapy with any of these agents, the continuous infusion of heparin is reinstituted once the measured aPTT is less than 2.5 times control. Streptokinase and urokinase activate plasminogen bound to both fibrinogen and fibrin, but tissue plasminogen activator, a genetic recombinant product, is somewhat more specific for activation of plasminogen bound to fibrin. This finding suggested that tissue plasminogen activator may be associated with fewer bleeding complications than urokinase or streptokinase, but clinical bleeding has so far been found to be similar for all three agents.

C. Inferior Vena Cava Interruption

There are no data supporting the routine use of an inferior vena cava (IVC) filter in patients with deep venous thrombosis or pulmonary emboli. A study comparing anticoagulation to anticoagulation plus placement of an IVC filter demonstrated a slight reduction in early symptomatic or asymptomatic pulmonary embolism. There was no effect on mortality. After 3 years, a significant increase in recurrent deep venous thrombosis was found in the IVC filter group.

These data, however, support the effectiveness of IVC interruption in reducing near-term embolization. Therefore, three main indications have evolved for interruption of the inferior vena cava in patients with deep venous thrombosis and pulmonary embolism. First, patients who are at high risk for pulmonary embolism (proximal deep venous thrombosis) in whom heparin is contraindicated should be strongly considered for the procedure. The contraindication may be a strong likelihood of bleeding prior to anticoagulation or moderate to severe bleeding during heparin therapy. For example, in trauma patients admitted to the ICU who were treated for deep venous thrombosis or pulmonary embolism with heparin, 36% developed complications requiring termination of the drug, whereas no serious complications or deaths were reported in 34 other patients who underwent placement of an IVC filter. A second indication is failure of anticoagulation to prevent recurrent pulmonary embolism despite an adequate dose and duration of therapy. However, early embolism after initiation of heparin should not generally be considered as necessitating inferior vena cava interruption, because poorly organized thrombi may detach themselves from the venous wall or from other parts of the clot regardless of heparin. Finally, a clinical indication for inferior vena cava interruption is identified in the rare patient whose cardiac and pulmonary reserves are so low that even a single small additional pulmonary thromboembolus may be life-threatening.

The decision to proceed with interruption of the inferior vena cava should be based on evidence that the thromboemboli are coming from deep veins that flow into that vessel. The right atrium and ventricle and the upper extremities should be excluded as sources. If an upper extremity is identified as the continued source of emboli, some centers are capable of placing superior vena cava filters. Contrast venography or other proof of existing clot below the site of planned interruption should be obtained.

The Greenfield filter or other type of intravenous device is most often used, and surgical ligation of the inferior vena cava is rarely needed. The filter can be placed via percutaneous venous access under fluoroscopic guidance either from an internal jugular vein or from a femoral vein. The filter is usually positioned below the level of the renal veins, but there are reports of its being placed above the renal veins in patients with inferior vena cava and renal vein thrombosis. If the filter is placed because of recurrent pulmonary emboli during anticoagulation, anticoagulation is usually continued to prevent additional thrombi from forming on the filter and elsewhere. If the filter is placed because of a contraindication or adverse reaction to anticoagulation, anticoagulation therapy is not given. The risk of recurrent pulmonary emboli after interruption of the vena cava with this device is low (2–3%). Other reported problems include procedural complications, filter malposition and migration, caval occlusion, and sepsis due to device infection.

D. Other Treatment

In some centers, emergent pulmonary embolectomy can be performed in selected patients. Mortality is high, and special experience and expertise are needed. Other modalities currently being investigated include local instillation of thrombolytics directly into the embolus; intravascular catheter disruption systems, including fragmentation and rotor devices that break the clot into smaller pieces that can then be removed; suction catheter removal of the clot; and balloon angioplasty of the embolus.

E. Supportive Care

Abnormal pulmonary gas exchange may require supplemental oxygen. Severe respiratory distress, because of involvement of large portions of the lungs or because of underlying heart or lung disease, may necessitate mechanical ventilatory support. Some patients may have bronchospasm that benefits from bronchodilators. Hemodynamic compromise in pulmonary embolism usually indicates severe obstruction of the pulmonary circulation with failure of the right ventricle. Volume loading of the right ventricle may be helpful. However, volume overexpansion can lead to increasing right ventricular myocardial oxygen consumption and subsequent deterioration of function. Inotropic and vasoactive drugs are generally of little value in severe hemodynamic compromise, but dopamine, dobutamine, and norepinephrine may be tried.

Prevention

Prevention of deep venous thrombosis and, thereby, pulmonary embolism has become a major goal in the management of critically ill patients, who are at high risk of development of deep venous thrombosis as a consequence of bed rest, immobility, critical illness, or trauma. It has been pointed out, however, that many intensive care unit patients are not receiving thromboembolism prophylaxis despite this high risk. For example, patients with hip fracture, total hip replacement, or total knee replacement have a 40–70% chance of developing deep venous thrombosis. Other surgical and medical patients have approximately a 15–50% risk. It is estimated that patients with myocardial infarction have about a 24% overall incidence of deep venous thrombosis, and patients with stroke may have up to a 55% risk.

Prevention of deep venous thrombosis depends on reversal of predisposing conditions (eg, the local hypercoagulable state and venous stasis). Antithrombotic therapy can interfere with thrombus formation either by preventing the platelet nidus from forming or by preventing activation of the coagulation cascade. The type of preventive therapy is closely linked to the underlying condition and the bleeding risk. For example, patients at moderate risk (minor surgery, age under 40, no additional risks) will benefit from low-dose unfractionated heparin, low-molecular-weight heparin, or intermittent pneumatic compression of the legs. On the other hand, hip fracture or total knee replacement patients must be treated with LMW heparin or adjusted-dose warfarin. A summary of recommendations is presented in Table 24–9.

Low-dose unfractionated heparin, 5000–7500 units subcutaneously every 8–12 hours, has been shown to be effective and safe in several groups of patients, including those immediately postoperative from general or gynecologic surgery and medical patients with heart failure, myocardial infarction, respiratory failure, and stroke. At these doses, the activated partial thromboplastin time is not usually prolonged, and there is little increased risk of bleeding. Low-molecular-weight heparins have also been shown to have reliably favorable dose-response properties and turn out to be superior for prophylaxis of deep venous thrombosis in a number of clinical settings. Warfarin is effective in certain clinical situations and, for example, is one of the choices of prophylactic treatment for patients with hip fractures as well as elective hip and knee replacement surgeries. Finally, external compression of the legs can be provided by rhythmic intermittent pneumatic compression devices shown to have comparable effectiveness in preventing deep venous thrombosis with no risk of hemorrhage. These mechanical devices can be combined with medical means of prophylaxis in very high risk patients or used alone in patients at risk of bleeding complications from medical therapy.

However, in patients with trauma—especially to the brain or spinal cord—or those undergoing surgical procedures of the eye, brain, or spinal cord, even low-dose heparin may be contraindicated because of the increased risk of bleeding. External pneumatic compression of the legs is effective in these patients. Neurosurgical patients and patients with heparin-induced thrombocytopenia

Table 24–9. Prophylaxis of deep vein thrombosis and pulmonary embolism.

	Medical Conditions
Acute myocardial infarction	Prophylactic or therapeutic anticoagulant therapy with subcutaneous LDUH or IV heparin
Ischemic stroke with impaired mobility	LDUH, LMWH, or danaparoid. If anticoagulation is contraindicated: ES or IPC device
General medical patients with risk factors	LDUH or LMWH
Critically ill patients	Consider combining pharmacologic method (LDUH or LMWH) with mechanical device (ES or IPC device)
	General Surgery
Low risk	Early ambulation
Moderate risk	LDUH, LMWH, ES, or IPC device
High risk	LDUH, LMWH, or IPC device
Higher risk with greater than usual risk for bleeding	Mechanical prophylaxis with ES or IPC
Very high risk	Effective pharmacologic method (LDUH or LMWH) combined with mechanical method (ES or IPC)
	Gynecologic Surgery
Major surgery for benign disease	LDUH twice daily; LMWH or IPC started before surgery and continued at least several days postoperatively
Extensive surgery for malignant disease	LDUH three times daily. Additional protection: LDUH plus mechanical prophylaxis with ES or IPC device; or higher doses of LMWH
	Urologic Surgery
Major open procedure	LDUH, ES, IPC device, or LMWH
Highest risk patients	ES with or without IPC device added to LDUH or LMWH
	Orthopedic Surgery
Elective total hip replacement	LMWH or adjusted-dose warfarin therapy (goal INR 2.5). Alternative option: adjusted-dose heparin therapy; adjuvant prophylaxis with ES or IPC device may improve efficacy
Elective total knee replacement	LMWH or adjusted-dose warfarin (goal INR 2.5). Alternative: optimal use of IPC device
Hip fracture surgery	LMWH or adjusted-dose warfarin (goal INR 2.5). Possible alternative: LDUH
	Neurosurgical Procedures, Trauma, or Spinal Cord Injury
Intracranial neurosurgery	IPC device with or without ES; LUDH or postoperative LMWH may be acceptable alternative
Trauma, with identifiable risk factor	LMWH as soon as considered safe. If delayed or contraindicated because of bleeding concerns: initial use of ES or IPC device or both
Acute spinal cord injury	LMWH; ES and IPC device may be offered in combination with LMWH or LDUH; LDUH as sole prophylaxis is not recommended.

LDUH = low-dose unfractionated heparin (5000–7500 units); LMWH = low-molecular-weight heparin; ES = elastic graded stockings; IPC = intermittent pneumatic compression.
Modified from the Sixth (2000). ACCP Guidelines for antithrombotic therapy for prevention and treatment of thrombosis.

should also be considered for prevention of deep venous thrombosis by pneumatic compression. This therapy is generally well tolerated, but patients may require sedation due to discomfort from the cyclic compression or heat generated by the apparatus.

Hip fractures, major orthopedic surgery, and some types of urologic surgery enhance the thrombogenic state, probably by increased contact with and release of tissue thromboplastin. While low-dose unfractionated heparin does decrease the risk of deep venous thrombosis in some of these patients, it is less effective than LMW heparin. Current guidelines recommend the use of LMW heparin, adjusted-dose heparin (given every 8 hours to achieve a goal aPTT of 1.5 times control), or adjusted-dose warfarin (goal: INR 2.5) in these patients. Adjunctive prophylaxis with mechanical devices such as elastic stockings and intermittent pneumatic compression devices can add additional benefit with little risk. The duration of prophylaxis, especially in the orthopedic patient population, is being investigated. There is some evidence that prolonging the period of prophylaxis to 2–3 weeks postoperatively has reduced the incidence of deep venous thrombosis and subsequent pulmonary embolism. The ACCP Consensus Guidelines recommend outpatient prophylaxis with LMW heparin for 7–10 days after surgery for these high-risk patients.

Inferior vena cava filters have also been studied for their use in the prevention of complications from deep venous thrombosis, primarily in the surgical population. Four studies evaluating high-risk surgical patients without current evidence of deep venous thrombosis using historical controls found a decreased incidence of pulmonary emboli in the following patients who had an inferior vena cava filter placed: those with high injury severity scores, head or spinal cord trauma, pelvic or lower extremity fractures, prolonged immobility, and mechanical ventilatory support. This means of prophylaxis has not been studied in direct comparison with heparin or mechanical devices. Other patient populations that may benefit from prophylactic filter placement include patients with advanced malignancy, orthopedic surgical patients, and patients with limited cardiopulmonary reserve such as those with severe COPD. The use of these filters as prophylaxis remains controversial and requires larger studies to determine their exact role.

Current Controversies & Unresolved Issues

The diagnosis of pulmonary embolism in the critically ill patient with multiple preexisting diseases can be very difficult. The incidence of pulmonary embolism complicating critical illness is unknown, but 5–10% of deaths may be associated with unsuspected pulmonary emboli. Abnormal pulmonary gas exchange and hemodynamic compromise resulting from new pulmonary emboli may not be identified in patients who already have underlying lung or heart disease. Defects on perfusion lung scans may or may not represent pulmonary emboli in patients with abnormal chest x-rays, and ventilation scans cannot be performed without special arrangements for patients receiving mechanical ventilation. The helical or spiral CT scan requires a degree of patient cooperation and breathholding in order to achieve adequate imaging. Again, this may be difficult for critically ill patients to perform. Magnetic resonance imaging may not be possible in the patient who is mechanically ventilated. Finally, treatment issues are complex, with some patients having relative contraindications to anticoagulation while others may have diseases in which adequate anticoagulation is difficult to achieve.

Patients with worsening hypoxemia or increased physiologic dead space, increased pulmonary artery pressure (in the absence of other causes), unexplained tachycardia or hypotension, or other features of unclear cardiopulmonary insufficiency should be suspected of having pulmonary thromboembolic disease. The use of end-tidal CO_2 monitors in the ICU may be a noninvasive means for detecting an acute change in dead space ventilation that may be an early clue for pulmonary embolism.

Ventilation-perfusion scans in patients with COPD are generally considered to be of limited value because airway obstruction causes falsely positive perfusion defects. A study of such patients suspected of having a pulmonary embolism found that high-probability scans were rare but had high predictive value for pulmonary embolism; similarly, a normal perfusion scan was highly predictive of a normal pulmonary angiogram. However, 90% of the group had *intermediate-probability* (60%), or low-probability (30%) scans, of which only 17% had pulmonary embolism confirmed by angiography. The authors of the study concluded that ventilation-perfusion lung scans were helpful only if they were high-probability or normal. In all others, they concluded, sufficient clinical suspicion should lead to pulmonary angiography.

Ansell J et al: Heparin-induced thrombocytopenia: A prospective study. Thromb Haemost 1980;43:61–5.

Arcasoy SM, Kreit JW: Thrombolytic therapy of pulmonary embolism. A comprehensive review of current evidence. Chest 1999;115:1695–1707.

Becker DM et al: D-dimer testing and acute venous thromboembolism. A shortcut to accurate diagnosis? Arch Intern Med 1996;156:939–46.

Decousus H et al: A clinical trial of vena caval filters in the prevention of pulmonary embolism in patients with proximal deep-vein thrombosis. N Engl J Med 1998;338:409–15.

Freyburger G et al: D-dimer strategy in thrombosis exclusion. A gold standard study in 100 patients suspected of deep venous thrombosis or pulmonary embolism: 8 DD methods compared. Thromb Haemost 1998;79:32–37.

Geerts WH et al: Prevention of venous thromboembolism. Chest 2001;119:132S–75S.

Goodman LR et al: Subsequent pulmonary embolism: Risk after a negative helical CT pulmonary angiogram-prospective comparison with scintigraphy. Radiology 2000;215:535–42.

Gould MK et al: Low-molecular-weight heparins compared with unfractionated heparin for treatment of acute deep venous thrombosis: A cost-effectiveness analysis. Ann Intern Med 1999;130:789–99.

Grant BJB: Noninvasive tests for acute venous thromboembolism. Am J Respir Crit Care Med 1994;149:1044–7.

Hirsh J et al: Heparin and low-molecular weight-heparin: Mechanisms of action, pharmacokinetics, dosing, monitoring, efficacy, and safety. Chest 2001;119:64S–94S.

Hull RD et al: A noninvasive strategy for the treatment of patients with suspected pulmonary embolism. Arch Intern Med 1994;154:289–97.

Hull RD et al: Low-molecular-weight heparin vs. heparin in the treatment of patients with pulmonary embolism. Arch Intern Med 2000;160:229–36.

Hyers TM et al: Antithrombotic therapy for venous thromboembolic disease. Chest 2001;119:176S–206S.

Hyers TM: Venous thromboembolism: State of the art. Am J Respir Crit Care Med 1999;159:1–14.

Kearon C et al: Noninvasive diagnosis of deep venous thrombosis. Ann Intern Med 1998;128:663–77.

Kutinsky I, Blakley S, Roche V: Normal D-dimer levels in patients with pulmonary embolism. Arch Intern Med 1999; 159:1569–72.

Levine MN et al: Hemorrhagic complications of anticoagulant treatment. Chest 2001;119:108S–21S.

Loud PA et al: Combined CT venography and pulmonary angiography in suspected thromboembolic disease: Diagnostic accuracy of deep venous evaluation. AJR Am J Roentgenol 2000;174:61–65.

Low-molecular-weight heparin in the treatment of patients with venous thromboembolism. The Columbus Investigators. N Engl J Med 1997;337:657–62.

Lualdi JC, Goldhaber SZ: Right ventricular dysfunction after acute pulmonary embolism: Pathophysiologic factors, detection, and therapeutic implications. Am Heart J 1995;130:1276–82.

Mayo JR et al: Pulmonary embolism: Prospective comparison of spiral CT with ventilation-perfusion scintigraphy. Radiology 1997;205:447–52.

Miniati M et al: Accuracy of clinical assessment in the diagnosis of pulmonary embolism. Am J Respir Crit Care Med 1999; 159:864–71.

Rathbun SW, Raskob GE, Whitsett TL: Sensitivity and specificity of helical computed tomography in the diagnosis of pulmonary embolism: A systematic review. Ann Intern Med 2000;132:227–32.

Remy-Jardin M et al: Clinical value of thin collimation in the diagnostic work up of pulmonary embolism. AJR Am J Roentgenol 2000;175:407–11.

Ribeiro A et al: Echocardiography doppler in pulmonary embolism: Right ventricular dysfunction as a predictor of mortality rate. Am Heart J 1997;134:479–87.

Ryu JH et al: Diagnosis of pulmonary embolism with use of computed tomographic angiography. Mayo Clin Proc 2001;76:59–65.

Seligsohn U, Lubetsky A: Genetic susceptibility to venous thrombosis. N Engl J Med 2001;344:1222–31.

Simonneau G et al: A comparison of low-molecular-weight heparin with unfractionated heparin for acute pulmonary embolism. N Engl J Med 1997;337:663–9.

Spence LD et al: Acute upper extremity deep venous thrombosis: Safety and effectiveness of superior vena caval filters. Radiology 1999;210:53–8.

Tapson VF et al: The diagnostic approach to acute venous thromboembolism. Clinical Practice Guideline. Am J Respir Crit Care Med 1999;160:1043–66.

Value of the ventilation/perfusion scan in acute pulmonary embolism. Results of the prospective investigation of pulmonary embolism diagnosis (PIOPED). The PIOPED Investigators. JAMA 1990;263:2753–59.

Wells PS et al: Use of a clinical model for safe management of patients with suspected pulmonary embolism. Ann Intern Med 1998;129:997–1005.

ANAPHYLAXIS

ESSENTIALS OF DIAGNOSIS

- *Follows reexposure to foreign antigens such as food, drug, nonhuman protein, or other substances.*
- *Respiratory tract: rhinitis, edema, laryngeal edema, asthma.*
- *Hypotension, light-headedness, collapse.*
- *Generalized erythema, pruritus, and urticarial skin lesions with or without angioedema.*

General Considerations

Anaphylaxis is a severe allergic reaction that occurs after reexposure to a foreign substance such as food, a drug, serum, venoms, or nonhuman proteins but occasionally occurs after exercise. Approximately 72 hours after initial exposure to a foreign antigen, IgE antibody synthesis begins. Reexposure to the antigen promotes cross-linking of mast cell- and basophil-bound IgE molecules and causes the subsequent release of stored mediators of anaphylaxis such as histamine and other substances. These factors cause increases in capillary permeability, mucosal edema, and smooth muscle contraction; activate the classic complement pathway and components of the clotting cascade; and cause the release of other mediators.

Anaphylactoid (anaphylaxis-like) reactions are clinically similar to anaphylaxis but are not mediated by antigen-antibody interactions. Many of the same mediators are involved, so that treatment is identical to that for anaphylaxis. Mechanisms include (1) activation of the complement cascade by immune complexes or other substances that cause release of anaphylatoxins (eg, C3a and C5a), resulting in mediator release from mast cells and basophils; and (2) direct activation by certain agents of mast cells and basophils, resulting in mediator release (eg, effect of hyperosmolar solutions such as mannitol and radiocontrast media).

Patients with anaphylaxis may be admitted to the ICU because of severe respiratory or cardiovascular compromise, or they may develop anaphylaxis in the ICU from exposure to blood products or drugs.

Clinical Features

The onset of a systemic anaphylactic reaction, which may develop over minutes to 1–2 hours, depends on the sensitivity of the person as well as the route, rate, and quantity of the precipitating agent. The clinical signs and symptoms can differ greatly depending on the severity of the anaphylactic reaction, and clinical findings may be present in various combinations. Severe systemic reactions are characterized by respiratory failure and cardiovascular collapse. Recurrence of symptoms can occur 2–24 hours after onset despite initial stabilization and treatment.

A. History

A history of recent use of medication, ingestion of new or unusual foods (notably peanuts and other nuts, shellfish), and exposure to toxic products such as venoms or insect bites should be sought, but treatment should be initiated immediately if necessary. An increasingly recognized cause of allergy and anaphylaxis is exposure to latex rubber. About half of patients will have a history of atopy, and only about 70% of patients who develop anaphylaxis outside of the hospital will have an identifiable precipitating cause. In the ICU, intravenous contrast agents, antibiotics, NSAIDs, aspirin, and other drugs are the most likely causes.

B. Symptoms and Signs

Anaphylaxis is often associated with severe anxiety and apprehension. Patients may experience any combination of the following symptoms: itching of skin and mucosal surfaces, swelling of the lips and tongue, hoarseness, coughing, shortness of breath, wheezing, vomiting, abdominal cramps, diarrhea, and palpitations.

Physical findings in severe systemic reactions include hypotension, upper airway obstruction resulting in stridor, and bronchospasm with impaired gas exchange, hypercapnia, and wheezing. Loss of consciousness may result from poor cerebral perfusion. Urticaria may be present, and there may be evidence of angioedema.

Allergens injected systemically—eg, insect stings, intravenous drugs, blood products, and allergy desensitization treatments—often cause a predominantly cardiovascular reaction with hypotension. Food and inhaled allergens may cause more facial and respiratory edema, associated with respiratory problems.

Differential Diagnosis

Anaphylaxis may be confused with syncopal episodes associated with metabolic or vascular disturbances, acute respiratory failure secondary to epiglottitis, status asthmaticus, obstruction due to foreign body aspiration, and pulmonary embolism. Similar disorders with cutaneous and respiratory manifestations—eg, mastocytosis, carcinoid syndrome, hereditary angioedema, and other specific adverse pharmacologic (allergic and nonallergic) reaction to drugs—should be considered if appropriate.

Treatment

Treatment is based on early recognition of features of anaphylaxis combined with a history of exposure to an inciting agent. The suspected agent should be discontinued if possible (eg, a drug, blood products, contact with latex rubber); the extent and severity of the reaction should be assessed; and treatment should be initiated as soon as anaphylaxis is suspected.

A. General Measures

The patient should be positioned supine or head down with the feet elevated. The airway must be maintained by proper positioning. If necessary, endotracheal intubation, tracheostomy, or cricothyroidotomy should be performed. Because of the need for intravenous fluid infusion and medications, a large-bore intravenous catheter should be inserted.

B. Initial Treatment

Epinephrine should be given first in a dosage of 0.3–0.5 mL of 1:1000 dilution (0.3–0.5 mg) subcutaneously every 10–20 minutes as needed. In severe anaphylaxis with suspicion of poor perfusion, intramuscular epinephrine (0.5 mg; 0.5 mL of 1:1000 dilution) or slow intravenous injection (5 mL of 1:10,000 dilution) should be considered. Other initial treatment includes oxygen, inhaled beta-adrenergic agonists for bronchospasm, and airway management.

C. Other Medications

Medications are directed toward blocking further mediator action on target organs, preventing further release of mediators, reversing the physiologic effects of the mediators, and supporting vital functions. Antihistamines (histamine H_1-antagonists) such as diphenhydramine hydrochloride, 25–50 mg intravenously every 6 hours, are useful. Some studies show additional benefit of histamine H_2-receptor antagonists, so cimetidine or ranitidine may be given as well. Excessive antihistamine dosages may cause impaired central nervous system function, anticholinergic symptoms (dry mouth, urinary retention), and drowsiness, especially in elderly patients.

Hydrocortisone, 100 mg intravenously every 8 hours for several doses, is recommended, especially if there is bronchospasm or airway compromise.

Patients who are receiving beta-blockers may have a poor response to treatment directed at hypotension. These patients may have some response to glucagon, which has both inotropic and chronotropic effects on the heart.

D. Intravenous Fluids

Adults should receive 0.9% NaCl solution, 0.5–1 L intravenously over 30 minutes, if hypotensive. Additional fluid therapy is dependent on blood pressure, heart rate, urine output, and clinical response.

E. Prevention of Anaphylaxis

The patient should be instructed to avoid the offending agent in future if possible. For patients who have a likelihood of reexposure to an identified antigen, a kit containing epinephrine for self-administration should be considered.

ANGIOEDEMA

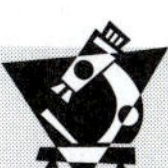

ESSENTIALS OF DIAGNOSIS

- *Subcutaneous swelling of skin or mucous membranes, possibly with laryngeal or lower airway compromise.*
- *May present with urticaria.*
- *Acute angioedema: May have history of ACE inhibitor, aspirin, or NSAID therapy, or a history of allergies.*
- *History of recurrent transient episodes of swelling may be present in allergic or hereditary forms.*

General Considerations

Angioedema is produced by mechanisms similar to those that cause anaphylaxis and anaphylactoid reactions. In addition, these mechanisms can be triggered by various physical forces, exercise, and other medical conditions such as endocrine disorders, infections, malignancies, allergic phenomena, and collagen-vascular diseases. Severe angioedema involving the upper or lower airways is a medical emergency similar to anaphylaxis.

Acute angioedema, which may occur once or on multiple occasions, is often idiopathic or associated with allergic phenomena. Among identified causes, the most common are related to ACE inhibitor therapy, aspirin, and NSAIDs.

Hereditary angioedema is caused by an autosomal dominant inherited deficiency or functional abnormality of C1 esterase inhibitor. Without this inhibitor, the complement cascade is activated, and a kinin-like fragment and other mediators are released that produce the angioedema.

Acquired C1 esterase inhibitor deficiency is very rare and seen in adults with autoimmune or lymphoproliferative disorders. Patients have unexplained recurrent angioedema, and the diagnosis is confirmed by low levels of C1q and low C1 esterase inhibitor activity.

Clinical Features

A. Symptoms and Signs

Angioedema is characterized by the presence of nonpruritic subcutaneous swelling of the skin and mucous membranes. Lesions of the skin are poorly demarcated and reddish. These may occur in conjunction with urticarial lesions. Involvement of the upper airway can result in hoarseness, stridor, shortness of breath, and even death. Likewise, gastrointestinal involvement is associated with abdominal pain, nausea, and diarrhea. Patients may or may not have associated urticaria, characterized by evanescent pruritic lesions.

Because of widespread use of ACE inhibitors for hypertension, diabetic proteinuria, and congestive heart failure, these agents are a common cause of acute angioedema. This disorder may present after recent initiation of ACE inhibitor therapy but may occur even after prolonged use. It is said that urticaria is unusual in ACE inhibitor-induced angioedema. Angiotensin receptor blockers, sometimes given to patients instead of or in addition to ACE inhibitor, have been rarely associated with angioedema, but some experts have cautioned against use of these agents in patients with ACE inhibitor-induced angioedema. Hereditary or acquired angioedema has been precipitated by ACE inhibitors.

In hereditary angioedema, episodes can be precipitated by trauma, emotional upset, infections, and exposure to sudden temperature changes. The disorder is usually apparent in childhood, and attacks tend to be recurrent and usually are of 2–4 days' duration. The physical findings are similar to those described above. Similar features are present in acquired forms of angioedema.

B. Laboratory Findings

In patients with angioedema or urticaria, investigation should include a complete blood count, erythrocyte sedimentation rate, and urinalysis. Other laboratory tests should be ordered depending upon the underlying medical condition. In patients with abdominal symptoms, edema of the bowel wall may be seen on CT imaging.

When hereditary angioedema is suspected, C4, C3, CH50 or total complement, and C1 esterase inhibitor (by immunochemical and functional assay) should be measured. C4 and C2 are always low, and CH50 is usually diminished or absent during an attack. C1 esterase will be reduced but may be normal in persons with a functional abnormality. Acquired angioedema (acquired C1 inhibitor deficiency) is due to increased catabolism of C1 esterase inhibitor and C1q. Laboratory findings in allergic angioedema and that induced by ACE inhibitors and NSAIDs are rarely specific or helpful.

Treatment

Patients may require long-term treatment and should avoid precipitating conditions and situations. In some patients, the underlying cause may not be identifiable.

A. General Measures

Acute angioedema is treated initially much the same way as anaphylaxis. The underlying cause should be treated or removed, especially if ACE inhibitors have been implicated. Hypotension and shock should be treated with intravenous fluids. The airway should be protected, and endotracheal intubation may become necessary. If there is severe upper airway obstruction, tracheostomy should be considered.

B. Specific Treatment

1. Epinephrine—Epinephrine is indicated for patients with severe acute urticaria or angioedema with airway involvement. It can be given subcutaneously or intravenously. One recommendation is to give 0.3–0.5 mL of 1:1000 solution subcutaneously and repeat every 10–20 minutes as necessary. Epinephrine may be life-saving in angioedema, but it should be noted that many patients with ACE inhibitor-induced angioedema are elderly or have heart disease or hypertension. Epinephrine may cause excessive tachycardia, may increase myocardial oxygen demand, may provoke myocardial ischemia, and may raise blood pressure excessively.

2. Antihistamines—Antihistamines are usually effective against urticaria and can be helpful for some forms of angioedema. H_1 blockers such as diphenhydramine, 50 mg orally or intravenously every 6 hours, are helpful for an acute episode of urticaria. Patients may have dry mouth, drowsiness, and excessive sedation with these agents. In patients with angioedema, in addition to H_1 blockers, an H_2 blocker such as ranitidine, 50 mg intravenously two or three times daily or 150 mg orally twice daily, or cimetidine, 300 mg orally or intravenously every 6 hours, may be helpful.

3. Corticosteroids—Corticosteroids are usually not necessary for acute urticaria alone but can be very helpful in refractory acute urticaria or chronic urticaria. A recommended initial dosage is prednisone, 2 mg/kg/d orally, or methylprednisolone, 60 mg intravenously every 6 hours.

C. Hereditary Angioedema

Clinical trials of recombinant C1 inhibitor concentrate for acute hereditary angioedema are under way. C1 inhibitor concentrates from pooled plasma are available in Europe but not in the United States. Fresh frozen plasma may be given (two units) as treatment to prevent angioedema or in preparation for surgery. Long-term preventive treatment of angioedema can be tried using androgen derivatives such as danazol, 200 mg orally three times daily, or stanozolol, 2–4 mg/d.

Bochner BS, Lichtenstein LM: Anaphylaxis. N Engl J Med 1991;324:1785–90.

Bork K, Barnstedt SE: Treatment of 193 episodes of laryngeal edema with C1 inhibitor concentrate in patient with hereditary angioedema. Arch Intern Med 2001;161:714–8.

Brady WJ Jr, Luber S, Joyce TP: Multiphasic anaphylaxis: report of a case with prehospital and emergency department considerations. J Emerg Med 1997;15:477–81.

Ewan PW: Anaphylaxis. BMJ 1998;316:1442–5.

Kleiner GI et al: Unmasking of acquired autoimmune C1-inhibitor deficiency by an angiotensin-converting enzyme inhibitor. Ann Allergy Asthma Immunol 2001;86:461–4.

Lin RY et al: Improved outcomes in patients with acute allergic syndromes who are treated with combined H_1 and H_2 antagonists. Ann Emerg Med 2000;36:462–8.

Endocrine Problems in the Critically Ill Patient

25

Shalender Bhasin, MD, Laurie K. S. Tom, MD, & Phong Mac, MD

Several endocrine problems may require management in the ICU, including severe thyroid disease, acute adrenal insufficiency, and diabetic ketoacidosis. While these problems are usually encountered in patients in whom a diagnosis of endocrine dysfunction has already been made, they are occasionally the presenting manifestation in an undiagnosed patient. If these endocrine disorders are not identified, specific treatment such as endocrine replacement therapy may be delayed and significant complications or death may ensue.

In this chapter, severe thyrotoxicosis (thyroid storm or decompensated hyperthyroidism), severe hypothyroidism (myxedema coma), and acute and chronic adrenal insufficiency are discussed. Diabetic ketoacidosis and other manifestations of severe diabetes mellitus are covered in Chapter 26. In this chapter we discuss also the problem of assessing thyroid function in severe nonthyroidal illness ("sick euthyroid syndrome").

THYROID STORM

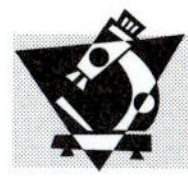

ESSENTIALS OF DIAGNOSIS

- *Long-standing hyperthyroidism, uncontrolled or poorly controlled.*
- *Breakdown of the body's thermoregulatory mechanisms, resulting in hyperpyrexia.*
- *Altered mental status.*
- *Precipitating illnesses or events such as thyroid surgery, infection, trauma, acute abdominal problems, or anesthesia.*
- *Signs and symptoms of severe hyperthyroidism—usually marked wasting.*

General Considerations

Thyroid storm—or thyrotoxic crisis—results from the eventual failure of the body's compensatory mechanisms in severe hyperthyroidism. Clinically, thyroid storm has been defined as "a life-threatening augmentation of the manifestations of hyperthyroidism." There are no pathognomonic laboratory markers of thyroid storm. However, because of its high mortality rate, one should be vigilant for its diagnosis and provide aggressive and prompt management. This is especially true because the features of thyroid storm are common findings in other critically ill patients.

A. Incidence

The incidence of thyroid storm has decreased markedly since the advent of antithyroid drugs. Some studies suggest that the incidence is 2–8% of all patients admitted to the hospital for management of hyperthyroidism. Thyroid storm occurs nine to ten times more commonly in women than in men, probably a reflection of the higher incidence of thyroid diseases in women in general. No race- or age-related differences in incidence have been reported. An association between thyroid storm and medically underserved poorer populations has been suggested. One explanation is that control of chronic hyperthyroidism with antithyroid drugs is very effective in preventing decompensation, but poorer populations may be less likely to receive adequate treatment.

Pathophysiology

The pathophysiology of thyrotoxic crisis is not well understood. Indices of thyroid gland overactivity (levels of total and free thyroxine or tri-iodothyronine) are not significantly higher than in usual cases of hyperthyroidism.

Although the signs and symptoms of hyperthyroidism suggest sympathetic overactivity, plasma levels and secretion rates of epinephrine and norepinephrine are actually normal in patients with thyroid storm. Because of this, increased sensitivity to catecholamines has been suggested, and elevated cAMP levels in these patients have been cited as evidence of increased adrenergic activity. The mechanisms that lead to the decompensated state characteristic of thyroid storm have not been well studied. The basal metabolic rate and thermogenesis are increased, and there is a net degradation of proteins. Although both protein synthesis and degradation are increased, hyperthyroidism results in negative nitrogen balance, muscle wasting, and reduced albumin concentrations. Although cortisol clearance is increased, its production rates are also increased, so that the cortisol levels remain essentially unchanged. Thyroid hormones have direct cardiostimulatory effects, resulting in tachycardia and increased contractility. Increased thermogenesis results in vasodilation as part of the compensatory response to increased body temperature.

Clinical Features

Thyroid storm is usually seen in patients with known hyperthyroidism but may be the presenting feature in a patient with previously undiagnosed thyrotoxicosis. Thyroid storm is often seen in association with one of a long list of precipitating conditions, but the two most common conditions are surgical procedures of any kind—but particularly thyroid surgery in an uncontrolled or poorly prepared hyperthyroid patient—and infections. Thyroid storm is now quite uncommon following thyroid surgery because of preoperative preparation and control of hyperthyroidism with antithyroid drugs.

Other precipitating factors include cardiovascular disease (including acute myocardial infarction), systemic illness, trauma, diabetic ketoacidosis, vigorous palpation of an untreated hyperthyroid gland, administration of iodinated contrast material, stroke, and preeclampsia-eclampsia. Exacerbation of hyperthyroidism may occur following radioactive iodine treatment of Graves' disease, but thyroid storm is unusual because most hyperthyroid patients are well controlled by antithyroid drug therapy. In contrast, thyroid storm may occur in hyperthyroid patients who discontinue antithyroid medications prematurely or inadvertently. Patients who accidentally or deliberately ingest an excessive amount of thyroid hormone may present with severe hyperthyroidism but usually without the complete picture seen in thyroid storm.

A. Symptoms and Signs

Thyroid storm is characterized by clinical features of severe thyrotoxicosis with fever and altered mental status. Mental status changes may include confusion, agitation, overt psychosis, or, in extreme cases, even coma. Common cardiovascular manifestations include tachycardia that is out of proportion to fever, cardiac arrhythmias (sinus or supraventricular tachycardia, including atrial fibrillation), and congestive heart failure. Patients presenting with congestive heart failure are usually elderly and have an underlying history of heart disease. However, it is well documented that hyperthyroidism causes congestive heart failure even in the absence of underlying heart disease. Hypotension and shock may be late manifestations. Gastrointestinal manifestations include nausea, vomiting, diarrhea, and abdominal pain. Weight loss and cachexia are common.

Goiter is almost always present and may be diffuse or multinodular. Since many of these patients have Graves' disease, the goiter is more often diffuse and nontender. Patients often have marked muscle weakness due to proximal myopathy and generalized cachexia. Tremor is present. The skin is warm, moist, flushed, soft, and "velvety." The reflexes may be brisk. Graves' disease patients may also have ophthalmopathy and dermopathy.

B. Laboratory Findings

Abnormalities of liver function, including elevated aminotransferases, hyperbilirubinemia, and hepatomegaly, are common. Alkaline phosphatase levels are also increased, but this usually represents an increase in the bone fraction rather than the liver fraction. Serum calcium may be elevated as a reflection of increased bone resorption.

The diagnosis of thyroid storm is essentially a clinical one. The presence of high fever and altered mental status in a severely ill patient with hyperthyroidism should warrant aggressive treatment for thyrotoxic crisis. Therefore, laboratory tests of thyroid function merely confirm the presence of hyperthyroidism, ie, high total and free thyroxine (T_4) and triiodothyronine (T_3) and a reduced and nearly undetectable thyrotropin (TSH) level. However, T_3 and T_4 levels may be decreased by concurrent nonthyroidal illness. In fact, the levels of T_4 and T_3 may not correlate with the patient's clinical picture.

Treatment

The management of thyroid storm can be discussed under three broad categories: (1) control of hyperthyroidism, (2) treatment of the precipitating illness, and (3) other supportive measures. Treatment is summarized in Table 25–1.

A. Control of Hyperthyroidism

Several therapeutic agents that act by different mechanisms to block the synthesis, secretion, activation, or action of thyroid hormones can be used together for rapid control of hyperthyroidism.

1. Thioureas—Propylthiouracil, methimazole, and carbimazole inhibit thyroid hormone synthesis primarily by inhibiting reactions catalyzed by the thyroid peroxidase enzyme. These reactions include oxidation, organification, and iodotyrosine coupling. Propylthiouracil is also a weak inhibitor of peripheral conversion of T_4 to T_3. Methimazole is generally considered to be more potent than propylthiouracil. In comatose patients with thyroid storm, propylthiouracil or methimazole may be given

Table 25–1. Treatment of thyroid storm.

Mechanism of Action	Treatment
Measures to reduce thyroid hormone synthesis or peripheral conversion of T_4 to T_3	Propylthiouracil,[1] 200–300 mg orally or through a nasogastric tube every 6 hours. *or* Propylthiouracil, 600 mg loading dose orally, followed by 200–300 mg every 8 hours. *or* Methimazole, 20–30 mg orally or through a nasogastric tube every 6 hours. *plus* Ipodate,[2] 1–1.5 g/d for the first 24 hours, then 500 mg twice daily.
Measures to inhibit the release of thyroid hormones	Lugol's solution, 10 drops three times daily, or saturated solution of sodium iodide, 3 drops three times daily, after antithyroid therapy (above) has been instituted. Lithium carbonate, 300 mg every 8 hours, may be used in patients with iodine allergy.
Sympathetic blockade	Propranolol, 0.5–1 mg IV slowly over 5-10 minutes. Repeat every 3–4 hours as indicated. Contraindicated in COPD and asthma; should be very carefully administered in patients with congestive heart failure.
Glucocorticoids	Dexamethasone, 2–4 mg IV every 6–8 hours.
Supportive measures	Identify and treat the precipitating event. Provide fluid and electrolyte replacement as needed. Hyperpyrexia: Cooling blankets, ice, or cool sponges as necessary. Other supportive measures.

[1]Both propylthiouracil and methimazole may be administered rectally.
[2]If the patient is allergic to iodine, lithium may be used: lithium carbonate, 300–400 mg every 8 hours. Serum lithium levels to be maintained at approximately 1 meq/L.

through a nasogastric tube because these drugs are not available in parenteral formulations.

There is no agreement about the optimum dosage of antithyroid drugs. One regimen is to start propylthiouracil at an initial dose of 600–1200 mg/d in four divided doses. Alternatively, 60–120 mg/d of methimazole can be given in four divided doses. Should the patient be unable to take medication orally, these medications can be administered rectally. Others have advocated giving a loading dose of 600–1200 mg of propylthiouracil followed by 200–300 mg every 8 hours. However, some investigators have questioned whether additional inhibition of thyroperoxidase is achievable at dosages of propylthiouracil in excess of 300 mg daily. Methimazole is given at one-tenth the above dosage. The serum half-life of propylthiouracil is 75 minutes; of methimazole, 240–360 minutes. However, the intrathyroidal residence time of methimazole is 20 hours, and its duration of action is believed to be as long as 40 hours. These data have been used to support once-daily administration of methimazole. However, in the life-threatening situation of thyroid storm, it may be preferable to give methimazole three or four times daily. Propylthiouracil is also a weak inhibitor of 5′-deiodinase, the enzyme that converts T_4 to T_3, and this may be a minor advantage over methimazole—though the two drugs have never been directly compared.

Resistance to the effects of antithyroid drugs is extremely uncommon. Most cases of apparent resistance turn out to be problems of noncompliance. Acute side effects of these drugs are uncommon, but allergic reactions, leukopenia, and hepatotoxicity may occur.

2. Ipodate sodium—Ipodate sodium is an iodine-containing radiocontrast agent used for gallbladder imaging. It is one of the most potent inhibitors of 5′-deiodinase. Clinical studies with ipodate in hyperthyroidism have shown that the drug has an extremely rapid onset of action, resulting in marked lowering of serum T_3 levels within 4–6 hours and normalization of serum T_3 levels within 24–48 hours. The mechanism of antithyroid effect of ipodate is complex. Besides inhibiting conversion of T_4 to T_3, ipodate also lowers serum T_4 levels, albeit to a lesser degree, indicating additional direct effects on thyroid hormone synthesis. Reverse T_3 levels are higher in ipodate-treated patients, an observation consistent with drug-induced inhibition of 5′-deiodinase. Although ipodate is an iodine-containing contrast agent, radioiodine uptake studies in patients with Graves' disease treated with ipodate for more than a year reveal normal uptake a week after discontinuation of ipodate therapy.

Ipodate sodium is administered orally as capsules containing 500 mg. Recommended dosages range from 1–3 g/d. In obtunded patients, ipodate can be administered via the intragastric route. Ipodate sodium has replaced oral administration of potassium iodide in the treatment of severe hyperthyroidism. It has been recommended that propylthiouracil or methimazole be given prior to administration of iodine-containing medications to prevent an iodide-mediated exacerbation of hyperthyroidism.

3. Lithium—Lithium can be used in patients unable to tolerate iodine. Lithium is concentrated by the thyroid and inhibits iodine uptake by the thyroid. It also inhibits thyroid hormone release. A dosage of 300–400 mg every 8 hours can be used to temporarily control the thyrotoxic patient allergic to iodine. The dose should be adjusted as necessary to maintain a serum lithium level of approximately 1 meq/L.

4. Iodide—Iodide blocks the release of thyroid hormones from the gland. Iodide also has an inhibitory effect on thyroid hormone synthesis. However, this inhibitory effect on thyroid hormone synthesis is transient, and in most patients an escape from this inhibition occurs with time—a phenomenon referred to as the Wolff-Chaikoff effect.

Iodide should only be administered after the synthesis of thyroid hormones has been inhibited by prior administration of thioureas. Intravenous sodium iodide can be administered at a dosage of 1 g daily. Alternatively, if the patient is able to take medication orally, Lugol's solution at a dosage of 10 drops three times a day, or saturated potassium iodide solution at a dose of 3 drops three times daily can be used.

Administration of a large dose of inorganic iodide will predictably reduce radioiodine uptake by the thyroid gland for several weeks. Therefore, prior administration of inorganic iodide will preclude subsequent treatment with radioactive iodine for several weeks.

5. Propranolol—Beta-adrenergic blockers attenuate many of the peripheral manifestations of hyperthyroidism. Thus, these agents can reverse the thyroid hormone-induced increase in heart rate, cardiac output, and muscle tremor. However, weight loss is not affected by beta-blockers. Propranolol, in addition to its antiadrenergic properties, is also a weak inhibitor of 5′-deiodinase and thus lowers T_3 levels. The advantage of the 5′-deiodinase inhibition property of propranolol over other beta-adrenergic blockers is unclear given the similar action of propylthiouracil and ipodate sodium. Other beta-adrenergic blocking agents such as esmolol and labetalol have also been used successfully.

The responses to propranolol vary from patient to patient, and dosages should be titrated to the clinical response. The initial dose usually is 0.5–1 mg intravenously given slowly over 5–10 minutes for a total of up to 10 mg. This can be followed by 40–60 mg orally every 6 hours. If the patient is unable to take medication orally, propranolol can be administered intravenously in doses of 1–2 mg every 3–4 hours. It is worth emphasizing that these dosage recommendations are only general guidelines to be used initially. Subsequent dosage adjustments should be dictated by the clinical response. Propranolol blood levels in the range of 50–100 μg/mL have been shown to provide effective beta blockade. However, blood levels of propranolol have not been extensively utilized in clinical practice; it is much simpler to follow the clinical heart rate and blood pressure responses. Side effects of beta-adrenergic blockade in patients with thyroid storm include heart failure, bradycardia, hypotension, and increased airway resistance.

6. Glucocorticoids—The older literature warned that adrenal insufficiency might ensue in patients with thyroid storm because of accelerated cortisol degradation. However, this hypothesis has never been validated, and the routine use of glucocorticoid replacement has declined. Glucocorticoids do, however, have several salutary effects on thyroid function in thyroid storm. In patients receiving thyroxine replacement, glucocorticoids lower serum T_3 concentrations, probably by inhibition of peripheral 5′-deiodinase. In addition, glucocorticoids lower serum T_4 levels in patients with Graves' disease. Finally, glucocorticoids in pharmacologic doses inhibit TSH secretion. One recommended regimen is 2–4 mg of dexamethasone every 6 hours intravenously. Patients suspected of having adrenal insufficiency should be treated accordingly with higher doses of hydrocortisone (see below).

7. Extracorporeal therapy—Exchange transfusion and plasmapheresis have been advocated as ways of removing large amounts of thyroid hormones from the circulation. Experience with these techniques is limited. Furthermore, with the availability of potent antithyroid drugs, they are not likely to be needed.

B. General Supportive Measures

General measures include fluid and electrolyte replacement and control of hyperpyrexia. The latter may require the use of cooling blankets. Salicylates should be avoided because these drugs can inhibit T_4 and T_3 binding to the binding proteins and increase the concentrations of the free T_4 and T_3. In addition, specific measures for prompt treatment of the precipitating illness, cardiac arrhythmias, and congestive heart failure should be initiated if indicated.

Prognosis

Most data on mortality statistics in thyroid storm are old, and there are no recent series. Survival figures vary from 24–66% in older series. The precipitating illness is clearly an important determinant of prognosis.

Cooper DS: Antithyroid drugs for the treatment of hyperthyroidism caused by Graves' disease. Endocrinol Metab Clin North Am 1998;27:225–47.

Ringel MD: Management of hypothyroidism and hyperthyroidism in the intensive care unit. Crit Care Clin 2001;17:59–74.

Roth RN, McAuliffe MJ: Hyperthyroidism and thyroid storm. Emerg Med Clin North Am 1989;7:873–83.

Sherman SI, Simons L, Ladenson PW: Clinical and socioeconomic predispositions to complicated thyrotoxicosis: a predictable and preventable syndrome? Am J Med 1996;101:192–8.

Tietgens ST, Leinung MC: Thyroid storm. Med Clin North Am 1995;79:169–84.

MYXEDEMA COMA

ESSENTIALS OF DIAGNOSIS

- *Features of severe hypothyroidism (myxedema): dry, rough, cold skin; nonpitting doughy edema; loss of eyebrows and scalp hair; and delayed relaxation phase of deep tendon reflexes.*
- *Hypothermia.*
- *Altered mental status or coma.*
- *Hypercapnic respiratory failure.*

General Considerations

Myxedema coma represents a breakdown of the body's compensatory mechanisms during the course of longstanding severe hypothyroidism. Development of an intercurrent illness such as an infection on top of the underlying severe myxedema usually leads to this decompensation. Myxedema coma is primarily a clinical diagnosis. While laboratory tests confirm hypothyroidism, the diagnosis is based on the constellation of clinical findings of myxedema, altered mental status, and hypothermia. The physician must remain alert for the possibility of myxedema coma because the consequences of missing the diagnosis can be devastating. In addition, the usual clinical signs of infection such as fever and leukocytosis may be masked in patients with severe hypothyroidism. Therefore, one must also actively search for infection or other precipitating factors and aggressively treat these illnesses.

Pathophysiology

Hypothyroidism is a common endocrinopathy, but myxedema coma is encountered much less commonly because of thyroid hormone replacement therapy. Myxedema coma is associated with poor outcome. Patients with myxedema most often have a history of hypothyroidism, but the precipitating condition is almost always a combination of failure to take an adequate amount of thyroid replacement therapy and the presence of some comorbid condition. Because the serum half-life of T_4 is quite long, hypothyroidism is a subacute condition characterized by decreased metabolic rate, accumulation of edema fluid, deterioration of cardiac function from structural and physiologic changes, hyperlipidemia, and inability to manifest an appropriate response to hypothermia. Ventilatory drive is diminished from central mechanisms and, because of respiratory muscle weakness and pleural effusions and ascites, can result in hypercapnia. Hyponatremia is common and results from the inability to maximally dilute urine.

Clinical Features

Myxedema coma almost always occurs in patients with known hypothyroidism but can rarely present as the initial finding in hypothyroidism. A precipitating event can usually be identified along with absent or inadequate thyroid replacement therapy. The majority of cases of myxedema coma are reported in winter months in regions with cold climates. Thus, cold exposure appears to be an important antecedent factor. Other precipitating factors include sedative or anesthetic drugs, congestive heart failure, cerebrovascular accidents, trauma, infections, and a variety of other illnesses.

A. Symptoms and Signs

Most patients with myxedema are elderly women. The classic signs of myxedema are present, including puffy expressionless face; dry, rough, and cold skin; nonpitting doughy edema; loss of eyebrows and scalp hair; delayed relaxation phase of the tendon reflexes; and enlarged tongue. Hypothermia is a hallmark of myxedema coma, with core body temperatures as low as 21 °C but more often in the range of 32–35 °C. Severe hypothermia (temperature < 32 °C) is associated with a poor prognosis. However, hypothermia can be easily overlooked if a thermometer that can register temperatures below the usual range is not used. Blood pressure may be normal, high, or low. The heart rate is classically slow. Respirations may be slow and shallow, depending on the level of ventilatory drive and respiratory muscle weakness. Mental status changes may include confusion, somnolence, hallucinations, or coma. The thyroid gland may not be palpable because of idiopathic atrophy, prior radiation, or surgery.

Drug metabolism is significantly reduced in hypothyroidism, and administration of the usual doses of sedatives may significantly depress ventilation and compromise mental status. In critically ill patients, the diagnosis of hypothyroidism may sometimes be hard to make on clinical grounds.

B. Laboratory Findings

Hyponatremia is often present. Arterial blood gases may reveal respiratory acidosis, hypercapnia, and hypoxemia. Hypoglycemia may occur, particularly if there is deficiency of pituitary hormones as well. Chest x-ray may reveal an enlarged cardiac silhouette and pleural and pericardial effusions. The ECG may demonstrate low voltage, sinus bradycardia, diffuse T wave depression, nonspecific ST changes, and prolonged QT and PR intervals. There may be conduction blocks as well. Cerebrospinal fluid pressure and protein concentrations may be increased.

Although myxedema coma is a clinical diagnosis, thyroid function tests reveal low thyroxine (T_4), low T_3 resin uptake, and a high thyrotropin (TSH) level. It may at times be difficult to distinguish sick euthyroid syndrome from primary hypothyroidism by thyroid function tests. Very high serum TSH levels (> 20 μU/mL) favor the diagnosis of primary hypothyroidism. Moderately elevated TSH levels (up to 20 μU/mL) may be seen in the course of sick euthyroid syndrome. Severe nonthyroidal illness decreases the TSH response, and inappropriately low TSH is seen in secondary hypothyroidism (hypothalamic or pituitary disorders).

C. Adrenal Insufficiency

In patients with hypothyroidism, the manifestations of adrenal insufficiency may be masked. This is important because adrenal insufficiency can coexist with hypothyroidism in two clinical situations. First, in patients with autoimmune thyroid disease, there is a higher incidence of autoimmune adrenalitis and adrenal insufficiency than in the general population. Second, patients with panhypopituitarism may have absence of both TSH and ACTH. These patients with secondary adrenal insufficiency lack the skin and mucosal hyperpigmentation that is characteristic of primary adrenal insufficiency. For these reasons, it is easy to miss adrenal insufficiency in this setting, and the clinician must keep alert to the possibility of concomitant adrenal insufficiency. A rapid ACTH stimulation test should be performed in patients with myxedema. However, it should be recognized that the cortisol response to ACTH may be attenuated by hypothyroidism.

Treatment

Treatment consists of thyroid hormone replacement, replacement of other necessary hormones, and supportive measures (Table 25–2), including treatment of hypothermia and of the precipitating illness.

A. Thyroid Hormone Replacement

While all commentators assert the need for prompt thyroid hormone replacement in myxedema coma, there is disagreement about what constitutes an optimal regimen. The major controversy relates to which regimen of thyroid hormone replacement to use: T_4 alone, T_3 alone, or a combination of T_4 and T_3. The use of T_3 alone has been advocated by some on physiologic grounds. This is because the activity of 5′-deiodinase is diminished in hypothyroidism and the conversion of T_4 to T_3 may be limited. On the other hand, a rapid increase in T_3 may be detrimental to the patient because of cardiac arrhythmias and too rapid an increase in myocardial oxygen demand. Large doses of T_3 (> 75 μg) have been associated with increased mortality. Because of its potential adverse effects, the use of this regimen has been discouraged by some.

Intravenous administration of T_4 is considered safe and has been the standard for the past 3 decades. One traditional regimen comprises 500 μg of levothyroxine (T_4) given slowly intravenously followed by 100–150 μg every 24 hours. The rationale for the large initial dose is that it restores the total thyroxine pool. However, it is not clear if this regimen is any better than 150 μg given intravenously daily. The rate of fall in serum TSH levels is not significantly different between the two regimens. In fact, a dose of 100 μg of levothyroxine daily would correct the thermoregulatory, respiratory, cardiac, and mental status changes over 24–48 hours.

A third regimen consists of a combination of both T_4 and T_3. It is suggested that 200–300 μg of T_4 be given simultaneously with 25 μg of T_3 intravenously. This is followed by administration of another 25 μg of T_3 12 hours later and 100 μg of T_4 at 24 hours. Starting the third day, 100 μg of T_4 is given daily until the patient regains consciousness.

There is no strong basis for advocating any one regimen. The rapid restoration of thyroid hormone levels

Table 25–2. Treatment of myxedema coma.

Mechanism of Action	Treatment
Thyroid hormone replacement	Levothyroxine (T_4), 500 μg by slow intravenous infusion, followed by 100–150 μg every 24 hours. *or* T_4, 200–300 μg, and triiodothyronine (T_3), 25 μg IV; 25 μg of T_3 12 hours later; and 100 μg of T_4 at 24 hours.
Glucocorticoid	Hydrocortisone, 100 mg IV every 8 hours.
Supportive measures	Maintain adequate ventilation. Institute endoctracheal intubation and mechanical ventilation if necessary. Identify and treat the precipitating event. Provide fluid and electrolyte replacement as needed. Correct core body temperature.

must be balanced against the known mortality of prolonged myxedema coma. However, most authorities would agree that high-dose thyroxine would be a reasonable and safe choice.

B. Glucocorticoids

As discussed above, signs of adrenal insufficiency may be masked in hypothyroid patients. On the other hand, initiation of levothyroxine therapy without concomitant glucocorticoid replacement may precipitate adrenal crisis if the patient has adrenal insufficiency. Therefore, one must be on guard against the possibility of adrenal insufficiency in appropriate patients. If in doubt, it is better to err on the side of treatment with corticosteroids (see Adrenal Insufficiency, below), since the consequences of delayed or no replacement can be serious.

C. Supportive Measures

These patients may need transient endotracheal intubation and mechanical ventilation for hypercapnic respiratory failure. Intravenous fluids, electrolytes, and pressor agents may be needed to maintain blood pressure. Rapid rewarming through the use of heating blankets is not generally recommended because it may provoke or worsen peripheral vasodilation and hypotension. However, in patients with severe hypothermia, thermogenic shivering mechanisms may become impaired, and these patients may not be able to raise their body temperatures. Therefore, gradual but active rewarming may be required. In most patients with mild hypothermia, wrapping the patient in blankets in a warm room is sufficient to restore body temperature provided thyroid replacement therapy has been initiated. Treatment of hypothermia is discussed in Chapter 38. A search for infection or other precipitating factors should be mounted. In many instances, empiric antibiotic therapy may be justified. Because of decreased metabolic rate, many drugs are cleared more slowly in patients with severe hypothyroidism.

Prognosis

Myxedema coma may be fatal if unrecognized and left untreated. Poor prognostic indicators include severe hypercapnia and hypothermia. If infection or other precipitating illness is present, outcome is dependent on treatment and response to these problems. Complications of thyroxine (T_4) and triiodothyronine (T_3) replacement therapy may include serious cardiac morbidities.

Hylander B, Rosenqvist U: Treatment of myxedema coma: Factors associated with fatal outcome. Acta Endocrinol (Copenhagen) 1985;108:65–71.

Jordan RM: Myxedema coma: Pathophysiology, therapy, and factors affecting prognosis. Med Clin North Am 1995;79:185–94.

Menendez CE, Rivlin RS: Thyrotoxic crisis and myxedema coma. Med Clin North Am 1973;57:1463–70.

Nicoloff JT: Thyroid storm and myxedema coma. Med Clin North Am 1985;69:1005–17.

Ridgeway EC et al: Metabolic responses of patients with myxedema to large doses of intravenous L-thyroxine. Ann Intern Med 1972;77:549–55.

Ringel MD: Management of hypothyroidism and hyperthyroidism in the intensive care unit. Crit Care Clin 2001;17:59–74.

Yamamoto T, Fukuyama J, Fujiyoshi A: Factors associated with mortality of myxedema coma: Report of eight cases and literature survey. Thyroid 1999;9:1167–72.

ACUTE ADRENAL INSUFFICIENCY

ESSENTIALS OF DIAGNOSIS

- *Hypotension, volume depletion, hypovolemic shock.*
- *Hyperkalemia, hyponatremia.*
- *Weakness, abdominal pain, nausea, vomiting, fever.*
- *Acute infectious illness or trauma, recent cessation of corticosteroid therapy, or inadequate replacement in chronic adrenal insufficiency.*
- *Abnormal cosyntropin stimulation test.*

General Considerations

Critical illness, whether from sepsis, trauma, surgery, or any condition associated with hemodynamic compromise, stimulates the hypothalamic-pituitary-adrenal axis with a resultant increased production of cortisol. This hormone, synthesized in the adrenal cortex under the influence of ACTH, maintains vascular integrity and tone, stimulates neoglucogenesis, helps free water clearance, and influences fluid and electrolyte balance. Lack of aldosterone—a mineralocorticoid—is associated with inability to conserve sodium in the face of hypovolemia and hyperkalemia. Deficiency of cortisol—a glucocorticoid—on the other hand is associated with inability to clear free water and with hemodynamic compromise mimicking hypovolemic or septic shock. Patients with adrenal insufficiency become hypotensive due to a combination of factors including hypovolemia and impaired vascular response to catecholamines and due also to loss of a direct inotropic effect of cortisol. Cortisol stimulates hepatic neoglucogenesis, and it is therefore not surprising that patients with adrenal insufficiency may present with hypoglycemia. Serum cortisol levels in acutely ill patients are usually increased.

Acute adrenal insufficiency is the result of inadequate cortisol production with life-threatening cardiovascular collapse and potentially severe electrolyte and fluid abnormalities. Acute insufficiency can occur as a result of an acute insult to the adrenal glands from infection or trauma or may be seen in a patient with chronic adrenal insufficiency who has critical illness. Patients who receive corticosteroids for treatment of inflammatory diseases will have chronic suppression of pituitary-adrenal function. Abrupt cessation of therapy may precipitate acute adrenal insufficiency, especially if there is intercurrent illness. Suspecting the diagnosis of adrenal crisis is the key. Because delay in instituting treatment can be fatal, acute adrenal insufficiency should be suspected in any patient presenting with hypotension, fever, abdominal pain, hyponatremia, or hyperkalemia, especially if hyperpigmentation is present. In many clinical situations, empiric therapy may be appropriate even before a definitive diagnosis has been made.

Idiopathic or autoimmune adrenalitis accounts for about 80% of cases of chronic adrenal insufficiency in outpatients. Tuberculosis used to be a major cause of adrenal insufficiency, but that disease is relatively uncommon now in developed countries. Other less common causes include adrenal hemorrhage; fungal infections such as histoplasmosis, coccidioidomycosis, blastomycosis, and candidiasis; hemochromatosis; irradiation; surgical removal of the adrenal glands, drug toxicity, and congenital disorders such as synthetic enzyme deficiencies. Patients with HIV infection often have abnormalities in the adrenal glands at autopsy but appear to have only a slightly increased incidence of adrenal insufficiency (about 5–10%). The impaired immune status resulting from HIV infection increases the likelihood of adrenal involvement with cytomegalovirus (the most common finding), fungi (cryptococcus, histoplasma), or mycobacteria (both tuberculous and nontuberculous). HIV, however, directly affects the adrenal glands only in a small number of patients. Other causes include metastatic disease and hemorrhage. Although metastases to the adrenal gland are relatively common, adrenal insufficiency as a result of metastatic disease is uncommon. Adrenal hemorrhage may occur during the course of sepsis, anticoagulants, trauma, pregnancy, or surgery. Adrenal infarction may occur as a result of thrombosis, embolism, or arteritis. Infiltrative disorders include amyloidosis, sarcoidosis, and hemochromatosis. Congenital disorders leading to adrenal insufficiency include congenital adrenal hyperplasia. This is due to a genetic defect in one of the steroidogenic enzymes or hypoplasia. Secondary adrenal insufficiency can occur in HIV-infected patients because of direct involvement of the hypothalamus or the pituitary gland, opportunistic infections (tuberculoma, histoplasmosis), or lymphoma.

A number of drugs directly inhibit the enzymes involved in steroidogenesis. For example, metyrapone inhibits β-hydroxylase, aminoglutethimide inhibits side chain cleavage enzymes, ketoconazole inhibits a number of P450-linked steroidogenic enzymes, and mitotane is an adrenolytic cytotoxic agent. Fluconazole has also been implicated. Relatively common medications such as rifampin and seizure medications (phenytoin, carbamazepine) increase hepatic cytochrome P450 activity, thus increasing cortisol metabolism. These medications should be used with caution in patients with limited adrenal reserve.

In patients with autoimmune adrenalitis, there is an increased incidence of other endocrinopathies. For example, Hashimoto's thyroiditis, Graves' disease, pernicious anemia, hypoparathyroidism, premature ovarian or testicular failure, and type 1 diabetes occur with a greater frequency than in the general population. It is now clear that multiple endocrine organs may be affected by organ-specific autoimmune disease. These polyendocrine autoimmune syndromes are classified into two major groups: type I and type II. Type I patients usually present in early childhood with hypoparathyroidism and mucocutaneous candidiasis; adrenal insufficiency may develop later. Disease is usually limited to one generation of siblings. In contrast, type II patients usually present with adrenal insufficiency in the third or fourth decade. Diabetes occurs in almost half of patients. There is a strong association with HLA-DR3 or -DR4 haplotypes. Hyperthyroidism (Graves' disease), Hashimoto's thyroiditis, primary ovarian failure, myasthenia gravis, celiac disease, and pernicious anemia occur much more commonly in patients with type 2 polyendocrine autoimmune syndrome than in the general population. Multiple generations in the same family are usually affected.

Acute Adrenal Crisis

Acute adrenal crisis refers to the collapse and shock syndrome that occurs in a patient with inadequate adrenal cortical function. This can occur in chronic adrenal insufficiency because of stress imposed by a serious illness such as infection, trauma, or surgery without adequate replacement. In other patients, acute bilateral adrenal hemorrhage (Waterhouse-Friderichsen syndrome), originally described in association with meningococcemia, is the cause of acute adrenal insufficiency. Acute adrenal hemorrhage can complicate the course of systemic sepsis from other pathogens as well. In fact, *Pseudomonas aeruginosa* is a common organism in children dying with sepsis and adrenal hemorrhage. Other common antecedent factors include anticoagulant therapy, disseminated intravascular coagulation, and the perioperative state.

Clinical Features

The clinical manifestations of adrenal insufficiency depend (1) on whether the patient has primary or secondary adrenal failure; (2) on the presence or absence of other endocrinopathies (eg, coexistence of hypothyroidism may significantly attenuate the manifestations of adrenal insufficiency); and (3) on the presence of superimposed nonendocrinologic illness or stress. In the ICU, symptoms and signs of the acute illness may overshadow the features of concomitant adrenal insufficiency, making clinical suspicion the key to diagnosis.

A. Symptoms and Signs

Patients with chronic adrenal insufficiency may not come to medical attention for some time because of the nonspecific nature of symptoms, such as fatigue, anorexia, weight loss, nausea, and vomiting. Other manifestations include weakness, salt craving, and postural dizziness. Patients with primary adrenal insufficiency usually have hyperpigmentation of the skin and mucous membranes because of increased ACTH production by the pituitary. Patients often develop a "tan" in exposed parts, especially in areas that suffer chronic friction and trauma such as elbows, knees, knuckles, and the beltline. The buccal mucosa may show hyperpigmentation, especially along sites of dental occlusion. The "tan" appearance of these patients often conveys a misleading impression of good health. Scars acquired during the course of adrenal insufficiency also become hyperpigmented, while those acquired before or after remain unpigmented.

The hallmarks of acute adrenal insufficiency (adrenal crisis) include severe hypotension and vascular collapse, nausea, vomiting, abdominal pain, and fever. Hypotension is due largely to volume depletion, and there may be other evidence of volume depletion. Abdominal symptoms may lead to an erroneous diagnosis of acute abdomen resulting in unwarranted and potentially catastrophic surgical exploration. Confusion and altered mental status may also occur. Petechiae may be found if meningococcemia is the cause of acute adrenal hemorrhage. Hyperpigmentation, if present, indicates chronic primary adrenal insufficiency. Infection, surgical stress, and trauma may precipitate acute adrenal crisis in patients with chronic adrenal insufficiency. Patients should be questioned about receiving chronic corticosteroid therapy, especially if they have a history of asthma, interstitial lung disease, rheumatologic diseases such as systemic lupus erythematosus, or lymphoproliferative disorders. Patients with HIV infection and autoimmune endocrinopathies should be suspected of adrenal insufficiency if they present with intractable hypotension and hyponatremia.

A degree of clinical suspicion may be necessary in evaluating critically ill patients who may present in atypical fashion. Patients with hemodynamic instability that cannot be easily explained—in association with fever with no identified source and alteration in mental status—should be considered for adrenal insufficiency.

B. Laboratory Findings

Laboratory data may reveal hyponatremia, hyperkalemia, and azotemia. Hypoglycemia occurs more often in children but may be seen in adults as well, especially in those who have been vomiting. Corticosteroids play an important role in regulating gluconeogenesis and have potent anti-insulin actions. Hypercalcemia and eosinophilia may also be found. Hyponatremia is usually multifactorial. Patients with primary adrenal insufficiency are unable to conserve sodium because of mineralocorticoid deficiency. However, these patients become hyponatremic even in the face of positive sodium balance. This is mainly because of inability to clear free water due to corticosteroid deficiency. The exact pathophysiology of the defect in free water clearance in primary adrenal insufficiency is not known, but there is lack of adequate suppression of ADH levels in the face of hyponatremia. In addition, corticosteroids are also felt to exert a permissive effect directly at the kidney level in modulating ADH action. In the evaluation of volume depletion and hyponatremia, low urinary sodium usually reflects volume depletion; in adrenal insufficiency, however, urinary sodium may be elevated because of inability of the kidneys to conserve sodium maximally in the absence of cortisol and aldosterone.

C. Adrenal Function Tests

A patient in whom acute adrenal insufficiency is suspected should be treated immediately. However, diagnosis can be made rapidly and reliably by an ACTH stimulation test. A random serum cortisol level greater than 20 μg/dL makes the diagnosis of adrenal insufficiency unlikely.

The traditional protocol for the rapid ACTH stimulation test is as follows: 250 μg of cosyntropin (containing amino acids 1–24 of ACTH) is administered intravenously or intramuscularly, and plasma samples are obtained at 0, 30, and 60 minutes for measurement of cortisol. In addition, it is helpful to save contingency samples for plasma aldosterone measurement. Studies had suggested that an increment of > 7 μg/dL after cosyntropin administration or peak levels > 17 μg/dL would exclude adrenal insufficiency. However, other data indicate that any cortisol value ≥ 20 μg/dL before or after the cosyntropin test is consistent with normal adrenal function. Concern about adrenal insufficiency should be raised if any of these criteria are not met. A normal response excludes primary adrenal insufficiency. A small incremental increase in plasma cortisol after cosyntropin despite a baseline value in the normal range may be associated with a poor outcome and increased mortality.

Some studies have suggested that the supraphysiologic dose of corticotropin used may cause false-negative readings in patients with partial or secondary adrenal insufficiency. This is because patients with acute adrenal insufficiency may have some reserves left and using the relatively large dose of corticotropin would lead to a normal response. Some have advocated using the low-dose ACTH stimulation test with 1 μg of corticotropin. A normal response is a rise in cortisol level to 20 μg/dL or more at 30 minutes or 60 minutes.

If the cortisol response to cosyntropin is subnormal, the contingency samples can be used for aldosterone and endogenous ACTH measurements in order to distinguish primary from secondary adrenal insufficiency. Aldosterone responses to cosyntropin are impaired in primary adrenal insufficiency but are preserved in secondary adrenal insufficiency (decreased endogenous ACTH secretion). ACTH levels are elevated in primary adrenal insufficiency and low normal or below normal in secondary adrenal insufficiency. Certain clinical features can also be useful in distinguishing primary from secondary adrenal insufficiency. For example, hyperpigmentation and hyperkalemia are observed only in primary but not in secondary adrenal insufficiency. The presence of other endocrine hormone deficiencies does not necessarily indicate panhypopituitarism, since these could also be a consequence of autoimmune polyendocrinopathy.

Treatment

Once the diagnosis of adrenal insufficiency has been made, treatment is relatively straightforward (Table 25–3).

A. Corticosteroid Replacement

Promptness in instituting corticosteroid therapy is very important. Corticosteroid therapy can be given as hydrocortisone sodium succinate, 75–100 mg intravenously every 6–8 hours. If the patient is hypotensive, performance of the diagnostic ACTH stimulation test may unduly delay institution of therapy. Under these circumstances, an equivalent dose of dexamethasone (3–4 mg every 6–8 hours) can be given intravenously contemporaneously with ACTH administration. Dexamethasone does not cross-react in the cortisol assay, and the diagnostic procedure can therefore be done without concern about the delay in instituting replacement therapy. The dose of hydrocortisone sodium succinate can be reduced to the replacement level (10–20 mg in the morning and 5–10 mg in the evening) as the patient's condition improves.

Some studies cast doubt on the need for large pharmacologic doses of corticosteroids during stress. Studies in adrenalectomized monkeys suggest that physiologic replacement doses of corticosteroids are sufficient in this primate model to tolerate stress of surgical laparotomy. Supraphysiologic doses of corticosteroids conferred no survival advantage on these adrenalectomized monkeys over physiologic replacement doses during the period of surgical stress. Other studies have shown that patients receiving steroids prior to undergoing surgery did not require additional glucocorticoids during the perioperative period.

Empiric recommendations for glucocorticoid administration in surgical patients are to estimate the degree of stress and give 25 mg/d of hydrocortisone for mild stress, 50–75 mg/d for 2–3 days for moderate stress, and 100–150 mg/d for 2–3 days for severe stress. After recovery from acute illness, patients with adrenal insufficiency should be placed on chronic replacement therapy with hydrocortisone. Traditionally, a dose of

Table 25–3. Management of acute adrenal insufficiency (adrenal crisis).

Diagnostic testing	If you are considering a diagnosis of acute adrenal insufficiency, perform a rapid ACTH test (see text) immediately and initiate treatment pending return of laboratory results. If a patient is highly likely to have adrenal insufficiency, give dexamethasone immediately while the ACTH test is being conducted.
Glucocorticoid	Hydrocortisone sodium succinate, 75–100 mg IV immediately and then every 6–8 hours. *or* Dexamethasone, 3–4 mg IV every 6–8 hours.
Mineralocorticoid	Not required when large doses of hydrocortisone (> 50–60 mg/d) are used. Consider adding fludrocortisone acetate, 0.05–0.1 mg orally daily if dexamethasone is used.
Supportive measures	Identify and treat the precipitating illness. Correct fluid and electrolyte abnormalities. Intravenous NaCl 0.9% is usually given initially. Monitor blood glucose and electrolytes and administer glucose if necessary.

30 mg hydrocortisone administered in two divided doses—20 mg in the morning and 10 mg in the evening—has been widely used. However, recent assessments using more accurate isotope dilution and mass spectrometric methods suggest that the daily cortisol production rates are 5–6 mg/m^2 body surface area rather than the 12–15 mg/m^2 body surface area, as was previously thought. Therefore, the traditional regimen of 30 mg hydrocortisone daily probably represents excessive glucocorticoid replacement, and may increase the risk of osteoporosis. A more appropriate regimen may be 15 mg of hydrocortisone administered in two divided doses: 10 mg in the morning and 5 mg in the afternoon.

B. Mineralocorticoid Replacement

Most patients with primary adrenal insufficiency require mineralocorticoid replacement. In chronic adrenal insufficiency, this can be administered as fludrocortisone acetate. The usual starting dosage is 0.05–0.1 mg by mouth daily. Some patients may develop leg edema upon initiation of therapy. This will usually abate if the dose is reduced. Hydrocortisone by itself has some mineralocorticoid activity, so that when patients are receiving more than 50–60 mg/d of hydrocortisone, no additional mineralocorticoid replacement is necessary. However, if dexamethasone, which has little or no mineralocorticoid activity, is used instead of hydrocortisone, a mineralocorticoid should be added.

C. Fluid and Electrolytes

Patients with adrenal insufficiency often have an enormous salt and water deficit. It is important to correct these deficits aggressively by administration of 0.9% NaCl solution intravenously. However, patients with adrenal insufficiency may continue to be hypotensive even after adequate fluid and electrolyte replacement. Blood pressure may only be restored by corticosteroid administration. It is often not recognized that corticosteroids have an inotropic effect on the myocardium. Patients with adrenal insufficiency may present with hyperkalemia, so routine potassium replacement should be postponed until serum potassium measurements are obtained.

D. Glucose

Corticosteroids are important regulators of gluconeogenesis. In adults (unlike children), hypoglycemia is not a common manifestation of adrenal insufficiency. However, patients who have been vomiting for a few days may present with hypoglycemia or develop hypoglycemia during the course of evaluation or treatment. Therefore, plasma glucose levels should be monitored and glucose given intravenously to correct or prevent hypoglycemia.

E. Other Treatment

It is crucial to identify and treat the antecedent illness precipitating acute adrenal insufficiency. This may include administration of antibiotics to treat an infection. Many patients with adrenal insufficiency have one or more endocrinopathies. It is important to recognize and treat these when identified.

Lamberts SWJ, Bruining HA, De Jong FH: Corticosteroid therapy in severe illness. N Engl J Med 1997;337:1285–92.

Laureti S et al: Low dose (1 μg) ACTH test in the evaluation of adrenal dysfunction in pre-clinical Addison's disease. Clin Endocrinol (Oxf) 2000;53:107–15.

May ME, Carey RM: Rapid adrenocorticotropic hormone test in practice: Retrospective review. Am J Med 1985;79:679–84.

Peacey SR et al: Glucocorticoid replacement therapy: are patients over treated and does it matter? Clin Endocrinol (Oxf) 1997;46:255–61.

Rivers EP et al: Adrenal insufficiency in high-risk surgical ICU patients. Chest 2001;119:889–96.

Salem M et al: Perioperative glucocorticoid coverage: a reassessment 42 years after emergence of a problem. Ann Surg 1994;219:416–25.

Schroeder S et al: The hypothalamic-pituitary-adrenal axis of patients with severe sepsis: altered response to corticotropin-releasing hormone. Crit Care Med 2001;29:310–16.

Shenker Y, Skatrud JB: Adrenal insufficiency in critically ill patients. Am J Resp Crit Care Med 2001;163:1520–3.

Udelsman R et al: Adaptation during surgical stress. A reevaluation of the role of glucocorticoids. J Clin Invest 1986;77:1377–81.

Zaloga GP, Marik P: Hypothalamic-pituitary-adrenal insufficiency. Crit Care Clin 2001;17:25–41.

SICK EUTHYROID SYNDROME

ESSENTIALS OF DIAGNOSIS

- *Low T_3 suggestive of hypothyroidism in a patient with acute or chronic nonthyroidal illness.*
- *But patient is euthyroid, as shown by clinical appearance, normal TSH, usually normal or blunted TSH response to TRH, and normal free T_4 by equilibrium dialysis.*
- *In extremely ill patients, free T_4 may fall to subnormal levels.*

General Considerations

Alterations in thyroid function occurring with nonthyroidal illness are usually associated with changes in other hormonal systems and can be thought of as part of a complex and multifaceted response of the endocrine system to illness. A variety of nonthyroidal illnesses produce alterations in thyroid function in patients in whom no intrinsic thyroid disease is present and the patient is judged to be euthyroid. These low T_3 and low T_3-T_4 syndromes seen with nonthyroidal illness represent a continuum probably reflecting severity of the disease process rather than discrete conditions. The syndromes must be distinguished from hypothyroidism, as their treatment requires correction of the underlying disorder rather than thyroid hormone replacement.

Pathophysiology

The sick euthyroid syndrome is essentially a laboratory diagnosis (Table 25–4). Patients are clinically euthyroid, but because they have acute or chronic nonthyroidal illness, clinical features of the underlying disease may make assessment of thyroid status difficult or unclear. The syndrome may be divided into three patterns: low T_3, low T_3 and T_4, and low thyroid-stimulating hormone (TSH).

A. Low T_3

This is the most common presentation. In the early stages of nonthyroidal illness, serum T_3 (bound and free) decreases and reverse T_3 (rT_3) is increased. T_4 and TSH levels are within the normal range. The low T_3 state results in part from decreased conversion of T_4 to T_3 because of inhibition of peripheral tissue 5′-monodeiodinase activity and reduced T_3 production. Contrary to earlier belief that the elevated rT_3 resulted from increased conversion of T_4 to rT_3, the elevated rT_3 results from decreased rT_3 clearance secondary to decreased 5′-monodeiodinase activity. Circulating T_3 levels can fall below normal within 24 hours after onset of any systemic illness, major trauma, surgery, or caloric deprivation, and T_3 concentrations generally become normal as the underlying illness resolves. It has been postulated that decreased T_3 may be a protective mechanism during acute illness because it is associated with decreased urine urea nitrogen excretion and decreased protein breakdown.

In the early recovery phases from illness, there may be a transient increase in serum TSH concentrations to levels seen in patients with primary hypothyroidism. Although these levels rarely exceed 20 μU/L, there have been several case reports of sick euthyroid patients having TSH values exceeding this commonly used cutoff value. This elevation of TSH has been proposed to stimulate the thyroid gland to increase its secretion of T_4. Nonetheless, a TSH level > 20 μU/mL in a sick patient is suggestive of primary hypothyroidism.

B. Low T_3 and T_4

Free T_4 (FT_4) is almost always normal early in the course of nonthyroidal illness. In more severe illness of longer duration, the decreased serum T_3 levels are accompanied by a reduction in serum T_4. This portends a poor prognosis: the greater the reduction in T_4, the worse the outcome. This condition may occur in up to 50% of medical patients admitted to an ICU. In patients with T_4 concentrations less than 3 μg/dL, the mortality rate may reach 80%. The fall in free T_4 to subnormal levels is multifactorial; decreased TSH resulting in decreased T_4 secretion from the thyroid, alterations in T_4 binding to plasma proteins, and alterations in binding protein concentrations all contribute to low T_4 concentrations. Despite the finding of very low T_4, these patients are not generally considered as having hypothyroidism; replacement of thyroid hormone does not improve outcome.

C. Low TSH

Low T_3 or low T_3 and T_4 are also seen in hypothyroidism, but a euthyroid state in these patients with nonthyroidal illness is suggested by the clinical appearance, the normal TSH, and the normal free T_4 by equilibrium dialysis. Also, the TSH response may be blunted to TRH stimulation.

TSH values < 0.1 μU/mL are commonly encountered in euthyroid hospitalized patients, though most patients will have only marginally depressed values > 0.1 μU/mL. The availability of more sensitive third-generation TSH assays has made it possible to distinguish between marginally depressed TSH concentrations in euthyroid patients and the suppressed levels seen with hyperthyroidism (< 0.01 μU/mL). If necessary, a TRH (thyrotropin-releasing hormone) stimulation test can be used to confirm the result. Euthyroid patients with nonthyroidal illness and depressed TSH will show detectable responses of TSH (> 0.1 μU/mL) to TRH stimulation, whereas hyperthyroid patients will show the expected absence of response to TRH stimulation.

Table 25–4. Profile of thyroid hormone indices during different phases of acute illness.

Phases of Illness	T_3	T_4	FT_4	rT_3	TSH
Mild, early	D	N	N	I	N
Moderate	D	N, D	N	I	N
Severe	D	D	D	I	N, D
Early recovery	D	D, N	D, N	I	N, I

Key: D = decreased; I = increased; N = normal

A. Laboratory Findings

When assessing thyroid dysfunction in the critically ill, perhaps the best initial screening tests are total T_4, T_3 resin uptake, T_3, and sensitive TSH levels. Low T_3 is always seen in sick euthyroid syndrome and can fall from normal values within 24 hours after onset of acute illness. The rT_3 level may be increased. The euthyroid state is confirmed if total T_4 and T_3 resin uptake are normal or if free T_4 by equilibrium dialysis is normal, along with normal TSH values.

As described above, a more difficult situation arises when T_3 and T_4 are reduced in more severe or prolonged illness. Free T_4 by equilibrium dialysis is often normal but may be misleadingly low despite the patient being clinically euthyroid. A low TSH generally confirms the finding of a euthyroid state, while TSH > 20 μU/L make hypothyroidism a strong possibility. If there is any doubt about the TSH response, then evaluation of pituitary function may be helpful.

B. Disorders Associated With Altered Thyroid Function Tests

A variety of conditions can produce alterations in thyroid function tests suggesting thyroid hormone deficiency (Table 25–5).

1. Malnutrition or caloric deprivation—Caloric deprivation such as is seen during fasting can produce a significant fall in serum T_3 concentrations and rise in serum rT_3 within the first 24 hours. Hypocaloric diets as low as 600 kcal/d can produce these same changes. T_4 concentrations are usually normal, but the TSH response to TRH is blunted. Free T_4 may rise transiently and then stabilize. It has been suggested that caloric deprivation causes the starving body to conserve energy by reducing the amount of metabolically active T_3. Administering T_3 to starving subjects induces greater muscle catabolism. Refeeding with as little as 50 g carbohydrate (200 kcal) will normalize serum T_3 and rT_3. However, the TSH response to TRH may remain reduced, suggesting a difference in recovery time between peripheral 5′-monodeiodination and pituitary responsiveness.

2. Chronic liver disease—Liver disease may have profound effects on thyroid function. The liver is the main organ for thyroid hormone metabolism and the major site for extrathyroidal (peripheral) conversion of T_4 to T_3. Serum T_3 levels are low, rT_3 elevated, and TSH normal in patients with liver disease. The serum T_4 is usually normal, though low levels are found in the most severely ill. Very low T_3 predicts a poor outcome.

3. Renal disease—Patients with chronic renal failure tend to have multiple factors that may affect thyroid function tests. These include poor nutrition, metabolic disturbances, medications, and hemodialysis. A reduced serum T_3 is found in many patients, and T_3 does not increase with thyroxine replacement. However, rT_3 is normal rather than elevated because of increased uptake in tissues. Secondary hyperparathyroidism, which often accompanies renal failure, may also be partly responsible for this pattern of thyroid function tests because a low T_3 and normal rT_3 is also seen in states of elevated parathyroid hormone. Free T_4 may be elevated transiently during hemodialysis, probably representing a heparin effect. TSH levels are usually normal. Extensive metabolic studies of patients with renal failure and low serum T_3 concentrations indicate that they are euthyroid.

Patients with nephrotic syndrome may lose significant amounts of thyroid-binding globulin (TBG) from urinary protein losses, resulting in decreased serum T_4 levels. The T_3 resin uptake is increased in proportion to the lowered TBG levels, and the free T_4 index is usually normal. A variety of other conditions are associated with increased and decreased TBG levels (Table 25–6).

4. Diabetes mellitus—Diabetes and thyroid disorders are linked at several levels. The association of autoimmune thyroid disease with type 1 diabetes mellitus as part of the autoimmune polyendocrinopathy syndrome is well recognized. Diabetic ketoacidosis produces a similar pattern of altered thyroid function tests seen in other severe illnesses. With treatment, most patients normalize thyroid function tests within a few days. Insulin deficiency mimics a fasting state because carbohydrate is not properly utilized. Poorly controlled diabetes causes a marked reduction in conversion of T_4 to T_3; T_3 levels increase with improved glycemic control.

5. Infection—Infection also produces changes in thyroid hormone parameters similar to those seen in sick euthyroid patients. These alterations are corrected by successful treatment of the infection. Because malnutrition often accompanies severe infection, it is thought to

Table 25–5. Conditions that produce thyroid function test patterns suggesting thyroid hormone deficiency (sick euthyroid syndrome).

Malnutrition, caloric deprivation
Chronic liver disease
Renal disease
Diabetes mellitus
Infection
Acute myocardial infarction
Cancer
Surgery
Medications
AIDS

Table 25–6. Conditions associated with altered throxine binding globulin (TBG) concentrations.

Increased TBG	Decreased TBG
Physiologic conditions	Nonthyroidal illness
Pregnancy	Nephrotic syndrome
Newborn state	Chronic liver disease, cirrhosis
Nonthyroidal illness	Acromegaly
Acute hepatitis	Cushing's syndrome
Chronic liver disease	
Acute intermittent porphyria	Drugs
Hydatidiform mole	Androgens
Lymphosarcoma	Anabolic steroids
Estrogen-producing tumor	Glucocorticoids
Drugs	
Estrogens	Familial disorders
Heroin and methadone	
Clofibrate	
Fluorouracil	
Familial disorders	

play a role in the changes observed. Fever alone may also be a factor in altering thyroid function tests. A negative correlation between temperature and serum T_3 has been observed.

6. Acute myocardial infarction—A consistent pattern of thyroid function abnormalities has been observed in acute myocardial infarction. Serum T_3 concentrations fall after an acute myocardial infarction, reaching a nadir at 1–3 days with a reciprocal increase in rT_3. Serum TSH levels increase at day 4–5, followed by a rise in T_4. The severity and size of the infarct are correlated with the degree of fall in T_3 and the increase in rT_3.

7. Cancer—Most cancer patients show a pattern of thyroid studies similar to other nonthyroidal illness. Malnutrition and cachexia are contributing factors. Some antitumor chemotherapeutic agents such as fluorouracil and asparaginase alter TBG levels.

8. Surgery—Elective and emergency surgeries typically cause significant changes in thyroid hormone levels. Serum T_3 concentrations fall during surgery and may take up to a week to recover. This is accompanied by a reciprocal rise in rT_3. Serum T_4 levels usually remain stable unless there is a prolonged recovery period. TSH may be unchanged or reduced intraoperatively but returns to normal within a couple of days.

9. Medications—The patient in the intensive care unit is commonly taking multiple medications, some of which may have profound effects on thyroid function parameters. Some common drugs and their effects are listed in Table 25–7. Patients in the ICU commonly receive dopamine for blood pressure support or high-dose corticosteroids for various reasons. These drugs suppress TSH secretion, but not usually to the levels seen in hyperthyroidism. However, in patients with primary hypothyroidism, dopamine may suppress an elevated TSH into the normal range.

Other drugs likely to be encountered in the ICU that may confuse interpretation of thyroid function tests include octreotide, amiodarone, and beta-adrenergic antagonists. Octreotide decreases TSH secretion at high doses. Amiodarone, an antiarrhythmic drug containing iodide, may induce hypothyroidism or hyperthyroidism but more commonly results in low serum T_3 and normal or high T_4. Amiodarone inhibits 5′-deiodinase. Large doses of propranolol, atenolol, and metoprolol decrease serum T_3 levels but do not result in hypothyroidism.

10. AIDS—In patients with AIDS, direct infection of the thyroid gland by opportunistic organisms such as cytomegalovirus, cryptococcus, and *Pneumocystis carinii*

Table 25–7. Effect of drugs on thyroid function.

TSH suppression
Dopamine
Glucocorticoids
Bromocriptine
Apomorphine
Pyridoxine
Octreotide
Impaired thyroid hormone production or secretion
Thionamides (propylthiouracil, methimazole, carbimazole)
Lithium
Iodide
Amiodarone
Impaired T_4 to T_3 conversion
Propylthiouracil
Glucocorticoids
Propranolol
Ipodate sodium
Iopanoic acid
Amiodarone
Increased hepatic uptake and metabolism of T_4
Phenobarbital
Phenytoin
Carbamazepine
Rifampin
Impaired protein binding
Salicylates
Phenytoin

may rarely occur in addition to infiltration by Kaposi's sarcoma. Patients with *P carinii* thyroiditis may have hypo- or hyperthyroidism depending on the degree of involvement and disruption of the gland. Cytomegalovirus thyroiditis is usually associated with sick euthyroid syndrome rather than hypothyroidism. Some of the medications used for treating patients with AIDS may alter thyroid function. For example, rifampin increases T_4 clearance by hepatic microsomal enzyme induction. Hypothyroidism has been reported after ketoconazole treatment. One would expect to see a sick euthyroid pattern with AIDS, but this occurs infrequently and usually at later stages of HIV infection due to decreased extrathyroidal conversion to T_3. A unique pattern of thyroid function tests in AIDS has been observed that includes a progressive elevation in TBG, decreased rT_3, and normal T_3 levels. These alterations are felt to be part of the abnormal immunoregulation in HIV-infected individuals and may be mediated by tumor necrosis factor or other cytokines. The normal T_3 is felt to be a failure of the normal adaptive response to illness, but whether this causes the cachexia associated with AIDS remains to be proved.

Treatment

It is important to distinguish the sick euthyroid state from intrinsic thyroid disease, since the former does not require thyroid hormone replacement therapy. Studies show that treating patients with the low T_3-T_4 syndromes with T_4 was not beneficial and had no effect on mortality rates. In fact, there was no increase in T_3 levels, suggesting that peripheral conversion was not enhanced. To exclude inhibition of peripheral conversion as a factor in nonthyroidal illness, some investigators have administered T_3, but—once again—these studies have not demonstrated a beneficial effect on outcome. Supportive measures such as adequate nutrition and specific and successful treatment of the underlying illness should result in eventual normalization of the thyroid function alterations.

Current Controversies & Unresolved Issues

Two major issues related to sick euthyroid syndrome are the subject of some controversy. First, the pathogenesis of the syndrome remains unclear. The only thing that appears certain is that the mechanisms are complex and multifactorial and involve changes at multiple levels of the thyroid loop, including changes in TSH and thyroid hormone secretion, 5′-deiodinase, and thyroid hormone binding to proteins due to a variety of inhibitors.

Second, the physiologic significance of these changes in the thyroid function tests remains unclear. We do not know whether these abnormalities signal a functionally hypothyroid state or whether they are part of the body's adaptation to the stress of acute illness. The answer to this question will determine whether these patients should receive thyroid hormone replacement therapy. Unfortunately, there are no clinically practical markers that reflect the biologic action of thyroid hormones in tissues rather than their levels in the blood. Several studies in small numbers of patients have failed to reveal any benefit of thyroid hormone replacement therapy. On the contrary, in patients with burns, T_3 replacement increased urinary nitrogen excretion. Furthermore, thyroid hormone replacement therapy may inhibit TSH secretion and thereby delay recovery of thyroid function as the acute underlying illness abates. Only a large prospective study randomizing administration of thyroid hormone can answer this question.

Brent GA, Hershman JM: Thyroxine therapy in patients with severe nonthyroidal illnesses and low serum thyroxine concentration. J Clin Endocrinol Metab 1986;63:1–8.

Burman K, Wartofsky L: Thyroid function in the intensive care unit setting. Crit Care Clin 2001;17:43–57.

de los Santos ET, Mazzaferri EL: Sensitive thyroid-stimulating hormone assays: Clinical applications and limitations. Compr Ther 1988;14:26–33.

de los Santos ET, Mazzaferri EL: Thyroid function tests: Guidelines for interpretation in common clinical disorders. Postgrad Med 1989;85:333–40, 345–52.

Lopresti JS et al: Unique alterations of thyroid hormone indices in the acquired immunodeficiency syndrome (AIDS). Ann Intern Med 1989;110:970–5.

Ross DS: New sensitive immunoradiometric assays for thyrotropin. Ann Intern Med 1986;104:718–20.

Surks MI, Sievert R: Drugs and thyroid function. N Engl J Med 1995;333:1688–94.

Vasa FR, Molitch ME: Endocrine problems in the chronically critically ill patient. Clin Chest Med 2001;1:193–208.

Diabetes Mellitus & The Critically Ill Patient

26

Eli Ipp, MD, & Tricia L. Westhoff, MD

Patients with diabetes mellitus are frequently seen in the critical care unit because of complications of poorly controlled disease, including diabetic ketoacidosis, hyperglycemic hyperosmolar nonketotic diabetic coma, and hypoglycemia. In addition, diabetic patients with critical illness often will exhibit instability and poor control of blood glucose, including hyper- and hypoglycemia.

DIABETIC KETOACIDOSIS

ESSENTIALS OF DIAGNOSIS

- *Acute illness in a patient with known type 1 (insulin-dependent) diabetes mellitus, especially if the patient is vomiting.*
- *Evidence of precipitating illness, including infection.*
- *Clinical symptoms and signs of volume depletion.*
- *Clinical features of metabolic acidosis.*
- *Laboratory features: hyperglycemia, anion gap acidosis, ketonemia, and acidemia.*

General Considerations

Diabetic ketoacidosis is the most serious metabolic complication of type 1 (insulin-dependent) and, to a smaller extent, type 2 (non-insulin-dependent) diabetes mellitus. There has been little change in the mortality rate associated with diabetic ketoacidosis in recent decades despite great improvements in our understanding of its pathophysiology and treatment. The most effective means of reducing deaths due to diabetic ketoacidosis consists of teaching patients to recognize its early signs. Close clinical and biochemical observation of every patient during treatment of diabetic ketoacidosis remains the cornerstone of effective management.

A. Pathophysiology

The pathophysiology of diabetic ketoacidosis is based primarily upon an abnormal hormonal setting: insulin deficiency combined with an excess of hormones that increase the blood glucose level. This situation is similar to the physiologic state seen during normal fasting and is probably best considered as an abnormal and extreme expression of the fasting state. During the fed state, insulin is the predominant hormone, required for disposal and storage of ingested nutrients. During fasting, the body converts to a state in which endogenous sources of fuels need to be tapped for ongoing support of metabolism in the brain and in muscle tissue, and the hormonal milieu therefore begins to change. Plasma insulin concentrations fall, and glucagon concentrations rise. This change in the insulin:glucagon ratio permits the liver to become the major source for glucose during fasting. At the same time, decreased insulin concentrations lead to lipolysis in fat depots, providing a source of free fatty acids as a fuel for muscle and thus sparing glucose for use by the brain. Furthermore, free fatty acids are converted by the liver to ketones under the influence of glucagon. Ketones constitute another alternative (nonglucose) energy source for brain and muscle tissues. Glycerol released by lipolysis and alanine from protein catabolism in muscle also provides substrate for gluconeogenesis in the liver.

In diabetic ketoacidosis, this picture is greatly exaggerated because of severe insulin deficiency. Insulin deficiency need not be absolute, and in several studies measurable concentrations of serum insulin have been observed during diabetic ketoacidosis within what would be considered a "normal" range. However, these insulin levels are markedly deficient relative to the high glucose concentrations that are found in these patients. The effectiveness of circulating insulin is also reduced because patients with diabetic ketoacidosis also have considerable insulin resistance. Historically, this resistance to insulin action was thought to require massive doses of insulin during treatment of diabetic ketoacidosis. Although since the 1970s "low-dose" continuous insulin infusion has replaced the large intermittent doses previously used, a high level of resistance to insulin action remains an important feature of diabetic ketoacidosis. Some of the known causes of insulin resistance in diabetic ketoacidosis are listed in Table 26–1.

Table 26–1. Mechanisms of insulin resistance in diabetic ketoacidosis.

Elevated counterregulatory hormones
Acidemia
Hypertonicity
Phosphate depletion
Elevated plasma free fatty acids
Hyperaminoacidemia
Glucose toxicity

In contrast to the low levels of insulin, glucagon concentration is markedly elevated, with a high glucagon:insulin ratio more striking than that seen during fasting. In addition, diabetic ketoacidosis is characterized by large increases in the levels of stress hormones, including the glucose counterregulatory hormones cortisol, growth hormone, and catecholamines. These hormones help to define diabetic ketoacidosis and are responsible for its two major features: hyperglycemia and ketonemia. Glucagon has its predominant effects upon the liver, enhancing long-chain fatty acid transport into mitochondria by decreasing levels of malonyl-CoA and increasing activity of carnitine acyltransferase I. Cortisol enhances gluconeogenesis by increasing delivery of gluconeogenic substrates to and transamination in the liver. Prolonged hypersecretion of cortisol also decreases sensitivity to insulin. Catecholamines enhance lipolysis, providing substrate for ketogenesis, and accelerate glycogenolysis and gluconeogenesis. Finally, growth hormone also contributes to increased lipolysis and insulin resistance.

B. Hyperglycemia

Hyperglycemia in diabetic ketoacidosis results from several mechanisms. These mechanisms include both excessive and deficient secretion and action of a variety of hormones as well as involvement of their different target organs. Using glucose turnover studies, it has been shown that the major physiologic aberration that results from the combination of mechanisms described above is excessive hepatic glucose production. This in turn is primarily responsible for hyperglycemia in patients with diabetic ketoacidosis. Glucose clearance by insulin-sensitive tissues is also reduced, though some increase in glucose utilization is associated with the mass action effect of high blood glucose levels. Another important factor that determines the degree of hyperglycemia in diabetic ketoacidosis is the extent of renal glucose losses. As long as the kidneys are well perfused, they act as a continuing source of glucose leak from the extracellular space and thereby prevent severe hyperglycemia.

In Figure 26–1, mechanisms for hyperglycemia are illustrated, with emphasis on a quantitative estimate of their contributions in diabetic ketoacidosis. The numbers presented in this diagram are drawn from mean values reported in patients with diabetic ketoacidosis. Insulin deficiency associated with glucose counterregulatory hormone excess gives rise to highly exaggerated hepatic glucose production. Although some increase in glucose utilization due to severe hyperglycemia may occur, glucose clearance remains low and utilization is insufficient to match the rise in glucose production by the liver. In an average 70-kg patient in diabetic ketoacidosis with a hypothetical stable glucose concentration of 450 mg/dL, hepatic glucose production would be approximately 18 g/h. Average glucose utilization at the same time is estimated to be about 7 g/h. The square in the diagram represents the extracellular space, in which there is a total of 81 g of glucose at this time. Considering that the input into the system (hepatic glucose production) exceeds the output (glucose utilization), stable glucose concentrations can only persist if there is another source of glucose loss. In fact, renal losses of glucose are an important component

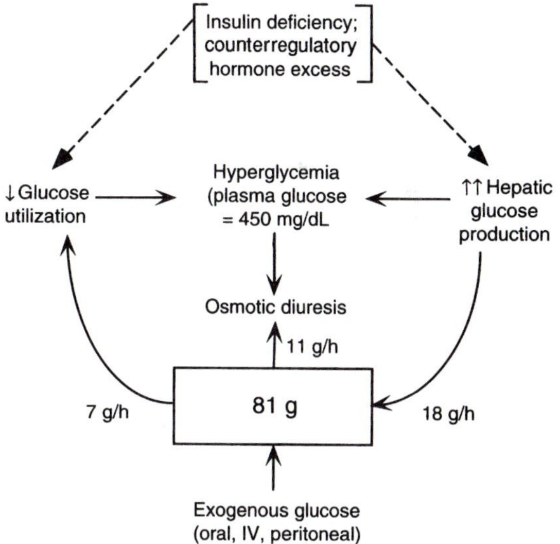

Figure 26–1 Mechanisms contributing to hyperglycemia in a 70-kg patient with a plasma glucose of 450 mg/dL. Values are from mean values obtained in patients with diabetic ketoacidosis. The box represents the extracellular glucose compartment. Lack of insulin and increased counterregulatory hormones result in decreased glucose utilization (7 g/h) and increased hepatic glucose production (18 g/h). Renal glucose losses may delay development of severe hyperglycemia.

of the protection from severe hyperglycemia afforded patients with developing diabetic ketoacidosis. The average amount of glucose lost through the kidneys in this example would be approximately 11 g/h.

If, without any increase in hepatic glucose production, the leak of glucose in the urine were diminished by only one-fifth—eg, as a result of diminished perfusion of the kidney due to volume depletion—considerable net accumulation of glucose would rapidly occur in the extracellular space. In this example, a reduction of about 2 g/h of urinary glucose losses would result in a further accumulation of about 50 g of glucose added to the 81 g in the extracellular space over 24 hours. If the rate of glucose utilization were unchanged—and with contraction of the extracellular space due to fluid losses—this could result almost in a doubling of serum glucose concentrations within a 24-hour period. The features of this diagram therefore accentuate the important role of the kidneys as well as the liver in the generation of hyperglycemia in diabetic ketoacidosis. Although not demonstrated in this diagram, these factors will be discussed later as an important mechanism for reduction of hyperglycemia once treatment begins.

The amount of volume depletion has an important effect on the development of hyperglycemia. In a study of insulin withdrawal in type 1 diabetes, volume depletion (> 3% of weight) increased plasma glucose concentrations compared with control subjects, while a 32-hour fast resulted in reduced plasma glucose. Glucose production and disposal were increased during the volume depletion study and decreased during fasting compared with the control study. Although the study did not evaluate renal perfusion, a likely explanation of the increased glycemia is a reduction of glucose excreted due to reduced glomerular filtration during volume depletion. Much of the variability of glycemia in ketoacidosis may be the result of lack of fluid or energy intake prior to or during metabolic decompensation. Given the common occurrence of both anorexia and volume depletion in patients who present with diabetic ketoacidosis, it is probable that the variability in severity of these two factors—as well as in the severity of insulin deficiency and underlying illness—explain much of the glycemic variability observed in diabetic ketoacidosis.

C. Ketosis and Metabolic Acidosis

Ketosis is the second major manifestation of diabetic ketoacidosis, and results from the accumulation of keto acids generated by the liver. Ketosis is predominantly a disorder of increased synthesis of ketones, though inability of peripheral tissues to utilize the excess ketones probably plays a small role. The keto acid measured in the blood during diabetic ketoacidosis is predominantly beta-hydroxybutyrate rather than acetoacetate. This reflects an altered redox state in the liver.

The increase in keto acids results in an increase in the serum anion gap that develops because of buffering by bicarbonate of hydrogen ion. If the acidosis in diabetic ketoacidosis is due only to ketosis, the fall in serum bicarbonate is equal to the increase in anion gap. It is evident, however, that acidosis in diabetic ketoacidosis may have additional mechanisms. Many patients have a reduction in serum bicarbonate concentration that is greater than the increase in anion gap, indicating, in addition, the presence of a non-anion gap hyperchloremic acidosis. Previously, hyperchloremic acidosis was recognized as a common manifestation of the later treatment stages in diabetic ketoacidosis. It is now appreciated that it may also be present at initial presentation, where it appears to occur in patients who are less severely volume-depleted. Recognition of hyperchloremic acidosis is important because hyperchloremic acidosis takes longer to resolve during treatment than ketoacidosis. This is because keto acids are metabolized to generate bicarbonate in equimolar amounts, whereas hyperchloremic acidosis depends for its correction on regeneration of bicarbonate by the kidneys. Another cause of acidosis in diabetic ketoacidosis is lactic acidosis. Lactic acidosis also contributes to the increase in the anion gap, with a corresponding further decrease in serum bicarbonate.

In the study referred to above, it is interesting to note that the rates of development of ketosis and metabolic acidosis were increased when the insulin withdrawal period was preceded by a period of fasting or volume depletion. This implies that variation in the nutritional or hydration status of patients before the onset of insulin deficiency may not only determine the glycemic variability but may also accelerate the development of both ketosis and metabolic acidosis.

D. Fluid and Electrolyte Imbalance

Extensive losses of fluids and electrolytes comprise the third important feature of diabetic ketoacidosis and are a consequence of the foregoing abnormalities. Fluid and electrolytes are lost in the osmotic diuresis caused by glycosuria that occurs as a result of marked hyperglycemia in diabetic ketoacidosis. Fluid losses are generally about 5–8 L in a 70-kg person, and depletion of sodium, potassium, and chloride may be 300–500 mmol or more at presentation (Table 26–2). Magnesium and phosphate are also lost but in smaller quantities. While water losses are usually easily appreciated clinically, serum electrolyte concentrations do not generally reflect the large losses that occur in these patients. This is especially true for potassium because, despite large urinary losses, normal or even high serum levels are seen at presentation as a result of a shift of potassium from the intracellular to the extracellular fluid—a consequence of acidosis and the loss of water from the extra-

Table 26–2. Approximate fluid and electrolyte deficits in patients with diabetic ketoacidosis.

Water	5–8 L
Sodium	400–700 mmol
Chloride	300–500 mmol
Potassium	300–1000 mmol
Calcium	100 mmol
Magnesium	50 mmol
Phosphate	50 mmol
Bicarbonate	350–400 mmol

cellular space. The water shift is in response to the hyperosmolar extracellular space brought on by hyperglycemia; intracellular potassium accompanies the water shift. This fluid shift also plays a role in determining serum sodium concentration. Because osmotic diuresis is associated with greater water loss than sodium or chloride, hypernatremia might be expected to occur, but this is not commonly seen because of the fluid shift from the intracellular space. This mechanism explains the mild hyponatremia often found at diagnosis. In contrast, normal serum chloride concentrations are the rule, for the reason that chloride losses are less than sodium losses. This is because sodium is also lost as the cation accompanying ketones excreted in the urine.

E. Altered Mental Status

The altered state of consciousness observed in diabetic ketoacidosis has not been explained. The closest correlation with impaired consciousness is the serum osmolarity. There appears to be an almost linear relationship between the degree of mental obtundation and the level of serum osmolarity, and most patients with mental impairment have been found to have serum osmolarities > 350 mosm/L (Figure 26–2). If a patient has altered consciousness in association with a serum osmolarity of less than 340 mosm/L, another cause for the neurologic problems should be considered.

F. Precipitating Disease

Although diabetic ketoacidosis can occur in the absence of any coexisting disease, in all patients with diabetic ketoacidosis (or even milder metabolic decompensation in diabetes mellitus) a precipitating factor should be looked for. The most commonly identified precipitating factors are withdrawal of insulin, infection, and undiagnosed diabetes during the initial presentation of the disease. Intercurrent illnesses increase the requirements for insulin by increasing insulin resistance, a consequence of the hormonal mechanisms outlined above. In the absence of an appropriate increase in the dose of insulin, patients become acutely insulin-deficient; the effects of stress increase the counterregulatory hormones; and the stage is set for the development of diabetic ketoacidosis.

Clinical Features

A. Symptoms and Signs

Most patients present with a history of polyuria and polydipsia, weakness, and weight loss. Duration is often as short as 24 hours, but the history usually extends over several days, and, in newly diagnosed diabetes, symptoms often go on for weeks. Patients are usually anorexic and may have vomiting and abdominal pain. Abdominal pain associated with ketosis is most common in children, though it may occur in adults as well, and occasionally has features of an acute abdomen. Fatigue and muscle cramps are also presenting features of diabetic ketoacidosis.

Signs of volume depletion are characteristic. Decreased skin turgor, dry mucous membranes, sunken eyeballs, tachycardia, orthostatic hypotension, and even supine hypotension may be present. If severe acidosis is present, deep and slow Kussmaul respirations may be noted as well as the characteristic odor of ketones on the breath. Additional findings include alteration in central nervous system function, ranging from drowsiness to coma. Only about 10% of patients who present with diabetic ketoacidosis are actually in coma, and about 20% have clear mentation. The rest have various

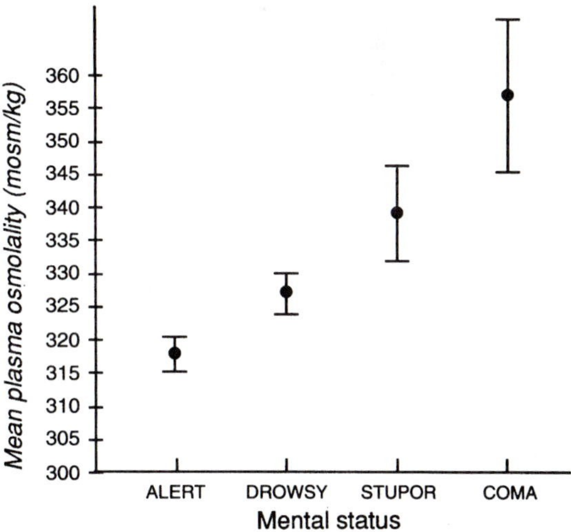

Figure 26–2 Mean calculated plasma osmolarity in 122 patients with diabetic ketoacidosis plotted against mental status at time of admission. (Reproduced, with permission, from data from Kitabchi AE: Low dose insulin therapy in diabetic ketoacidosis: Fact or fiction? Diabetes Metab Rev 1989;5:337–63.)

degrees of altered consciousness. Abdominal tenderness may be noted. Hypothermia may be present, but fever is not associated with diabetic ketoacidosis alone. The features of an associated precipitating illness often dominate the clinical picture.

Precipitating factors for diabetic ketoacidosis are listed in Table 26–3. The most commonly recognized causes fall into three groups. (1) First, undiagnosed type 1 diabetes mellitus. (2) Second, reduction of insulin dose may be associated with intercurrent illness (particularly patients who have anorexia and vomiting and reduce insulin dose for fear of hypoglycemia) or noncompliance. In recent times, interruption of nonconventional, nondepot insulin delivery—eg, insulin infusion pumps—may also be responsible for an unintended reduction in insulin dose. (3) The third precipitating factor is infection, where two important and potentially confounding features of diabetic ketoacidosis should be recognized: Fever is not caused by diabetic ketoacidosis alone and therefore suggests the presence of infection; and a white blood cell count of 15,000–40,000/μL may be seen in the absence of any infection. In some patients, precipitating factors cannot be identified.

Unusual presentations of patients with diabetic ketoacidosis must be recognized in order to make the correct diagnosis and provide appropriate therapy (Table 26–4). Diabetic ketoacidosis should be considered in any patient with type 1 diabetes who develops an acute illness. The need to rule out diabetic ketoacidosis in a patient with type 1 diabetes who is becoming ill applies equally in the outpatient or inpatient setting. When patients are at home, ketosis can be easily tested by checking urine ketones. The possibility of developing diabetic ketoacidosis provides a rationale for teaching patients to test their urine for glucose and ketones even though urine glucose measurement has not been an acceptable approach for routine monitoring for many years. In inpatients, urine or serum ketones will help exclude diabetic ketoacidosis as the cause of a change in a patient's condition. Effective bedside methods for measurement of serum beta-hydroxybutyrate have now been developed, and this should contribute to more rapid diagnosis of ketosis in hospitalized patients.

Table 26–3. Precipitating factors in patients with diabetic ketoacidosis.

1. New-onset type 1
2. Reduction of insulin dosage
   - Anorexia and vomiting
   - Noncompliance
   - Failure of nondepot insulin delivery
3. Infection
4. Acute disease
   - Trauma
   - Pancreatitis
   - Myocardial infarction
   - Cerebrovascular accident
5. Treatment
   - Steroids
   - Pentamidine
   - Peritoneal dialysis
6. Endocrine disorders
   - Hyperthyroidism
   - Pheochromocytoma
   - Somatostatinoma

Table 26–4. Typical and atypical features of diabetic ketoacidosis.

Typical	Exceptions
Acute illness in a patient with (suspected) type 2 diabetes	Diagnosis of diabetic ketoacidosis may be delayed in older patients with new-onset type 2 diabetes.
Clinical symptoms and signs of volume depletion	Absence of volume depletion in patient with diabetic ketoacidosis and oliguric renal failure.
Laboratory features	
Hyperglycemia	Less severe hyperglycemia in pregnancy or after alcohol intake.
Increased anion gap	Hypertiglyceridemia may mask increase in anion gap by interfering with serum Cl^- and HCO^{3-} measurements.
Metabolic acidemia	Vomiting may cause concurrent metabolic acidosis, decreasing severity of metabolic acidosis.
Ketonemia	Beta-hydroxybutyrate is not detected by nitroprusside reaction. If this ketone predominates, ketonemia may be underestimated or absent.

B. Laboratory Findings

(Table 26–5.)

1. Hyperglycemia—Serum glucose usually ranges from 500 to 800 mg/dL in patients with diabetic ketoacidosis. Although it is often the blood glucose measurement that alerts the staff to the possibility of diabetic ketoacidosis in an undiagnosed patient, it is important to keep in mind that severe hyperglycemia does not always occur. The diagnosis should be suspected even if serum glucose levels are not greatly elevated. This is particularly important in patients who are fasting and may recently have imbibed alcohol (which inhibits gluconeogenesis), or in pregnant

Table 26–5. Mean laboratory values in patients with diabetic ketoacidosis on admission to hospital.[1]

	Foster (n=88)	Kitabchi (n=123)	Ipp and Linfoot[2] (n=511)	Normal
Glucose (mg/dL)	476	606	542	75–110
Sodium (meq/L)	132	135	132	136–145
Potassium (meq/L)	4.8	5.7	4.9	3.5–5.0
Bicarbonate (meq/L)	<10	6.3	16	24–29
Anion gap (meq/L)	...	...	20	8–16
Blood urea nitrogen (mg/dL)	25	29	25	10–20
Acetoacetate (mmol/L)	4.8	3.1	...	<0.3
β-hyroxybutyrate (mmol/L)	13.7	9.8	9.1	<0.5
Lactate (mmol/L)	4.6	2.5	2.0	0.5–1.2
Blood pH	...	7.11	7.26	7.37–7.43

[1]Adapted with persmission from Foster and McGarry (personal communication).
[2]Unpublished.

women, whose serum glucose levels can be normal or only slightly elevated during severe diabetic ketoacidosis.

2. Metabolic acidosis—Total keto acids average 10–20 mmol/L; lactate is often elevated. As shown in Table 26–5, however, less severe acidosis may be seen, based on the bicarbonate and pH measurements at initial presentation. This may in part be a result of possible earlier access to medical care, but it may also be due to a shift in the strictness of the criteria used to classify acute metabolic decompensation in diabetes.

Absence of acidemia or only mild acidemia in diabetic ketoacidosis may occur if the patient has had vomiting severe enough to result in a mixed metabolic alkalosis and acidosis. Absence of ketones in a patient with acidosis, hyperglycemia, and volume depletion should make one suspect a predominance of the beta-hydroxybutyrate component of the serum ketones. With an altered redox state—in particular in the presence lactic acidosis—acetoacetate is converted to beta-hydroxybutyrate. The nitroprusside reagent that is used to measure ketones semiquantitatively in most laboratories recognizes only acetoacetate. A predominantly beta-hydroxybutyrate acidosis may therefore be missed because it will not be picked up by this method. Use of bedside methodology for beta-hydroxybutyrate measurement should help to eliminate this factor as a source of confusion in the diagnosis of diabetic ketoacidosis.

3. Serum electrolytes—Table 26–6 summarizes electrolyte abnormalities seen at the time of presentation in diabetic ketoacidosis. Mild hyponatremia is the most common abnormal finding and is due to a shift of water from the intracellular compartment into the hypertonic extracellular fluid. In addition, a total sodium deficit occurs as a result of the osmotic diuresis and the obligate cations accompanying ketones excreted in the urine. Hypochloremia is less common because chloride is not lost with urinary ketones and because of the high incidence of hyperchloremic acidosis mentioned earlier. Despite total body losses of other electrolytes, serum chloride concentrations are usually normal or low-normal at presentation. Most patients have normokalemia or hyperkalemia at presentation, but it is important to recognize that up to 20% will be hypokalemic at that time. Ten percent of patients have hypophosphatemia at diagnosis, and less than 10% of patients present with hypomagnesemia. Hypocalcemia occurs in almost 30% of patients. Serum osmolarity is rarely directly measured but instead calculated from the electrolytes. Hyperosmolarity of varying degree is a typical feature.

4. Interference with other laboratory tests—Abnormalities observed in diabetic ketoacidosis may contribute to artifactual interference with other laboratory tests. Acetoacetate cross-reacts in the automated methods for measuring creatinine and thus may artificially elevate creatinine concentrations; if due to this mechanism, elevated serum creatinine concentrations rapidly diminish as acetoacetate levels are cleared with therapy.

Hypertriglyceridemia occurs quite frequently in diabetic ketoacidosis. This is of importance not only because of the clinical manifestations of hypertriglyceridemia (eg, acute pancreatitis) but also because high

Table 26–6. Serum electrolyte concentrations in patients with diabetic ketoacidosis at presentation (% of patients).

	Low	Normal	High	Comment
Sodium	67	26	7	Bodystores depleted; serum [Na^+] depends on [glucose] and relative water loss.
Chloride	33	45	22	
Potassium	18	43	39	Body stores depleted.
Magnesium	7	25	68	
Phosphate	11	18	71	Decreases with insulin treatment.
Calcium	28	68	4	

triglyceride levels interfere with accurate measurement of sodium, chloride, and bicarbonate. When hypertriglyceridemia is present, pseudohyponatremia may be seen (serum is composed of a sodium-containing water phase and a large lipid—triglyceride—phase that contributes non-sodium-containing volume). What is less well recognized is that hypertriglyceridemia can interfere with the colorimetric measurement of chloride and bicarbonate, though there is no interference with more commonly used ion-specific electrode assays. The effect is to report falsely high serum chloride and bicarbonate concentrations that may mask the increase in anion gap expected in ketoacidosis and lead to incorrect evaluation of the patient. This possibility should be considered whenever the anion gap is not elevated in an otherwise typical clinical situation suggestive of diabetic ketoacidosis.

Differential Diagnosis

Clinical manifestations of diabetic ketoacidosis, such as dyspnea, nausea, vomiting, or abdominal pain, may mimic nondiabetic acute disease. In known diabetics with coma or altered mental status, diabetic ketoacidosis must be distinguished from hypoglycemia. This is usually not difficult clinically, since the circumstances and clinical findings are usually quite different. The patient with diabetic ketoacidosis is volume-depleted and may be acidotic, whereas the hypoglycemic patient is usually cold and clammy. In either case, bedside diagnosis of these conditions by direct measurement of blood glucose can be made quickly, so that clinical differentiation is less relevant. In comatose patients with diabetic ketoacidosis in whom serum osmolarity is < 340 mosm/L, another cause of coma should be considered.

A common difficulty arises when differentiating alcoholic ketosis from diabetic ketoacidosis in a patient with diabetes who has ingested alcohol. In such situations, whatever the cause of ketosis, the management is that of diabetic ketoacidosis. Severe abdominal pain from diabetic ketoacidosis, often accompanied by vomiting, may mimic an acute abdomen. Acute pancreatitis is often in the differential diagnosis, and its diagnosis is complicated by the fact that serum amylase levels are often elevated in diabetic ketoacidosis as a result of an increase in the amount of salivary amylase isoenzyme in the blood.

Treatment

The principles of management of diabetic ketoacidosis are to replace losses of water and electrolytes, give sufficient insulin (ie, stop ketogenesis, lipolysis, and gluconeogenesis), correct blood pH, closely monitor the patient through all stages of management, and eliminate or treat precipitating causes.

Rapid initial evaluation takes place in the emergency room in most patients with diabetic ketoacidosis, though at times diabetic ketoacidosis does develop in the hospital. Table 26–7 sets forth the initial steps in management when diabetic ketoacidosis is suspected.

A. Monitoring

Close monitoring is the key to successful management of diabetic ketoacidosis. Most management decisions are fairly straightforward if the data are available in timely fashion. Errors in management occur most often when there is a lapse in monitoring, so that a "catch-up" situation develops or the effects of overtreatment need to be corrected.

Blood glucose should be monitored hourly at the bedside. This provides information about whether the insulin dose is adequate to cause a fall in blood glucose at the expected rate of about 100 mg/dL per hour. Later, glucose measurement prevents overshooting the

Table 26–7. Initial diagnosis and management of diabetic ketoacidosis.

Rapid clinical examination.
Bedside blood glucose and urine ketone determinations.
Obtain blood for laboratory determination of glucose, ketones, electrolytes, urea nitrogen, creatinine, phosphorus, magnesium.
Obtain arterial blood for blood gases.
Chest x-ray.
ECG (also to monitor K^+ levels).
Search for precipitating factor.
Monitoring: Hourly bedside glucose and two-hourly measurement of anion gap, serum electrolytes, serum ketones, serum phosphorus. Obtain arterial blood gases as needed.

target serum glucose of 250–300 mg/dL, at which time infusion of dextrose should be started. Serum electrolytes and ketones should be monitored every 2 hours, and this should include measurement of serum phosphorus as well. Arterial blood gases should be repeated as necessary if progress in the clearing of acidosis is slow or if there are associated pulmonary problems. If phosphate therapy is used, serum calcium should be measured at least once (after an initial measurement) during the first 12 hours to detect any large decrease in serum calcium. All of the data obtained, including fluid balance measurements, should be maintained on a flowchart for easy review and evaluation.

1. Correction of hyperglycemia—Correction of hyperglycemia occurs by four different mechanisms (Table 26–8). First, the concentration of the extracellular glucose is diluted by fluid replacement, expanding the extracellular space. The second is by continuing—and usually increased—urinary loss of glucose that occurs with improved renal perfusion following expansion of the intravascular space. Third is the effect of insulin to diminish the hepatic glucose production rate. Considering that this is one of the important pathophysiologic mechanisms producing hyperglycemia in diabetic ketoacidosis, inhibition of this process must be one of the management goals. Indeed, it has been demonstrated that insulin at the routine doses infused is very effective in reducing glucose production by the liver during recovery from diabetic ketoacidosis. Increased glucose utilization is the fourth mechanism and is also an insulin-dependent process.

2. Correction of ketosis—Ketosis is corrected more slowly than hyperglycemia, so that while serum glucose levels will usually reach 250–300 mg/dL within an average of 6–8 hours, it can take up to 12 hours or more for ketosis to clear. It is particularly important to continue insulin infusion during this period despite the fact that one major goal of therapy (reduction of hyperglycemia) has been attained. Intravenous insulin should therefore be stopped only when ketosis has cleared.

It is not always easy to decide when a patient is no longer in a state of ketoacidosis. Serum ketone measurements do not provide the entire answer because they can remain positive for many hours after the acidosis is resolved, probably because acetone is cleared much more slowly than the two keto acids. Acetone is, however, measured by the nitroprusside reaction and can give rise to persistently positive serum ketone measurements even though it does not alter acid-base balance. For this reason, monitoring the anion gap is a better way of determining when ketosis has cleared. Serum bicarbonate concentrations are not useful when used alone because they are slow to return to normal after diabetic ketoacidosis. This is because of the slowly resolving hyperchloremic acidosis that accompanies saline therapy in almost all patients and because slight hyperventilation persists after the patient is no longer acidotic. Arterial blood pH measurement can be useful when it is difficult to decide whether ketosis has cleared—particularly if the anion gap has normalized and hyperglycemia is resolved yet the patient still appears to be ill.

B. Fluid Replacement

Fluid losses in an adult with diabetic ketoacidosis average 5–7 L and may be as much as 10–15% of body weight. Fluid replacement should be initiated immediately after diagnosis in order to prevent further deterioration of hemodynamic status. Fluid therapy is begun with intravenous 0.9% NaCl solution. A rough guide to volume replacement is as follows: (1) 2 L are given over the first 2 hours; (2) this can be followed by 2 L over the next 4 hours using 0.9% or 0.45% NaCl solution; and (3) over the next 8 hours, another 2 L can be given using either 0.9% or 0.45% NaCl. This schedule should be modified according to ongoing assessment of volume replacement needs and serum sodium levels. In hemodynamically compromised patients and the elderly, close monitoring of volume status may be necessary, and consideration should be given to use of a cen-

Table 26–8. Correction of hyperglycemia: Mechanisms.

Dilution by expansion of extracellular volume
Urinary losses
Diminished glucose production rates
Increased glucose utilization

tral venous pressure or pulmonary artery catheter. If severe hypotension is present, maintaining intravascular volume with albumin or other plasma expanders should also be considered.

When plasma glucose reaches 250–300 mg/dL, 5% dextrose solution should be started with an appropriate amount of NaCl according to the needs of the patient at that time.

There is disagreement about the best approach when serum sodium exceeds 150 meq/L at presentation. Some give 0.45% NaCl at the outset, but in some cases this has been associated with hypotension during treatment. This is because when insulin is given and glucose moves intracellularly, water will follow and deplete the intravascular space. When hypotonic saline is used, there is less addition of solute that will remain in the intravascular and extracellular spaces. Therefore, a greater proportion of the infused fluid will be ineffective in expanding the intravascular volume.

Administering 0.9% NaCl solution provides a greater osmotic load, and thus it is more likely to protect intravascular volume in the face of fluid shifts in diabetic ketoacidosis patients who are strikingly volume-depleted. The concern with infusing 0.9% NaCl (normal saline) is that hyperosmolarity will not be corrected. However, this approach conforms to the physiologic principle that during states of severe volume depletion, volume maintenance takes precedence over maintaining normal serum osmolarity. Thus, 0.9% NaCl is recommended as the volume replacement fluid of first choice even when the patient is initially hypernatremic, and 0.9% NaCl is hypo-osmolar relative to serum when serum osmolarity > 308 mosm/L. Once volume depletion has been corrected, administration of 0.45% NaCl or 5% dextrose in water to correct hypernatremia is indicated.

Fluid replacement has been given without insulin therapy to test its effects in the absence of insulin. In a few studies there has been considerable improvement in hyperglycemia but with no consistent effect on serum ketones. The improvement in serum glucose concentrations in the absence of insulin is probably the result of increased renal glucose losses and a dilution effect (Table 26–8).

C. Insulin

1. Initial therapy—Insulin is started at the time of diagnosis at a rate of 0.1 unit/kg/h by continuous intravenous infusion. A bolus dose of 0.1 unit/kg may be administered initially. Blood glucose levels should be checked at hourly intervals using bedside (glucometer) measurements, and laboratory serum glucose determinations can be obtained every 2 hours along with serum electrolytes to provide confirmation of the glucometer measurements.

In most patients, the recommended starting dose is sufficient to treat diabetic ketoacidosis because the serum free insulin levels achieved with this infusion rate are seven to ten times normal basal concentrations. However, some patients do require even faster infusion rates. Therefore, if serum glucose concentrations have not begun to fall after the first hour, the rate of insulin infusion should be doubled—and doubled once again if the same should happen during continuing therapy. The insulin infusion should cause blood glucose to fall at a rate of about 75 mg/dL/h. The rate of insulin infusion should be continued—if glucose is falling appropriately—until serum glucose has reached 230–300 mg/dL. At that time, a 5% dextrose infusion should be started, but the insulin infusion must continue until ketosis clears. Because considerable insulin resistance remains even though some of the factors described in Table 26–1 have normalized, insulin infusion should be maintained at the same rate and 10% dextrose infused, if necessary, to maintain serum glucose levels while awaiting clearance of ketones. Decreasing insulin infusion rates at this time may result in slower resolution of ketosis. Clearing of ketosis should be monitored using a combination of the anion gap, bicarbonate and serum ketone measurements, and, if necessary, arterial blood gas pH measurement.

2. After resolution of ketosis—Once ketosis has cleared—and if the patient is eating—a subcutaneous insulin regimen can be started. The patient should be given a subcutaneous injection of regular insulin about 30 minutes before stopping the insulin infusion. This allows some of the subcutaneously injected insulin to be absorbed before the insulin infusion is halted. Because intravenous insulin has a half-life of only 5–6 minutes, stopping the intravenous insulin prior to giving subcutaneous insulin can result in temporarily inadequate serum insulin concentrations. Low serum insulin levels can in turn cause rebound into diabetic ketoacidosis, particularly if there is significant delay in delivering the subcutaneous regular insulin injection. Subcutaneous insulin is also best injected 30 minutes before a meal, and the insulin infusion can be halted once the meal begins. The bolus of regular insulin will thus be delivered at a physiologically appropriate time, and the meal will help compensate for any error of excess in estimating the regular insulin dosage at that time.

Split-dose insulin therapy with a combination of regular and NPH insulin before breakfast and dinner can be started as soon as diabetic ketoacidosis has resolved and the patient is able to eat. The total daily dose can be similar to prehospital doses in patients with known diabetes; in newly diagnosed patients, regular insulin can be given before meals and at 12 midnight using a sliding scale for 24 hours. The total dose required can then be used to calculate split-dose therapy, giving two-thirds of the total dose in the morning and one-third in the evening. NPH insulin usually constitutes two-thirds of the morning dose and three-fourths of the evening dose with the remainder in each case being regular insulin.

D. Potassium Replacement

Usual potassium deficits in diabetic ketoacidosis have been estimated to be approximately 300 meq, but the deficit may be as much as 1000 meq. This total body potassium deficit is the result of combined renal losses due to osmotic diuresis and potassium shifts from intracellular to extracellular fluid that lead to further loss through the kidneys.

If the patient is normokalemic or hypokalemic at presentation, potassium replacement should be started when insulin therapy is initiated. If serum potassium is high, potassium therapy should only be started after insulin therapy is begun and with the second bottle of fluid replacement. If treatment is necessary before the serum potassium level is reported, epidemiologic data provide a basis for determining the frequency of serum potassium abnormalities (Tables 26–5 and 26–6). Most patients initially have either normal or high serum potassium; however, up to 20% of patients will have hypokalemia at the outset. In this last group of patients, insulin infusion alone (without potassium replacement) will exacerbate the hypokalemia, with potentially severe consequences. In contrast, the fear of giving potassium to normokalemic or hyperkalemic patients is mitigated by the effects of the concomitant insulin infusion, intracellular rehydration, and rise in pH. Thus, if the serum potassium concentration is unknown, the ECG does not demonstrate hyperkalemic changes, and the patient is producing adequate amounts of urine, potassium infusion should be started at the same time insulin therapy is begun.

Potassium replacement is started by addition of potassium chloride 20–40 meq/L to the fluid replacement solution. Potassium phosphate may also be given (alternating with potassium chloride) if phosphate repletion is necessary. Subsequent potassium replacement is dependent on the results of serum potassium, which should be done at 2-hour intervals throughout the period of management of diabetic ketoacidosis. In addition, electrocardiographic follow-up with single-lead measurement is a useful way of monitoring serum potassium for gross hyperkalemia or hypokalemia, so that emergency treatment can be initiated if necessary. It should be kept in mind that even while replacement of potassium is taking place, continuing potassium losses occur in the kidney throughout the period of management of diabetic ketoacidosis. For this reason, serum potassium measurement should also be obtained daily once the patient is no longer ketotic. A total body deficit of potassium may persist despite initial correction of serum potassium, and oral potassium replacement therapy should be given to patients who continue to be hypokalemic.

E. Bicarbonate

Acidosis generally resolves with insulin therapy and metabolism of keto acids. In most cases of diabetic ketoacidosis, it is not necessary to treat acidemia with bicarbonate. Recent studies have demonstrated that bicarbonate therapy does not alter the eventual outcome of diabetic ketoacidosis nor does it increase the rate at which pH is corrected. In fact, some studies have found a counterproductive effect of sodium bicarbonate in the treatment of diabetic ketoacidosis. Clinical and animal studies have shown that bicarbonate administration may actually increase ketone production. Recent data suggest also that in children with diabetic ketoacidosis, the mean duration of hospitalization for those receiving bicarbonate was 23% longer than that of children who did not receive bicarbonate. Lastly, a multicenter retrospective study of the risk factors associated with cerebral edema in children with diabetic ketoacidosis found that the relative risk of cerebral edema was 4.2 in children treated with bicarbonate as compared with a matched control group who did not receive bicarbonate. Bicarbonate therapy has also been associated with hypocalcemic tetany, decreased tissue oxygen delivery, a paradoxical fall in pH of the cerebrospinal fluid, rebound alkalosis, greater potassium needs, and sodium overload.

However, when pH values are extremely low, concern about the hazards of acidemia begin to outweigh the concerns with alkali therapy. Therefore, at a pH of less than 7.0, particularly in a patient who is very ill, many clinicians will administer bicarbonate. The effects of low pH are a negative inotropic effect on the heart, vasodilation, cerebral depression, insulin resistance, and depression of enzyme activity. If treatment with bicarbonate is begun, recent American Diabetes Association recommendations suggest that 100 mmol of sodium bicarbonate should be added to 400 mL of sterile water and given at a rate of 200 mL/h in severe acidosis (pH < 6.9). In patients with a pH of 6.9–7.0, 50 mmol of sodium bicarbonate should be diluted in 200 mL of sterile water and infused at a rate of 200 mL/h.

In general, taking into account the hazards of treatment, the hazards of acidemia, and the probable benefits of bicarbonate administration, it is not necessary to treat routinely with bicarbonate.

F. Phosphate Replacement

The routine administration of phosphate in the management of diabetic ketoacidosis remains controversial. Although there are theoretical reasons requiring the replacement of phosphate during treatment, most studies have not demonstrated any beneficial effect. Despite depletion of erythrocyte 2,3-diphosphoglycerate and the concern about decreased oxygen delivery to the tissues resulting from a leftward shift in the oxyhemoglobin dissociation curve, there are no deleterious clinical consequences of mildly low serum phosphorus. For most patients with diabetic ketoacidosis, routine administration of phosphate is unnecessary.

However, it is important to separate out one group of patients in whom phosphate therapy is essential—those with low serum phosphorus levels at presentation, which includes about 10% of patients (Table 26–6). Serum phosphorus decreases in all patients with treatment, sometimes dramatically after institution of insulin therapy. But if initial serum phosphorus is ≤ 1.5 mg/dL, it may fall with treatment into the range of concentrations that are associated with the hypophosphatemia syndrome (Table 26–9). This syndrome may include decreased myocardial contractility, respiratory muscle weakness and respiratory failure, hemolysis, and rhabdomyolysis. It is important to note that none of the studies evaluating the efficacy of phosphate therapy in diabetic ketoacidosis included patients with severely depressed serum levels at presentation, so that a conclusion to the effect that phosphate therapy is unnecessary should not be extended to include the group with low serum phosphate at diagnosis.

Severe hypophosphatemia may not be recognized unless frequent serum phosphorus measurements are made. These should be obtained every 2 hours during treatment of diabetic ketoacidosis in all patients whose serum phosphorus is ≤ 2 mg/dL at presentation. Patients with hypophosphatemia should be given supplemental phosphorus in the form of potassium phosphate.

Potassium phosphate can be added to the fluid replacement solution, alternating with potassium chloride. Hypophosphatemic patients will generally require 500–1000 mg of elemental phosphorus given over 12–24 hours depending on the severity of phosphorus depletion.

Table 26–9. Hazards of hypophosphatemia and phosphorus repletion in diabetic ketoacidosis.

Hypophosphatemia
Decreased red cell 2,3 diphosphoglycerate with decreased O_2 delivery
Muscle weakness
Hypophosphatemia syndrome ([P] < 1.0 mg/dL) with respiratory insufficiency, decreased myocardial contractility, rhabdomyolysis, hemolysis
Phosphorus administration
Hypocalcemia and tetany

This is equivalent to about 15–30 mmol of phosphate, or a total of 5–10 mL of potassium phosphate solution (3 mmol/mL) to be added to the fluid replacement solutions (1–4 mL potassium phosphate solution per liter of replacement fluid). A concern about phosphate administration in patients with diabetic ketoacidosis is hypocalcemic tetany, which has been described in some patients who receive phosphate therapy. It should be kept in mind that calcium levels may fall during the management of diabetic ketoacidosis. Small decreases in serum calcium may therefore not be a contraindication to continued phosphate repletion in patients who are phosphorus-depleted, but they do require more frequent monitoring of serum calcium to prevent hypocalcemia.

Patients with normal or high serum phosphorus at diagnosis will have a decrease in serum phosphorus during therapy but only to levels that do not usually require treatment.

Complications of Diabetic Ketoacidosis

A number of complications of diabetic ketoacidosis may occur during treatment. Hypocalcemia, hypokalemia or hyperkalemia, hypophosphatemia, and hypoglycemia need to be watched for during continuous monitoring of patients with diabetic ketoacidosis (Table 26–10). An-

Table 26–10. Complications of diabetic ketoacidosis.

Complication	Possible Mechanism
Hypokalemia	Bicarbonate therapy, inadequate replacement, insulin
Hyperkalemia	Anuria, excessive replacement
Hypophosphatemia	Insulin therapy (if [P] starts out < 1.5 mg/dL)
Hypoglycemia	Inadequate glucose infusion with insulin therapy
Other	
Thromboembolism	Increased platelet adhesiveness, hyperviscosity, poor perfusion
Aspiration	Gastric stasis, vomiting; lack of nasogastric suction
ARDS	Use of hypotonic replacement fluids or excess crystalloid infusion or increased pulmonary epithelial permeability
Cerebral edema	Excessive correction of hyperglycemia Use of hypotonic replacement fluids(?)
Mucormycosis	Acidemia

other recognized complication is thromboembolism that occurs as a result of increased platelet adhesiveness and hyperviscosity. Aspiration of gastric contents is associated with gastroparesis and vomiting. Nasogastric suction should be initiated in all patients who have altered consciousness to prevent this complication. Cerebral edema and acute respiratory distress syndrome are other complications that will be discussed below.

One of the rare but significant conditions that should be kept in mind in the management of diabetic ketoacidosis is mucormycosis. This rare condition associated with ketoacidosis is a treatable yet severe infection by the fungus rhizopus. Early diagnosis is essential so that therapy can be instituted in order to prevent the severe morbidity associated with this rapidly invasive infectious process. The hallmark of mucormycosis is the finding of black necrotic debris in the area of the eye, nose, or nasal cavity and histologic evidence of vascular thrombosis or tissue infarction on biopsy. These findings result from the propensity for invasion by mucormycosis into the vascular system. This diagnosis is considered to be a medical emergency.

Current Controversies & Unresolved Issues

A. Fluid Replacement

Fluid replacement remains a controversial issue from two different points of view. The first is volume replacement. A study comparing the effects of providing 3 L of volume replacement over the first 8-hour period of treatment versus giving 6 L over the same period of time showed very little difference in outcomes in the two groups of patients. The conclusion is that smaller volumes of fluid may safely be administered to patients in diabetic ketoacidosis. It needs to be emphasized that patients with severe volume deficits were excluded from study, but patients with moderate fluid deficits may do well with slower replacement of their losses. One approach provides a more flexible regimen for fluid replacement that recognizes the unique requirements of each patient but consequently requires careful monitoring. Fluid is replaced at a rate of 15–20 mL/kg/h for 1 hour, then 4–14 mL/kg/h thereafter according to need as determined by careful monitoring of fluid balance.

The type of fluid replacement has also been an issue of controversy. Some investigators feel that colloid therapy would be better than crystalloid infusion in the management of diabetic ketoacidosis. Their concern is that insufficient fluid is maintained in the intravascular space during therapy and that much of the fluid when given as crystalloid finds its way into the interstitial space, where edema is the result. It has been suggested that the syndromes of cerebral edema and pulmonary edema may be a consequence in part of the sequestration of fluid outside of the intravascular space. However, no controlled studies of colloid infusion have been performed. Colloid solutions should be considered in the management of hypotension in patients who present with diabetic ketoacidosis, but at this time crystalloid infusion remains the management of choice.

B. Cerebral Edema

This serious complication is fortunately quite rare. Cerebral edema manifests as a deteriorating level of consciousness at a time when other parameters of diabetic ketoacidosis are improving in response to treatment. Clinical evidence for this complication generally appears early in the course of treatment; almost two-thirds of patients who develop neurologic deterioration begin to do so within 12 hours after initiation of therapy. Cerebral edema occurs mainly in children and young adults and is associated with a greater than 90% mortality. However, despite its rarity, this complication has influenced one of the basic aspects in our management of diabetic ketoacidosis because of its catastrophic consequences. As mentioned above, it is accepted practice to start glucose infusion to prevent serum glucose concentrations from falling below 250–300 mg/dL. This recommendation derives from studies of experimentally induced cerebral edema in diabetic dogs that demonstrated an association of cerebral edema with greater decrements in plasma glucose concentrations during treatment.

On the other hand, in a study of children who developed cerebral edema with diabetic ketoacidosis, only treatment with bicarbonate was associated with cerebral edema. Neither the initial serum glucose concentration nor the rate of change in the serum glucose concentration during therapy was associated with the development of cerebral edema. In addition, symptomatic cerebral edema developed in a few children with diabetic ketoacidosis before the initiation of therapy. This observation suggests that cerebral edema may not necessarily be caused by therapy per se. They also found that children with diabetic ketoacidosis who have low partial pressures of arterial carbon dioxide (relative risk 2.7 per decrease of 7.8 mm Hg), and high serum urea nitrogen concentrations (relative risk 1.8 per increase of 9 mg/dL) at presentation were at increased risk for cerebral edema. This supports the hypothesis that cerebral edema in children with diabetic ketoacidosis is related to decreased perfusion of the brain. Both hypocapnia, which causes cerebral vasoconstriction, and extreme dehydration would be expected to decrease brain perfusion. Furthermore, because the developing brains of children are more sensitive to hypoxia, this may explain the greater incidence of cerebral edema in children as compared with adults.

Subclinical cerebral edema appears to be quite common in patients with diabetic ketoacidosis, as compression of the subarachnoid and ventricular spaces during treatment has been observed by CT scan without any obvious clinical manifestations. The high frequency of subclinical edema has raised questions about the rate and composition of fluid replacement discussed earlier in this section.

C. Acute Respiratory Distress Syndrome (ARDS)

Another unusual but serious complication of ketoacidosis is ARDS. Patients present with progressive dyspnea and hypoxemia; the earliest sign appears to be an increased $P(A{-}a)O_2$, and pulmonary edema is found on chest x-ray. ARDS in diabetic ketoacidosis tends to occur most often in patients under 50 years of age, and the mortality rate associated with this syndrome is extremely high. The pathogenesis of ARDS in diabetic ketoacidosis is unknown, but it has also been suggested that the syndrome may be associated with crystalloid infusion and perhaps with excess volume replacement. It is unlikely that either of these factors is the sole cause of ARDS, because it is too unusual a complication of diabetic ketoacidosis to be simply fluid-dependent given the wide range of replacement regimens that are used. However, it is possible that there is an association with excessive fluid replacement in patients who have some underlying pulmonary disease process associated with increased pulmonary epithelial permeability.

Adrogue HJ et al: Plasma acid base patterns in diabetic ketoacidosis. N Engl J Med 1982;307:1603–10.

Adrogue HJ, Barrero J, Eknoyan G: Salutary effects of modest fluid replacement in the treatment of adults with diabetic ketoacidosis. JAMA 1989;262:2108–13.

Burge MR et al: Differential effects of fasting and dehydration in the pathogenesis of diabetic ketoacidosis. Metabolism 2001;50:171–7.

Glaser N et al: Risk factors for cerebral edema in children with diabetic ketoacidosis. N Engl J Med 2001;344:264–9.

Kitabchi AE: Low dose insulin therapy in diabetic ketoacidosis: fact or fiction? Diabetes Metab Rev 1989;5: 337–63.

Kitabchi AE et al: Management of hyperglycemic crises in patients with diabetes. Diabetes Care 2001;24:131–53.

Ennis ED, Stahl EJ, Kreisberg RA: Diabetic ketoacidosis. In: *Ellenberg & Rifkin's Diabetes Mellitus,* 5th ed. Appleton & Lange, 1997.

HYPERGLYCEMIC HYPEROSMOLAR NONKETOTIC COMA

This disorder is probably not a distinct entity but rather a variant of the diabetic ketoacidosis syndrome because a large overlap exists in the clinical presentation and pathogenesis of diabetic ketoacidosis and nonketotic coma. Management of the two conditions is essentially identical. However, there are clearly major differences in clinical presentation between typical patients with nonketotic coma and diabetic ketoacidosis, who probably represent opposite extremes of this metabolic syndrome.

The patient with nonketotic coma is typically an elderly person who presents with diabetes for the first time, is severely dehydrated, is more often in coma, and has severe associated diseases and a poor outcome. In contrast, the common first presentation of diabetic ketoacidosis is in a teenager who is otherwise healthy, not often in coma, and has an excellent chance of recovery. Biochemically, the typical patient with hyperglycemic hyperosmolar nonketotic coma has more severe hyperglycemia (serum glucose often > 1000 mg/dL) and hyperosmolarity, more pronounced electrolyte abnormalities, and no ketosis. Between these two extremes are a large number of patients in whom the clinical syndromes overlap, so that some degree of ketosis is often present in a patient who otherwise would be classified as having typical nonketotic coma; on the other hand, hyperosmolarity and severe hyperglycemia occur in what otherwise appears to be typical diabetic ketoacidosis.

The pathogenesis of hyperglycemic hyperosmolar nonketotic coma is not well understood. The severity of the hyperosmolarity can be ascribed to a greater degree of volume depletion. Indeed, severe volume depletion is the most important common feature and can best be explained by the degree of hyperglycemia and thus the extreme hyperosmolarity found in these patients. Figure 26–1 provides an explanation for this severe hyperglycemia. Since volume depletion is a characteristic feature, renal blood flow and the glomerular filtration rate are reduced, thus diminishing the urinary escape of glucose. However, the hormonal setting ensures a continuing high rate of hepatic glucose production (see above for further discussion of Figure 26–1), and this has the capacity to rapidly increase blood glucose levels. If this sequence of events is not halted, severe hyperglycemia and hyperosmolarity ensue.

The other major feature of nonketotic coma—the relatively low level of serum keto acids—may also play an important role in the development of severe hyperglycemia. It has been suggested that in diabetic ketoacidosis, acidosis makes the patients feel more ill and thus prevents the syndrome from going undiagnosed for prolonged periods. The lack of ketosis in hyperglycemic hyperosmolar nonketotic coma may delay presentation, resulting in ongoing osmotic diuresis that results in more severe volume depletion. The mechanism for the lower levels of ketosis is unexplained. The hormonal picture at presentation is not helpful because concentrations of circulating counterregulatory hormones do not appear to be different from those seen in diabetic ketoacidosis, nor do insulin levels seem to differ. Nevertheless, it is thought that a restraining effect upon lipolysis by small increases of circulating insulin—and, as a result, less availability of substrate for ketogenesis—may explain low ketone concentrations in this syndrome. It appears also that hyperosmolarity may itself play a role in diminishing ketosis; this is based on in vitro studies in which hyperosmolarity was shown to suppress lipolysis.

Management is not different from that of diabetic ketoacidosis. Plasma glucose concentrations should be allowed to decrease at a rate of about 100 mg/dL/h, and fluid replacement should begin with normal saline as discussed earlier. Early aggressive volume replacement is important to prevent hypotension that may result from fluid shifts which accompany insulin-mediated glucose transport into the intracellular compartment. Many of these patients are elderly, and monitoring fluid balance with central venous or pulmonary artery catheters is therefore advised. Because of the massive osmotic diuresis that precedes presentation in these patients, electrolyte losses may be severe. It is particularly important to monitor serum potassium carefully during early management and in subsequent days so as to provide potassium supplements if they become necessary. The mortality rate is high, with deaths often due to concurrent illnesses or thrombotic and infectious complications.

Kitabchi AE, Murphy MB: Diabetic ketoacidosis and hyperosmolar hyperglycemic nonketotic coma. Med Clin North Am 1988;72:1545–63.

Wachtel TJ, Silliman RA, Lamberton P: Predisposing factors for the diabetic hyperosmolar state. Arch Intern Med 1987; 147:499–501.

MANAGEMENT OF THE ACUTELY ILL PATIENT WITH DIABETES MELLITUS

Maintenance of glucose control in a diabetic patient in whom intercurrent illness has acutely altered metabolic homeostasis can be a challenging problem. One must also consider how diabetes or its complications may affect the management of an unrelated acute illness. This continuing interaction must be kept in mind while managing patients with diabetes in an intensive care setting.

Acute illness frequently alters metabolic control in patients with diabetes. Most often this is associated with excessive hyperglycemia; however, hypoglycemia may also occur.

HYPERGLYCEMIA

Pathophysiology

The most frequent pathophysiologic abnormality induced by acute illness is an increase in insulin resistance. This occurs as a result of increased secretion of glucose counterregulatory hormones in the acutely ill patient. The mechanisms are not entirely clear, but it is assumed that these patients are under considerable physiologic stress. In a previously well-controlled diabetic, glucose control worsens as a result of increased concentrations of cortisol, catecholamines, growth hormone, and glucagon, leading to increased hepatic glucose production by gluconeogenesis and glycogenolysis as well as insulin resistance. Hyperglycemia develops in patients with type 2 diabetes from a lack of ability of the B cell to increase insulin secretion appropriately despite rising serum glucose concentrations; in type 1 diabetes, hyperglycemia occurs because the normal insulin doses are insufficient to match the increasing insulin needs.

When infused alone into patients with diabetes mellitus, each of the glucose counterregulatory hormones can exaggerate hyperglycemia, and when all are infused together in experimental studies, there is a synergistic effect resulting in destabilization of blood glucose concentrations. In addition, in patients with type 2 diabetes who have residual insulin secretion, catecholamines may have an inhibitory effect on insulin secretion. This may also play a role in deteriorating glucose tolerance in ill patients. Even though they are suppressed, insulin levels tend to rise along with increasing serum glucose concentrations in patients with type 2 diabetes. This ability to continue to secrete increasing (though inadequate) amounts of insulin in response to elevated serum glucose is probably what prevents the development of ketoacidosis in most patients with type 2 diabetes when acute illness supervenes, though insulin levels are insufficient to prevent hyperglycemia. The presence of even low levels of insulin may be sufficient to inhibit lipolysis in adipose tissue and suppress ketogenesis in the liver. Indeed, it is unusual for patients with type 2 diabetes to develop diabetic ketoacidosis even though they may have the same pattern of glucose counterregulatory hormone release. It has therefore been suggested that if diabetic ketoacidosis occurs in type 2 diabetes, it is due to more severe insulin deficiency, though there is no evidence that this is directly related to an effect of catecholamines.

Clinical Features

Many acute illnesses unrelated to diabetes may have an impact upon glucose control, including infection, pancreatitis, acute renal failure, myocardial infarction, and trauma. Diabetic patients undergoing surgery usually require adjustment of diet and insulin or oral hypoglycemic medications. Alcohol ingestion, medications, and administration of glucose-containing solutions during intravenous hyperalimentation or peritoneal dialysis may also affect serum glucose.

There are also other conditions that are diabetogenic in nature and can initiate hyperglycemia or diabetes. These should be considered in the differential diagnosis of patients with diabetes and acute illness, because diabetes in some of these conditions may be previously unrecognized or could be transient, resolving with treatment of the acute illness. Examples include cerebrovascular accidents or brain lesions that involve the hypothalamic area and may cause hyperglycemia by activating or destroying brain centers that play a role in the regulation of glucose homeostasis; acute pancreatitis with destruction or edema of the islets of Langerhans, which may be associated with transient (or permanent) exacerbation of hyperglycemia; and endocrine disorders such as Cushing's syndrome (spontaneous or iatrogenic) or acromegaly, which can induce marked insulin resistance.

Patients who have inadequate insulin secretory reserve but who are not frankly diabetic are at greatest risk for severe metabolic decompensation due to intercurrent disease. These patients are unable to respond to increasing insulin needs, but, unlike previously diagnosed diabetics, may not necessarily recognize the symptom complex associated with hyperglycemia. Situations may occur in which large quantities of glucose are introduced into the patient and result in precipitation or exacerbation of diabetes. For example, unexpectedly high blood glucose levels may be seen in patients who ingest a large amount of sucrose from sugar-containing soft drinks because of extreme thirst induced by diuresis or diarrhea. Development or exacerbation of osmotic diuresis can make this a self-perpetuating disorder. Similarly, peritoneal dialysis using solutions with high glucose concentrations, used in an attempt to remove excess extracellular fluid, may be associated with hyperglycemia, and indeed this has resulted in hyperosmolar diabetic coma.

An example of how control of diabetes influences the management of another disorder is when diabetes insipidus and diabetes mellitus (or diminished insulin reserves) occur together. Diabetes insipidus causes the patient to lose a large volume of free water in the urine because of inability to concentrate urine appropriately. During treatment, equally large quantities of electrolyte-poor solutions—usually 5% dextrose—are infused to match the urine output. Vasopressin at first leads to reduction in urine output, but inexplicably, despite increasing doses of vasopressin, urine outflow may begin to increase. An explanation can be found in the 6–10 L of 5% dextrose that may be given within a 24-hour period, representing a load of 300–500 g of glucose into the extracellular pool compared with about 20 g in the extracellular pool in a patient with normal serum glucose. The enormous impact that this load may have in a patient with poor insulin reserves can be appreciated by referring to Figure 26–1. Normal subjects can handle this additional quantity of glucose by increasing the secretion of insulin, but in patients who have underlying or overt diabetes and a poor insulin response, serum glucose will be extremely high. As a result, glycosuria develops, with an osmotic diuresis that antagonizes the action of vasopressin. This results in the administration of even larger volumes of 5% dextrose, perpetuating a vicious circle. Proper management consists of preventing glycosuria by tightly controlling blood glucose. This can be achieved using an intravenous insulin infusion in an ICU while simultaneously treating the diabetes insipidus.

HYPOGLYCEMIA

Some diabetic patients appear to have decreased insulin requirements or a decreasing need for oral hypoglycemic agents when acute illness supervenes. A decrease in insulin requirements may result from a number of different mechanisms.

Pathophysiology

A. Decreased Insulin Resistance

Weight loss may occur prior to or during the acute illness. It is well known that weight loss reduces insulin resistance in diabetes mellitus, and small decreases in weight are often sufficient to produce a substantially decreased requirement for insulin or other hypoglycemic agents. Another cause of decreased insulin resistance is a deficiency of one of the glucose counterregulatory hormones. Adrenal or pituitary insufficiency may occur as part of an intercurrent disease process. Decreased growth hormone or cortisol can diminish the need for hypoglycemic agents by enhancing peripheral insulin sensitivity and decreasing gluconeogenesis.

B. Decreased Clearance of Insulin or Oral Hypoglycemic Agents

Because the liver and the kidneys are the primary organs involved in metabolism of insulin and the sulfonylurea drugs, development of renal or hepatic failure may delay drug clearance and result in hypoglycemia. In the case of the sulfonylureas, this may be associated with the onset of severe, prolonged hypoglycemia and coma. Concomitant use of other drugs may also influence the metabolism of sulfonylurea agents (Table 26–11). A relatively common cause of unexpected hypoglycemia occurs during acute episodes of congestive heart failure in insulin-treated patients. As a result of liver congestion and possibly impaired hepatic blood flow, insulin requirements are transiently diminished. If the insulin dose is not reduced, hypoglycemia may occur.

Table 26–11. Pharmacokinetic and pharmacodynamic interactions that augment the hypoglycemic actions of sulfonylurea drugs.

Interaction	Drug
Displacement of sulfonylureas from plasma proteins	Clofibrate, phenylbutazone, salicylates, sulfonamides
Reduced hepatic sulfonylurea metabolism	Dicumarol, chloramphenicol, monoamine oxidase inhibitors, phenylbutazone.
Decreased urinary excretion of sulfonylureas or metabolites	Allopurinol, probenecid, phenylbutazone, salicylates, sulfonamides
Intrinsic hypoglycemic activity	Insulin, alcohol, beta-adrenergic agonists, salicylates, guanethidine, monoamine oxidase inhibitors

C. Drug Interactions

Drug interactions are of particular importance with the first generation of oral hypoglycemic agents that are tightly protein-bound and may be displaced by other protein-bound drugs. Table 26–11 summarizes possible interactions between drugs used in management of diabetes and therapeutic agents that may affect glucose control. Because multiple drugs are often used in acutely ill patients, particularly the elderly, the possibility of drug interactions giving rise to hypoglycemia always needs to be considered.

Clinical Features

Hypoglycemia in hospitalized patients occurs most commonly in patients with diabetes, and this is usually due to a decrease in caloric intake related to illness or hospital routine with continued administration of hypoglycemic drugs. Some of the causes of hypoglycemia observed in hospitalized patients with diabetes are presented in Table 26–12. Concomitant diseases play an important role in increasing the risk of hypoglycemia in patients with diabetes, eg, renal insufficiency, malnutrition, and sepsis—three disorders known to be associated with hypoglycemia even in nondiabetic hospitalized patients—as well as alcohol ingestion, liver disease, shock, pregnancy, and malignancy. A high mortality rate has been reported in nondiabetic critically ill patients who develop hypoglycemia, and in some this may represent a terminal phenomenon associated with malnutrition or kidney and liver disease.

Pentamidine, used for treatment for *Pneumocystis carinii* infection, is associated with hypoglycemia probably due to destruction of pancreatic islet cells with acute increase in insulin release. Some of these patients will eventually develop hyperglycemia with insufficient insulin release.

Treatment

Several factors determine appropriate management for patients with diabetes mellitus and acute illness to avoid the consequences of hyperglycemia and hypoglycemia.

A. Goal for Serum Glucose

Target glucose concentrations in acutely ill patients should not be set as low as those desired in stable patients. When mean glucose concentrations are < 200 mg/dL, diabetes can often be managed with an oral hypoglycemic agent, but glucose should be closely monitored in case insulin is required. When more severe hyperglycemia occurs (serum glucose > 250 mg/dL), insulin treatment is required. The goal of treatment in acutely ill patients with diabetes is to maintain the blood glucose level in a range between 150 mg/dL and 250 mg/dL.

B. Fasting Patients

Patients who for any reason are not being fed require a different approach to insulin management. These patients do not need the bolus injections of regular insulin that are required to maintain glucose homeostasis post-

Table 26–12. Proximate causes of hypoglycemia in 42 diabetic patients receiving insulin (60 episodes) or oral hypoglycemia drugs (four episodes).

Cause	% Episodes
Decreased intake of calories	45
Nausea, vomiting, anorexia, lethargy	23
NPO because of diagnostic test or surgical procedures	14
Enteral tube feedings held for measurement of residual	5
Meals not delivered	3
Adjustment of insulin dosage	39
Treatment of diabetic ketoacidosis or nonketotic coma	17
Attempt at tighter metabolic control	9
Sliding scale insulin doses too high for patient with renal insufficiency	6
Failure to reduce insulin dose after one hypoglycemia episode	5
Less insulin needed as infection resolved	2
Incorrect dose of insulin given	8
No cause identified	8

prandially; a continuous intravenous insulin infusion is more appropriate. Intravenous insulin is routinely given if a patient is receiving total parenteral nutrition because of the large load of calories given to patients during this therapy. However, even in the absence of an exogenous source of glucose such as total parenteral nutrition, it is important to recognize that hyperglycemia in patients with diabetes is the result of a continuous supply of large amounts of glucose from an endogenous source, ie, the liver. It is logical, therefore, that serum glucose be controlled by continuous levels of insulin, and this can be done with intravenous insulin infusion. The response should be evaluated by monitoring blood glucose at the bedside at 2- to 3-hour intervals.

C. Patients With Intermittent Food Intake

Patients who are acutely ill, have some vomiting, or have decreased food intake can be managed somewhat differently. Under these circumstances, longer-acting insulins may be inappropriate because it is difficult to predict insulin needs for more than a few hours in advance. Thus, even if NPH insulin were administered in an appropriate dose, inability to eat a meal hours later could put the patient at risk for hypoglycemia. Regular insulin given before each meal and at midnight is preferable.

Regular insulin can be given to patients four times a day using a variable insulin dosage (2–10 units) based on the bedside blood glucose determination ("sliding scale"). Glucose is measured about 30 minutes preprandially, immediately before each insulin dose is to be administered, and at midnight. This provides insulin coverage for the expected glucose excursion with each meal, and the dose can be reduced if the patient is not going to eat the next meal. As soon as the patient begins to stabilize and is able to eat consistently, an attempt should be made to convert the patient to morning and evening split-dose insulin injections using a combination of NPH and regular insulin.

D. Patients Eating Regularly

Patients who are eating meals or receiving feeding in bolus fashion in reasonably consistent fashion can be treated with a split-dose regimen of NPH and regular insulin. If necessary, a sliding scale of supplementary preprandial regular insulin doses set to operate at high glucose levels only (> 300 mg/dL) can be added to ensure that excessive hyperglycemia is prevented. There is no need for prolonged use of sliding scales in this situation, because by the sliding scale approach the doses of insulin are variable from day to day, and more stable patients will do better if managed with a more constant regimen.

Most patients will be released from the critical care area once they are receiving NPH or another intermediate-acting insulin and the medical condition has stabilized. In addition to preprandial glucose measurements, which are the basis for the sliding scale, measurements should also be performed 2 hours after breakfast and dinner in order to evaluate whether the dose of regular insulin given prior to those meals is appropriate for adequate glucose control. These 2-hour postprandial glucose measurements are most useful for determining the required dose of regular insulin. Regular insulin dosages can be increased or decreased depending on the change in glucose concentration from that obtained immediately prior to the meal (keeping in mind that there is a normal rise in blood glucose levels of about 50 mg/dL after a meal).

OTHER COMPLICATIONS OF DIABETES MELLITUS

In addition to disordered glucose control, it is important to consider the interaction between the complications of diabetes and unrelated acute illness. Some of the complications are clinically obvious, such as renal failure or nephrotic syndrome with hypoalbuminemia. Others are less obvious, such as defects in vision (short of total blindness), which may make it difficult for the patient to be totally compliant with management.

Renal and retinal complications are routinely looked for if the patient is known to have diabetes. However, consequences of autonomic neuropathy may not be well addressed in clinical evaluation. In patients with long-standing diabetes, these may be devastating effects. For example, orthostatic hypotension is usually not symptomatic in most patients with autonomic neuropathy yet may become dramatically important when other causes of hypotension are present, such as volume depletion, cardiac disease, or drug-related causes. Another overlooked problem that can interfere with management is gastroparesis diabeticorum, which should be considered in patients who are vomiting or have diabetes that is difficult to control. With this disorder, poor glucose control results from a lack of coordination between insulin injection and absorption of meals due to delay in food exiting the stomach. Recurrent urinary tract infections may result from a neurogenic bladder. Lastly, patients with symptomatic autonomic neuropathy are also at increased risk for sudden death from cardiorespiratory arrest.

Another not uncommon phenomenon that can cause an acute problem in patients with long-standing diabetes is the syndrome of hyporeninemic hypoaldosteronism. This disorder is commonly seen in older patients with type 2 diabetes and mild renal insufficiency. With administration of angiotensin-converting enzyme inhibitors or in the presence of other acute illness, severe hyperkalemia may be seen. Hyperkalemia may occur in patients whose serum potassium may be only mildly elevated or at the upper limit of normal under usual circumstances due to hyporeninemic hypoaldosteronism.

Fischer KF, Lees JA, Newman JH: Hypoglycemia in hospitalized patients: Causes and outcomes. N Engl J Med 1986; 315:1245–50.

Gerich JE: Oral hypoglycemic agents. N Engl J Med 1989; 321:1231–45.

HIV Infection in the Critically Ill Patient

27

Mallory D. Witt, MD, & Darryl Y. Sue, MD

Since acquired immunodeficiency syndrome (AIDS) was first described in 1981, much has been learned about the spectrum of diseases associated with the progressive immunosuppression caused by the human immunodeficiency virus (HIV). Malignancies and opportunistic infections are the most common sequelae of HIV infection, but HIV can also directly and indirectly affect the pulmonary circulation, kidneys, heart, and adrenal glands. Sepsis, respiratory failure, and neurologic complications are common problems that will often require management in the intensive care unit. The advent of highly active antiretroviral therapy (HAART) and the success of prophylaxis against several common opportunistic infections have led to prolonged survival and improved quality of life of patients with HIV infection. In turn, there have been changes in the characteristics of patients with HIV who are admitted to the ICU, as well as reconsideration of the benefits of ICU care. However, widespread use of HAART has led to new problems and complications of treatment, some of which require ICU care or complicate the treatment of other disorders.

The benefits of ICU care for HIV-infected patients have been questioned because of early studies reporting poor outcomes for patients with respiratory failure due to *Pneumocystis carinii* pneumonia. However, the prognosis in patients with pneumocystis pneumonia has improved since the early 1980s. In the early stages of the HIV epidemic, respiratory failure due to pneumocystis pneumonia was responsible for about one-third to one-half of ICU admissions for patients with HIV infection, with a mortality approaching 80–90%. By the mid 1990s, the incidence of pneumocystis pneumonia with respiratory failure declined significantly, accounting for only 18% of ICU admissions, and mortality rates were considerably lower (50–60%).

With the decline in ICU admissions due to pneumocystis pneumonia, the most common indications for admission for patients with HIV are respiratory failure (47%, including PCP), sepsis (12%), and neurologic disease (11%), followed by smaller percentages of patients requiring postoperative care and those with heart disease, gastrointestinal bleeding, trauma, and drug overdoses. In one study, 63% of patients with HIV infection admitted to the ICU for any reason survived hospitalization, though 1-year survival was only 27%. Patients with ICU admission for sepsis had the worst outcomes. Low serum albumin, low CD4 count, and use of mechanical ventilation were independent predictors of poor long-term survival. In another study, elevated serum creatinine and respiratory infections were associated with ICU mortality. End-stage liver disease is an increasingly common cause of death in HIV-infected patients as deaths from opportunistic infections decline and the complications of hepatitis C are seen.

Patients with HIV infection may be admitted to the ICU for a number of reasons. Conditions such as trauma, infections, and organ system failure unrelated to HIV disease may necessitate admission. Patients may have complications of advanced HIV disease, such as opportunistic infections or malignancies. Examples include pulmonary hypertension, renal failure, or heart failure associated with HIV, pneumocystis pneumonia, cryptococcal meningitis, disseminated histoplasmosis or coccidioidomycosis, and mycobacterial or viral infections. These patients may present with unique complications of HAART such as lactic acidosis, impaired glucose tolerance, hyperlipidemia, and adverse drug reactions and interactions.

Characteristics of HIV Infection

Acute HIV infection is associated with a syndrome of fever, rash, headache, and lymphadenopathy in over 50% of patients, though some patients are only mildly symptomatic. Seroconversion is followed by a highly variable period of clinical quiescence followed by progressive disease as the consequences of worsening immunosuppression and organ damage are manifested. During the asymptomatic stage, the presence of antibody to HIV may be the only evidence of HIV infection.

The primary cause of immunosuppression is the decrease in the number and percentage of CD4 lymphocytes, resulting in decreased cellular immunity as well as impairment of B lymphocyte function. Increased likelihood of infections caused by bacterial, protozoal, mycobacterial, fungal, and viral pathogens can occur throughout the entire course of HIV infection. However, infections with opportunistic organisms, malignancies, certain neurologic disorders, and severe wasting are associated with advanced HIV infection.

The use of HAART has greatly modified the course of HIV disease. HAART regimens are often complex, consisting of multiple drugs from as many as three different classes of antiretroviral agents; their success depends on strict compliance with dosage regimens, careful attention to the effects of food on absorption of antiretroviral drugs, and patient willingness to tolerate adverse effects of the medications. Side effects and toxicities of HAART drugs are relatively common, and adjustments in dosage and substitution of different agents may be necessary. As described below, a number of antiretroviral agents preclude prescription of other commonly used medications, and there are several drugs for which important dose modification is necessary.

Although the presentation of patients with HIV infection can be highly variable, a number of general principles have evolved. First, the level of immunosuppression must be considered when evaluating any disorder in an HIV-infected patient. In general, the likelihood of opportunistic infection and malignancy increases as the number of CD4+T lymphocytes decreases. In addition to its immunosuppressive effects, HIV also affects some organ systems directly. Examples include HIV nephropathy, a variety of central nervous system disorders, dilated cardiomyopathy, pulmonary hypertension, biliary tract disorders, thrombotic thrombocytopenic purpura-hemolytic uremic syndrome, pancytopenia, and adrenal insufficiency.

In the presence of waning cellular and humoral immunity, reactivation of latent infections may occur. For example, one-third of HIV-infected patients who have evidence of past exposure to toxoplasma (positive serum titer of IgG antibody to toxoplasma) will develop active cerebral toxoplasmosis when they reach a sufficient level of immunosuppression. In the absence of appropriate prophylaxis, an HIV-infected individual with a positive tuberculin skin test has a 7–10% chance per year of developing active tuberculosis—compared with an individual without HIV infection with a positive skin test, who has less than a 10% lifetime risk. Endemic fungal infections, such as histoplasmosis and coccidioidomycosis, may reactivate with declining immune status, presenting as disseminated infections.

However, the most common infectious agents encountered in patients with HIV are traditional bacterial pathogens. Common infectious syndromes include pneumonia, tuberculosis, bacteremia, sepsis, and sinusitis. For some common infections, the presentation may be atypical. In HIV-infected patients with tuberculosis, chest x-ray findings may include infiltrates located in the mid and lower lung zones, interstitial infiltrates, and hilar adenopathy or may show no abnormalities—rather than the typical cavitary lesions or upper lobe and apical disease usually seen in immunocompetent HIV-negative patients.

Patients with severe immunosuppression marked by low CD4 lymphocyte counts benefit substantially from prophylaxis against infections with *P carinii* and *Mycobacterium avium* complex (MAC). Other prophylaxis should be given to selected patients, including those with positive PPD skin tests for tuberculosis and those with antitoxoplasma antibodies.

Afessa B, Green B: Clinical course, prognostic factors, and outcome prediction for HIV patients in the ICU. Chest 2000; 118:138–45.

Bica I et al: Increasing mortality due to end-stage liver disease in patients with human immunodeficiency virus infection. Clin Infect Dis 2001;32:492–7.

Nickas G, Wachter RM: Outcomes of intensive care for patients with human immunodeficiency virus infection. Arch Intern Med 2000;160:541–7.

Valdez H et al: Changing spectrum of mortality due to human immunodeficiency virus: analysis of 260 deaths during 1995–1999. Clin Infect Dis 2001;32:1487–93.

SEVERE COMPLICATIONS OF ANTIRETROVIRAL THERAPY

Beginning with zidovudine (azidothymidine; AZT), antiretroviral therapy has been used to slow the progression of HIV infection. In the mid 1990s, protease inhibitors in combination with other antiretroviral therapy demonstrated potent effects on HIV, termed highly active antiretroviral therapy (HAART). Antiretroviral therapy can be divided into several drug classes: nucleoside analog reverse transcriptase inhibitors (NRTIs), nonnucleoside reverse transcriptase inhibitors (NNRTIs), and protease inhibitors (PIs). These drugs demonstrate both class and individual adverse drug reactions as well as important and common interactions with each other and with other drugs used to treat heart failure, anxiety, infection, depression, and hyperlipidemia. In the ICU, patients with HIV may have recently received antiretroviral therapy that can complicate current management or present with unique adverse reactions.

Lactic Acidosis & Hepatic Steatosis

This uncommon complication of NRTIs is associated with high mortality as well as features that may suggest septic or cardiogenic shock, hepatitis, or drug-induced liver failure. Clinical features include hepatomegaly, variably abnormal liver function tests, mild to severe lactic acidosis, and evidence of fatty liver on ultrasound or CT imaging. All NRTIs have been associated with this disorder. One proposed mechanism is inhibition of mitochondrial DNA synthesis leading to impaired oxidative phosphorylation with ensuing lactic acidosis and evidence of dysfunction in the liver as well as other organs.

Hyperglycemia

Evidence of diabetes, including hyperglycemia and ketoacidosis in some patients, has been associated with protease inhibitor use and resulting insulin resistance after a median of 60 days from initiation of therapy. It is not clear whether discontinuation of therapy is necessary unless hyperglycemia is poorly controlled.

Other Complications

Increased bleeding has been suggested in patients with hemophilia A and B who are given protease inhibitors. Hyperlipidemia is a common problem associated with some protease inhibitors. These patients have elevated triglycerides and cholesterol, with evidence for accelerated atherosclerosis in some reports. Dietary management may be useful; lipid-lowering drugs may be difficult to use because drugs such as simvastatin and lovastatin are contraindicated when protease inhibitors are used because of potential increase in statin levels. Rashes are not uncommon side effects of antiretroviral therapy, especially NNRTIs. In the ICU, these rashes may be confused with other dermatologic disorders.

Didanosine, stavudine, lamivudine, ritonavir, and pentamidine have been associated with pancreatitis. The hypertriglyceridemia associated with protease inhibitors is not usually severe enough to cause pancreatitis alone.

Antiretroviral drugs that commonly cause adverse effects are zidovudine (headaches, gastrointestinal symptoms, bone marrow suppression), various NRTIs (peripheral neuropathy, gastrointestinal symptoms), and most protease inhibitors (nausea, vomiting, diarrhea).

Drug Interactions & Toxicity

Potential adverse drug interactions can be divided into (1) those due to combining drugs that should not be used together and (2) those calling for dose modifications or additional caution. Drugs that should not be used together are listed in Table 27–1. Some drug interactions may prompt dosage modification, as shown in Table 27–2. Toxic potentials of drugs used in patients with HIV infection are set forth in Table 27-3.

Bartlett JG, Gallant JE: *Medical Management of HIV Infection,* 2000 ed. Johns Hopkins Univ Press, 2000.

Table 27–1. Drugs that should not be used for patients taking protease inhibitors or nonnucleoside reverse transriptase inhibitors.[1]

	Protease Inhibitors						NNRTIs	
	Lopinavir/r	**Indinavir**	**Ritonavir**	**Saquinavir**	**Nelfinavir**	**Amprenavir**	**Efavirenz**	**Delavirdine**
Midazolam, triazolam	✓	✓	✓	✓	✓	✓	✓	✓
Dihydroergotamine, ergotamine	✓	✓	✓	✓	✓	✓	✓	✓
St. John's wort	✓	✓	✓	✓	✓	✓	✓	✓
Rifampin	✓	✓	✓	✓	✓	✓		✓
Rifabutin			✓				✓	
Clozapine, pimezide		✓						
Astemizole, terfenadine	✓	✓	✓	✓	✓	✓	✓	✓
Simvastatin, lovastatin	✓	✓	✓	✓	✓	✓		✓
Amiodarone, encainide, flecainide, propafenone, quinidine, bepridil	✓		✓					
Cisapride	✓	✓	✓	✓	✓	✓	✓	✓

[1]Modified from Bartlett J.G., and Gallant J.E.: *Medical Management of HIV Infection,* 2001-2002 ed. Johns Hopkins Univ Press, 2001.

Table 27–2. ICU drug interactions with antiretroviral therapy that may require avoidance, dose modification, or monitoring.[1]

	Indinavir	Ritonavir	Saquinavir	Nelfinavir	Delavirdine	Elfavirenz	Amprenavir
Ketoconazole	↑ Indinavir levels	↑ Ketoconazole levels	↑ Saquinavir levels				↑ Amprenavir and ketoconazole levels
Rifampin	Do not use	↓ Ritonavir levels	Do not use. ↓ Saquinavir levels	Do not use. ↓ Nelfinavir levels	Do not use. ↓ Delavirdine levels	↓ Efavirenz levels	Do not use. ↓ Amprenavir levels
Rifabutin	↓ Indinavir; ↑ rifabutin levels	↑ Rifabutin levels	Do not use. ↓ Saquinavir levels	↓ Nelfinavir levels; ↑ rifabutin levels	Do not use. ↑ Delavirdine; increases rifabutin	↓ Rifabutin levels	↓ Amprenavir; ↑ rifabutin levels
Clarithromycin	↑ Clarithyromycin levels	↑ Clarithyromycin levels	↑ Clarithyromycin levels		↑ Clarithyromycin levels	↓ Clarithyromycin levels	↑ Amprenavir levels
Phenobarbital, phenytoin, carbamazepine	Avoid. ↓ indinavir levels	Unknown	↓ Saquinavir levels	↓ Nelfinavir levels	↓ Delavirdine levels	Unknown	↓ Amprenavir levels
Methadone		↓ Methadone levels		↓ Methadone levels		↓ Methadone levels	
Others		↓ Theophylline levels	Dexamethasone ↓ Saquinavir levels		↑ Levels of dapsone, warfarin, quinidine	Monitor warfarin	

[1]Modified from Bartleet JH, Gallant JE: *Medical Management of HIV infection,* 2001–2002 ed. John Hopkins Univ Press, 2001.

Table 27–3. Drug toxicity for some medications used in HIV-patients.

Bone marrow suppression
Dapsone
Flucytosine
Ganciclovir
Pentamidine
Pyrimethamine
Ribavirin
Sulfadiazine
Trimethoprim-sulfamethoxazole
Zidovudine
Pancreatitis
Co-trimoxazole
Didanosine
Lamivudine
Zalcitabine
Hepatotoxicity
Delavirdine
Efavirenz
Nevirapine
Nucleoside reverse transcriptase inhibitors
Protease inhibitors
Fluconazole
Isoniazid
Ketoconazole
Rifabutin
Rifampin
Diarrhea
Didanosine
Nelfinavir
Ritonavir
Clindamycin
Nephrotoxicity
Indinavir
Aminoglycosides
Amphotericin B
Foscarnet
Pentamidine

Max B, Sherer R: Management of the adverse effects of antiretroviral therapy and medication adherence. Clin Infect Dis 2000;30(Suppl 2):S96–S116.

PULMONARY COMPLICATIONS OF HIV INFECTION

Infection is by the far the most common pulmonary complication of HIV infection. The approach to an HIV-infected patient with suspected pulmonary infection is challenging because of the great variety of potential pathogens. The likelihood of certain pathogens causing pulmonary infection depends on several factors. First, the number and kind of pathogens that must be considered are directly related to the degree of immunosuppression (CD4 count). For example, bacterial organisms that cause community-acquired pneumonia may infect patients irrespective of CD4 count, while *Pneumocystis carinii* is uncommon unless the CD4 count is < 200/μL. Second, patients receiving prophylaxis for *P carinii* infection have a significantly lower incidence of pneumocystis pneumonia. Third, a history of prior or latent infection may be important, such as the presence of a positive tuberculin skin test, a history of exposure to endemic fungi, or prior pneumocystis pneumonia. Finally, the pattern on the chest x-ray may provide important clues, including evidence of localized infection or findings consistent with disseminated infection.

Pulmonary Infections

A. Symptoms and Signs

Important clues include the duration of symptoms, the presence or absence of sputum and the quality of sputum, hemoptysis, dyspnea, cyanosis, recent travel, geographic place of residence, history of tuberculin skin testing results, and recent adherence to prophylaxis.

B. Laboratory and Imaging Studies

Evaluation should include chest x-ray, sputum Gram stain, sputum acid-fast stain, complete blood count, blood cultures for bacteria, liver function tests, serum lactic dehydrogenase, creatinine, and arterial blood gases. In some cases, additional studies may be warranted, including serum crypotcoccal antigen, fungal and mycobacterial blood cultures, and CD_4 lymphocyte count (if not known). Chest CT scan may be helpful to identify additional foci of infection, demonstrate cavities, or confirm disseminated infection as well as to evaluate hilar or mediastinal involvement. Urinary histoplasma antigen should be measured in patients from endemic areas or with known or potential exposure. In the appropriate geographic area or with known or suspected prior exposure, the presence of antibody to *Coccidioides immitis* should be determined, but antibody is absent in up to 25% of patients with advanced HIV infection and disseminated coccidioidomycosis.

C. Fiberoptic Bronchoscopy

For patients with pneumocystis pneumonia (see below), fiberoptic bronchoscopy with bronchoalveolar lavage is diagnostic, and lavage may be useful for diagnosis of tuberculosis and nontuberculous mycobacterial infections.

D. Empiric Therapy

If the patient is critically ill, empiric therapy is indicated before results of laboratory studies are available. Because bacterial pneumonia is the most common infection leading to focal or diffuse infiltrates, antibacterial antibiotics should be initiated. For ICU patients, recommended treatment includes a third-generation cephalosporin plus a macrolide such as azithromycin. the patient is at risk for *Pseudomonas aeruginosa,* treatment should be adjusted to cover this pathogen.

The decision to start empiric treatment for pneumocystis pneumonia depends on clinical suspicion. Patients likely to have pneumocystis pneumonia have more severe hypoxemia, may have diffuse lung disease (though x-ray abnormalities vary widely), often have elevated serum LDH, and have a CD4 lymphocyte count under 200/μL. Treatment should consist of trimethoprim-sulfamethoxazole unless contraindicated; high-dose corticosteroids are indicated if severe hypoxemia is present (see below).

Empiric antituberculous therapy should be considered in patients at high risk, but the chest x-ray pattern may be atypical. Another important consideration is the need for isolation of patients to prevent nosocomial spread of tuberculosis.

PNEUMOCYSTIS CARINII PNEUMONIA

ESSENTIALS OF DIAGNOSIS

- *Nonproductive cough, fever, anorexia, progressive dyspnea.*
- *Hypoxemia with increased* $P(A-a)O_2$.
- *Focal, diffuse, or patchy infiltrates on chest x-ray; on occasion, the chest x-ray appears normal.*
- *Finding of* P carinii *on bronchoalveolar lavage.*

General Considerations

Despite the widespread use of primary and secondary prophylaxis, pneumocystis pneumonia remains the most common pulmonary infection associated with respiratory failure in persons with AIDS. Early recognition and treatment as well as the use of adjunctive corticosteroid therapy have resulted in improved survival and less morbidity for patients with moderate to severe disease.

Decreased survival of patients with pneumocystis pneumonia and respiratory failure has been associated with severity of illness at hospital admission and prior use of pneumocystis pneumonia prophylaxis. Decreased survival with pneumocystis pneumonia prophylaxis has been attributed to more severe immunosuppression or potential resistance to antibiotics.

Clinical Features

A. Symptoms and Signs

Common symptoms include nonproductive cough, fever, anorexia, and progressive dyspnea. There may be tachypnea, cyanosis, rales, and decreased basilar breath sounds.

B. Laboratory Findings

The white blood cell count is often normal. The CD4 lymphocyte count is generally < 200/μL. Patients have moderate to severe hypoxemia with increased $P(A-a)O_2$. Serum LDH is in nearly all cases elevated.

C. Imaging Studies

The chest radiograph may occasionally be normal but more often shows bilateral interstitial or alveolar infiltrates. Pleural effusions are absent.

D. Fiberoptic Bronchoscopy With Bronchoalveolar Lavage

The diagnosis is confirmed by finding the organism using modified Giemsa or methenamine silver stains or immunofluorescent antibody. In most patients, the diagnosis is made by bronchoalveolar lavage using fiberoptic bronchoscopy. Sensitivity is 85–95%. On occasion, patients may be too hypoxemic to undergo fiberoptic bronchoscopy. Sputum obtained by suctioning from the endotracheal tube (or expectorated sputum) may be stained and examined for *P carinii,* but the sensitivity is considerably lower.

Differential Diagnosis

In a patient with known or suspected HIV infection and pulmonary infiltrates consistent with pneumocystis pneumonia, the differential diagnosis includes bacterial and viral pneumonia, tuberculosis, other opportunistic infections (including fungal pneumonia), congestive heart failure with pulmonary edema, and ARDS.

Treatment

Patients with hypoxemic respiratory failure from pneumocystis pneumonia are generally managed in somewhat the same way as patients with ARDS. Patients will require oxygen supplementation and may require endotracheal intubation and mechanical ventilation.

A. Antipneumocystis Therapy

1. Trimethoprim-sulfamethoxazole (TMP-SMZ)— This agent is the treatment of choice for patients with pneumocystis pneumonia. It is given as a fixed combination that delivers 15 mg/kg per day of trimethoprim in divided doses every 8 hours intravenously or orally for 21 days. Side effects include fever, a spectrum of exfoliative skin eruptions, eosinophilia, leukopenia, thrombocytopenia, nausea, vomiting, and hepatitis. The dose must be decreased if the creatinine clearance is < 40 mL/min.

2. Pentamidine isethionate—This drug may be given to patients with moderate to severe pneumocystis pneumonia who are unable to take TMP-SMZ because of serious allergic reactions. It is given in a dose of 4 mg/kg per day intravenously for 21 days. Side effects include renal insufficiency, pancreatitis, and orthostatic hypotension. Hypoglycemia may occur during or after treatment and is exacerbated by renal insufficiency. Serum glucose should be monitored at least every 8 hours. In some patients, hypoglycemia may be followed by protracted hyperglycemia requiring insulin. If any of these side effects occur, alternative treatment must be chosen.

3. Clindamycin and primaquine—Clindamycin, 600 mg intravenously or 300–450 mg orally every 6 hours, can be given with primaquine, 30 mg base orally once daily, for 21 days. Side effects include pseudomembranous *(Clostridium difficile)* colitis, rash, hemolytic anemia in persons deficient in glucose-6-phosphate dehydrogenase, liver function test abnormalities, and methemoglobinemia.

4. Dapsone and trimethoprim—Dapsone is given in a dosage of 100 mg orally once daily along with trimethoprim, 15 mg/kg per day in three or four divided doses for 21 days. Side effects include hemolytic anemia in glucose-6-phosphate dehydrogenase deficiency, methemoglobinemia, liver function test abnormalities, rash, fever, leukopenia, and thrombocytopenia.

B. Corticosteroids

In patients with pneumocystis pneumonia who present with respiratory failure of moderate to severe degree, adjunctive therapy with corticosteroids is indicated. Corticosteroids have been shown to reduce the incidence of severe respiratory failure and decrease mortality in patients with severe hypoxemia. Candidates for corticosteroids have a $P(A-a)O_2$ of ≥ 35 mm Hg or an arterial PO_2 of ≤ 70 mm Hg.

These patients should be given prednisone, 40 mg orally twice daily for 5 days, 40 mg orally once daily for 5 days, and then 20 mg orally once daily for the remainder of the 21-day course of treatment. To achieve maximum benefit, prednisone should be started within 72 hours after beginning therapy. In patients unable to take oral medications, intravenous methylprednisolone can be substituted using the same dosage regimen.

C. Follow-Up Care

Response to therapy occurs within 5–7 days, marked by improvement in gas exchange and decrease in fever. For patients who initially respond to therapy and then develop fever, a search for another source of infection should be undertaken. Drug fever, often caused by TMP-SMZ, should be considered when no other pathogens are recovered and the patient is clinically improving.

Twenty-one days of antipneumocystis therapy should be followed by secondary prophylaxis with TMP-SMZ, one tablet (double-strength) orally three times per week. In patients unable to tolerate TMP-SMZ, acceptable alternative prophylactic regimens include using dapsone, atovaquone, and other agents.

PULMONARY INFECTION WITH *MYCOBACTERIUM TUBERCULOSIS*

ESSENTIALS OF DIAGNOSIS

- *Fever, night sweats, weight loss, cough, hemoptysis.*
- *Chest radiograph showing focal infiltrates with cavitation (CD4 lymphocytes > 500/μL); focal or generalized infiltrates (CD4 lymphocytes < 500/μL); hilar and mediastinal lymphadenopathy.*
- *Positive sputum for acid-fast bacilli or positive culture for* M tuberculosis. *Positive acid-fast stain or culture from nonpulmonary site.*

General Considerations

Tuberculosis is common in HIV-infected individuals. Both primary infection and reactivation occur with great frequency in this highly susceptible population. The clinical presentation of tuberculosis in HIV-infected individuals is often atypical compared with non-HIV-related tuberculosis. Patients may have symptoms more consistent with acute pneumonia than with a long-standing pulmonary problem. Chest x-ray findings may include mid and lower lung field infiltrates rather than apical fibronodular infiltrates with cavities. Disseminated tuberculosis with lymphatic, bone marrow, and liver involvement is much more common in persons with HIV infection than in those with normal immune function. Mycobacterial blood cultures are much more frequently positive in HIV-infected patients. The tuberculin skin test (PPD) is unreliable as a marker of tuberculous infection because of its low sensitivity in HIV-infected patients.

Clinical Features

A. Symptoms and Signs

Patients with tuberculosis and HIV infection may present with fever, productive cough, shortness of breath, night sweats, lymphadenopathy, and weight loss similar to that observed in non-HIV-infected patients. Alternatively, they may be minimally symptomatic. Physical examination findings include loss of lean body mass (wasting); some patients may have hepatosplenomegaly and lymphadenopathy.

B. Laboratory Findings

Liver function tests may be abnormal in patients with tuberculosis, especially with dissemination; elevated alkaline phosphatase, LDH, and γ-glutamyl transpeptidase are commonly seen. Anemia is frequently present, and pancytopenia may be present if there is bone marrow infection with tuberculosis.

Smears for acid-fast bacilli from sputum and culture of sputum for mycobacteria are the key to diagnosis. Three or more sputum samples should be submitted to the laboratory. If the patient is unable to cough or produce adequate samples, sputum can be induced by breathing aerosolized hypertonic saline. Negative acid-fast smears do not exclude tuberculosis; in selected patients, empiric treatment should be continued until cultures are negative. In patients undergoing fiberoptic bronchoscopy with bronchoalveolar lavage for diagnosis of pneumocystis pneumonia, fluid should be sent for acid-fast staining and mycobacterial culture. Urine cultures and blood isolators for mycobacteria may be positive. Drug susceptibility studies should be done on all *M tuberculosis* isolates, as drug-resistant strains are emerging in many areas.

Patients suspected of having disseminated tuberculosis should be considered for lumbar puncture, bone marrow examination, and liver biopsy to assist in the diagnosis.

C. Imaging Studies

Almost any chest x-ray pattern can be seen in tuberculosis with HIV. These range from classic apical fibronodular infiltrates with cavitation to—in some patients—normal lung parenchyma. A pattern consistent with primary tuberculous infection is more often seen with HIV infection. These consist of mid to lower lung field infiltrates, sometimes with hilar adenopathy. Disseminated tuberculous infection may be accompanied by a miliary pattern on chest x-ray.

Treatment

Patients with HIV infection and tuberculosis with susceptible strains of *M tuberculosis* are usually successfully treated with conventional antituberculous drug regimens. The ideal duration of therapy is not known. The initial use of rifampin, isoniazid, ethambutol, and pyrazinamide is recommended if organisms are likely to be sensitive. However, if multidrug-resistant tuberculosis is suspected, five- and six-drug regimens should be considered. Absorption of antituberculous drugs may be impaired in critically ill patients, and parenteral agents may be necessary. Liver aminotransferase levels should be monitored because isoniazid, rifampin, and pyrazinamide are hepatotoxic. Tuberculosis and HIV coinfection is an indication for instituting directly observed therapy (DOT) of tuberculosis.

A. Isoniazid, Rifampin, Pyrazinamide, and Ethambutol

This combination of drugs is highly effective against susceptible tuberculous organisms. The duration of treatment in the HIV patient consists of 2 months of all four drugs followed by 18 weeks of isoniazid and rifampin. Isoniazid is given in a dosage of 300 mg orally or intramuscularly daily. Common side effects include hepatitis, peripheral neuropathy from pyridoxine deficiency, alteration in sensorium, fever, and rash. Patients receiving isoniazid should be given pyridoxine, 50 mg daily.

The usual dose of rifampin is 600 mg/d orally or intravenously. Side effects include hepatitis, discoloration of urine, rash, fever, and alteration in other drug levels (oral contraceptives, warfarin, corticosteroids, digoxin, and methadone). Pyrazinamide is given as 15 mg/kg orally daily. Elevation of aminotransferases, hepatitis, hyperuricemia, and arthralgias may be seen as side effects of this drug. Ethambutol is given orally at a dosage of 15 mg/kg per day. Ethambutol is generally well tolerated, but loss of color vision or visual acuity may occur.

Rifampin is contraindicated in patients receiving protease inhibitors such as indinavir and ritonavir and nonnucleoside reverse transcriptase inhibitors (NNRTIs) such as nevirapine and delavirdine because of significant drug interactions. If concurrent use of protease inhibitors or NNRTIs is necessary, rifabutin can be substituted. Dose modifications of both antiretrovirals and rifabutin may be needed.

B. Other Antituberculous Drugs

Patients in the ICU who must receive parenteral medications may be given isoniazid and rifampin, but because only two antituberculous drugs are insufficient, intravenous amikacin and ciprofloxacin can be added. The usual dose for amikacin is 7.5 mg/kg every 12 hours intravenously or intramuscularly. Serum levels should be followed to avoid nephrotoxicity. Side effects may include renal failure, ototoxicity, and rare neuromuscular blockade. Alteration in dose for renal impairment is necessary. Ciprofloxacin is usually given as 750 mg orally twice daily or 200–400 mg intravenously twice daily. Common side effects include gastrointestinal intolerance, rash, and altered sensorium. The dose is decreased in patients with renal function abnormalities.

FUNGAL PNEUMONIA

Fungal pneumonias should be considered in patients with pulmonary infiltrates, negative cultures and smears for mycobacteria, negative stains and cultures for bacteria, and clinical progression with antibacterial treatment. Fungal infections may also present as disseminated processes with multiple organ involvement. Tissue biopsies and serologic tests are most helpful, since fungal cultures can take weeks to become positive.

A. Cryptococcal Pneumonia

Cryptococcal pneumonia is the most commonly encountered fungal pneumonia in patients with HIV infection, usually in the setting of advanced disease (CD4 lymphocyte count < 200/μL.). Patients present with fever (95%) and cough (70%). The chest radiograph usually shows diffuse interstitial opacities, but focal infiltrates, alveolar infiltrates, pleural effusions, and cavitary lesions may occur. Diagnosis can be made by culture of *C neoformans* from sputum, bronchoalveolar lavage fluid, or pleural fluid or by the finding of cryptococcal antigen in bronchoalveolar lavage fluid. Lumbar puncture must be performed to rule out central nervous system cryptococcal infection even if patients are asymptomatic. Serum cryptococcal antigen measurement is insensitive in the absence of dissemination.

Cryptococcal pneumonia may present with respiratory failure. In one study, respiratory failure was associated with dyspnea, LDH > 500 units/L, the presence of interstitial infiltrates, cachexia, and cutaneous lesions. Disseminated cryptococcosis was more commonly associated with respiratory failure. Patients at risk for respiratory failure from cryptococcal pneumonia should be considered for pneumocystis pneumonia as well. Mortality for those with respiratory failure from cryptococcal pneumonia is very high despite aggressive treatment.

Although mild to moderate cryptococcal pneumonia alone can be treated with fluconazole, HIV patients with severe cryptococcal pneumonia admitted to the ICU should receive amphotericin B, 0.7–1 mg/kg per day intravenously, plus flucytosine, 100 mg/kg daily, until symptoms are controlled, followed by fluconazole, 200–400 mg/d indefinitely. This regimen is recommended for central nervous system disease as well except that amphotericin B and flucytosine are given for at least 2 weeks.

B. Other Fungal Pneumonias

Endemic mycoses caused by such fungi as *Histoplasma capsulatum* and *Coccidioides immitis* usually present in patients with advanced immunodeficiency as a disseminated process of which pulmonary disease is one component. Fever, cough, and progressive dyspnea are common and may be accompanied by signs and symptoms of sepsis or other organ system involvement.

Chronic or subacute pneumonia caused by *C immitis* occurs in up to 10% of AIDS patients living in endemic areas such as Arizona and the San Joaquin Valley of California. Any findings may be seen on chest x-ray, including cavities, infiltrates, nodules, or pleural effusions. Dissemination is associated with low CD4 lymphocyte counts. Sputum, bronchoalveolar lavage fluid, or bronchial washings should be sent for stain and culture. Complement fixation titers of ≥ 1:16 are diagnostic of disseminated coccidioidomycosis but may be insensitive in HIV-infected patients. Intravenous amphotericin B, 0.5–1 mg/kg/d, should be used for initial treatment to a total dose of 30–40 mg/kg, followed by fluconazole, 200 mg/d orally. Patients with suspected dissemination should have a lumbar puncture to look for meningitis, largely because fluconazole is preferred treatment for meningitis caused by *C immitis.*

Pneumonia due to histoplasma can be seen in up to 15% of AIDS patients living in endemic areas. Dissemination occurs in patients with advanced disease and low CD4 lymphocyte counts. Chest x-ray findings are nonspecific, including diffuse infiltrates, nodules, focal infiltrates, cavities, and hilar adenopathy. Urine histoplasma polysaccharide antigen assay is moderately sensitive (50–70%) in cases of pneumonia. Histoplasma serum and bronchoalveolar lavage antigen, serologic studies (immunodiffusion M or H precipitin bands and complement fixation antibody at a titer of > 1:8), the presence of intracellular organisms on peripheral blood smear (30% sensitivity for disseminated histoplasma infection), and tissue biopsy and culture may be helpful in diagnosis. In severe or disseminated disease for patients in the ICU, intravenous amphotericin B should be given initially (for 3–14 days depending on response), followed by itraconazole, 200 mg orally twice daily indefinitely.

Invasive and obstructing aspergillosis has been described in patients with HIV infection and advanced immunodeficiency but is less common than other infections. Factors related to aspergillus infection include recent corticosteroid use, neutropenia, pneumonia with other pathogens, marijuana smoking, and the use of broad-spectrum antibiotics. Chest x-ray abnormalities may include focal infiltrates, cavities, pleura-based densities, or diffuse infiltrates. Because aspergillus organisms may colonize these patients without causing infection, sputum culture and staining may be unreliable. A tissue biopsy showing aspergillus in tissue or invading blood vessels is the most reliable diagnostic test. Treatment consists of a prolonged course of intravenous amphotericin B, but itraconazole may be substituted later for prolonged treatment in milder cases if there has been a good clinical response to initial treatment. The failure rate of itraconazole for serious aspergillus infection is unacceptably high.

VIRAL PNEUMONIA

Cytomegalovirus (CMV) is commonly isolated from sputum or bronchoscopic specimens but is rarely an important cause of pulmonary disease in patients with HIV infection. The likelihood of CMV pneumonia increases with severity of immunodeficiency, especially at very low CD4 lymphocyte counts (<20/μL). CMV may coexist with other pathogens, including pneumocystis. Because isolation of CMV does not indicate pulmonary infection, a more definitive diagnosis is made by finding intracellular inclusion bodies or evidence of invasive disease on cytologic specimens or lung biopsy. CMV retinitis or other organ involvement with CMV may be present. Treatment with ganciclovir is started at a dosage of 5 mg/kg intravenously every 12 hours for 14–21 days, then 5 mg/kg/d intravenously. Side effects include neutropenia, thrombocytopenia, central nervous system toxicity, and hepatotoxicity. A number of significant drug interactions may occur with ganciclovir, and zidovudine should not be used with this drug. Dosage must be modified in renal failure. Influenza, measles, herpes simplex virus, and varicella can also present with respiratory involvement.

KAPOSI'S SARCOMA

Pulmonary involvement with Kaposi's sarcoma occurs in about 35% of patients with this disorder and HIV infection. It may or may not be associated with cutaneous disease and can occasionally be found incidentally on postmortem examination without any other evidence of disease. Chest x-ray abnormalities vary but most commonly show a bilateral interstitial pattern with or without nodular lesions or linear perihilar densities. Abnormal gas exchange, hemoptysis, and superinfection with bacteria may be seen. A diagnosis of Kaposi's sarcoma involving proximal bronchi can sometimes be made by fiberoptic bronchoscopy. Bronchoalveolar lavage is useful for ruling out the presence of other pathogens. Transbronchial biopsy may be helpful but may miss the tumor because of sampling problems. Transthoracic and open lung biopsy are possible diagnostic maneuvers for patients without cutaneous lesions in whom Kaposi's sarcoma is suggested. Response of Kaposi's sarcoma to chemotherapy or radiation therapy is generally poor; however, potent antiretroviral therapy may arrest or even reverse the course of Kaposi's sarcoma.

BACTERIAL PNEUMONIA

In HIV-infected individuals, community-acquired pneumonias due to *Streptococcus pneumoniae, Haemophilus influenzae, Legionella pneumophila,* and *Mycoplasma pneumoniae* are still the most common pulmonary infections. Hospitalized or neutropenic patients are at increased risk for infection with *Staphylococcus aureus* and gram-negative aerobic bacilli, including *Pseudomonas aeruginosa.* Bacterial infections may occur alone or may be superimposed on an opportunistic infectious process such as pneumocystis pneumonia. HIV-infected patients with pneumonia have a higher incidence of bacteremia than non-HIV-infected patients—especially if they have pneumococcal pneumonia, which is associated with positive blood cultures in up to 90% of cases. Unusual bacteria may be responsible for pneumonia, including *Rhodococcus equi,* an aerobic intracellular gram-positive coccobacillus causing cavitary lung disease. For patients admitted to the ICU with community-acquired pneumonia, recommended initial therapy includes a third-generation cephalosporin (eg, ceftriaxone, 2 g intravenously once daily) plus azithromycin, 500 mg intravenously once daily, unless there is suspicion of pseudomonas infection (substitute a beta-lactam with antipseudomonal efficacy such as ceftazidime or piperacillin-tazobactam).

Afessa B, Green B: Bacterial pneumonia in hospitalized patients with HIV infection: the Pulmonary Complications, ICU Support, and Prognostic Factors of Hospitalized Patients with HIV (PIP) Study. Chest 2000;117:1017–22.

Curtis JR et al: Improvements in outcomes of acute respiratory failure for patients with human immunodeficiency virus-related *Pneumocystis carinii* pneumonia. Am J Respir Crit Care Med 2000;162:393–8.

Gallant JE, Chaisson RE, Moore RD: The effect of adjunctive corticosteroids for the treatment of *Pneumocystis carinii* pneumonia on mortality and subsequent complications. Chest 1998;114:1258–63.

Meyohas MC et al: Pulmonary cryptococcosis: localized and disseminated infections in 27 patients with AIDS. Clin Infect Dis 1995;21:628–33.

Navin TR et al: Risk factors for community-acquired pneumonia among persons infected with human immunodeficiency virus. J Infect Dis 2000;181:158–64.

Park DR et al: The etiology of community-acquired pneumonia at an urban public hospital: influence of human immunodeficiency virus infection and initial severity of illness. J Infect Dis 2001;184:268–77.

Prevention and treatment of tuberculosis among patients infected with human immunodeficiency virus: principles of therapy and revised recommendations. Centers for Disease Control and Prevention. MMWR Morb Mortal Wkly Rep 1998;47:1–58.

Saag MS et al: Practice guidelines for the management of cryptococcal disease. Clin Infect Dis 2000;30:710–8.

Schluger NW. Issues in the treatment of active tuberculosis in human immunodeficiency virus-infected patients. Clin Infect Dis 1999;28:130–5.

Visnegarwala F et al: Acute respiratory failure associated with cryptococcosis in patients with AIDS: analysis of predictive factors. Clin Infect Dis 1998;27:1231–7.

CARDIAC DISEASE IN HIV-INFECTED PATIENTS

Cardiac involvement in HIV-infected patients can occur as an unusual manifestation of common infections or opportunistic infections, or it may be due to HIV itself.

Myocardial Disease

Patients may have subtle subclinical evidence of myocardial disease noted on echocardiography or may have severe dilated cardiomyopathy. Infectious causes include CMV, toxoplasma, *Cryptococcus neoformans,* and *Mycobacteria tuberculosis.* A diagnosis of HIV-related cardiomyopathy is made when no defined agent is identified. Patients with congestive heart failure should receive treatment for dilated cardiomyopathy, including afterload reduction using vasodilators such as ACE inhibitors, and diuretics and digoxin.

Right heart failure due to pulmonary hypertension is seen in HIV-infected patients. In some cases, pulmonary hypertension occurs as a result of vasculitis, injection drug use, or chronic thromboembolic disease. However, primary pulmonary hypertension without a discernible cause occurs more commonly in persons with HIV infection than in the general population.

Myocarditis and dilated cardiomyopathy have been reported in association with zidovudine. Other drugs with rare adverse cardiac effects include pentamidine, ganciclovir, and amphotericin B.

Endocarditis

Bacterial endocarditis should be considered in HIV patients who have a history of injection drug use.

Pericardial Disease

Pericardial effusion has been found in 11–39% of HIV-infected patients, many of whom are asymptomatic. Causes of pericardial effusions to be considered include infections (mycobacteria, CMV, fungi), malignancies (widespread non-Hodgkin's lymphoma, Kaposi's sarcoma), and uremia. In one study, pericardial effusion may indicate a poor short-term prognosis, though patients with pericardial effusions had lower CD4 lymphocyte counts as a confounding variable.

Rerkpattanapipat P et al: Cardiac manifestations of acquired immunodeficiency syndrome. Arch Intern Med 2000;160:602–8.

Heidenreich PA et al: Pericardial effusions in AIDS: incidence and survival. Circulation 1995;92:3229–34.

Petitpretz P et al: Pulmonary hypertension in patients with human immunodeficiency virus infection: comparison with primary pulmonary hypertension. Circulation 1994;89:2722–7.

ACUTE RENAL FAILURE IN HIV-INFECTED PATIENTS

HIV-associated nephropathy consists of focal and segmental glomerulosclerosis, nephrotic syndrome, and rapid progression to renal failure in 1–4 months. In the ICU, HIV-infected patients may have HIV-associated nephropathy or may develop acute tubular necrosis as a result of hypotension from sepsis, heart failure, or volume depletion. Other causes of acute renal failure include drug toxicity from antibiotics (especially aminoglycosides, amphotericin B, trimethoprim-sulfamethoxazole, pentamidine), antiretroviral therapy (indinavir, ritonavir), and radiocontrast agents. There is an increased incidence of thrombotic thrombocytopenic purpura-hemolytic uremic syndrome in HIV-infected patients, and acute renal failure is part of this syndrome.

Renal insufficiency requires dosage adjustment of many drugs that are normally eliminated by the kidneys. Besides usual drugs encountered in the ICU, other medications that need dosage adjustment due to kidney disease include didanosine, stavudine, lamivudine, trimethoprim-sulfamethoxazole, ganciclovir, and amphotericin B.

Humphreys MH: Human immunodeficiency virus-associated glomerulosclerosis. Kidney Int 1995;48:311–20.

Rao TK: Acute renal failure syndromes in human immunodeficiency virus infection. Semin Nephrol 1998;18:378–95.

SEPSIS IN HIV-INFECTED PATIENTS

ESSENTIALS OF DIAGNOSIS

- *Fever or hypothermia, hypotension, hyperventilation, change in mental status.*
- *Complications of organ failure, such as alteration in gas exchange, renal insufficiency or failure, lactic acidosis, disseminated intravascular coagulation, or liver failure.*
- *Bacteremia, fungemia, or features arousing a high clinical suspicion of infection.*
- *Previous evidence or suspicion of bacterial, fungal, or mycobacterial infection may be helpful in differential diagnosis.*

General Considerations

Sepsis is discussed in Chapter 15. Important considerations in patients with HIV infection include increased risk of sepsis from any infection site, the potential for some unusual microbial organisms to be involved, and differences in diagnostic strategy and empiric therapy.

Because HIV infection is associated with disruption of both cellular and humoral immunity, disseminated infection is seen in a large proportion of patients; the rate of dissemination is proportionate to the degree of immunosuppression. Furthermore, there is phagocytic cell dysfunction and skin and mucosal membrane disruptions that increase the likelihood of microorganism translocation. Compared with age-matched cohorts, bacteremia is more commonly seen in HIV-infected patients with an identified focal bacterial infection. In addition, *M tuberculosis* spreads more rapidly, actively replicates in all tissues, and causes active disease more often in patients with HIV infection and immunosuppression than in normals. Treatment with zidovudine, trimethoprim-sulfamethoxazole, pyrimethamine, and ganciclovir—and HIV itself—can cause leukopenia.

A. Bacterial Sepsis

Most of these infections are associated with an identifiable source such as the lungs, gastrointestinal tract, urinary tract, central nervous system, or intravascular catheter. Clinically silent sites of bacterial infection include the sinuses, prostate, biliary tract, skin lesions, endocardium, and gastrointestinal tract. Sepsis may be caused by enteric diarrhea-associated pathogens and listeria. The most commonly isolated gram-positive organism from the blood is *S pneumoniae,* while *E coli* is the most common gram-negative organism found in blood, suggesting that common infections such as pneumonia and urinary tract infection are still the most likely sources of bacterial infection. Neutropenia should alert one to the possible presence of *P aeruginosa* and staphylococci, both community- and hospital-acquired. In particular, *P aeruginosa* infection is reported to be increasing in incidence, with risk factors including neutropenia, antibiotic use, corticosteroid use, and low CD4 lymphocyte count.

Two unusual bacterial infections are seen with increased frequency in HIV-infected individuals. Staphylococcal nontropical pyomyositis is described in patients with advanced HIV infection. It results from hematogenous spread of the organism (in rare instances, bacteria other than staphylococci). Patients complain of progressive myalgias and low-grade fever over several weeks. There may be palpable lesions in muscle, but these occur late because the initial foci of infection are deep in the muscle tissue. Laboratory findings include elevated skeletal muscle creatine kinase and aldolase, neutropenia or left shift of the differential count, and gallium scan or MRI showing areas of abscess and muscle infiltration. Needle aspiration of the muscle and blood cultures may yield the organism.

Bacillary angiomatosis was originally thought to be found only in association with HIV infection and involved skin and lymph nodes, but it can be seen in other immunocompromised hosts and in immunocompetent patients as well. Involvement of the liver, spleen, bone, brain, lungs, and gastrointestinal tract has been described. Focal lesions show areas of neovascular proliferation. *Bartonella henselae* and *Bartonella quintana* are the etiologic agents. Bacillary peliosis is a related disorder caused by *B henselae.* These lesions consist of blood-filled cysts involving the liver, spleen, and lymph nodes.

B. Disseminated Mycobacterial Infections

A subacute course of fever, weight loss, night sweats, cough, headache, or lymphadenopathy suggests a fungal or mycobacterial pathogen. The initial symptoms are often nonspecific and the clinical picture benign. Findings suggestive of disseminated fungal or mycobacterial infections include hepatosplenomegaly, lymphadenopathy, and the presence of skin or oral lesions. There may be laboratory findings of pancytopenia (bone marrow replacement) and elevated LDH and alkaline phosphatase.

Tuberculosis can present as a widely disseminated process. The clinical picture is characterized by weight loss, anorexia, and fever and sometimes by cough, dyspnea, and night sweats. Disseminated tuberculosis may be associated with tuberculous meningitis, and a lumbar puncture should be done if there is any suspicion. Disseminated *M avium* complex (MAC) is a late sequela of HIV infection and is seen in patients with CD4 lymphocyte counts $< 50/\mu L$. The clinical picture is similar to that of late-stage tuberculosis and is associated also with severe diarrhea. The course is protracted, and the diagnosis is often made by demonstration of the organisms in the blood, using the lysis-centrifugation method, or on tissue biopsy. MAC grows in approximately 3–6 weeks and can be identified using a DNA-specific probe.

C. Disseminated Fungal Infections

C neoformans, C immitis, and *H capsulatum* are primarily acquired through the respiratory tract and are hematogenously disseminated to multiple organs. Because of impaired cellular immunity, infections with these organisms may progress rapidly in HIV-infected persons. Progressive disseminated histoplasmosis is characterized by an initial mild course with minimal symptoms of 4–5 weeks' duration followed by a syndrome of hypotension, disseminated intravascular coagulation, renal insufficiency, severe pancytopenia, abnormal liver function tests (especially LDH), and respiratory failure. Central nervous system involvement is common. Intracellular organisms may be seen on the peripheral blood smear. Early initiation of amphotericin B therapy is critical while awaiting diagnostic studies. Disseminated coccidioides infection presents in a similar manner. Diagnosis and treatment of coccidioidomycosis are discussed in the section on pulmonary infection in HIV-infected patients.

Although oral and esophageal candidiasis occurs with great frequency in patients with symptomatic HIV infection, disseminated candidiasis is rare except in the usual settings of intravascular catheters, broad-spectrum antibiotics, or intravenous hyperalimentation.

Clinical Features

A. Symptoms and Signs

In addition to features that may localize the primary site of infection, additional information useful for planning empiric therapy include the travel history, tuberculin skin test status, history of exposure to or previous infection with mycobacteria or fungi, and recent use of antibiotics, both for treatment and for prophylaxis. Besides the primary infection site, examination should focus on potential sites of dissemination, including a careful funduscopic examination, inspection of skin and mucous membranes, and a search for lymphadenopathy and hepatosplenomegaly.

B. Laboratory and Imaging Studies

This should include initially complete blood count; peripheral blood smear (intracellular histoplasma organisms may be seen); blood cultures (two sets each for aerobic and anaerobic bacteria); liver function tests, LDH; urinalysis; chest x-ray; and creatine kinase.

Any potential site of infection should be cultured for suspected pathogens. Special culture techniques—such as urine culture after prostatic massage or aspiration of skeletal muscle in suspected pyomyositis—may be indicated. Imaging of specific sites may include CT scan, ultrasonography, MRI, or x-rays.

Septic patients with no obvious site of infection require more generalized investigation. Urine culture for fungi and mycobacteria, blood cultures using the lysis-centrifugation method for mycobacteria and fungi, serum antigen for *Cryptococcus neoformans,* sputum for acid-fast smear and mycobacterial culture, and urine and serum histoplasma antigen tests should be considered in appropriate patients. Patients with sepsis may have subtle central nervous system, pulmonary, abdominal, soft tissue, or mucosal sources of infection. In these patients, CT scan of the head, abdomen, and pelvis may be indicated. Lumbar puncture should be performed in any patient with unexplained sepsis or fever with or without alteration in mental status or abnormal neurologic findings. Cryptococcal meningitis and fungal and mycobacterial infections of the central nervous system may be associated with no findings or only very subtle ones.

Biopsy of skin or mucosal lesions, lymph nodes, spleen, liver, or bone marrow should be performed expeditiously in patients with suggestive symptoms or signs if results of other studies are negative or indeterminate. Special stains for microorganisms are necessary as well as histologic examinations of the usual sort. Cultures from biopsy specimens for many potential organisms may take 4–6 weeks to yield results.

Treatment

Patients with sepsis in whom there is hypotension, altered mental status, severe localized infection, or any organ system dysfunction should be treated immediately after appropriate cultures have been obtained. Empiric antibiotic treatment is generally directed initially at possible bacterial pathogens unless there is a suspicion of fungal or mycobacterial dissemination. The likelihood of bacterial infection is enhanced in patients who have leukocytosis or neutropenia; in those who have an acute onset of chills and fever or who have an identifiable infectious site; and in those who have higher CD4 lymphocyte counts. Patients with very low CD4 lymphocyte counts are prone to all types of infections, including bacteria, fungi, and mycobacteria. In these patients, antifungal and antimycobacterial agents should be considered early, but these antibiotics should be considered also in any patient who is deteriorating clinically on antibacterial therapy alone. Filgrastim (G-CSF) is indicated in patients with severe neutropenia (< 500–750 cells/μL).

Patients with disseminated tuberculosis can be treated initially with regimens used for pulmonary tuberculosis (see above), usually including multiple drugs, especially if drug resistance is likely. In general, MAC is not sensitive to the usual antimycobacterial agents, but various multiple drug regimens have shown promise in decreasing symptoms and reducing quantitative cultures. These regimens contain macrolides such as clarithromycin, which show excellent activity against MAC. Combination therapy with clarithromycin, 500 mg orally twice daily, plus ethambutol, 15 mg/kg per day orally, with or without rifabutin, 300 mg/d orally, can be started in patients with severe MAC if oral medications can be taken. If intravenous therapy is necessary, azithromycin plus amikacin or ciprofloxacin should be considered.

Afessa B, Morales I, Weaver B: Bacteremia in hospitalized patients with human immunodeficiency virus: a prospective, cohort study. BMC Infect Dis 2001;1:13.

Frank U et al: Incidence and epidemiology of nosocomial infections in patients infected with human immunodeficiency virus. Clin Infect Dis 1997;25:318–20.

Keiser P, Higgs E, Smith J: Neutropenia is associated with bacteremia in patients infected with the human immunodeficiency virus. Am J Med Sci 1996;312:118–22.

Moore RD, Keruly JC, Chaisson RE: Neutropenia and bacterial infection in acquired immunodeficiency syndrome. Arch Intern Med 1995;155:1965–70.

HEPATIC & BILIARY DISEASE IN HIV-INFECTED PATIENTS

Calculous and acalculous cholecystitis (gangrenous) have been reported in HIV-infected patients. Cryptosporidium, *Isospora belli,* microsporidia, cytomegalovirus, Kaposi's sarcoma, and lymphoma have been associated with these entities as well as sclerosing cholangitis, papillary stenosis, and papillitis.

Parenchymal hepatic disease is common in HIV-infected patients, including viral and drug-induced hepatitis (ketoconazole, zidovudine, delavirdine, efavirenz, nevirapine, isoniazid, rifampin, rifabutin, protease inhibitors, NRTIs, trimethoprim-sulfamethoxazole); infiltrative processes with MAC, *M tuberculosis,* and nontuberculous mycobacteria; Kaposi's sarcoma, lymphoma, or disseminated fungal infection. Hepatitis C virus (HCV) infection has a more rapid progression in the HIV-infected population, and injection drug users have an increased incidence of HCV infection. Imaging of the liver and biliary tract, endoscopic retrograde cholangiography, viral serology, liver function tests, and liver biopsy with special stains and cultures can be helpful in evaluation.

Bica I et al: Increasing mortality due to end-stage liver disease in patients with human immunodeficiency virus infection. Clin Infect Dis 2001;32:492–7.

Cappell MS: Hepatobiliary manifestations of the acquired immune deficiency syndrome. Am J Gastroenterol 1991;86:1–15.

Cohen J, West AB, Bini EJ: Infectious diarrhea in human immunodeficiency virus. Gastroenterol Clin North Am 2001;30: 637–64.

Kartalija M, Sande MA: Diarrhea and AIDS in the era of highly active antiretroviral therapy. Clin Infect Dis 1999; 28:701–5.

Tacconelli E et al: Clostridium difficile-associated diarrhea in human immunodeficiency virus infection: a changing scenario. Clin Infect Dis 1999;28:936–7.

CENTRAL NERVOUS SYSTEM DISORDERS IN HIV-INFECTED PATIENTS

HIV is neurotropic, and infection of the central and peripheral nervous systems is likely to occur very early in the disease course. Nevertheless, major central nervous system manifestations due to HIV occur late, and disorders related to immunosuppression are more commonly found. Neurologic disorders may result from autoimmune phenomena (vasculitis, demyelinating inflammatory polyneuropathy), immunosuppression (opportunistic infections, central nervous system lymphoma), and direct effects of HIV (meningitis, dementia). In the ICU patient, neurologic problems are the third most common single reason for admission. Severe central nervous system problems leading to ICU admission include delirium and coma; status epilepticus (structural lesion of the brain); intracranial mass lesions from tumor, lymphoma, or toxoplasmosis; meningitis (bacterial, cryptococcal, tuberculous, aseptic, viral); and respiratory failure due to severe neuropathy or myopathy.

Focal central nervous system disorders include cerebral toxoplasmosis, primary central nervous system lymphoma, and progressive multifocal leukoencephalopathy. Mass lesions can present in a variety of ways, including symptomatic neurologic deficits, altered mental status, or even frank psychosis alone. Toxoplasmosis of the central nervous system characteristically develops much faster than lymphoma or progressive multifocal leukoencephalopathy. Central nervous system imaging with CT or MRI may be able to distinguish among the causes. Other studies that may be necessary include antibodies to toxoplasma. Empiric therapy for toxoplasmosis may be started in critically ill patients, largely because other likely causes of central nervous system mass lesions have a very poor prognosis and little response to therapy. Patients with these lesions may require endotracheal intubation, ventilatory support, corticosteroids to decrease cerebral edema, antiseizure medications, and frequent neurologic evaluation.

CRYPTOCOCCAL MENINGITIS IN HIV-INFECTED PATIENTS

Meningitis caused by *Cryptococcus neoformans* is very unusual in nonimmunocompromised patients but is a relatively common development in HIV-infected patients. These patients may develop fever, headache, and nonspecific neurologic findings, including weakness, fatigue, dizziness, lack of alertness, visual changes, and seizures. Importantly, HIV patients with cryptococcal meningitis have very little or no meningeal irritation. Therefore, meningismus is rare, and clinical suspicion leading to lumbar puncture is necessary. Cerebrospinal fluid may occasionally be normal but more often has mildly elevated protein, decreased glucose, and a mild lymphocytic response (up to 100/μL). In contrast to these mild abnormalities, India ink preparations are positive in 60–80%; culture of cryptococcus is very often positive; and cerebrospinal fluid cryptococcal antigen is nearly 100% sensitive and specific. Opening pressure should always be measured because it has important prognostic significance. For example, elevated opening pressure of the cerebrospinal fluid (> 250 mm H_2O) correlates with high cryptococcal polysaccharide antigen, poorer clinical response, and poorer short-term survival. With treatment, failure of cerebrospinal fluid opening pressure to fall was associated with poor outcome. Patients with cryptococcal meningitis should be treated with amphotericin B, 0.7–1 mg/kg per day intravenously, plus flucytosine, 100 mg/kg daily orally for 2 weeks, followed by fluconazole 400 mg/d orally for 8–10 weeks.

Graybill JR et al: Diagnosis and management of increased intracranial pressure in patients with AIDS and cryptococcal meningitis. Clin Infect Dis 2000;30:47–54.

Price RW: Neurological complications of HIV infection. Lancet 1996;348:445–52.

Weisberg LA: Neurologic abnormalities in human immunodeficiency virus infection. South Med J 2001;94:266–75.

Dermatologic Problems in the Intensive Care Unit

28

Arnold W. Gurevitch, MD, & Kory Zipperstein, MD

The skin plays an important role in maintaining homeostasis. Thermoregulation, containment of body fluids, and protection of internal organs and structures from environmental insults are some of the vital functions performed by the skin. The skin is readily available for examination, so that inspection often provides important clues to underlying diseases. This chapter focuses on the following categories of cutaneous disorders in the critically ill patient: common skin disorders, drug eruptions, purpura, life-threatening dermatoses, and cutaneous manifestations of infections.

Common Skin Disorders

Contact dermatitis, miliaria (heat rash), and candidiasis are common in the critically ill patient as well as in the general population. These conditions, as well as graft-versus-host disease, which is seen in the ICU with increasing frequency because of the dramatic increase in allogeneic transplantations, are discussed in this section.

CONTACT DERMATITIS

ESSENTIALS OF DIAGNOSIS

- *Circumscribed vesiculobullous eruptions on a base of erythema, confined to the area of the contact.*
- *Especially linear or sharply angulated pattern suggesting external contact.*
- *Pruritus may be a prominent symptom.*
- *History of exposure or contact in involved areas.*

General Considerations

Contact dermatitis is an eczematous eruption caused by allergens or irritants coming in contact with the skin. The latter type is more common and results from exposure to irritating substances. Allergic contact dermatitis is a delayed hypersensitivity reaction that affects individuals previously exposed to the antigen. Any substance applied to the skin, including tape, cleansing agents, and topical medications, may be the offender. Even some topical steroids contain sensitizing chemicals. An eruption that appears to improve but subsequently becomes worse may be due to a contact dermatitis from an applied medication. Occasionally, candida or bacteria are secondary invaders.

Clinical Features

The morphology and distribution of the lesions, as well as the history of exposure, are diagnostic. Clinically, a circumscribed vesiculobullous eruption on a base of erythema, confined to the area of the contact, is the hallmark of contact dermatitis. Pruritus may be prominent. Contact dermatitis often has a characteristic configuration—eg, linear or sharply angulated patterns—that suggest the eruption is caused by external rather than internal stimuli. Marked erythema, often with an eroded surface, suggests an irritant contact dermatitis. Constant exposure to moisture, urine, or fecal matter in areas such as the groin, perineum, the backs of bedridden patients, and around a colostomy site may produce such an eruption. The differential diagnosis of contact dermatitis includes other eczematous eruptions, impetigo, and candidiasis.

Treatment

The suspected irritant or allergen should be removed, and cool tap water compresses can be applied to alleviate discomfort and remove crusts. Apply a high-potency topical steroid such as fluocinonide cream twice daily to the affected area. Eruptions on the face or intertriginous areas should be treated with low-potency to medium-potency topical steroids. Antihistamines may be administered to control itching. The involved area should be observed for the development of secondary infection.

Rietschel RL, Fowler JF Jr: *Fisher's Contact Dermatitis,* 5th ed. Lippincott Williams & Wilkins, 2001.

MILIARIA (HEAT RASH)

ESSENTIALS OF DIAGNOSIS

- *Seen in bedridden patients with fever.*
- *Miliaria crystallina: small, superficial sweat-filled vesicles without surrounding inflammation, giving the appearance of clear dewdrops. The vesicles rupture with the slightest frictional trauma.*
- *Miliaria rubra (prickly heat): discrete, pruritic, erythematous papules and vesiculopustules, especially on the back, the antecubital and popliteal fossae, the chest, and other regions prone to sweating and occlusion. Burning, itching, superficial aggregated small vesicles, papules, or pustules on covered areas of the skin.*

General Considerations

Miliaria is a common disorder characterized by retention of sweat. It is seen in individuals exposed to warm or humid climates and in bedridden patients with fever and increased sweating. Increased moisture causes swelling of the stratum corneum, with resulting occlusion of eccrine sweat ducts and pores and eventual disruption of the sweat gland or duct. Leakage of sweat into the surrounding tissue produces the lesions of miliaria.

Clinical Features

Two forms of miliaria may be seen in the febrile patient. In **miliaria crystallina,** the sweat duct is occluded at the skin surface, producing small and very superficial sweat-filled vesicles without surrounding inflammation, giving the appearance of clear dewdrops. The vesicles rupture with the slightest frictional trauma. The eruption is asymptomatic and self-limited.

A second form, **miliaria rubra (prickly heat),** is due to occlusion of the intraepidermal portion of the sweat duct. The eruption consists of discrete, pruritic, erythematous papules and vesiculopustules. The erythema may be broad and diffuse depending on the degree of inflammation. Areas such as the backs of patients lying in bed, the antecubital and popliteal fossae, the chest, and other regions prone to sweating and occlusions are the sites of predilection; the palms and soles are spared.

Miliaria crystallina is clinically distinct. However, miliaria rubra may resemble folliculitis, which usually can be distinguished by its follicular papulopustules with penetrating hair shafts. A Gram stain or culture of the pustular contents may help in distinguishing the two conditions.

Treatment

The patient should be kept cool and dry. The pruritus associated with miliaria rubra may respond to oral antihistamines, such as hydroxyzine; medium-potency topical steroids, such as triamcinolone acetonide 0.1%; or a topical antipruritic lotion containing phenol and menthol (eg, Sarna) or pramoxine hydrochloride.

CANDIDIASIS (MONILIASIS)

ESSENTIALS OF DIAGNOSIS

- *Oral candidiasis: white curd-like plaques on the oral mucosa, including the tongue, with a red, macerated base and painful erosions.*
- *Easily ruptured pustules commonly found in the groin, between the buttocks, under overhanging abdominal folds or pendulous breasts, and in the umbilicus. If ruptured, a bright red base with a fringe of moist scale at the border and satellite pustules. Intense pruritus, irritation, and burning are common.*
- *In systemic candidiasis, may have acneiform pustules or petechiae that may progress to necrotic ulcerative lesions on the trunk and extremities.*

General Considerations

The yeast-like fungus *Candida albicans* may cause infections limited to the skin and mucous membranes in addition to severe disseminated disease. Superficial candidiasis affects warm, moist areas such as the vagina (vulvovaginitis), the mouth (thrush), the uncircumcised penis (balanitis), the intertriginous areas, and sites around fistulas and artificial openings. Other predisposing factors include endocrine abnormalities (especially diabetes), malignancies, and immune-impaired states. Broad-spectrum antibiotics, pregnancy, incontinence, and skin maceration may also allow the yeast to become pathogenic.

Clinical Features

A. Symptoms and Signs

Oral candidiasis, or thrush, commonly consists of white curd-like plaques on the oral mucosa, including the tongue. The base of these plaques is red and macerated, and painful erosions may also be seen. Frequently, the infection will spread to the angles of the mouth (angular cheilitis; perlèche), resulting in maceration and fissuring of the oral commissures.

Candidiasis also tends to develop in intertriginous regions, including the groin, between the buttocks, under overhanging abdominal folds or pendulous breasts, and in the umbilicus. In these areas, pustules form but are easily ruptured by the friction of opposing surfaces, leaving a bright red base with a fringe of moist scale at the border. Coalescence of individual lesions results in spreading of the erythema with satellite pustules at the edges. Intense pruritus, irritation, and burning are common.

Oral candidiasis may spread to the esophagus or lungs. Candidal proctitis may develop with or without concurrent perianal infection. Systemic candidiasis is an opportunistic infection that tends to occur in patients with AIDS, hematologic malignancies, indwelling intravenous catheters, or malnutrition. Widespread dissemination may produce fever and proximal muscle tenderness, but any organ may be affected. Skin findings occur in about 10% of patients with candidal sepsis and consist of acneiform pustules or petechiae that may progress to necrotic ulcerative lesions on the trunk and extremities. Ophthalmoscopy may be helpful to look for candidal endophthalmitis. Concurrent superficial candidiasis may not be present and, by itself, is not helpful in establishing the diagnosis of systemic infection.

Superficial candidiasis is usually distinctive, but it may be confused with eczematous eruptions, dermatophytosis, and pus-producing bacterial skin infections (pyodermas). Systemic candidiasis must be distinguished from other septicemias.

B. Laboratory Findings

For superficial candidiasis, a potassium hydroxide preparation demonstrating budding yeast or spores and pseudohyphae establishes the diagnosis. Culture on Sabouraud's agar shows growth in 3–4 days. The diagnosis of systemic candidiasis is made by discovery of microorganisms in cutaneous biopsy or a positive culture from fluids (eg, blood, cerebrospinal fluid) or tissues normally sterile for candida in a patient in whom clinical findings are compatible.

Treatment

A. Superficial Candidiasis

Moist areas should be kept clean and dry. If the skin is weeping, a wet compress should be applied for 10–20 minutes twice daily. Topical anticandidal creams (eg, clotrimazole) applied twice daily are effective. Adding a low-potency topical steroid to the anticandidal agent may reduce the inflammatory component and speed healing. Creams should be rubbed into the area gently but thoroughly. This should be followed with an anticandidal powder (eg, miconazole).

The patient should be evaluated for predisposing factors such as diabetes, fecal and urinary incontinence, and immunosuppression.

B. Systemic Candidiasis

Systemic candidiasis requires more aggressive therapy with systemic agents such as amphotericin B, fluconazole, or itraconazole.

Bodey GP (editor): *Candidiasis,* 2nd ed. Raven Press, 1993.

GRAFT-VERSUS-HOST DISEASE

ESSENTIALS OF DIAGNOSIS

- *Prior allogeneic transplant containing immunologically competent cells, particularly bone marrow.*
- *Acute (days to weeks after transplant): Pruritic macular and papular erythema, frequently progressing to a generalized erythroderma with bullae in severe cases.*
- *Chronic (50–100 days after transplant): Widespread scaly plaques and desquamation. Cicatricial alopecia and dystrophic nails. In severe forms, sclerodermatous changes supervene.*

General Considerations

Graft-versus-host disease occurs when tissues containing immunologically competent cells (blood products, bone marrow, and solid organs) are introduced into an antigenically foreign person who is incapable of mounting an effective response to destroy the transplanted cells. It is the chief complication of allogeneic transplantation. Two forms are recognized: an acute form that can occur within days or as late as 1–2 months after transplantation and a chronic form that typically presents from 50–100 days or more after transplantation. Both forms are associated with significant morbidity and a high mortality rate.

Clinical Features

A. Symptoms and Signs

In acute graft-versus-host disease, the skin is the most commonly affected organ. The cutaneous eruption is characterized by a pruritic macular and papular erythema, often on the palms, soles, ears, and upper trunk, frequently progressing to a generalized erythroderma. In severe cases, bullae may develop, resembling the lesions of toxic epidermal necrolysis. The intestines, liver, and immune system are the other principally involved organs in acute graft-versus-host disease, with manifestations of diarrhea, hepatitis, and delayed immunologic recovery usually appearing after the skin eruption. The incidence of acute graft-versus-host disease ranges from 10–80%.

Chronic graft-versus-host disease may occur with or without preceding acute disease. However, any manifestation of acute graft-versus-host disease increases the chance of developing the chronic form. The incidence ranges from 30–60%. Cutaneous abnormalities occur in about 80% of patients with chronic graft-versus-host disease and usually resemble lichen planus, with widespread scaly plaques and desquamation. Destruction of skin appendages leads to cicatricial alopecia and dystrophic nails. In severe forms, sclerodermatous changes supervene. This may remain localized but more often is generalized, producing induration, dyspigmentation, atrophy, telangiectases, and chronic skin ulcers. Vitiligo may also occur. Other target organs include the mucosal surfaces, the eyes, the hematopoietic and immune systems, the liver, and the lungs.

B. Laboratory Findings

Laboratory studies are not specific but are important for monitoring other organ system involvement, the severity of illness, and the response to treatment. Key values are total bilirubin and stool output, which, when evaluated with the extent of rash and stage of disease, are prognostic for early acute graft-versus-host disease. Circulating autoantibodies and elevated immunoglobulins may be present in chronic graft-versus-host disease.

Differential Diagnosis

The skin abnormalities in acute graft-versus-host disease may be confused with toxic epidermal necrolysis, drug-induced eruptions, infectious exanthems, and other causes of palmar erythema—including cirrhosis, pregnancy, and other hyperestrogen states—and chemotherapy-related acral erythema. Of these, drug eruptions may be the most difficult to exclude. The skin in chronic graft-versus-host disease may have the appearance of collagen-vascular diseases such as scleroderma, lupus erythematosus, and dermatomyositis. The diagnosis is suspected when a characteristic skin eruption occurs in the presence of typical involvement in other organs.

Treatment

Over the past several years, major efforts have been focused on prophylaxis against graft-versus-host disease, utilizing corticosteroids, cyclosporine, azathioprine, mycophenolate mofetil, and methotrexate. Posttransfusion graft-versus-host disease can be prevented by irradiating blood products prior to transfusion. The immunosuppressive agents used for preventing graft-versus-host disease are also useful in treating established acute disease.

Patients with localized chronic graft-versus-host disease do well without intervention. In generalized chronic disease, immunosuppressive agents are the mainstays of treatment. In addition, photochemotherapy with oral PUVA (psoralen) or UVA is sometimes used.

Darmstadt GL et al: Clinical, laboratory, and histopathologic indicators of progressive acute graft-versus-host disease. J Invest Dermatol 1992;99:397–402.

Ferrara JL, Deeg HJ: Graft-versus-host disease. N Engl J Med 1991;324:667–74.

Grundmann-Kollmann M et al: Chronic sclerodermic graft-versus-host disease refractory to immunosuppressive treatment responds to UVA phototherapy. J Am Acad Dermatol 2000;42:134–6.

DRUG REACTIONS

A drug reaction is defined as any adverse response temporally related to the administration of a drug. Unwanted drug reactions have been estimated to occur in 15–30% of hospitalized patients. Cutaneous eruptions are among the most common adverse reactions to drugs, affecting 2–3% of hospitalized patients. Patients receiving many different drugs, such as the critically ill, are more likely to develop a drug eruption. The cutaneous manifestations vary in severity from mild and transient to the occasional development of severe systemic disease and even death, and often mimic other dermatoses, both clinically and histologically. In this section, drug eruptions with distinctive morphologic characteristics will be discussed, with emphasis on some common or life-threatening conditions encountered in critically ill patients. Special forms of drug reactions are also discussed in the sections on contact dermatitis, vasculitis, anticoagulant necrosis, and exfoliative erythroderma.

MORBILLIFORM, URTICARIAL, & BULLOUS DRUG ERUPTIONS

ESSENTIALS OF DIAGNOSIS

- *Exposure to drugs commonly associated with drug eruptions, especially antibiotics, anticonvulsants, and blood products— but may be due to any medication.*

- *Onset of rash temporally related to drug administration, most often 5–10 days after exposure to a new drug or 1–2 days as a reaction to a drug to which the patient has been previously sensitized.*
- *Eruptions are usually symmetric and widespread, appear suddenly, and are not associated with systemic symptoms other than pruritus and mild fever.*
- *Improvement with cessation of drug supports diagnosis.*

General Considerations

Adverse reactions that involve immune mechanisms, such as IgE-mediated urticaria and anaphylaxis, and cell-mediated contact reactions are true drug allergies. Reactions involving suspected immune mechanisms of unknown or mixed pathogenesis include the erythematous maculopapular or morbilliform rashes, bullous eruptions, erythema multiforme and Stevens-Johnson syndrome, and exfoliative erythrodermas. Nonimmune mechanisms and idiosyncratic reactions may lead to skin abnormalities via activation of effector pathways, direct toxicity, drug interactions, and overdosage. Drug-induced urticaria can be produced by several mechanisms: IgE-mediated anaphylactic hypersensitivity, immune complex-induced urticaria associated with serum sickness-like reactions (urticaria, fever, hematuria, and arthralgias), nonimmunologic release of mast cell mediators, and direct stimulation of the complement cascade.

Unfortunately, the pathogenic mechanisms in the majority of drug eruptions remain unknown.

Clinical Features

A. History of Medications

When a drug eruption is suspected, it is important to document each medication currently being given or recently discontinued, the duration of its use, and the timing of drug exposure in relation to onset of the rash. As a rule, a recently started medication is more apt to be responsible for a drug eruption. Rarely will a medication that has been taken regularly for months to years stimulate the immune system to produce an eruption. It typically takes 5–10 days following exposure to a new drug—or 1–2 days after previous sensitization—for a drug eruption to appear. However, the rash may appear suddenly, as seen in urticaria and anaphylaxis. Prior history of an adverse reaction is the only clinically helpful risk factor.

B. Symptoms and Signs

The morphology of the rash and the reported frequency of adverse cutaneous reactions to a given drug may assist in identifying the offending agent. Some drugs are rarely associated with skin eruptions (Table 28–1). In the ICU setting, the most frequently implicated medications are antibiotics (eg, ampicillin, semisynthetic penicillins, and trimethoprim-sulfamethoxazole), anticonvulsants, and blood products. Certain drugs are more commonly associated with specific morphologic patterns, thus helping identify the causative agent when multiple drug exposures have occurred (Table 28–2).

Morbilliform eruptions, or toxic erythemas, are the most common type of drug-induced rashes. These eruptions are usually symmetric, widespread, and consist of erythematous macules or papules that often become confluent. The rash typically begins on the trunk or in dependent areas; involvement of the palms and soles is variable. Pruritus and mild fever may accompany the reaction. Signs and symptoms usually regress within a few days after treatment is stopped. Exceptionally, the eruption fades despite continued intake of the drug.

Urticaria represents the second most common type of drug eruption. Urticaria is a vascular reaction of the skin characterized by wheals, which are pinkish, edematous, pruritic lesions that vary in size and shape. Individual lesions are transient, rarely lasting longer than 24 hours. Angioedema refers to urticarial swelling of deep dermal and subcutaneous tissues. Angioedema may involve the mucous membranes and may be life-threatening. Urticaria may occur alone or in conjunction with angioedema or anaphylaxis. The reaction is usually self-limited, lasting a few days to a few weeks.

Blisters may accompany a variety of drug-induced eruptions including fixed-drug eruptions, erythema

Table 28–1. Drugs infrequently associated with adverse skin reactions.

Acetaminophen	Isosorbide dinitrate
Aminophylline	Laxatives
Antacid	Lidocaine
Atropine	Meperidine
Chloral hydrate	Morphine
Chloramphenicol	Multivitamins
Chlorpromazine	Nitroglycerin
Dexamethasone	Potassium iodide
Digoxin	Prednisolone
Diphenhydramine	Prednisone
Ferrous sulfate	Promethazine
Flurazepam	Propranolol
Folic acid	Spironolactone
Hydrochlorothiazide	Tetracycline
Hydroxyzine	Theophylline
Insulin	Thyroid hormones

Table 28–2. Some morphologic patterns of drug eruptions and commonly incriminated agents.

Maculopapular eruptions
- Ampicillin
- Barbiturates
- Blood products
- Captopril
- Gentamicin
- Isoniazid
- Phenytoin
- Sulfonamides

Urticaria
- Allopurinol
- Aminoglycosides
- Barbiturates
- Blood products
- Chlorpromazine
- Hydralazine
- Morphine
- NSAIDs
- Penicillins
- Phenytoin
- Radiographic contrast
- Salicylates
- Sulfonamides

Bullous eruptions
- Barbiturates (coma bullae)
- Captopril
- Heparin
- Pencillamine (pemphigus-like)
- Piroxicam
- Phenytoin
- Sulfonamides
- Warfarin

Erythema multiforme
- Barbiturates
- NSAIDs
- Penicillins
- Phenytoin
- Rifampin
- Sulfonamides
- Sulfonylureas

Toxic epidermal necrolysis
- Barbiturates
- Carbamazepine
- Dapsone
- Phenytoin
- Sulfonamides
- Allopurinol

Purpura
- ***Thrombocytopenic***
  - Carbamazepine
  - NSAIDs
- ***Vasculitis***
  - Allopurinol
  - Barbiturates
  - Clindamycin
  - Furosemide
  - Hydralazine
  - Penicillins
  - Phenytoin
  - Salicylates
  - Sulfonamides
- ***Miscellaneous***
  - Corticosteroids
  - Heparin
  - Warfarin

Serum sickness
- Antithymocyte globulin
- Blood products
- Cephalosporins
- Penicillins
- Phenytoin
- Radiographic contrast
- Sulfonamides

Exfoliative erythroderma
- Barbiturates
- Captopril
- Carbamazepine
- Cefoxitin
- Cimetidine
- Furosemide
- Isoniazid
- Phenytoin
- Salicylates
- Sulfonamides
- Sulfonylureas

multiforme, Stevens-Johnson syndrome, toxic epidermal necrolysis, vasculitis, and anticoagulant necrosis. Some drugs can produce blistering eruptions that are indistinguishable from primary bullous dermatoses such as bullous pemphigoid and porphyria cutanea tarda. Coma bullae—blisters over pressure areas—are seen in patients in coma from various causes, including narcotics, barbiturates, and carbon monoxide poisoning. Some bullous drug eruptions do not fit into any of these diagnostic classes.

C. Laboratory Findings

Laboratory tests are rarely helpful in diagnosis. Morbilliform reactions are occasionally associated with eosinophilia; antinuclear antibody titers are positive in drug-induced lupus; and there may be evidence of liver, kidney, and hematologic abnormalities in the phenytoin hypersensitivity syndrome (see below). Skin biopsy findings are usually nonspecific. Tissue eosinophils may help differentiate drug eruptions from the dermatoses they mimic. However, a few specific eruptions, including coma bullae, fixed drug eruptions, erythema multiforme, toxic epidermal necrolysis, and vasculitis, may show distinctive histopathologic changes.

Differential Diagnosis

Drug eruptions may sometimes be distinguished clinically from the dermatoses they simulate by their sudden appearance, symmetry, widespread distribution, and paucity of associated systemic symptoms. Medication history and improvement of the skin after the medication is stopped may support the diagnosis.

The principal causes of morbilliform eruptions are drug reactions and infections, especially viral exanthems. Occasionally, a morbilliform drug rash may be confused with a bacterial or rickettsial infection or collagen-vascular disease. Although the diagnosis of urticaria is usually apparent because of the presence of evanescent wheals, the cause may be difficult to discern. In addition to drugs, other common causes of urticaria include food allergies, insect bites and stings, and parasitic infections. If the urticarial lesions persist longer than 24–36 hours, are tender, or have a purpuric component, an urticarial vasculitis or serum sickness-like reaction should be considered. Bullous drug eruptions may resemble primary blistering dermatoses.

Treatment

The challenges to the clinician faced with a suspected drug rash are to consider alternative explanations for the rash, identify the offending drug, predict progression to serious or life-threatening eruptions, and decide whether or not to intervene.

A. Review Medications

When feasible, discontinue likely causative agents and substitute chemically unrelated drugs. If the medication is not essential, it may be stopped without substitution. If the eruption is mild and relatively asymptomatic and a particular drug is necessary, the drug may be continued with cautious observation. However, urticaria, erythema multiforme, vasculitis, or generalized erythema (erythroderma) requires a search for alternative therapy.

B. General Measures

Treatment of drug eruptions is usually supportive and symptomatic, since the majority of eruptions resolve within 2–5 days after stopping the offending drug. Pruritus can be treated with oral antihistamines, such as hydroxyzine, and a topical antipruritic lotion (eg, Sarna, Pramosone). Treatment of severe urticarial reactions associated with angioedema or anaphylaxis consists of supportive measures to maintain vital functions, epinephrine, antihistamines, and, if all else fails, systemic corticosteroids. Blistering eruptions may require decompression of large bullae, topical antibiotics to denuded areas, and baths or wet compresses to remove exudate or crusts. Drug-induced erythroderma may require systemic corticosteroid therapy.

Bigby M, Jick S, Arndt K: Drug-induced cutaneous reactions: A report from the Boston collaborative drug surveillance program on 15,438 consecutive inpatients, 1975 to 1982. JAMA 1986;256:3358–63.

Litt JZ: *Drug Eruption Reference Manual 2001.* Parthenon, 2001.

ERYTHEMA MULTIFORME & STEVENS-JOHNSON SYNDROME

ESSENTIALS OF DIAGNOSIS

- *Prodrome of low-grade fever, malaise, and upper respiratory symptoms, followed by a nonspecific symmetric eruption of erythematous macules, papules, and urticarial plaques.*
- *Evolves into concentric rings of erythema with papular, dusky, necrotic, or bullous centers ("target lesions") over 1–2 days, but may also be annular, polycyclic, or purpuric (multiforme).*
- *Stevens-Johnson syndrome marked by high fever, headache, myalgias, and sore throat, with more than one mucosal surface affected. Stomatitis is conspicuous, beginning with vesicles on the lips, tongue, and buccal mucosa. The vesicles rapidly evolve into erosions and ulcers covered by hemorrhagic crusts.*

General Considerations

Erythema multiforme is an acute, self-limited inflammatory disease of the skin or mucous membranes. It represents a hypersensitivity reaction pattern to a variety of stimuli, most commonly drugs and infectious agents (Table 28–3). The cause is not found in about half of cases. Stevens-Johnson syndrome (erythema multiforme major) is a severe and occasionally fatal form characterized by marked oral and ocular mucosal involvement. Erythema multiforme occurs in all age groups, while Stevens-Johnson syndrome most often affects children and young men.

The pathogenesis of erythema multiforme and Stevens-Johnson syndrome is not fully understood. According to one hypothesis, foreign antigens are sequestered in the epithelium, leading to immune-mediated epithelial damage. Although circulating immune complexes have been documented in some cases and direct immunofluorescence may show deposits of IgM and C3 in the superficial dermal vessels, vasculitis does not appear to be the primary event in these disorders. Polymerase chain reaction studies have demonstrated herpes simplex virus DNA in the skin lesions of some patients.

Clinical Features

A. Symptoms and Signs

Within hours to weeks after exposure to an inciting agent, a prodrome of low-grade fever, malaise, and upper respiratory symptoms may appear. This is followed by a nonspecific symmetric eruption of erythematous macules, papules, and urticarial plaques that evolve into tar-

Table 28–3. Common causes of erythema multiforme and Stevens-Johnson syndrome.

Drugs: See Table 28–2.
Infection
Herpes simplex
Mycoplasma pneumoniae
Streptococcus
Yersinia
Tuberculosis
Histoplasmosis
Other conditions
Irradiation of tumors
Sarcoidosis
Pregnancy
Carcinomas
Leukemias
Collagen-vascular diseases
Inflammatory bowel disease
Idiopathic

get lesions over a 1- to 2-day period. The classic target or "iris" lesions are concentric rings of erythema with papular, dusky, necrotic, or bullous centers. The lesions may also be annular, polycyclic, or purpuric, demonstrating the polymorphous ("multiforme") nature of the eruption. The extensor surfaces of the forearms, the face, the neck, the legs, and the palms and soles are the most commonly involved sites. The lesions appear in crops over 1–2 weeks and usually resolve within 4 weeks, often with residual hyperpigmentation. The mucous membranes commonly reveal hemorrhagic crusting of the lips, painful oral erosions, and purulent conjunctivitis.

In Stevens-Johnson syndrome, high fever, headache, myalgias, and sore throat develop abruptly, often associated with coryza, vomiting, diarrhea, and joint pains. Patients appear extremely ill and may have tachycardia and tachypnea. More than one mucosal surface is affected. Stomatitis is conspicuous, beginning with vesicles on the lips, tongue, and buccal mucosa. The vesicles rapidly evolve into erosions and ulcers, covered by hemorrhagic crusts. Bilateral catarrhal conjunctivitis, corneal ulcers, erosive rhinitis, balanitis, and vulvovaginitis may develop. The urethra, larynx, esophagus, trachea, and bronchi may also be involved. Occasionally the skin is spared, but in most instances a vesiculobullous or erythematous eruption appears on the face and distal extremities. Complications include dehydration resulting from the ulcerative stomatitis and blindness resulting from the corneal ulcers. Pneumonia, nephritis, hepatitis, pericarditis, cardiac arrhythmias, arthritis, and myositis may occur, though it has not been determined if these are manifestations of Stevens-Johnson syndrome or due to the underlying causative factor. In patients with extensive disease, the mortality rate approaches 10–15%, with deaths usually a result of sepsis.

B. Laboratory Findings

There are no specific laboratory abnormalities. Leukocytosis, elevated erythrocyte sedimentation rate, abnormal liver function tests, proteinuria, and, occasionally, hematuria are seen. The diagnosis is based on characteristic clinical features with histopathologic confirmation.

Underlying causative factors should be sought. Evaluation of the patient should include the following: complete blood count, erythrocyte sedimentation rate, urinalysis, and PPD test. Other tests may include cold agglutinin titers; chest, sinus, and dental x-rays; hepatitis B serologic tests; cultures for bacteria, viruses, and fungi; and ANA and rheumatoid factor determinations. Other tests for the evaluation of diseases such as sarcoidosis or occult malignancies should also be considered.

Differential Diagnosis

Erythema multiforme may resemble many other skin disorders, especially when the classic target lesions are absent. The presence of target lesions and characteristic histopathologic features helps distinguish erythema multiforme and Stevens-Johnson syndrome from urticaria, viral exanthems, and vasculitis as well as from other mucocutaneous disorders such as Reiter's syndrome, Behçet's syndrome, herpes gingivostomatitis, and Kawasaki's disease. When blisters are present, erythema multiforme and Stevens-Johnson syndrome must be differentiated from bullous impetigo, bullous pemphigoid, pemphigus vulgaris, and toxic epidermal necrolysis.

Treatment

If the specific cause is identified, treatment directed at that cause is indicated. In most cases, therapy is supportive and symptomatic. Incriminated drugs should be discontinued and the patient monitored closely for potential progression to secondary infection and sepsis or to toxic epidermal necrolysis. Cool compresses, followed by the application of mupirocin ointment, are useful for crusting and secondary infection.

For patients with compromised oral intake or extensive erosions, proper attention must be paid to fluids, electrolytes, and nutrition. An antiseptic mouthwash or hydrogen peroxide should be used to keep the oral cavity clean. Viscous lidocaine or a mixture of equal parts of diphenhydramine hydrochloride and an oral antacid may alleviate pain on swallowing.

Eye involvement should be managed in consultation with an ophthalmologist. Avoid sulfonamide-containing eye drops, since they can cause or exacerbate sulfonamide-induced reactions. Topical or systemic steroids have not been proved to prevent ocular sequelae or progression of cutaneous disease, and they may be harmful. However, some authorities advocate systemic steroids early in the course of the reaction (within 48 hours).

Rzany B et al: Risk of Stevens-Johnson syndrome and toxic epidermal necrolysis during first weeks of antiepileptic therapy. Lancet 1999;353:2190–4.

Strom BL et al: A population-based study of Stevens-Johnson syndrome: Incidence and antecedent drug exposures. Arch Dermatol 1991;127:831–8.

TOXIC EPIDERMAL NECROLYSIS

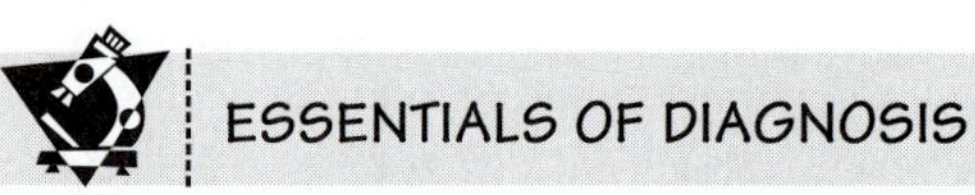
ESSENTIALS OF DIAGNOSIS

- *Tender, discrete, erythematous macules.*
- *Red, scalded appearance of skin; bullae and epidermal sloughing.*

- *Often a recent history of drug ingestion.*
- *Subepidermal separation of skin (Nikolsky's sign).*
- *Features of erythema multiforme major (Stevens-Johnson syndrome): stomatitis, blotchy eruption with target lesions.*

General Considerations

Toxic epidermal necrolysis is a rare, life-threatening syndrome characterized by skin tenderness, erythema, and exfoliation of the epidermis and mucous membranes reminiscent of a scald injury. The pathophysiology is not known, but the disorder is believed to be immunologically mediated. The majority of cases are drug-induced by such agents as antiepileptics (phenytoin, phenobarbital, carbamazepine), sulfonamides, sulfones, nonsteroidal anti-inflammatory drugs (especially pyrazolone derivatives), allopurinol, and ampicillin. Identification of the causative drug is often difficult, since many patients are treated with multiple medications. In general, the interval between initial dose of the drug and onset of the disease is 1–3 weeks, except for phenytoin-induced cases, which may occur as late as 8 weeks following the start of therapy. If the patient has a history of toxic epidermal necrolysis from previous exposure to a drug, the time period may be reduced to 24–48 hours.

Patients with AIDS appear to have an increased risk for toxic epidermal necrolysis.

Clinical Features

A. Symptoms and Signs

Fever, malaise, upper respiratory symptoms, and conjunctivitis usually precede the skin lesions by 2–3 days. Cutaneous involvement appears acutely as tender, discrete, symmetric erythematous macules and urticarial plaques with dusky centers on the face and upper trunk. Coalescence and extension to the entire body rapidly ensue. Subsequently, large flaccid bullae develop within the areas of erythema, and the necrotic epidermis sloughs in sheets. Pressure applied directly over an intact blister produces lateral spread of the lesion. Gentle rubbing of erythematous areas induces separation of the epidermis (Nikolsky's sign). The palms and soles may be involved, but the hairy part of the scalp characteristically is spared. Mucous membrane involvement is extensive, with erosions or ulcers of the conjunctiva, lips, oropharynx, trachea, esophagus, and anogenital area.

Sepsis is the most frequent cause of death and may be heralded by a sudden drop in temperature. Pulmonary embolism, pulmonary edema, and gastrointestinal bleeding are other important causes of death. Pneumonia superimposed on sloughing of the tracheobronchial mucosa may require ventilatory assistance. Fluid loss, thermoregulatory impairment, and increased energy expenditure result from extensive skin loss, as in burn victims. The mortality rate ranges from 25–75% and is higher in elderly patients. Disabling ocular sequelae affect up to 50% of survivors. Cutaneous reepithelialization requires 2–3 weeks, while the mucous membrane lesions persist longer.

B. Laboratory Findings

Routine laboratory studies reflect the extent and severity of the disease but are not specific. There may be evidence of electrolyte depletion and dehydration. Serum creatinine may be elevated owing to prerenal azotemia or acute tubular necrosis. Serum aminotransferase levels are often slightly increased. In virtually all patients, anemia is present; lymphopenia, neutropenia, and thrombocytopenia are sometimes seen and may indicate a poor prognosis. Biopsy of involved skin may be very helpful, revealing full-thickness epithelial necrosis.

Differential Diagnosis

Clinically, toxic epidermal necrolysis and staphylococcal scalded skin syndrome are quite similar. The latter disorder is caused by an epidermolytic toxin produced by *Staphylococcus aureus.* The toxin produces superficial (subcorneal) skin separation. Nikolsky's sign is present, but skin tenderness and mucous membrane lesions usually are absent. Staphylococcal scalded skin syndrome more frequently affects neonates and toddlers, is rare in adults, and has a much better prognosis than toxic epidermal necrolysis.

Other differential diagnostic considerations include pemphigus vulgaris and other blistering diseases, toxic shock syndrome, chemical or thermal burns, and Kawasaki's disease. Toxic epidermal necrolysis shares many features with—and is considered by some to be a severe form of—Stevens-Johnson syndrome.

Treatment

The principles of therapy are similar to those for major second-degree burn victims. Ideally, patients should be managed in a burn unit.

A. General Measures

Discontinue the most likely offending medication, provide pain control as necessary, and attend to fluids, electrolytes, and nutrition. Aggressive nutritional support should be started early; nasogastric feeding is preferred to parenteral nutrition.

B. Infection Control

Prophylactic antibiotics may promote the emergence of resistant strains of bacteria or candida and should be avoided. Obtain blood, urine, and skin cultures frequently and start empiric broad-spectrum antibiotics at the earliest sign of infection. Consider acyclovir in HIV-infected patients, since secondary herpes simplex virus infection may be clinically undetectable.

C. Skin and Mucous Membrane Care

Ophthalmologic consultation is essential to prevent blindness and other ocular sequelae. Oral hygiene and antisepsis are important. Intact bullae should be left in place, since they provide a natural dressing. Nonviable, necrotic, and loosely attached areas of epidermis should be debrided. Apply biologic dressings, such as porcine xenografts and cryopreserved cadaveric allografts, or synthetic coverings, such as hydrogel dressing or paraffin gauze, to denuded areas. Silver sulfadiazine must be avoided in patients suspected of sulfonamide sensitivity.

Current Controversies & Unresolved Issues

Toxic epidermal necrolysis has been considered by some to be at the most severe end of the spectrum of erythema multiforme and Stevens-Johnson syndrome, but the two disorders may instead be distinct reactional states with clinicopathologic similarities. Supporting the latter view is the observation that the three do not have the same etiologic spectrum.

Although corticosteroids have been used for decades, recent studies suggest that systemic steroid therapy is more detrimental than useful in toxic epidermal necrolysis. Claims for a reduction of morbidity and mortality in response to a large dose of systemic steroids in the first 24–48 hours have not been substantiated. Plasmapheresis, cyclophosphamide, and cyclosporine have likewise been claimed to be beneficial on the basis of case reports and uncontrolled studies, but again there is no proof.

Avakian R et al: Toxic epidermal necrolysis: A review. J Am Acad Dermatol 1991;25:69–79.

Birchall N et al: Toxic epidermal necrolysis: An approach to management using cryopreserved allograft skin. J Am Acad Dermatol 1987;16:368–72.

Parsons JM: Toxic epidermal necrolysis. Int J Dermatol 1992;31: 749–68.

Saiag P et al: Drug-induced toxic epidermal necrolysis (Lyell syndrome) in patients infected with the human immunodeficiency virus. J Am Acad Dermatol 1992;26:567–74.

Tong P, Mutasim DF: Toxic epidermal necrolysis in the elderly. J Geriatr Dermatol 1996;4:63–70.

PHENYTOIN HYPERSENSITIVITY SYNDROME

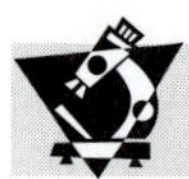

ESSENTIALS OF DIAGNOSIS

- *High spiking fever, malaise, and rash 2–3 weeks after starting phenytoin therapy—or sooner if prior exposure to drug.*
- *Patchy erythematous rash, evolving into extensive pruritic maculopapular rash, occasionally with follicular papules and pustules.*
- *Exfoliative erythroderma, erythema multiforme, Stevens-Johnson syndrome, or toxic epidermal necrolysis may develop, especially in those with prior adverse reactions to phenytoin. Edema of palms, soles, and face.*
- *Tender localized or generalized lymphadenopathy. Mild to severe hepatic injury. Sometimes conjunctivitis, pharyngitis, diarrhea, myositis, and reversible acute renal failure. Eosinophilia.*

General Considerations

A variety of adverse skin reactions, ranging from morbilliform eruptions to vasculitis, exfoliative erythroderma, erythema multiforme and Stevens-Johnson syndrome, and toxic epidermal necrolysis, occur in up to 3–15% of patients receiving phenytoin. In a small percentage of these patients, a distinctive syndrome occurs, characterized by an extensive rash, fever, eosinophilia, and hepatic injury. The disorder is believed to be immune-mediated. All age groups are affected. The incidence is highest in blacks.

Clinical Features

A. Symptoms and Signs

Onset is usually 2–3 weeks after initiation of therapy—or within days if prior exposure has occurred—heralded by high spiking fevers, malaise, and a rash. The cutaneous eruption is variable. It often begins as patchy erythema that evolves into an extensive pruritic maculopapular rash. Some patients have follicular papules and pustules. The rash may generalize into an exfoliative erythroderma. Erythema multiforme, Stevens-Johnson syndrome, and toxic epidermal necrolysis may occur, especially in patients with previous adverse reactions to the drug and in those who continue to receive the drug after developing signs of hypersensitivity. Erythema and edema of the palms and soles and prominent facial edema are common. The eruption usually resolves with desquamation.

Tender localized or generalized lymphadenopathy is a consistent finding. Virtually all patients with this syndrome have hepatic injury, which varies from mild and transient to severe and fulminant, resulting in massive hepatic necrosis. Hepatosplenomegaly is found in most patients. Other features of the syndrome, not uniformly present, are conjunctivitis, pharyngitis, diarrhea, myositis, and reversible acute renal failure. In general, the signs and symptoms resolve rapidly once the medication is discontinued; however, multiorgan abnormalities may progress even after the phenytoin has been stopped. Some patients endure a prolonged and complicated course of exacerbations and remissions. The mortality rate approaches 20% in patients with severe liver damage.

B. Laboratory Findings

Laboratory studies are important for monitoring the severity and progression of the reaction. Leukocytosis with eosinophilia (5–50%) is common. Coombs-negative hemolytic anemia and atypical circulating lymphocytes may be seen. The degree of elevation in serum aminotransferases and alkaline phosphatase levels reflects the severity of liver injury, and renal function may be abnormal. It is of note that the erythrocyte sedimentation rate and serum complement levels are normal in this disorder.

Differential Diagnosis

Other anticonvulsant medications, particularly phenobarbital, may cause reactions indistinguishable from phenytoin hypersensitivity disorder. Infectious mononucleosis may resemble this syndrome.

Treatment

The medication must be discontinued. Data regarding cross-reactivity among the anticonvulsants is scanty, but if anticonvulsant therapy is still necessary, valproic acid or carbamazepine may be safe alternatives.

General supportive care is vital because of the multisystem involvement. Systemic corticosteroids are sometimes used, but their effectiveness has not been documented.

Silverman AK, Fairley J, Wong RC: Cutaneous and immunologic reactions to phenytoin. J Am Acad Dermatol 1988;18:721–41.

PURPURA

Purpura results from hemorrhage into the skin or mucous membranes. Incomplete blanching on pressure is characteristic. Purpuric lesions may be a clue to acutely life-threatening diseases but are seen in benign conditions as well. An important step in evaluating the patient with purpura is to determine whether the lesions are macular (flat) or palpable. **Nonpalpable purpura,** the result of bleeding into the skin without inflammation, is due to disorders of hemostasis and vessel wall integrity. In these cases, small petechial hemorrhages (< 3 mm) occur. Common causative factors are thrombocytopenia or disorders of platelet function. Petechiae may also be a clue to diseases that affect the integrity of blood vessels, eg, scurvy or amyloidosis. In contrast, disorders of coagulation cause bleeding from larger vessels, producing ecchymoses (hemorrhagic macules larger than 3 mm). **Palpable purpura,** the expression of inflammatory damage to the vasculature and consequent extravasation of blood, is the hallmark of small vessel vasculitis but may also be seen with septic emboli.

Purpura occasionally develops as a secondary manifestation in an inflammatory dermatosis. For example, macular drug eruptions or exanthematous infectious diseases such as measles and scarlet fever can become purpuric as a result of increased permeability of the blood vessels and extravasation of red cells into the surrounding tissue. Causes of purpura are classified arbitrarily in Table 28–4. In this section, leukocytoclastic vasculitis, disseminated intravascular coagulation, and purpura fulminans are discussed.

LEUKOCYTOCLASTIC VASCULITIS

ESSENTIALS OF DIAGNOSIS

- *Palpable purpura. Hemorrhagic bullae, purpuric plaques, vesicles, pustules on a purpuric base, and urticaria-like papules may be present.*
- *Systemic symptoms occur in 40–50%, including fever, myalgias, and arthralgias. Abdominal pain, gastrointestinal bleeding, and pulmonary disease (pneumonitis, pleuritis, or hemoptysis) occur less frequently.*
- *Biopsy of involved skin shows necrotizing vasculitis with prominent neutrophilic infiltrates in and around the vessel walls, extravasated red blood cells, and deposition of fibrin.*

Table 28–4. Causes of purpura.

Vascular Disorders	Abnormal distribution
Inflammatory disorders	Diseases associated with splenomegaly
Palpable purpura	Kasabach-Merritt syndrome
Vasculitis	***Purpura with normal platelet counts***
Septic emboli	Platelet function defects
Nonpalpable purpura	Drugs (eg, salicylates, NSAIDs)
Viral infections	Uremia
Rickettsial infections	Coagulopathies
Drugs and chemicals	***Purpura with high platelet counts***
Pigmented purpuric dermatoses	Myeloproliferative syndromes
Noninflammatory disorders	Postsplenectomy
Trauma	Various neoplasms and inflammatory diseases
Amyloidosis	**Disorders of Coagulation**
Scurvy	***Acquired***
Dysproteinemic states	Vitamin K deficiency
Solar purpura	Disseminated intravascular coagulation
Abnormalities of Platelet Number and Function	Parenchymal liver disease
Thrombocytopenic purpuras	Cardiopulmonary bypass surgery
Increased platelet destruction	Lupus anticoagulant syndrome
Microangiopathic diseases	***Inherited***
Infections	Classic hemophilia
Immunologic disorders	von Willebrand's disease
Idiopathic thrombocytopenic purpura (ITP)	***Thrombotic disorders***
Drug-induced thrombocytopenia	Protein C and S deficiency
Autoimmune diseases (eg, SLE)	Antithrombin III deficiency
Decreased platelet production	Drugs (eg, aminocaproic acid, estrogen compounds)
Neoplastic replacement of bone marrow	Nephrotic syndrome
Myelosuppressive disorders	Anticoagulant necrosis
Radiation	
Chemotherapy	
Infections	

General Considerations

Vasculitis is defined as inflammation and subsequent necrosis of the vessel wall. Various clinical syndromes share vasculitis as a feature and may be classified according to the size and type of involved vessels (postcapillary venule, arteriole, vein, or artery), the type of inflammatory infiltrate (necrotizing or granulomatous), and the organs affected (Table 28–5). Some forms of vasculitis are confined to the skin, whereas others involve internal organs and may cause severe and potentially fatal disease. When the small vessels of the skin are involved, the most common finding is palpable purpura. Involvement of larger vessels produces subcutaneous nodules, stellate-shaped purpura, or necrosis.

Pathophysiology

Most of the vasculitic diseases are immunologically mediated and are probably due to immune complex deposition. The evidence for immune complex-mediated damage is most compelling for small vessel or "leukocytoclastic" vasculitis. The pathologic process involves the following sequence of events: deposition of circulating soluble antigen-antibody complexes in postcapillary venule walls; activation of the complement cascade; chemotaxis of neutrophils to the sites of immune complex deposition; and release of lysosomal enzymes and other products from neutrophils resulting in necrosis of the vessel wall. Hemorrhage, thrombosis, and surrounding tissue necrosis follow. The inflammatory cell infiltrate and edema in and around the vessels cause the lesions to become palpable. In some situations, vasculitis may result from direct invasion of vessels by infectious agents. Cell-mediated immune damage may be involved in granulomatous vasculitis.

Clinical Features

A. Symptoms and Signs

As noted, the classic cutaneous finding in leukocytoclastic vasculitis is palpable purpura (though the palpability may be subtle). However, hemorrhagic bullae,

Table 28–5. Classification of vasculitis.

Leukocytoclastic (hypersensitivity) vasculitis
Systemic-cutaneous vasculitis
Variants of leukocytoclastic vasculitis
Urticarial (hypocomplementemic) vasculitis
Serum sickness
Henoch-Schönlein purpura
Rheumatic vasculitis
Systemic lupus erythematosus
Rheumatoid vasculitis
Sjögren's syndrome
Scleroderma and dermatomyositis
Polyarteritis nodosa
Cutaneous type
Systemic type
Granulomatous vasculitis
Churg-Strauss syndrome (allergic granulomatosis)
Wegener's granulomatosis
Giant cell arteritis
Temporal arteritis
Takayasu's arteritis
Miscellaneous
Degos' disease (malignant atrophic papulosis)
Kawasaki's disease
Lucio phenomenon

purpuric plaques, vesicles, pustules on a purpuric base, and urticaria-like papules may be present. Affected patients may also have ulcerative, infarcted, or reticulated lesions. The lesions arise in crops, predominantly on the lower extremities and in dependent areas. Edema of the lower legs is common. About 40–50% of patients with leukocytoclastic vasculitis have systemic symptoms. Fever, myalgias, and arthralgias may accompany the cutaneous manifestations. Kidney involvement may be transient, with hematuria or proteinuria, or may lead to glomerulonephritis or renal failure. Abdominal pain, gastrointestinal bleeding, and pulmonary disease (pneumonitis, pleuritis, or hemoptysis) occur less often. Peripheral neuropathies occur infrequently and portend a poor prognosis.

B. Laboratory Findings

The definitive diagnosis of cutaneous vasculitis depends on compatible cutaneous lesions plus histopathologic confirmation of blood vessel damage. Necrotizing vasculitis is characterized by a prominent neutrophilic infiltrate in and around the vessel wall, associated with nuclear fragments ("nuclear dust"), extravasated red blood cells, and deposition of fibrin. Furthermore, granulomatous vasculitis shows fibrinoid necrosis of the blood vessels associated with intravascular and extravascular granulomas.

Evaluation of lesions by direct immunofluorescence for the presence of immunoglobulins and complement may help confirm the diagnosis. However, negative results are common, and this test is often of little clinical value.

Once the diagnosis of cutaneous vasculitis is established, a comprehensive evaluation is necessary to determine the presence and extent of internal involvement and to identify potential underlying causes (Table 28–6). Some recommended screening studies include the following: complete blood count and erythrocyte sedimentation rate; chemistry profile; serum protein electrophoresis and cryoglobulin titer; hepatitis B and C screens; antinuclear antibody titer, anti-Ro titer, total hemolytic complement, and VDRL; urinalysis and stool occult blood; throat culture and antistreptolysin O titer; and chest x-ray. Depending on the clinical situation, other tests may include antineutrophilic cytoplasmic antibody titer, direct immunofluorescence, biopsy of affected organs, radiographic studies (including angiograms) of affected organs, and nerve conduction studies.

Table 28–6. Causes of vasculitis.

Drugs: See Table 28–2.
Chemical
Insecticides
Petroleum products
Weed killers
Foreign proteins
Heterologous serum
Snake antivenin
Hyposensitization antigens
Infections
Group A beta-hemolytic streptococci
Hepatitis B
Mycobacterial diseases
Influenza
Abnormal immunoglobulins
Multiple myeloma
Cryoglobulinemia
Macroglobulinemia
Rheumatic diseases
Rheumatoid arthritis
Systemic lupus erythematosus
Dermatomyositis
Sjögren's syndrome
Miscellaneous diseases
Ulcerative colitis
Lymphomas and leukemias
Malignant tumors
Idiopathic

Differential Diagnosis

Palpable purpura occurs in both vasculitis and septicemia. Certain clinical patterns favor the diagnosis of sepsis and sometimes can provide clues to the causative organism. The skin lesions associated with staphylococcal sepsis are acrally located, asymmetric, and fewer in number than those associated with vasculitis. The characteristic lesions of gonococcal bacteremia are discrete, tender pustules on a hemorrhagic base, often accompanied by polyarthralgias, tenosynovitis, or septic arthritis. The well-known skin findings in infective endocarditis are painful nodules on the volar surfaces of the fingers and toes (Osler's nodes), nontender hemorrhagic macules on the palms and soles (Janeway's lesions), and subungual splinter hemorrhages. Petechiae, ecchymoses, hemorrhagic vesicles and pustules, and ulcerated nodules may all be seen with sepsis. The diagnosis is confirmed by a positive blood culture or a positive culture or Gram stain from the skin lesions. Palpable purpura can also occur in nonseptic embolic disorders such as atheromatous emboli or left atrial myxoma.

Treatment

The therapy of vasculitis is based on the extent and severity of the disease. Any associated disease, infection, chemical, or drug should be treated or removed. For vasculitis limited to the skin, conservative therapy is appropriate since most cases are acute and self-limited. Bed rest, antihistamines, and nonsteroidal anti-inflammatory drugs may effectively suppress or control cutaneous lesions. For necrotic or highly symptomatic eruptions, colchicine, dapsone, or prednisone may be useful.

For systemic vasculitis, therapy with immunosuppressive and cytotoxic agents such as corticosteroids, azathioprine, cyclosporine, and methotrexate is usually necessary. Plasmapheresis may be tried in patients refractory to other therapeutic modalities. Monoclonal antibody therapy may be of value in the future.

Cutaneous ulcers or bullae are treated with debridement, tap water soaks, topical antibiotics, and vapor-permeable membranes.

Callen JP et al. Azathioprine: an effective corticosteroid-sparing therapy for patients with recalcitrant cutaneous lupus erythematosus or with recalcitrant cutaneous leukocytoclastic vasculitis. Arch Dermatol 1991; 127:515–22.

Callen JP: Cutaneous vasculitis: relationship to systemic disease and therapy. Curr Probl Dermatol 1993;5:50–80.

Conn DL: Update on systemic necrotizing vasculitis. Mayo Clinic Proc 1989;64:535–43.

Daoud MS et al: Chronic hepatitis C, cryoglobulinemia, and cutaneous necrotizing vasculitis. J Am Acad Dermatol 1996; 34:219–23.

Michel BA et al. Hypersensitivity vasculitis and Henoch-Schönlein purpura: a comparison between the two disorders. J Rheumatol 1992;19:721–8.

DISSEMINATED INTRAVASCULAR COAGULATION & PURPURA FULMINANS

ESSENTIALS OF DIAGNOSIS

- *Extensive skin necrosis, fever, and hypotension associated with evidence of disseminated intravascular coagulation.*
- *Sudden appearance of large, irregular areas of purpura, especially over the extremities.*
- *Skin lesions are tender, enlarge rapidly, and may evolve into hemorrhagic bullae with subsequent necrosis and black eschar formation. Necrosis of an entire extremity may develop.*
- *May be associated with pulmonary, hepatic, or renal failure, gastrointestinal bleeding, and hemorrhagic adrenal infarction.*

General Considerations

Disseminated intravascular coagulation (DIC) is a dynamic process associated with a variety of underlying diseases and is the result of uncontrolled activation of coagulation and fibrinolysis. Purpura fulminans is an acute, severe, often rapidly fatal syndrome characterized by extensive necrosis of the skin associated with fever and hypotension. Purpura fulminans represents the extreme end of the spectrum of DIC.

Pathophysiology

The central pathogenic events in DIC are excessive generation of thrombin and formation of intravascular fibrin clots, secondary activation of the fibrinolytic system, and consumption of platelets and coagulation factors. Abnormalities of the endogenous anticoagulants protein C and protein S may be directly related to the pathogenesis of purpura fulminans by contributing to the thrombotic tendency in patients with DIC. Neonates with homozygous protein C deficiency present with massive thrombosis of skin capillaries and veins, resulting in cutaneous necrosis, secondary sepsis, and death (purpura fulminans neonatalis). Acquired deficiencies of proteins C and S have been reported in liver disease and sepsis. Purpura fulminans occurs most commonly in children and often follows an infectious process such as scarlet fever or streptococcal pharyngitis, meningococcemia, varicella, rubeola, or Rocky Mountain spotted fever. Adults may be affected also, and the syndrome may occur without a preceding illness.

Clinical Features

A. Symptoms and Signs

Cutaneous findings of DIC may range from insignificant bruising and oozing from venipuncture sites to massive hemorrhage and necrosis of skin and vital organs.

Purpura fulminans is characterized by the sudden appearance of large, irregular areas of purpura, especially over the extremities. The lesions are tender, enlarge rapidly, and may evolve into hemorrhagic bullae with subsequent necrosis and black eschar formation. The trunk, ears, and nose may be involved. Necrosis of an entire extremity may develop. Fever, chills, and hypotension almost always accompany the disorder. Complications may include pulmonary, hepatic, and renal failure as well as gastrointestinal bleeding and hemorrhagic adrenal infarction (Waterhouse-Friderichsen syndrome). Mortality rates range from 20% to 40%. The differential diagnosis of purpura fulminans encompasses the entire spectrum of purpuric conditions.

B. Laboratory Findings

Because of the dynamic balance between intravascular clot deposition and dissolution, serial laboratory studies may be required to diagnose and monitor DIC. The blood count usually shows thrombocytopenia, and anemia may result from bleeding or microangiopathic hemolysis. Consumption of coagulation factors and fibrinogen cause prolongation of the prothrombin time and partial thromboplastin time. There is hypofibrinogenemia, and increased fibrin degradation products (fibrin split products) are present. More specific tests, such as measurement of the D-dimer fragment, a breakdown product of cross-linked fibrin, may be helpful.

Treatment

Immediate attention must be directed toward stabilizing the patient and treating the underlying cause. Heparin may prevent further clot formation but should be avoided in patients with suspected or documented intracranial bleeding. Surgical debridement of necrotic eschars, grafting, and even amputation are sometimes necessary.

Levi M et al. Pathogenesis of disseminated intravascular coagulation in sepsis. JAMA 1993;270:975–9.

Levin M et al: Postinfectious purpura fulminans caused by an antibody directed against protein S. J Pediatr 1995;127:355–63.

Moake JL: Hypercoagulable states: New knowledge about old problems. Hosp Pract (Off Ed) 1991;26:31–42.

LIFE-THREATENING DERMATOSES

PEMPHIGUS VULGARIS

ESSENTIALS OF DIAGNOSIS

- *Flaccid, easily ruptured blisters on noninflamed skin. After rupture, nonhealing crusted erosions remain.*
- *Superficial detachment of the skin after pressure or trauma variably present (Nikolsky's sign).*
- *Skin biopsy shows characteristic intraepidermal cleft just above the basal cell layer, with separation of keratinocytes from one another (acantholysis).*
- *Direct immunofluorescence of normal-appearing skin shows intercellular IgG and complement throughout the epithelium.*

General Considerations

Pemphigus vulgaris is a rare life-threatening autoimmune disease characterized by intraepithelial vesicles and bullae. Stratified squamous epithelium of both skin and mucosal surfaces is involved. The pathogenic process involves circulating IgG autoantibodies directed against the intercellular substance of the epidermis. The mean age at onset is the sixth decade.

Clinical Features

A. Symptoms and Signs

Nonhealing oropharyngeal erosions are common and often precede the skin findings by weeks or months. The primary cutaneous lesion is a flaccid blister on noninflamed skin. These blisters rupture easily, leaving nonhealing erosions that ultimately develop crusts. A positive Nikolsky sign (tractional pressure adjacent to a lesion causes skin separation) is characteristic but not pathognomonic. With treatment, the lesions generally heal without scarring. The sites of predilection are the scalp, face, axillae, and oral cavity. The conjunctival, vaginal, and esophageal mucosa and the vermilion border of the lips may also be involved. The process may become generalized. Oropharyngeal involvement causes difficulty in swallowing, and laryngeal involvement produces hoarseness.

Prior to the availability of corticosteroids, the mortality rate of pemphigus approached 60–90%, due primarily to protein, fluid, and electrolyte losses or to sepsis. More recently, the mortality rate has dropped to the range of 5–15%; the most common causes of death today are infection and complications of treatment.

B. Laboratory Findings

The diagnosis is based on pathologic findings, including skin biopsy showing a characteristic intraepidermal cleft just above the basal cell layer, with separation of keratinocytes from one another (acantholysis). The acantholytic cells line the vesicle and also lie free within the cavity. A Tzanck smear from the base of a bulla may show acantholytic epidermal cells. Direct immunofluorescence of normal-appearing skin near a lesion shows intercellular IgG and complement throughout the epithelium. Indirect immunofluorescence of the patient's serum demonstrates circulating intercellular autoantibodies in about 80–90% of patients. However, titers of the circulating autoantibodies do not correlate with disease severity but often parallel disease activity.

Fluid, electrolyte, and nutritional disturbances may occur but are less pronounced than in disorders involving loss of the entire thickness of the epidermis (eg, toxic epidermal necrolysis).

Differential Diagnosis

Histopathologic examination, immunofluorescent microscopy, and bacterial cultures permit differentiation from erythema multiforme, Stevens-Johnson syndrome, toxic epidermal necrolysis, bullous drug eruptions, and bullous impetigo, as well as from other primary blistering diseases such as bullous pemphigoid and dermatitis herpetiformis.

Treatment

Discontinue drugs known to cause pemphigus (eg, penicillamine and captopril).

A. Specific Treatment

Prednisone, 60–120 mg/d, in combination with azathioprine, 100–150 mg/d, is usually effective. Prior to initiation of therapy, the patient should be evaluated for contraindications to systemic steroids. Patients with a history of tuberculosis or a positive skin test for tuberculosis need concomitant isoniazid while receiving immunosuppressive therapy. When control of the blistering is achieved, prednisone is gradually reduced as tolerated. Methotrexate, cyclophosphamide, mycophenolate mofetil, cyclosporine, gold, and plasmapheresis are alternative modalities, as is pulse corticosteroid therapy.

B. Topical Therapy

Silver sulfadiazine or mupirocin ointment may reduce secondary infection. Whirlpool treatments are helpful in removing crusts from lesions. Oral mucosal erosions may benefit from topical steroids, antiseptics, viscous lidocaine, and attention to oral hygiene.

Becker BA, Gaspari AA: Pemphigus vulgaris and vegetans. Dermatol Clin 1993;11:429–52.

Udey MC, Stanley JR: Pemphigus—diseases of antidesmosomal autoimmunity. JAMA 1999;282:572–6.

GENERALIZED PUSTULAR PSORIASIS

ESSENTIALS OF DIAGNOSIS

- *Acute onset of widespread sterile pustules arising on tender, warm, erythematous skin that coalesce into lakes of pus. The tongue and mouth are commonly involved.*
- *Recurrent waves of pustulation and remissions occur. Fever and leukocytosis are often present. Bacterial infections and sepsis may be complications.*
- *Arthritis and pericholangitis are sometimes present. Rarely, there is associated hypotension, high-output heart failure, and renal failure. A history of psoriasis may or may not be present.*
- *Characteristic subcorneal pustules are seen on histologic examination.*

General Considerations

In addition to the exfoliative erythrodermic form of psoriasis, another serious and sometimes fatal type is generalized pustular psoriasis. It is characterized by the acute onset of widespread erythematous areas studded with many sterile pustules and associated with fever, chills, and leukocytosis. The disease may develop either de novo or in individuals with a history of psoriasis. The exact pathogenesis is unclear; however, precipitating events include topical and systemic corticosteroid therapy and their subsequent withdrawal, other medications (eg, sulfonamide drugs, penicillin, lithium, and pyrazolones), infections, pregnancy, and hypocalcemia. Pustular psoriasis tends to occur in patients over 40 years of age.

Clinical Features

A. Symptoms and Signs

The primary lesions are sterile pustules that arise on tender, warm, erythematous skin and coalesce into lakes of pus. Lesions typical of psoriasis vulgaris may coexist. The tongue and mouth are commonly involved, with geographic tongue and superficial erosions. These patients appear ill and complain of itching and burning. The course is punctuated by recurrent waves of pustulation and remissions. Arthritis and pericholangitis sometimes occur. Circulatory shunting through the skin may lead to significant edema and, rarely, hypotension, high-output heart failure, and renal failure. Superimposed bacterial infections or sepsis can complicate the clinical picture.

B. Laboratory Findings

Laboratory data are nonspecific but may be helpful. Leukocytosis, hypoalbuminemia, and hypocalcemia are often seen during flares of this disorder, though Gram stains and bacterial cultures of lesions are negative. HIV serology should be checked, since severe exacerbations of psoriasis can be seen in HIV-infected individuals.

Histologic examination of a lesion shows a characteristic subcorneal pustule.

Differential Diagnosis

The diagnosis of pustular psoriasis is generally clear-cut on clinical and histologic grounds. Other diagnostic considerations include miliaria rubra, acneiform secondary syphilis, pustular drug eruptions, and folliculitis. Cellulitis may be suggested by the marked edema and erythema of the legs.

Treatment

A. Specific Treatment

The drugs of choice in this severe form of psoriasis are the retinoids, acitretin and isotretinoin. These drugs should not be used in patients with lipid abnormalities or active hepatitis, and effective contraception must be assured during and for at least 3 years after treatment in women of child-bearing potential. Most patients show significant improvement in 5–7 days. Methotrexate and cyclosporine are alternatives in carefully selected cases; methotrexate is absolutely contraindicated in HIV-infected patients. Systemic steroids are best avoided.

B. General Measures

A medium-potency topical steroid applied twice daily to affected areas, emollient creams, cool compresses, and baths alleviate discomfort. Attention must be paid to fluid and electrolyte imbalances. The patient should be monitored for secondary infection and sepsis.

Feldman SR, Clark AR: Psoriasis. Med Clin North Am 1998;82: 1135–44.

EXFOLIATIVE ERYTHRODERMA

ESSENTIALS OF DIAGNOSIS

- *Generalized or nearly generalized diffuse erythema with desquamation.*
- *Pruritus, malaise, fever, chills, and weight loss may be present.*
- *There may be a history of primary dermatologic disease, or the erythroderma may be a sign of malignancy (T cell lymphoma). The cause in many cases remains undetermined.*

General Considerations

Exfoliative erythroderma is a clinical syndrome characterized by generalized or nearly total diffuse erythema of the skin accompanied by variable degrees of desquamation. Exfoliative erythroderma is a nonspecific end point of skin reactivity; multiple conditions can lead to it (Table 28–7). Approximately half of all cases are due to exacerbation of a primary dermatologic condition. Underlying skin diseases such as psoriasis and various forms of eczema may become generalized through neglect, the abrupt discontinuation of therapy, or intercurrent cutaneous or systemic infection (eg, HIV-infected individuals are at risk of development of erythrodermic psoriasis). Less commonly, exfoliative erythroderma is the initial manifestation of a dermatosis. The remaining cases are nearly equally divided among undetermined causes, drug reactions, and underlying malignancies, most commonly cutaneous T cell lymphoma.

Clinical Features

A. History

A careful history with attention to preexisting dermatoses, family history of skin conditions, medication history, and clues to occult malignancy may suggest a specific cause.

Table 28–7. Causes of exfoliative erythroderma.

Underlying dermatosis
Eczematous conditions
Contact dermatitis
Atopic dermatitis
Seborrheic dermatitis
Psoriasis
Pityriasis rubra pilaris
Pemphigus foliaceus
Norwegian scabies
Others
Drugs: See Table 28–2.
Malignancies
Cutaneous T cell lymphoma
Hodgkin's disease
Miscellaneous lymphomas and leukemias
Idiopathic

B. Symptoms and Signs

Most patients complain of pruritus. The entire skin surface is red, scaly, and indurated. Excoriations, peripheral edema, and moderate symmetric lymph node enlargement are common; massive or asymmetric lymphadenopathy and splenomegaly are suggestive of an underlying lymphoma. The mucous membranes usually are spared. There may be symptoms of orthostatic hypotension due to increased insensible water loss. Congestive heart failure due to marked circulatory shunting through the skin may develop in patients with preexisting cardiac disease.

Thermoregulatory dysfunction can result in relative hypothermia and chills, thereby concealing the fever of sepsis. Nevertheless, patients with erythroderma due to drugs or lymphoma—or patients with secondary infections—often present with fever. Secondary bacterial infection manifests as purulent exudate or crusting. Sepsis, pneumonia, and complications of malignancy are the leading causes of death.

C. Laboratory Findings

Laboratory studies are usually of limited value in establishing the underlying cause but are necessary for assessing response to the skin disease. Leukocytosis and anemia are common, while eosinophilia suggests a drug offender. Atypical circulating lymphocytes (Sézary cells) if present in sufficiently high numbers, suggest Sézary's syndrome, the leukemic phase of cutaneous T cell lymphoma. Hypoalbuminemia and negative nitrogen balance result from protein loss by desquamation and an elevated metabolic rate. Serologic testing for HIV is recommended for patients with erythrodermic psoriasis.

Other tests should include urinalysis and stool occult blood, chest x-ray, and ECG. Skin biopsy results are usually nonspecific but may be diagnostic in leukemia, cutaneous T cell lymphoma, or Norwegian crusted scabies. Routine biopsy of superficial lymph nodes is even less helpful, since the pathologic findings are usually reactive (dermatopathic lymphadenopathy). However, biopsy of unusually prominent or asymmetric lymph nodes may yield a diagnosis of lymphoreticular malignancy.

Differential Diagnosis

Exfoliative erythroderma should be differentiated from other conditions associated with diffuse erythema such as common morbilliform drug eruptions, various viral and bacterial exanthems, early phases of toxic epidermal necrolysis, toxic shock syndrome, and graft-versus-host disease.

Treatment

Irrespective of the underlying cause, all exfoliative erythrodermas may be treated initially in a similar manner. The goals of therapy are relief of symptoms and reduction of cutaneous inflammation.

A. Specific Treatment

Once the cause is established, specific treatment may be initiated. Systemic steroids should be avoided unless indicated as specific therapy for the underlying disease.

B. General Measures

Patients must be monitored closely for complications of erythroderma, including anemia, electrolyte imbalances, high-output heart failure, hypothermia, pneumonia, and sepsis. Administer systemic antibiotics to patients with cutaneous or systemic infection. Adequate nutrition is essential. One should stop any potentially offending medications and keep the patient warm. Daily whirlpool treatments aid in removing scale and decreasing bacterial colonization. Baths and wet compresses may also be used. After each whirlpool treatment, apply a medium-potency topical steroid such as fluocinolone acetonide 0.025% ointment. Antihistamines are helpful in controlling pruritus.

Inspect the skin regularly for morphologic changes that may be diagnostic of an underlying dermatitis as the erythroderma subsides.

Sigurdsson V et al: Erythroderma: a clinical and follow-up study of 102 patients, with special emphasis on survival. J Am Acad Dermatol 1996;35:53–7.

CUTANEOUS MANIFESTATIONS OF INFECTION

The febrile patient with a rash often presents a clinical dilemma in that both noninfectious and infectious causes must be considered. Among the noninfectious causes already discussed are drug eruptions, vasculitis, and exfoliative erythroderma. In addition, systemic lupus erythematosus, juvenile rheumatoid arthritis, and Kawasaki's disease may be manifested as eruptions associated with fever.

Systemic viral, bacterial, rickettsial, and fungal diseases may involve the skin, producing a multiplicity of cutaneous reactions which, in general, are not pathognomonic either for infection or for a specific organism. The following discussion focuses on life-threatening infections with sufficiently distinctive skin findings to facilitate early diagnosis. Cutaneous manifestations of sepsis were addressed earlier.

VARICELLA-ZOSTER

ESSENTIALS OF DIAGNOSIS

Primary infection—Varicella:

- *After a prodromal period of 1–3 days, small erythematous macules appear and evolve into clear vesicles. Pruritus is intense. New crops appear at 3- to 5-day intervals.*
- *Vesicles form crusted erosions. Oropharyngeal vesicles rupture quickly to form superficial mucosal ulcers.*
- *In normal adults as well as immunosuppressed individuals, varicella may be complicated by life-threatening pneumonia, hepatitis, myocarditis, encephalitis, and disseminated intravascular coagulation.*

Reactivation infection—Herpes zoster:

- *Acute, usually painful unilateral eruption in dermatomal distribution, with clusters of vesicles occurring on a background of erythema. In persons with compromised immune systems, the lesions may become severe and necrotic.*

General Considerations

Varicella-zoster virus (VZV) is a herpesvirus that typically causes a self-limited infection but is capable of producing life-threatening illness. Primary infection produces varicella; reactivation of latent virus in sensory ganglia results in herpes zoster (shingles). Varicella is spread by direct person-to-person contact or inhalation of infected droplets. Contact with the lesions of herpes zoster may produce varicella in a person not previously infected with VZV.

Clinical Features

A. Symptoms and Signs

After primary exposure to VZV, the incubation period ranges from 11 days to 21 days but may be shorter in immunocompromised persons. The prodromal symptoms in children are minimal and consist of low-grade fever and malaise. In adults, the symptoms are more severe and include prolonged fever, malaise, and arthralgias. One to a few days after onset of illness, small erythematous macules appear on the trunk, face, and proximal extremities. The primary lesion evolves rapidly into a clear vesicle which, if left undisturbed, becomes cloudy. The vesicles eventually rupture to form crusted erosions. New crops appear at irregular intervals over the next 3–5 days, giving the characteristic finding of lesions in various stages of development. Pruritus is often intense. Healing with scarring is not uncommon, particularly in excoriated or secondarily infected lesions. Oropharyngeal vesicles rupture quickly to form superficial mucosal ulcers. In normal adults as well as immunosuppressed individuals, varicella may be especially severe and complicated by life-threatening pneumonia. Hepatitis, myocarditis, encephalitis, and disseminated intravascular coagulation may also occur along with extensive hemorrhagic skin lesions.

In the normal host, herpes zoster is an acute self-limited, usually painful unilateral eruption in a dermatomal distribution. Characteristically, clusters of vesicles occur on a background of erythema. Occasionally—especially in persons with compromised immune systems—herpes zoster may become severe and necrotic. Wide dissemination of multiple small varicella-like vesicles may develop. In such patients, secondary bacterial infection is an added risk.

B. Laboratory Findings

A Tzanck smear demonstrates diagnostic multinucleated epithelial giant cells. This test is performed by scraping the base of a vesicular lesion with a scalpel blade, transferring the material to a glass slide, and staining with Giemsa's or Wright's stain. The Tzanck smear is also positive in herpes simplex infections. Culture of a lesion may confirm the diagnosis but requires approximately 10 days of growth. An immunofluorescent antibody test, utilizing materials from a lesion, is also available.

Differential Diagnosis

Varicella may be confused with widespread impetigo, disseminated herpes zoster, disseminated herpes simplex, and eczema herpeticum. Eczema herpeticum is a widespread cutaneous infection with herpes simplex virus occurring in patients with preexisting skin disorders such as atopic dermatitis.

Treatment

Systemic acyclovir in the doses listed is recommended in the following situations: (1) All VZV infections in immunocompromised individuals (10 mg/kg intravenously every 8 hours for 7–10 days). (2) Varicella in teenage and adult patients (800 mg orally five times a day for 5–7 days). (3) Elderly patients and patients with severe, painful, or destructive zoster when seen within 48–72 hours after onset (800 mg orally five times a day for 7 days). Alternative drugs for acute herpes zoster are famciclovir, 500 mg three time daily for 7 days; or valacyclovir, 1 g three times daily for 7 days.

Secondary bacterial infection should be treated aggressively. Cool compresses and antihistamines may help remove crusts and alleviate pruritus. Analgesics should be provided as necessary.

Drugs for viral infections. Med Lett Drugs Ther 1994;36:27–32.

Glesby MJ, Oobre RD, Chaisson RE: Clinical spectrum of herpes zoster in adults infected with human immunodeficiency virus. Clin Infect Dis 1995;21:370–375.

RUBEOLA (MEASLES)

ESSENTIALS OF DIAGNOSIS

- *Incubation period of 7–14 days, followed by high fever, malaise, cough, coryza, and conjunctivitis with photophobia.*
- *Three to 5 days later, discrete erythematous macules and thin papules appear on the forehead and behind the ears, spreading to the trunk and extremities, with coalescence and increased redness.*
- *Koplik's spots usually appear on buccal mucosa 1–2 days before exanthem.*
- *Complications include secondary bacterial infection, otitis media, pneumonia, viral myocarditis, liver function abnormalities, and thrombocytopenia.*

General Considerations

Rubeola is an acute epidemic disease characterized by marked upper respiratory symptoms and a widespread erythematous maculopapular rash. It is caused by a paramyxovirus transmitted by inhalation of infected droplets. The severity of the illness varies with the age and immunologic status of the patient.

Clinical Features

A. Symptoms and Signs

After an incubation period of 7–14 days, a prodrome of high fever develops, associated with malaise, cough, coryza, and conjunctivitis with photophobia. In 3–5 days, discrete erythematous macules and thin papules appear on the forehead and behind the ears. Over the next few days, the lesions spread to the trunk and extremities (including the palms and soles), coalesce on the face and upper trunk, and intensify in color to a deeper red. The eruption fades after 5–10 days in the order of its appearance, often with fine desquamation and postinflammatory hyperpigmentation. Koplik's spots—blue-white pinpoint macules with a red halo—usually appear on the buccal mucosa 1–2 days before the exanthem and remain for several days. Up to 40% of immunocompromised patients with measles have no rash; the remainder have either typical or unusual skin findings, including urticarial plaques, petechiae, and palpable purpura. Rubeola must be distinguished from cutaneous drug reactions as well as other viral exanthems.

Complications may arise from viral dissemination, secondary bacterial infection, or hypersensitivity phenomena. Otitis media, sinusitis, pneumonia, and liver function abnormalities are common. Viral myocarditis and thrombocytopenic purpura (due to immune-mediated platelet destruction) may occur. Death, resulting from pneumonitis or encephalitis, occurs in about 0.1% of cases in the United States. The complication and case fatality rate for the very young, the elderly, the malnourished, and patients with malignancies or HIV infection is significantly higher. The clinical presentation in immunocompromised patients is frequently atypical. One-third of such patients present with no rash.

B. Laboratory Findings

Serologic studies of paired specimens are the most practical method of confirming the diagnosis. Measles virus may be isolated from the blood, urine, nasopharyngeal washings, and throat or from conjunctival secretions.

Treatment

Therapy is supportive, since no proven antiviral agent is available. Aerosolized ribavirin may be beneficial for the treatment of measles pneumonitis, but its effectiveness has not yet been proved. Intravenous immunoglobulin and interferon are other treatment options for measles pneumonitis and encephalitis. Isolation precautions must be observed.

Kaplan LJ et al: Severe measles in immunocompromised patients. JAMA 1992;267:1237–41.

MENINGOCOCCEMIA

ESSENTIALS OF DIAGNOSIS

- *Petechial (or, less commonly, urticarial or morbilliform) rash on the trunk and lower extremities; also on the palms, soles, and mucous membranes. Petechiae are frequently palpable, with gun-metal gray centers and irregular borders.*
- *If complicated by purpura fulminans, extensive hemorrhagic bullae and areas of necrosis.*
- *Other features of meningococcal meningitis or disseminated meningococcemia, including meningeal signs, arthritis, myocarditis, pericarditis, and acute adrenal infarction. Hypotension and shock are often present.*
- *Confirmation of* Neisseria meningitidis *by culture, Gram stain, or immunologic tests.*

General Considerations

Neisseria meningitidis is a gram-negative diplococcus responsible for a spectrum of illnesses ranging from a mild upper respiratory infection to fulminant septicemia. Disease occurs most often in children under 15, with the attack rate highest in infants 6–12 months of age. Peak incidence of infection is in the winter and spring. Asymptomatic colonization of the nasopharynx is common and provides a source of person-to-person transmission through infected droplets. People with deficiencies of the terminal components of the complement cascade (C5–9) are particularly susceptible to invasive and recurrent meningococcal disease. The cutaneous lesions are a consequence of damage to small dermal blood vessels both by direct bacterial involvement of skin vessels and by lipopolysaccharide endotoxins.

Clinical Features

A. Symptoms and Signs

Invasive meningococcal disease usually results in meningitis or meningococcemia. The incubation period varies from 2 days to 10 days. The onset may be insidious, following a flu-like illness; or abrupt, with fever, chills, malaise, signs of meningeal irritation, prostration, and shock. A rash that is characteristically petechial or, less commonly, urticarial or morbilliform is often among the earliest signs of generalized infection. The petechiae typically appear on the trunk and lower extremities but can also be found on the palms, soles, and mucous membranes. They are frequently palpable, with gun-metal gray centers and irregular borders.

Extensive hemorrhagic bullae and areas of necrosis develop in patients with meningococcemia whose disease is complicated by purpura fulminans. Obtundation, hypotension, and death may ensue within hours despite appropriate antimicrobial therapy. Absence of meningeal signs is a feature of this acute fulminant form of meningococcal disease. Children under age 2 have the highest mortality rate, perhaps as a consequence of immaturity of the protein C system.

Other complications of invasive meningococcal disease are arthritis, myocarditis, pericarditis, cervicitis, and Waterhouse-Friderichsen syndrome. More rare meningococcal diseases include occult bacteremia and chronic meningococcemia.

B. Laboratory Findings

Confirmation of the diagnosis depends on demonstration of the organism. This may be by culture, Gram stain, or immunologic tests. Blood and cerebrospinal fluid cultures are indicated in all patients suspected of having invasive disease. Nasopharyngeal and synovial cultures are positive in some cases. Counterimmunoelectrophoresis or latex agglutination with group-specific antisera of cerebrospinal fluid, urine, or tears can facilitate rapid diagnosis. A Gram stain of material from purpuric lesions may reveal the organism. Other laboratory studies are otherwise nonspecific but should be performed as indicated to assess and monitor the illness, including evaluation for disseminated intravascular coagulation.

Differential Diagnosis

Meningococcal infection must be considered in patients with the combination of fever and a petechial rash, especially in association with meningitis. Depending on the clinical presentation, other infections, such as gram-negative septicemia, Rocky Mountain spotted fever, echovirus and coxsackievirus infections, and atypical measles, must be excluded. Vasculitis and other causes of purpura also are diagnostic possibilities.

Treatment

Intravenous penicillin G or ampicillin is the therapy of choice. Ceftriaxone is an acceptable alternative. (See

Chapter 15.) Hemodynamic and other supportive measures must be provided as necessary to maintain organ system function. Respiratory isolation is mandatory. Close contacts of patients with meningococcal disease should be given rifampin prophylaxis and closely monitored.

Marzouk O et al: Features and outcome in meningococcal disease presenting with maculopapular rash. Arch Dis Child 1991;66:485–7.

ROCKY MOUNTAIN SPOTTED FEVER

ESSENTIALS OF DIAGNOSIS

- *Potential exposure to ticks in endemic area.*
- *After incubation period of 1–14 days, sudden onset of fever, headache, myalgia, and nausea or vomiting.*
- *Appearance on days 2–4 of blanchable pinkish red macular rash over ankles, wrists, and forearms, spreading to involve the soles, palms, extremities, trunk, and face within hours. Bilaterally symmetric petechiae of the palms and soles are a major finding.*
- *May be complicated by central nervous system, cardiac, pulmonary, renal, or other organ involvement. Disseminated intravascular coagulation and shock leading to death may occur.*
- *Diagnosis can be confirmed by serologic tests, but these are not reliable before the second week of illness.*

General Considerations

Rocky Mountain spotted fever is an acute systemic illness characterized by fever and a purpuric eruption. The disease is transmitted to humans by the bite of a tick infected with the causative organism, *Rickettsia rickettsii.* Transmission reflects the tick season in a particular geographic area, with highest incidence in spring and summer. The disease is widespread in the United States and Canada; most cases are from the southeastern and the Rocky Mountain states. All age groups are affected, but most are between 5 and 9 years old.

Clinical Features

The incubation period is usually about 1 week, ranging from 1–14 days.

A. Symptoms and Signs

Sudden onset of fever, headache, myalgia, and nausea or vomiting are initial features. On the second to fourth days of illness, a blanchable pinkish red macular rash appears over the ankles, wrists, and forearms, spreading to involve the soles, palms, extremities, trunk, and face within hours. Over the next 1–2 days the eruption becomes papular and nonblanchable (purpuric) and may evolve into gangrene of the digits, nose, earlobes, scrotum, or vulva. Bilaterally symmetric petechiae of the palms and soles is a major finding. The illness can persist up to 3 weeks and may be complicated by central nervous system, cardiac, pulmonary, renal, or other organ involvement. Disseminated intravascular coagulation and shock leading to death may occur.

B. Laboratory Findings

The diagnosis of Rocky Mountain spotted fever can be established retrospectively by one of many serologic techniques, including complement fixation, latex agglutination, or microagglutination tests. However, these tests are not reliably positive before the second week of the illness.

Skin biopsy reveals a necrotizing vasculitis. A Giemsa-stained smear of tissue sections may occasionally demonstrate the organism. Immunofluorescent microscopic examination of skin biopsy specimens may confirm the diagnosis as early as the fourth day of illness.

Differential Diagnosis

Rocky Mountain spotted fever must be differentiated from other serious febrile illnesses such as viral and bacterial meningitis, meningococcemia, measles, vasculitis, and thrombotic thrombocytopenic purpura.

Treatment

Treatment should be initiated as soon as the diagnosis is suspected. Chloramphenicol and tetracycline are the agents of choice. Gangrene of the earlobes, digits, nose, etc, requires additional antibiotics if secondarily infected.

Weber DJ, Walker DH: Rocky mountain spotted fever. Infect Dis Clin North Am 1991;5:19–35.

NECROTIZING FASCIITIS

ESSENTIALS OF DIAGNOSIS

- *Typically occurs following surgery or penetrating trauma; diabetes may be a predisposing condition.*

- *Erythema, edema, and pain develop 1–2 days following surgery or trauma with central areas of dusky gray-blue discoloration, occasionally in association with serosanguineous blisters.*
- *Involved areas become gangrenous within a few days; culture frequently grows multiple aerobic and anaerobic bacteria.*
- *Severe systemic toxicity is usually present.*

General Considerations

Necrotizing fasciitis is a rare, life-threatening soft tissue infection characterized by acute and widespread fascial necrosis. It typically occurs following surgery or penetrating trauma. Diabetes may be a predisposing condition. The pathogenesis involves the introduction of organisms into the subcutis with subsequent spread through fascial planes. Many different virulent bacteria have been isolated in association with necrotizing fasciitis, including beta-hemolytic streptococci, staphylococci, coliforms, enterococci, pseudomonas, and bacteroides. Rhizopus and *Candida albicans* have been cultured from tissue. The process is often fatal unless diagnosed quickly and treated aggressively.

Clinical Features

A. Symptoms and Signs

Erythema, edema, and pain develop 1–2 days following introduction of the organism into the subcutis. The infection spreads rapidly and deeply, resulting in local tissue ischemia. Clinically, there are central areas of dusky gray-blue discoloration, occasionally in association with serosanguineous blisters. Crepitus is usually absent in necrotizing fasciitis. Within a few days these areas become gangrenous; liberation of toxins and organisms into the bloodstream leads to severe systemic toxicity. The extremities are the most commonly affected site, but the trunk, perineum, and abdomen may also be affected. **Fournier's gangrene** is necrotizing fasciitis of the perineum, scrotum, or penis that spreads rapidly to the anterior abdominal wall. Necrotizing fasciitis may be confused with cellulitis, angioedema, eosinophilic fasciitis, and clostridial myonecrosis.

B. Laboratory Findings

Incisional biopsy of both the advancing edge and the involved tissue should be performed early, looking for necrotic fascia and the causative organism. Tissue cultures frequently grow multiple aerobic and anaerobic bacteria as well as fungi. Radiographs of soft tissue may rarely reveal tissue gas.

Treatment

Radical surgical debridement, intravenous broad-spectrum antibiotics, and general supportive care are the mainstays of therapy. The major indication for operative treatment is fasciitis spreading in spite of empiric antibiotics in an acutely ill patient.

Stamenkovic I, Lew PD: Early recognition of potentially fatal necrotizing fasciitis: The use of frozen-section biopsy. N Engl J Med 1984;310:1689–93.

Ward RG, Walsh MS: Necrotizing fasciitis: 10 year's experience in a district general hospital. Br J Surg 1991;78:488–9.

TOXIC SHOCK SYNDROME (TSS)

ESSENTIALS OF DIAGNOSIS

- *Highest incidence in menstruating women, persons with focal staphylococcal infection or colonization, and women using a diaphragm or contraceptive sponge—but may occur in others.*
- *Rapid onset of fever, vomiting, watery diarrhea, sore throat, and profound myalgias, with hypotension.*
- *Diffuse, blanching erythema appears early, predominantly truncal, with accentuation in the axillary and inguinal folds and spreading to the extremities. Desquamation of the involved skin and of the palms and soles is seen during the second or third week.*
- *Acute renal failure, acute respiratory distress syndrome, refractory shock, ventricular arrhythmias, and disseminated intravascular coagulation may occur.*

General Considerations

Toxic shock syndrome is a multisystem illness characterized by the acute onset of high fever associated with myalgias, vomiting, diarrhea, headache, pharyngitis, and hypotension. Mucocutaneous findings are prominent. Staphylococcal pyogenic toxin superantigens (TSST-1) and enterotoxins B and C are involved in the pathogenesis. Streptococcal toxic shock syndrome is caused mainly by toxin-producing group A strains but also by strains of groups B, C, F, and G. In the 1980s, most cases occurred in menstruating women using superabsorbent tampons. Currently, most cases are caused by nonmenstrual *S aureus* infection—postsurgical, influenza-associated, or recalcitrant erythematous desquamating syndrome—or by colonization of contraceptive diaphragms or sponges. Streptococcal toxic shock syndrome may or may not be associated with necrotizing fasciitis or myositis.

Clinical Features

The CDC case definition of toxic shock syndrome is based on six major criteria: high fever, rash, desquamation, hypotension, involvement of three or more organ systems (gastrointestinal, muscular, mucous membrane, renal, hepatic, hematologic, and central nervous system), and exclusion of other causes.

A. Symptoms and Signs

Patients usually present with rapid onset of fever, vomiting, watery diarrhea, sore throat, and profound myalgias. Significant hypotension develops during the first 48–72 hours of illness. Multisystem organ involvement probably results both from poor tissue perfusion and from toxin-induced damage. Potentially devastating complications include acute renal failure, acute respiratory distress syndrome with pulmonary edema, refractory shock, ventricular arrhythmia, and disseminated intravascular coagulation. Some patients have relatively mild episodes.

The cutaneous and mucous membrane findings are prominent but not diagnostic. A diffuse, blanching erythema ("scarlatiniform" exanthem) appears early. The rash is predominantly truncal, with accentuation in the axillary and inguinal folds and spreading to the extremities. Erythema and edema of the palms and soles may develop. Generalized nonpitting edema is also common. Intense hyperemia of the conjunctival, oropharyngeal, and vaginal surfaces are frequent findings. Desquamation of the involved skin and of the palms and soles is seen during the second or third week of illness. Toxic shock syndrome recurs in approximately 30% of untreated cases. Mortality is higher (12%) in patients with nonmenstrual causation.

B. Laboratory Findings

Laboratory studies are useful for assessing and monitoring the severity and progression of the illness. Patients often have leukocytosis with a left shift and thrombocytopenia. If disseminated intravascular coagulation is suspected, coagulation studies should be obtained. Serum electrolytes, calcium, phosphorus, creatine kinase, renal function and liver function tests, albumin, total serum protein, and amylase may be abnormal. Urinalysis may show proteinuria and pyuria.

Chest x-ray, arterial blood gas determinations, and echocardiography may provide useful information. Cultures of blood, soft tissue sites of infection, and all mucosal surfaces (including the trachea if intubation is performed) should be obtained. Serologic tests should be ordered for Rocky Mountain spotted fever, leptospirosis, or measles as indicated in individual patients to exclude alternative diagnoses.

Differential Diagnosis

Toxic shock syndrome is a clinical diagnosis. Appropriate laboratory tests help to distinguish it from several serious and potentially life-threatening exanthematous diseases including streptococcal toxic shock-like disease, scarlet fever, Kawasaki's disease, Rocky Mountain spotted fever, Stevens-Johnson syndrome, drug eruptions, bacterial sepsis, measles, and leptospirosis.

Treatment

Tampons or other contraceptive devices must be removed immediately, followed by irrigation of the vagina. Any surgical packings should also be removed. Soft tissue abscesses, empyema, and other sites of infection require surgical drainage and irrigation.

An antistaphylococcal antibiotic should be administered intravenously based on a presumptive diagnosis, though its effect on the outcome of the acute episode is unclear. Antibiotics do reduce the recurrence of menses-related toxic shock syndrome. Treatment of group A streptococcal toxic shock syndrome includes penicillin or ceftriaxone plus clindamycin or erythromycin.

Supportive care, including management of organ system failure and treatment of hypotension, is the mainstay of therapy. Systemic corticosteroids, if given within 3 or 4 days after onset of disease, reduce its severity and shorten the duration of fever.

Kain KC et al: Clinical spectrum of non-menstrual toxic shock syndrome (TSS). Clin Infect Dis 1993;16:100–6.

REFERENCES

Arnold HL, Odom RB, James WD (editors): *Andrew's Diseases of the Skin: Clinical Dermatology,* 8th ed. Saunders, 1990.

Fitzpatrick TB et al (editors): *Dermatology in General Medicine,* 4th ed. McGraw-Hill, 1993.

Habif TP: *Clinical Dermatology: A Color Guide to Diagnosis and Therapy,* 3rd ed. Mosby, 1996.

Provost TT, Flynn JA (editors): *Cutaneous Medicine: Cutaneous Manifestations of Systemic Disease.* BC Decker, 2001.

Critical Care of Vascular Disease & Emergencies

29

James T. Lee, MD, & Frederic S. Bongard, MD

The critical care of patients with peripheral vascular disease requires considerable diagnostic skill and clinical acumen. Associated medical comorbidities—diabetes, renal insufficiency, coronary artery disease, many others—necessitate admission to an ICU for preoperative optimization and postoperative observation. Acute arterial occlusion, pulmonary embolism, and—with the advent of endovascular interventions—pseudoaneurysm formation are among the more common vascular-related complications encountered in the otherwise routine care of medical and surgical patients. This chapter addresses acute vascular emergencies in critically ill patients and discusses the management of complications following both elective and emergency vascular surgical procedures.

VASCULAR EMERGENCIES IN THE ICU

ACUTE ARTERIAL INSUFFICIENCY

ESSENTIALS OF DIAGNOSIS

- *The "six Ps": pain, paralysis, paresthesia, pallor, pulselessness, and poikilothermia.*
- *Loss of light touch and position sense followed by paralysis.*
- *Absence of previously palpable distal pulses and slow capillary refill.*
- *Cool extremity with skin mottling, often with a detectable line of demarcation.*
- *Collapse of the superficial venous system and development of venous thrombosis and rigid muscular compartments in prolonged ischemia.*

General Considerations

The management of acute limb ischemia continues to challenge today's critical care specialist. Patients often present in a severely compromised state with unclear symptomatology and may have multiple associated medical illnesses. Despite improved therapeutic options in recent years, outcome remains poor. In a review of 35 reported series, a mortality rate of 26% and an amputation rate of 37% were documented.

Decreased arterial inflow in a previously normal limb may be due to embolization from a remote origin (due to in situ thrombosis from preexisting occlusive disease) or may occur in association with a low-flow state. Although thrombosis occurs more frequently than embolic occlusion in the general population, progression to complete occlusion of an atherosclerotic thrombus is an unusual cause of acute arterial insufficiency in a critically ill patient admitted for other reasons. Depending on the artery affected and the adequacy of collateral circulation, clinical presentation may be along a continuum from subtle to overt limb threat.

The most common site of origin of an embolus is the heart, with atherosclerotic disease the predominant underlying factor. Other sources include aortic and peripheral aneurysms, atherosclerotic debris from ulcerating plaques, and, less commonly, paradoxical embolus through a cardiac anomaly, arteritis, or vascular trauma. Atrial fibrillation, often seen in the postoperative setting, is currently associated with two-thirds to three-quarters of peripheral emboli.

Acute arterial insufficiency in the ICU is most commonly caused by intrinsic obstruction produced by the embolization of clot from distant sites. Atherosclerotic cardiac vascular disease accounts for 60–70% of all arterial emboli. The majority arise in patients with atrial fibrillation and stasis in the left atrial appendage. Those who have sustained a recent myocardial infarction may also develop mural thrombi, most commonly at the cardiac apex or in a trabeculation of the left ventricle. No clear temporal relationship exists between the time of the myocardial infarction and when embolization occurs. When congestive heart failure or cardiomyopathy is present, dyskinetic segments again result in areas of

Table 29–1. Sites of peripheral arterial emboli.[1]

Segment	Incidence (%)
Femoral	36
Aortoiliac	22
Popliteal-tibial	15
Upper extremity	14
Visceral	7
Other	6

[1]Data complied from 1303 embolic events at the Massachusetts General Hospital and Stanford University. Adapted from Rutherford RB (editor): *Vascular Surgery*. Saunders, 2000.

relative stasis that lead to the formation of thrombi. After separation from its site of origin, an embolus may be swept into the innominate or left subclavian artery and travel distally in an upper extremity until the arterial tree narrows sufficiently to trap it. If it is carried into either of the internal carotid or vertebral arteries, a bland (dry) stroke results. Distal emboli typically lodge where vessels taper or branch and consequently are seen in the superior mesenteric artery, resulting in visceral ischemia; or in the iliac, femoral, or popliteal arteries. Peripheral emboli travel to the lower extremities ten times more often than to the upper extremities. Commonly involved arterial segments are listed in Table 29-1.

Other intrinsic sources of arterial emboli are atherosclerotic debris from aneurysms, fibrin plugs, or collections of platelets. It is unusual for atherosclerotic emboli to present de novo in a patient admitted to the ICU for another reason. The exception to this is the blue toe syndrome, which results from occlusion of digital vessels by atherosclerotic emboli. However, when the possibility of an expanding aneurysm or symptomatic chronic aortic dissection was the reason for admission, acute limb ischemia should arouse concern that the atherosclerotic plaque or the grumous clot lining the aneurysm has embolized.

Patients with atherosclerotic microemboli frequently have transient focal ischemia associated with minor tissue loss. The clinical distinction between arterial embolism and arterial thrombosis is often difficult to make, though an effort should be made to confirm the diagnosis because of the differences in therapeutic approach and outcome (Table 29–2). Fibrin plugs and platelet emboli occur most commonly in patients with disseminated intravascular coagulation or in those anticoagulated with heparin who develop antiheparin antibodies.

Extrinsic emboli are produced when foreign material such as catheter tips, balloon fragments, or endovascular occluding devices migrate to distant sites. Bullet emboli should be remembered as a possible cause of acute arter-

Table 29–2. Differentiation of emoblism from thrombosis.[1]

Characterisitics of Occlusion	Embolus	Thrombosis
Onset of symptons	Rapid or immediate	Slower or insidious
Prior symptoms: claudication	Rare	Frequent
Length of time to presentation	Acute	Chronic
Identifiable source	Recent cardiac disease (eg, artial fibrillation, myocardial infarction)	None
Physical findings	Normal contralateral extremity	Bilateral peripheral vascular disease
Angiography	Multiple sharp cutoffs, "reversed meniscus", scant collateral	Diffuse peripheral vascular disease, irregular cutoff, many collaterals
Goal of immediate therapy	Eliminate embolus	Correct disease
Long-term pharmacologic treatment	Anticoagulation	Platelet inhibition
Results of thromboembolectomy	Good	Poor
Amputation risk	Lower	Higher
Causes of mortality	Cardiac disease	Limb ischemia

[1]Adapted from Young JR et al (editors): *Peripheral Vascular Disease*. Mosby Year Book, 1991; and from Rutherford RB (editor): *Vascular Surgery*. Saunders, 2000.

ial insufficiency in a trauma victim in whom the missile was not recovered or was unreachable at the time of surgery. Other penetrating injuries, such as stab wounds, may partially disrupt the vascular intima and begin the process of dissection and thrombotic occlusion.

Once arterial flow is halted, three pathophysiologic events occur, each worsening the overall ischemic insult. Initially, propagation of thrombus can occlude potential collateral vessel orifices and lend to the "no-reflow" phenomenon once large vessel revascularization is established. Second, cellular swelling due to local hypoxia may cause red cell trapping and effectively increase the ischemic period even after adequate inflow is restored. The cause of cellular swelling is debated but may consist of failure of the sodium pump. This inability to reperfuse after ischemic intervals is termed the "no-reflow" or "low-reflow" phenomenon. As fluid leaves the interstitium and enters the cellular matrix, the effective viscosity of the blood increases, raising the pressure required to overcome the blood's inertia (yield stress) and causing significant narrowing and occlusion of the arterioles, capillaries, and venules. The more protracted the ischemic period, the greater the fluid loss and the higher the yield stress. Muscle damage produced by ischemia and reperfusion is more related to "reflow" than to the absolute period of ischemia. Animal models have shown that graded return of inflow over a period of time did result in improved postischemic muscle function and less edema. The mediators of capillary endothelial injury are highly active oxygen metabolites such as superoxide (O_2^-) and hydroxyl (–OH) radicals. Upon reperfusion, the lactic acid, potassium, myoglobin, and cardiodepressants such as thromboxane, which have accumulated in the ischemic limb, are systemically released. The resultant metabolic acidosis and biochemical insult can have profound consequences in an already fragile patient.

Peripheral nerve fibers that mediate light touch and position sense are much more vulnerable than skin and subcutaneous tissue. Thus, deficits in these areas, although subtle, present an illusion of surface viability while masking the presence of complete functional loss.

Table 29–3. Demarcation of physical findings in relation to site of arterial occlusion.[1]

Site of Occlusion	Line of Demarcation
Infrarenal aorta	Mid abdomen
Aortic bifurcation and common iliac arteries	Groin/pelvis
External iliac arteries	Proximal thigh
Common femoral artery	Lower third of thigh
Superficial femoral artery	Upper third of calf
Popliteal artery	Lower third of calf

[1]Adapted from Way LW (editor): *Current Surgical Diagnosis and Treatment,* 10th ed. Originally published by Appleton & Lange. Copyright © 1994 by The McGraw-Hill Companies, Inc.

Clinical Features

A. Symptoms and Signs

Acute ischemia is often manifested by some or all of the six cardinal signs known as the "six Ps." Ischemic pain is profound, and most patients require large doses of opioid analgesics before they obtain relief. The diagnosis of acute arterial ischemia is usually entertained because of the localized nature of the pain. The level of the obstruction is typically in the artery lying one joint above the area of discomfort (Table 29–3). Emboli to the axillary artery, which has excellent collateral flow, are either asymptomatic, detected primarily by a pulse deficit, or noted only with physical activity. Conversely, emboli to the common femoral or popliteal arteries typically produce profound ischemia, and symptoms appear rapidly. On examination, the extremity is pallid and cool. Unlike venous thrombosis, arterial ischemia produces a white rather than a violaceous limb. Occasionally, the sensorial perception of numbness and paresthesias predominates and may mask the primary component of pain. A late sign, paralysis is the result of motor nerve ischemia followed by muscle necrosis. Distal pulses are usually absent, though profound ischemia may occur in the presence of a normal pulse when the embolus is lodged distally in the small arteries of the hand or foot. In some patients—especially those with chronic disease and generalized edema or anasarca—pulses may be difficult or impossible to detect. The extremity may be firm because of muscle swelling. A compartment syndrome occurs when muscle swelling limits venous outflow from within a fascial compartment. An indurated and hard compartment is an indication for release of the pressure by fasciotomy.

Although indicative of arterial insufficiency, these symptoms are in essence nonspecific. They serve to alert the clinician to the presence of ischemia but do not lend themselves to grading or quantification. It is of paramount importance to assess the degree of ischemia, which is stratified into three categories based on the physical findings: viable, threatened, and irreversible. Symptoms depend on the location of the embolus and the adequacy of the collateral circulation. The Joint Council of the Society for Vascular Surgery and the North American Chapter of the International Society for Cardiovascular Surgery have developed a consensus describing severity of limb ischemia into three categories (Table 29-4). Category I (viable) limbs usually present as an acute on chronic process. Patients in this category have abundant collaterals and develop an acute femoral artery thrombosis overlying a chronic stenosis.

Table 29–4. Clinical categories of acute limb ischemia.[1]

Category	Description	Sensory Loss	Muscle Weakness	Arterial Doppler	Venous Doppler
I. Viable	No immediate threat	None	None	+	+
II. Threatened					
Marginal	Salvage with prompt treatment	Minimal	None	–	+
Immediate	Salvage with immediate treatment	Rest pain	Mild to moderate	–	+
III. Irreversible	Permanent tissue loss	Anesthetic	Paralysis	–	–

[1]Adapted from Rutherford RB, Baker JD, Ernst C, et al: Recommended standards for reports dealing with lower extremity ischemia: Revised version. J Vasc Surg 1997;26:517.

The prognosis of category II patients is dictated by the time interval between diagnosis and revascularization. Prompt versus immediate intervention is dictated by the severity of presentation. Amputation is the only recourse in category III patients.

B. Noninvasive Diagnostic Studies

1. Doppler examination—A Doppler flow probe is useful in patients who are edematous or in whom a pulse may not be detectable for other reasons. Evidence of flow by Doppler examination indicates only that obstruction is not complete–*it does not mean that flow is adequate.* One should guard against grading "Doppler pulses," since they are influenced by several factors including the angle of insonation, the gain of the system, and the flow in the artery. The more superficial the vessel under consideration, the higher the frequency of the probe that should be used.

2. Ankle-brachial index (ABI)—Although used primarily in patients with chronic arterial disease, the ABI may be useful in patients who complain of subtle changes in their extremities. The ABI is also useful in postoperative vascular patients for monitoring graft patency. The index is calculated by placing a blood pressure cuff at the high calf position, just below the knee, where it will occlude the tibial arteries. A Doppler probe is placed over either the posterior tibial or the dorsalis pedis artery, and the cuff is then deflated. The pressure at which flow resumes is documented to obtain an opening pressure. The brachial artery pressure is measured in a similar manner, taking the arm with the higher systolic pressure. The ankle-brachial index is then calculated (by dividing ankle Doppler pressure by brachial Doppler pressure). An index of > 1.0 is normal, and an index < 0.4 signifies a threat to the limb. Of greatest value are changes in the index from previous values or a discrepancy between the two extremities.

3. Duplex scanning—In equivocal cases or when angiography is not available, noninvasive color-flow duplex ultrasonography has been a major advance in the diagnosis and treatment of vascular diseases. It has several components. A two-dimensional real-time image is projected in the B mode, which can locate vessels in soft tissues, measure vessel diameters, and reveal irregularities within the lumen. This may be helpful in locating the position of the embolus. Pulsed-wave Doppler technology determines the velocity of blood flow at a specified location that is superimposed on the B mode image. Turbulent flow is seen with a mosaic pattern, while a color-flow void signifies occlusion. Although duplex scanning can be performed conveniently at the bedside, it has the disadvantage of being highly operator-dependent. Duplex scanning can provide essentially the same information as arteriography with respect to localization of arterial segments with either stenosis or total occlusion.

4. Air plethysmography—Although it is seldom used, air plethysmography remains a valuable noninvasive diagnostic technique. Several types are available but all measure the same physiologic parameter: change in volume. A blood pressure cuff is placed around the affected extremity and inflated to 65 mm Hg. A pressure wave form tracing is then recorded, and occlusive disease is graded based on pulse contour. An advantage of this application is that the recording obtained is not affected by vessel wall stiffness. In conjunction with segmental pressure measurements, an accurate assessment in patients with peripheral occlusive disease can be made. However, in the setting of acute limb ischemia, other more specific modalities are necessary.

C. Angiography

Radiographic studies are best obtained in consultation with a vascular surgeon to avoid unnecessary delays. Arteriography remains the standard and is extremely useful in the planning of operative procedures and is recommended in all but the most straightforward cases. Only when the location of the occlusion is apparent (eg, femoral embolus) and coupled with an acutely ischemic limb is preoperative angiography required. However, when symptoms are atypical in a threatened limb, arteriography is helpful in determining the surgical strategy or in the institution of catheter-directed thrombolytic therapy. The major disadvantage of radiologic studies in this setting is the time required to obtain them. Delayed can lead to irreversible soft tissue ischemic injury.

Differential Diagnosis

Acute arterial insufficiency due to an embolus may be mimicked by low-flow states produced by congestive heart failure and hypovolemic shock. In the latter conditions, however, global ischemia is present, and the localizing symptoms associated with an embolus are lacking. Acute stroke or transient ischemic attacks may produce muscle weakness but are seldom associated with pain. Aneurysmal disease or aortic dissection may not only be the source of emboli but may also result in rupture. If a dissection extends distally, it may become thrombotic, producing acute ischemia of the organs that receive blood from its false channel. Diabetic neuropathy and neuritis may produce hypesthesias in the extremities but seldom are a diagnostic dilemma.

Treatment

Prompt restoration of inflow is the most important management priority. In general, the extent of tissue necrosis and the resultant disability are directly proportionate to the duration of ischemia. Tolerance of ischemia varies widely between different tissues, extremities, and individuals. Thus, a safe upper limit for arterial compromise cannot be established, though most authorities cite 4–6 hours as the usual time limit beyond which irreversible injury of muscles and nerves may have occurred, though the overlying skin may still be viable. For this reason, once a threat to limb survival has been recognized, prompt treatment is paramount.

A. Anticoagulation

Systemic anticoagulation with heparin is used unless life-threatening contraindications such as active gastrointestinal or cerebral bleeding are present. Heparin prevents the distal propagation of thrombus, protects the distal vascular bed, and preserves the extremity's outflow. The usual dose of heparin is 100 units/kg given as a bolus, followed by 10–20 units/kg/h. Before heparin is started, one should record a baseline partial thromboplastin time (aPTT), prothrombin time (PT), and platelet count. Heparin is cleared when bound to receptors on endothelial cells and macrophages, where it is depolymerized. Consequently, its half-life is dependent on the initial bolus. The half-life increases from approximately 30 minutes following an intravenous bolus of 25 units/kg, to 60 minutes with a bolus of 100 units/kg, and to 150 minutes with a bolus of 400 units/kg. Based on the standard dosage, most authors recommend titrating a continuous heparin drip to lengthen the aPTT to twice baseline. Heparin should be started before any diagnostic maneuvers and may be continued through to the time of surgery. Titration of the heparin dosage should not substitute for or delay appropriate surgical management. The use of heparin should be followed by oral anticoagulation to prevent recurrent embolism in patients undergoing thromboembolectomy.

Some surgeons recommend nonoperative management for acute arterial ischemia, in which case heparin in "high" doses (20,000 units as intravenous bolus followed by 4000 units/h) is used as the sole form of treatment. Extreme caution must be exercised in recommending such therapy, however, and only patients without signs of limb threat should be treated with anticoagulation alone. This therapy is best reserved for upper extremity lesions where collateral flow is good—or, in lower extremity cases, for patients whose neural function is not diminished or in whom it improves quickly after institution of therapy.

B. Rheologic Agents

The increase in blood viscosity associated with acute ischemia has led some vascular surgeons to recommend the use of either mannitol or low-molecular-weight dextran (dextran 40; MW 40,000) to reduce cellular swelling. An additional benefit of these agents is that they produce an osmotic diuresis and may help prevent renal failure due to myoglobin released from ischemic and necrotic muscle. Mannitol is started with an intravenous bolus dose of 25–50 g. Care must be exercised in patients with congestive heart failure because the increased intravascular volume may worsen cardiac symptoms.

C. Platelet-Active Agents

Aspirin, the agent most commonly prescribed for this purpose, has been thoroughly evaluated and found to prevent vascular death by approximately 15% and nonfatal vascular events by about 30% in a meta-analysis of over 50 secondary prevention trials in various groups of patients. The role of aspirin in acute limb ischemia is more restricted to postoperative adjunctive cardiac prophylaxis.

Integrin glycoprotein IIb/IIIa receptor antagonists (eg, abciximab) inhibit the final common pathway of platelet aggregation. Their development objective was to prevent restenosis in patients undergoing percutaneous coronary intervention. Three large randomized trials involving approximately 27,000 patients resulted in a higher mortality and excessive bleeding complications when compared with aspirin. The role of this class of medications is evolving.

Thienopyridines such as clopidogrel inhibit ADP-induced platelet aggregation with no direct effects on arachidonic acid metabolism. Use of this agent in the acute setting has not been studied; however in a comparison trial with aspirin involving a subset of 6400 patients, virtually all of the benefit associated with clopidogrel was observed in the group with symptomatic peripheral vascular disease. As a group, these patients had fewer myocardial infarctions and fewer vascular-related deaths than did the aspirin-treated group. The main disadvantage is the permanent platelet defect encountered, which can only be replaced with platelet turnover.

D. Thrombin Inhibitors

Direct thrombin inhibitors (hirudin, bivalirudin) have been used successfully to treat arterial and venous thrombotic complications of heparin-induced thrombocytopenia. Hirudin has a half-life of 40 minutes after intravenous administration and approximately 120 minutes after subcutaneous injection. The drug is predominantly cleared by the kidneys, with little hepatic metabolism. Despite producing a more predictable anticoagulant response than heparin, direct thrombin inhibitors have yet to find a place in the treatment of acute arterial thrombosis. Potential disadvantages include the irreversible nature of this complex, as no antidote is available should bleeding occur, and its narrow therapeutic window when combined with thrombolytic therapy.

E. Thrombolytic Agents

Thrombolytic agents such as urokinase, streptokinase, and recombinant tissue plasminogen activator (rt-PA; alteplase) have been evaluated in numerous clinical trials for safety and efficacy and in comparison with operative management. Initially, an intense thrombolytic state was induced with systemic therapy sustained by constant intravenous infusion. In ten uncontrolled studies involving 1800 patients, best results were obtained within 72 hours after onset of symptoms. Lysis was observed in 40%, with no difference in success rates between embolic or thrombotic occlusions. Unfortunately, serious hemorrhagic complications occurred in one-third of patients.

Regional or intra-arterial thrombolysis has become an alternative to systemic therapy. The rate of successful reperfusion (50–85%) appears to be higher than what is reported with systemic infusion. Local infusion coupled with arteriography conferred an additional advantage in delineating the cause of the arterial occlusion (thrombosis versus embolus). Vessel wall morphologic characteristics that may lead to early recurrent thrombosis were also unmasked and further directed appropriate management (surgery versus angioplasty). Prolonged arterial catheterization (hours to days) resulting in major bleeding (6–20%) remains the main disadvantage of this approach. Current thrombolytic agents include streptokinase, urokinase, alteplase, reteplase, and tenecteplase.

Urokinase, a relatively inexpensive trypsin-like protease, directly converts plasminogen to plasmin. Initially, the main advantages of urokinase over streptokinase were its direct action on plasminogen and its nonantigenicity. However, pyretic reactions have been observed and attributed to interleukins present during the manufacturing process. As a result, urokinase is currently not available in the United States.

Alteplase is now the only thrombolytic agent available for peripheral arterial thrombolysis. A naturally occurring activator of plasminogen, it is produced and released by the endothelium. Manufactured through recombinant DNA techniques, it is nonantigenic, has a half-life of 3.5–4 minutes, and has a high affinity for fibrin, which enhances lysis at the thrombus level. Similar to urokinase, the primary route of metabolism is hepatic.

Reteplase is a new plasminogen activator approved for treatment of acute myocardial infarction and is used anecdotally in the peripheral vasculature. Designed for use as bolus therapy through recombinant DNA technology, experience with reteplase in arterial and venous thromboembolic disease is limited.

An inert zymogen activated by the presence of fibrin clot, prourokinase is converted to an active two-chain urokinase which is highly fibrin-specific. Availability of this agent is also limited.

Tenecteplase, a genetically engineered variant of alteplase, has a prolonged half-life, increased fibrin specificity, and higher resistance to inhibition by circulating plasminogen activator inhibitor-1. A three-amino-acid substitution resulted in a 14- to 19-minute half-life and more specific fibrinolysis in comparison with alteplase. Pending approval by the FDA for treatment of acute myocardial infarction, the role of tenecteplase in the management of peripheral arterial and venous thrombotic occlusion has yet to be explored.

Because of the lack of evidence demonstrating the benefits of improved limb salvage, lower mortality, or cost-effectiveness, thrombolytic therapy cannot be regarded as first-line treatment in the management of acute limb ischemia. However, it remains a reasonable alternative in a select group of patients, especially those with distal thromboembolic occlusions in surgically inaccessible small arteries of the hands and feet and in those patients who are at high risk for surgery.

F. Surgery

Operation is the best treatment of acute extremity ischemia, achieving both life and limb salvage. Adequate preoperative support is essential. In the presence of active cardiac risk, use of local anesthesia must be considered and adequate intravenous hydration provided to minimize renal insufficiency. At the time of surgery, placement of the incision is guided by the cause of occlusion, the presence of a palpable pulse, and a history of previous revascularization.

In patients with embolic occlusion, exploration of the femoral artery is considered in the presence of femoral and distal pulses. A below-the-knee approach is preferred in patients presenting with a palpable popliteal pulse and distal embolization. Patients with acute ischemia and a previous bypass graft are usually explored through the distal anastomosis.

A transverse incision is often sufficient for passage of a Fogarty catheter. Longitudinal arteriotomy is considered if the cause is not certainly known or if bypass is necessary. Removal of the entire embolic material is essential, and success is confirmed through an intraoperative arteriogram to ensure patency of the arterial runoff distal to the embolus. Approximately 35–40% of completion angiograms will identify residual thrombus.

Although highly successful in embolic occlusion, blind thromboembolectomy in patients with acute on chronic thrombosis is highly dangerous and risks further intimal disruption to an already diseased vessel. Often these patients require further surgical revascularization (bypass or endarterectomy) or endovascular management (thrombolysis, angioplasty, or stent placement in debilitated patients).

Intraoperative lytic therapy has been reported in several series for the following indications: residual thrombus on angiography, slow flow despite the absence of an angiographic defect, prolonged ischemia with evidence of thickened blood on retrograde bleeding, and persistent ischemia despite restoration of sufficient proximal inflow. In a series of 78 patients, limb salvage was achieved in 73% of the 67% treated successfully.

A new approach to intraoperative thrombolysis undergoing recent investigation is high-dose isolated limb perfusion. Surgical cutdowns of the femoral vessels are performed, with intra-arterial insertion of standard infusion pumps. A tourniquet is applied proximal to the exposed vessels, and venous effluent is drained by gravity or through the use of extracorporeal pump support with concomitant dialysis.

Fasciotomy should be considered in all cases following successful revascularization in the setting of prolonged ischemia. Common clinical indications are pain out of proportion to findings, pain on passive stretch, tense muscular compartments with elevated pressures, and compartmental hypesthesia and paralysis.

G. Supportive Care

Perioperative care of the patient following revascularization of an acutely ischemic limb can vary from simple to extremely complex. Reperfusion of an ischemic extremity can lead to the release of toxic cellular products, the generation of oxygen free radicals, hyperkalemia, increased intracellular calcium overload, myoglobinuria, and altered arachidonic acid metabolism. Critical care is therefore directed toward ameliorating the damage done by cellular breakdown.

Appropriate hemodynamic monitoring is essential. Correction of electrolyte abnormalities and prompt treatment of hyperkalemia through brisk diuresis and administration of insulin and glucose can prevent fatal cardiac arrhythmias. Adequate fluid volume and the administration of mannitol—a free radical scavenger and osmotic diuretic—is the best strategy to correct acidosis and to prevent acute renal failure caused by myoglobin precipitates.

Local mechanical factors are also important to prevent skin and soft tissue breakdown. The extremity should be kept warm but must not be heated in an effort to restore flow, as this will increase the metabolic rate, further the lactic acidosis, and contribute to tissue destruction. Similarly, cooling is inappropriate. Care must be taken to prevent pressure on an ischemic extremity. Heel pads and cushions should be used as needed. Other vascular precautions include keeping linens suspended with a bed cradle and positioning the patient in reverse Trendelenburg.

In patients who have not undergone fasciotomy, frequent and careful assessment of the lower extremities is warranted. In the event that a compartment syndrome is diagnosed, prompt decompression is required to preserve tissue viability.

Pain control typically requires high doses of an opioid such as morphine. Analgesia must not be increased to the point that symptoms are masked and a reliable neurologic examination cannot be obtained. Short-acting intravenous agents such as fentanyl have been used with success provided that the dose is regulated so as not to obscure worsening of symptoms.

Prognosis

Despite recent advances in perioperative critical care, the mortality rate after acute leg ischemia remains relatively high. Both the mortality rate and the need for amputation are directly related to the duration of ischemia. A recent study found that no amputations were required when surgery was undertaken within 2 hours, as compared to a 44% amputation rate when operation was delayed up to 7 days. The mortality rate was 10% in patients with symptoms for less than 2 hours and 32% in those whose symptoms were present for up to 8 hours. Coexistent cardiopulmonary complications were the underlying cause of most fatalities, especially in patients with acute arterial thrombosis in contrast to peripheral embolism.

Current Controversies & Unresolved Issues

The cause of ischemic injury remains unclear. While it is logical to assume that hypoxia is the culprit, investigations have shown that the majority of tissue damage actually occurs during the time of reperfusion. Even short periods of ischemia followed by reperfusion can cause cell damage. A recent canine study found that 3 hours of partial ischemia resulted in more tissue damage than the same period of complete ischemia. Furthermore, the extent of postreperfusion damage can be decreased by graded reflow. These investigations suggest that scavengers of free radicals may be useful in the treatment of acute vascular insufficiency.

Although numerous investigations have been undertaken, little improvement has been made over the last 2 decades in morbidity and mortality associated with surgical thrombectomy in this fragile patient group. The advantage of surgery stems from rapid restoration of blood flow. On the contrary, pharmacologic thrombolysis is much less invasive. The main disadvantage is the time lag involved for revascularization. What is needed is an ideal therapeutic option that achieves rapid blood flow and is minimally invasive. The advent of endovascular surgery has spurred the development of percutaneous mechanical thrombectomy devices to answer this need. Current devices in various stages of clinical trials include rheolytic, clot aspiration, and microfragmentation catheters.

Andaz S et al: Thrombolysis in acute lower limb ischaemia. Eur J Vasc Surg 1993;7:595–603.

Comerota AJ, Schmieder FA: Intraoperative lytic therapy: Agents and methods of administration. Semin Vasc Surg 2001;14: 132–42.

Davies MG et al: Upper limb embolus: A timely diagnosis. Ann Vasc Surg 1991;5:85–7.

Eslami MH, Ricotta JJ: Operation for acute peripheral arterial occlusion: Is it still the gold standard? Semin Vasc Surg 2001;14:93–9.

Friedl HP et al: Ischemia-reperfusion in humans: Appearance of xanthine oxidase activity. Am J Pathol 1990;136:491–5.

Greenberg RK, Ouriel K: Arterial thromboembolism. In: *Vascular Surgery,* 15th ed. Rutherford R (editor). Saunders, 2000.

Jackson MR, Clagett GP: Antithrombotic therapy in peripheral arterial occlusive disease. Chest 2001;119(1 Suppl):283S–9S.

Kubaska SM, Greenberg RK: Techniques for percutaneous treatment of acute arterial occlusion. Semin Vasc Surg 2001;14: 114–22.

Kasirajan K, Marek JM, Langsfeld M: Mechanical thrombectomy as first-line treatment for arterial occlusion. Semin Vasc Surg 2001;14:123–31.

Lyden SP, Shortell CK, Illig KA: Reperfusion and compartment syndromes: Strategies for prevention and treatment. Semin Vasc Surg 2001;14:107–13.

Ouriel K, Veith FJ, Sasahara AA: A comparison of recombinant urokinase with vascular surgery as initial treatment for acute arterial occlusion of the legs. Thrombolysis or Peripheral Arterial Surgery (TOPAS) Investigators. N Engl J Med 1998;338:1105–11.

Ouriel K, Vieth FJ: Acute lower limb ischemia: Determinants of outcome. Surgery 1998;124:336–41.

Patrono C et al: Platelet-active drugs: The relationship among dose, effectiveness, and side effects. Chest 2001;119(1 Suppl): 39S–63S.

Singh S et al: Thrombo-embolectomy and thrombolytic therapy in acute lower limb ischemia: A five-year experience. Int Angiol 1996;15:6–8.

Thrombolysis in the management of lower limb peripheral arterial occlusion—a consensus document. Working Party on Thrombolysis in the Management of Limb Ischemia. Am J Cardiol 1998;81:207–18.

Weaver FA et al: Surgical revascularization versus thrombolysis for nonembolic lower extremity native artery occlusions: Results of a prospective randomized trial. The STILE Investigators: Results of a prospective randomized trial evaluating surgery versus thrombolysis for ischemia of the lower extremity. J Vasc Surg 1996;24:513–21.

Weitz JI, Hirsh J: New anticoagulant drugs. Chest 2001;119(1 Suppl):95S–107S.

DEEP VENOUS THROMBOSIS

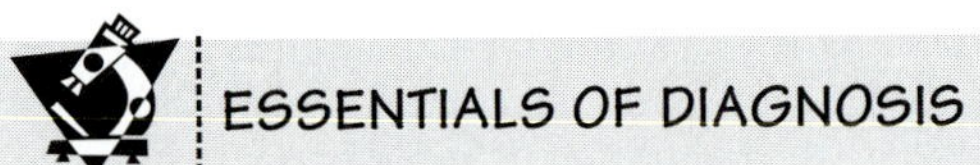
ESSENTIALS OF DIAGNOSIS

- *Multiple risk factors.*
- *Aching pain exaggerated by motion.*
- *Calf and thigh swelling.*
- *Tenderness to palpation and dorsiflexion.*
- *Erythema, cyanosis, or venous distention.*

General Considerations

Three factors (Virchow's triad) contribute to the development of venous thrombosis: stasis, increased coagulability, and vessel wall damage. Contrary to former belief, low flow alone is not sufficient to cause thrombosis. Thrombophlebitis is venous thrombosis that follows inflammation of the vessel wall. Because of underlying intimal irregularities, the clot adheres firmly and is unlikely to become dislodged. Phlebothrombosis occurs without vessel wall injury and results in minimal clot adherence.

Patients at risk for the development of deep venous thrombosis may be divided into three groups: (1) Low-risk patients are under 40 years of age and are free of systemic disease. Surgery lasts less than 60 minutes and is uncomplicated. Overall risk for the development of deep venous thrombosis is less than 2%, and the chance of proximal progression is less than 1%. (2) Moderate-risk patients are over age 40 and have undergone general anesthesia for more than 60 minutes. They may also have risk factors such as cancer, obesity, varicose veins, bed rest, or cardiac failure. If prophylaxis is not given, the risk for development of deep venous thrombosis is between 10% and 40% and that of proximal propagation is between 2% and 8%. The risk of fatal pulmonary embolism is almost 1%. (3) High-risk patients have a history of deep venous thrombosis or of pulmonary embolism. They undergo extensive abdominal or pelvic procedures for advanced disease or for some orthopedic indication. The risk of calf vein thrombosis is between 40% and 80% without prophylaxis. Proximal extension occurs in 10–20%, leading to fatal pulmonary embolism in up to 5%. Risk factors for the development of venous thrombi and recommended prophylaxis are listed in Table 29–5. Most deep venous thrombi are initiated by platelet adhesion either to endothelial tissue or to exposed collagen of damaged vascular walls. As platelet aggregation continues, the clot becomes organized and begins to trap circulating white and red blood cells. Deposition of fibrin organizes the clot and allows it to build a stable matrix.

Activation of either the intrinsic or the extrinsic clotting system contributes to thrombus formation. Adhesion of factor XII to exposed endothelium results in progressive activation of factor X. Activated factor X (Xa), along with factor V, converts prothrombin to thrombin and fibrinogen to fibrin, producing an insoluble clot. Platelets accumulate within the matrix and provide a surface for further fibrin deposition. Thromboxane A_2, produced and released by platelets, aids the process by contributing to vasoconstriction and further platelet aggregation. Prostacyclin, which is produced by vascular intima, limits the process by causing vascular dilation and by inhibiting platelet aggregation. Antithrombin III inhibits the action of factors IX, X, XI, and XII. Proteins C and S, produced by the liver, inhibit coagulation by destroying factors V and VII and provide negative feedback to control the generation of thrombin (Figure 29–1).

The velocity of blood flow is inversely proportionate to the propensity for intravascular clotting. However, the threshold for thrombus formation is decreased in the face of vascular endothelial injury. Such injury may be caused

Table 29–5. Risk stratification for venous thrombosis and recommended prophylaxis.[1]

	Low-Risk	Moderate-Risk	High-Risk
Event or condition			
General surgery	Age < 40 years or time < 60 minutes	Age > 40 years or time > 60 minutes	Age > 40 years or time > 60 minutes plus risk factor
Orthopedic surgery	–	–	Elective hip or knee surgery
Trauma	–	–	Extensive soft tissue injury; major fractures; multiple trauma
Medical conditions	Pregnancy	Myocardial infarction postpartum, especially with previous deep venous thrombosis; estrogen use; varicose veins	Stroke, paraplegia, spine fracture, prolonged bed rest, burns, hypercoagulable state, obesity
Incidence of thromboembolism without prophylaxis (%)			
Distal calf veins	2	10–40	40–80
Proximal veins (pelvis, thigh, popliteal veins)	0.4	2–8	10–20
Symptomatic pulmonary embolism	0.2	1–8	5–10
Fatal pulmonary embolism	0.002	0.1–0.4	1–5
Recommended prophylaxis	Graduated compression stockings; early ambulation	Heparin (5000 units SC twice daily), LMWH, external or pneumatic compression	Heparin (5000 units SC three times daily), LMWH, external pneumatic compression, inferior vena caval filter, warfarin

[1]Adapted from Colman RW et al (editors): *Hemostasis and Thrombosis: Basic Principles and Clinical Practice.* Lippincott, 1994; and from

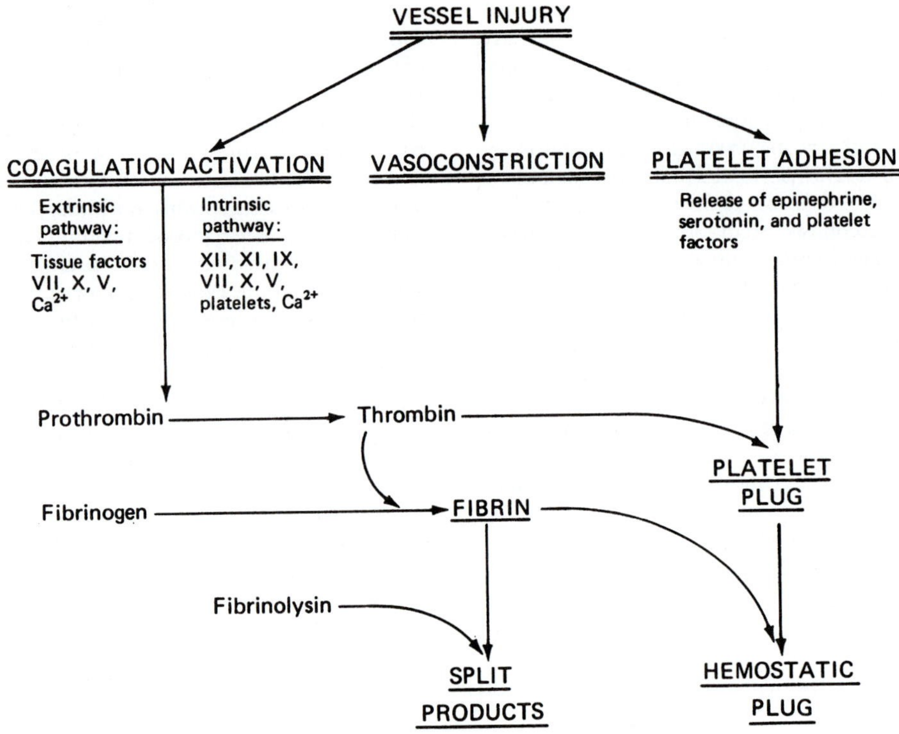

Figure 29–1. Factors involved in arrest of hemorrhage. Injury to the blood vessel wall initiates a series of reactions that arrest hemorrhage. The exposed subendothelial collagen initiates formation of the platelet plug (primary hemostasis). The coagulation system is activated, leading to production of fibrin, which interacts with the platelet aggregate to form a hemostatic seal. These relationships are also involved in spontaneous thrombus formation, although the inciting event is usually not identifiable. (Reproduced, with permission, from Way LW [editor]: *Current Surgical Diagnosis & Treatment,* 10th ed. Originally published by Appleton & Lange. Copyright © 1993 by The McGraw-Hill Companies, Inc.)

by catheters, infection, or external influences. In normal veins, the endothelium is well supplied with prostacyclin and plasminogen, which prevent thrombus formation even at low flow rates. However, when intimal damage is present—or in the face of a hypercoagulable state—thrombus accumulates rapidly. Red clots predominate in the venous system and consist of platelets, red cells, and fibrin. White thrombi, which contain chiefly platelets, are usually found in the arterial system.

Hypercoagulable states are common in postoperative critical care patients. The plasma concentration of clotting factors rises after surgery. Maximum procoagulant activity corresponds temporally with the peak incidence of thromboembolism. Detection of hypercoagulability remains difficult except in certain pathologic conditions such as decreased concentrations of antithrombin III, protein C, and protein S. Use of some medications, such as oral contraceptives, is known to increase the risk of thromboembolic disease. Ill-defined alterations in the clotting mechanism that predispose to clotting accompany some severe systemic diseases such as cancer and sepsis.

Most deep venous thrombi begin in the veins of the calf. When limited to this location, they are usually asymptomatic except for mild calf pain and minimal swelling. Extension into the deep venous system of the thigh produces more swelling, pain, and purpura. Proximal propagation involves the veins of the pelvis (iliofemoral thrombosis). As outflow is restricted, the lower extremity swells and causes obstruction of lymphatic channels, producing a blanched "milk leg" (phlegmasia alba dolens). If patency is not restored, cyanosis and venous gangrene result. This condition, known as phlegmasia cerulea ("blue") dolens, is more common in the left lower extremity than in the right from compression of the left iliac vein as it passes under the right iliac artery. Phlegmasia cerulea dolens is usually associated with disseminated malignancies or sepsis. It is accompanied by hypotension and hypovolemia, which result from venous pooling in the leg.

Thrombosis of the deep veins of the thigh and pelvis dramatically increases the risk of pulmonary embolism. Approximately 85% of clinically significant pulmonary emboli arise from the thighs and pelvis. Eighty percent of deep venous thrombi remain confined to the calf, while 20% extend proximally. In the latter group, 40–50% will result in pulmonary embolism if not treated appropriately. Unfortunately, only 30% of those with confirmed pulmonary embolism have objective signs consistent with deep venous thrombosis.

Venous thrombosis of the upper extremities is becoming increasingly prevalent in the intensive care unit as a result of chronic indwelling central venous catheters. Patients being maintained on long-term parenteral nutrition, hemodialysis, antibiotics, or chemotherapy or those with poor peripheral access are some of those at risk. Other predisposing factors include exertion, thoracic outlet syndrome, congenital malformations, and trauma (see Table 29–6). Approximately 3–6% of all pulmonary emboli and 1–2% of fatal pulmonary emboli have been reported to originate from clots in the deep veins of the upper extremity.

Superficial venous thrombi typically present as a small lump or cord. These are usually of no systemic significance except in the saphenous vein of the thigh, where they can propagate through the saphenofemoral junction and gain access to the deep iliofemoral system. When such proximal extension is noted, ligation of the saphenous vein just distal to its origin is warranted.

Clinical Features

A. Symptoms and Signs

Patients may complain of a vague aching sensation or tightness in the calf or thigh. This is worsened by active motion of the calf or foot. When superficial thrombosis is present, localized tenderness is usually present also.

Physical examination is notoriously unreliable for deep venous thrombosis and accurately detects only 50% of cases. Areas with increased tenderness to palpation include the sole, the region deep to Achilles' tendon, the groove between the tibia and fibula, the regions over the soleus and gastrocnemius muscles, in the popliteal fossa, over the adductor muscles of the thigh, and at the femoral vein near the inguinal ligament. Tenderness induced by compression of the calf muscles anteriorly against the interosseous membrane or with passive dorsiflexion of the ankle (Homans' sign) is present in less than 30% of patients. Inflation of a sphygmomanometer cuff (40 mm Hg) placed above the knee may provoke pain at the site of the thrombosis. A difference of 1.5 cm in diameter between the swollen and the contralateral leg supports the diagnosis.

Deep venous thrombosis of the axillary and subclavian veins of the upper extremity results in swelling of the entire arm. Pitting edema is usually absent. Percussion over the clavicle and the course of the axillary vein often elicits tenderness.

B. Noninvasive Diagnostic Techniques

Hand-held continuous wave Doppler devices test for continuity between the deep system of the leg and the intrathoracic vena cava. The probe is placed initially at the popliteal fossa and subsequently over the femoral vein. The patient is instructed to inspire, at which time an augmentation of flow should be heard. The increased flow is due to transmission of the negative intrathoracic pressure to the deep system. This is a useful screening test that can be performed at the bedside, but it has a sensitivity of only about 75% when compared with venography. Duplex scans and color-coded Doppler examinations have accuracy rates between 90% and 100% for detecting large thrombi of the femoral veins in symptomatic patients. The sensitivity decreases to 59%, though the sensitivity remains at 98% in asymptomatic patients. Accuracy also diminishes when examining the distal veins of the calf due to poor visualization. Isolated instances of iliac vein thrombosis are also not detectable by ultrasound imaging but may be diagnosed by simple Doppler examination. Multiple studies have shown that repeat duplex scanning has an improved negative predictive value in patients suspected of DVT but who have negative initial scans. Pressure on the underlying vein by the ultrasound probe helps to establish the age of the clot, since fresh thrombi are poorly organized and easily compressible. This is the diagnostic test of choice for most patients, though it requires an experienced technician to perform and interpret.

Impedance plethysmography relies on changes in electrical resistance associated with alteration in limb

Table 29–6. Etiology of upper extremity venous thrombosis.

Source	Incidence (%)
Catheter-associated	30–40
Spontaneous (effort-induced)	20–30
Miscellaneous	30–40
Intravenous drug use	
Thoracic tumors	
Trauma	
Radiation	

volume. Deep venous thrombosis impedes venous outflow and causes a slower change in impedance when a proximally occluding cuff is deflated. This technique is very accurate in ambulatory patients but should be interpreted cautiously in those with congestive heart failure or hypervolemia. It is more sensitive for iliac and femoral vein thrombosis than for calf thrombi and generally cannot be used in patients with fractures or bandages that prevent proper electrode positioning. A positive test correctly indicates the presence of thrombosis in 90% of patients. Recently, however, the sensitivity for plethysmography in symptomatic patients was found to be much less than earlier studies reported. In asymptomatic patients, the specificity also falls. Impedance plethysmography can overlook sizable thrombi which are not totally occlusive and can interpret any pelvic venous outflow obstruction (ie. enlarged nodes, pregnancy) as a venous thrombus. It may also be falsely negative in patients with well-developed collaterals.

Computed tomography and magnetic resonance venography have successfully diagnosed thrombi in the proximal veins and have proved to be superior to conventional phlebography in visualizing the great veins, identifying intraluminal thrombi, distinguishing new thrombi, and delineating adjacent abnormalities. Ongoing prospective trials are confirming these initial findings.

C. Invasive Diagnostic Studies

Contrast venography is the gold standard with which all noninvasive modalities are compared. It is the most reliable technique for detecting thrombi in any location. Positive findings on venography include constant filling defects, abrupt termination of the dye column, nonfilling of the entire deep venous system or portions thereof, and diversion of flow through collaterals. The venogram catheter may be exchanged for one capable of delivering thrombolytic agents if that therapeutic route is chosen. Overall accuracy is better than 90%. A negative study virtually eliminates the possibility of venous thrombosis. Complications include foot pain at the site of injection and a 2–3% incidence of thrombosis due to contrast-induced endothelial cell injury. Not routinely used for primary diagnosis, phlebography has been advocated in the diagnosis of symptomatic recurrent venous thrombosis and after hip operations in suspected patients where noninvasive means lack sensitivity.

D. Laboratory Findings

Several blood tests are available that detect activation of the clotting cascade, including measurement of fibrinopeptide A, fibrin monomers, and fibrin degradation products. Plasma D-dimer, a degradation product of plasmin digestion of mature cross-linked fibrin, is elevated in patients with venous thrombosis. The sensitivity measured by enzyme-linked immunosorbent assay approaches 97%. Although highly accurate, confirmation of venous thrombosis with an elevated D-dimer concentration are necessary, with objective imaging tests.

Differential Diagnosis

See Table 29–7.

Prevention

All critically ill patients should be considered for thromboembolic prophylaxis. Particular attention should be paid to those with preexisting risk factors (see Table 29–5).

A. Physical Measures

Early ambulation or exercise of the lower extremity muscles is probably the best and most cost-effective prophylactic measure for preventing subsequent venous thrombosis. Lower extremity elevation and active flexion-extension exercises of the ankle will prevent stasis. Prolonged standing in one position should be discouraged as it promotes venous pooling. Use of thigh-high antiembolism stockings is encouraged when they are properly fitted. Casual application of stockings that extend only to the knee are unlikely to be of value.

Of the compression techniques available, intermittent compression garments are best. Garments with single compartments for the calves or multiple sequential compartments are available. Maximum benefit is realized when they are applied prior to surgery. Direct sequential compression promotes blood flow and also stimulates systemic fibrinolytic activity. Therefore, benefit still accrues even with only unilateral application can be achieved because of bandages or casts. Studies have shown a reduction in the incidence of thrombosis from 23% to 7% in patients so treated.

B. Anticoagulation

When used properly, preoperative anticoagulation decreases the incidence of postoperative deep venous thrombosis and secondary pulmonary embolism.

Table 29–7. Differential diagnosis of deep venous thrombosis.

Lymphatic obstruction
Cellulitis
Baker's cyst
Traumatic contusion
Tendon rupture
Congestive heart failure
Nephrosis
Arterial occlusion

1. Warfarin—Coumarin derivatives act by suppressing the formation of vitamin K-dependent clotting factors (II, VII, IX, and X). When these agents are initiated before and continued after operation, they are safe and effective. Coumarins require several days to reach full effect because of the time interval required for clearance of normal coagulation factors. These agents are usually started after the patient has already been systemically anticoagulated with unfractionated heparin. Initiation of therapy with warfarin alone can have deleterious effects. Protein C and protein S—natural anticoagulants—are similarly reduced (especially protein C) with factor VII, thereby shifting the hemostatic balance toward coagulation. In patients with underlying protein C and protein S deficiency, warfarin-induced skin necrosis can occur from thrombotic occlusion of small vessels in the subcutaneous tissue. This effect is manifested within 3–8 days after administration of the initial dose. Patients with protein C and protein S deficiency should not receive a loading dose of warfarin, and heparin should be continued until the INR is therapeutic for 2 consecutive days.

Several drug interactions are known to occur with warfarin. Of particular importance are those that increase hepatic degradation (barbiturates) and those that displace warfarin from albumin (aspirin, nonsteroidal anti-inflammatory agents). Coumarins are also teratogenic and should not be given to expectant patients.

2. Heparin—Unfractionated heparin binds with antithrombin III to prevent the conversion of prothrombin to thrombin. A "low-dose" regimen is customarily used prior to surgery and in the postoperative period while the patient is still at risk. The postulated mechanism of action is enhancement of antithrombin III. The usual regimen consists of 5000 units given subcutaneously 2 hours before surgery and every 8–12 hours during the postoperative period. No changes in the usual coagulation parameters can be detected at this dosing level. Increased bleeding at the time of surgery generally does not occur. Heparin prophylaxis is unlikely to be effective when started in the postoperative period. It is not effective for patients undergoing hip surgery and should not be used in those with bleeding disorders or for scheduled intracerebral procedures.

An adjusted-dose heparin regimen has been described for patients undergoing total hip replacement. Two days prior to surgery, the patient receives 3500 units of heparin subcutaneously every 8 hours, with the dose adjusted to elevate the activated partial thromboplastin time (aPTT) to the high normal range. This regimen has been shown to reduce the incidence of deep venous thrombosis in hip replacement patients from 39% to 13%.

3. Low-molecular-weight heparin (LMWH)—LMWH has several advantages over unfractionated heparin. First evaluated in the 1980s in high-risk surgical patients, one daily dose administered subcutaneously is as effective as two or three doses of unfractionated heparin for DVT prophylaxis. It has become the anticoagulant of choice for preventing DVT in most orthopedic procedures, causes less bleeding, and may have some antineoplastic effects. Its long half-life precludes the need for laboratory monitoring, and it is more effective than unfractionated heparin in preventing recurrence of venous thrombosis. Inpatient and outpatient uses of LMWH have equivalent safety and efficacy.

4. Low-molecular-weight dextran—Dextran 40 acts by coating platelet surfaces to reduce adhesion. It also increases plasma volume and decreases the viscosity of blood. An important mechanism of action may be the prevention of platelet adhesion to venous valve cusps. The usual dose of dextran 40 is 100–200 mL as an intravenous bolus (intraoperatively), followed by 30–40 mL/h for 2–3 days after surgery. Because dextran 40 is a volume expander, patients with congestive heart failure or respiratory distress should be monitored carefully for hypervolemia. Dextran potentiates the effects of heparin, reducing the dosing requirements of the latter by up to 50%.

Management of Deep Vein Thrombosis

The objectives of treatment are to limit further accumulation of thrombus, prevent embolization, and minimize injury to venous valves.

A. Supportive Therapy

Treatment of calf vein thrombi remains largely controversial, with the majority of centers recommending supportive care. In several large trials, anticoagulation was safely withheld in patients with suspected DVT and normal results on serial examinations with compression ultrasonography. Only supportive therapy is required, consisting of bed rest, leg elevation, and mild analgesics. Although some advocate the use of warm soaks, this measure can macerate the overlying skin and promote infection. Early ambulation should be encouraged, with elastic stockings as required. Anticoagulation is indicated in patients with symptomatic DVT identified by duplex scanning and those with recurrent venous thrombosis.

B. Anticoagulation

Thrombi of the proximal veins (popliteal vein, femoral vein, iliac veins) or of the axillary and subclavian veins require anticoagulation. Heparin is the agent of choice because it limits further propagation of the thrombus. For most patients, an initial bolus dose of 100 units/kg followed by a continuous infusion of 10 units/kg/h is adequate. Larger doses (200 units/kg as bolus injection) may be given if the clot extends into the iliac or femoral system, if there is profound edema of the leg, or if imaging studies indicate the presence of a long tail extending proximally. Anticoagulation should be assessed by monitoring either the aPTT or the activated clotting time (ACT). The heparin infusion should be titrated to keep the aPTT between 1.5 and 2.5 times normal. Failure to achieve a therapeutic level of anticoagulation within 24 hours carries a 25% risk of recurrent deep venous thrombosis. Bleeding complications are reduced if dosage is regulated by monitoring of anticoagulation and if the heparin is given by continuous infusion rather than by intermittent bolus administration. Five days of intravenous heparin therapy followed by oral warfarin is usually effective and is generally regarded as conventional therapy.

Although warfarin therapy can be started concomitantly with heparin, most prefer to wait several days before starting oral anticoagulation. Titration of the dose to achieve an INR of 2.0–3.0 is adequate. Oral anticoagulation is continued for 3–6 months following discharge from the hospital based on risk factors (see Table 29–8).

Platelet counts should be obtained initially and every other day to detect the development of heparin-induced antiplatelet antibodies. Immune heparin-induced thrombocytopenia (HIT) is suspected when the platelet count falls below 100,000/μL or less than 50% of the baseline value. This IgG-mediated platelet deficiency is seen in 3% of patients and occurs 5–15 days after heparin therapy is initiated. Management of patients with persistent thrombosis and HIT can be difficult. Some have advocated the use of LMWH, but others are apprehensive about the slight chance of cross-reactivity. Historically treated with snake venom (ancrod), the current shift is toward the use of thrombin inhibitors. Two agents, argatroban and lepirudin, have been approved for patients with HIT needing anticoagulant therapy. Argatroban is begun with a continuous intravenous infusion at 2 μg/kg/min and titrated to keep the aPTT 1.5–3 times the initial baseline. Lepirudin (recombinant hirudin) achieves rapid anticoagulation with a loading dose of 0.4 mg/kg followed by an infusion of 0.15 mg/kg/h. It is adjusted to maintain an aPTT 1.5–3 times normal. Oral warfarin is then instituted for the appropriate duration.

Approximately 3% of patients receiving oral anticoagulation will present with recurrent deep venous thrombosis. These patients should be assessed for a deficiency in antithrombin III and proteins C and S. Bleeding is the major complication of anticoagulation and occurs in 5–10% of patients. This often presents as oozing from wounds, melena, or a heme-positive gastric aspirate. If bleeding continues in spite of discontinuation of heparin, protamine sulfate, a heparin inhibitor, may be required. Infusion of fresh frozen plasma and vitamin K can counteract the effects of warfarin.

C. Thrombolytic Therapy

There are currently two available thrombolytic agents for use in venous thrombosis. Multiple investigations

Table 29–8. Recommendations for long-term management of venous thromboembolism.[1]

Patient Characteristic	Recommendation
Calf vein thrombosis	Up to 3 months of anticoagulant therapy
Proximal venous thrombosis or pulmonary embolus without previous episode	
a. Transient clinical risk factor—major orthopedic surgery or trauma	Anticoagulant therapy for 4–6 weeks or until risk factor is resolved and patient is mobile, whichever is later.
b. Metastatic cancer	Long-term anticoagulation (indefinite)
c. Hypercoagulable risk factors[2] *or* Idiopathic thromboembolism	Either 3–6 months of therapy *or* Lifelong anticoagulation
Recurrent venous thromboembolism	1 year or lifelong anticoagulation
Any venous thromboembolism during pregnancy	Unfractionated intravenous heparin for 5 days, followed by adjusted-dose subcutaneous heparin every 12 hours;[3] or low-molecular-weight heparin until delivery followed by oral warfarin for 4–6 weeks.

[1]Adapted from Ginsberg JS: Management of venous thromboembolism. N Engl J Med 1996;335:1816.
[2]Hypercoagulable risk factors include protein C and S, antithrombin III, plasminogen deficiencies; resistance to activated protein C; hyperhomocystinemia, and antiphospholipid antibodies.
[3]aPTT should be checked 6 hours after initial subcutaneous dosing.

have determined that streptokinase and recombinant tissue plasminogen activator (rt-PA; alteplase) are superior to intravenous heparin in preserving venous patency and valvular function. Approximately 50% of patients treated with thrombolytic agents retain valve function, compared with 7% of those treated with heparin alone. If complete thrombolysis is achieved, the incidence of postphlebitic syndrome is reduced. However, due to the variable nature of this syndrome, further investigation is warranted to confirm these early findings.

Thrombolytic agents followed by heparin result in more rapid resolution of lower extremity and pulmonary emboli, restoring hemodynamic homeostasis. The main disadvantage is the additional 1–2% risk of intracranial hemorrhage. Because the incidence and mortality of pulmonary embolism is the same in the two treatment modalities, systemic thrombolysis is reserved for acute massive pulmonary embolus in an unstable patient with no bleeding dyscrasias. Young patients with massive ileofemoral venous thrombosis (eg, phlegmasia cerulea dolens) may also benefit from thrombolysis.

Neither streptokinase nor alteplase directly dissolves the clot but rather requires activation of the fibrinolytic system. Absolute contraindications to the use of lytic therapy include active bleeding, recent (less than 2 months) cerebrovascular accident, or intracranial disease. Major contraindications include recent surgery and evidence of gastrointestinal hemorrhage. Prior to institution of therapy, the fibrinogen level, thrombin time, PT and aPTT, platelet count, and hematocrit should be determined. Heparin administration should be discontinued. Dosing regimens vary widely, but common doses are as follows: (1) streptokinase, 250,000 units over 30 minutes, followed by an infusion of 100,000 units/h up to 72 hours; or (2) alteplase, 100 mg infusion over 2 hours. Within 4 hours after commencing therapy, thrombin time, fibrinogen level, and fibrin degradation products should be assessed. A lytic state is documented by an elevated thrombin time and the presence of fibrin degradation products. Hematocrit should be assessed every 6 hours. Elevation of fibrin degradation products is anticipated. Infusion for more than 24 hours seldom produces additional results. Lytic therapy should be instituted as early as possible, because thrombi older than 3–5 days are less likely to respond. Bleeding, both superficial and internal, is the most common complication. When a severe coagulopathy develops, transfusion with fresh frozen plasma may be necessary to correct the deficit.

The use of thrombolytic agents in the treatment of venous thromboembolism continues to be highly individualized. In general, patients with hemodynamically unstable pulmonary embolus or massive iliofemoral thrombosis, who are at low risk to bleed, are the most appropriate candidates. Endovascular placement of stents for residual iliac stenosis after venous thrombolysis has also been reported. In a small group of patients, patency was shown to be superior compared with conventional heparin and warfarin. Survival rates on Kaplan-Meier life table analysis, however, were equivalent.

D. Vena Caval Interruption

Historically, ligation of the vena cava was performed to prevent thrombi arising in the lower extremities and pelvis from reaching the pulmonary bed. Plication with a clip has also been attempted. Avoidance of complete occlusion maintained circulatory stability and resulted in a lower frequency of recurrent pulmonary emboli than complete ligation. In the latter, dilation of collateral vessels in the retroperitoneum became a potential route for pulmonary emboli.

Placement of a stainless steel filter, such as the Greenfield filter, is now the preferred procedure. Absolute indications for filter placement include recurrent thromboembolism in spite of adequate anticoagulation and deep venous thrombosis in patients at risk for hemorrhage. Relative indications include the presence of a propagating iliac or femoral vein thrombus despite adequate anticoagulation and a high-risk patient with a large free-floating iliac or femoral vein thrombus demonstrated on venography. Sepsis is not a contraindication to filter placement.

Filters are usually placed percutaneously through the uninvolved femoral vein or through a jugular vein and positioned below the renal veins. The long-term patency rate of the device is 98%, with a recurrent embolism rate of 4%. Up to 80% of the filter may become filled with thrombus before it loses its efficacy. Recurrent embolism is an indication for inferior venacavography to evaluate the filter for the presence of proximal thrombus. The most common complication is displacement, which occurs in 7% of patients.

E. Operative Embolectomy

Operative removal of a deep venous thrombus is usually reserved for cases of phlegmasia cerulea dolens with limb threat. The highest success rate is achieved when the procedure is performed within 24 hours after onset of symptoms. Although early postoperative results may be encouraging, subsequent venograms usually show rethrombosis. This is often due to incomplete thrombus removal and injury to the venous endothelium. Reocclusion is often well tolerated as long as it occurs after the formation of sufficient venous collaterals. Mechanical thrombectomy with creation of a temporary arteriovenous fistula can improve early patency and allow collaterals to develop. A recent study that examined long-term results after embolectomy found fewer instances of venous hypertension, valvular incompetency, and restrictions in activity among patients who had embolectomy performed for deep venous thrombosis of less than 3 days' duration.

Postthrombotic Syndrome

Venous thrombosis is often accompanied by symptoms of pain, swelling, and skin ulceration occurring immediately or years after an episode of DVT. It is present in over 50% of patients with proximal thrombosis and has been reported in one third of patients with calf thrombosis. The symptoms are thought to stem from the development of venous hypertension caused by valvular dysfunction. Residual venous obstruction may also contribute to the syndrome to a lesser extent. Thrombolytic therapy preserves valvular function and can potentially reduce the incidence of this phenomenon. Early results are promising. Standard treatment involves the use of graduated compression stockings and sequential compression devices.

Venous Thromboembolism in Pregnancy

Care of the pregnant patient focuses on avoiding teratogenic injury to the fetus. Patients can be treated with continuous unfractionated heparin and gradually switched over to multiple daily subcutaneous doses or low-molecular-weight heparin until delivery. Warfarin, reportedly safe for infants of nursing mothers, is continued for 4–6 weeks postpartum. Supplemental calcium should be given in cases of prolonged heparinization (longer than 1 month) to prevent heparin-induced osteoporosis. In the event of a bleeding contraindication or a documented pulmonary embolus, a vena caval filter can be placed. The procedure should be performed in the third trimester through an internal jugular approach. The site of deployment—contrary to what is done for a nonpregnant patient—is above the renal veins. This avoids kinking and displacement of the device by a gravid uterus.

AbuRahma AF et al: Iliofemoral deep vein thrombosis: conventional therapy versus lysis and percutaneous transluminal angioplasty and stenting. Ann Surg 2001;233:752–60.

Decousus H et al: A clinical trial of vena caval filters in the prevention of pulmonary embolism in patients with proximal deep-vein thrombosis. N Engl J Med 1998;338:409–15.

Erdman WA et al: Deep venous thrombosis of extremities: Role of MR imaging in the diagnosis. Radiology 1990;174:425–31.

Geerts WH et al: Prevention of venous thromboembolism. Chest 2001;119(1 Suppl):132S–75S.

Ginsberg JS: Management of venous thromboembolism. N Engl J Med 1996;335:1816–28.

Hingorani A et al: Upper extremity deep venous thrombosis and its impact on morbidity and mortality rates in a hospital-based population. J Vasc Surg 1997;26:853–60.

Hoyt DB, Swegle JR: Deep venous thrombosis in the surgical intensive care unit. Surg Clin North Am 1991;71:811–30.

Hull R, Raskob GE, Hirsh J: Continuous intravenous heparin compared with intermittent subcutaneous heparin in the initial treatment of proximal-vein thrombosis. N Engl J Med 1986;315:1109–14.

Hyers TM et al: Antithrombotic therapy for venous thromboembolic disease. Chest 2001;119(1 Suppl):176S–93S.

Kerr TM: Analysis of 1084 consecutive lower extremities involved with acute venous thrombosis diagnosed by duplex scanning. Surgery 1990;108:520–7.

Lensing AWA et al: Detection of deep-vein thrombosis by real-time B mode ultrasonography. N Engl J Med 1989;320:342–5.

Levine M et al: A comparison of low-molecular-weight heparin administered primarily at home with unfractionated heparin administered in the hospital for proximal deep-vein thrombosis. N Engl J Med 1996;334:677-81.

Levine MN et al: Hemorrhagic complications of anticoagulant treatment. Chest 1995;108(4 Suppl):276S–290S.

Levine MN et al: Optimal duration of oral anticoagulant therapy: a randomized trial comparing four weeks with three months of warfarin in patients with proximal deep vein thrombosis. Thromb Haemost 1995;74:606–11.

Markel A, Manzo RA, Strandness DE Jr: The potential role of thrombolytic therapy in venous thrombosis. Arch Intern Med 1992;152:1265–7.

Martinelli I et al: Risk factors for deep venous thrombosis of the upper extremities. Ann Intern Med 1997;126:707–11.

Plate G et al: Venous thrombectomy for iliofemoral vein thrombosis: 10-year results of a prospective randomized study. Eur J Vasc Endovasc Surg 1997;14:367–74.

Porteous MJ et al: Thigh length versus knee length stockings in the prevention of deep vein thrombosis. Brit J Surg 1989;76:296–7.

Prandoni P et al: A simple ultrasound approach for detection of recurrent proximal-vein thrombosis. Circulation 1993;88:1730–5.

Schulman S et al: The duration of oral anticoagulant therapy after a second episode of venous thromboembolism. N Engl J Med 1997;336:393–8.

Siragusa S et al: Low-molecular weight heparins and unfractionated heparin in the treatment of patients with acute venous thromboembolism: results of a meta-analysis. Am J Med 1996;100:269–77.

Wakefield TW: Treatment options for venous thrombosis. J Vasc Surg 2000;31:613–20.

Warkentin TE et al: Heparin-induced thrombocytopenia in patients treated with low-molecular weight heparin or unfractionated heparin. N Engl J Med 1995;332:1330–5.

Weinmann EE, Salzman EW. Deep-vein thrombosis. N Engl J Med 1994;331:1630–41.

Wells PS et al: Accuracy of clinical assessment of deep-vein thrombosis. Lancet 1995;345:1326–30.

ACUTE MESENTERIC ISCHEMIA

ESSENTIALS OF DIAGNOSIS

- *Severe acute abdominal pain out of proportion to the physical examination.*
- *Gastrointestinal symptoms—nausea, emesis, forceful evacuation.*
- *Abdominal distention and gastrointestinal hemorrhage.*
- *Leukocytosis, acidosis, and hyperamylasemia.*
- *Mesenteric arterial occlusion with minimal collateralization on angiography.*

General Considerations

Acute mesenteric ischemia of the bowel is an uncommon but dramatic occurrence among ICU patients, with an estimated overall incidence of 0.1% of all hospital admissions. Predisposing factors include age, cardiovascular disease, atherosclerosis, systemic disorders (collagen-vascular disease), hypercoagulable states, malignancy, portal hypertension, inflammation, and trauma. Semiacute and chronic syndromes have been described, but they are rare among ICU patients admitted for other reasons.

The consequences of vascular occlusion depend on the vessel involved, the extent of collateral flow, and the time period over which the occlusion took place. Acute occlusion of vascular inflow or outflow quickly causes ischemia and leads to transmural necrosis within 6–12 hours. The seromuscular layer is particularly sensitive and begins to slough within 4 hours. Xanthine oxidase, found in high concentrations within the villi, is responsible for the production of superoxides that mediates many of the toxic reactions. Ulceration and bacterial overgrowth follow ischemic sloughing. Bacterial proliferation leads to increased edema and further thrombosis of small vessels. Increased capillary permeability and the absorption of toxic products across the compromised mucosa causes remote complications such as respiratory distress syndrome. Continued ischemia leads to intraluminal sequestration of fluid which ultimately results in hypovolemia and hypotension.

Four general categories of acute mesenteric ischemia are recognized.

A. Acute Embolic Occlusion

Emboli to the superior mesenteric artery account for 40–50% of all cases. Because these are almost always mural thrombi of cardiac origin, up to 20% of patients have synchronous emboli to other arteries. In the majority of cases, the embolus lodges just distal to the origin of the superior mesenteric artery. Occasionally, the emboli fracture and travel into the distal arcades of the artery before they become lodged. Initially, collateral flow is adequate to maintain viability of the intestine. However, after a period of partial occlusion, vasoconstriction develops both proximal and distal to the embolus and produces profound ischemia.

B. Mesenteric Thrombosis

Progressive atherosclerotic narrowing of the origin of the superior mesenteric artery is responsible for mesenteric thrombosis. Conditions that compromise flow through the stenotic orifice can lead to thrombotic occlusion. Between 20% and 50% of patients with mesenteric thrombosis will give a history of postprandial pain and weight loss within the 6 months prior to admission. Many have severe and diffuse atherosclerosis, with a history of coronary, cardiac, or peripheral vascular arterial insufficiency. Mesenteric thrombosis occurs in 10–15% of all cases of acute mesenteric ischemia.

C. Venous Thrombosis

Once thought to be the major cause of acute mesenteric ischemia, venous thrombosis is diagnosed in 8–10% of patients. Hypercoagulable states including neoplasms, cirrhosis and portal hypertension, pancreatitis, peritonitis, diverticular disease, trauma, and splenectomy are precipitating factors. Presentation can be either acute or protracted, developing over a period of several weeks. Up to 60% of patients have a history of deep venous thrombosis in an extremity.

D. Nonocclusive Intestinal Ischemia

Hypoperfusion or a low flow state is the inciting event of acute mesenteric ischemia in 25% of cases. Coexistent conditions—predominantly cardiac pump failure—lead to prolonged visceral arterial spasm and subsequent tissue infarct. Shunting of arterial blood away from the seromuscular layer and the villi causes activation of toxic intermediates. The vasoconstriction may persist long after the inciting cause or agent has been removed. Pharmacologic agents such as ergotamine derivatives, digitalis, cocaine, and peripheral vasocontrictors administered for sepsis or postcardiovascular surgery are also associated with acute mesenteric ischemia. In 4% of patients undergoing repair of an aortic coarctation, postoperative hypertension may lead to a necrotizing vasculitis from reperfusion injury.

Clinical Features

A. Symptoms and Signs

Acute abdominal pain is the most common finding. Peritoneal signs are often absent on physical examination despite the complaint of sharp excruciating pain—thus the sine qua non of "pain out of proportion." Shortly thereafter, many patients experience rapid and forceful evacuation of the bowels. Nausea and vomiting—seen in 50% of patients—hematochezia, hematemesis, abdominal distention, back pain, and shock are late signs that usually accompany progression of intestinal necrosis. The presence of peritoneal signs often heralds the onset of systemic toxicity. Up to 30% of elderly patients develop mental confusion. The duration of symptoms, however, does not correlate with the reversibility of injury. A history of weight loss and an acute exacerbation of chronic abdominal pain are suggestive of acute thrombosis due to underlying chronic occlusive disease.

Mesenteric venous thrombosis also presents with pain as the initial finding, but only two-thirds of patients manifest clear signs of peritonitis. Occult blood is often present, though frank hematochezia or hematemesis is found in 15% of patients, usually from bleeding esophageal varices. The most common findings are abdominal pain (90%), vomiting (77%), nausea (54%), diarrhea (36%), and constipation (14%). Most patients have temperatures higher than 38 °C. Hemorrhage resulting from gastric varices due to isolated splenic vein thrombosis is termed sinistral portal hypertension. In this case, intestinal ischemia is not expected.

A variant of splanchnic venous disease has recently been described. Mesenteric inflammatory veno-occlusive disease results in unexplained acute mesenteric ischemia. Diagnosis is based on the presence of venulitis or phlebitis with a lymphocytic, necrotizing, granulomatous mural infiltrate on pathologic specimen examination.

B. Laboratory Findings

A marked leukocytosis, often greater than 15,000/μL, is usually present, although 10% of patients have a normal white cell count. The smooth muscle fraction (BB) of creatine kinase (CK) is elevated in the presence of intestinal infarction. Elevations of lactate dehydrogenase (LDH) may also be seen. Serum inorganic phosphate is often elevated, due either to spillage from phosphate-rich intestinal cells or from degradation of intracellular ATP. Approximately 80% of patients with intestinal infarction have high serum levels of inorganic phosphate, and 50% demonstrate hyperamylasemia. Fluid sequestration results in hemoconcentration and oliguria. Increased base deficit may occur but was found in only 18 of 43 patients in a retrospective study. Peritoneal fluid analysis typically reveals leukocytosis and bacteria proportionate to the extent of necrosis. It may not be helpful in the early stages.

C. Imaging Studies

Plain films of the abdomen should be obtained as an initial screening procedure. Nonspecific findings consistent with the diagnosis include air-fluid levels, dilated and thickened bowel wall, blunted plicae circulares, and distention of the bowel to the level of the splenic flexure. Specific findings of bowel necrosis include transmural air, pneumatosis intestinalis, or gas in the portal system. Barium contrast studies may reveal decreased motility and thumbprinting due to necrosis.

Angiography is the mainstay of the diagnosis and should be individualized. The presence of peritoneal signs and systemic toxicity requires immediate operative treatment to remove devitalized tissue. Mesenteric angiography can be performed early in hemodynamically stable patients suspected of having the disease with a sole complaint of abdominal pain. Radiographic findings will vary depending on the cause. When an embolus is present, early truncation of the superior mesenteric artery is observed. With acute thrombosis, complete obliteration of the trunk of the artery is common. The findings of nonocclusive ischemia are (1) tapered narrowing of the origins of multiple branches of the superior mesenteric artery, (2) segmental irregularities of the intestinal branches, (3) spasm of the arcades, and (4) impaired filling of the intramural branches. Findings consistent with mesenteric venous thrombosis include (1) demonstration of a thrombus in the superior mesenteric vein with partial or complete occlusion, (2) failure to visualize the superior mesenteric vein or portal vein, (3) slow or absent filling of the mesenteric veins, (4) arterial spasm, (5) failure of the arterial arcades to empty, (6) reflux of contrast into the artery, and (7) a prolonged blush phase. Abdominal CT scanning can establish the diagnosis in more than 90% of patients with venous occlusion. Thrombus with enhanced venous wall opacification is a highly indicative finding. Hypodensity of the superior mesenteric vein, thickening of the bowel wall, and the presence of peritoneal fluid are a diagnostic triad seen on CT suggesting probable bowel infarction. Scintiangiography with ^{99m}Tc sulfur colloid-labeled leukocytes has been described but is too unreliable for general use. Recently, the use of duplex scanning has been proposed as a bedside screening test, though the technique is limited by intestinal gas overlying the vessels of interest and the need for a skilled technician.

D. Special Studies

Laparoscopy can be useful in diagnosis, though complete exploration of the abdomen with the laparoscope is difficult. Furthermore, abdominal insufflation to more than

20 mm Hg reduces mesenteric blood flow and may exacerbate the condition. Preliminary evidence indicates that if CO_2 is used for insufflation at lower pressures, it may provide some mesenteric vasodilation. Colonoscopy may be useful if the large intestine is involved, though nonspecific colitis may be the only finding. Esophagogastroduodenoscopy can be used to detect and sclerose bleeding varices but does not treat the underlying venous thrombosis. Both modalities avail little in small bowel ischemia, the most common location of acute mesenteric ischemia. Bowel tonometry using an inflatable balloon to provide information about intramucosal pH (pH_i) may be helpful, though decreased motility may prevent proper peroral placement.

Differential Diagnosis

Other conditions associated with abdominal pain in the ICU such as a perforated ulcer, pancreatitis, acalculous cholecystitis, appendicitis, and gynecologic pathology in women must be investigated. These can often be identified by ultrasound and specific serum tests. Renal calculi produce colicky pain radiating to the groin. Aortic dissection and rupture of an abdominal aortic aneurysm are rare occurrences in patients admitted to the ICU for other reasons.

Treatment

Optimal outcome depends on rapid recognition and treatment. Initial therapy consists of fluid resuscitation, correction of electrolyte and acid-base abnormalities, and management of cardiac arrhythmias. Systemic heparinization is instituted in patients with suspected superior mesenteric artery thrombosis or venous occlusion. If time permits, demonstration of the offending lesion by angiography is ideal. When arterial spasm is present, 25 mg of tolazoline may be injected, followed by repeat angiography. If an embolus is the cause, an infusion of papaverine into the superior mesenteric artery orifice should be instituted immediately. The dose customarily used is 30–60 mg/h. Some also use papaverine in the face of mesenteric thrombosis, though catheter placement is difficult owing to the occluded arterial orifice. Papaverine infusion should be continued while the patient is readied for surgery. Because arterial spasm and the hypercoagulable state may persist even after successful surgery, papaverine and heparin infusions should be continued following operation. Broad-spectrum antibiotics are indicated both before and after surgery. Nonoperative therapy is appropriate (1) if there are significant contraindications to surgery, (2) if there are no peritoneal signs, and (3) if there is adequate perfusion of the vascular beds distal to the site of partial obstruction.

Infusion of thrombolytic agents has been anecdotally successful in both venous and arterial thrombosis. The presence of gastroesophageal varices—once thought to be a contraindication to this practice—were seen to resolve with successful venous clot lysis. Problems with access to the splanchnic venous system have limited this approach. In arterial thrombosis, lytic therapy should be instituted only in the most stable patients because of the time required for clot lysis. When patients are treated without operation, repeat angiography at 6- to 8-hour intervals is required to monitor the progress of therapy. Any worsening in the patient's condition is an indication for immediate operation.

Surgical management is aimed at restoration of flow and resection of nonviable bowel. Arterial inflow may be restored either by bypass, endarterectomy, or embolectomy. When venous thrombosis is present, extensive bowel resections may be required. Assessment of intestinal viability is often difficult, and adjuncts such as Doppler flow probes and tissue fluorescence are often used, though no method is always reliable in separating viable from ischemic bowel. A wide resection is usually undertaken as long as more than 6 feet of normal bowel remain. Sixty percent of recurrent infarcts occur in the area adjacent to the anastomosis. If the majority of the intestine is compromised, resection is more conservative, and second-look procedures to determine the viability of unresected bowel are commonly performed within 12–24 hours after the initial procedure.

Nonocclusive ischemia is best managed through treatment of the underlying disorder causing the low-flow state. Resuscitation and optimization of the patient's hemodynamic status are essential. Vasopressors should be discontinued if possible. An alternative to digoxin should be sought, especially in patients with portal hypertension. Digitalis derivatives promote mesenteric vasoconstriction in patients with hepatic congestion from congestive heart failure. Ergotamine poisoning is treated with selective infusion of vasodilators (eg, papaverine), sympatholytics, and anticoagulants. Angiotensin-converting enzyme inhibitors (eg, captopril) also serve to assuage the vasoconstrictive effects of the renin-angiotensinogen axis in hypovolemic patients. Surgery is reserved for resection of nonviable intestine. In addition to careful hemodynamic support, perioperative anticoagulation has been shown to improve survival in patients with mesenteric venous thrombosis. In one study, half of patients receiving no postoperative anticoagulation died. Without anticoagulation, one-third of patients will also experience a recurrence. Most centers recommend continuing anticoagulation indefinitely unless there is a contraindication or the factor responsible for the venous thrombosis has been corrected. Recently, intravenous glucagon administered during the early phase of reperfusion of ischemic intestinal segments has been shown experimentally to improve mucosal recovery, suggesting possible adjunctive use in the clinical setting.

Prognosis

Acute mesenteric ischemia carries a high mortality rate—in some series approaching 70%. When more than half of the small bowel must be resected, the death rate increases to as high as 85%. The cause of death in most cases is irreversible shock or advanced intestinal necrosis. Reconstruction is attempted in less than 10% of patients because findings at laparotomy often show advanced disease. Patients diagnosed with superior mesenteric artery thrombosis have an overall worse prognosis than those in whom distal embolization has occurred. Acute venous thrombosis has a 30% mortality rate, while nonocclusive intestinal ischemia has been associated with death rates as high as 90%. Early recognition of low-flow states, resuscitation, and aggressive therapy have lowered mortality.

Abd RA, Achor BG, Dallies DJ: Mesenteric venous thrombosis 1911 to 1984. Surgery 1987;101:383–8.

Bakau CW, Spray regen S, Wolf EL: Radiology in intestinal ischemia: Angiographic diagnosis and management. Surg Clin North Am 1992;72:125–41.

Boley JS, Alyea RN, Brandt LDI: Mesenteric venous thrombosis. Surg Clin North Am 1992;72:183–201.

Gangadharan SP, Wagner RJ, Cronenwett JL: Effect of intravenous glucagons on intestinal viability after segmental mesenteric ischemia. J Vasc Surg 1995;21:900–7.

Geelkerken RH, van Bockel JH: Mesenteric vascular disease: A review of diagnostic methods and therapies. Cardiovasc Surg 1995;3:247–60.

Greene FL, Ariyan S, Stansel HC Jr: Mesenteric and peripheral vascular ischemia secondary to ergotism. Surgery 1977;81:176–9.

Harward TR et al: Mesenteric venous thrombosis. J Vasc Surg 1989;9:328–33.

Jona J et al: Recurrent primary mesenteric venous thrombosis. JAMA 1974;227:1033–5.

Kaleya RN, Sammartano RJ, Boley SJ: Aggressive approach to acute mesenteric ischemia. Surg Clin North Am 1992;72: 157–82.

Kazmers A: Operative management of acute mesenteric ischemia. Ann Vasc Surg 1998;12:299–308.

Kurland B, Brandt LJ, Delaney HM: Diagnostic tests for intestinal ischemia. Surg Clin North Am 1992;72:85–105.

Leo PJ, Simonian HG: The role of serum phosphate level and acute ischemic bowel disease. Am J Emerg Med 1996;14:377–9.

Lilly MP et al: Duplex ultrasound measurements of changes in mesenteric blood flow. J Vasc Surg 1989;9:18–25.

Moneta GL et al: Mesenteric artery duplex scanning: A blinded, prospective study. J Vasc Surg 1993;17:79–84.

Myers SI et al: Chronic intestinal ischemia caused by intravenous cocaine use: Report of two cases and review of the literature. J Vasc Surg 1996;23:724–9.

Rhee RY, Gloviczki P: Mesenteric venous thrombosis. Surg Clin North Am 1997;77:327–38.

Robin P et al: Complete thrombolysis of mesenteric vein occlusion with recombinant tissue-type plasminogen activator. Lancet 1988;1:1391.

Sachs SM, Morton JH, Schwartz SI: Acute mesenteric ischemia. Surgery 1982;92:646–53.

Serreyn RF et al: Laparoscopic diagnosis of mesenteric venous thrombosis. Endoscopy 1986;18:249–50.

Wilson C et al: Acute superior mesenteric ischemia. Br J Surg 1987;74:279–81.

CRITICAL CARE OF THE VASCULAR SURGERY PATIENT

Atherosclerosis affects one in four Americans and constitutes a major international health problem. There are over 600,000 episodes of stroke and 1.5 million myocardial infarctions each year in the United States alone. Medical care of these patients is complicated by advanced age and additional medical comorbidities which create a challenge in preoperative and postsurgical management.

This section will address specific problems encountered when caring for vascular surgery patients.

RESPIRATORY MANAGEMENT

Vascular surgery patients often have an extensive smoking history. COPD, bronchitis, and asthma are therefore not unexpected. A room air arterial gas measurement often determines whether more extensive pulmonary workup is necessary. Formal pulmonary function tests are useful to determine the nature and extent of respiratory compromise. Encouragement in cessation of smoking for a minimum of 2 weeks prior to elective surgery and maximization of pulmonary reserve with adequate pharmacologic support for patients with obstructive or restrictive airway disease is ideal. Instruction in the use of incentive spirometry and deep breathing exercises is also helpful in restoring postsurgical lung function. Mechanical ventilator support is the rule in patients undergoing intracavitary aortic operations. An aggressive attempt at weaning should be instituted once the patient is sufficiently awake to cooperate and maintain airway patency. This should be followed by aggressive incentive spirometry, adequate pain control, and early ambulation. The details of ventilator management are presented in Chapter 12.

NUTRITIONAL MANAGEMENT

Nutritional support is a mandatory but frequently neglected aspect of postoperative care. The catabolic response following aortic surgery is pronounced. Because most vascular surgery patients are well-nourished prior to surgery, immediate institution of nutritional support is not necessary. However, if resumption of oral intake is not anticipated within 5–7 days after surgery, enteral nutrition should be started through a nasoenteric feeding tube. Extensive manipulation of the small bowel may cause mechanical ileus, though absorptive capacity is maintained. Transient pancreatitis can also be encountered in aortic surgery from retractor blade pancreatic irritation. Feeding with an elemental formula can be instituted at low rates (30 mL/h) and increased in volume as tolerated. Enteral feedings reduce the risk of septicemia associated with hyperalimentation catheters. This is of particular importance in vascular disease patients who have unincorporated graft surfaces exposed to the circulation. If nutritional support is required for more than 1 week, a nitrogen balance study should be completed to ensure that protein needs are being met.

MANAGEMENT OF ISCHEMIC HEART DISEASE

Atherosclerosis is a systemic disease that affects both the peripheral vasculature and the coronary arteries. An analysis of pooled data from 50 studies composed of more than 10,000 patients demonstrated the presence of coronary artery disease in 50% of patients who had operations for aortic aneurysms, carotid artery disease, and lower extremity ischemia. In another series of patients with known coronary artery disease undergoing vascular surgery, 63% were found to have ischemic cardiac events. In the Cleveland Clinic series, fatal myocardial infarction accounted for a 3.3% mortality rate after lower extremity procedures and a 6% mortality rate after aortic aneurysm resection. A study from the same institution utilizing routine coronary angiography before aortic surgery found that 85% of patients had some degree of coronary artery disease while 31% had severe disease consisting of either two- or three-vessel involvement or stenosis of the left anterior descending artery. In a study of 1000 patients undergoing routine coronary angiography, 14–22% of patients without any prior clinical history of coronary artery disease had severe coronary disease on angiography. It should be remembered, however, that demonstration of an anatomic lesion does not necessarily equate with physiologic compromise.

The pathophysiology of acute perioperative infarction is not completely understood, though multiple factors are certainly involved. These include catechol release, increased myocardial sensitivity to catechols, fluid sequestration, alterations in oxygen transport, hypercoagulable states, and tachycardia. Because elevations in heart rate and blood pressure increase the tension-time index, they result in increased oxygen consumption. Tachycardia further limits oxygen delivery by decreasing the diastolic filling time, during which the myocardium receives its perfusion.

Valvular heart disease also increases morbidity after vascular procedures. In the presence of aortic stenosis, up to 20% mortality may be expected for abdominal or thoracic operations and up to 10% for peripheral procedures.

Preoperative Assessment of Risk Due to Coronary Artery Disease

The high incidence of cardiac ischemia after vascular surgery frequently occasions preoperative admission of these patients to the ICU for hemodynamic evaluation and optimization of cardiac status. Several scales have been devised to predict surgical risk based on clinical assessment. The American Association of Anesthesiologists score is based on assessment of overall health and chronic disease. While generally useful, it is not sufficiently specific for use in patients with critical illnesses. An evaluation developed by Goldman employs nine variables to predict cardiac risk. Unfortunately, it underestimates cardiac complications in vascular patients and is able to predict cardiac mortality in only 50% of cases. An alternative scale includes a history of previous myocardial infarction, congestive heart failure, unstable angina, diabetes, and age over 70. Patients classified as intermediate-risk or high-risk were expected to have an event rate of 10–15%. Those in the low-risk group had a less than 5% incidence of cardiac ischemia.

A. Ambulatory Electrocardiographic (Holter) Monitoring

Continuous ambulatory monitoring of the ECG is used to detect clinically silent ischemia. A positive finding consists of six or more episodes in a 24-hour period of ST segment depression of more than 2 mm. A significantly greater incidence of perioperative cardiac morbidity and mortality occurs in those with abnormal results. A recent study found that 38% of patients with preoperative ischemia had postoperative cardiac events while less than 1% of patients without ischemia suffered cardiac morbidity. Continuous preoperative monitoring identifies those patients with clinically silent ischemia who might benefit from therapy. Although this method is simple, noninvasive, and inexpensive, it suffers from low sensitivity and has a positive predictive value of only 38%.

B. Exercise Electrocardiographic Testing

Exercise stress-induced alterations in the ECG have been used extensively to assess cardiac risk. Because they typically require walking or running, they are not suitable for use in dysvascular patients whose exercise tolerance is limited by claudication. Submaximal effort may yield false-negative results.

C. Dipyridamole-Thallium Scintigraphy

In this test, a pharmacologic agent is substituted for exercise to increase coronary artery blood flow. Intravenously administered dipyridamole promotes coronary artery blood flow without increasing myocardial oxygen consumption by increasing the intracellular concentration of adenosine. Blood flow increases through normal arteries that dilate maximally. Stenotic arteries do not respond because of fixed anatomic lesions. Prior to administration of dipyridamole, thallium-201 is injected to demonstrate areas of myocardial ischemia. Because thallium-201 is preferentially taken up by the normal myocardium, areas of hypoperfusion appear as "cold" spots. If homogeneity improves after dipyridamole is given, thallium redistribution is said to have occurred, and the scan is considered positive. Redistributed areas consist of viable but ischemic myocardium that are at risk for infarction. Areas that fail to improve after dipyridamole infusion probably consist of previously infarcted muscle that is not at risk for a future ischemic event. Thallium redistribution is associated with a 30–50% risk of some postoperative cardiac event. The positive predictive value of the test is only 22%. A negative scan indicates a low likelihood of perioperative infarction, but a positive scan is of ambiguous import. The specificity of thallium scans can be increased by combining them with other risk factors for myocardial ischemia, including age, a history of angina, the presence of Q waves on ECG, the presence of type 1 diabetes, and a history of therapy-dependent ventricular ectopy. The risk of a cardiac event in intermediate-risk patients (one or two predictors) is as high as 30%. This finding has since been challenged by reports from several centers finding little use for dipyridamole-thallium scanning in moderate-risk patients and suggesting that a new procedure be investigated.

D. Radionuclide Ventriculography

Multiple-gated acquisition (MUGA) blood pool scans provide quantitative information about the left ventricular ejection fraction (LVEF) and ventricular wall motion. The normal LVEF is 55% or greater. Those with a normal LVEF are at low risk for postoperative cardiac events. Those with LVEF values between 36% and 55% are at intermediate risk with a perioperative infarction risk of 20%. High-risk patients have LVEF values less than 35% and had an 80% risk of myocardial infarction. Unfortunately, the test has a low sensitivity (44%), which means that a negative study does not necessarily eliminate the risk of myocardial infarction.

E. Dobutamine Stress Echocardiography

Dobutamine stimulates myocardial contractility and increases heart rate through β_1 activity. Administration of this pharmacologic agent results in higher oxygen demand. Two-dimensional echocardiography is then used to visualize regional wall dysfunction from myocardial ischemia. Compared with dipyridamole-thallium scanning, this test was also initially more successful in predicting perioperative cardiac events. However, ensuing studies reported inconsistent results with a sensitivity ranging from 54–96% and specificity in the range of 57–95% in comparison with cardiac catheterization.

F. Coronary Angiography

Coronary angiography should be used only in selected patients whose noninvasive studies place them at high risk for coronary events. The results of angiography can be used to plan further procedures such as angioplasty or coronary artery bypass.

Postoperative Cardiac Management

Postoperative cardiac ischemia and myocardial infarction are caused by an increased myocardial oxygen requirement in the face of inadequate supply. Myocardial oxygen consumption is related to the "tension-time" index, which is the product of systolic blood pressure and heart rate. Animal studies have shown that cardiac work and myocardial oxygen consumption both increase when the heart pumps against elevated diastolic pressures. Prolonged work against increased afterload results in myocardial hypertrophy, which also increases oxygen consumption. Tachycardia has two adverse effects on myocardial oxygen balance. First, it directly increases oxygen demand by increasing the time-tension index; and second, it reduces the diastolic filling time, thereby limiting the period during which myocardial blood flow occurs. Pharmacologic management is frequently necessary to improve myocardial oxygenation by decreasing the heart rate and lowering blood pressure.

Antihypertensive Therapy

Postoperative hypertension occurs in up to 50% of patients after aortic or carotid surgery. Pain is one of the most common causes and should be addressed initially. Small intravenous doses of morphine sulfate should be titrated to effect. Hypotension and respiratory depression are the major complications of opioid administration. Opioids should be given to carotid surgery patients only after they have recovered from their anesthetic and a postoperative neurologic examination has been completed. Lorazepam is a relatively short-acting benzodiazepine that provides sedation. It may be used as an adjunct to the analgesic effect of morphine.

Lorazepam is particularly useful in aortic surgery patients who require mechanical ventilation after operation. The initial intravenous dose is usually 2–3 mg titrated to effect at intervals of 4–6 hours.

Excessive intraoperative volume administration may cause postsurgical hypertension. This is particularly true among patients who have received epidural anesthetics that cause vasodilation. Resolution of the block and return of normal vascular tone may result in hypertension. Hypervolemia may also follow mannitol administration and excessive volume loading instituted prior to removal of the aortic cross-clamp. Postoperative volume status should be evaluated and optimized with the aid of a pulmonary artery flotation catheter. Careful administration of diuretics is required to avoid inadvertent iatrogenic hypervolemia.

Once remediable causes of hypertension have been eliminated, persistent hypertension should be treated to reduce myocardial oxygen demand due to increased wall stress. The threshold for treatment will vary with the patient, the type of procedure performed, the duration of hypertension, and preoperative risk factors. Elevation of systolic blood pressure above 120% of baseline is a reasonable point at which therapy should be instituted. Agents with shorter half-lives allow more precise titration of blood pressure, while longer-acting agents have the advantage of decreased dosing requirements. Nitroprusside and nitroglycerin are both fast-acting agents which can be given intravenously. Nitroprusside has a balanced effect because it dilates both arterioles and veins. As an arterial vasodilator, it lowers blood pressure by decreasing arteriolar vascular resistance without increasing venous capacity. The decreased afterload reflexively increases cardiac sympathetic stimulation that may result in undesirable tachycardia. Nitroglycerin is preferred because it produces coronary artery vasodilation in addition to decreasing preload. Because nitroglycerin can precipitously decrease filling pressures, it is imperative to ensure normal PCWP prior to the institution of therapy. Intravenous doses are started near 5 μg/min and increased by this amount every 5–10 minutes until the desired effect is reached. The normal vasodilatory dose is between 50 and 100 μg/min, though some patients require doses as high as 400 μg/min. High doses can be tolerated for several days, though methemoglobin concentration should be monitored.

Agents that provide beta-adrenergic blockade may also be used to treat postoperative hypertension. Labetalol is particularly useful because it provides not only nonspecific beta blockade but prevents reflex increases in vasoconstriction by its alpha-adrenergic blocking activity. Labetalol has a relatively long half-life of 6–8 hours and should be used with caution in patients with hepatic and renal insufficiency because of its route of elimination. The initial intravenous dose is 10–25 mg, supplemented every half-hour to desired effect. Angiotensin-converting enzyme inhibitors, initially used to decrease afterload in heart failure, were recently demonstrated to significantly reduce mortality, myocardial infarction, stroke, cardiac arrest and heart failure. The Heart Outcomes Prevention Evaluation Study investigators found that treating 1000 patients with ramipril (long-acting ACE-inhibitor) for 4 years prevented approximately 150 events in 70 patients.

Tachycardia

Fever, pain, and hypovolemia are the most common causes of tachycardia (heart rate > 100 beats/min) in postoperative patients. Hypovolemia may be caused by inadequate volume replacement or by continued volume loss such as hemorrhage or osmotic diuresis. Unrecognized causes of obligatory osmotic diuresis include hyperglycemia and intravenous contrast material administered prior to or during surgery. Pulmonary artery flotation catheters facilitate the evaluation of tachycardia by providing information on relative volume status. After inciting causes have been addressed, primary tachycardia should be treated if the heart rate remains elevated. Esmolol is an agent that is relatively β_1-selective and has a half-life of only 9–10 minutes. A loading dose of 500 μg/kg is administered over 1 minute, followed by a continuous infusion of 50 μg/kg/min. The infusion rate is decreased as tachycardia resolves.

RENAL FAILURE

The incidence and prognosis of acute renal failure occurring after vascular surgery depends upon the overall preoperative status of the patient, the nature of the surgery performed, and associated complications such as cardiac failure or sepsis. The reported incidence of acute renal failure after elective aortic surgery ranges from 1–15%. Following surgery for ruptured aortic aneurysms, it is between 21% and 100%, with associated mortality rates between 50% and 95%. In spite of improved intraoperative and postsurgical management, the incidence of acute renal failure after vascular surgery has not changed appreciably in the past 20 years. Several factors contribute to the development of renal failure, including suprarenal aortic cross-clamping, renal artery occlusion, declamping hypotension, and embolization of atherosclerotic debris to the kidneys. Autopsy studies of patients with postischemic acute renal failure have found minimal alterations of glomerular architecture in the face of profound disruption of tubular morphology. Acute tubular necrosis or luminal obstruction caused by sloughing of tubular cells is thought to be the inciting event.

Intraoperative maneuvers aimed at protecting renal function are directed mainly at reducing the severity and duration of renal ischemia. Circulating blood volume and cardiac output should be optimized prior to interruption of renal blood flow. The intravenous infusion of 12.5–25 g of mannitol prior to aortic occlusion is common practice. Mannitol offers a protective effect by (1) expanding circulating blood volume, (2) acting as an osmotic diuretic to promote urine flow and prevent stasis, (3) attenuating the reduction in cortical blood flow, and (4) serving as a free radical scavenger. Intraoperative contrast angiography produces a postoperative osmotic diuresis and makes absolute urine output an unreliable indicator of renal perfusion. When dye has been used, sufficient fluid should be administered to reduce urine specific gravity below 1.015. In the postoperative period, maintenance of adequate blood volume and cardiac output are the best defenses against renal failure. A pulmonary artery catheter should be used to assess venous return and cardiac function in patients who have had intra-abdominal surgery. Sufficient maintenance and replacement fluid must be given to ensure adequate cardiac preload. Inotropic agents such as dopamine or dobutamine may also be required. Dopamine in doses below 5 μg/kg/min promotes diuresis by dilating renal afferent arterioles. Recently, the administration of oral acetylcysteine along with hydration has been shown to prevent the reduction in renal function caused by low-osmolarity contrast agents in patients with chronic renal insufficiency. Its vasodilatory and antioxidant properties are speculated to be the mechanisms of action. Acetylcysteine is given in a dosage of 600 mg twice on the day prior to and on the day of contrast administration.

Reperfusion of severely ischemic muscle beds may cause the release of myoglobin into the circulation. A positive dipstick reaction for urine hemoglobin without the presence of red blood cells on microscopic analysis is evidence of myoglobinuria. Administration of sodium bicarbonate (100 meq/L) admixed with maintenance intravenous solutions should be instituted to alkalinize the urine. Urine volume must be maintained above 1–2 mL/kg/h. The myonephrotic syndrome of renal failure in the face of progressive rhabdomyolysis carries a mortality rate of more than 50%.

Other causes of oliguria include aminoglycoside toxicity and postrenal obstruction. The latter may be caused by a kinked urinary catheter or by inadvertent intraoperative ureteral ligation. After other causes of oliguria have been excluded, radionuclide imaging is reasonable to assess renal blood flow and urinary excretion. If concern about postrenal obstruction exists, bedside ultrasound can be used to identify hydronephrosis.

COMPLICATIONS OF VASCULAR SURGERY

Infection

Prosthetic graft infection is a devastating complication that occurs in 1–6% of cases depending on comorbid factors, location, and type of graft. The organism usually responsible is *Staphylococcus aureus,* though others, including yeasts, anaerobic bacteria, and mycobacteria, have been identified. Most graft infections are diagnosed after discharge (> 4 months) rather than in the early postoperative period. Perioperative antibiotic prophylaxis usually consists of a first-generation cephalosporin with good activity against *S aureus* and *Staphylococcus epidermidis.* It should be noted that comparable rates of graft infection have been reported both with and without the use of perioperative antibiotics.

Antibiotic administration should be continued until all indwelling intravenous and urinary catheters have been removed. Patients who have undergone reconstruction following vascular trauma should be observed closely for evidence of necrosis at wound sites. Devitalized tissue is an excellent culture source for bacteria. Early debridement and sufficient autologous coverage can prevent the late sequelae of graft infections—namely, thrombosis, rupture, and the development of para-anastomotic pseudoaneurysms.

Gastrointestinal Complications

Ischemic colitis and mesenteric ischemia are feared complications following resection of an abdominal aortic aneurysm. Interruption of the blood supply to the left colon following ligation of the inferior mesenteric artery is the usual cause, especially after repair of a ruptured aneurysm. In patients with severe chronic occlusive disease or those who have had previous abdominal procedures, interruption of vital visceral collaterals can also contribute to bowel ischemia. Early nonspecific harbingers of this complication include an acute fever spike with increased white cell count, lactic acidosis, and bloody diarrhea. Antibiotics, intravenous fluid administration, and immediate sigmoidoscopy and colonoscopy are undertaken. Once the diagnosis is verified, a transmural infarct requires operative resection. Expectant management is justified in cases where ischemia does not involve the full thickness of the bowel wall.

Acalculous cholecystitis occurs in 1% of all patients undergoing aortic surgery. Right upper quadrant abdominal pain, fever, leukocytosis, and hyperbilirubinemia are common. Bedside ultrasonography is preferred over ^{99m}Tc-HIDA scanning to establish the diagnosis.

Immediate cholecystectomy or cholecystostomy is usually required. Ischemic pancreatitis may be confused with cholecystitis. Elevation of the serum amylase and lipase allows separation of the two. A mild pancreatitis is caused by exposure of the aorta and retractor injury. It is usually self-limiting.

COMPLICATIONS OF COMMON VASCULAR PROCEDURES

Carotid Endarterectomy

Either hypotension or hypertension may occur early in the postoperative course. Hypertension may lead to the formation of neck hematomas and hemorrhagic stroke. Hypotension can lower the cerebral perfusion pressure that a hypertensive patient is normally accustomed to and thus result in cerebral infarct. Judicious use of fast-acting vasodilators (eg, nitroglycerin, nitroprusside), beta-blockers (eg, esmolol), or vasoconstrictors (eg, dopamine) in the immediate perioperative period to maintain a constant and stable blood pressure is a sound management stratagem. Effective weaning from these agents is accomplished once sufficient volume is infused.

The incidence of postoperative strokes ranges from 1–3%. Although the majority result from intraoperative embolization or cerebral ischemia, up to 19% may be due to acute thrombosis of the carotid artery. Transient ischemic attacks within the first week have been reported to be as high as 8%. When a patient is first noted to have a neurologic deficit, determining internal carotid artery patency is important since prospects for neurologic recovery are directly related to the speed with which flow is restored. If no intraoperative completion studies were performed, initial diagnostic evaluation should be via noninvasive bedside imaging such as Doppler ultrasound or duplex scanning. Patients with abnormal or equivocal findings require immediate reexploration. If noninvasive studies are normal, emergency carotid angiography is indicated to identify small defects that can be repaired. If the patient had a normal intraoperative completion arteriogram or duplex scan, the source of deficit is embolic and reoperation offers little benefit.

Headaches after carotid surgery are not uncommon. Severe headaches in the face of hypertension should be carefully monitored and the blood pressure expeditiously controlled. A CT scan of the brain is obtained, and a diagnosis of cerebral hyperperfusion syndrome is then entertained. This can happen in patients undergoing endarterectomy for chronic severe occlusive disease or in patients with an acute cerebrovascular accident. The common denominator is reactive hyperemia or cerebral reperfusion injury. Lesser forms of this condition result in symptoms consistent with mild cerebral edema, headache, and seizures. A more severe presentation results in catastrophic intracerebral hemorrhage from vessel rupture. Prompt recognition and treatment with antihypertensives, osmotic diuretics, and anticonvulsants can be lifesaving. If intracerebral hemorrhage has occurred, the prognosis is poor.

Aortic Operations

Abdominal aortic aneurysm repair in the elective setting has a mortality rate of 1–3%. Repaired emergently, mortality is often greater than 50%. Predictors that herald poor survival include the duration and severity of perioperative shock, hypothermia, and cardiac reserve. Postoperatively, myocardial infarction, coagulopathy, renal failure, respiratory insufficiency, ischemic bowel, poor nutrition, and infection often contribute to morbidity. Meticulous intensive care monitoring with a pulmonary catheter and aggressive treatment are mandatory. Adequate intravascular volume replacement is necessary to maintain organ perfusion. Patients often require a significant amount of volume for the first 24–48 hours due to shifts of intravascular fluid into the interstitium. On the third or fourth day, reentry into the vascular system occurs and a brisk diuresis ensues. At this stage, electrolytes are carefully replaced and urine output maintained, with diuretics if necessary. Prolonged mechanical ventilation is required for respiratory failure and hemodialysis for renal compromise. Mesenteric ischemia and ischemic colitis may result, and the first sign is often an uncorrectable metabolic acidosis, fever, and rapid leukocytosis. Melena and hematochezia are late signs and portend bowel necrosis. Prolonged shock and ischemia of the spinal cord result in paraplegia in 2% of patients. Corticosteroids may be used once other causes of spinal shock have been eliminated.

Peripheral Operations

The most common cause of morbidity in lower extremity bypass operations is cardiac insufficiency. Preoperative optimization and dosing with beta-blockers have been shown to decrease postoperative events. Prolonged hypotension or hypovolemia may lead not only to myocardial ischemia but also to thrombosis of the bypass graft. Careful hemodynamic monitoring and support can prevent these complications. If a palpable pulse is present distal to the graft, it should be monitored regularly for any change in strength or character. An abrupt decline or absence of the pulse is highly suggestive of graft occlusion. In patients who are admitted to the ICU without palpable pulses, a Doppler probe or piezoelectric pulse monitor can be used to evaluate graft patency. A pulse oximeter probe placed on a finger or toe distal to the bypass site is another convenient technique for monitoring graft patency. Revascularization for traumatic injury or chronic ischemia may cause limb swelling that resolves with elevation. The development of a compartment syndrome should be immediately recognized and promptly treated with fasciotomies. In patients with prolonged ischemia, myoglobinuria may occur after revascularization and may lead to renal failure unless recognized and treated with adequate hydration and diuresis.

Angevine PD et al: Significant reductions in length of stay after carotid endarterectomy can be safely accomplished without modifying either anesthetic technique or postoperative ICU monitoring. Stroke 1999;30:2341–6.

Bjorek M, Bergqvist D, Troeng T: Incidence and clinical presentation of bowel ischemia after aortoiliac surgery—2930 operations from a population-based registry in Sweden. Eur J Endovasc Surg 1996;12:139.

Davila-Roman VG et al: Dobutamine stress echocardiography predicts surgical outcome in patients with an aortic aneurysm and peripheral vascular disease. J Am Coll Cardiol 1993; 21:957–63.

Eagle KA et al: Combining clinical and thallium data optimizes preoperative assessment of cardiac risk before major vascular surgery. Ann Intern Med 1989;110:859–66.

Eagle KA et al: Guidelines for perioperative cardiovascular evaluation for noncardiac surgery. Report of the American College of Cardiology/American Heart Association Task Force on Practice Guidelines. Committee on Perioperative Cardiovascular Evaluation for Noncardiac Surgery. Circulation 1996; 93:1278–317.

Farkas JC et al: Acute colorectal ischemia after aortic surgery: Pathophysiology and prognostic criteria. Ann Vasc Surg 1992;6:111–8.

Frishman WH et al: Beta-adrenergic blockade and calcium channel blockade in myocardial infarction. Med Clin North Am 1989;73:409–36.

Goldman L et al: Multifactorial index of cardiac risk in noncardiac surgical procedures. N Engl J Med 1977;297:845–50.

Hertzer NR et al: Coronary artery disease in peripheral vascular patients: A classification of 1000 coronary angiograms and results of surgical management. Ann Surg 1984;199:223–33.

Jamieson WR et al: Influence of ischemic heart disease on early and late mortality after surgery for peripheral occlusive vascular disease. Circulation 1982;66(2 Part 2): I92–7.

Jayr C et al: Preoperative and interoperative factors associated with prolonged mechanical ventilation: A study in patients following major vascular surgery. Chest 1993;103:1231–6.

Mangano DT et al: Dipyridamole thallium-201 scintigraphy as a preoperative screening test: A reexamination of its predictive potential. Circulation 1991;84:493–502.

Miller DC, Myers BD: Pathophysiology and prevention of acute renal failure associated with thoracoabdominal or abdominal aortic surgery. J Vasc Surg 1987;5:518–23.

Nicholson ML et al: Randomized control trial of the effect of mannitol on renal reperfusion injury during aortic aneurysm surgery. Br J Surg 1996;83:1230–3.

O'Donnell D, Clarke G, Hurst P: Acute renal failure following surgery for abdominal aortic aneurysm. Aust N Z J Surg 1989;59:405–8.

Pasternack PF et al: The value of radionuclide angiography as a predictor of perioperative myocardial infarction in patients undergoing abdominal aortic aneurysm resection. J Vasc Surg 1984;1:320–5.

Perry MO, Fantini G: Ischemia: Profile of an enemy. Reperfusion injury of skeletal muscle. J Vasc Surg 1987;6:231–4.

Poldermans D et al: The effect of bisoprolol on perioperative mortality and myocardial infarction in high-risk patients undergoing vascular surgery. N Engl J Med 1999;341:1789–94.

Powell RJ et al: Effect of renal insufficiency on outcome following infrarenal aortic surgery. Am J Surg 1997;174:126–30.

Raby KE et al: Correlation between preoperative ischemia and major cardiac events after peripheral vascular surgery. N Engl J Med 1989;321:1296–300.

Tepel M et al: Prevention of radiographic-contrast-agent-induced reductions in renal function by acetylcysteine. N Engl J Med 2000;343:180–184.

Samson RH et al: A modified classification and approach to the management of infections involving peripheral arterial prosthetic grafts. J Vasc Surg 1988;8:147–53.

Yusuf S et al: Effects of an angiotensin-converting-enzyme inhibitor, ramipril, on cardiovascular events in high-risk patients. The Heart Outcomes Prevention Evaluation Study Investigators. N Engl J Med. 2000;342:145–53.

Critical Care of Neurologic Disease 30

Hugh B. McIntyre, MD, PhD, Linda Chang, MD, & Bruce L. Miller, MD

Alterations of consciousness, including coma, seizures, and neuromuscular disorders account for many of the neurologic problems in patients admitted to intensive care units. Therefore, this chapter emphasizes encephalopathy and coma, seizures and status epilepticus, and problems associated with neuromuscular disorders. A comprehensive review of cerebrovascular disease and stroke syndromes is beyond the scope of this book, but since the critical care physician will undoubtedly have to deal with cerebrovascular diseases, some fundamental aspects of these disorders are described. In addition, certain aspects and complications of central nervous system infectious diseases are included.

ENCEPHALOPATHY & COMA

COMA

The brain controls the individual's ability to breathe, obtain food and water, and avoid noxious stimuli in the environment. When the individual slips into coma, the ability to perform these functions is lost, and the patient will not survive unless coma is reversed. In this sense, coma represents a global failure of brain function. There are many causes of coma, some of them reversible. The first responsibility of the physician caring for a patient in coma is to ensure that breathing, circulation, and nutrition are maintained. The cause of coma must then be determined and reversible causes treated appropriately.

Normal consciousness has two main components: content and arousal. They have different anatomic substrates, with the former localized largely in the cerebral cortex and the latter dependent upon the brain stem reticular activating system. Injury to the dominant cortical hemisphere leads to impairment or loss of language function, but bilateral cortical injury is required for complete loss of consciousness. Furthermore, the cortex is responsible for interpreting incoming signals. This includes encoding and assigning "meaning" to emotional and sensory inputs. When the cortex is diffusely injured, the ability to reflect upon and interpret experience is lost, and for that reason the content of consciousness is lost as well.

The major role of the brain stem reticular activating system is to arouse and alert the cortex so that the organism can reflect upon and react to stimuli from the environment. A patient can lose consciousness by two different mechanisms: diffuse dysfunction of the cerebral cortex or injury to the reticular activating system. Coma often develops as a result of injury to both areas. However, cortical neurons are extremely sensitive to a variety of metabolic and toxic injuries, including hypoxia, hypercapnia, hyponatremia, hypernatremia, hypoglycemia, hyperglycemia, and many drugs, while the brain stem is more resistant to these injuries. Thus, toxic and metabolic injuries tend to first cause dysfunction in cortical neurons and only with increasing severity influence the brain stem. In contrast, coma due to primary brain injury affects the reticular activating system. These major anatomic differences allow the clinician to distinguish metabolic from structural causes of coma.

Neuroimaging techniques suggest that there may be a fundamental pathophysiologic basis for many of the metabolic causes of coma, perhaps explaining why so many cases with different causes present with such similar clinical profiles. In comas due to metabolic encephalopathy, a profound and diffuse decrease in cerebral glucose metabolism has been shown using positron emission tomography. Similarly, severe and diffuse cerebral hypoperfusion as measured with ^{133}Xe appears in patients in coma due to sepsis, hepatic encephalopathy, hypoxia, head trauma, and cocaine intoxication. Studies in comatose patients utilizing ^{31}P magnetic resonance spectroscopy have shown dramatic decreases in the brain's energy-containing phosphorus compounds, including ATP and phosphocreatine. This work suggests that any process which compromises cortical neuronal energy production may lead to a comatose state.

Clinical Features

One key issue in the evaluation of any unconscious patient is whether the unconscious state is due to metabolic, toxic, or structural brain injury. Because there are only minor differences in the clinical characteristics of comatose states due to varying types of metabolic and toxic insults, the clinical examination cannot definitively distinguish one metabolic cause from another;

thus, the cause must be sought or confirmed with laboratory investigations. In contrast, if the clinical examination suggests structural brain injury, emergency imaging tests must be performed to determine the cause so that appropriate treatment can be initiated.

Simultaneously with the assessment of the neurologic examination, it is critical that the physician obtain an accurate history. Although a comatose patient cannot give a history, relatives, housemates, and others can often describe the onset of coma and provide information regarding medications and preexisting illnesses. Even when information from these sources is not available, paramedics usually can provide details about the circumstances in which the patient was found. In all cases, a check of the patient's pockets and purse or wallet may help to elicit important medical data, and some patients wear medical bracelets or necklaces that will alert the examiner to potential causes of coma.

Rapidity of onset is an important clue to the cause of coma. Certain metabolic insults such as hypoxia, ischemia, or hypoglycemia may come on suddenly, while others such as hyponatremia, hypernatremia, and hyperglycemia develop subacutely. Similarly, subarachnoid hemorrhage or brain stem ischemic stroke can lead to sudden coma, while coma related to chronic subdural hematoma, cortical ischemic stroke, or brain tumor usually develops slowly.

The five main areas that need to be assessed in the evaluation of a patient in coma are the following: (1) level of consciousness, (2) pupillary responses and ophthalmoscopic examination, (3) oculomotor system, (4) motor systems, and (5) respiratory and circulatory systems.

Based upon the findings in these domains, it is usually possible to accurately localize the specific regions in the brain that are impaired. Table 30–1 lists changes that occur with injury at different anatomic areas of the brain. A precise anatomic localization of the area of dysfunction in the brain often helps to elucidate the cause of coma. Although coma scales are helpful in assessing prognosis, they are not a substitute for neurologic examination since they neither localize the area of dysfunction nor help in determination of the cause.

A. Level of Consciousness

Many terms such as stuporous, lethargic, drowsy, and semicomatose have been used to characterize degrees of altered consciousness. However, it is better to describe the patient's spontaneous activity, response to verbal stimuli, and reaction to painful stimuli in precise terms that do not have different meanings to different observers. A carefully recorded description of the patient's level of consciousness upon entry into the hospital will be invaluable in following the progression of the comatose state. With herniation from a large unilateral cerebral hemisphere mass, drowsiness occurs when the reticular activating system in the thalamus is compressed; coma ensues when injury to the reticular activating system reaches the midbrain.

The best places to apply painful stimuli to determine arousability are over the sternum or the nail beds; these maneuvers also help to determine whether the patient responds with evidence of focality, eg, if there is no movement of one side while the other hand attempts to remove the painful stimulus.

B. Pupillary and Ophthalmoscopic Evaluation

Perhaps no component of the neurologic examination is as valuable for differentiating metabolic or toxic coma from coma due to structural brain disease as inspection of the pupils. Pupillary size is determined by the relative contributions of the parasympathetic and sympathetic autonomic fibers. Coma associated with brain injury usually exhibits changes in the pupillary response. These changes occur because most structural comas are associ-

Table 30–1. Localization of brain lesions in a comatose patient.

Anatomic Level	Mental Status	Pupillary Size and Position	Eye Movement	Motor Responses	Respiration and Circulation
Diencephalon	Drowsy	Small (1–2 mm)	Normal	Abnormalities of flexion	Cheyne-Stokes
Midbrain	Coma	Fixed in mid position	Dysconjugate	Abnormalities of extension	Hyperventilation
Pons	Coma	1 mm in primary pontine injury; fixed and 4–5 mm with prior midbrain injury	Complete paralysis	Abnormalities of extension	Hyperventilation
Medulla	Variable	Variable	Variable	Flaccid	Apnea, circulatory collapse

ated with injury to the reticular activating system in the brain stem, where the Edinger-Westphal and sympathetic autonomic fibers are located. With acute injury to the midbrain, the pupils become fixed in mid position as a result of simultaneous injury of sympathetic and parasympathetic fibers. In contrast, injury to the pons often is associated with pinpoint, minimally reactive pupils. Lateral tentorial herniation of the temporal lobe may result in compression of the third cranial nerve and the parasympathetic fibers traveling with it, causing dilation of the pupil on the side of the herniation. In some lateral herniations, there will be compression of the contralateral third nerve against the edge of the tentorium.

A major characteristic of coma due to metabolic diseases is sparing of the pupillary response. This occurs because metabolic coma causes selective dysfunction of the cortex while the centers in the brain stem that control the pupils are spared. Many comas due to drugs spare the pupils, though some commonly used drugs do influence the pupillary response (Table 30–2).

The ophthalmoscopic examination can provide valuable information. Papilledema usually implies increased intracranial pressure, while subhyaloid hemorrhage, which appears as a fresh, red flame-shaped hemorrhage between the retina and vitreous, is virtually pathognomonic of subarachnoid hemorrhage.

Despite the importance of the ophthalmoscopic evaluation, under no circumstances should the pupil be dilated in a comatose patient, since changes in the pupils are often the most reliable clinical indication of deterioration following brain injury.

Table 30–2. Physical findings in drug-induced comas.

Drug Type	Pupillary Response	Other Changes
Opioids	Pinpoint	None
Barbiturates and benzodiazepines	Reactive	None
Anticholinergics (scopolamine, etc.)	Pupils dilated	Tachycardia, seizures
Anticholinesterases (organophosphates)	Pupils constricted	Bradycardia, sweating, salivation
Cocaine and amphetamine	Pupils dilated	Tachycardia, hypertension, hypotension, arrhythmia
Neuroleptics	Pupils variable	Motor rigidity, hypotension, hyperthermia
Antidepressants	Pupils dilated	Rarely seizure

C. Oculomotor System

Like the pupillary responses, changes in the oculomotor system often occur with primary neurologic injury. The system responsible for moving the eyes is located between the sixth nerve in the pons and the third nerve in the midbrain. Closely adjacent to the sixth nerve is a gaze center known as the pontine paramedian reticular formation (PPRF). Just prior to moving one of the eyes laterally, which is accomplished with the sixth nerve, there is rapid firing in the PPRF. The contralateral eye will deviate medially via fibers that travel from the PPRF, cross in the pons, and travel medially to the contralateral third nerve nucleus in the medial longitudinal fasciculus.

The simplest way to test the viability of this system is the oculocephalic ("doll's eye") reflex. For this test, the patient is positioned with 30-degree neck extension and the head is moved from side to side. If the brain stem PPRF and the vestibular system are intact, the eyes should move smoothly in the direction opposite to that in which the head is moved. A more precise test is the caloric oculovestibular response. For this test, the comatose patient is elevated to a 30-degree angle and one tympanic membrane is irrigated with ice-cold water. Ten milliliters usually is sufficient to produce a response. Within 1–2 minutes, both eyes should deviate laterally toward the side where the cold water was instilled. In metabolic or toxic coma, this system is spared, while in many structural comas the oculovestibular system is impaired; in brain death, it is absent. In the normal, awake patient, slow deviation toward the side of the stimulus is lost, and nystagmus in the contralateral direction is observed.

D. Motor Systems

Primary brain lesions often are associated with focal motor deficits, but in metabolic or toxic states, focal motor findings are normally absent. With lateral cortical or internal capsular injury, the examination shows contralateral motor deficit. Posturing in flexion (decorticate posturing) supervenes when diffuse dysfunction of the diencephalon occurs. Injury of the brain stem motor systems between the red nucleus in the midbrain and the vestibulospinal nuclei in the medulla leads to an abnormal extensor response in the arms with flaccid or flexor response in the legs (decerebrate posturing). Injury to motor systems at or below the level of the vestibulospinal nuclei results in flaccidity. With progressive neurologic injury, moving from higher to lower centers, one sees a progression from paralysis to flexor posturing to extensor posturing to flaccidity.

E. Respiratory and Circulatory Changes

With injury at the level of the pons, abnormal respirations may occur. Once the medulla is injured, there is loss of respiratory function, and apnea ensues. Similarly, in the beginning stages of medullary compression, abnormalities in blood pressure—usually hypertension—can present. As the medullary injury progresses, hypotension intervenes.

The first manifestation of a compressive lesion of the medulla is often respiratory or circulatory collapse. Severe hypertension is sometimes the first or main manifestation of posterior fossa lesions. For these reasons, posterior fossa lesions are difficult to diagnose and can be catastrophic when missed.

Differential Diagnosis

The major group of diseases that cause coma include metabolic, toxic, and primary neurologic injury. The cause usually can be determined by neurologic examination.

A. Metabolic Coma

In any patient with unexplained coma suggesting metabolic dysfunction, it is important to measure serum sodium, glucose, urea nitrogen, and creatinine; to determine PaO_2 and $PaCO_2$; and to perform liver and thyroid function tests. A toxicology screen also is mandatory. Sepsis can lead to coma, and evidence for infection should be sought in any delirious or comatose patient. The physician should have a low threshold for obtaining lumbar puncture for cerebrospinal fluid analysis in a patient with unexplained coma. Comas due to various metabolic factors have more similarities than differences. Table 30–3 lists the major metabolic causes of coma and comments on subtle differences in coma due to these various metabolic abnormalities.

Elderly people are particularly vulnerable to the effects of metabolic insults and poorly tolerant of mild fluctuations in metabolic status. Therefore, it is common to observe an elderly patient in coma due to relatively mild metabolic abnormalities, whereas this same combination of metabolic changes might not lead to coma in a young, healthy individual. One typical example is the elderly patient who develops delirium or even coma associated with a pulmonary or urinary tract infection. In fact, elderly patients' changes in mental status are often the first manifestation of sepsis. Many patients with primary brain injury, however, demonstrate mild metabolic abnormalities, and one should not automatically assume that subtle metabolic changes explain why a patient is in coma.

B. Toxic Coma

Coma secondary to drugs often resembles coma from metabolic processes. However, respiratory suppression may be more common in patients with drug-induced coma than with metabolic coma. Similarly, some

Table 30–3. Metabolic comas: mechanisms and treatment.

Disease	Coma	Mechanisms and Features	Treatment
Hyponatremia	Acutely: < 120 meq/dL Chronically: < 110 meq/dL	Leads to true cytotoxic edema. Skin can be doughy.	Hypertonic saline. Overly rapid correction may lead to central pontine myelinolysis.
Hypernatremia	> 155 meq/dL	Loss in brain water. Seizures common.	Slow rehydration.
Hypoglycemia	< 30 meq/dL	Deprivation of brain glucose for energy metabolism. Seizures are common.	Needs urgent glucose replacement.
Hyperglycemia	Ketotic or nonketotic	Changes in brain water and pH contribute to both. Nonketotic coma often has focal findings.	Slow correction.
Hypoxia	PaO_2 usually < 40 mm Hg	Loss of brain O_2 for aerobic metabolism.	Need urgent correction.
Renal failure	Variable	Brain acidosis is a factor.	Renal dialysis.
Hepatic failure	Variable. Often precipitated by medications or gastrointestinal bleeding.	Brain ammonia and changes in glutamine or dopamine hypothesized as causes. Hyperventilation and decerebrate posturing.	Treat precipitating factor. Lactulose administration.
Hypothyroidism	Chronic low levels.	Clinical findings of myxedema.	Slow thyroid hormone replacement.

groups of drugs have specific effects on the pupils. The drugs that can cause coma are too numerous to list in this chapter. Table 30–2 lists some commonly abused drugs and emphasizes the characteristics of coma associated with drug overdose.

C. Primary Brain Injury

Central nervous system infection, trauma, and stroke can lead to coma. Massive rises in intracranial pressure such as those seen with severe head injury, subarachnoid hemorrhage, or blockage of cerebrospinal fluid flow by a ventricular mass cause sudden coma. Coma also occurs with acute injury to the reticular activating system in the brain stem due to basilar artery thrombosis or pontine hemorrhage. In any patient with altered consciousness and focal motor findings, it should be assumed that a focal brain lesion is present.

Once it has been determined that a primary neurologic event is a possible cause of the coma, emergency scan of the brain is required. CT generally can be done quickly, is very sensitive for acute hemorrhage, and demonstrates most focal injuries. However, many patients with coma secondary to ischemic brain injury, isodense subdural hematomas, encephalitis, and meningitis will not show changes on CT unless contrast is used. If readily available, MRI is a good choice though the scanning process takes longer than CT and is more expensive. Cerebral blood flow imaging, single-photon emission computerized tomography (SPECT), and diffusion MRI also may be helpful in the evaluation and management of patients with acute brain injury.

D. Brain Death

The diagnosis of brain death is an unavoidable issue in the practice of critical care medicine and must be approached with sensitivity to the patients' close associates and an awareness of the possibility of organ donation. When brain death appears likely, a frank discussion with family members usually is indicated. It should be recognized that spinal reflexes and even myoclonus may persist in the brain-dead patient and can be misunderstood both by medical personnel and by family members. Declaration of brain death requires the demonstration of irreversible loss of both brain stem and cerebral function and should be done in consultation with a neurologist. Permanent loss of cerebral function with preservation of brain stem function is termed the chronic vegetative state, and current practice requires that such patients be given appropriate supportive care.

Treatment

The first step in the management of a patient in coma is to secure the airway and ensure adequate oxygenation. This may require intubation. Furthermore, intubation should be considered when control of Pa_{CO_2} is necessary. Hypercapnia causes cerebral vasodilation, and hypocapnia causes vasoconstriction; the former can increase intracranial pressure, and the latter can reduce it. In addition, aspiration is a common problem in the patient with altered consciousness and another reason to consider intubation.

Just as important in the management of coma is the quick assessment and control of the circulatory system. Even in patients with initially normal blood pressures, sudden loss of systemic perfusion can occur and can lead to irreversible brain injury. Therefore, a large-bore intravenous catheter should be placed in all comatose patients so that circulatory access is assured. Following this and when dealing with an unknown cause, 100 mg of thiamine and then a bolus of dextrose should be administered as treatment for potential cases of Wernicke's encephalopathy or hypoglycemia. In many patients with brain lesions and increased intracranial pressure, reflex systemic hypertension occurs. In the case of cerebellar or ventricular mass lesions, focal findings may be subtle or even absent and can lead to the incorrect assumption that the coma is due to hypertension and the primary problem ignored. Unexpected herniation can occur in such patients. Irrespective of the cause of increased intracranial pressure, lowering of systemic blood pressure could result in loss of cerebral perfusion.

Once respiration and circulation are maintained, the focus is on treatment appropriate to the diagnosis. The next chapter outlines the management of coma due to increased intracranial pressure. Many metabolic causes of coma such as hypernatremia, hyponatremia, hyperglycemia, and hepatic encephalopathy have protocols that demand meticulously organized treatments which often require days. Similarly, drug-induced comas may require specific treatment. In coma due to barbiturate or benzodiazepine toxicity, simply maintaining respiratory and circulatory support until the drug is cleared will be sufficient, whereas other poisons may require administration of specific antidotes (see Chapter 37).

SEIZURES

All physicians in critical care medicine will on occasion have to manage seizures, which may be seen as the patient's primary problem or as a problem complicating other illnesses. Prompt recognition and treatment of seizures are important because prolonged or frequently repeated generalized seizures may lead to permanent brain injury.

The basic functional property of neurons is electrochemical, and the basic disturbance of this property that underlies all seizures is termed the **paroxysmal depolarization shift.** The various lesions that produce seizures result in a paroxysmal production of synaptic potentials, which brings neurons above their threshold and causes repetitive action potentials. Thus, the electrochemical disturbance is propagated, and clinical seizures result.

Seizures may occur as a result of substrate deprivation, synaptic dysfunction, or brain injury or as a manifestation of primary generalized epilepsy. The brain depends upon two major substrates—oxygen and glucose—and deprivation of either may result in seizures. Similarly, sodium is required to maintain the electrochemical property of neurons, and extreme changes in sodium concentration also can lead to seizures. In general, the magnitude of hypoglycemia, hypoxia, and hyponatremia must be great enough to result in alteration of consciousness, following which seizures occur. Similarly, various toxic insults can result in seizures by altering synaptic function.

Direct brain injury may cause seizures, both acutely and in delayed fashion. In acute head injury, mechanical factors probably disturb membrane function, and the resulting seizures are seen within minutes to hours following the trauma. These seizures may be limited and do not typically recur. Brain injury from laceration in open head wounds or direct tissue damage in closed head injury may result in posttraumatic seizures. Pathologically, this occurs after healing and gliosis have taken place at the injured site. Typically, these seizures begin a few months to a year following trauma. The precise nature of this "ripening" process is unclear, but dendritic abnormalities have been observed on surviving neurons in the areas of gliosis. Direct electric shock can cause seizures also and is a classic method for testing the effectiveness of proposed anticonvulsant medications in animal models.

Finally, a common cause of seizures is primary generalized epilepsy. The precise pathophysiologic mechanisms are unknown, but most investigators believe the disturbance probably is related to neurotransmitter and synaptic dysfunction. Potential insights into the pathophysiology of primary generalized epilepsy are provided by the proposed mechanism of action of anticonvulsant medications. Phenytoin and carbamazepine are thought to act at sodium channels, while valproic acid is thought to act at sodium and calcium channels. In addition, a great deal of investigation with valproic acid concerns its action on gamma-aminobutyric acid (GABA) receptors. Phenobarbital has been found to block posttetanic potentiation produced by electroshock and may act also at calcium and chloride channels.

Classification of Seizures

Recognition and understanding of the seizure type is the first step in the evaluation process and serves as a guide for workup and management. The types of seizures are summarized in Table 30–4.

A. Partial Seizures

Partial seizures are those that arise from a focal area of the cortex. The clinical nature of the seizure is dictated by the functional specialization of the cortical area from which it arises. Focal motor seizures are a good example. Note that a seizure is an activation of function and not a loss of function as occurs in a transient ischemic attack. Partial seizures that are limited and not associated with alteration of consciousness are termed simple partial seizures. Impairment of consciousness coupled with a partial seizure is called a complex partial seizure.

Complex partial seizures generally arise from the temporal lobe or other limbic structures. At the onset of this type of seizure, the patient commonly experiences some autonomic or emotional symptoms, such as a feeling of fear, associated with a rising or breathless sensation within the chest or a sense of being "startled." Abdominal sensations are commonly reported. The patient may experience other phenomena such as déjà vu or may experience visual or olfactory hallucinations. These altered perceptions tend to be stereotyped from seizure to seizure in any given patient and are usually brief in duration. Following this type of onset, the patient has an alteration of consciousness and usually has little memory of what occurs until the seizure is completed.

To an observer, the onset of a complex partial seizure may appear only as a motionless stare. After the onset, the patient may develop some type of automatic and repetitive movements. Examples are lip smacking or movements of one or both extremities, or repetitive picking at some part of the body or a piece of clothing. During this time, the patient is poorly responsive to the

Table 30–4. Classification of seizures.

Simple partial (focal seizure with preservation of consciousness)
Complex partial (focal seizure with alteration of consciousness)
Secondarily generalized tonic-clonic
Primarily generalized tonic-clonic (grand mal)
Absence (petit mal)
Status epilepticus
Convulsive tonic-clonic
Nonconvulsive
Absence
Partial (epilepsia partialis continua)

environment but may still have some limited interaction. The patient then seems to recover but remains confused for variable periods, usually only a few minutes. Most seizures last from a few minutes to about 15 minutes. In repetitive frequent complex partial seizures, the patient seems to be in a twilight state, awake yet poorly responsive to the examiner and the environment.

B. Generalized Tonic-Clonic Seizures

These were at one time called "grand mal" seizures. Such seizures are sometimes preceded by a cry. They are always accompanied by loss of consciousness, but the tonic and clonic phases are variable. The tonic phase usually precedes the clonic phase, and all of the extremities are involved with both phases. During the tonic phase there is expression of extensor motor dysfunction, while throughout the rhythmic clonic phase there is flexor motor predominance. The duration of a single generalized seizure is measured in minutes, and there will always be a period of postictal confusion that is likewise usually brief.

Generalized tonic-clonic seizures may develop as a consequence of spread from a partial seizure; in this instance, it would be designated as secondarily generalized. Tonic-clonic seizures generalized at onset may be caused by metabolic abnormalities, poisons, or other pathologic states that affect overall brain function. Primary generalized epilepsy is a major cause of generalized tonic-clonic seizures. However, the essential pathogenesis of primary generalized epilepsy is poorly understood. In general, the primary generalized epilepsies (both generalized and absence) have their onset in childhood.

C. Absence Seizures

Typical absence seizures were formerly called "petit mal" seizures. They are due to another type of primary generalized epilepsy and always begin abruptly with the patient losing contact. There may be some fluttering of the eyelids, but body tone is maintained and the patient does not fall. Typically, after a few moments (occasionally up to 1 minute or longer), the patient abruptly regains contact and will continue the interrupted activity. Some patients are aware of the period of absence, but others are not. This type of seizure is not associated with a postictal state. The EEG shows generalized, 3/s spike-and-wave discharges during the seizure. Characteristically, the discharges are provoked by hyperventilation. Absence seizures can be very frequent and prolonged—a condition referred to as "absence status."

D. Status Epilepticus

Status epilepticus exists whenever seizures are persistent or there is incomplete recovery between seizures. Generalized tonic-clonic status epilepticus is a medical emergency. The consequences of status can include aspiration pneumonia, hypoxia, hypotension, hyperthermia, autonomic instability with cardiac arrhythmias, hyperkalemia, lactic acidosis, myoglobinuria, decreased cerebral perfusion, and death. Furthermore, prolonged generalized tonic-clonic seizures can result in permanent neuronal injury, particularly in the hippocampus, cerebellum, and neocortex.

In **nonconvulsive status,** the patient has impairment or loss of consciousness without generalized motor seizures. These can be quite subtle and difficult to recognize in the critical care setting. The patient may show an occasional twitch of an extremity or a facial twitch. Sometimes the only evidence for seizure activity involves eye movements, which can be observed only by lifting the eyelids. Nonconvulsive status of this type often is associated with significant metabolic encephalopathy and sometimes with underlying structural brain disease. Electroencephalography is required for diagnosis.

Another type of generalized nonconvulsive status is absence status, also called spike-wave status. Absence status most often occurs in children who have generalized epilepsy. In adults it is rare, but it may occur suddenly in elderly patients and present as a confusional state with minor automatisms such as eye blinking or facial twitching.

Status epilepticus also can occur with partial seizures. This has been called **epilepsia partialis continua,** and focal motor seizures are the type most apt to be seen by the critical care physician. Complex partial status presents with a patient in a confusional state, often with various automatisms as described previously.

Clinical Features

A. History and Examination

The history is critical in the diagnosis of seizures, and a comprehensive review of the history and the hospital course is required. Patients may describe their symptoms, particularly in the case of complex partial seizures; however, many patients are unaware of activity during the episode because consciousness has been impaired. In fact, patients are sometimes even unaware that they have had a lapse of consciousness. Thus, it is important to obtain a history from the patient and from witnesses such as nurses, other patients in the room, family members, or other attending physicians. Neurologic examination should be directed toward signs of metabolic encephalopathy, increased intracranial pressure, and lateralized findings indicative of focal brain disease. An EEG will help to clarify the nature of the seizure, particularly if it is obtained during or soon after the seizure activity. Unless an obvious cause for seizure is found, brain imaging is necessary to see if structural brain disease is present. If an infectious cause is suspected and there is no contraindication due to intracranial mass effect, lumbar puncture should be performed to obtain cerebrospinal fluid for examination. If mass effect is present, neurosurgical consultation should be obtained.

With new-onset seizures in the critical care setting, a useful approach is to consider reversible causes first. In most instances, these seizures will be generalized tonic-clonic in nature. Hypoxic-ischemic events are a common cause of such seizures. The magnitude and duration of brain oxygen deprivation will determine the severity of the seizure disorder as well as the ultimate outcome. A brief seizure or several brief seizures with rapid resolution may require no anticonvulsant therapy. If the hypoxia-ischemia is severe, the seizures may be prolonged and difficult to treat. This also may be a cause of nonconvulsive status epilepticus.

The most common causes of drug withdrawal seizures are ethanol, barbiturates, and opioids. Ethanol withdrawal seizures usually occur after 24–72 hours of abstinence and rarely lead to status epilepticus unless there are other underlying diseases. Theophylline is probably the most common pharmacologic cause of seizures in the ICU. Lithium toxicity may cause an encephalopathy that may include seizures. Penicillin toxicity causes seizures but is a rare occurrence usually associated with kidney failure.

Seizures occurring with acute neurologic disease often are partial, or partial with secondary generalization, and the partial onset may not be clinically apparent. Herpes simplex encephalitis tends to be focal, while encephalitis from other causes is more generalized. Electroencephalography and imaging studies are helpful in differential diagnosis. Seizures usually do not occur with uncomplicated meningitis. If they occur in bacterial meningitis, one should suspect a complicating cortical venous thrombosis. Brain abscesses commonly cause seizures.

The EEG is very useful in critical care neurology. To obtain the maximum information from the EEG, the clinician should provide the electroencephalographer with a brief history that includes the patient's age, a description of the level of consciousness, and a list of the medications being administered. One syndrome that can be defined with the EEG is called periodic lateralized epileptiform discharges (PLEDS). Affected patients are stuporous or comatose, may have occasional epileptiform twitching movements of one side of the face, and show the characteristic lateralized epileptiform discharges. PLEDS usually is associated with some underlying structural brain disease, such as an old infarct, and a superimposed metabolic encephalopathy. In general, the prognosis is hopeful with correction of the metabolic disturbance and, usually, administration of anticonvulsant medication.

In the case of seizures, the EEG is diagnostic if obtained during the seizure, but also it may show interictal discharges and abnormalities supportive of the diagnosis and indicate any focal aspect. Sometimes it is helpful to employ closed-circuit TV and an electroencephalographic monitoring system to fully evaluate the seizure as well as the progress of therapy. The EEG also is helpful in establishing the diagnosis of a generalized toxic-metabolic encephalopathy whether or not seizures are present.

Differential Diagnosis

Seizures may be associated with many different pathologic states, including structural injuries due to neoplasms, vascular anomalies, old strokes, past trauma, or metabolic encephalopathies. Other common problems leading to seizures include poisoning, drug withdrawal, infections such as viral encephalitis, and primary generalized epilepsies. Poor compliance with the anticonvulsant regimen is a common reason for a patient with epilepsy to develop status epilepticus as well as to have poor seizure control. Drug level monitoring in these patients is essential.

Partial seizures of any type imply an underlying structural brain disease. Likewise, a postictal paresis (Todd's paresis) implies underlying focal disease.

Treatment

The management of seizures in critical care practice requires first the removal or correction of precipitating causes and second the administration of anticonvulsant medication. Often it will seem prudent to administer anticonvulsant medication on a temporary basis while causative conditions are resolving. Whether anticonvulsants are administered orally or intravenously, it is critical to monitor serum concentrations in order to ensure a therapeutic range. The available medications that can be administered either intravenously or orally are phenytoin (fosphenytoin IV preparation fully converted to phenytoin after injection), phenobarbital, and valproate. Lorazepam and diazepam are useful anticonvulsants only when given intravenously.

Table 30–5 lists the doses and average half-lives of intravenously administered anticonvulsant medicines. Since these half-lives are variable, the information provides an approximation of the duration of action.

The major limiting factor for diazepam is that it peaks into the therapeutic range for only a brief time; seizures may recur 15–20 minutes after it is given. On the other hand, it is rapidly effective. There may be some risk of apnea when diazepam and phenobarbital are given together. Lorazepam also is rapidly effective and has a longer duration of action. The dose of lor-

Table 30–5. Intravenous anticonvulsants.

Drug	Average Half-Life	Dose[1]
Diazepam	1 hour	10–30 mg
Lorazepam	3 hours	2–10 mg
Phenytoin	12 hours	18–20 mg/kg
Fosphenytoin	12 hours[2]	20 mg phenytoin equivalents (PE)/kg
Phenobarbital	99 hours	15–20 mg/kg
Valproate sodium injection[3]	10 hours	250–500 mg

[1]Status epilepticus or loading.
[2]Converted to phenytoin in 10–15 minutes.
[3]T_{MAX} = 1 hour.

azepam is usually 2–10 mg or 0.1 mg/kg. It can be administered in 2 mg increments at intervals of a few minutes until the seizures are controlled or the maximum dose is reached.

Both fosphenytoin or phenytoin and phenobarbital are effective anticonvulsants, though their onset of action may be slower than that of the benzodiazepines. Both phenytoin and phenobarbital can be continued orally. Phenytoin must be administered at a rate no faster than 50 mg/min because of the risk of cardiac arrhythmia. Electrocardiographic monitoring is advised while phenytoin is given. Phenytoin should not be mixed in a dextrose solution because it will precipitate. The initial intravenous dose is 18–20 mg/kg of body weight; the maximum dose is 30 mg/kg. Fosphenytoin is dosed in phenytoin equivalents (PE); it can be mixed in normal saline or a 5% dextrose solution and infused at a rate up to 150 mg PE per minute. Extravasated phenytoin solution often is harmful to surrounding tissues, while extravasated fosphenytoin usually results in no damage.

The intravenous dose of phenobarbital is 300–1000 mg (or 15–20 mg/kg) for seizure control. Usually it is supplied in 60 mg units, so an initial dose of 300 mg is convenient and can be repeated every 10–20 minutes until seizure control occurs or the maximum dose is reached.

Valproate sodium injection is a broad-spectrum anticonvulsant; it has complete bioequivalence with oral valproate and may be mixed in normal saline or 5% dextrose solution. The recommended infusion rate is up to 20 mg/min. Valproate is the drug of choice for absence seizures. Intravenous valproate, lorazepam, and diazepam are effective in absence status.

Seizures from metabolic encephalopathies, nonconvulsive status, and PLEDS often do not respond fully and quickly to anticonvulsive medications. In this circumstance, it is best to maintain therapeutic anticonvulsant blood concentrations while pursuing therapy of underlying diseases. Partial seizures or partial status likewise may be resistant to treatment. In such cases, two anticonvulsant drugs can be tried, but it is best to maintain them in the usual therapeutic range and determine if with time there is greater benefit.

Generalized tonic-clonic status epilepticus does constitute an emergency and must be controlled. Ventilation and cardiac function must be supported. If hypoglycemia is a consideration, 50 mL of a 50% dextrose solution should be promptly administered. If there is any possibility that the patient is alcoholic, dextrose should be preceded by 100 mg of thiamine to prevent Wernicke's encephalopathy. Anticonvulsant medication for status epilepticus is always administered intravenously and must always be given in full loading doses. A common mistake is to give inadequate amounts of several different drugs.

If generalized tonic-clonic seizures persist in spite of the patient's being given intravenous anticonvulsants, pentobarbital anesthesia is recommended. This should be accomplished with neurologic consultation and under electroencephalographic control. Pentobarbital is given in a dosage of 5 mg/kg for induction of anesthesia and 0.5–2 mg/kg/h for maintenance. The drug is administered so as to titrate the EEG to a burst-suppression pattern. When it is judged that an appropriate interval of time has lapsed (about 24–48 hours), the pentobarbital dose may be reduced to test for seizure recurrence. If the seizures are controlled, the pentobarbital may be withdrawn, but therapeutic levels of an anticonvulsant such as phenytoin must be present and maintained.

Current Controversies & Unresolved Issues

Resistant partial or lateralized seizures and nonconvulsive generalized status epilepticus remain problems in management, and there is some controversy about how vigorous the physician should be in the administration of medications.

No clear indication exists for the choice of first medication to treat generalized tonic-clonic status; rather, it is a matter of local practice and personal choice.

In the past few years, the number of available oral antiepileptic drugs has increased dramatically, and experience with them in common practice is not yet great. Use of these drugs and the management of chronic seizure disorders is mostly beyond the scope of critical care practice. Neurology consultation is recommended when newly prescribing or switching oral antiepileptic medicine.

NEUROMUSCULAR DISORDERS

Respiratory and cardiac failure are the most serious potential complications of neuromuscular diseases and can lead to death if not appropriately treated. Diseases directly affecting respiration include Guillain-Barré syndrome, myasthenia gravis, amyotrophic lateral sclerosis, and Duchenne's muscular dystrophy. Less commonly, botulism, tetanus, porphyria, and diphtheritic polyneuropathy cause neuromuscular failure. Similarly, a variety of neuronal poisons can lead to severe weakness and even respiratory failure. Chronic neuromuscular diseases can lead to secondary pulmonary problems, including phrenic nerve injury, kyphoscoliosis, pulmonary emboli, atelectasis, and, most frequently, aspiration pneumonia. Another potential problem associated with neuromuscular diseases involves cardiac complications such as arrhythmias, as seen in Guillain-Barré syndrome; or conduction blocks with sudden death, as in myotonic dystrophy. Advances in the intensive care treatment of these patients have decreased morbidity and mortality rates, avoiding sudden death in some instances.

Pathophysiology

Progressive weakness may result from disorders anywhere along the motor tract (Figure 30–1). Lesions in the brain, particularly the upper motor neuron pathways (site A) or brain stem (site B), may lead to progressive weakness. Likewise, disorders at the level of the spinal cord or the lower motor neurons (site C), either at the anterior horn cell bodies, motor axons, or myelin (site D) or at the pre- or postsynaptic terminals (site E), may lead to weakness. Furthermore, many of the muscle diseases (site F) can directly impair effective ventilation. Table 30–6 lists some examples of diseases that can occur at each site.

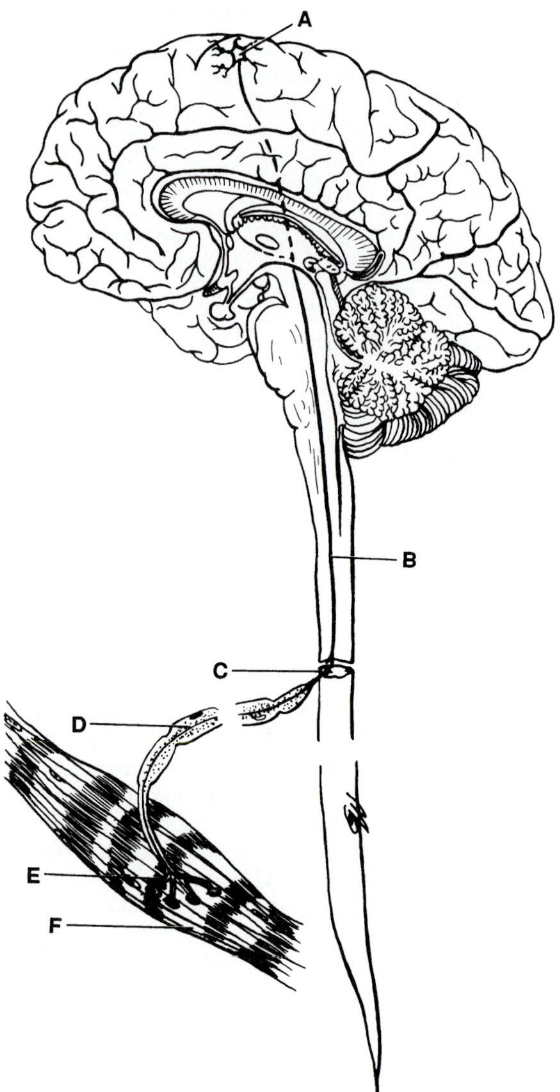

Figure 30–1. Localization of lesions causing neuromuscular diseases. ***A:*** cortex (upper motor neuron); ***B:*** spinal cord; ***C:*** anterior horn cell; ***D:*** peripheral nerve (axon or myelin); ***E:*** neuromuscular junction; ***F:*** muscle.

One general rule associated with respiratory failure secondary to neuromuscular disorders is that unlike primary pulmonary illnesses, where dysfunction in gas exchange often results predominantly in **hypoxemia,** respiratory failure secondary to neuromuscular dysfunction usually leads to hypoventilation. Arterial blood gases often demonstrate CO_2 retention, or **hypercapnia,** with relatively mild hypoxemia. By the time $PaCO_2$ begins to increase, hypoventilation has gone beyond the safe limit. Decrease in vital capacity is associated with predictable signs of pulmonary dysfunction (Figure 30–2). Therefore, the single most important parameter to measure in patients with neuromuscular diseases is the vital capacity.

In order to make an etiologic diagnosis of neuromuscular disease leading to weakness and respiratory failure, specific clinical symptoms and signs as well as laboratory diagnostic studies are used to localize the lesions. Measurements of vital capacity and cardiac monitoring are essential in patients admitted to the ICU due to exacerbation of neuromuscular diseases, since respiratory compromise and cardiac arrhythmias can develop rapidly. The clinical presentation of the illness depends on the site of the lesion.

Table 30–6. Neuromuscular diseases affecting respiration.

Motor cortex and pyramidal tract
Amyotrophic lateral sclerosis
Brain stem
Progressive bulbar palsy
Spinal cord and lower motor neuron
Spinal muscular atrophies
Amyotrophic lateral sclerosis
Poliomyelitis
Toxins: mercury
Infections: tetanus, spinal cord and epidural abscesses
Peripheral neuropathies
Axonal types (including critical illness polyneuropathy)
Diabetes
Alcohol-related
Uremia
Hypothyroidism
Sarcoidosis
Collagen-vascular diseases
Paraproteinemias
Drugs
Heavy metals
Industrial toxins
Amyloidosis
Carcinoma (remote effect)
Tick paralysis
Demyelinating neuropathies
Guillain-Barré syndrome
Diphtheria
Porphyria
Hereditary: Charcot-Marie-Tooth disease
Neuromuscular junction disorders
Myasthenia gravis
Botulism
Eaton-Lambert syndrome
Pseudocholinesterase deficiency
Organophosphate intoxication
Other drugs and toxins: neomycin, penicillamine
Disease of muscles
Muscular dystrophies
Inflammatory myopathies
Endocrine and metabolic myopathies
Toxic myopathies: alcohol, carbon monoxide
Inherited metabolic myopathies: periodic paralysis; glycogen or lipid enzymatic defect
Neuroleptic malignant syndrome, malignant hyperthermia

SPINAL CORD COMPRESSION

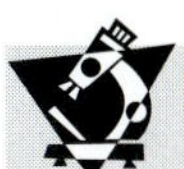

ESSENTIALS OF DIAGNOSIS

- *Back pain, limb paresis, and spasticity.*
- *Sensory loss below the level of the spinal cord lesion.*
- *Bowel or bladder incontinence.*
- *Neuroimaging studies of the clinically suspected spinal levels.*
- *Blood cultures and PPD test if an abscess is suspected.*
- *Biopsies to evaluate tumors and abscesses.*

General Considerations

Back pain can be caused by a variety of diseases such as local structural disorders, retroperitoneal disease, trauma, infection, and neoplasms. However, tumors, abscesses, or disk fragments in the spinal canal may produce an acute syndrome of spinal cord compression. This is a neurologic emergency that may lead to permanent paralysis if not rapidly treated. Diagnostic signs or symptoms vary depending on the spinal level of the compression.

Intra- and extramedullary spinal cord malignancies, as well as various infections with parasitic (cysticercosis), bacterial (anaerobes, tuberculomas, gummas), or viral (varicella-zoster, poliomyelitis) organisms, may produce direct or compressive lesions to the spinal cord. Most abscesses are in the thoracic or lumbar areas, and the agent is usually *Staphylococcus aureus.* Tuberculosis also may infect the vertebral column (Pott's disease), causing kyphosis, which may then cause cord compression or respiratory difficulties.

Clinical Features

A. Symptoms and Signs

Diagnosis of a spinal cord lesion depends upon clinical examination and neuroimaging studies. Limb weakness and the presence of a sensory level (particularly to pinprick and vibratory senses) are useful in approximating the level of involvement. Tendon reflexes below the level of the lesion may be increased, and Babinski signs may be present. Fever associated with back pain and myelophthisic signs should arouse suspicion of epidural abscess.

B. Laboratory Findings

When an infectious cause is suspected, blood cultures and a tuberculin test will help to direct specific antibiotic therapies. Biopsy examination is indicated for suspected tumor or abscess.

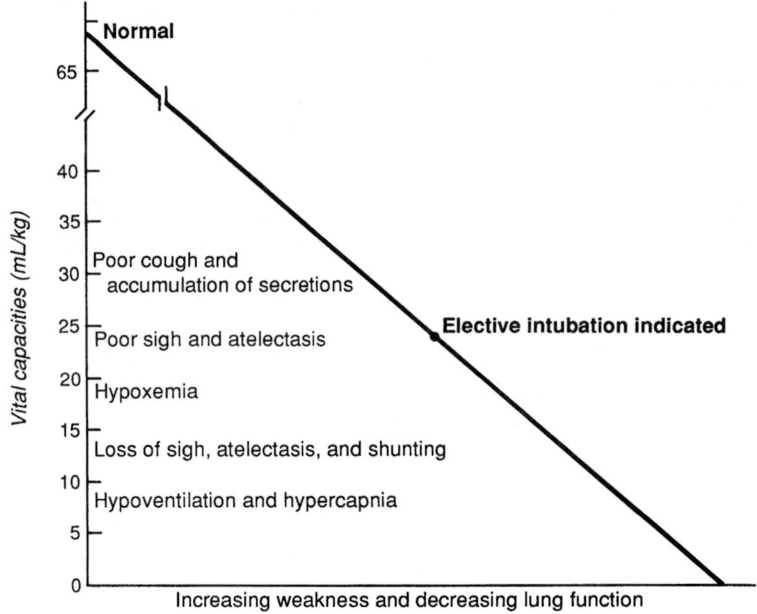

Figure 30–2. Effects of decreasing vital capacities secondary to weakness from neuromuscular diseases.

C. Imaging Studies

MRI or CT is necessary to accurately localize the lesion.

Treatment

Early recognition and treatment can prevent irreversible neurologic damage. Tumors generally respond to surgical removal or radiotherapy. High-dose corticosteroid therapy also may be indicated. Selection of antibiotic therapy for epidural abscess depends upon biopsy or culture results.

GUILLAIN-BARRÉ SYNDROME

ESSENTIALS OF DIAGNOSIS

- *Antecedent flu-like illness.*
- *Acute or subacute ascending flaccid paralysis.*
- *Early loss of tendon reflexes.*
- *Subjective distal paresthesias and pain.*
- *Occasional cranial nerve deficits.*
- *Elevated protein in cerebrospinal fluid with no cells.*

General Considerations

Guillain-Barré syndrome is an acute or subacute, primarily motor polyneuropathy that is usually idiopathic, though a variety of etiologic factors, including *Mycoplasma pneumoniae* and hepatitis B, have been implicated in rare cases. In more than 50% of patients with Guillain-Barré syndrome, an antecedent flu-like illness or vaccination occurred within 4 weeks prior to the neurologic symptoms.

Acute or subacute ascending muscle weakness develops over 2–4 weeks, followed by gradual recovery over a few weeks to many months. Eighty-five percent of patients will have complete functional recovery.

Clinical Features

A. Symptoms and Signs

Cranial nerve deficits, especially of those controlling eye movements and facial muscles, can be present either alone or associated with limb weakness. Deep tendon reflexes are absent, while pupils and eyelids often are spared. Miller-Fisher syndrome is a variant of Guillain-Barré syndrome characterized by absent reflexes, gait ataxia, and ophthalmoparesis. The prognosis for complete recovery of this form of Guillain-Barré syndrome is excellent.

B. Laboratory Findings

Lumbar puncture can be diagnostic by the second week, when cerebrospinal fluid shows an elevated protein concentration without pleocytosis ("albuminocytologic dissociation").

C. Nerve Conduction Studies

Nerve conduction studies show segmental demyelination and reduction of velocity in 85–90% of patients by the second week. Up to 40% of patients develop respiratory muscle weakness and/or autonomic instability. Therefore, ICU admission is best for most patients, and frequent vital capacity measurements and cardiac monitoring are necessary for timely detection of these complications.

Treatment

A. Respiratory Care

Respiratory weakness requiring ventilatory support develops in 40% of patients and may be rapidly progressive in the early phases. Intubation may be required. Bulbar muscle weakness can lead to aspiration pneumonia, which is potentially preventable by placement of a nasogastric tube as well as by intubation.

B. Cardiac Care

In up to 40% of patients with Guillain-Barré syndrome, autonomic dysfunction may occur and accounts for much of the morbidity and most of the deaths in this group of patients. The cardiac abnormalities frequently include sinus tachycardia, and asystole can occur. Therefore, it is essential to maintain cardiac monitoring and to administer antiarrhythmic drugs as necessary.

C. Other Treatment

When the weakness is progressive and severe, plasmapheresis or intravenous immune globulin (IGIV) is recommended. Because most of these patients experience a significant amount of pain (which may be difficult to recognize when the patient is intubated), use of opioids as needed is indicated.

CRITICAL ILLNESS POLYNEUROPATHY

ESSENTIALS OF DIAGNOSIS

- *Associated with multiorgan failure, often with sepsis.*
- *Difficulty weaning from respirator due to weakness.*
- *Distal limb weakness with diminished or absent reflexes.*
- *EMG nerve conduction studies characteristic.*

General Considerations

Critical illness polyneuropathy has been recognized in association with sepsis and multiorgan failure in the ICU setting. Sometimes it is first identified because of difficulty weaning a patient from the ventilator due to respiratory muscle weakness. It is an axonal sensorimotor polyneuropathy of obscure origin; there is no inflammation or demyelination of the nerves.

Clinical Features

A. Symptoms and Signs

The typical findings on examination are distal limb weakness with flaccidity and hyporeflexia or areflexia as well as respiratory muscle weakness or even quadriplegia in severe cases. Mild facial weakness sometimes occurs, but ophthalmoparesis is uncommon. Distal sensory loss may be expected, but under the usual circumstances of this condition sensory deficits are difficult or impossible to assess accurately. Superimposed entrapment or compression neuropathies, because of positioning problems, should be considered in the differential diagnosis. Also to be differentiated is **critical illness myopathy,** which is a syndrome of weakness that develops in some critically ill patients after the use of corticosteroids, often in combination with neuromuscular blocking agents. Creatine kinase usually is elevated, many times to very high levels, and can be associated with rhabdomyolysis and myoglobinuria. Another condition to be differentiated is prolonged neuromuscular blockade, which may occur in critically ill patients after neuromuscular blocking agents have been discontinued; the duration can range from hours to days.

B. Laboratory Findings

Electromyographic and nerve conduction studies show reduced motor and sensory amplitudes but preserved conduction velocities and distal latencies. This is distinguished from Guillain-Barré syndrome, in which conduction block and segmental slowing are found. The cerebrospinal fluid protein is normal in critical illness polyneuropathy.

Treatment

Treatment consists of correction and management of underlying illnesses. The neuropathy often improves after weeks or months as sepsis and organ failure resolve. Patients who have mild or moderate neuropathy may have complete recovery, while those severely affected will probably have residual and permanent weakness. It is prudent to minimize the use of neuromuscular blocking agents, especially in patients who are receiving corticosteroids.

TOXIC NEUROPATHIES

There are three anatomic locations where toxins can affect the peripheral nerve: the cell body, the nerve sheath myelin, and the axon. Diphtheria toxin, tetanus toxoid, and antibiotic treatments may lead to acute sensory neuropathy secondary to myelin loss, while the most common toxic neuropathies result in axonal injuries. Many drugs and industrial chemicals can be neurotoxic. Examples of such drugs are isoniazid, chloramphenicol, metronidazole, disulfiram, amiodarone, gold, cisplatin, vincristine, lithium, nitrofurantoin, nitrous oxide, and pyridoxine.

Exposure to industrial chemicals such as arsenic, acrylamide, carbon disulfide, mercury, the organophosphate parathion, and vinyl chloride can cause distal axonal neuropathy. The clinical course depends upon the concentration of the offending agent. Chronic exposure to these agents leads to an insidious onset of paresthesia in glove-stocking distribution. With more acute exposure, patients develop other systemic signs along with a more rapid onset of neuropathy. Two important ubiquitous toxins, lead and arsenic, both have characteristic clinical presentations.

Lead Poisoning

Lead poisoning can occur via the gastrointestinal tract, the lungs, or the skin and is associated with abdominal cramps and encephalopathy (particularly in infants). Blood smears show basophilic stippling in the erythrocytes. The elevated lead level can be measured in serum. Though other nerves may be affected, lead has a peculiar predilection for radial nerves resulting in weakness of wrist and finger extension. Sensory symptoms are unusual.

Arsenic Poisoning

Arsenic poisoning often results from accidental ingestion of rat poisons or industrial sprays, though intentional poisonings do occur. These patients often develop an acute polyneuropathy several weeks after exposure. The nail beds show pale bands called Mees's lines. After exposure, urine, hair, and nails may all contain arsenic. With higher exposure, a painful sensory neuropathy may evolve to a flaccid paralysis beginning in the lower extremity but eventually affecting the respiratory muscles and the upper extremities.

Urine and serum for a heavy metal screen along with a careful drug and toxin exposure history are mandatory in any patient presenting with an acute neuropathy. Finally, nerve conduction studies will help to differentiate demyelinating versus axonal types of neuropathy.

MYASTHENIA GRAVIS

ESSENTIALS OF DIAGNOSIS

- *History of fluctuating weakness and fatigability.*
- *Positive edrophonium (Tensilon) test.*
- *Decremental responses on nerve conduction studies.*
- *Positive serologic tests for acetylcholine receptor antibodies.*
- *Chest CT or MRI may show thymoma.*

General Considerations

Myasthenia gravis appears to be an autoimmune disease, primarily a disorder of the postsynaptic neuromuscular junction. Acetylcholine receptor antibodies are found in 85–90% of patients. Other immunologic diseases such as thyroid disease, polymyositis, rheumatoid arthritis, and systemic lupus erythematosus all have been associated with myasthenia gravis.

Repetitive stimulation of a motor nerve at 3 Hz shows a decremental response of electromyographic motor units in up to 85% of patients with myasthenia gravis, whereas diseases affecting the presynaptic nerve terminal such as Lambert-Eaton syndrome or botulism demonstrate an incremental response at a higher rate of stimulation.

Clinical Features

A. Symptoms and Signs

Myasthenia gravis is characterized by variable weakness and easy fatigability. The motor weakness worsens with exercise and improves after rest. Diplopia often is an early symptom, and over 90% of patients develop ocular muscle involvement. Patients feel strongest in the morning and weakest at night, as their muscles tire during the day.

B. Laboratory Findings

The edrophonium test demonstrates that an increase in peripheral acetylcholine improves motor function. It is performed as follows: (1) Stop other anticholinesterase medications 24 hours prior to the test if possible. (2) Atropine sulfate, 0.4 mg (1 mL), which blocks muscarinic "side effects" of edrophonium but not the nicotinic effect at the neuromuscular junction, and normal saline (1 mL) are used first as control injections. (3) Edrophonium should elicit a response in 30–60 seconds which should last for 10–30 minutes. Draw up 10 mg and give 2 mg for the first dose; if there is no response, follow with 8 mg. (4) Assess strength of affected muscles 1–2 minutes after each intravenous dose.

The absence of acetylcholine receptor antibodies does not exclude the diagnosis, but their presence is confirmatory. Antistriational antibodies are found in 90% of myasthenic patients with thymoma.

C. Imaging Studies

Approximately 10% of patients develop thymoma, and 70% will have thymic hyperplasia. Therefore, chest CT or MRI is performed to search for mass lesions.

Treatment

A. Oral Therapy

Pyridostigmine often is successful first-line therapy. The usual initial dose is 30 mg or 60 mg. The interval of dosing can be adjusted in individual patients depending upon observed duration of action but is usually on the order of 4 hours. Prednisone and other immunosuppressive drugs also are used in difficult cases.

B. Intravenous Therapy

Plasmapheresis, 2–3 L per exchange three times a week over 2 weeks, has been successful in some patients who do not respond to anticholinesterase medications. Intravenous immune globulin (IGIV) is an alternative to plasmapheresis, and both are useful in preparing patients for thymectomy.

C. Thymectomy

Thymectomy improves long-term outcome in patients with myasthenia gravis, and all patients undergoing thymectomy should be carefully monitored pre- and postoperatively in the ICU under the supervision of a neurologist. Postoperatively, immunosuppression with high-dose prednisone is helpful in many patients.

D. Exacerbations

When a myasthenic patient presents with increased weakness, it is important to differentiate between myasthenic versus cholinergic crisis. A myasthenic crisis requires treatment with additional anticholinesterase medications, whereas weakness due to cholinergic crisis only improves if the medication is withheld. An edrophonium test may be helpful in differentiating the two. In myasthenic crisis, look for causes such as infection (especially aspiration pneumonia), drugs with a potential for blocking neuromuscular transmission, and excessive use of sedative drugs. In general, if vital capacity is less than one liter, it is best to intubate and stop all myasthenic medication until the cause of the exacerbation is determined.

BOTULISM

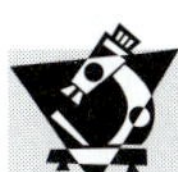

ESSENTIALS OF DIAGNOSIS

- *Gastrointestinal symptoms with dry mouth.*
- *Blurred vision, dilated pupils, and diplopia.*
- *Respiratory distress.*
- *Incremental response with repetitive nerve conduction studies.*
- *Stool examination positive for* Clostridium botulinum *and its exotoxin.*

General Considerations

Unlike myasthenia gravis, the neuromuscular junction defect in botulism results primarily from presynaptic cholinergic conduction blockade. It is an acute poisoning resulting from ingestion of *C botulinum* exotoxin. The organism is found in inadequately cooked or defectively canned food. It may be found also in clostridial wound infections, which is a source of the disease in people injecting illicit drugs. In infants between the ages of 1 and 38 weeks, the toxin may be found in the gastrointestinal tract.

Clinical Features

A. Symptoms and Signs

Symptoms begin within 5–50 hours after eating the contaminated food or exposure to the toxin. Dry mouth and gastrointestinal symptoms such as cramps, nausea, vomiting, and diarrhea or constipation as well as malaise and headaches are noted initially. Extraocular muscle weakness and dilated, sluggishly reactive pupils cause diplopia and blurred vision. These patients may rapidly develop dysphagia and respiratory distress. Respiratory failure and aspiration pneumonia may be the principal causes of death from botulism. The nervous system is involved in descending fashion, beginning with muscles innervated by the cranial nerves. Consciousness and sensation remain intact, however.

B. Laboratory Findings

Botulinus toxin can be isolated from infected serum, stool, or contaminated food. Since cultures of the organism or evaluation for the toxin may take several days, repetitive nerve stimulation should be performed as soon as possible in patients suspected of having botulism. Cerebrospinal fluid is normal.

C. Nerve Conduction Studies

Diagnostic studies with high-rate (40 Hz) repetitive nerve stimulation demonstrate incremental responses of the compound action potentials in the motor nerves.

Treatment

A. Antitoxin

Type E antitoxin has the greatest clinical efficacy and should be administered as quickly as possible. The dose may be repeated in 4 hours if the condition worsens. Skin testing to exclude hypersensitivity should precede administration of the antitoxin. One vial of antitoxin should be given orally and one intravenously.

B. Antibiotics

When botulism occurs from a wound infection, antibiotic therapy with penicillin, 300,000 units/kg/d intravenously, is preferred. Other useful drugs include clindamycin (30 mg/kg/d intravenously), chloramphenicol (50 mg/kg/d intravenously), and guanidine hydrochloride (50 mg/kg/d orally), which may improve muscle function.

INFLAMMATORY MYOPATHIES

The majority of the inflammatory myopathies result from autoimmune processes, though some result from infections. Typical examples include dermatomyositis, polymyositis, secondary involvement with lupus erythematosus, and viral myositis. In 20% of older patients (> 50 years), polymyositis and dermatomyositis may be associated with an occult malignancy.

Myalgia and proximal muscle weakness are the most common complaints in patients with inflammatory myopathies. Most forms are self-limited, lasting 2–3 weeks. However, fulminant myositis may lead to rhabdomyolysis, which can be fatal. Occasionally, when the swallowing muscles are involved, the patient requires nasogastric tube feedings.

Laboratory studies often reveal an elevated creatine kinase and sedimentation rate. Electromyography shows signs of muscular irritability with fibrillation potentials and small polyphasic waveforms—all characteristic of inflammatory myopathies. Perivascular infiltrates and perifascicular atrophy are seen in muscle biopsy specimens, and this information may be necessary for definitive diagnosis.

NEUROLEPTIC MALIGNANT SYNDROME

ESSENTIALS OF DIAGNOSIS

- *Encephalopathy.*
- *Markedly elevated core temperature.*
- *Autonomic dysfunction.*
- *"Lead pipe" muscular rigidity with elevated creatine kinase*

General Considerations

Neuroleptic malignant syndrome is a life-threatening idiosyncratic reaction to neuroleptic agents. The drugs that produce this syndrome typically include phenothiazines, butyrophenones, and other postsynaptic dopamine blocking agents. Failure to recognize the syndrome may lead to a rapidly fatal course over hours to several days. Even brief exposure to the drug may produce the syndrome.

Clinical Features

A. Symptoms and Signs

The clinical presentation may be variable but frequently consists of encephalopathy, markedly elevated core temperature, and muscular rigidity. Fever and increased muscle activity are the main features. Mental status changes may vary from confusion or agitation to coma. Involuntary movements such as tremor or dyskinesia occasionally accompany muscular rigidity—so-called "lead pipe rigidity." When severe rigidity occurs, rhabdomyolysis may result and in turn lead to myoglobinuria and acute renal failure.

B. Laboratory Findings

There is no unequivocal diagnostic test or criterion for neuroleptic malignant syndrome. Creatine kinase elevations may range from several hundred to over 10,000 units per liter.

Differential Diagnosis

Many nonneuroleptic drugs can produce similar disorders. Examples include cocaine, amphetamines, reserpine, metoclopramide, and tricyclic antidepressants in combination with lithium or monoamine oxidase inhibitors. The differential diagnosis also includes many causes of encephalopathy and fever, catatonia, and malignant hyperthermia.

Malignant hyperthermia is a genetically determined hypermetabolic state with onset shortly after the use of certain anesthetics. Although it is similar to neuroleptic malignant syndrome in the markedly elevated temperature and creatine kinase concentrations, it can be distinguished by the lack of encephalopathy or autonomic dysfunction. Furthermore, the generation of fever is most likely peripheral in malignant hyperthermia and central in neuroleptic malignant syndrome. The genetic trait for malignant hyperthermia does not appear to impose any risks for development of neuroleptic malignant syndrome.

Treatment

A. General Measures

Effective treatment requires early recognition and critical care monitoring of possible multiple organ failure. Fever must be controlled, and vigorous intravenous hydration is necessary to lower the body temperature and to minimize the effects of possible rhabdomyolysis. Blood pressure and urinary output must be monitored carefully. Most importantly, dopamine-blocking agents must be discontinued.

B. Drug Therapy

Centrally acting bromocriptine, 7.5–100 mg/d, has been used to control the high temperature and rigidity; effects may be seen within hours. Dantrolene, a peripherally acting muscle relaxant, also is highly effective. It can be given intravenously at a dosage of 0.25 mg/kg twice daily and increased as needed to control the rigidity. When the patient is able to take oral medications, 25–600 mg/d may be effective.

MUSCULAR DYSTROPHIES

ESSENTIALS OF DIAGNOSIS

- *Proximal extremity weakness.*
- *Pseudohypertrophy of the gastrocnemius muscles.*
- *Muscle fiber necrosis and minor regeneration on biopsy.*

General Considerations

There are a variety of inherited muscular diseases that may have respiratory or cardiac complications which ultimately require management in the ICU. Duchenne's muscular dystrophy and myotonic dystrophy are the commonest diseases of this type.

Muscular dystrophy patients have an increased rate of adverse reactions to many anesthetics and frequently have respiratory complications and prolonged postoperative courses if they undergo general anesthesia. When possible, surgery or general anesthesia should be avoided in these patients. In general, sedatives also are contraindicated because of their adverse effects on weakened muscles.

Clinical Features

A. Symptoms and Signs

Diagnosis of Duchenne's muscular dystrophy can be made by the family history (X-linked recessive, but one-third can be spontaneous mutations), clinical examination showing characteristic proximal extremity weakness, and pseudohypertrophy of the gastrocnemius muscles by age 3–4.

B. Laboratory Findings

Muscle biopsies demonstrate progressive muscle fiber necrosis and minor degrees of regeneration. These patients pursue a steady downhill course and develop lumbar lordosis and scoliosis. Laboratory studies will show markedly elevated (10–50 times normal) serum creatine kinase and characteristic abnormalities on electrocardiography, electromyography, and muscle biopsies. New findings from molecular genetic studies show absent dystrophin protein in muscles of patients with Duchenne's muscular dystrophy, whereas patients with the Becker variant (clinically similar but a later age at onset) have a slightly lower than normal level or an altered protein. Genetic linkage analysis, though inaccurate, usually provides a carrier status or prenatal diagnosis as a "percentage risk" rather than a definite yes or no.

Treatment

A. Respiratory Care

Elective intubation is recommended when vital capacity falls below 15–20 mL/kg. Ventilator settings should be monitored along with arterial blood gases. Baseline blood gases can be obtained after 20 minutes of F_{IO_2} at 100%, after which inspired oxygen concentration can be decreased to maintain the Pa_{O_2} between 75 and 85 mm Hg. Positive end-expiratory pressure (PEEP) should be set at 3–5 cm H_2O and tidal volume at 12 mL/kg. The intermittent mandatory ventilation (IMV) rate should be approximately 12/min with 30–40 L/min inspiratory flow. If the patient requires prolonged intubation—more than 2–3 weeks—a tracheostomy should be performed to maintain a stable airway.

Criteria for weaning a neuromuscular patient from a ventilator include several parameters, the most important of which is the vital capacity, which should be greater than 15 mL/kg. Inspiratory pressure should be greater than −25 cm H_2O and expiratory pressure greater than 40 cm H_2O. PaO_2 should be greater than 80 mm Hg and $PaCO_2$ less than 42 mm Hg at FIO_2 of 40%. Spontaneous respiration should be less than 20/min, and there should be no other adverse medical conditions such as fulminant pneumonia or serious cardiac problems.

All patients presenting with weakness should be followed carefully for respiratory status. Good pulmonary toilet is mandatory. It is helpful to have an accurate diagnosis so that special precautions can be taken to anticipate or prevent the progression of symptoms. A superimposed infection may exacerbate the weakness of many neuromuscular diseases, and temporary life support will enable the patient to return to baseline strength. Therefore, it is imperative to exclude the possibility of a reversible cardiopulmonary complication.

B. Cardiac Care

Between 70% and 90% of patients with Duchenne's muscular dystrophy will develop electrocardiographic abnormalities consisting of tall right precordial R waves and precordial Q waves. Arrhythmias and persistent tachycardia are frequently noted in Duchenne's muscular dystrophy. Patients with myotonic dystrophy also develop cardiac arrhythmias secondary to conduction abnormalities and can present with sudden death if not detected early.

Differential Diagnosis

There are many central nervous system disorders that can mimic neuromuscular diseases. For example, a brain stem lesion may produce bulbar symptoms or diplopia that may be mistaken for amyotrophic lateral sclerosis or myasthenia gravis. Neuroleptic malignant syndrome often is difficult to differentiate from other causes of fever and encephalopathy. Blood cultures, drug screens, and brain imaging may be necessary to exclude systemic infections, drug exposures, or disorders producing changes in autonomic control and temperature such as injury to the hypothalamic region.

A careful history (including family history) and physical examination will generally distinguish the major groups of illnesses. However, electrophysiologic studies or laboratory evaluations sometimes are necessary to differentiate the specific types of diseases. Nerve conduction studies with repetitive stimulation will help to differentiate presynaptic from postsynaptic diseases, and serum creatine kinase will help to distinguish a primary myopathy from neurogenic weakness.

CURRENT CONTROVERSIES & UNRESOLVED ISSUES

A particularly difficult problem is whether to intubate a patient who has an irreversible advanced neuromuscular disease. If possible, the issue of code status should be discussed with the patient and the family prior to clinical deterioration. Perhaps the patient already has a living will or a family member has power of attorney to help with the decision-making process.

In cases of spinal cord compression, some clinicians prefer CT for diagnosis while others favor MRI.

CEREBROVASCULAR DISEASES

ESSENTIALS OF DIAGNOSIS

- *Stepwise impairment, usually produced by occlusive disease.*
- *Emboli produce sudden deficits.*
- *Intracerebral hemorrhage causes rapid onset of symptoms, often with increased intracranial pressure.*

General Considerations

Brain stem and cerebral infarctions occur as a result of either progressive occlusive vascular disease, usually hypertensive and atherosclerotic, or as a result of embolism. In occlusive disease, infarcts are bland, and in embolic disease infarcts are hemorrhagic if the embolus fragments and the vascular territory is reperfused. A hemorrhagic infarct implies embolism. Spontaneous intracerebral hemorrhage occurs as a result of hypertensive vascular disease, but in elderly people it also can be caused by amyloid angiopathy.

Clinical Features

A. Symptoms and Signs

Stroke due to occlusive vascular disease, or **thrombosis,** tends to have its onset in a stepwise or progressive fashion. It commonly occurs while the patient is sleeping. An **embolic stroke** is sudden in onset and produces maximum neurologic deficit at the outset. **Transient ischemic attacks** can precede either thrombotic or embolic infarction but are probably more frequent in association with thrombotic disease. An intracerebral hemorrhage also is sudden in onset and may cause an acute rise in intracranial pressure due to mass effect. The location of a stroke is clinically helpful; for example, a small lacunar infarct in the internal capsule is almost certainly due to occlusive disease. The first step in localizing the lesion is a careful neurologic examination.

B. Imaging Studies

Brain imaging will confirm the location of the infarct and determine whether hemorrhage has occurred. This information is required before anticoagulation therapy can be started. Typically, a bland infarct will not show on CT scan in the first few hours up to about 24 hours after onset. CT imaging, however, is very sensitive for the detection of fresh bleeding. Magnetic resonance—especially with diffusion studies—images acute infarction. MR angiography can demonstrate occluded or stenotic large- and medium-sized arteries.

Differential Diagnosis

A history of hypertension, diabetes mellitus, or tobacco smoking and a family history of stroke or myocardial infarction are common in occlusive disease. A history of hypertension is to be expected in intracerebral hemorrhage. If an embolic infarction is present, a source should be found; this may be clots arising in the heart or clots from the periphery reaching the brain as a result of right-to-left cardiac shunting. Artery-to-artery embolization, usually from an internal carotid artery, also may be considered. Strokes secondary to cocaine abuse currently are a problem not to be overlooked. Also occasionally encountered are strokes caused by carotid artery dissection or vertebral artery dissection. These are traumatic in origin, and symptomatic onset usually is 24–72 hours following trauma. Often a history of neck extension is obtained. An intimal tear and flap is demonstrated by either endovascular or MR angiography. A brain CT is very sensitive for demonstrating intracerebral hemorrhage or hemorrhagic infarction, but an acute bland infarct does not show until density of the infarcted tissue has decreased and edema occurs. MRI is sensitive in all cases. Occlusion of large vessels supplying the brain can be demonstrated with Doppler ultrasound as well as with magnetic resonance angiography. Selective contrast angiography is indicated when the diagnosis is in doubt and a surgically treatable vascular lesion could be present. The workup for an embolic source should include electrocardiography and, if a rhythm disturbance such as atrial fibrillation is not found, echocardiography. An embolic source can sometimes be demonstrated only on the transesophageal echocardiogram.

Rarer causes of stroke include polycythemia, sickle cell disease, collagen-vascular diseases, lupus anticoagulant, and hypercoagulable states. Infrequent causes of stroke also are moyamoya disease, fibromuscular hyperplasia, Takayasu's disease, and tuberculous or other arteritis. Infarction caused by arterial spasm associated with ruptured berry aneurysm and subarachnoid hemorrhage is well known in neurosurgical practice.

Treatment

In general, the management of an acute stroke consists of supportive care and control of blood pressure. In this circumstance, autoregulation of cerebral blood flow is impaired or lost, and regional brain perfusion is passive and essentially dependent upon systemic blood pressure. Therefore, hypotension is to be avoided. Edema characteristically develops 24–72 hours following infarction and can lead to complications due to mass effect; this is especially critical in the posterior fossa, where obstruction of cerebrospinal fluid flow and secondary hydrocephalus can result (Figure 30–3). Fluid balance in acute stroke patients should therefore be watched carefully and kept on the "dry side" to minimize the risk of hyponatremia and further brain swelling. Inappropriate antidiuretic hormone secretion can sometimes complicate this problem. When progressive mass effect with secondary hydrocephalus occurs, management is as described in Chapter 28 and will require consultation with a neurosurgeon. Since many stroke patients develop dysphagia or have poor mental status, aspiration precautions should be taken and a nasogastric tube should be placed. Swallowing evaluations often are necessary before allowing oral intake.

Anticoagulation is clearly indicated in embolic disease but usually must be delayed in the presence of a significant hemorrhagic infarct because of the risk of further bleeding. However, this factor must be weighed against what one judges to be the risk for repeated embolization. Common practice is to delay for about 10–14 days. The efficacy of anticoagulation in occlusive vascular disease is less clear, but it is common practice at this time to anticoagulate patients with strokes in progression or frequently repeated **transient ischemic attacks.** In the critical care situation, initial anticoagulation for cerebrovascular disease is accomplished with intravenous heparin.

Antiplatelet therapy has been shown to reduce the incidence of future stroke in patients at risk, including those with present or prior stroke, and it can be initiated in the acute phase of a new stroke. The available agents are aspirin or enteric-coated aspirin, 81–325 mg/d; clopidogrel bisulfate, 75 mg/d; or aspirin and extended-release dipyridamole, one 25/200 mg capsule twice daily. Ticlopidine, 250 mg twice daily, also is available but is associated with a higher incidence of adverse reactions than the others.

Treatment of acute ischemic stroke with intravenous recombinant tissue plasminogen activator (rt-PA; al-

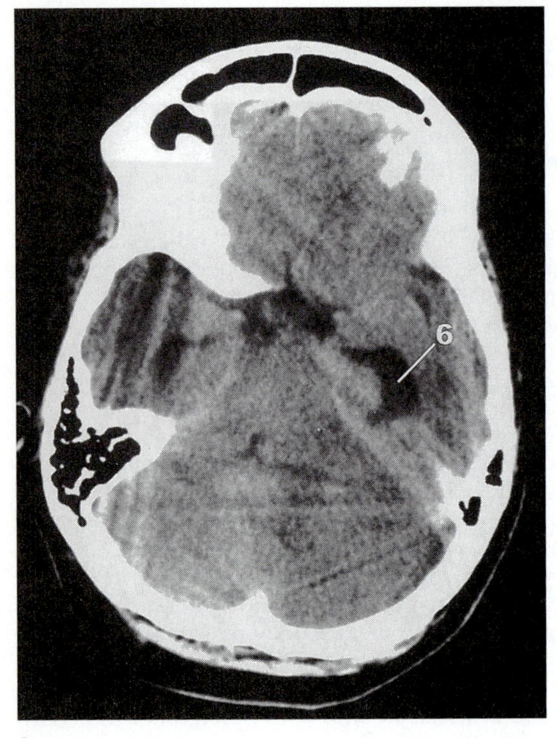

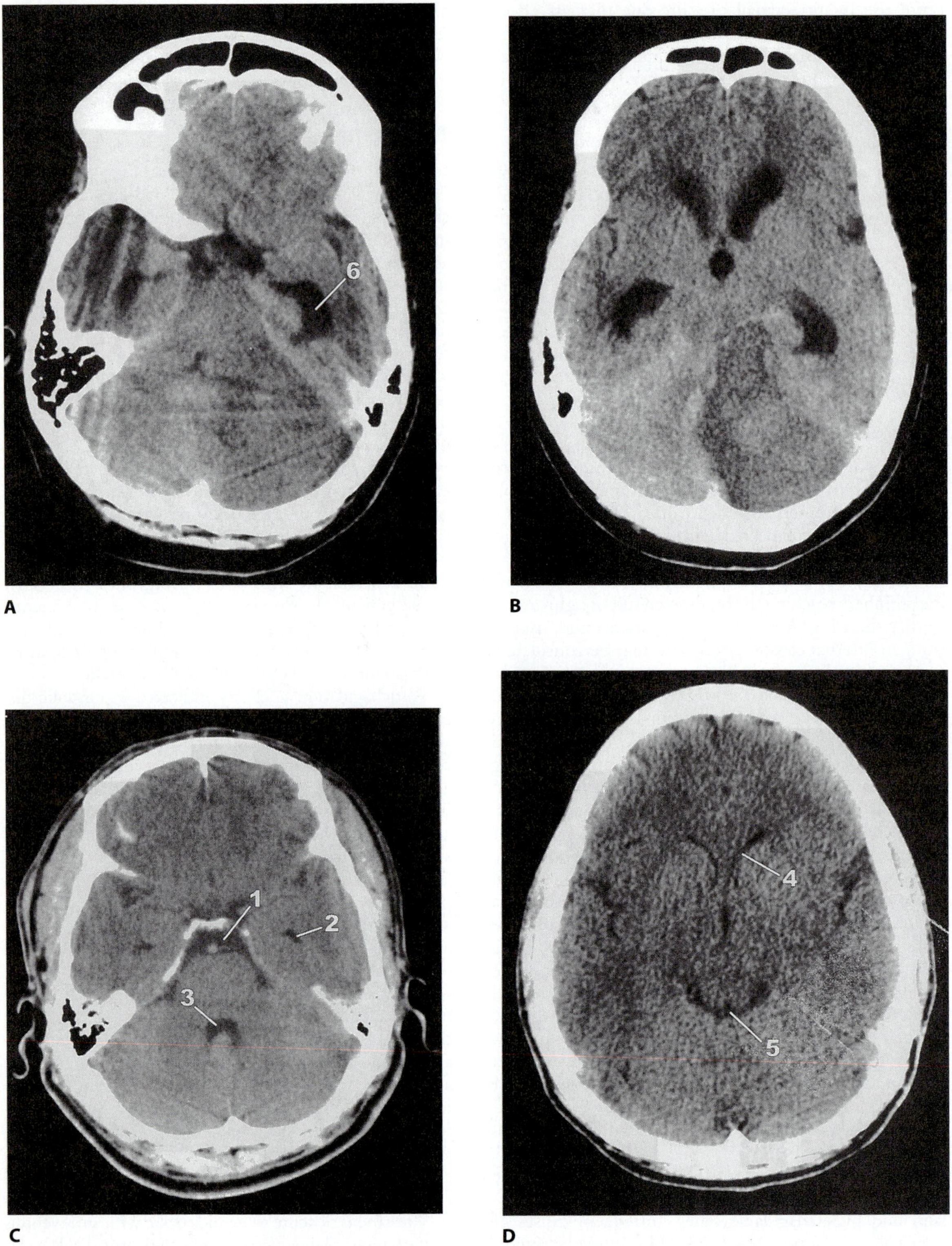

A

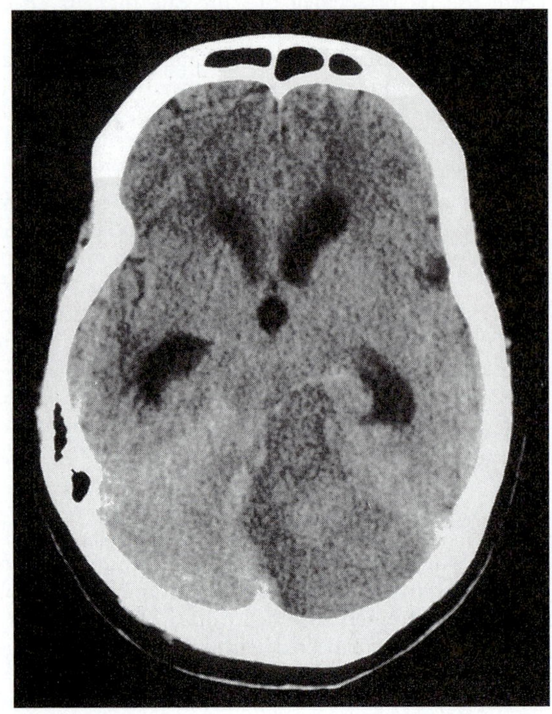

B

C

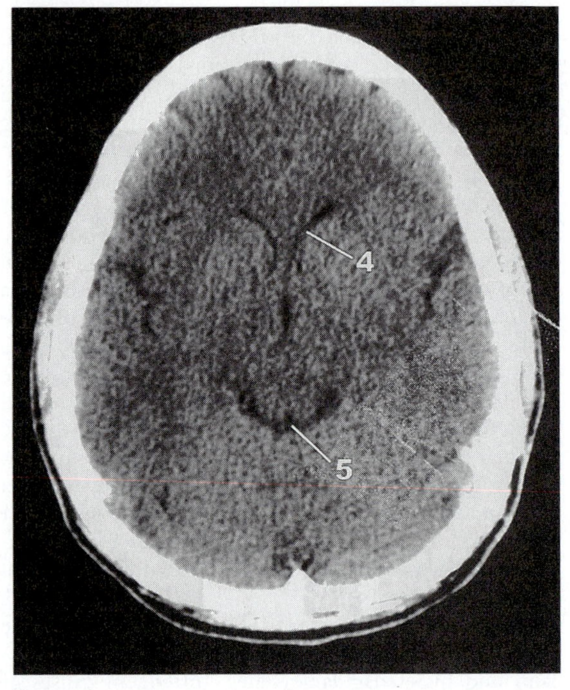

D

teplase) has been shown to be beneficial but only if initiated within 3 hours after stroke onset; thus, a clear history of time of onset and prompt transportation to a treatment facility are crucial. The benefit realized is reduction in long-term disability; improvement taking place in the acute phase is not clearly attributable to the treatment. Nevertheless, many specialists in this area believe that within the 3-hour time window, the sooner the better is the rt-PA treatment. The major adverse event of this treatment is intracerebral hemorrhage, but even so the long-term outcome may be improved if the patient survives. Overall, the most frequently reported hemorrhage rate is in the 3–6% or more range. It is essential that the treating institution establish a system for immediate patient evaluation and have a protocol in place. Table 30–7 lists the inclusion and exclusion criteria adopted by the authors' institution, and Table 30–8 gives the protocol for evaluation and treatment.

Current Controversies & Unresolved Issues

Carotid endarterectomy is generally recommended to reduce the risk of future stroke when 70% or more of stenosis is present in a symptomatic artery (it is contraindicated in an occluded artery). Some data exist indicating that endarterectomy on an asymptomatic, high-grade stenotic carotid artery is beneficial, but this remains controversial.

Work is in progress to better assess outcome of patients treated with rt-PA and to refine selection criteria for identifying those more likely or less likely to respond.

COMPLICATIONS OF CENTRAL NERVOUS SYSTEM INFECTIONS

ESSENTIALS OF DIAGNOSIS

- *History: Neurologic symptoms, exposures.*
- *Examination: Level of consciousness, neck stiffness, focal neurologic findings, seizures.*
- *Brain imaging with and without contrast.*
- *Cerebrospinal fluid analysis.*

Table 30–7. rt-PA (alteplase) criteria.

Inclusion criteria
- Age 18 or older
- Clearly defined time of onset (*very important!*)
- Ability to initiate rt-PA within 180 minutes from time of onset

Exclusion criteria
- Minor stroke or rapidly improving symptoms
- Hemorrhage or edema on noncontrast head CT
- Suspected subarachnoid hemorrhage
- Stroke or serious head trauma within 3 months prior to current stroke
- Major surgery or trauma within 14 days prior to current stroke
- History of intracranial hemorrhage
- Systolic blood pressure > 185 mm Hg or diastolic blood pressure > 110 mm Hg
- Gastrointestinal or urinary tract hemorrhage within 21 days prior to current stroke
- Arterial puncture at a noncompressible site within 7 days prior to current stroke
- Acute myocardial infarction or pericarditis
- Patient taking anticoagulants or has received heparin within the 48 hours preceding the onset of stroke and has elevated aPTT
- Platelet count < 100,000/μL
- PT > 15 seconds (INR > 1.7) or aPTT > 34 seconds
- Glucose < 50 mg/dL or > 400 mg/dL
- Seizure at onset of stroke
- Known or suspected pregnancy or lactating woman
- Aggressive treatment required to maintain blood pressure below indicated parameters
- Lumbar puncture within 7 days prior to current stroke
- Occult blood in urine or stool

General Considerations

The initial patient examination should lead to an etiologic diagnosis and selection of appropriate therapy. Infectious disease consultation may be necessary in the process. Beyond this, the critical care physician should be alert to certain aspects and complications of central nervous system infections. Viral, granulomatous, parasitic, and bacterial infections each have special features requiring consideration, and all have some common features.

Figure 30–3. ***A, B:*** Hypotense lesion in the right cerebellar hemisphere with swelling and mass effect resulting in obliteration of the fourth ventricle and cisterns surrounding the brain stem and secondary enlargement of the third ventricle and the temporal and lateral ventricles. Approximately $2^1/_2$ hours after this CT scan was obtained, the patient became comatose and lost brain stem function due to progressive obstructive hydrocephalus and brain stem compression. Also, intracranial pressure may exceed cerebral perfusion pressure in this circumstance. Timely neurosurgical intervention can prevent this sequence of events and thus be life saving. ***C, D:*** Normal studies for comparison. 1 and 5, cistern; 3, fourth ventricle; 2 and 6, temporal ventricle; 4, lateral ventricle (third ventricle, unlabeled).

Table 30–8. rt-PA (alteplase) protocol.

1. When notified of a possible rt-PA candidate, call designated medical personnel immediately.
2. Get the time of onset, a medication list, and complete neurologic examination. Patient needs a monitored bed in the emergency room.
3. Obtain stat head CT scan (noncontrast) to rule out hemorrhage; stat labs: CBC, PT/aPTT/glucose; stat ECG.
4. Go through all exclusion criteria (Table 30–7) and put sheet on chart.
5. Dose: Alteplase (Activase) 0.9 mg/kg (maximum 90 mg total dose) IV. Give 10% as bolus over 1 minute, remainder by continuous infusion over 60 minutes.
6. If patient get rt-PA, needs ICU bed.
7. Order vital signs and neurologic checks (specify what you want checked):
   - –every 15 minutes for 2 hours
   - –every 30 minutes for 6 hours
   - –every 1 hour for 16 hours
8. Strict blood pressure control (185/95 mm Hg or less). Use IV labetalol or nitroprusside drip.
9. Urgent: No anticoagulants and no antiplatelet agents whatsoever for 24 hours after rt-PA given.
10. If there is any worsening on neurologic or mental status examination, *stop rt-PA* if still being infused and order stat head CT (noncontrast) to rule out hemorrhage.

Clinical Features

A. Viral Infections

Meninges and neurons are the site of most central nervous system viral infections; human immunodeficiency virus (HIV), which infects microglia and leads to the formation of multinucleated cells in the brain, is a notable exception. **Viral meningitis** usually runs a self-limited course with supportive therapy only, and the specific virus usually is not identified—no more than headache, fever, neck stiffness, and abnormal cerebrospinal fluid findings are expected clinical features. On the other hand, **viral encephalitis** reflects neuronal dysfunction. Altered mental status, seizures, and even focal neurologic signs are common. Early recognition is especially important in herpes simplex type I (HSV) encephalitis because early and prompt treatment with acyclovir improves outcome. This virus has a predilection for temporal lobes; thus, presenting features commonly are confusion, change of usual behavior patterns, memory disturbance, and complex partial seizures, which may secondarily generalized (see section on seizures). Inflammation, sometimes with a hemorrhagic component, and edema may be enough to affect nearby cortex, giving rise to additional focal features such as hemiparesis, sensory deficit, or language disturbance. If HSV encephalitis is suspected, acyclovir should be started immediately and not postponed awaiting confirmatory workup. HIV infection of the central nervous system may result in mental and motor slowing (AIDS dementia complex) by mechanisms not yet understood, but—aside from the acute phase of infection—the occurrence of seizures, focal neurologic symptoms, and findings or symptoms and signs of meningitis indicate a superimposed complication such as infection with toxoplasma, cryptococcus, fungus, mycobacteria, or an intracerebral lymphoma.

B. Parasitic Infections

Cysticercosis is the most common parasitic central nervous system infection encountered in the United States. It is most common in states bordering Mexico and is most often seen in Mexican immigrants. It is a major public health problem in other parts of the world as well. It is acquired by ingestion of eggs of the tapeworm, taenia, which are shed in the feces of human carriers. Three forms of the disease exist. The most common site of infection is the parenchyma of the cerebral hemispheres, and the natural course of this form of the disease is eventual death of the organisms and subsequent calcification of the lesion, which is readily identified as punctate calcifications present on CT scans. This process often is entirely asymptomatic, but sometimes the tissue reaction and associated edema caused by the organisms' death produce focal neurologic symptoms and signs and imaging studies may not clearly distinguish such a lesion from a primary or metastatic neoplasm. In this instance, neurologic consultation is indicated. The characteristic locus of parenchymal cysticercosis is at the gray-white junction, and the usual clinical manifestation is a seizure disorder, which is sometimes limited in time and sometimes chronic. The seizures are partial, often with secondary generalization, which may be so rapid that the partial onset is unrecognizable. Treatment with antiepileptic medication is indicated.

Another form of this disease is intraventricular cysticercosis, in which the organism remains cystic and is located within the ventricular system. It is asymptomatic unless it causes obstructive hydrocephalus with headaches as the initial symptom. This is a very dangerous situation as the cysts often are free to move within a ventricle and thus can cause acute hydrocephalus and relatively sudden and unexpected death of the patient. A high degree of suspicion is necessary and should lead to brain imaging studies, which could include CT brain scan, intraventricular positive contrast CT brain scan to outline a cyst, and MRI of the brain. Neurosurgical intervention for shunting of cerebrospinal fluid or cyst removal is required.

Finally, the organism may reside in the subarachnoid space, where it exists in the racemose form and can cause meningeal inflammation. This is an indolent and chronic form, and racemose membrane formation with cystic loculations usually is slowly progressive. If this occurs around the base of the brain, it also may result in obstructive hydrocephalus and require placement of a cerebrospinal fluid shunt. Nonsteroidal anti-inflammatory medication is indicated for relief of headache due to the meningeal reaction and may decrease the inflammatory response.

Praziquantel or albendazole will kill the organism in the parenchymal form and perhaps the racemose form, but no controlled evidence exists that treatment with these agents changes the natural course of the disease. Furthermore, the increased rate of organism death and the subsequent brain tissue reaction has increased patient morbidity and in some instances, particularly when the disease was present in the posterior fossa and around the brain stem, has contributed to the death of the patient.

Amebic meningoencephalitis occurs but is rare in the United States. Usually it is acquired from swimming or bathing in infected fresh warm water springs. Fever, headache, and seizures are the presenting signs. Amphotericin B has been recommended for treatment.

Toxoplasmosis—infection with *Toxoplasma gondii,* an obligate intracellular parasite—is one of the most frequent opportunistic infections in patients who have AIDS and as a consequence is much more frequently encountered than it used to be. Symptoms are those of meningoencephalitis and often include headache, confusion, delirium, obtundation, and, less often, seizure. Brain imaging studies and cerebrospinal fluid examination, including serum toxoplasma IgG antibody titer, are useful in diagnosis, but sometimes a favorable response to treatment with pyrimethamine and sulfadiazine (usually judged by reduction of lesions seen on imaging studies) is necessary for diagnostic confirmation. Brain biopsy will be diagnostic if response to treatment is uncertain or fails.

C. Granulomatous Infections

Among fungi and yeast infections, coccidioidomycosis and cryptococcosis are most frequently encountered. While they and mycobacteria may form parenchymal lesions, a chronic progressive meningitis is the rule and it has a predilection for meninges at the base of the brain. A common complication is the development of hydrocephalus due to blockage of cerebrospinal fluid flow from the foramina of Luschka and Magendie. It is usually a relatively slow and progressive process, occurring in the mid to later stages of these diseases, and it often requires placement of a cerebrospinal fluid shunt. Brain CT scan or MRI will show the presence and progression of hydrocephalus. With contrast, those studies also show the presence of the inflammatory basilar meningitis. Other complications are cranial nerve deficits and infarctions caused by inflammation and constriction from the proliferative meningitis around arteries. Fluconazole and intravenous amphotericin B are the primary drugs for treatment of coccidioidomycosis and cryptococcosis, but sometimes the response is insufficient and intrathecal administration of amphotericin B is necessary. One must be aware that if the drug is delivered into a lateral ventricle in the presence of hydrocephalus and a shunt, it will not reach the site of infection but rather be diverted away. Under these circumstances, placement of a reservoir for delivery into the foramen magnum or lumbar subarachnoid space may be possible. This will require neurosurgical consultation.

D. Bacterial Infections

Central nervous system infection with *Listeria monocytogenes* is here singled out because it is unusual in that it can cause a rhombencephalitis with prominent brain stem findings—and it may also cause meningitis. Persons with chronic illness are predisposed to this disease. In general, prompt diagnosis and appropriate therapy of bacterial infections can prevent or reduce complications.

When seizures or focal neurologic deficits occur in the course of bacterial meningitis, one should suspect **cortical vein thrombosis,** which can be demonstrated by brain imaging studies. In the case of seizures, an antiepileptic drug such as phenytoin or phenobarbital should be administered and probably will have to be given intravenously (see section on seizures). Acute **sagittal sinus thrombosis** is a life-threatening complication because of brain swelling and bleeding into the parenchyma; neurologic findings can include obtundation and signs of increased intracranial pressure, seizures, and perhaps focal neurologic deficits—typically paresis of the legs because of the functional localization of the area of brain drained by the sinus. CT or MR imaging will confirm the diagnosis. Administration of an anticoagulant may only serve to increase bleeding from veins feeding the sinus. Seizures should be treated with an antiepileptic drug. As prompt a resolution as possible of the underlying infection will improve outcome.

Hydrocephalus can be an early or late complication of bacterial meningitis. Impairment of cerebrospinal fluid absorption at the arachnoid granulations, caused by purulent accumulation, inflammation, and adhesions, is a significant factor in this case. Cerebrospinal fluid shunting may be necessary.

Neurologic features of bacterial **brain abscesses** characteristically are focal neurologic findings and seizures. These abscesses often develop because of cardiac or pulmonary right-to-left shunting or extension of a sinus infection. In addition to antibiotic therapy, neurosurgical drainage and excision may be necessary. The dreaded complication is rupture of an abscess into the ventricles; this results in an acute ventriculitis, which almost always is fatal. Because of post-infectious scarring and gliosis, a chronic seizure disorder can develop.

Lastly, it is notable that a partially treated bacterial meningitis can mimic viral meningitis.

E. Laboratory Findings

The EEG should be normal in viral meningitis but it is highly likely to be abnormal in viral encephalitis, showing generalized slowing and, sometimes, epileptiform events. Characteristic of herpes encephalitis are periodic seizure discharges, predominant over the affected temporal area; absence of this finding does not rule out herpes encephalitis. Hydrocephalus, especially from disease in the posterior fossa, can show background disorganization and slowing with intermittent runs of high-voltage slow waves. Any focal brain disease may result in focal slow activity in the EEG, and often it is especially prominent in brain abscesses. The presence of epileptiform discharges will confirm the diagnosis of seizures and, if focal, indicate the site of the epileptogenic process.

The cerebrospinal fluid examination will show an increased cellular content in all active meningeal infections, although rarely the specimen may be obtained just preceding the cellular response; in this case, another specimen after a day or so should show increased cells. In general, bacterial infections will show polymorphonuclear leukocytes (PMNs) and the other infections predominantly mononuclear cells. Some viral infections, notably herpes simplex, may show a significant proportion of PMNs early in the course of the disease. It is typical in herpes encephalitis for the cerebrospinal fluid to contain red blood cells, but their absence does not rule it out. Partially treated bacterial meningitis can show predominantly mononuclear cells. Eosinophils are occasionally found in cases of cysticercosis. The organism can be demonstrated by India ink preparation in cryptococcosis and by wet preparation in amebic infection, but not finding them does not rule out either one. The Gram stain may find bacteria and the acid-fast stain mycobacteria. Low cerebrospinal fluid glucose results from infections interfering with its transport into the cerebrospinal fluid, and it is characteristically quite low in bacterial, fungal, and tuberculous meningitis. It is usually little altered in viral meningitis. Since the cerebrospinal fluid glucose level is normally close to half the blood glucose level, significantly high or low blood glucose can confuse the issue. Cerebrospinal fluid glucose concentration lags behind blood glucose 1–2 hours, but a blood glucose measured near the time of obtaining the cerebrospinal fluid specimen is usually satisfactory for judging the cerebrospinal fluid level. In viral infections, the cerebrospinal fluid protein content, like the glucose, is little altered, whereas it is elevated in the other infections. If the protein content is very high, blockage and impairment of cerebrospinal fluid flow should be suspected. Culture of cerebrospinal fluid can provide a definitive diagnosis in most infections other than viral, in which it is unusual to recover the agent. Anaerobic organisms are common in brain abscesses. Frequently the best management is to initiate appropriate therapy while awaiting the results of culture. Serologic tests of cerebrospinal fluid include latex agglutination or other techniques for detection of bacteria-specific antigens (usually available as a panel), measurement of cryptococcal antigen, and assay of coccidioidal antibody titer—the latter two are useful to follow as an index of response to treatment. False-negative immunologic tests frequently are encountered in neurocysticercosis, and a positive test may be found in extraneural cysticercosis, so the practical value of such testing is limited. Serum-specific herpes simplex antibody titers rising over the course of the illness can confirm the diagnosis, but usually in retrospect. Toxoplasma IgM titer is helpful if positive; a negative result does not exclude the disease in AIDS. HIV infection of the central nervous system can be accurately followed by assaying the cerebrospinal fluid viral load.

REFERENCES

Albers GW et al: Supplement to the guidelines for the management of transient ischemic attacks. Stroke 1999;30:2502–11.

Barohn RJ: Approach to peripheral neuropathy and neuronopathy. Semin Neurol 1998;18:7–18.

Brew BJ: *HIV Neurology,* Oxford Univ Press, 2001.

Broderick JP et al.: Guidelines for the management of spontaneous intracerebral hemorrhage. Stroke 1999;30:905–15.

Brott T, Bogousslavsky J: Treatment of acute ischemic stroke. N Engl J Med 2000;343:710–22.

Drachman DB: Myasthenia gravis. (Medical Progress.) N Engl J Med 1994;330:1797–1810.

Hamel MB et al: Identification of comatose patients at high risk for death or severe disability. JAMA 1995;273:1842–8.

Keys PA, Blume RP: Therapeutic strategies for myasthenia gravis. DICP 1991;25:1101–8.

Medical Consultants to the President's Commission for the Study of Ethical Problems in Medicine and Biomedical and Behavioral Research: Guidelines for the determination of death. Neurology (New York) 1982;32:395–99. (Also in JAMA 1981;246:2184–86.)

Plum F, Posner JB: *The Diagnosis of Stupor and Coma,* 3rd ed. Davis, 1982.

Ropper AH: *Neurological and Neurosurgical Intensive Care,* 3rd ed. Raven, 1993.

Rowland L: *Merritt's Neurology,* 10th ed. Lippincott Williams & Wilkins, 2000.

Shah SM, Kelly KM: *Emergency Neurology: Principles and Practice,* Cambridge Univ Press, 1999.

Status Epilepticus in Perspective. Neurology Supplement 2 1990; 40(5).

Van Ness PC: Pentobarbital and EEG burst suppression in treatment of status epilepticus refractory to benzodiazepines and phenytoin. Epilepsia 1990;31:61–67.

Victor M: *Adams & Victor's Principles of Neurology,* 7th ed. McGraw-Hill, 2001.

Wilson W: *Current Diagnosis and Treatment of Infectious Diseases,* McGraw-Hill, 2001.

Wylie E: *Treatment of Epilepsy,* 3rd ed. Lippincott Williams & Wilkins, 2000.

Neurosurgical Critical Care

31

Chris A. Lycette, MD, Curtis Doberstein, MD, Gerald E. Rodts, Jr., MD, & Duncan Q. McBride, MD

Neurosurgical critical care covers a wide array of disorders with varying pathophysiologic features. These conditions may also be associated with unique complications that must be recognized and promptly treated. Physicians involved in the ICU management of neurosurgical patients must therefore be familiar with the clinical features, complications, and treatment of central nervous system disorders.

This chapter focuses on the management of patients with head injuries, aneurysmal subarachnoid hemorrhage, brain tumors, and cervical spinal cord injury—disorders that comprise the majority of neurosurgical ICU admissions.

Following injury, the central nervous system is vulnerable to a variety of secondary insults that can occur minutes, hours, or days following the primary injury. Systemic conditions such as hypoxia, hypotension, and electrolyte disorders may contribute to morbidity in severely injured patients. Cerebral abnormalities such as elevated intracranial pressure, seizures, hemorrhage, and ischemia also have the potential to cause neurologic impairment. The main focus of modern intensive care is to avoid or quickly reverse any conditions that can lead to secondary injury. Therefore, meticulous management in all aspects of critical care is required to prevent neurologic damage and improve patient outcome.

HEAD INJURIES

ESSENTIALS OF DIAGNOSIS

- *Signs depend on severity and anatomic location.*
- *Concussion: Transient loss of consciousness, memory loss, headache, autonomic dysfunction.*
- *Herniation: Depressed level of consciousness, anisocoria, abnormal motor findings.*

General Considerations

Injuries to the brain remain the most common cause of trauma-related death and disability. More than 500,000 people suffer some degree of head trauma annually in the United States. In the past, patients with traumatic brain injuries were viewed with some pessimism because both surgical and medical therapeutic resources were limited. However, with recent advances and prompt and intensive management of head-injured patients, the outcome has improved. One of the major reasons for the better results has been improved critical care management, particularly the recognition and prevention of disorders that can cause secondary brain injury. The need for evidence-based standards led to the publication in 1995 of *Guidelines for Management of Severe Head Injury* by the Brain Tumor Foundation. This document provided the first set of uniform and effective protocols that were based on scientific evidence and supported various treatments demonstrated to improve survival and outcome of brain injury patients. The second edition in 2000 included updates in each category as well as a section on early indicators of the prognosis for patients with severe brain trauma. These guidelines have been incorporated into this chapter and should be referred to for guidance in the treatment of head injuries.

Classification

A. Primary Injuries

By definition, primary traumatic brain injury occurs at the time of impact. This may lead to irreversible damage from cell disruption depending on the mechanism and severity of the inciting event. Head trauma may cause damage to the scalp, skull, and underlying brain. Scalp lacerations can cause significant hemorrhage, but in most cases hemostasis can be achieved easily. Fractures are classified as linear, depressed, compound, or involving the skull base. Linear or simple skull fractures require no specific treatment. Depressed skull fracture occurs when the outer table of the skull is depressed below the inner table and may result in tearing of the dura or laceration of the brain. Operative repair may be required, especially if the depressed fracture involves the posterior wall of the frontal sinus or is associated with intracranial hematoma. Compound depressed fractures are defined as those associated with laceration of the overlying scalp and are treated by surgical wound debridement and fracture elevation, if severe. Basal skull fractures, which may be diagnosed by the clinical findings of periorbital ecchymosis ("raccoon eyes"), ecchymosis of the postauricular area

(Battle's sign), hemotympanum, or cerebrospinal fluid leak, may be complicated by meningitis or brain abscess. Patients suffering from skull fractures have an increased risk of delayed intracranial hematoma and should be observed for 12–24 hours after the initial injury.

Brain injury can occur directly under the injury site (coup injury), but because the brain may move relative to the skull and dura, compression of the brain remote from the site of impact can also occur. This explains why brain injury can occur in intracranial regions opposite the point of impact (contrecoup injury). Craniocerebral trauma can cause concussion, cerebral contusion, intracranial hemorrhage, or diffuse axonal injury.

1. Concussion—Concussion is an episode of transient loss of consciousness following craniocerebral trauma. There is no evidence of pathologic brain damage. Patients may suffer from variable degrees of memory loss, autonomic dysfunction, headaches, tinnitus, and irritability.

2. Cerebral contusions—Cerebral contusions are heterogeneous areas of hemorrhage into the brain parenchyma and may produce neurologic deficits depending upon their anatomic location. The anterior portions of the frontal and temporal lobes are particularly vulnerable because of the rough contour of the skull in these regions. Contusions are often associated with disruption of the blood-brain barrier and may be complicated by extension of the hemorrhage, edema formation, or seizure. Large contusions can cause a mass effect resulting in elevation of intracranial pressure or brain herniation.

3. Intracranial hematomas—Head injury may cause hemorrhage into the epidural, subdural, or subarachnoid spaces. This bleeding, which may require surgical evacuation depending upon its size and location, is usually diagnosed prior to admission to the ICU. However, delayed intracranial hematomas or postoperative hematomas are not uncommon following craniocerebral trauma and can develop and progress during ICU observation. Intracranial bleeding may result in a mass effect that can cause intracranial pressure elevation (see below) and brain herniation with compression of vital cerebral structures.

a. Epidural hematomas—These lesions are typically due to skull fracture and laceration of a meningeal vessel, most commonly the posterior branch of the middle meningeal artery. This may occur following low-velocity impact injuries. Because the dura is firmly attached to the inner table of the skull, the hematoma usually takes on a homogeneous lentiform configuration (Figure 31–1A).

b. Subdural hematomas—Subdural hematomas can be secondary to tearing of the cortical vessels, such as the bridging veins that drain from the cortex to the superior sagittal sinus. They are commonly associated with other injuries such as cerebral contusions and have a worse prognosis than epidural hematomas. Because it is not contained by dural attachments, the hemorrhage often spreads diffusely across the cortical surface (Figure 31–1B).

c. Subarachnoid hemorrhage—Subarachnoid hemorrhage is most commonly caused by craniocerebral trauma. The subarachnoid bleeding itself does not usually cause neurologic damage, but hydrocephalus and cerebral vasospasm, which are delayed complications typically seen days to weeks following subarachnoid hemorrhage, can lead to neurologic impairment. Subarachnoid hemorrhage as a result of a ruptured intracranial aneurysm should always be considered as a possible causative factor in trauma and needs to be ruled out with an angiogram if there is reasonable concern.

4. Diffuse axonal injury—Diffuse axonal injury is shearing of brain tissue with disruption of neuronal axon projections in the cerebral white matter. This diffuse injury to axons occurs microscopically and can result in severe neurologic impairment. Evidence of diffuse axonal injury is often not demonstrable on CT scans. However, macroscopic hemorrhagic lesions can occur in the deep brain such as the corpus callosum or brain stem in association with diffuse axonal injury.

B. Secondary Injuries

Many studies have observed that cerebral autoregulation is impaired after traumatic brain injury. This causes patients with head injuries to be unusually vulnerable to secondary ischemic insults such as hypotension, intracranial hypertension, and hypoxia. Further ischemic damage can be prevented with an understanding of the pathophysiology of these secondary insults and an aggressive targeted management protocol. These conditions can be conveniently divided into intracranial and systemic disorders (Table 31–1). Following traumatic brain injury, some cells are directly and irreversibly damaged. However, other cells may be functionally compromised and not mechanically disrupted. These may recover if provided with an optimal environment for survival. Compromised cells are vulnerable to the pathophysiologic challenges imposed by secondary insults. Prevention or rapid recognition and treatment of secondary insults is the primary focus of modern critical care management of head injury patients.

1. Secondary intracranial insults (raised intracranial pressure)—Intracranial hypertension following craniocerebral trauma may be caused by intracranial hematomas, cerebral edema, or cerebral hyperemia. The Monro-Kellie doctrine proposes that small changes in intracranial volume may ultimately cause intracranial pressure to increase because of the rigid and inelastic

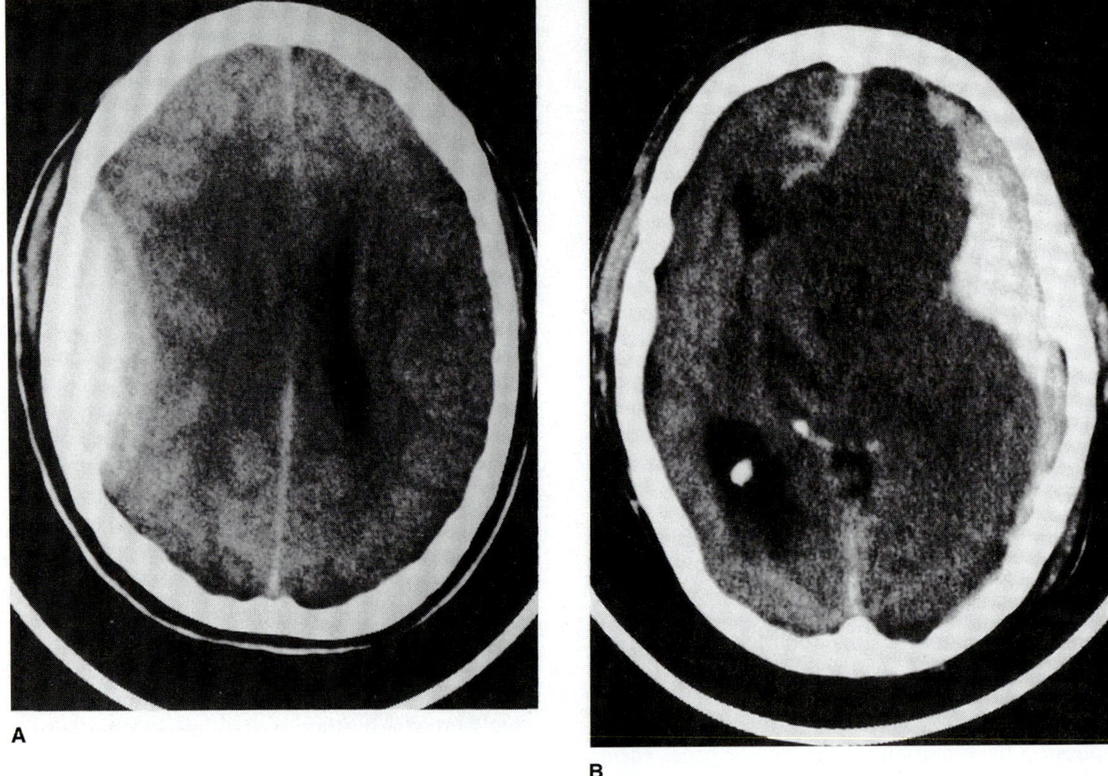

Figure 31–1. ***A:*** Left temporoparietal epidural hematoma with obliteration of the left lateral ventricle and midline shift. ***B:*** Right frontoparietal and interhemispheric subdural hematoma with massive right-to-left midline shift.

properties of the skull. Under normal circumstances, intracranial volume is composed of roughly 80% brain tissue, 10% cerebrospinal fluid, and 10% blood. An increase in volume of one of these compartments—or the addition of a new pathologic compartment (eg, intracranial hematoma)—must be compensated for by a reduction in the volume of another compartment. Compensatory mechanisms that "buffer" such volume changes include increased cerebrospinal fluid absorption, redistribution of cerebrospinal fluid from the intracranial cavity into the spinal subarachnoid space, and a reduction in cerebral blood volume. Cerebral compliance relates the change in intracranial volume to the resulting change in intracranial pressure (Figure 31–2). High compliance signifies a brain that can utilize buffering mechanisms to keep intracranial pressure stable with changes in intracranial volume. However, when the buffering becomes saturated, large pressure elevations result from small volume changes (poor compliance; arrow Figure 31–2). Therefore, although intracranial pressure may lie within a relatively normal range (up to 20 mm Hg), a low-compliance state may exist and rapid elevations in intracranial pressure may result from small increases in intracranial volume.

The falx cerebri, tentorium cerebelli, and foramen magnum are relatively rigid structures that compartmentalize regions of the brain. Because many pathologic processes are focal, pressure gradients can be generated between the intracranial compartments. Elevated intracranial pressure may exert its deleterious effects by causing pressure gradients between different brain compartments. If this pressure gradient is of sufficient magnitude, shifting or herniation of brain tissue occurs and can result in compression of vital structures. For example, transtentorial herniation occurs when increased supratentorial volume and pressure are sufficient to shift the uncus and the medial portion of the temporal lobe through the tentorial notch, causing compression and dysfunction of the midbrain and oculomotor nerve. Compression of the medulla occurs when in-

Table 31–1. Secondary insults.

Intracranial
Raised intracranial pressure
Delayed intracerebral hematoma
Edema
Hyperemia
Carotid artery dissection
Seizures
Vasospasm
Systemic
Hypoxia
Respiratory arrest
Airway obstruction
ARDS
Aspiration pneumonia
Pneumonia and hemothorax
Pulmonary contusion
Hypotension
Shock
Excessive bleeding
Myocardial infarction
Cardiac contusion or tamponade
Spinal cord injury
Tension pneumothorax
Electrolyte imbalance
Diabetes insipidus
SIADH
Others
Anemia
Hyperthermia
Hypercapnia
Hypoglycemia

tracranial pressure is elevated and the cerebellar tonsils herniate through the foramen magnum. This condition, known as tonsillar herniation, can prove fatal because of the location of vital respiratory and vasomotor centers in this area of the brain stem.

Alternatively, since cerebral perfusion pressure is inversely related to intracranial pressure,* elevations in intracranial pressure may cause impaired cerebral perfusion. If cerebral perfusion pressure is greatly reduced (< 40–50 mm Hg), cerebral ischemia or infarction can occur. Therefore, maintenance of systemic blood pressure is of paramount importance when intracranial pressure is elevated.

2. Secondary systemic insults—Of the various systemic secondary insults, hypoxia and hypotension are the most significant. Prospective clinical studies have demonstrated that these two variables independently have a deleterious influence on the outcome in severe head injury. Hypotension alone is associated with a 150% increase in mortality rate. In patients with significant head injuries, hypoxemia may be due to upper airway obstruction, pneumothorax, hemothorax, pulmonary edema, or hypoventilation. Whatever the cause, hypoxemia must be corrected rapidly to avoid potential damage to nervous tissues. Hypotension reduces cerebral perfusion, which promotes cerebral ischemia and infarction. This is particularly harmful in the face of elevated

* CPP = MABP—MICP, where CPP = cerebral perfusion pressure, MABP = mean arterial blood pressure, and MICP = mean intracranial pressure.

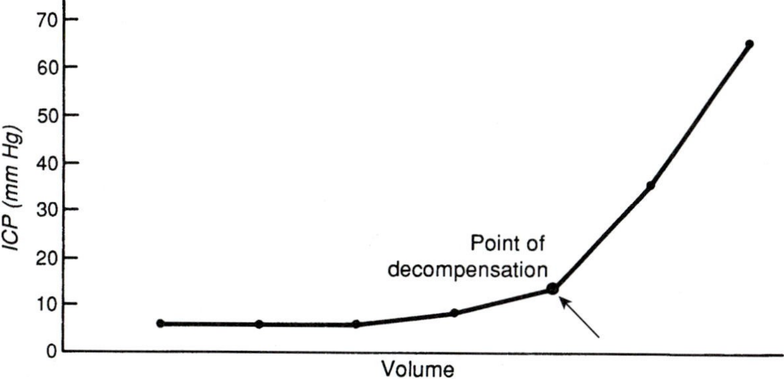

Figure 31–2. Intracranial pressure (ICP) remains normal with increased volume until the point of decompensation is reached. Above this critical volume, intracranial pressure increases quickly.

intracranial pressure. In addition, impaired cerebral autoregulation can occur after brain injury. With normal autoregulation, cerebral blood flow remains constant despite fluctuation in mean arterial pressure between 60 and 180 mm Hg (Figure 31–3). Rapid arteriolar constriction or dilation occurs in response to pressure changes. However, when this normal response is impaired, cerebral blood flow is directly related to systemic arterial pressure. Thus, if hypotension occurs, reduced tissue perfusion and ischemia may result. Surgery for extracranial injuries should be delayed as long as possible because of this issue. Surgery-related hypotensive episodes can have a very negative impact on brain perfusion and ultimately the quality of overall outcome. Other preventable systemic causes of secondary brain injury include electrolyte disturbances, anemia, hypoglycemia, hyperthermia, coagulopathies, and seizures.

Clinical Features

A. Symptoms and Signs

Clinical examination remains the best method for rapidly identifying neurologic deterioration. The Glasgow Coma Scale, which is based on eye opening as well as verbal and motor responses, is widely used to assess head injury patients (Table 31–2). Other important components of an initial neurologic examination assessments of brain stem function, including level of consciousness, respiratory pattern, and pupillary size and reactivity as well as oculocephalic, oculovestibular, and gag reflexes. Eye movements, extremity motor and sensory function, and speech should also be evaluated. Following this initial brief examination, a more thorough neurologic assessment can be performed.

Table 31–2. Glasgow Coma Scale.

Eye opening (E)	
Spontaneous	4
To voice	3
To pain	2
None	1
Motor responses (M)	
Obeys commands	6
Localizes pain	5
Withdraws	4
Abnormal flexion	3
Abnormal extension	2
None	1
Verbal responses (V)	
Oriented	5
Confused	4
Inappropriate words	3
Incomprehensible sounds	2
None	1
TOTAL SCORE	**(3 to 15)**

Transtentorial herniation, usually secondary to an expanding supratentorial mass, produces a classic triad of clinical signs: (1) depressed level of consciousness due to compression of the midbrain reticular activating system, (2) anisocoria and loss of the pupillary light reflex due to ipsilateral third nerve compression, and (3) abnormal motor findings. In the early stages of herniation, the ipsilateral third nerve is compressed; however, if pressure on the brain stem increases, both pupils may become dilated and unreactive. Contralateral hemiparesis due to com-

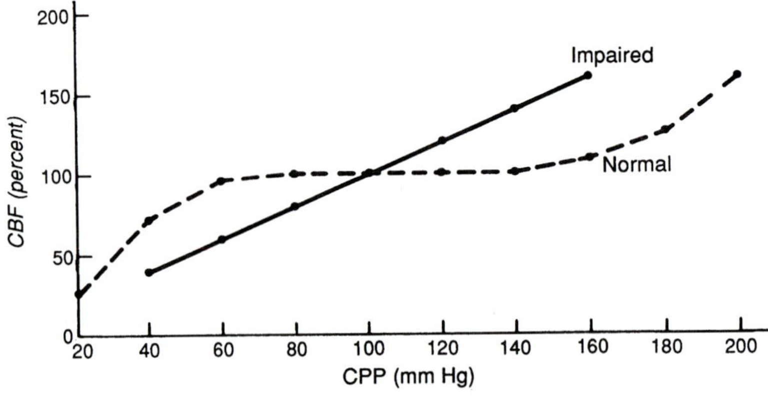

Figure 31–3. Cerebral blood flow (CBF) remains normal over a wide range of cerebral perfusion pressures in normal patients. Under pathologic conditions, cerebral blood flow varies directly with cerebral perfusion pressure (CPP).

pression of the ipsilateral cerebral peduncle is the most frequent abnormal motor response. However, in about 25% of cases, hemiparesis may occur on the same side as the mass lesion because the brain stem is displaced away from the mass, compressing the opposite cerebral peduncle against the free edge of the tentorium (Kernohan's notch phenomenon). The posterior cerebral artery can be compressed during transtentorial herniation and result in infarction of the brain tissue it supplies.

Signs of tonsillar herniation include respiratory irregularities, Cushing's response (elevated blood pressure associated with bradycardia), nuchal rigidity, and abnormal gag and cough reflexes due to medullary compression. During early herniation, the patient's level of consciousness may be normal because the upper brain stem and reticular activating system remain intact.

Neurologic deterioration in the ICU warrants immediate and thorough evaluation in an effort to elucidate the cause. Vital signs, serum electrolytes, and arterial blood gas values should be determined if the deterioration is nonfocal in nature. However, if the examination suggests a focal lesion, an intracranial hematoma, elevated intracranial pressure with a herniation syndrome, cerebral edema, or cerebral ischemia is probably present. Studies validate that aggressive medical management can reverse herniation and improve outcome.

B. Imaging Studies:

1. CT scan—Computed tomography is significantly more accurate than conventional radiographs and has replaced them in the evaluation of head injuries. CT can delineate parenchymal contusions, epidural and subdural hematomas, cerebral edema, hydrocephalus, and cerebral infarction. An intracranial lesion is said to exert a "mass effect" on the brain when there is CT evidence of effacement of the cerebral ventricles, subarachnoid cisterns, or cortical sulci signifying redistribution of cerebrospinal fluid. Further CT evidence of a mass effect includes a shift of midline structures away from the lesion and herniation of tissues. The outlet of the contralateral ventricle can become "trapped" as a result of midline shifting, and this can further increase intracranial pressure. Because MRI is slower and generally not available emergently, it is not commonly used to assess acute neurologic deteriorations. The availability of portable CT scanners enables the diagnostic study to be performed without transporting an unstable patient and risking harmful respiratory or cardiovascular events.

2. Cerebral angiography—Prior to the advent of CT scanning, angiography was the primary diagnostic study for evaluating head injury patients because it detects the mass effect from intracranial lesions. Currently, however, the main role for angiography is the assessment of vascular disorders such as dissection or traumatic pseudoaneurysm of the internal carotid or vertebral arteries and cerebral vasospasm.

3. Transcranial Doppler ultrasonography—Transcranial Doppler ultrasonography is a noninvasive technique that measures blood flow velocity in the basal cerebral arteries. It can be performed serially at the bedside in the ICU and can reliably detect arterial narrowing due to vasospasm, which causes increased flow velocity. It can also aid in the confirmation of absent blood flow due to brain death.

C. Monitoring of Intracranial Pressure

Measurement of intracranial pressure through an open catheter placed in the lateral ventricle (ventriculostomy) is the standard with which all other methods of intracranial pressure measurement must be compared. An additional advantage is that cerebrospinal fluid may be drained via the ventriculostomy to treat elevated pressures, if present. Ventricular catheters may be placed in the operating room during surgery or can be inserted at the bedside in the emergency room or ICU. Because of the risk of infection, patients with ventriculostomies should be given prophylactic antibiotics with gram-positive coverage such as cefazolin or vancomycin, and the catheters must be changed every 4–6 days. Measurement of ICP can also be determined using a fiberoptic or strain gauge device. These monitors are usually more expensive, have a tendency to drift, and are unable to drain cerebrospinal fluid as needed.

D. Lumbar Puncture

Lumbar puncture should not be performed in the initial evaluation of head trauma patients because of the risk of tonsillar herniation. The only role for lumbar puncture is to examine cerebrospinal fluid in patients who may have meningitis. In such cases, intracranial pressure must be thought to lie within the normal range prior to the procedure, or patients should receive mannitol to induce diuresis prior to a small-volume tap with a thin (eg, 22-gauge) spinal needle.

Treatment

A. Surgery

Patients who show neurologic deterioration require rapid intervention to prevent irreversible tissue damage. Cerebral contusions, intracranial hematomas, and foreign bodies may require emergent evacuation depending upon their size and location.

B. Reduction of Intracranial Pressure

Raised intracranial pressure should be treated using the following measures.

1. Removal of cerebrospinal fluid by ventricular drainage.

2. The use of mannitol prior to intracranial pressure monitoring should be reserved for signs of transtentorial herniation or progressive neurologic deterioration not attributable to extracranial explanations. Serum osmolarity should be maintained below 320 mosm/L in order to avoid renal failure, and volume should be replaced with colloid agents or blood if necessary to avoid hypotension or reduced cerebral perfusion. A Foley catheter is essential.

3. Hyperventilation results in cerebral vasoconstriction and can help reduce intracranial pressure for brief and specific periods. The vasoconstrictive effects assist in the management of an intracranial hypertensive crisis; however, the long-term influence can produce permanent injury by reducing blood flow below critical levels in an already injured brain. Therefore, the Brain Trauma Foundation standard is that in the absence of high intracranial pressure, chronic hyperventilation ($Pa_{CO_2} < 25$ mm Hg) should be avoided in the first 24 hours after traumatic brain injury. In addition, the use of prophylactic hyperventilation ($Pa_{CO_2} < 35$ mm Hg) during the first 24 hours should be avoided because it can compromise cerebral perfusion during a time of reduced cerebral blood flow (CBF).

4. Head elevation should be maintained to promote cerebral venous drainage. The head should be kept straight, and tape from the endotracheal tube should not cross the jugular area.

5. Sedation and neuromuscular paralysis are recommended in intubated patients. Noxious stimuli may increase intracranial pressure, which can be alleviated by sedation. Narcotics are useful because they can be rapidly reversed. Neuromuscular paralysis can reduce intracranial pressure in intubated patients by preventing increases in venous pressure associated with Valsalva's maneuver during ventilatory support. Benzodiazepines or propofol can be used as first-line agents for the sedation of head injury patients.

6. Anticonvulsant therapy (usually with phenytoin) can be used to prevent or control seizure activity that increases cerebral blood flow and subsequently intracranial pressure. Available evidence does not indicate that the prevention of early posttraumatic seizures improves outcome following head injury, so these agents should be used with discretion.

7. Fever increases intracranial pressure and should be prevented when possible. Cooling blankets are helpful for the management of refractory temperature elevations.

8. Barbiturate (pentobarbital) coma is useful if all other medical therapies fail because it reduces intracranial pressure by decreasing cerebral metabolism and therefore cerebral blood flow. Care must be taken to prevent hypotension.

9. In selected cases where maximum medical therapy has failed to reduce intracranial pressure, bony decompression or temporal lobectomy can be performed surgically. A randomized clinical trial is being organized to evaluate hemicraniectomy with duraplasty versus traditional craniotomy and removal of grossly contused brain.

C. Electrolytes

Cerebral salt wasting is a recognized phenomenon following brain injury. It is defined as renal loss of sodium during intracranial disease leading to hyponatremia and a decrease in extracellular fluid volume. Hyponatremia produces increased brain swelling, and the volume depletion that accompanies cerebral salt wasting must be aggressively treated to avoid hypotension and reduced cerebral perfusion. Therefore, cerebral salt wasting should be recognized promptly and treated with hypertonic saline solutions.

Traumatic brain injury can also result in a variety of other electrolyte disturbances requiring treatment, including hypomagnesemia, hypophosphotemia, and hypokalemia.

Becker DP, Gudeman SK (editors): *Textbook of Head Injury.* Saunders, 1989.

Chesnut RM, Marshall LF: Treatment of abnormal intracranial pressure. Neurosurg Clin North Am 1991;2: 267–84.

Cooper PR: Delayed brain injury: Secondary insults. In: *Central Nervous System Trauma Status Report—1985.* Becker DP, Povlishock JT (editors). Prepared for the National Institute of Neurological and Communicative Disorders and Stroke, National Institutes of Health, 1986.

Guidelines for the Management of Severe Head Injury, 2nd ed. Brain Tumor Foundation, 2000.

Marshall LF, Smith RW, Shapiro HM: The outcome with aggressive treatment in severe head injuries. J Neurosurg 1979;50:20–5.

Seelig JM et al: Traumatic acute subdural hematoma: Major mortality reduction in comatose patients treated under four hours. N Engl J Med 1981;304:1511–8.

Temkin NR et al: A randomized double-blind study of phenytoin for prevention of post-traumatic seizures. N Engl J Med 1990;323:497–502.

ANEURYSMAL SUBARACHNOID HEMORRHAGE

ESSENTIALS OF DIAGNOSIS

- *Headache.*
- *Nausea and vomiting.*
- *Photophobia.*
- *Nuchal rigidity.*
- *Depressed level of consciousness.*
- *Cranial nerve palsies, motor abnormalities.*

General Considerations

Rupture of an intracranial aneurysm is a devastating event, since roughly half of these patients die. Of the remainder, almost half are left with significant neurologic deficits as a result of their initial hemorrhage or due to delayed complications such as rebleeding, vasospasm, or hydrocephalus. In order to optimize outcome following subarachnoid hemorrhage, both good technical surgical intervention and meticulous ICU care are required.

Intracranial aneurysms usually occur at bifurcation sites of major arteries at the base of the brain and usually point in the direction of blood flow. It is believed that at these bifurcation sites a defect in the medial elastic lamina is present that predisposes to aneurysm formation. Aneurysms are associated with a variety of conditions, including hypertension, polycystic kidney disease, coarctation of the aorta, Ehlers-Danlos syndrome, pseudoxanthoma elasticum, and cerebral arteriovenous malformations. Approximately 85% are located in the anterior circulation, with the most common sites being the junction of the anterior cerebral and anterior communicating arteries, the junction of the internal carotid and posterior communicating arteries, the bifurcation or trifurcation of the middle cerebral artery, and the bifurcation of the internal carotid artery. Fifteen percent of aneurysms lie within the posterior circulation; the basilar artery apex is the most common site. Multiple aneurysms can be identified in 15–20% of patients. Since the cerebral arteries course within the subarachnoid space, rupture typically produces subarachnoid hemorrhage. However, intraparenchymal and intraventricular bleeding may occur depending upon the location of the aneurysm and the extent of bleeding.

The three major complications following aneurysmal subarachnoid hemorrhage are rebleeding, vasospasm, and hydrocephalus. Rebleeding from a ruptured intracranial aneurysm occurs in 20% of cases during the first 2 weeks after the initial hemorrhage if the aneurysm is untreated. The highest risk is in the first 24 hours, and treatment with surgery or interventional embolization techniques is required. Cerebral vasospasm is a common delayed complication of subarachnoid hemorrhage and is related to the amount of blood located within the subarachnoid space. Arterial narrowing is thought to result from degradation of subarachnoid blood, which produces breakdown products that cause smooth muscle constriction. If this smooth muscle constriction is prolonged, morphologic alterations such as fibrosis can occur in the vessel wall, further enhancing arterial narrowing. Communicating hydrocephalus is another complication that can occur after subarachnoid hemorrhage and is secondary to blockage of cerebrospinal fluid reabsorption by platelets, erythrocytes, and their breakdown products. Hydrocephalus may present in an acute, subacute, or delayed fashion.

In addition to the previously described neurologic complications, several systemic medical disorders can occur. Cardiac arrhythmias and myocardial ischemia are frequently observed. Respiratory complications such as pulmonary edema, ARDS, and pneumonia are common. Other disorders such as anemia, gastrointestinal bleeding, deep vein thrombosis, and hyponatremia occur with varying frequency.

Clinical Features

A. Symptoms and Signs

Symptoms such as headache, nausea and vomiting, photophobia, nuchal rigidity, depressed level of consciousness, cranial nerve palsies, and motor abnormalities can occur. The severity of symptoms is related to the site and extent of the bleeding. Following aneurysmal subarachnoid hemorrhage, the patient is categorized by grade using the Hunt and Hess classification system (Table 31–3). This system has been widely accepted and is the equivalent of the Glasgow Coma Score in trauma patients.

B. Imaging Studies

1. CT scanning—Ninety percent of patients with subarachnoid hemorrhage have evidence of subarachnoid blood on initial CT scans obtained within the first 48 hours after rupture. Scanning also detects intraparenchymal and intraventricular bleeding. The extent and location of subarachnoid hemorrhage can help determine the location of the aneurysm and identify patients at highest risk for developing cerebral vasospasm. Rebleeding, hydrocephalus, and cerebral infarction can also be verified using this technique.

2. Angiography—Once the diagnosis of subarachnoid hemorrhage has been established, four-vessel cerebral angiography should be performed unless a surgical le-

Table 31–3. Hunt and Hess grades for the assessment of patients with subarachnoid hemorrhage.

Grade 1	Asymptomatic, or minimal headache and slight nuchal rigidity.
Grade 2	Moderate to severe headache, nuchal rigidity, no neuroligic deficit other than a cranial nerve palsy.
Grade 3	Drowsiness, confusion, or mild focal deficit.
Grade 4	Stupor, moderate to severe hemiparesis, early decerebrate rigidity and vegetative disturbances.
Grade 5	Deep coma, decerebrate rigidity, moribund rigidity.

sion such as a significant intraparenchymal hematoma is present and requires emergent life-saving evacuation. Angiography is required prior to aneurysm surgery to localize the aneurysm, define its anatomy, and identify areas of cerebral vasospasm that may require postponement of surgery. Vasospasm typically occurs 3 days post hemorrhage and can continue for 3 weeks. All cerebral vessels should be imaged because of the occurrence of multiple aneurysms in 15–20% of patients.

3. Transcranial Doppler ultrasonography—Transcranial Doppler ultrasonography has become a useful technique for monitoring patients at risk for developing vasospasm. With progressive arterial narrowing, blood flow velocity increases through the constricted segment and can be detected by this procedure. Since this technique is noninvasive and portable, it can be performed at the bedside in the ICU. It can detect arterial narrowing prior to the development of ischemic symptoms so that therapy aimed at improving cerebral blood flow can be instituted.

C. Lumbar Puncture

In cases where no subarachnoid hemorrhage is present on CT and the history is suggestive of rupture of an intracranial aneurysm, lumbar puncture should be performed. Bloody or xanthochromic fluid is the most sensitive indicator of subarachnoid hemorrhage. However, lumbar puncture should never be performed prior to CT scanning because patients with elevated intracranial pressure are at risk for herniation following removal of fluid from the spinal subarachnoid space.

D. Laboratory Findings

Coagulation parameters, including a platelet count, bleeding time, and prothrombin and partial thromboplastin times should be obtained. If abnormal clotting parameters are present, they should be rapidly corrected because of the increased risk of rebleeding.

E. Electrocardiography

The ECG is abnormal in most cases of subarachnoid hemorrhage and may identify cardiac arrhythmias or ischemia that may require treatment.

Treatment

A. Surgery or Embolization

Most centers advocate early intervention (within 24 hours of rupture) with either surgery or embolization. Early treatment of the aneurysm has the advantage of preventing rebleeding and allowing aggressive therapy for vasospasm should it develop. Because of the risk of exacerbating ischemia by brain retraction, surgery may be delayed in patients who are medically unstable or who have severe vasospasm.

B. Preoperative ICU Therapy

Prior to surgery, treatment is aimed at reducing the risk of rebleeding and preventing ischemic complications related to vasospasm.

Patients should remain at bed rest in a quiet setting. Mild analgesics (not aspirin because of its antiplatelet properties) are used if headache or neck pain is severe. Stool softeners are useful to prevent straining, which can increase intracranial pressure and promote rerupture.

C. Blood Pressure Control

Systolic blood pressure should be maintained below 150 mm Hg; however, hypotension must be avoided so that cerebral perfusion pressure is not reduced to ischemic levels. Intravenous administration of sodium nitroprusside has the advantage of being rapidly reversible. Mild intravascular fluid augmentation using intravenous colloid infusion (5% albumin, 250 mL every 6–8 hours) helps maintain adequate cerebral perfusion.

D. Reduction of Ischemic Deficits Due to Vasospasm

Vasospasm is the most frequent cause of morbidity and mortality in patients admitted after subarachnoid hemorrhage and occurs in 22–44% of cases. Arterial narrowing may lead to diminished perfusion and cause infarction. Vasospasm is induced by products of erythrocyte breakdown, and the risk of developing this complication is related to the quantity of blood in the subarachnoid space. There is a peak incidence 4–12 days after subarachnoid hemorrhage, and vasospasm then gradually resolves. Prophylactic therapy using calcium channel blockers and mild volume expansion are only partially effective. Once vasospasm has been diagnosed by transcranial Doppler ultrasonography or angiography, more intense therapy is warranted. If ischemic neurologic symptoms are evident, aggressive treatment should be immediately instituted.

Induced hypervolemia, hemodilution, and hypertension ("triple-H" therapy) may augment cerebral blood flow and prevent ischemic cellular damage. Because cerebral autoregulation can be impaired after subarachnoid hemorrhage, hypertension and hypervolemia may directly increase cerebral blood flow. Decreased blood viscosity by induced hemodilution can improve cerebral blood flow in regions of hypoperfusion. The optimal hematocrit is between 31% and 33%. Oxygen-carrying capacity of the blood is not significantly reduced in this range. Since aggressive therapy is often required, placement of an indwelling pulmonary artery catheter is needed to monitor hemodynamics. Therapy should be titrated to ameliorate ischemic symptoms. In addition, cerebral blood flow measurements may aid in documenting adequate perfusion following treatment.

It should be noted that a recent study demonstrated a poor outcome despite triple-H therapy in almost all patients with a low Glasgow Coma Score and evidence of hydrocephalus at onset of vasospasm.

Oral administration of the calcium channel antagonist nimodipine (60 mg orally every 4 hours for 21 days) has been shown to reduce ischemic neurologic deficits attributable to vasospasm following aneurysmal subarachnoid hemorrhage.

E. Prevention of Seizures

Patients who have sustained aneurysmal subarachnoid hemorrhage are at risk for seizures and should receive anticonvulsants (phenytoin, 18 mg/kg intravenously initially followed by 300–400 mg daily) because of the risk of seizure-induced arterial hypertension, intracranial pressure alterations, and local increased cerebral blood flow requirements.

F. Respiratory Management

Intubation and mechanical ventilation are required in comatose patients and those with respiratory compromise. Mild hyperventilation can be useful to control elevations of intracranial pressure.

G. Correction of Electrolyte Disturbances

Hyponatremia is common following subarachnoid hemorrhage and can lead to harmful cellular volume changes in the central nervous system. (Please refer to the discussion of cerebral salt wasting.) Correction of hyponatremia should be done carefully so that abrupt sodium changes do not occur. Administration of hypertonic saline (3%) is often necessary to improve the sodium level and volume depletion.

H. Intracranial Pressure Monitoring

Placement of a ventricular catheter is necessary to monitor intracranial pressure in comatose patients and to treat hydrocephalus if present. This also helps clear erythrocyte breakdown products, which are associated with the development of hydrocephalus. Care should be taken to avoid rapid overdrainage of cerebrospinal fluid because abrupt reduction in intracranial pressure may induce aneurysm rebleeding. Many patients will eventually require a permanent ventriculoperitoneal shunt.

I. Antifibrinolytic Therapy

Agents such as aminocaproic acid that inhibit dissolution of the fibrin clot have been shown to reduce the incidence of rebleeding. However, this positive effect is offset by an increased risk of permanent ischemic sequelae and systemic venous thrombosis. Treatment with antifibrinolytic agents does not improve clinical outcome following aneurysmal hemorrhage and should not be used.

J. Angioplasty

Even though treatment using hypervolemic hemodilution and induced arterial hypertension is effective, a significant number of patients do not respond to these techniques. Balloon dilation angioplasty can mechanically increase vessel diameter and has been shown to dramatically improve cerebral blood flow and relieve symptoms. Cerebral angioplasty is a new technique and is indicated, where available, in subjects who do not respond to medical therapy.

Adams HP et al: Predicting cerebral ischemia after aneurysmal subarachnoid hemorrhage: Influences of clinical condition, CT results, and antifibrinolytic therapy. A report of the Cooperative Aneurysm Study. Neurology 1987;37:1586–90.

Barker FG, Heros RC: Clinical aspects of vasospasm. Neurosurg Clin North Am 1990;1:277–88.

Kassell NF et al: Treatment of ischemic deficits from vasospasm with intravascular volume expansion and induced arterial hypertension. Neurosurgery 1982;11:337–43.

Newell DW et al: Angioplasty for the treatment of symptomatic vasospasm following subarachnoid hemorrhage. Neurosurgery 1989;71:654–60.

Ojemann RG, Heros RC, Crowell RM: *Surgical Management of Cerebrovascular Disease.* Williams & Wilkins, 1988.

Qureshi AI et al: Early predictors of outcome in patients receiving hypervolemic and hypertensive therapy for symptomatic vasospasm after subarachnoid hemorrhage. Crit Care Med 2000;28:824–34.

TUMORS OF THE CENTRAL NERVOUS SYSTEM

ESSENTIALS OF DIAGNOSIS

- *Generalized signs of mass effect.*
- *Aphasia.*
- *Memory disturbance.*
- *Hemiparesis.*
- *Sensory impairment.*
- *Seizure may be the presenting sign.*

General Considerations

The critical care of patients harboring brain tumors requires an understanding of intracranial mass effect, cerebral edema and the blood brain barrier, progression of neurologic symptoms, seizures, and serum electrolyte abnormalities. Careful serial neurologic examination and physiologic monitoring can result in optimal care for the patient with a brain tumor.

The signs of either a primary or metastatic brain tumor are the result of the tumor's mass effect, location, and rate of growth and of metabolic disturbances. The Monro-Kellie doctrine describes the relationship between intracranial volume (composed of brain, cerebrospinal fluid, and blood) and intracranial pressure. The brain can accommodate enlarging mass lesions until a critical volume is reached. At this point, the intracranial pressure increases dramatically (Figure 31–2). Normally, the endothelial tight junctions of cerebral vessels (blood-brain barrier) prevent the leakage of large solutes and water into the brain. Vessels in cerebral tumors tend to have less constant tight junctions and may lack certain enzymes that degrade vasoactive substances in the brain such as leukotrienes. Reactive edema fluid thus accumulates in the extracellular space adjacent to the tumor. Edema can cause neurologic deterioration by increasing intracranial pressure and causing a midline shift of brain structures. Hyponatremia can occur in patients with a central nervous system neoplasm and may cause cytotoxic edema and seizures. This can occur secondary to cerebral salt wasting as described on page 736. Conversely, hypernatremia can result from hypothalamic dysfunction and lack of ADH response and is referred to as diabetes insipidus. These patients lose excessive amounts of free water. Any serum sodium abnormality can result in altered mental status, coma, and neuronal death.

Clinical Features

A. Symptoms and Signs

In contrast to the generalized symptoms of mass effect, edema, and sodium imbalance (which include headache, nausea and vomiting, and mental status changes), the precise location of a tumor can cause specific neurologic deficits. These deficits include aphasia, memory disturbances, hemiparesis, or sensory impairment. In many patients, no neurologic deficit is present on initial presentation, and a seizure is the first indication of a central nervous system neoplasm. In the awake patient, the history should be taken carefully to determine the exact initial symptoms and the rate at which the problems have advanced. This information can indicate the approximate location in the nervous system and serves as a clue to the rate of tumor growth. Neurologic examination in the ICU should include ophthalmoscopy; mental status assessment; cranial nerve tests; motor, sensory, and reflex tests; and testing of cerebellar function.

B. Imaging Studies

A chest x-ray should be performed to evaluate whether a metastatic source of central nervous system disease is present. The study of choice for a suspected central nervous system mass lesion is CT or MRI. The latter technique gives finer detail and subtracts the image of cortical bone. It is particularly helpful in evaluating the posterior fossa and skull base. SPECT-thallium scans are useful in differentiating high-grade versus low-grade gliomas.

C. Electroencephalography

Electroencephalography can localize dysfunctional cortex and epileptogenic foci related to neoplastic growths.

Differential Diagnosis

Several disease processes should be considered when evaluating a patient who presents with confusion, headache, dysphasia, motor or sensory deficits, seizures, hyponatremia, or any combination of these findings. Stroke usually presents with a sudden onset of fixed neurologic signs and differs from the progressive course of a central nervous system neoplasm. The gradual progression of a degenerative disease can result in symptoms similar to those caused by a mass lesion, but preliminary CT or MRI can rule out this lesion. Infections such as meningitis, encephalitis, and especially cerebral abscess can result in global or focal neurologic dysfunction and seizures but are frequently accompanied by fever, leukocytosis, and (in the case of cerebral abscess) characteristic findings on CT or MRI. An important distinction to be made is whether the mass represents a primary or metastatic lesion. In the latter, a general physical examination with radiologic studies and metastatic evaluation is required.

Treatment

A. Immediate ICU Intervention

Treatment of the patient with altered mental status and findings of papilledema should begin with protection of the airway and elevation of the head. The neck should be neither flexed nor the head turned so that optimal venous drainage of the brain via the jugular veins can be ensured. Hyperventilation, systemic arterial hypertension, and bradycardia are signs of Cushing's response (to raised intracranial pressure) and identify a patient in great danger. Mannitol, 1 g/kg, should be infused rapidly via an intravenous catheter. This can be followed by a 0.25–0.5 g/kg every 4 hours accompanied by frequent testing of serum osmolarity. If seizure activity has been observed or reported, a loading dose of phenytoin (18 mg/kg) should be infused intravenously at a rate not to exceed 50 mg/min. A daily dose of 300–400 mg/d can be started the next day. An immediate CT or MRI scan should be obtained. If a tumor is diagnosed and significant mass effect is present, one can consider placement of a ventricular catheter in patients at risk of critical elevation in intracranial pressure (> 20 mm Hg). Ventricular catheters allow continuous intracranial pressure monitoring and drainage of cerebrospinal fluid. If a neurologic deficit or significant cerebral edema is present, dexamethasone should be administered. The initial dose is 20–24 mg intravenously followed by 10 mg every 6 hours. This steroid can stabilize endothelial cell membranes and reduce the accumulation of cerebral edema. For the severely ill or deteriorating patient, endotracheal intubation should be performed with hyperventilation to achieve an arterial P_{CO_2} of 30–35 mm Hg. Lowering the arterial P_{CO_2} constricts cerebral arterioles and reduces the volume of blood in the brain, thereby alleviating one component of intracranial volume and increased intracranial pressure.

B. Nonoperative Therapy

For patients in poor medical condition, with multiple metastatic lesions, or with a solitary tumor in an inaccessible location, stereotactic or CT-guided biopsy followed by radiation or chemotherapy (or both) should be instituted. Patients should be weaned from ventilator support and ventricular drainage whenever possible. This may be difficult in a deteriorating patient because of ethical and family considerations.

C. Surgery

The goals of surgery are to obtain a tissue diagnosis and decrease the mass effect by safely removing as much of the lesion as possible. Craniotomy (removal of a replaceable bone flap) or craniectomy (removal of sections of the base of the skull that are not replaced) with microscope-assisted removal of the tumor can be accomplished with very satisfactory morbidity and mortality results. Bipolar coagulation forceps, suction and irrigation, ultrasonic aspirators, and (less frequently) lasers can be used to precisely remove tumor while limiting damage to surrounding brain. For tumors in the sellar region, a transnasal, transsphenoidal approach is most useful. The risks of operation include increased neurologic deficit, bleeding, deep vein thrombosis, pulmonary embolism, and death. Mortality rates in most large centers for patients undergoing removal of intracranial tumors are under 5%.

Current Controversies & Unresolved Issues

Several aspects of the care of critically ill patients harboring brain tumors remain controversial. It is still unclear what the roles of surgery and radiation are in the patient with a low-grade primary brain tumor. The risk of slow progression of tumor growth over many years may not outweigh the ill effects of operation or postirradiation angiopathy and neuronal death. Another debatable aspect of care is the role of chemotherapy for high-grade primary tumors. Prolongation of survival of 3–6 months with chemotherapy (beyond the 6- to 12-month survival of surgery and radiation alone) may not outweigh the short-term morbidity associated with intravenous antineoplastic therapy.

Deep vein thrombosis and pulmonary embolism represent a considerable risk to the patient with a brain tumor who is less mobile or bedridden, yet the role of perioperative anticoagulation remains an unresolved issue. The duration of prophylactic anticonvulsant therapy following craniotomy remains debatable. The range in practice is between 1 month and 12 months.

Future issues that are likely to make a major impact on the therapy for critically ill patients with brain tumors include advances in stereotactic radiation, manipulation of the blood-brain barrier for selective delivery of antineoplastic agents to the tumor, and molecular engineering to selectively transfect tumor cells with gene fragments capable of inducing differentiation and stopping cellular proliferation. At the present time, however, surgical reduction of the total malignant cell mass and radiation remain standard therapy for malignant brain tumors. Frameless image-guided neurosurgery has improved intraoperative visualization of these tumors and provides hope for improved outcomes in the future.

Brennan RW: Differential diagnosis of altered states of consciousness. In: *Neurological Surgery: A Comprehensive Reference Guide to the Diagnosis and Management of Neurosurgical Problems,* vol 1. Youmans JR (editor). Saunders, 1990.

Plum F, Posner JB: *The Diagnosis of Stupor and Coma,* 3rd ed. Davis, 1985.

Wilkinson HK: Intracranial pressure. In: *Neurological Surgery: A Comprehensive Reference Guide to the Diagnosis and Management of Neurosurgical Problems,* vol 2. Youmans JR (editor). Saunders, 1990.

CERVICAL SPINAL CORD INJURIES

ESSENTIALS OF DIAGNOSIS

- *Neck pains.*
- *Motor or sensory deficits.*
- *Hypoventilation.*
- *Neurogenic shock.*
- *Priapism.*

General Considerations

Approximately 10,000 new cervical and thoracic spinal cord injuries occur each year in the United States. Most result from motor vehicle accidents, falls, gunshot wounds, and sporting accidents. Improved acute management has permitted many patients to survive the initial injury and to have a near-normal life expectancy. Adolescents and young adults suffer the highest incidence of spinal cord injuries, with the majority occurring in young males. Although the loss of motor and sensory function imposes a catastrophic physical and emotional handicap, many spinal cord injury patients are able to return to a nondependent functional state.

Most spinal cord injuries occur in the mobile cervical region. The cervical cord contains lower motor neurons as well as long tracts conveying motor and sensory fibers which, if damaged, can result in variable neurologic dysfunction. In addition, the cervical cord also conducts vital respiratory and sympathetic functions that can be damaged following trauma and lead to devastating respiratory or circulatory collapse. Secondary events such as hypotension, hypoxia, and reinjury of the cord can cause further neurologic deterioration. Because of these unique features, all patients with cervical cord injuries should be admitted to an ICU staffed by personnel experienced with the complex care of spinal cord injuries.

Pathophysiology

There are a number of anatomic, chemical, and vascular changes that occur in response to blunt injury of the spinal cord. Within 3–5 hours after injury, there is focal swelling of the cord due to disruption of blood vessels and their endothelial tight junctions. This leads to localized bleeding and leakage of albumin, neurotransmitters, extracellular calcium, lactate, and prostaglandins. There is a decrease in local blood flow beginning in the central regions of the cord and spreading to the surrounding white matter (centripetal decrease in blood flow). This leads to worsening edema over the first 2–3 days and central cavitary necrosis over the ensuing week. The level of injury may rise as much as two vertebral levels in response to these secondary events. Diminished swelling followed by cord atrophy becomes evident after the first week after injury. Experimental and clinical treatment strategies are aimed at blocking this cascade of secondary events following spinal cord contusion. Calcium channel blockers, diuretics, corticosteroids, and other free radical scavengers may be helpful, though their true efficacy is debated.

Clinical Features

A. History

The key to the initial diagnosis of cervical spine injuries is maintaining a high level of suspicion for an underlying bony or ligamentous injury. This is especially true in patients involved in motor vehicle accidents or significant falls, particularly if they have other associated injuries such as head trauma or extremity fractures.

Many trauma patients are conscious and may complain of neck pain, numbness, or weakness suggestive of spinal cord injury. In trauma patients with altered mental status, it is best to assume that an unstable cervical spine injury is present until proved otherwise by radiography.

B. Symptoms and Signs

Several complications of cervical cord injuries may require immediate attention and therefore must be diagnosed promptly. Hypoventilation and respiratory compromise secondary to injury of cord segments supplying the phrenic nerve (C3–5) usually can be diagnosed easily and require immediate assisted ventilation. Although respiratory dysfunction may not be apparent immediately after a high cervical injury, respiratory status may deteriorate during the first few days in the ICU. This can be secondary to primary muscle fatigue or "ascending" cord involvement from edema or ischemia. Neurogenic shock may be encountered following cervical cord injury. This results from interruption of sympathetic fibers which are descending to the T1–L2 spinal cord segments and can lead to hypotension, bradycardia, and hypothermia. Priapism may also occur in males due to unopposed parasympathetic impulses. Although neurogenic shock patients do not appear to be hypovolemic (eg, the skin is warm and the pulse is slow), their hypotension responds to rapid administration of intravascular colloid or crystalloid solutions. Central venous pressure and cardiac monitoring may be required along with the frequent assessment of temperature.

After initial resuscitation, meticulous neurologic assessment should be performed to determine the level and severity of spinal cord damage. Evaluation should include assessment of motor strength; sensory testing; assessment of reflexes, including abdominal cutaneous, cremasteric, and bulbocavernosus reflexes; rectal and perirectal examination; and palpation of the entire spine while the patient is carefully log-rolled to maintain spinal alignment.

A complete spinal cord lesion is defined as total loss of motor and sensory function below the level of injury. One must not be confused by spinal mass reflexes such as reflex withdrawal of an extremity in response to pain, which is not representative of true motor function and may mistakenly lead to classification of the injury as incomplete. Figure 31–4 portrays the motor and sensory levels of the spinal cord, and Table 31–4 lists the important motor findings associated with injuries at different cervical levels. Patients with complete cervical cord lesions initially present in a state of spinal shock defined as a total loss of motor and sensory function associated

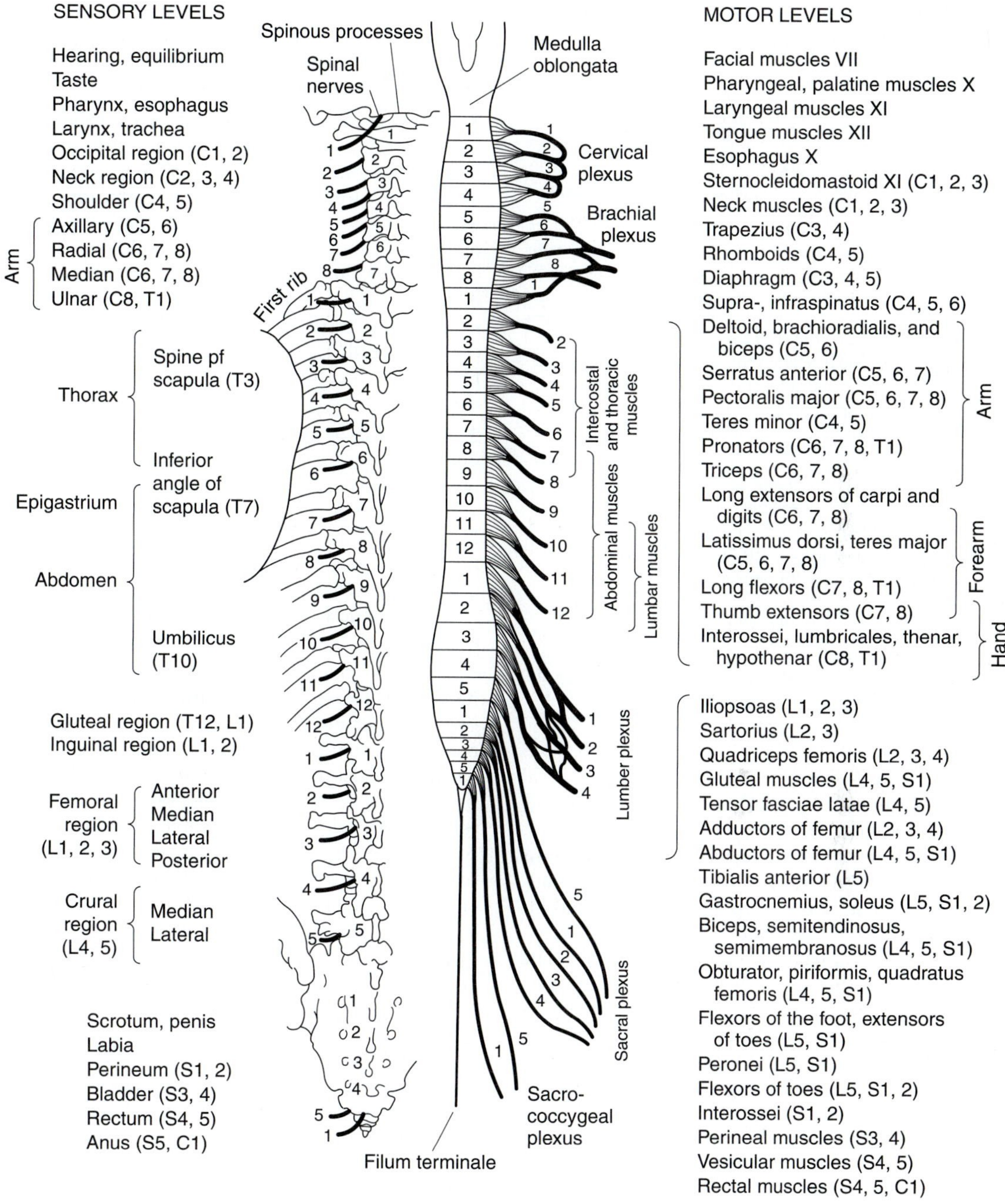
SENSORY LEVELS
Hearing, equilibrium
Taste
Pharynx, esophagus
Larynx, trachea
Occipital region (C1, 2)
Neck region (C2, 3, 4)
Shoulder (C4, 5)
Arm
Axillary (C5, 6)
Radial (C6, 7, 8)
Median (C6, 7, 8)
Ulnar (C8, T1)
Thorax
Spine pf scapula (T3)
Inferior angle of scapula (T7)
Epigastrium
Abdomen
Umbilicus (T10)
Gluteal region (T12, L1)
Inguinal region (L1, 2)
Femoral region (L1, 2, 3)
Anterior
Median
Lateral
Posterior
Crural region (L4, 5)
Median
Lateral
Scrotum, penis
Labia
Perineum (S1, 2)
Bladder (S3, 4)
Rectum (S4, 5)
Anus (S5, C1)
Spinous processes
Spinal nerves
First rib
Medulla oblongata
Cervical plexus
Brachial plexus
Intercostal and thoracic muscles
Abdominal muscles
Lumbar muscles
Lumber plexus
Sacral plexus
Sacro-coccygeal plexus
Filum terminale
MOTOR LEVELS
Facial muscles VII
Pharyngeal, palatine muscles X
Laryngeal muscles XI
Tongue muscles XII
Esophagus X
Sternocleidomastoid XI (C1, 2, 3)
Neck muscles (C1, 2, 3)
Trapezius (C3, 4)
Rhomboids (C4, 5)
Diaphragm (C3, 4, 5)
Supra-, infraspinatus (C4, 5, 6)
Arm
Deltoid, brachioradialis, and biceps (C5, 6)
Serratus anterior (C5, 6, 7)
Pectoralis major (C5, 6, 7, 8)
Teres minor (C4, 5)
Pronators (C6, 7, 8, T1)
Triceps (C6, 7, 8)
Forearm
Long extensors of carpi and digits (C6, 7, 8)
Latissimus dorsi, teres major (C5, 6, 7, 8)
Long flexors (C7, 8, T1)
Thumb extensors (C7, 8)
Hand
Interossei, lumbricales, thenar, hypothenar (C8, T1)
Iliopsoas (L1, 2, 3)
Sartorius (L2, 3)
Quadriceps femoris (L2, 3, 4)
Gluteal muscles (L4, 5, S1)
Tensor fasciae latae (L4, 5)
Adductors of femur (L2, 3, 4)
Abductors of femur (L4, 5, S1)
Tibialis anterior (L5)
Gastrocnemius, soleus (L5, S1, 2)
Biceps, semitendinosus, semimembranosus (L4, 5, S1)
Obturator, piriformis, quadratus femoris (L4, 5, S1)
Flexors of the foot, extensors of toes (L5, S1)
Peronei (L5, S1)
Flexors of toes (L5, S1, 2)
Interossei (S1, 2)
Perineal muscles (S3, 4)
Vesicular muscles (S4, 5)
Rectal muscles (S4, 5, C1)

Figure 31–4. Motor and sensory levels of the spinal cord. (Reproduced, with permission, from Waxman SG: *Correlative Neuroanatomy,* 20th ed. McGraw-Hill, 2000.)

Table 31–4. Important motor characteristics associated with injuries at different cervical levels and T1.

Segment	Important Characteristics
C1 to C3	No arm motor function. Absent respiratory muscle contractions. If C3 is spared, patient can support neck.
C4	If the C4 segment is functional, patients may only require initial ventilatory support and then, after strengthening, may self-ventilate.
C5	Useful movements of the deltoid, biceps, and usually the brachialis muscles are present, permitting shoulder shrug, elbow flexion, and forearm pronation.
C6	Allows wrist extension.
C7	Functional upper extremity movements with maintained innervation of the triceps (elbow extension), extensor digitorum (finger extension), and flexor carpi ulnaris (wrist extension). Weak finger flexors with poor grasp.
C8	Improved hand function due to innervation of most hand intrinsic muscles.
T1	Complete hand strength maintained because of innervation of all hand intrinsic muscles.

with an areflexic, flaccid trunk and extremities below the level of the lesion. In a complete lesion, spinal shock occurs immediately after the injury and may persist for 1–2 weeks, after which time upper motor neuron findings develop with increased deep tendon reflexes and increased muscular tone associated with spasticity. However, abdominal cutaneous reflexes remain absent. The mass reflex may occur and is characterized by exaggerated involuntary extremity movement due to loss of descending cortical inhibition. Interruption of autonomic fibers results in bladder paralysis, urinary retention, poor gastric emptying, and intestinal ileus with abdominal distention.

An incomplete lesion is characterized by evidence of any motor or sensory function below the level of the lesion. In severe incomplete injuries, spinal shock may be present initially but begins to wear off within 24 hours. Patients with incomplete cervical cord injuries generally show some degree of neurologic recovery (up to 40% may make a functional recovery), whereas patients with true complete injuries demonstrate no significant neurologic recovery. Rectal examination is an essential part of a complete neurologic assessment, since any evidence of sacral sparing, such as voluntary sphincter contraction or sensation in the perianal region, classifies the injury as incomplete and implies the possibility of some functional recovery. Important incomplete spinal cord injury syndromes include the following.

1. Anterior cord syndrome—This syndrome is most often associated with cervical flexion injuries and results in loss of motor function and pain and temperature perception (corticospinal and spinothalamic tracts), with preservation of proprioception and of perception of vibration and light touch (dorsal columns) below the level of the lesion. This is thought to result either from direct anterior trauma or from injury to the anterior spinal artery, which supplies the anterior two-thirds of the spinal cord. The paired posterior spinal arteries supply the dorsal columns and the posterior one-third of the cord.

2. Central cord syndrome—This is most commonly due to a hyperextension injury in an older patient with preexisting cervical spondylosis or stenosis. The motor and sensory deficits are greater in the upper extremities (more pronounced distally) than in the lower extremities. Hemorrhagic necrosis in the central portions (eg, gray matter) of the cervical cord results in upper extremity weakness. Since the lumbar leg and sacral tracts are peripheral in the cervical cord, they are relatively spared.

3. Brown-Séquard's syndrome—This syndrome occurs with hemisection of the spinal cord, usually from penetrating injuries such as stab or gunshot wounds. The result is ipsilateral loss of motor and dorsal column function (vibration, proprioception, discriminatory touch) immediately below the level of injury associated with contralateral loss of pain and temperature sensation one or two levels below the injury (spinothalamic tracts decussate within one to two levels of their entry).

4. Posterior spinal cord syndrome—This rare syndrome results from disruption of the posterior columns, causing loss of vibration, proprioception, and discriminatory sense below the level of the lesion.

C. Imaging Studies

Radiographs are essential for the evaluation and diagnosis of cervical spine injuries. These should include a cervical spine series with lateral, anteroposterior, and odontoid (open mouth) views. Radiographs are inspected for the presence of prevertebral soft tissue swelling, alignment of the anterior and posterior aspects of the vertebral bodies, angulation of the bony spinal canal, and the presence of fractures. The odontoid view is essential to diagnose axis (C2) fractures or Jefferson fractures of the ring of the atlas (displacement of the lateral masses of C1). Ligamentous damage should be suspected in subjects with minimal subluxation or persistent neck pain without evidence of a fracture. Dynamic flexion and extension cervical radiographs, which should only be considered in awake and cooperative patients, are useful to detect instability secondary to ligamentous injury. These x-rays are typically performed several days after the initial injury so that muscle spasms, which can mask instability by limiting subluxation, may subside.

CT is excellent for visualizing the bony structures of the spinal canal and is the next step in evaluating a fracture or subluxation. In patients with neurologic symptoms or signs and no radiographic evidence of bony abnormalities, MRI should be obtained. MRI demonstrates the cord and soft tissue structures with outstanding clarity and can identify intra-axial contusions and cord compression from a herniated disk or hematoma. However, MRI images do not demonstrate bony structures very well.

The role of myelography in spinal cord injury is controversial. Myelography should be performed if there is a significant incomplete neurologic deficit that cannot be explained by bony abnormalities and if an MRI cannot be obtained.

D. Other Studies

Somatosensory evoked potentials are occasionally useful to confirm or dispute the diagnosis of complete spinal cord injury. This is especially true in patients who are difficult to examine, such as those with altered mental status.

Treatment

Optimal treatment of spinal cord injuries must be initiated at the scene of the accident. The spinal cord is susceptible to reinjury after the primary insult, making prevention of secondary injury one of the most important aims of therapy. This includes immediate spinal immobilization with sandbags or a hard collar and rapid correction of hypoxia, hypotension, shock, or hypothermia, if present. Early placement of a nasogastric tube and an indwelling urinary catheter are necessary because an atonic bladder and gastrointestinal tract commonly accompany cervical cord injuries.

Serial neurologic examinations are important to detect signs of deterioration so that corrective measures can be expeditiously taken. The patient must be maintained in optimal physiologic condition to maximize the chances of neurologic repair and recovery.

A. Respiratory Care

Patients with cervical cord injuries frequently develop worsening of their respiratory status in the ICU. This may be secondary to diaphragm fatigue or ascending neurologic damage from edema or ischemia and may require prompt respiratory support. Intubation in patients with unstable cervical injuries should be performed using fiberoptic nasotracheal intubation (see below for selection of neuromuscular blocking agents). Hypoventilation, particularly during sleep, is not uncommon in the early stages following high cervical cord injury and may require nighttime ventilation. This is probably due to an impaired respiratory drive to CO_2 or diaphragm fatigue. A high index of suspicion for this disorder, which usually resolves in 1–2 weeks, must be maintained in the early phases of ICU care.

Aggressive pulmonary toilet and aerosol bronchodilators should be utilized to avoid atelectasis, mucus plugs, and pneumonia. Prophylactic antibiotics should not be used to prevent pulmonary infections.

B. Hemodynamic Support

During spinal shock, decreased sympathetic outflow may be manifested by bradycardia or hypotension. However, one must not overlook a source of hemorrhage (eg, liver laceration, pelvic fracture), since such patients will not complain of pain. Hypotension from spinal shock usually responds well to intravenous infusions of crystalloid and colloid solutions. Vasopressors are not often required. Atropine, though short-acting, may rapidly reverse hypotension associated with bradycardia. Placement of a temporary cardiac pacemaker may be required for severe bradycardia. Following recovery from spinal shock, reflex hypertension, sweating, pilomotor erection, or, rarely, bradycardia or cardiac arrest (autonomic dysreflexia) may occur. This is usually precipitated by painful stimuli such as bladder catheterization, respiratory suctioning, or colorectal manipulation. Hypertensive crises, which can be life-threatening, should be treated by elimination of the precipitating stimulus and administration of rapid-acting intravenous antihypertensive agents. In recurrent severe attacks, prophylaxis with phenoxybenzamine may be useful.

C. Cervical Immobilization

Unstable malaligned cervical spine subluxations or fractures should be managed initially with external immobilization. This can be achieved by attaching tongs or a halo ring to the patient's skull and applying distraction force through a pulley system attached to weights. One must exclude the presence of atlanto-occipital dislocation, since traction in this condition can result in overdistraction and serious injury. Gentle application of 5–10 lb is used initially, gradually increasing by up to 5 lb per cervical level (eg, 20 lb for C4, 30 lb for C6). More weight may be required for reduction, but no more than 10 lb per level should be administered. After each weight increase, the lateral x-ray should be repeated to determine if realignment has been achieved. It is often necessary to administer muscle relaxants such as diazepam (10 mg intravenously every 8 hours) during skeletal traction to reduce muscle contractions or spasms that can hinder spinal realignment.

D. Surgery

The principal goal in the management of cervical spine injuries is prevention of secondary neurologic injury and provision of an optimal environment for recovery. Securing a stable cervical spine (bones, muscles, and ligaments) will prevent further neurologic injury and reduce the chance for persistent cervical pain resulting from instability. In general, bony lesions heal well if immobilized properly, whereas ligamentous injuries typically do not heal. The indications for operation are decompression of incompletely injured neural tissue or reduction and stabilization of malaligned or unstable cervical segments. Some of the basic features and treatment modalities for several common cervical injuries are outlined below.

1. Atlanto-occipital dislocation—These injuries, which are most commonly seen in children due to immature craniovertebral articulations, are often fatal. They involve extensive ligamentous disruption and can cause injury to the brain stem, cervical cord, nerve roots, or vertebral artery. Traction should not be utilized because it can increase the distraction and cause further central nervous system damage. These injuries are highly unstable and require operative bony fusion.

2. Jefferson fracture of the atlas—This is a burst fracture of the ring of the atlas resulting from an axial force and is usually asymptomatic. If combined displacement of the left and right lateral masses on open mouth x-ray is more than 6.9 mm, immobilization with a halo vest is suggested; otherwise, a hard cervical collar is sufficient.

3. Axis fractures—A type 1 odontoid fracture involves only the tip of the odontoid and can be treated with hard cervical collar immobilization. Fractures through the odontoid base are classified as type 2 and have a high incidence of nonunion. Current treatment recommendations are for surgical fusion if the fracture is displaced more than 6 mm or halo immobilization for fractures displaced less than 6 mm. However, new surgical techniques such as odontoid screw fixation may change these current treatment guidelines. Type 3 odontoid fractures involve the base of the odontoid with extension into the vertebral body and require only halo vest immobilization for fusion. Hangman fractures are bilateral fractures of the C2 pedicles with anterior displacement of C2 onto C3. They are usually due to hyperextension injuries such as automobile accidents when the head hits the windshield. Hangman fractures may be unstable and require traction initially if malalignment is present, followed by immobilization in a halo vest. Isolated laminal or spinous process fractures of the axis usually can be treated with a hard cervical collar. Treatment for combined atlas and axis fractures is usually based upon the type of axis fracture present.

4. Wedge compression fracture—This results from a hyperflexion force causing compression of one vertebra against an adjacent vertebra. The optimal management of these injuries is controversial. Simple wedge fractures without associated ligamentous injury or significant subluxation heal well in a hard cervical collar. If the kyphotic angulation is significant or if instability is present, early surgical fusion or closed realignment with skeletal traction followed by halo vest application may be warranted. Delayed instability may be present in 15% of patients treated by immobilization only and require subsequent operative surgical fusion. Care must be taken in patients with neurologic deficits to exclude a compressive lesion such as an extruded cervical disk that may require early operation.

5. Flexion teardrop fracture—This is secondary to severe hyperflexion with disruption of the intervertebral disk associated with ligamentous damage and a fracture through the anterior inferior vertebral body. This is a highly unstable injury often associated with devastating neurologic damage and requires early realignment by traction. Management after initial stabilization is controversial and may include halo vest immobilization or surgical fusion. Care must be taken to exclude any compressive lesions, such as bone or disk material, which may contribute to neurologic dysfunction and require removal.

6. Facet dislocation—Bilateral facet dislocation occurs when the inferior articular facet of the upper vertebra slides forward over the superior articular facet of the lower vertebra. This is due to severe hyperflexion injury and is unstable. Lateral cervical x-rays show anterior subluxation of the superior vertebra by over 50% of the length of the vertebral body. Anteroposterior views demonstrate alignment of the spinous processes. Immediate closed reduction using skeletal traction should be attempted; if this fails, open surgical reduction may be necessary. Surgical fusion is required in either case. Unilateral facet dislocation results from simultaneous flexion and rotation injuries. The lateral cervical spine x-ray shows anterior subluxation of the superior vertebra, but this is only 30% or less of the length of the vertebral body. The spinous processes on anteroposterior views are rotated and do not align. Although the unilateral locked facet is a stable injury, it is commonly associated with nerve root injury and chronic pain. In these cases, closed or open reduction may be beneficial.

E. Corticosteroids

A large multicenter randomized and controlled study demonstrated significant improvement in total motor score following incomplete or complete spinal cord injury with early administration of high-dose intravenous methylprednisolone (30 mg/kg loading dose followed by

5.4 mg/kg/h for the following 23 hours). This is now considered the standard of care and is started for spinal cord injury patients within 8 hours after injury. The most likely explanation for the beneficial effects of methylprednisolone is inhibition of lipid peroxidation and hydrolysis at the site of injury. This suppresses the breakdown of cellular membranes and the production of deleterious by-products of arachidonic acid metabolism and may thus lead to improved regional blood flow. A small study utilizing GM_1 ganglioside, a glycolipid found in central nervous system cells, appears promising, and a larger clinical trial is currently being conducted.

F. Pulmonary Embolism Prophylaxis

Pulmonary embolism is a constant threat to patients with weak limbs and should be combated using subcutaneous heparin (5000 units twice daily), pneumatic compression stockings, or both.

G. Gastrointestinal Considerations

Atony and paralytic ileus may occur for days to weeks following spinal cord injury. Early nasogastric decompression is required to reduce abdominal distention. Serum electrolytes should be regularly evaluated. Because these patients are in a catabolic state after injury, they often require early nutritional support. Reflex evacuation of the rectum occurs following the acute phase of spinal cord injury and can be aided by a regular regimen of laxative agents.

H. Urinary Care

Bladder atonia resulting in urinary retention occurs early after spinal cord injuries. Initial placement of an indwelling bladder catheter is required but should not be left in place for longer than 2–3 weeks. After this time, reflex emptying of the neurogenic bladder can occur spontaneously or in response to stimuli such as suprapubic compression. Many patients require intermittent bladder catheterization, and this can be self-administered using meticulous technique. Urologic consultation is frequently helpful to determine individual bladder care programs.

I. Skin Care

Prevention of decubitus ulcers is a primary concern in spinal injury patients. Patients should be turned at least every 2 hours; pressure points should be padded; and kinetic therapy beds should be utilized if available.

J. Avoidance of Depolarizing Neuromuscular Blocking Agents

Denervated muscles are hypersensitive to depolarization, and administration of a depolarizing agent (eg, succinylcholine) can result in rapid hyperkalemia that may be complicated by ventricular fibrillation.

Bracken MB et al: A randomized, controlled trial of methylprednisolone or naloxone in the treatment of acute spinal cord injury. N Engl J Med 1990;322:1405–11.

Janssen L, Hansebout RR: Pathogenesis of spinal cord injury and newer treatments: A review. Spine 1989;14:23–31.

McBride D: Spinal cord injury syndromes. In: *Handbook of Central Nervous System Trauma.*® Greenberg J (editor). Marcel Dekker, 1993.

Ogilvy CS, Heros RC: Spinal cord compression. In: *Neurological and Neurosurgical Intensive Care,* 2nd ed. Ropper AH, Kennedy SF (editors). Aspen, 1988.

Sonntag VKH, Hadley MN: Management of upper cervical instability. In: *Neurosurgery Update II.* Wilkins RH, Rengachary SS (editors). McGraw-Hill, 1991.

Sypert GW: Management of lower cervical instability. In: *Neurosurgery Update II.* Wilkins RH, Rengachary SS (editors). McGraw-Hill, 1991.

Acute Abdomen

32

Michael J. Stamos, MD

The term acute abdomen denotes an abdominal pathologic condition which, if left undiscovered and untreated, would have a deleterious effect on the patient's health status. Numerous factors make the diagnosis and treatment of abdominal conditions more difficult in intensive care patients.

Physiologic Considerations

The peritoneum is a complex mesothelium-lined organ that invests the intra-abdominal viscera (visceral peritoneum) and the abdominal cavity (parietal peritoneum). The peritoneum functions to maintain the integrity of the intra-abdominal organs and provides lubrication by peritoneal fluid (normally < 50 mL). For free movement of the viscera, the nondiaphragmatic peritoneal surface behaves as a passive semipermeable membrane that allows bidirectional exchange of water and electrolytes. The diaphragmatic surface is highly specialized, with numerous gaps in the peritoneal lining that serve as entrances to a plexus of lymphatic channels which drain via substernal lymph nodes into the thoracic duct. This diaphragmatic absorptive pathway is enhanced by respiratory excursion and normally accounts for at least 30% of the total lymphatic drainage of the abdomen, helping to maintain the balance between visceral parietal transudation and parietal peritoneal fluid uptake.

The omentum participates in absorption of peritoneal fluid and particulate material up to 10 μm in diameter. The omentum is highly mobile and can act to seal off a perforated viscus or contain a bacterial inoculum.

Pain from intra-abdominal disease is transmitted via somatic sensory and visceral autonomic pathways. Visceral pain, primarily elicited by distention, is referred in a logical fashion in the same order as embryologic development; the nerves accompany the major splanchnic vessels. Foregut sources (esophagus, stomach, liver, pancreas, biliary tract, duodenum, and spleen) elicit upper epigastric pain; midgut lesions (jejunum, ileum, appendix, and right colon) elicit periumbilical pain; and hindgut lesions (left colon, rectum) radiate to the hypogastrium. This visceral pain is typically colicky in nature and somewhat vague in location—in contrast to somatic pain, which is usually constant and well localized to the site of direct parietal peritoneal irritation.

Intra-abdominal disease can also cause pain to be referred to other areas through neural pathways or other anatomic constraints. Examples of referred pain include shoulder pain from splenic or hepatic hemorrhage, causing phrenic nerve irritation, or hip or thigh pain from a psoas abscess.

Pathophysiology

Critical care patients are susceptible to common causes of abdominal disease such as appendicitis, diverticulitis, and calculous cholecystitis with approximately the same frequency as the general population. More importantly, they are prone to develop more complex and unusual abdominal processes resulting from a variety of predisposing conditions. For example, recent surgery, especially involving enteric anastomoses, may lead to intra-abdominal abscess or small bowel obstruction.

Shock with associated low flow states leads to an increased risk of mesenteric ischemia, acalculous cholecystitis, and possibly gut translocation of bacteria. Present or previous antimicrobial therapy may also contribute to illness with overgrowth of resistant organisms, including *Clostridium difficile* (pseudomembranous) colitis. The fasting state of many critically ill patients may contribute to the development of acalculous cholecystitis or, along with opioid use, lead to a colonic pseudo-obstruction (Ogilvie's syndrome; see below).

Iatrogenic complications are common in patients undergoing multiple procedures and receiving several medications. Inadvertent visceral injury may occur during paracentesis or thoracentesis. Missed intra-abdominal disease in traumatized patients should be strongly considered in any patient not recovering as expected. The problem of stress gastritis and stress ulcers has been diminished with aggressive pH monitoring and pharmacologic prophylaxis but still presents a formidable challenge.

Clinical Features

A. Symptoms

While many patients in a critical care unit are unable to give a history because of intubation or altered mental status, a detailed review of recent symptomatology should be obtained whenever possible. Family members and friends should be interviewed. Patients may have been transferred from a hospital ward or may have had recent contact with the hospital or emergency room. However obtained, the history should describe any preexisting medical conditions, previous surgery, present medications, prior abdominal complaints, changes in eating or bowel habits, and recent weight loss. Exposure to toxic substances (including alcohol) and recent trauma should be noted. The obstetric and gynecologic history should include data about menses and sexual contacts.

Events leading to hospitalization need to be reviewed, and if pain is part of the symptomatology a history of its presentation and progression is helpful. In spite of efforts to elicit a detailed history, this is often not possible in critically ill patients.

1. Location of the pain—The location of pain can give valuable information about its cause. Even more important is an account of its progression and changes in location (Table 32–1). Knowing where the pain began occasionally means more than determining where it is at presentation. A perforated ulcer may cause lower abdominal pain from intestinal contents collecting in the pelvis due to gravitational effects or even due to a pelvic abscess, while a detailed history may reveal days or weeks of epigastric or right upper quadrant pain. Pain radiating to some other area of the body may also give valuable information. For example, epigastric pain that radiates through to the back is more likely to be due to pancreatitis than to reflux esophagitis.

2. Nature of the pain—Episodic or crampy pain is usually due to blockage or obstruction of a hollow viscus during contraction or attempted peristalsis such as in bowel obstruction or during an attack of acute cholecystitis. Questioning and observation will often determine what factors increase or relieve the pain. Patients with direct peritoneal inflammation will resist movement, whereas the patient with renal colic will writhe about with no apparent exacerbation from the movement itself.

3. Progression of the pain—Since virtually all patients subjected to abdominal operations have postoperative pain, progression of the pain gives important information about its source. Incisional pain usually begins to subside after the first 72 hours, whereas pain due to other causes such as an intra-abdominal abscess or bowel obstruction will often begin after 72 hours and become progressively worse.

B. Physical Examination

A comprehensive physical examination of the ICU patient can be difficult and frustrating, especially just after an operation. Nevertheless, a complete examination is essential on admission to the unit, starting with measurement of routine vital signs. Body temperatures should be obtained from a reliable site—rectal, bladder, or core measurements from a Swan-Ganz catheter probe will suffice. Oral and axillary temperatures are often unreliable. Fever with or without hypotension arouses suspicion of abdominal disease, and the presence of both will often suggest an acute abdomen. Examination to exclude an extra-abdominal source of sepsis should include inspection of old and existing intravenous sites, chest auscultation and percussion, and inspection of all wounds (traumatic and surgical).

1. Observation—Abdominal examination should begin with careful observation of not only the abdomen but also the patient's body position and general demeanor. Is the patient resting comfortably or in significant distress, with guarding of the abdominal area? Any distention, ecchymoses, and old surgical scars should be noted. Some abdominal distention is normal in the postoperative abdominal surgical patient, but any increase in distention postoperatively may signify problems such as a nonfunctioning nasogastric tube, prolonged ileus, small bowel obstruction, or development of ascites. Recent incisions should be inspected, and any erythema, edema, or fluid discharge should alert the examiner to a potential wound or intra-abdominal infection.

2. Auscultation—Auscultation is difficult in a noisy ICU environment and therefore frequently neglected. Absent bowel sounds may be normal in recent postoperative patients but in others may appropriately be viewed with suspicion. Hyperactive, high-pitched rushes may signify bowel obstruction. Abdominal bruits indicate the presence of aneurysms, arteriovenous fistulas, or severe atherosclerotic disease.

3. Percussion—Gentle percussion with close attention to grimacing or other movement by the patient can give subtle information about localized peritoneal irritation. The presence of a tympanic area in the right upper quadrant overlying the liver suggests pneumoperitoneum. Percussion can also help detect bowel obstruction (calling for nasogastric intubation) or ascites or may disclose a distended bladder due to a nonfunctioning or nonexistent Foley catheter.

4. Palpation—Palpation may reveal hepatomegaly or splenomegaly, an abdominal wall hernia, a distended gallbladder, an intra-abdominal tumor or abscess, or an aortic aneurysm. Rebound tenderness is intended to elicit peritoneal irritation. Gentle percussion is a good test for localized peritonitis. Gently bumping the patient or the bed or having the patient cough will cause enough peritoneal movement to exacerbate pain from peritoneal inflammation. Careful observation of the patient's facial expression and body position will be revealing. Deep palpation of the abdominal wall and sudden release to elicit rebound tenderness is often misleading and in the presence of peritonitis will often increase guarding and make subsequent examinations more difficult.

Table 32–1. Locations of common etiologies of acute abdomen.

Location	Etiologies
Epigastrium	Esophageal disease Peptic ulcer disease Pancreatitis (including pseudocyst) Cardiac disease Hiatal hernia (including paraesophageal)
Right Upper Quadrant	Cholecystitis Cholangitis Pancreatitis (including pseudocyst) Peptic ulcer disease Renal colic Hepatitis Appendicitis Cecal volvulus Hepatic abscess Subphrenic abscess Right lower lobe pneumonia
Right Lower Quadrant	Appendicitis Diverticulitis Crohn's disease Colonic obstruction Psoas abscess Pelvic inflammatory disease Ovarian cyst or torsion Ectopic pregnancy Inguinal hernia Epididymitis Pelvic abscess
Suprapubic and Pelvic	Cystitis Diverticulitis Proctitis Pelvic abscess Renal colic
Left Upper Quadrant	Pancreatitis (including pseudocyst) Splenic disease Hiatal hernia (including paraesophageal) Renal colic Left lower lobe pneumonia Colitis (especially ischemic) Subphrenic abscess
Periumbilical	Umbilical hernia Early appendicitis Small bowel obstruction Mesenteric ischemia Aortic aneurysm
Left Lower Quadrant	Diverticulitis Sigmoid volvulus Colitis (especially ischemic) Renal colic Inguinal hernia Pelvic inflammatory disease Ovarian cyst or torsion Ectopic pregnancy Epididymitis Pelvic abscess Psoas abscess

When cholecystitis is in the differential diagnosis, right upper quadrant palpation may reveal tenderness or even a positive Murphy sign (arrested inspiration during palpation of the right upper quadrant). Although the retroperitoneum and pelvis are less accessible to direct palpation, indirect evidence of inflammation can be elicited. Pain on hyperextension of the hip, stretching the iliopsoas muscle (psoas sign), and on flexion and internal rotation of the hip, stretching the obturator muscle (obturator sign), can indicate an adjacent inflammatory process. Gentle palpation or percussion of the posterior costovertebral angles should diagnose or exclude pyelonephritis.

5. Rectal and pelvic examination—Genitourinary and rectal examinations are essential to evaluate for incarcerated hernias, pelvic or rectal masses, cervical motion tenderness, prostatic or scrotal disease, and bloody stools. Stool may be guaiac-tested to confirm a clinical suspicion, but—at least in the ICU patient population—this test is too insensitive and nonspecific to be useful in making clinical decisions.

C. Laboratory Findings

A white blood cell count is nonspecific and relatively insensitive—its absolute level is less useful than its trend. A differential count indicating a left shift increases the sensitivity of this test. The hematocrit is helpful or even essential in diagnosing intra-abdominal or gastrointestinal bleeding.

Urinalysis should be performed with attention to the presence of white cells or white cell casts indicative of urinary tract infection. Urine specific gravity can give information useful in fluid resuscitation efforts, and the presence of glucose or ketones is of diagnostic and therapeutic importance.

Elevated liver enzymes (AST, ALT, and alkaline phosphatase) direct attention to the liver (hepatitis) and biliary system (cholangitis, cholecystitis). Bilirubin elevation is seen in hepatobiliary disease but can also be associated with sepsis, hemolysis, and cholestasis due to parenteral nutrition.

Serum amylase is neither sensitive nor specific, though markedly elevated values usually indicate pancreatitis. Elevated serum amylase is also seen with perforated ulcer, mesenteric ischemia, facial trauma, parotitis, and ruptured ectopic pregnancy. Lipase values may improve specificity in the diagnosis of pancreatitis.

Arterial blood gas measurements may demonstrate acidosis or hypoxia. Acidosis may reflect severe sepsis or ischemia, while hypoxia may reflect ARDS due to uncontrolled sepsis.

D. Imaging Studies

Although bedside studies are relatively risk-free, CT scans, MRI, arteriography, and nuclear medicine scans usually require patient transport. In this select group of critically ill patients, transfer to other areas of the hospital carries significant risks.

1. Bedside films—Radiographs of the chest can evaluate for pulmonary infections as well as free air when performed with the patient in a sitting position. Pleural effusions, especially when asymmetric, may signify an intra-abdominal process. Abdominal radiographs may show a colonic volvulus or obstructed bowel gas pattern, biliary or renal calculi, or (rarely) pneumobilia. Ultrasound can be useful as a diagnostic and therapeutic tool—intra-abdominal abscesses can be identified with this procedure and percutaneous drainage facilitated. Cholecystitis (calculous or acalculous) can be diagnosed and even treated (percutaneous cholecystostomy). In questionable cases, percutaneous aspiration with analysis of gallbladder contents (Gram stain, culture) can be invaluable.

2. Radiology department studies—CT scans have assumed a primary position in diagnosis of the acute abdomen. They should not be used indiscriminately, however, and are of little value in the first week after abdominal surgery, when normal postoperative findings (blood, air, seromas) make identification of an abscess difficult. In the critically ill patient with multiple system organ failure, transport to the radiology department may carry a greater risk than the potential benefit. These patients should perhaps be considered for early laparotomy. CT scanning for intra-abdominal abscesses has an accuracy rate greater than 95%. Studies that have looked specifically at critically ill surgical patients, however, are not so promising, with sensitivity rates as low as 50% and with only 25% of the scans actually providing beneficial information that perhaps altered the outcome of therapy. CT scans should be performed only when the information obtained is expected to have that result.

Gastrointestinal contrast studies can occasionally be useful in patients with recent anastomoses or in those with possible missed injuries (especially esophageal injuries). In general, water-soluble agents (eg, Gastrografin) should be utilized. Angiography is useful in patients with suspected mesenteric ischemia and should be performed early after initial resuscitation. In addition to securing the diagnosis, intra-arterial vasodilators (eg, papaverine) can be used as primary therapy or to demarcate and salvage marginally viable intestine. Angiography also plays a diagnostic role in selected patients with gastrointestinal bleeding, aiding in localization of the bleeding site; and it has therapeutic applications in the delivery of intra-arterial vasopressin or embolization. Blood loss of at least 0.5 mL/min is required before it can be detected by angiography. ^{99m}Tc-tagged red blood cell scans have a reported sensitivity of 0.05–0.1 mL/min and may play a role in screening patients for the more invasive angiographic approach.

Gallium- or indium-tagged white blood cell scans are occasionally useful in relatively stable patients. The poor specificity of the tests, especially in the postoperative patient, and the 24- to 48-hour time period for completion limit their usefulness.

E. Peritoneal Lavage

Extensively used in abdominal trauma, diagnostic peritoneal lavage also may be quite useful in selected ICU patients. The same factors that make assessment of critically ill patients difficult (altered mental status, intubation, etc.) make lavage an attractive alternative. Numerous studies have shown its utility in selected patients with white cell counts > 500/μL or red cell counts > 50,000–100,000/μL. Lavage has limited if any usefulness in the recent postoperative patient. In this setting, CT-guided or ultrasound-guided percutaneous aspiration is safer and more reliable.

F. Endoscopy

In the presence of active upper gastrointestinal bleeding, esophagogastroduodenoscopy is of proved diagnostic and therapeutic benefit. Flexible sigmoidoscopy and colonoscopy may also be of diagnostic value in the patient with possible ischemic colitis or pseudomembranous colitis. Up to one-third of patients with pseudomembranous colitis have negative *C difficile* toxic assays; visualization and biopsy will increase the diagnostic accuracy to over 95%. Ischemic colitis can occur as a result of embolic disease, shock (low flow state), or—not uncommonly in the ICU setting—after aortic surgery. Endoscopy can confirm the diagnosis and can allow observation of the progression of disease in selected cases. Endoscopic retrograde cholangiopancreatography has a proved therapeutic role in septic patients with cholangitis, allowing stone extraction or stenting.

Evaluation of the Postoperative Abdomen

Postoperatively, a number of potential intra-abdominal complications can occur in the ICU patient. These include such diverse problems as intraperitoneal bleeding, anastomotic dehiscence, early small bowel obstruction, and fascial dehiscence. Early recognition and aggressive corrective action are required.

In order to identify a failure to recover on schedule after laparotomy, one must understand the normal course following major abdominal surgery. Third-space fluid sequestration occurs in approximate proportion to the magnitude of the surgery. Mild to moderate abdominal distention and oliguria—frequently seen in the first 24–72 hours after surgery—can make identification of postoperative hemorrhage difficult. Not infrequently, a declining hematocrit is attributed to dilutional effects or to equilibration. The accompanying tachycardia may be falsely attributed to pain. Alert watchfulness for possible postoperative bleeding can avert a disastrous outcome.

Fever is the most commonly observed postoperative physiologic abnormality. The presence of fever suggests infection, but the approach to evaluation must be methodical. A single febrile episode should in most patients call for nothing more than a review of the history and a physical examination. Intermittent spikes of recurrent fever may warrant a more thorough investigation—again directed by a thorough physical examination. The goal should be to identify a complication early while intervention may still improve the outcome.

Other than missed injuries to hollow viscera (traumatic or iatrogenic), intra-abdominal sepsis—including abscess and anastomotic leaks or dehiscences—typically is manifested between 5 days and 10 days after surgery. Early recognition and treatment are critical. Subtle signs may aid in early diagnosis. Third-spacing should resolve within 48–96 hours, and observation of a vigorous postoperative diuresis during this period is a reliable sign of improvement. Leukocytosis following major surgery is frequently regarded as a normal finding (largely due to demargination), whereas failure of the white count to return to normal or an increase from a declining value should suggest the possibility of intra-abdominal sepsis. Other findings include glucose intolerance, continued tachycardia, prolonged ileus, or persistent diarrhea upon return of bowel function (due to adjacent pelvic abscess).

Treatment

Following the initial evaluation of an ICU patient for consideration of an acute abdomen, the primary decision is whether urgent surgery is required. Resuscitation with intravenous fluids is usually necessary to correct third-space losses or bleeding. A bladder catheter should be inserted to monitor urine output and, unless contraindicated, a nasogastric tube to decompress the stomach. Both H_2 blockers and antacids are effective, with greatest efficacy achieved by maintaining the gastric pH > 5.0. An arterial and a pulmonary artery flotation catheter may be necessary in some patients to monitor hemodynamic function and intravascular volume. Antibiotics should be given as indicated. Caution should be exercised in giving antibiotics to patients with undiagnosed but suspected sepsis because of concerns about obfuscating the clinical picture and frustrating further evaluation. Antibiotic therapy is largely adjunctive, though small abscesses or phlegmonous processes due to contained enteric leaks will often resolve with their use.

SPECIFIC PATHOLOGIC ENTITIES

BOWEL OBSTRUCTION

The diagnosis of early postoperative small bowel obstruction is frequently delayed, primarily because of the differential consideration of persistent adynamic ileus. The characteristic symptoms of obstruction include abdominal distention, obstipation, and vomiting. These symptoms also characterize adynamic ileus, and the first step in differentiation is consideration of the diagnosis. Further confusing the clinical picture is the side effect of opioid analgesics on decreasing gastrointestinal motility.

The clinical history and physical examination are often nondiagnostic, though the patient who has brief return of gastrointestinal function followed by its cessation probably has an adhesive obstruction. Plain radiographs likewise are frequently nondiagnostic in this setting.

A nasogastric tube should be inserted. Hypovolemia should be corrected and electrolytes checked, with special attention to hypokalemia and hypocalcemia. If there is a possibility of intra-abdominal abscess or sepsis, CT or ultrasonography is indicated. If the diagnosis is still in doubt, a water-soluble contrast study (eg, Gastrografin) can be diagnostic as well as therapeutic because of the cathartic effect of the hyperosmolar solution. Drainage of an abscess may relieve the localized ileus or obstruction. Patients who are receiving adrenal corticosteroids may develop adynamic ileus if the drug is withdrawn too quickly. High doses (300 mg of hydrocortisone daily or equivalent) intravenously will give prompt resolution.

Complete obstruction warrants reoperation as soon as resuscitation is complete. Partial obstruction will often resolve with conservative management.

ENTERIC FISTULA

Risk factors for enteric fistula include previous radiation, inflammatory bowel disease, and chronic corticosteroid administration. After initial resuscitation, the first maneuver is to determine the need for early operation. A controlled fistula is present when enteric contents are captured by a drain or when rapid egress from a wound results in little or no peritoneal contamination or irritation—such cases can be expected to resolve with nonoperative therapy. Percutaneous drainage of an associated abscess found by ultrasound or CT scan may allow closure of the fistula and improve the patient's physiologic status prior to definitive management. Complicating conditions include radiation damage, malignancy, inflammatory bowel disease, the presence of a foreign body, and distal intestinal obstruction. Water-soluble contrast studies are occasionally helpful to visualize the site of fistula, evaluate the adequacy of drainage, and rule out distal obstruction. Once a decision to attempt conservative management is made, useful therapeutic maneuvers may include restriction of oral intake, parenteral nutrition, octreotide acetate (50–200 μg subcutaneously twice to three times daily), and nasogastric suction. Elemental diets may be substituted for parenteral nutrition in selected patients—especially those with distal fistulas or with fistulas not in continuity (duodenal stump, pancreatic).

Conversely, an anastomotic leak or dehiscence that results in free peritoneal spillage requires emergent operation for patient survival. The clinical setting and physical examination will usually allow an accurate assessment. Oliguria and hypovolemia often portend extensive peritoneal contamination and third-spacing, while diffuse peritoneal irritation manifested by a rigid abdomen on examination offers no real dilemma. The patient with localized peritoneal signs, mild to moderate leukocytosis, and perhaps minimal additional fluid requirements presents a more difficult decision.

INTRA-ABDOMINAL ABSCESS

Intra-abdominal abscess is usually the result of contamination at the time of surgery or leakage of enteric contents. The process has been contained by the patient's immune system and defense mechanisms, including the omentum. Antibiotics—especially with smaller collections—may resolve the process. Larger abscesses—especially those with continued enteric communication—may require drainage or even intestinal resection to control the process. The exact role and limitations of percutaneous drainage seem to be more dependent on the availability of an experienced interventional radiologist than any absolute criteria, though multiloculated and interloop abscesses may be less amenable to this technique. Success rates range from 25–100%. Infected pancreatic necrosis and other phlegmonous processes are not amenable to the percutaneous approach. Of particular importance is appropriate attention to ensure continued success, including catheter irrigations, frequent rescanning, and contrast studies.

CHOLECYSTITIS

Patients in the ICU may develop calculous or acalculous cholecystitis as well as cholangitis or biliary pancreatitis. The diagnosis may already be known or suspected, as in the patient admitted for observation of acute pancreatitis; or may be a confounding factor, as in the recent cardiac surgical patient developing acalculous cholecystitis.

The typical findings of right upper quadrant pain, fever, and Murphy's sign may not be present even in an awake, responsive patient. Elevated liver enzymes or unexplained fever often prompt consideration of biliary-disease. Well-recognized risk factors for cholecystitis (NPO, parenteral nutrition, recent surgery, shock) should arouse suspicion. Perhaps the main difficulty is the lack of a reliable diagnostic examination in a critically ill patient, especially one with acalculous disease. The findings of sludge in the gallbladder by ultrasound and nonvisualization on ^{99m}Tc-HIDA scan are nonspecific and even expected in patients being maintained on long-term parenteral nutrition. The technique of percutaneous cholecystostomy (transhepatic) or aspiration of gallbladder contents with analysis (Gram stain, culture) can be useful and deserves consideration in the most unstable patients. The diagnosis remains largely a clinical one, and exploration is often required for confirmation and treatment. Surgical exploration is frequently based on clinical suspicion and nonexclusionary test results.

COLONIC PSEUDO-OBSTRUCTION (Ogilvie's Syndrome)

Typical findings include abdominal distention, abdominal pain, and obstruction. Plain abdominal radiographs are usually diagnostic, though contrast studies or endoscopy may be necessary to exclude volvulus and distal colonic obstruction. Predisposing factors include bed rest, spinal fractures and cord injuries, and prolonged opioid use. Treatment is required when the cecal diameter exceeds 10 cm on a plain film of the abdomen. Therapy should include correction of electrolyte disturbances (especially hypokalemia), cessation of narcotics, and nasogastric decompression to prevent further gaseous distention. Neostigmine has emerged as the treatment of choice. If the cecal diameter exceeds 12 cm and if there is no improvement with the above measures, colonoscopic decompression is usually effective, with 15–20% of patients requiring repeated procedures. Operative treatment (tube cecostomy, right colectomy) is reserved for patients with signs of present or impending perforation or a situation in which a skilled endoscopist is not available.

CURRENT CONTROVERSIES & UNRESOLVED ISSUES

Abdominal Compartment Syndrome

The concept of elevated intra-abdominal pressure having detrimental clinical sequelae was enunciated nearly two decades ago. Initially, renal "toxicity" was focused on, and oliguria remains one of the earlier clinical signs. Other sequelae include pulmonary compromise and mesenteric ischemia. The important factors to keep in mind are to have a high index of suspicion, to use bladder pressure measurements as a reflection of intra-abdominal pressure, and to consider or perform decompressive laparotomy early if indicated.

Bacterial Translocation & Enteral Feedings

The clinical picture of a critically ill patient succumbing to sepsis and multiple system organ failure without any apparent septic focus is a not infrequent clinical problem. A large volume of data—largely experimental or anecdotal—points to bacterial translocation across a dysfunctional gastrointestinal barrier as the cause. Attempts at correction or prevention have included selective gut decontamination, maintenance of intravascular volume, and enteral feedings. Adequate enteral feedings initiated early appear to maintain adequate gastrointestinal barrier function. Crucial to this effect seems to be the amino acid glutamine, a specific nutrient that supports intestinal mucosal cell growth and replication. Glutamine-containing enteral nutrition may prevent or at least lessen the severity of multisystem organ failure induced by bacterial translocation and bypass the difficulties inherent in enteral feedings in this group of patients.

Monoclonal Antibodies

Despite recent advances in critical care, patients continue to succumb to septic states. This may occur as a result of delayed recognition or presentation, diminished immune responses, or overwhelming insults.

Numerous monoclonal antibodies have been tested and show promise. These agents are targeted against mediators of sepsis and in no way obviate standard identification and treatment of the septic source. They include antibodies against gram-negative endotoxin as well as tumor necrosis factor and interleukin-1. Of these, monoclonal antibodies against tumor necrosis factor are the only ones with proven efficacy in human trials, albeit with a modest benefit (3.5–4% increase in survival). Appropriate selection of patients and timing of therapy are among the ongoing clinical issues. Additionally, their widespread use may be limited by the expected prohibitive costs.

Laparoscopy

The laparoscope has become a common tool of the general surgeon in the last 15 years, and it is only natural that its role in critical care patients has been explored. The laparoscope is likely to be mainly a diagnostic instrument for the near future because of the untoward cardiovascular and respiratory side effects of prolonged abdominal insufflation, especially in this group of high-risk patients. If anecdotal results are supported by further prospective investigations, laparoscopy may supplant peritoneal lavage for the bedside diagnosis of peritonitis or visceral perforation.

REFERENCES

Alverdy JC et al: Diagnostic peritoneal lavage in intraabdominal sepsis. Am Surgeon 1988;5:456–9.

Freischlag J, Busuttil RW: The value of postoperative fever evaluation. Surgery 1983;94:358–63.

Gerzof SG et al: Expanded criteria for percutaneous abscess drainage. Arch Surg 1985;120:227–32.

Gomez JA, Diehl AK: Admission stool guaiac test: Use and impact on patient management. Am J Med 1991;92:603–6.

Guttormson NL, Bubrick MP: Postoperative ileus versus intestinal obstruction. Probl Gen Surg 1992;9:683–97.

Machiedo GW et al: Reoperation of sepsis. Am Surg 1985;51: 149–54.

Marshall JC: Clinical trials of mediator-directed therapy in sepsis: what have we learned? Intensive Care Med 2000;26:S74–83.

Menzies D, Ellis H: Intestinal obstruction from adhesions. How big is the problem? Ann R Coll Surg Engl 1990;72:60–3.

Norwood SH, Civetta JM: Abdominal CT scanning in critically ill surgical patients. Ann Surg 1985;202:166–75.

Norwood SH, Civetta JM: Evaluating sepsis in critically ill patients. Chest 1987;92:137–44.

Panacek E eta l: Neutralization of TNF by a monoclonal antibody improves survival and reduces organ dysfunction in human sepsis. Results of the MONARCS trial. Chest 2000;118:88S.

Pitcher WD, Musler DM: Critical importance of early diagnosis and treatment of intra-abdominal infection. Arch Surg 1982;117:328–33.

Saggi BH et al: Abdominal compartment syndrome. J Trauma 1998;45:597–609.

Wilmore DW et al: The gut: A central organ after surgical stress. Surgery 1988;104:917–23.

Gastrointestinal Bleeding

33

Tracey D. Arnell, MD

Gastrointestinal bleeding is a common complaint and finding in both the inpatient and outpatient settings. There are a variety of causes, including upper intestinal sources such as peptic ulcer disease and lower intestinal causes such as diverticulosis. The diversity of the causes of gastrointestinal bleeding is reflected in the various presentations, which range from hematemesis to bright red rectal bleeding and from life-threatening hemorrhage to chronic, compensated blood loss. Management of the patient is based on the severity of the bleeding as well as its location and cause. Therefore, a deliberate approach to diagnosis is important, including the history, physical findings, and selected laboratory and other tests. This chapter will outline the initial assessment of all patients with acute intestinal bleeding followed by a more detailed discussion of the causes of gastrointestinal bleeding and their treatment.

PATIENT ASSESSMENT

Initial Approach

Evaluation of the patient presenting with complaints of gastrointestinal bleeding, regardless of whether it is vomiting or bleeding per rectum, begins with an assessment of the severity of the episode and the patient's hemodynamic status. The initial history should include details regarding the bleeding event, including the duration, amount, and color of the blood, the general medical history with emphasis on liver diseases and cardiac disease, and the presence of symptoms related to hemorrhage such as syncope or chest pain. The mnemonic HEMATOCRIT (Table 33–1) may be helpful in obtaining key information that will aid in evaluating patients.

Determining the severity of the bleeding is of primary importance for appropriate triage. Factors in the history suggesting severe bleeding include passage of clots, multiple episodes, light-headedness, chest pain, syncope, and hemodynamic instability. A patient with significant comorbidities—especially cardiac disease and liver disease—and a history of coagulopathies, both pharmacologic and related to disease states, is at increased risk for complications. The description of the color of the blood by both the patient and the physician has been found to be unreliable as evidence and should be interpreted with caution. The color of the blood may be more indicative of the time it has been in the gastrointestinal tract than of bleeding severity. Hematochezia occurs if the blood is present for less than 8 hours, and the color darkens, becoming melena with increasing transit time.

The next step in evaluating the patient is determining whether the source of bleeding is in the upper or lower intestinal tract. Upper intestinal bleeding is defined as that occurring proximal to the ligament of Treitz; and lower intestinal bleeding, distal to that ligament. The major historical questions outlined in Table 33–1 include hematemesis, hematochezia; history of liver disease, peptic ulcer, or inflammatory bowel disease; use of alcohol, aspirin, or steroids; and coagulopathies. Physical examination may also reveal clues to the cause of bleeding. Significant findings include evidence of liver disease such as ascites, caput medusae, and jaundice. Mucosal pigmentation in Peutz-Jeghers syndrome and skin telangiectasias in hereditary hemorrhagic telangiectasia (Rendu-Osler-Weber syndrome) are occasionally seen. Digital rectal examination is performed both to assess for rectal masses and to determine the presence and note the character of blood. In cases of a suspected colonic source of bleeding, proctoscopy can visualize actively bleeding hemorrhoids or proctitis. Placement of a nasogastric tube with aspiration to determine if there is blood in the stomach or duodenum gives positive results in 85–90% of patients with an upper intestinal source of bleeding. For improved sensitivity, the presence of bile should be documented to confirm that the duodenum was intubated.

Basic laboratory tests to be obtained are hematocrit, platelets, prothrombin time (PT) and partial thromboplastin time (aPTT), liver function tests, serum chemistries including sodium, BUN, and creatinine, type and screen or type and cross, and an electrocardiogram.

Treatment

Restoration of intravascular volume with crystalloids and blood products as needed is conducted concomitantly with evaluation. Large-bore intravenous lines are placed and fluid administration started. The use of fluids high in sodium such as normal saline and albumin should be used sparingly in patients with known liver disease because of their sodium avidity. Generally, if hemodynamic instability is severe or persists after the administration of 2 L of crystalloid, blood is transfused. The

Table 33–1. Hematocrit mnemonic for obtaining initial history of a patient presenting with gastrointestinal hemorrhage.

H	Hepatic disease
E	Ethanol
M	Medications
A	Angina pectoris
T	Time (duration of symptoms)
O	Orifice
C	Clots
R	Recent (last episode)
I	Illnesses (other medical history)
T	Transfusions (number)

adequacy of resuscitation is monitored by following hemodynamic parameters, urine output, and serial hemoglobin measurements. In patients with cardiac and renal insufficiency, central venous pressures or pulmonary artery catheters aid in following the course of resuscitation. It should be remembered that equilibration of hemoglobin with whole blood losses may take up to 72 hours. The trend of hemoglobin measurements is often more important than the absolute number.

Clotting factors are given in cases of known coagulopathy. The general rule of administering fresh frozen plasma and platelets after 4–6 units of packed red blood cells (PRBCs) has been shown to be unwarranted. Except for cases of overwhelming bleeding, clotting factors and platelets are given based on demonstrated laboratory deficiencies.

UPPER INTESTINAL TRACT BLEEDING

The rate of upper intestinal tract bleeding is approximately 0.1% of hospitalized patients per year. Stress ulcers and gastritis are frequent causes in the critically ill, although with improved critical care these numbers have significantly decreased. Mortality has remained relatively stable since the 1990s and is affected by patient age and comorbidities. Long-term mortality also remains high in patients with liver disease and esophageal variceal bleeding.

Diagnosis

The history and physical examination may be very suggestive of the cause of upper intestinal tract bleeding, especially in cases of esophageal and gastric varices related to liver disease and the use of agents that predispose to peptic ulcer disease. Definitive determination of the source is necessary using additional diagnostic tests and procedures. Causes of upper tract bleeding and their frequency in a large series are set forth in Table 33–2.

A. Endoscopy

Esophagogastroduodenoscopy has become the standard procedure for diagnosis of upper intestinal bleeding. Treatment can be given as well, as will be discussed further below. Prior to performing this procedure, an attempt should be made to irrigate the stomach using a nasogastric tube because the caliber of the suction port of the scope is of smaller caliber than the nasogastric tube and not as effective in clearing blood. In patients who are at risk for aspiration, unable to protect their airway, or combative, intubation is necessary prior to the procedure. When esophagogastroduodenoscopy is performed in the urgent or emergent setting, the source will be identified 90–95% of the time. If the examination is delayed more than 48 hours, the sensitivity drops to 33%. Esophagogastroduodenoscopy may be difficult in patients who are bleeding massively since blood obscures the mucosa. In these cases, continued resuscitation, correction of coagulopathy, and repeat esophagogastroduodenoscopy has been shown to be successful.

B. Angiography

Angiography is occasionally used in diagnosis, though more commonly it is undertaken with therapeutic intent. For angiography to be diagnostic, bleeding must be ongoing at a rate of 0.5–1 mL/min. Pertinent findings are bleeding from the gastroduodenal artery in patients with peptic ulcer hemorrhage, pooling of the contrast in cases of Mallory-Weiss tears, arteriovenous malformations, or Dieulafoy's erosions. If a venous phase is performed, esophageal or gastric varices are occasionally visualized.

Table 33–2. Causes of upper gastrointestinal tract bleeding.[1]

	% of Total Cases
Gastric erosions	21.9
Duodenal ulcer	16.8
Gastric ulcer	16.2
Varicies	11.4
Esophagitis	9.5
Erosive duodenitis	6.7
Mallory-Weiss tear	5.9
Neoplasm	2.8
Esophageal ulcer	1.6
Stomal ulcer	1.4
Rendu-Osler-Weber syndrome	0.4
Others	5.4

[1]Reproduced, with permission, from Silverstein FE et al: The national ASGE survey on upper gastrointestinal bleeding. II. Clinical prognostic factors. Gastrointest Endosc 1981;27:80–93.

Treatment

Specific therapies are discussed below for the common causes of upper intestinal bleeding, but the majority are managed endoscopically or angiographically, with surgery reserved for failures.

ESOPHAGEAL & GASTRIC VARICES

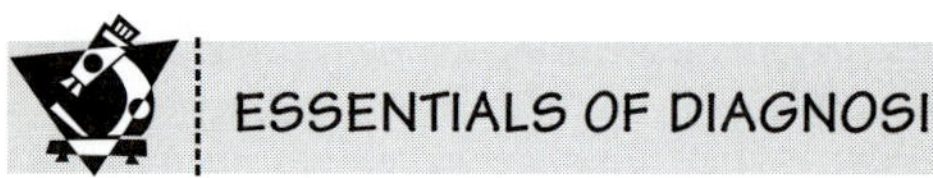

- *Hematemesis.*
- *Stigmas of liver disease.*
- *Endoscopic observation of varices.*

General Considerations

In the United States, alcoholic and viral cirrhosis are the most common causes of portal hypertension and subsequent varices. Esophageal variceal bleeding is a common complication of portal hypertension, occurring in 30% of patients with varices. Varices occur in the esophagus and stomach most commonly, and prognosis and treatment vary based on the location. The mortality rate is 30% for each episode of variceal bleeding, and rebleeding occurs in 70% of patients. Gastric varices occur with esophageal varices—or alone in the case of splenic vein thrombosis. Additionally, variceal patients have significant associated and coexisting morbidities such as malnutrition, coagulopathy, encephalopathy, and thrombocytopenia. The Child-Pugh classification of liver failure is useful in grading of liver disease severity and identification of operative risk (Table 33–3).

Table 33–3. Child-Pugh classification of functional status in liver disease.

	Class (Risk)		
	A (Low)	B (Moderate)	C (High)
Ascites	Absent	Slight to moderate	Tense
Encephalopathy	None	Grades I–II	Grades III–IV
Serum albumin (g/dL)	> 3.5	3.0–3.5	< 3.0
Serum bilirubin (g/dL)	< 2.0	2.0–3.0	> 3.0
Prothrombin time (seconds above control)	< 4.0	4.0–6.0	> 6.0

Clinical Features

A. Symptoms and Signs

Patients with variceal bleeding usually present with painless, massive hematemesis, often with hemodynamic compromise. A history of alcohol consumption, viral hepatitis, or liver disease may be elucidated. Confusion related to hypotension or encephalopathy may be present. On physical examination, stigmas such as evidence of malnutrition, caput medusae, ascites, or splenomegaly can be found.

B. Diagnosis

Following restoration of intravascular volume with fluid, packed red cells, and clotting factors as needed, urgent endoscopy is performed. It is important in diagnosis, as 50% of patients with known liver disease are bleeding from another source. Complete esophagoduodenoscopy is performed to assess for this as well as to identify gastric varices. Many patients will have stopped bleeding and may have only indirect signs such as clot or "cherry spots" on the varices.

Treatment

A. Medical Therapy

Variceal bleeding is directly related to elevated portal pressure, and therapy is aimed at lowering this. Octreotide and vasopressin decrease splanchnic and hepatic blood flow, effectively decreasing portal pressures. Vasopressin has significant systemic effects, including cardiac ischemia, and should be administered concomitantly with nitroglycerin. Octreotide has a much more benign side effect profile and has been found to be as effective as vasopressin, with a trend toward better survival. For this reason, it has become the agent of choice in variceal bleeding. Pharmacologic control of bleeding is achieved in 70% of patients, but nearly 45% develop rebleeding when therapy is stopped. Beta-blocking agents are generally not indicated in the acutely bleeding patient and have more relevance in prevention of bleeding. Commonly used medications, dosages, pharmacologic effects, and side effects are listed in Table 33–4.

B. Balloon Tamponade

Insertion of a balloon into the stomach to tamponade variceal bleeding may be indicated in patients with

Table 33–4. Commonly used medications in management of active variceal bleeding.

	Mechanism	Dose	Adverse Effects
Octreotide	↓ Splanchnic and hepatic blood flow	100 μg bolus IV 50 μg/h infusion IV	Minimal
Vasopressin	Splanchnic vasoconstrictor ↓ Portal flow	0.4 units/min IV	Intestinal ischemia Cardiac ischemia Arrhythmia
Nitroglycerin	Vasodilator Compensates cardiac ischemia from vasopressin	5 μg/min IV	Hypotension Headaches

continued bleeding despite pharmacologic therapy if endoscopic therapy is not immediately available. It is effective in about 50–90% of patients for short-term control of bleeding. There are three types of tubes with balloons: Linton, Sengstaken-Blakemore, and Minnesota. The Linton tube has a single balloon that is inflated in the stomach, the Sengstaken-Blakemore tube has an esophageal and gastric balloon with a gastric suction port, and the Minnesota tube has two balloons and two suction ports: esophageal and gastric. Patients are intubated; the tube is passed transorally or transnasally; gastric location is confirmed with instillation of air in the stomach port; the balloon is inflated with 200 mL of air; and approximately 0.5 kg of traction is placed cephalad. A radiograph is obtained to confirm position in the stomach. If bleeding continues in a patient for whom the Sengstaken-Blakemore or Minnesota balloon has been used, the esophageal balloon is inflated. Gastric tamponade can be continued for 48–72 hours, but esophageal balloon inflation is limited to 24 hours. Potential complications include aspiration and esophageal or gastric ulceration or rupture.

C. Sclerotherapy

Endoscopic injection of sclerosing agents into or around varices achieves control of bleeding in up to 90% of patients. Initial control occurs because of variceal thrombosis with ultimate fibrosis and obliteration of the varices. Cyanoacrylate glue has been used in gastric varices with improved results, but damage to the endoscope has occurred as well as cerebral emboli in patients with right-to-left shunts.

D. Band Ligation

Approximately three bands per varix are applied. The result is variceal thrombosis and obliteration. Banding is repeated in subsequent sessions until all varices have been treated. Band ligation is associated with fewer complications and the need for fewer sessions than sclerotherapy and is the preferred treatment for esophageal variceal bleeding. This modality as well as sclerotherapy are minimally effective with gastric varices.

E. Transjugular Intrahepatic Portosystemic Shunting (TIPS)

Prior to the introduction of the TIPS procedure in 1988, patients failing medical and endoscopic management of variceal bleeding underwent surgical portosystemic shunt procedures with high morbidity and mortality rates. The goal of treatment is to divert blood flow around the cirrhotic liver directly to the systemic caval system, and the TIPS procedure achieves this percutaneously through the internal jugular vein with local anesthesia. Under fluoroscopic guidance, a needle—and eventually an expandable metal stent—are placed from the hepatic vein to the portal vein through the liver parenchyma creating a portosystemic shunt. This method is effective in controlling bleeding in 90% of patients, though encephalopathy occurs in 25–40%. It has lower morbidity and mortality than surgery, especially in patients with advanced liver disease such as Child-Pugh C.

F. Surgery

Potential surgical options include portosystemic shunts such as portacaval, mesocaval, and splenorenal shunts, transplantation, and splenectomy in patients with gastric varices. Shunts have been shown to stop bleeding in 90% of patients, but the mortality for patients with advanced liver disease is as high as 85%. Generally, surgical shunts are reserved for patients with Child-Pugh A and B liver disease as prevention of future bleeding. TIPS is performed in most other patients who fail medical and endoscopic therapy.

PEPTIC ULCER DISEASE

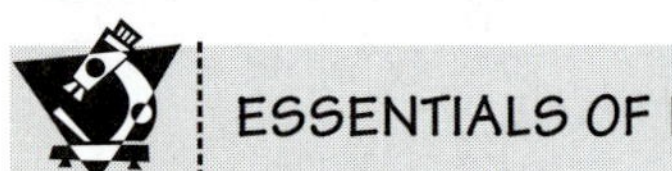

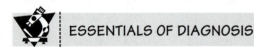

ESSENTIALS OF DIAGNOSIS

- *Epigastric abdominal pain.*
- *Use of aspirin, NSAIDs, steroids.*
- *Aspiration of blood via nasogastric tube.*
- *Endoscopic identification of ulcer.*

General Considerations

Despite the use of anti-ulcer medications such as histamine H_2 blockers and proton pump inhibitors, peptic ulcer disease remains the most common cause of upper intestinal bleeding, accounting for 50% of cases. Even in patients with varices, ulcers are responsible for 50% of bleeding episodes. The clinical presentation and risk factors are generally quite different for the outpatient peptic ulcer and the inpatient stress ulcer. Inpatients are frequently elderly and critically ill, with the primary risk factors for stress ulcers being ventilatory support, lack of enteral feeding, age, and burns or head injury. Gastric hypoperfusion with resultant mucosal ischemia predisposes to ulceration in these patients. With improved critical care support and end organ perfusion, the incidence of bleeding in the intensive care unit has decreased from 30% to less than 10%. Over 80% of patients will stop bleeding spontaneously, and the most common cause of mortality is related to comorbidities rather than bleeding.

Gastric ulcers are more common in elderly patients and generally occur along the lesser curvature. It is unusual for gastric cancers to bleed massively, but consideration should be given to the possibility that a gastric ulcer may be malignant. Most patients with ulcer disease—especially those with duodenal and prepyloric ulcers—will be found to be *Helicobacter pylori*-positive.

Clinical Features

A. Symptoms and Signs

Hematemesis occurs in 80% of patients with acute bleeding from ulcer disease. Approximately 11% of patients, usually those with exsanguinating hemorrhage, have hematochezia. Epigastric tenderness may be elicited on physical examination.

B. Diagnosis

Nasogastric tube aspiration usually reveals blood or coffee ground material. Duodenal bleeding can be missed unless the nasogastric tube is passed beyond the pylorus and bile obtained. As discussed previously, urgent endoscopy is performed and will identify the source in 90% of patients. Table 33–5 lists the stigmas associated with bleeding that can be visualized. It was previously believed that if a clot was seen, it should not be removed for fear of causing bleeding. It has been shown that removing the clot, visualizing the vessel, and treating it endoscopically is associated with lower rates of rebleeding.

Treatment

A. Medical Treatment

Traditional anti-ulcer medications such as antacids and histamine H_2 receptor antagonists have been shown to be ineffective in acid suppression. Proton pump inhibitors are efficacious, but an intravenous formulation (pantoprazole) has only recently become available. *H pylori* is found in more than 60% of patients with ulcer disease, and treatment of this entity will reduce the rate of rebleeding but has no effect on the acute bleeding episode. In the critically ill patient with stress ulcers, resuscitation and hemodynamic support with the goal of restoring end organ perfusion are vital therapeutic goals.

B. Endoscopy

Endoscopic management of ulcer bleeding is successful in 85–90% of patients and is most effective when a visible vessel or actively bleeding vessel is seen. Therapeutic options include injection with vasoconstrictive and sclerosing agents, thermal probes, bipolar coagulation, argon and laser coagulation, and application of hemostatic agents. Clinical trials have not shown a significant difference in efficacy with the varying techniques and agents. As stated previously, overlying clots should be removed and the underlying vessel treated, as this is associated with significantly lower rates of rebleeding. Ten to 20 percent of patients treated endoscopically will rebleed—most within 72 hours—and repeat endoscopy is effective in 50% of

Table 33–5. Endoscopic signs of peptic ulcer bleeding.

Spurting arterial bleeding
Oozing bleeding
Nonbleeding visible vessel
Clot
Blood or coffee ground material in the presence of an ulcer

patients. There is a significant reduction in morbidity and mortality in patients treated successfully with endoscopic therapy compared with those treated surgically, including those requiring a second endoscopic maneuver.

C. Angiography

Embolization of the gastroduodenal or gastric artery may be used as primary therapy or as an adjunct to endoscopic control of ulcer bleeding. Agents used include absorbable gelatin sponge, autologous clot, and small metal coils. The incidence of ischemia is very low because of the rich collaterals of the upper intestinal tract, especially with selective embolization.

D. Surgical Treatment

Surgery is now necessary in less than 10% of patients presenting with ulcer bleeding and is reserved for those failing endoscopic or angiographic management. Relative indications for surgery are listed in Table 33–6. The choice of operation includes simple oversewing of the ulcer with or without vessel ligation, ulcer excision, addition of vagotomy, or radical surgery, including vagotomy and antrectomy versus gastrectomy, depending on the ulcer location. In a recent review of surgical options, conservative therapy with oversewing of the ulcer is associated with a higher rate of rebleeding and with rates of morbidity and mortality similar to what is reported with more radical surgery. The recommendation based on a review of the available literature is for ulcer excision in patients with bleeding gastric ulcer. In the case of a large penetrating ulcer, gastric resection should be performed. Duodenal ulcers should be oversewn and vessel ligation performed. Because of effective medical regimens to prevent rebleeding, including anti-*H pylori* therapies, vagotomy is not recommended. With the availability of effective medical therapy, the goal of urgent and emergent surgery is not cure of the ulcer disease but control of the hemorrhage.

Table 33–6. Relative indications for surgical therapy in hemorrhage associated with peptic ulcer disease.

1. Severe hemorrhage unresponsive to initial resuscitative measures
2. Unavailability or failure of endoscopic or other nonsurgical therapies to control persistent or recurrent bleeding
3. Coexisting second indication for operation such as perforation, obstruction, or suspected malignancy

Figure 33–1 sets out a treatment algorithm for patients presenting with ulcer bleeding.

GASTRITIS

ESSENTIALS OF DIAGNOSIS

- *Evidence of gastrointestinal bleeding.*
- *Gastric erosions on endoscopy.*

General Considerations

Stress gastritis most commonly occurs in the critically ill patient. It may be a result of pharmacologic agents known to be injurious to the stomach or to hypoperfusion as a result of shock with diminished mucosal blood flow. It is usually self-limited and rarely life-threatening, requiring transfusions in fewer than 5% of events.

Treatment

Most patients will respond to proton pump inhibitors and treatment of the underlying cause of hypoperfusion and shock, with resolution of the gastritis. Those with continued bleeding can be managed by endoscopic treatments to punctate bleeding sites, intravenous infusion of vasopressin, or selective angiographic embolization of gastric vessels. In the rare patient failing these methods, emergent surgery with gastrectomy or gastric devascularization is warranted. The operative mortality rate is nearly 50%, and these procedures should be reserved for cases in which all other therapies have failed. Surgery is reserved for patients failing these maneuvers. In these rare cases, gastrectomy or gastric devascularization is performed. Operative mortality for these procedures is nearly 50%, often from the associated comorbid diseases.

UNUSUAL LESIONS

Less common entities associated with significant upper intestinal bleeding and their causes are listed in Table 33–7. Endoscopic therapy is effective in the treatment of most of these lesions. Surgery is occasionally indicated in those failing endoscopic management and generally involves oversewing of the lesion or wedge excision in cases of vessel malformations.

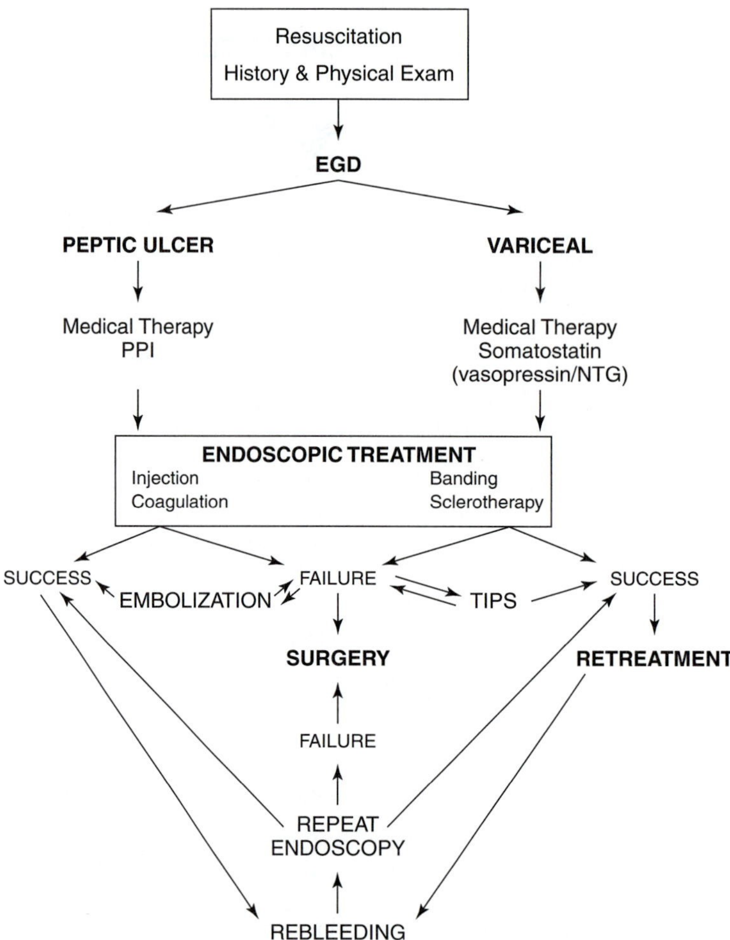

Figure 33–1. Algorithm for management of acute upper intestinal bleeding. (EGD, esophagogastroduodenoscopy; PPI, proton pump inhibitor; NGT, nasogastric tube; TIPS, transjugular intrahepatic portosystemic shunting.)

LOWER INTESTINAL TRACT BLEEDING

Lower intestinal bleeding—that occurring distal to the ligament of Treitz—is responsible for 25–30% of cases of gastrointestinal hemorrhage in most series. Most cases of acute hemorrhage are caused by diverticular bleeding or angiodysplasia. Common causes and treatments are summarized in Table 33–8. As compared with cases of upper intestinal bleeding, patients are nearly half as likely to present with shock (19%), or require blood transfusions (36%) and have a significantly higher hemoglobin concentration upon presentation. Spontaneous cessation of bleeding occurs in 75–85% of patients. This intermittent bleeding makes the source of bleeding difficult to localize. The history may be very helpful in cases of lower intestinal bleeding—specifically, previous pelvic radiation, a history of abdominal pain, diarrhea, weight loss, inflammatory bowel disease, and previous colonic screening examinations. Sources such as Meckel's diverticular bleeding are unusual in the adult population but do occasionally occur.

An algorithm for the evaluation and treatment of lower intestinal tract bleeding is presented in Figure 33–2.

Table 33–7. Uncommon causes of upper intestinal tract bleeding.

Diagnosis	General Information	Treatment
Esophageal ulcers	Esophagitis	Endoscopic
Mallory-Weiss tear	Vomiting Gastroesphageal junction	Endoscopic Vasopressin Surgical oversewing
Dieulafoy's erosions	Vascular malformation Large submucosal artery in proximal stomach area	Endoscopic Surgical wedge resection
Angiodysplasia	Arteriovenous malformation Small and superficial Rendu-Olser-Weber syndrome	Endoscopic

Table 33–8. Causes and treatment of lower intestinal tract bleeding.

Cause	Treatment
Diverticular disease	Endoscopic control Angiography Vasopressin Embolization Surgical treatment
Angiodysplasia	Endoscopic control Angiography Vasopressin Embolization Surgical treatment
Inflammatory bowel disease	Medical treatment Surgical treatment
Infectious colitis *E coli* O157 Salmonella Shigella Campylobacter Cytomegalovirus	Antibiotics
Radiation proctitis	Formaldehyde Endoscopic coagulation
Ischemic colitis	Resuscitation Surgical resection
Hemorrhoids	Ligation Surgical hemorrhoidectomy

Diagnosis

Lower intestinal bleeding is notoriously difficult to localize because of its intermittent nature. The sensitivity of most diagnostic modalities is increased if the patient is actively bleeding. The single best sign that there is active bleeding is passage of bright red blood. If this occurs, immediate attempts at localization using the available procedures should be performed.

A. Laboratory Findings

In addition to the usual laboratory tests, patients with suspected colitis should have stool sent for examination including fecal white blood cells, enteric pathogens, and ova and parasites.

B. Endoscopy

Limited endoscopy—primarily anoscopy and proctoscopy—can be performed easily in the emergent setting without preparation or sedation. For proctoscopy, suction and irrigation should be available and may identify colitis involving the rectum, actively bleeding hemorrhoids, or rectosigmoid neoplasms. If blood is seen more proximal to the proctoscopic examination, a colonic source is likely.

The use of colonoscopy in the acutely bleeding patient remains controversial. Initially, there was a theoretical concern that performing a bowel preparation might stimulate bleeding that has ceased. Several randomized studies have dispelled this misapprehension. The major limitation of colonoscopy in the acute setting is poor visualization because of inability to clear the blood in the lumen and the effect blood has on the optics of the scope. The use of high-volume pulsatile irrigation may improve visualization. Criteria for colonoscopic diagnosis of bleeding are shown in Table 33–9. Identification based on the distribution of blood must be interpreted with

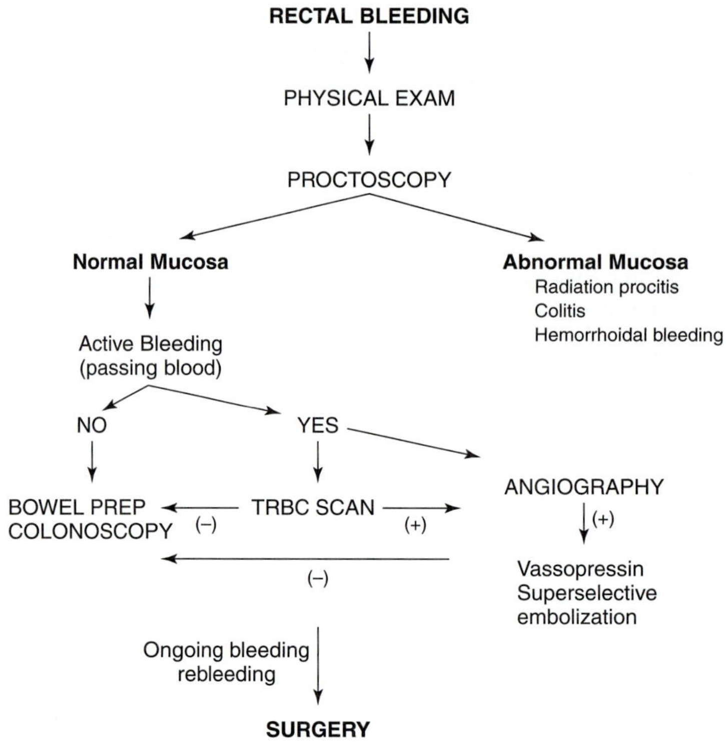

Figure 33–2. Algorithm for management of acute lower intestinal bleeding. (TRBC scan, tagged red blood cell scan.)

caution because of peristalsis. A review of 13 studies utilizing colonoscopy in the urgent setting reports a positive identification of the source of bleeding in 68% of patients. The accuracy of colonoscopy is dependent on the availability and dedication of endoscopists and will vary in different institutions.

Once the acute episode has resolved, colonoscopy should be performed and can identify arteriovenous malformations and the presence of diverticulosis. Its greatest utility after bleeding has ceased is to exclude mucosal lesions such as colitis and neoplasms.

Table 33–9. Diagnostic criteria for colonic bleeding observed endoscopically.

Active colonic bleeding site
Nonbleeding visible vessel
Adherent clot
Fresh blood localized to a colonic segment
Ulceration of a diverticulum with fresh blood in the immediate area
Absence of fresh blood in the terminal ileum with fresh blood in the colon

C. Nuclear Medicine

Labeling either a patient's red blood cells for a tagged red blood cell scan or sulfur colloid with agents such as technetium-99m can identify the location of blood extravasation into the gastrointestinal tract. This technique can identify bleeding as low as 0.1 mL/min. Red blood cells that are labeled with technetium-99m remain in the circulation for up to 48 hours and are not cleared by the liver and spleen—in contrast to sulfur colloid. Because of this, the tagged red cell scan is more sensitive and may be repeated within 48 hours in the case of an initially negative study if rebleeding occurs.

Potential findings include a "blush" or tuft of contrast and extravasation of contrast into the lumen of the bowel. Overall, nuclear medicine studies are positive in 50% of patients. This increases in the patients actively passing blood and is more specific if positive in the first 2 hours. When data were pooled from 16 studies, findings of a positive tagged red cell scan were inaccurate in 22% of patients. The relatively poor specificity and inaccuracy of localization has led to the recommendation that a confirmatory study such as colonoscopy or angiography be performed prior to surgery.

D. Angiography

Angiography is performed by cannulating the femoral artery (most commonly) and selectively injecting the mesenteric vessels with intravenous contrast. In cases of suspected lower intestinal bleeding, the most common causes are arteriovenous malformations and diverticulosis, both of which are more frequent on the right side of the colon. Therefore, the order of cannulation is ideally the superior mesenteric, then the inferior mesenteric, and then the celiac artery. Pooled data from 14 studies report a mean positive rate of diagnosis of 47%. Complications occurred in nearly 10% of patients and included renal failure, vessel injury, allergic contrast reactions, and transient ischemic attacks. Because of the low sensitivity of angiography and the risk for complications, the recommendation has been to first perform a nuclear medicine scan and, if positive, to proceed with angiography for more definitive localization. The studies that have evaluated this algorithm have not shown a decrease in negative angiograms. This suggests that angiography may be performed as the initial test in the actively bleeding patient, especially since therapeutic techniques such as superselective embolization and selective vasopressin infusion may be used.

Treatment

A. Medical Treatment

Other than resuscitation, effective medical therapy is limited to cases of infectious and inflammatory colitis. Primary treatment for flares of inflammatory bowel disease consists of intravenous steroids and bowel rest. If cultures demonstrate an infectious cause, appropriate antibiotic agents are administered.

B. Endoscopy

The same techniques available for upper intestinal bleeding—sclerosants, vasoactive agents, and thermal options—may be used for treatment of bleeding from colonic sources. These techniques are most commonly used in angiodysplastic lesions. The risk of perforation, especially in the thin-walled cecum, must be a consideration when using thermal, coagulation techniques.

C. Angiography

The vasa recta of the colon are end vessels, and the potential for ischemia with embolization is increased in that location compared with the stomach and duodenum. With current techniques of superselective embolization, the ischemic complications are minimal and the success of the procedure has improved. The experience of the angiographer should be taken into consideration and a period of observation of the patient following embolization is necessary. Selective infusion of vasopressin will lead to cessation of bleeding in 75% of patients, although half will rebleed when the infusion is stopped. Both techniques allow for resuscitation and preparation of the patient for a less emergent surgical procedure if one is needed.

D. Surgical Treatment

Surgery is recommended in patients with ongoing hemorrhage, transfusion requirement of 4 units packed red cells in less than 24 hours, and recurrent bleeding. Fewer than 10% of patients presenting with lower intestinal hemorrhage require emergent surgery because of ongoing hemorrhage. If bleeding has been localized preoperatively, segmental resection is performed with or without a stoma depending on the patient's overall medical condition. In cases of unlocalized bleeding, arrangements should be made for the availability of endoscopy and perhaps enteroscopy. A thorough exploration is performed, with examination and palpation of the entire small intestine for polyps or the presence of Meckel's diverticulum. If there is a significant amount of blood in the small intestine, esophagoduodenoscopy or enteroscopy (or both) must be performed. In the absence of an obvious source of hemorrhage, abdominal colectomy is undertaken with ileorectal anastomosis or ileostomy with Hartmann's pouch. Segmental colectomy in this situation is associated with an unacceptable 30% rate of rebleeding. Following an abdominal colectomy, patients can expect an average of two to four bowel movements a day. Mortality for this approach is less than 5%.

Diverticular Hemorrhage

The classic description of diverticular hemorrhage is painless bleeding with the passage of a large amount of blood or clots. Bleeding stops spontaneously in over 75%. Recent reports suggest that the use of NSAIDs increases the risk of diverticular bleeding, and these agents should be stopped if possible. The origin of bleeding is from erosion of a vasa recta artery at the neck of a diverticulum. Although most diverticula occur in the sigmoid colon, those that bleed are on the right side 70% of the time. The risk of rebleeding is 30% after the first episode and increases to 70% with a second episode. There is no evidence that the use of dietary fiber decreases the risk of this complication.

Arteriovenous Malformation (Angiodysplasia)

Bleeding from an arteriovenous malformation is venous, which means that the clinical presentation is more commonly one of chronic blood loss or melena rather than hematochezia. As is true also of diverticular hemorrhage, its incidence increases with age. At one time it was thought that patients with aortic stenosis had an increased risk of this lesion, but this does not appear to be the case. Diagnosis by endoscopy reveals a submucosal tortuous vessel. If the lesion is seen on routine colonoscopy, no endoscopic therapy is warranted. Angiographic findings include an early filling vein or a vascular tuft.

Radiation Proctitis

In a patient with a history of pelvic radiation, radiation proctitis may be the source of hemorrhage from arterioles made prone to trauma. The bleeding ranges from mild to hematochezia with significant transfusion requirements and is dependent on the severity of the proctitis. Treatment with corticosteroids and carafate enemas is ineffective. Topical 4% formaldehyde and endoscopic coagulation techniques have the greatest efficacy in this situation, and several treatments are often required. In cases of refractory severe bleeding, colostomy and/or proctectomy may be necessary.

Inflammatory Bowel Disease

Although ulcerative colitis commonly causes chronic ongoing rectal bleeding, it does not usually lead to acute hemorrhage because it is a mucosal process. Severe bleeding is more apt to be due to Crohn's disease since the deeper, larger submucosal vessels are the source. Treatment is targeted at controlling the acute flare with corticosteroids. Failure of medical therapy warrants urgent colectomy.

Ischemic Colitis

The most common cause of ischemic colitis is a low-flow state that frequently occurs in the absence of arteriosclerosis. Potential causes are many, and the disorder has been reported in critically ill patients, in marathon runners, in cocaine users, and in dialysis patients. Most patients present with abdominal pain and tenderness, which is not the case in other common causes of colonic bleeding. The primary therapy is volume support, cessation of exacerbating medications, and correction of hypotension. Colonoscopy is most sensitive if performed early, because resolution of mucosal abnormalities occurs within 1–2 weeks. The rectum is generally spared because of the dual mesenteric and systemic blood supply. Surgery is indicated if there is a suspicion of full-thickness ischemia or for complications such as stricture.

Hemorrhoids

Hemorrhoids are an uncommon source of significant lower intestinal bleeding and result in anemia less than 5% of the time. Patients complain of painless bleeding on the outside of the stool that drips into the toilet bowel. Hemorrhoidal bleeding is arterial and occasionally can be seen on anoscopy. Lower intestinal tract hemorrhage should not be attributed to hemorrhoids until evaluation for other colonic sources has been performed.

REFERENCES

Bhargava DK, Pokharna R: Endoscopic variceal ligation versus endoscopic variceal ligation and endoscopic sclerotherapy: A prospective randomized study. Am J Gastroenterol 1997;92:950–3.

Cello JP: Endoscopic management of esophageal variceal hemorrhage. injection, banding, glue, octreotide, or a combination? Semin Gastrointest Dis 1997;8:179–87.

Counter SF, Froese DP, Hart MJ: Prospective evaluation of formalin therapy for radiation proctitis. Am J Surg 1999;177:396–8.

Defreyne L et al: Embolization as a first approach with endoscopically unmanageable acute nonvariceal gastrointestinal hemorrhage. Radiology 2001;218:739–48.

El-Serag HB, Everhart JE: Improved survival after variceal hemorrhage over an 11-year period in the Department of Veterans Affairs. Am J Gastroenterol 2000;95:3566–73.

Fallah MA, Prakash C, Edmundowicz S: Acute gastrointestinal bleeding. Med Clin North Am 2000;84:1183–208.

Farner R et al: Total colectomy versus limited colonic resection for acute lower gastrointestinal bleeding. Am J Surg 1999;178:587–91.

Gonvers JJ et al: Appropriateness of colonoscopy: 8. Hematochezia. Endoscopy 1999;31:631–6.

Jensen DM: Current management of severe lower gastrointestinal bleeding. Gastrointest Endosc 1995;41:171–3.

Jensen DM et al: Urgent colonoscopy for the diagnosis and treatment of severe diverticular hemorrhage. N Engl J Med 2000;342:78–82.

Krige JE, Beckingham IJ: ABC of diseases of liver, pancreas, and biliary system. Portal hypertension—1: Varices. BMJ 2001;322:348–51.

Lai KC et al: Treatment of *Helicobacter pylori* in patients with duodenal ulcer hemorrhage—a long-term randomized, controlled study. Am J Gastroenterol 2000;95:2225–32.

Lau JY et al: Effect of intravenous omeprazole on recurrent bleeding after endoscopic treatment of bleeding peptic ulcers. N Engl J Med 2000;343:310–6.

Lau JY et al: Endoscopic retreatment compared with surgery in patients with recurrent bleeding after initial endoscopic control of bleeding ulcers. N Engl J Med 1999;340:751–6.

Lefkovitz Z et al: Radiology in the diagnosis and therapy of gastrointestinal bleeding. Gastroenterol Clin North Am 2000;29:489–512.

Ohmann C, Imhof M, Roher HD: Trends in peptic ulcer bleeding and surgical treatment. World J Surg 2000;24:284–93.

Orozco H, Mercado MA: The evolution of portal hypertension surgery. Lessons from 1000 operations and 50 years' experience. Arch Surg 2000:135;1389–94.

Pardi DS et al: Acute major gastrointestinal hemorrhage in inflammatory bowel disease. Gastrointest Endosc 1999;49:153–7.

Prakash C et al: Endoscopic hemostasis in acute diverticular bleeding. Endoscopy 1999;31:460–3.

American Society for Gastrointestinal Endoscopy: The role of endoscopy in the patient with lower gastrointestinal bleeding. Gastrointest Endosc 1998;48:685–8.

Stabile BE, Stamos MJ: Surgical management of gastrointestinal bleeding. Gastroenterol Clin North Am 2000;29:189–222.

Steffes C, Fromm D: The current diagnosis and management of upper gastrointestinal bleeding. Adv Surg 1992;25:331–61.

Suzman MS et al: Accurate localization and surgical management of active lower gastrointestinal hemorrhage with technetium-labeled erythrocyte scintigraphy. Ann Surg 1996;224:29–36.

Tam W, Moore J, Schoeman M: Treatment of radiation proctitis with argon plasma coagulation. Endoscopy 2000;32:667–72.

Yacyshyn BR, Thomson AB: Critical review of acid suppression in nonvariceal, acute, upper gastrointestinal bleeding. Dig Dis 2000;18:117–28.

Zuckerman GR, Prakash C: Acute lower intestinal bleeding: part I: clinical presentation and diagnosis. Gastrointest Endosc 1998;48:606–17.

Zuckerman GR, Prakash C: Acute lower intestinal bleeding: part II: etiology, therapy, and outcomes. Gastrointest Endosc 1999;49:228–38.

Hepatobiliary Disease

34

Hernan I. Vargas, MD

Liver disease is the ninth leading cause of death in the United States, resulting in approximately 30,000 deaths each year. Cirrhosis represents the final common pathway for a wide variety of chronic liver diseases. Cirrhosis is defined as a diffuse fibrotic process in the liver. Grossly, abnormal nodules replace the normally smooth hepatic parenchyma.

Patients with cirrhosis often develop complications from their underlying liver disease such as upper gastrointestinal bleeding, renal insufficiency, ascites, or encephalopathy and require critical care. In other circumstances, cirrhotic patients may require critical care due to unrelated problems such as trauma, cancer, or major surgery. Due to their fragile health and risk of morbidity and mortality also require critical care. The physician caring for patients in the ICU should therefore be knowledgeable about disorders of liver function. In this chapter, we address the diagnosis and management of serious conditions that affect liver function or complications that may occur in the care of patients with underlying liver disease.

ACUTE HEPATIC FAILURE

ESSENTIALS OF DIAGNOSIS

- *Acute onset.*
- *Jaundice.*
- *Encephalopathy.*

General Considerations

Acute hepatic failure is a rapid-onset, severe impairment of liver function. The natural history is that of progressive deterioration with multiple system organ failure. Prior to the availability of liver transplantation, the mortality was as high as 80%.

The interval between the development of jaundice and the onset of encephalopathy has been used to classify hepatic failure as hyperacute (0–7 days), acute (8–28 days), and subacute (28 days–12 weeks).

Acute viral hepatitis (HBV, HAV) and acetaminophen toxicity are the most common causes of acute hepatic failure in the United States. Other causes are as listed in Table 34–1.

Clinical Features

A. Symptoms and Signs

The onset of symptoms is usually abrupt, characterized by malaise, fatigue, and loss of appetite. Less frequently, patients complain of abdominal pain and fever. The physical examination is significant for the presence of jaundice, hepatomegaly, and right upper quadrant tenderness.

Signs of developing encephalopathy range from mild personality change to confusion and deep coma. The presence of encephalopathy is a precondition for a diagnosis of acute hepatic failure. The severity of encephalopathy is measured in four stages as set forth in Table 34–2.

Patients with encephalopathy stage III or stage IV commonly suffer from cerebral edema and increased intracranial pressure. Cerebral edema is a common finding in patients who die from acute hepatic failure. The pathogenesis of cerebral edema has not been clearly elucidated. However, investigators have proposed a breakdown of the blood-brain barrier as an important mechanism. Sodium accumulation in the brain cells secondary to inhibition of the Na^+-K^+ ATPase has also been proposed. Cerebral edema causes an acute rise in the intracranial pressure that decreases perfusion pressure and cerebral blood flow. Autoregulation of cerebral blood flow is lost.

Oliguria and generalized edema occur commonly and are associated with higher mortality. They are typically caused by hypovolemia, acute tubular necrosis, or hepatorenal syndrome.

Late in the course, patients may develop upper gastrointestinal bleeding and blood loss from the airway, puncture sites, and soft tissues.

The clinical course of acute hepatic failure is frequently complicated by bacterial and fungal infections. Infectious complications are a major contributor to increased morbidity and are the immediate cause of death in nearly half of fatal cases. The immune system is impaired by decreased function of the reticuloendothelial system and complement deficiency.

Coagulopathy may occur as a consequence of decreased production of coagulation factors by the liver, as a consequence of increased fibrinolysis, and from consump-

Table 34–1. Causes of acute hepatic failure.

Most common causes in USA
- Acute viral hepatitis (HBV, HAV)
- Acetaminophen toxicity

Less common causes
- Hepatitis D and E
- Herpes simplex virus
- Epstein-Barr virus
- Drug toxicity
  - Antimicrobials (eg, ampicillin-clavulanate, ciprofloxacin, erythromycin, isoniazid, tetracycline)
  - Sodium valproate
  - Lovastatin
  - Phenytoin
  - Tricyclic antidepressants
  - Halothane
- Other toxins
  - Ecstasy (methylenedioxymethamphetamine)
  - *Amanita phalloides* (mushrooms)
  - Organic solvents
  - Herbal medicines (eg, ginseng, pennyroyal oil, *Teucrium polium).*
- Miscellaneous causes
  - Acute fatty liver of pregnancy
  - Autoimmune hepatitis
  - Budd-Chiari syndrome
  - Reye's syndrome
  - Wilson's disease
  - Indeterminate

tion, such as in disseminated intravascular coagulation. Thrombocytopenia and platelet dysfunction are common.

Predictors of poor outcome are summarized in the King's College criteria (Table 34–3).

Treatment

Acute liver failure constitutes a medical emergency given the high incidence of multisystem organ failure and the high mortality. Patients with mild hepatic injury require maintenance therapy with adequate hydration, euglycemia, and electrolyte balance. Because the condition of patients with more severe liver damage may deteriorate rapidly, respiratory support is often needed—particularly when cerebral edema ensues.

A. Support Measures

1. Encephalopathy and intracranial hypertension—Herniation is a major cause of death if cerebral edema and hypertension are untreated. Intracranial pressure measurement is used for diagnosis of intracranial hypertension and monitoring of intracranial pressure dynamics. Other monitoring techniques are measurements of cerebral blood (with Xenon) and cerebral oxygen consumption (by calculating the arterial–jugular venous oxygen content difference).

The head of the bed is typically elevated 20–30 degrees to reduce intracranial pressure, though the cerebral perfusion pressure should be monitored to avoid an adverse impact from a decrease of systemic pressure. Patients being maintained on ventilatory support are subjected to mild hyperventilation to decrease cerebral hyperemia. Patient stimulation must be minimized by premedication prior to suctioning or postural changes in patients with severe intracranial hypertension. A number of other measures may decrease cerebral edema, such as mannitol (1g/kg). Serum osmolarity should be followed. Mannitol is contraindicated if the serum osmolarity is ≥ 320 mosm/L.

The use of barbiturates has been proposed as a means of lowering intracranial pressure in combination with hypothermia. Barbiturates decrease cerebral metabolism and further decrease cerebral blood flow and pressure. They also prevent seizures. Barbiturate use generates some controversy, however, because of its delayed metabolism due to liver insufficiency.

2. Cardiovascular support—Patients with acute liver insufficiency experience arteriovenous shunting and vasodilation that causes tachycardia and hypotension.

Table 34–2. Stages of encephalopathy.

Stage	Mental Status	Tremor	Electroencephalography
I	Euphoria, occasionally depression; fluctuating mild confusion; slowness of mentation and affect; slurred speech; disorder in sleep rhythm	Slight	Normal
II	Drowsiness; inappropriate behavior.	Present	Generalized slowing
III	Sleeps most of the time but is arousable, confused; incoherent speech.	Present	Abnormal
IV	Unarousable	Absent	Abnormal

Table 34–3. Predictors of poor outcome in patients with acute hepatic failure (King's College criteria).

Acetaminophen toxic patients
Blood pH < 7.30 (irrespective of grade of encephalopathy) or–
A combination of: encephalopathy stage III or IV, prothrombin time > 100 s (INR > 6.5), and serum creatinine > 300 mmol/L (>3.4 mg/dL)
Nonacetaminophen toxic patients
Prothrombin time > 100 s (INR > 6.5) (irrespective of stage of encephalopathy) or–
Any three of the following five variables (irrespective of stage of encephalopathy):
1. Age < 10 years or > 40 years
2. Etiology: hepatitis C, halothane hepatitis, idiosyncratic drug reactions
3. Duration of jaundice before onset of encephalopathy of > 7 days
4. Prothrombin time > 50 s (INR > 3.5)
5. Serum bilirubin level of > 300 μmol/L (> 17.5 mg/dL)

The decreased clearance of vasoactive metabolites causes decreased systemic vascular resistance and increased cardiac output. Therefore, volume resuscitation and vasoactive drugs may be necessary as support measures. With this hemodynamic profile, an important differential diagnosis is sepsis.

3. Coagulopathy—Transfusion therapy is in general reserved for patients with active bleeding. It is indicated also prior to invasive procedures such as the placement of intracranial pressure monitoring.

4. Renal failure—Renal failure is common in patients with acute liver insufficiency. Maintenance of euvolemia is critical. If renal azotemia ensues, dialysis may be needed. Continuous venovenous dialysis or arteriovenous dialysis methods are preferred to avoid hemodynamic changes and hypotension associated with standard hemodialysis.

5. Respiratory failure—Airway intubation and mechanical ventilation are frequently used as the encephalopathy progresses to stage III. ARDS occurs in one-third of patients, causing hypoxemia.

B. Liver Transplantation

The mortality of severe acute liver insufficiency in the absence of liver transplantation approaches 80%. Survival after orthotopic liver transplantation has improved in recent years from 50% to more than 80% in selected series. Unfortunately, only 40–60% of patients actually undergo transplantation due shortage of available organ donors.

Contraindications to liver transplantation are malignancy, extrahepatic sepsis, irreversible brain injury from intracranial hemorrhage, and unresponsive cerebral edema.

Bioartificial liver support is being investigated in selected centers as a bridge to transplantation. Reports of hemoperfusion, plasmapheresis, and extracorporeal perfusion abound in the literature, but there has been limited success. Most recently, the development of hybrid bioartificial support systems using hepatocytes from human or xenogeneic sources has been rewarded with some promising results.

ACUTE GASTROINTESTINAL BLEEDING FROM PORTAL HYPERTENSION

ESSENTIALS OF DIAGNOSIS

- *Hematemesis, melena.*
- *Stigmas of chronic liver disease.*
- *Endoscopic evidence of bleeding varices.*

General Considerations

Esophagogastric varices occur in 90% of patients with cirrhosis. Approximately one-third of these patients will experience gastrointestinal bleeding, and between 30% and 50% of them will die during each episode. It is not unexpected that bleeding from esophagogastric bleeding varices accounts for one-third of all deaths in patients with cirrhosis.

Esophagogastric varices are dilated intramural veins associated with an extensive and tortuous capillary network. They are alternative pathways of venous flow around the increased vascular resistance in the intrahepatic and portal system. They occur as a consequence of portal hypertension. The development of varices is facilitated by systemic vasodilation and decreased vascular resistance present in cirrhotics.

Clinical Features

A. Symptoms and Signs

Patients with acute bleeding present with hematemesis. Patients with more chronic bleeding present with melena and symptoms of anemia such as fatigue and weakness. Anemia may cause pallor and tachycardia.

B. Laboratory Findings

There is frequently evidence of anemia. Decreases in hemoglobin levels may not be detectable in an early assessment of the bleeding. Evidence of chronic hepatic dysfunction such as elevated serum aminotransferases, bilirubin, and alkaline phosphatase is commonly present.

Differential Diagnosis

Patients with cirrhosis may experience an upper gastrointestinal bleed from other causes such as gastritis, peptic ulcer disease, esophageal ulceration, or mucosal tears (Mallory-Weiss syndrome). Endoscopy is essential for diagnosis.

Treatment

Initial management is based on restoring blood volume through intravenous hydration and transfusion. Coagulopathy should be corrected as appropriate with fresh frozen plasma. In patients with significant bleeding or with altered sensorium, endotracheal intubation for protection of the airway may be necessary.

A. Medical Treatment

Vasoactive drugs may be started as soon as the diagnosis is suspected. These drugs have proven value in nonesophageal sites of bleeding, such as portal hypertensive gastropathy and gastric varices. Vasoconstrictors decrease portal flow and pressure by decreasing splanchnic arterial flow. Vasodilators decrease hepatic vascular resistance and cause peripheral vasodilation, causing reflex splanchnic vasoconstriction.

Vasopressin's main role is as a temporizing measure. It successfully controls acute variceal bleeding in half of patients. Unfortunately, the rebleed rate is high (approximately 50%). By decreasing the rate of bleeding it facilitates initial resuscitation and the performance of endoscopy for local definitive therapy of the bleeding varices. Secondary effects are significant vasoconstriction with hypertension, bradycardia, and a risk of myocardial infarction. Vasopressin is generally used in conjunction with nitroglycerin. The combination, which reduces cardiac ischemia, is superior to vasopressin alone in controlling acute variceal bleeding. Both are delivered via continuous infusion.

Somatostatin is an effective hormone in the control of acute variceal bleeding. It has been found to be as effective as vasopressin, balloon tamponade, and sclerotherapy in prospective randomized trials. Octreotide, the longer-acting form of somatostatin, is the agent of choice in the initial management of acute variceal bleeding because it is at least as effective as vasopressin but has fewer side effects. Octreotide has been found as effective as balloon tamponade of the esophagus in a clinical trial.

B. Endoscopic Management

Sclerotherapy is the treatment of choice in the management of acute variceal bleeding. Sclerotherapy is successful in 60–90% of cases during initial management and is superior to vasopressin and balloon tamponade. Complications of sclerotherapy are esophageal ulceration, bleeding, perforation, bacteremia, and mediastinitis. Complications can occur in 10–30% of cases.

Variceal ligation is an alternative to sclerotherapy. The efficacy is high and comparable to that of sclerotherapy. There seems to be a trend toward fewer complications with ligation.

Balloon tamponade is less frequently used. It is a temporizing measure with an efficacy of approximately 60–70%—comparable to that of vasopressin and sclerotherapy but associated with a high complication rate. However, the use of a Blakemore-Sengstaken tube or a Linton tube can be a lifesaving maneuver if medical and endoscopic measures fail to stop bleeding.

C. Nonsurgical Shunts (Transjugular Portosystemic Shunt [TIPS])

This technique is widely used in the setting of acute variceal bleeding because it offers a rapid decompressive shunt that does not require laparotomy. It is used as primary treatment for patients with bleeding gastric varices and for patients with hypertensive portal gastropathy—mainly because of the difficulty and poor results with endoscopic management.

D. Surgical Treatment

Surgery plays a role in the management of patients who fail medical, endoscopic, and TIPS management of acute variceal bleeding. The surgical options are either shunt or nonshunt operations.

Shunt procedures are either total (portacaval shunt, mesocaval shunt, central splenorenal shunt) or selective (distal splenorenal shunt). The most commonly used operation in the emergency setting is a portacaval shunt. It is very effective in controlling acute bleeding and preventing rebleeding, but the mortality rate is as high as 50%.

Gastroesophageal devascularization (Sugiura operation) is a nonshunt operation. It has fallen into disfavor because the recurrence rate of bleeding is high, but it is indicated in a selected subset of patients with portal vein thrombosis or segmental portal hypertension with an acute bleeding episode.

ASCITES

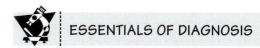

ESSENTIALS OF DIAGNOSIS

- *History: Abdominal distention.*
- *Physical examination: fluid wave, shifting dullness, and dullness to percussion.*

- *Abdominal ultrasound may detect up to 100 mL of ascitic fluid. Ultrasound is useful in the diagnosis of cases with minimal ascites.*
- *Paracentesis. Serum-ascites albumin gradient > 1.1 g/dL.*

General Considerations

A typical circulatory dysfunction characterized by arterial vasodilation and high cardiac output coupled with increased sinusoidal pressure and hepatic insufficiency is the cause of ascites in cirrhotic patients. In addition, there is renal sodium and water retention caused by stimulation of the renin-angiotensin-aldosterone axis and activation of ADH secretion by the relative underfilling of the arterial vascular compartment.

Over 50% of patients with cirrhosis will develop ascites. It is therefore one of the most common complications of cirrhosis. Once ascites develops, the median survival is approximately 1 year.

Clinical Features

A. Symptoms and Signs

Patients with large-volume ascites complain of increasing abdominal girth and abdominal pressure. Some patients complain of anorexia, early satiety, and nausea or flank pain. Clinical findings of abdominal distention, shifting dullness, and demonstration of a fluid wave support the diagnosis of ascites. Other stigmas of liver disease which aid in diagnosis are jaundice, spider angiomas, and large periumbilical collateral veins in the abdominal wall (caput medusae).

B. Laboratory Findings

Diagnostic paracentesis is essential in the evaluation and management of patients with ascites. Inspection of the fluid in patients with portal hypertension reveals clear, straw-colored fluid. Evaluation should includes cell count, cytologic examination, albumin and protein concentrations, and bacteriologic analysis. An initial determination is the serum-ascites albumin gradient (SAAG), which is done by subtracting the concentration of ascitic albumin from serum albumin. Patients with a gradient of ≥ 1.1 g/dL can be diagnosed as having portal hypertension with a reliability of 97%. If the gradient is less than 1.1 g/dL it is not related to portal hypertension. Further differentiation of the ascitic fluid as a transudate or exudate provides insight into the origin of ascites.

C. Imaging Studies

Ultrasonography may be helpful in the detection of small volumes of ascitic fluid. Duplex ultrasound of the portal and suprahepatic venous system is indicated if portal vein thrombosis or suprahepatic vein thrombosis is suspected. Computerized tomography is also helpful in the detection of small volumes of ascites, usually as an incidental finding when x-rays are requested for evaluation of intra-abdominal pathology.

Differential Diagnosis

Cirrhosis and chronic liver disease are the most common causes of ascites (approximately 70–80% of cases). The differential diagnosis of the most common causes of ascites is set forth in Table 34–4.

Spontaneous bacterial peritonitis is a frequent complication of cirrhotic patients with ascites. Because its inception can be subclinical; bacteriologic analysis should be done on every patient with new-onset ascites. Culture of ascitic fluid in blood culture bottles is more reliable and is successful in approximately 80% of cases.

Treatment

A. Medical Treatment

Patients with mild ascites may be managed with fluid (1.5 L/d) and sodium restriction (88 meq/d). Addition of an inhibitor of aldosterone (spironolactone) provides a slow sodium loss with preservation of potassium. Initial doses are 100 mg/d but may be progressively elevated up to 400 mg/d. Monitoring of weight and elec-

Table 34–4. Differential diagnosis of ascites.

Organ System	Cause
Hepatic	Cirrhosis Veno-occlusive disease
Cardiac	Right ventricular failure Constrictive pericarditis
Renal	Nephrotic syndrome Renal failure
Malignancy	Ovarian Gastric Colorectal Pancreatic
Immunologic	Tuberculosis
Pancreas	Pancreatitis
Lymphatic	Congenital anomaly Trauma
Digestive	Malnutrition
Endocrine	Myxedema

trolytes is important so that adjustments can be made to the initial therapy.

Patients with moderate ascites should in addition receive loop diuretics (furosemide). An initial dose of 40 mg/d is generally well tolerated and may be increased up to 160 mg/d in adults. Careful monitoring of weight, electrolytes, and serum creatinine may prevent complications from diuretic therapy. Any rise in serum creatinine or urea nitrogen warrants reduction of the diuretic dosage. An initial daily weight loss of 500 g/d is acceptable in patients with moderate ascites. If patients have peripheral edema, a weight loss of approximately 1 kg/d is acceptable.

Patients with tense ascites should in addition be treated with paracentesis. Up to 5 or 6 L may be removed safely. Attention to salt and water restriction is also a critical component of management. Patients who require large-volume paracentesis may develop rapid contraction of the intravascular space after fluid shifting. Clinical trials have documented a better outcome after large-volume paracentesis with the simultaneous infusion of intravenous albumin. Intravenous salt-poor albumin should be routinely used in patients undergoing large-volume paracentesis.

Spontaneous bacterial peritonitis must be suspected in patients with known liver disease who present with fever, leukocytosis, and abdominal pain. Cell count of the ascitic fluid is diagnostic if the polymorphonuclear neutrophil count is 250/μL in the absence of a visceral source of infection. Treatment should be initiated empirically upon diagnosis. A third-generation cephalosporin such as ceftriaxone or cefotaxime is generally the first-line therapy until a specific organism has been selected on the basis of ascitic fluid culture. A 5-day course is generally therapeutic. Most common organisms are *E coli,* klebsiella, and *Streptococcus pneumoniae.* Other organisms are enterococcus, bacteroides, and enterobacter.

B. Surgical Treatment

Ten percent of patients develop intractable ascites. If large-volume paracentesis fails to relieve ascites, operative therapy should be considered. In patients with otherwise mild, stable liver dysfunction, peritoneovenous shunting should be considered. Though shunting is a simple surgical procedure, the incidence of postoperative complications is high, related to infection, coagulopathy, congestive heart failure, and early shunt occlusion.

A more definitive procedure is portosystemic shunting. TIPS has been successfully used in the treatment of ascites.

Patients with severe or rapidly deteriorating liver dysfunction should be considered for liver transplantation.

HEPATORENAL SYNDROME

ESSENTIALS OF DIAGNOSIS

- *Chronic liver disease.*
- *Renal failure.*
- *Circulatory abnormalities (low systemic vascular resistance and blood pressure).*

General Considerations

Hepatorenal syndrome is a clinical condition that occurs in patients with chronic liver disease, advanced hepatic failure, and portal hypertension characterized by impaired renal function and marked abnormalities in the arterial circulation and activity of the endogenous vasoactive systems. In the kidney there is marked renal vasoconstriction that results in a low GFR, whereas in the extrarenal circulation there is predominance of arterial vasodilation, which results in reduction of total systemic vascular resistance and arterial hypotension.

Hepatorenal syndrome is caused by severe vasoconstriction of the renal circulation. A number of vasoactive mediators are implicated in the development of vasoconstriction, such as angiotensin II, norepinephrine, neuropeptide Y, endothelin, adenosine, and cysteine leukotrienes. The most commonly accepted explanation is the arterial vasodilation theory, which proposes that renal hypoperfusion represents the extreme manifestation of underfilling of the arterial circulation as a consequence of massive vasodilation of the splanchnic circulation. Splanchnic vasodilation is caused by nitric oxide, prostaglandins, and vasodilator peptides. In the early phase, urine output and renal function are maintained by renal vasodilator factors. Hepatorenal syndrome develops later, when vasoconstriction ensues from relative hypovolemia.

Hepatorenal syndrome may be precipitated by concomitant illnesses or may occur spontaneously. Spontaneous bacterial peritonitis is the most common precipitating factor of hepatorenal syndrome in patients with cirrhosis.

Clinical Features

A. Symptoms and Signs

Hepatorenal syndrome occurs as a complication of cirrhosis, more commonly in patients with ascites. Two types are recognized. Type I is characterized by rapid and progressive impairment of renal function. Dominant features are marked renal failure, oliguria or anuria, and high levels of urea and creatinine. Most patients have hyperbilirubinemia, coagulopathy, and encephalopathy. The median survival is only 2 weeks. Type II consists of mild and stable reduction in renal function. These patients typically present with diuretic-resistant ascites.

Four major criteria must be present to establish the diagnosis of hepatorenal syndrome: (1) low glomerular filtration rate (creatinine clearance < 40 mL/min or serum creatinine > 1.5 mg/dL); (2) absence of shock with ongoing bacterial infection, fluid loss, and current treatment with nephrotoxic drugs; (3) no improvement in renal function after withdrawal of diuretics; and (4) no evidence of obstructive uropathy and absence of proteinuria (< 500 mg/d).

B. Laboratory Findings

Laboratory findings in hepatorenal syndrome include creatinine clearance < 40 mL/min or serum creatinine > 1.5 mg/dL, urine sodium < 10 meq/L, urine osmolality > plasma osmolarity, urine red blood cells < 50/hpf, and serum sodium concentration < 130 meq/L.

Differential Diagnosis

Other causes of renal failure that must be excluded prior to making a diagnosis of hepatorenal syndrome include hypovolemia causing prerenal failure (use of diuretics, bleeding), acute tubular necrosis (following hypotension or sepsis), drug-induced nephrotoxicity (NSAIDs, aminoglycosides), and glomerulonephritis (commonly associated with proteinuria) secondary to autoimmune disease.

Treatment

Initial management requires volume replacement and reaching a euvolemic state. Once hepatorenal syndrome is suspected, medical management is difficult and more often than not unsuccessful.

Recent studies have documented a beneficial effect of vasopressin V_1 agonists (ornipressin, terlipressin). Other less selective splanchnic vasoconstrictors (vasopressin, catecholamines) have been used without significant success. Dopamine has been proposed as a selective vasodilator of the renal circulation in selected reports, but the literature suggests that there is only a very mild effect in increasing glomerular filtration rate.

Liver transplantation causes a dramatic improvement in renal function. Recovery of renal function is typically seen within 48–72 hours of transplantation. Long term survival after transplantation is very good—approximately 60% after 3 years. The perioperative phase may be more complicated due to a 30% requirement of temporary hemodialysis and the higher incidence of morbidity and mortality than in patients transplanted without hepatorenal syndrome.

PREOPERATIVE ASSESSMENT & PERIOPERATIVE MANAGEMENT OF PATIENTS WITH CIRRHOSIS

There is high perioperative morbidity and a high mortality risk in patients with cirrhosis undergoing abdominal surgery for any indication. Liver function may deteriorate from general anesthesia. Anesthesia reduces cardiac output, induces splanchnic vasodilation, and causes a 30–50%-reduction in hepatic blood flow.

The 30-day mortality for patients with cirrhosis undergoing celiotomy is 30%. A 60% major complication rate was also reported. The risk is dependent on a number of factors

A. Physiologic Status

The Child-Turcotte-Pugh classification of surgical risk is summarized in Table 34–5. This classification was first proposed (by Child) as a means of predicting the operative mortality associated with portacaval shunt surgery. The presence of ascites, encephalopathy, and coagulopathy predict mortality. There is a 10% mortality rate for patients with Child class A cirrhosis, 30% for Child class B, and 75% for Child class C.

B. Type of Surgery

The overall hospital mortality rate was estimated at 21% for biliary surgery, 35% for peptic ulcer disease, and 55% for colectomy. Newer techniques such as laparoscopy and better patient selection have contributed to a reduced mortality rate in recent reports of laparoscopic cholecystectomy and appendectomy.

C. Other Factors

Active infection, a higher number of blood transfusions, pulmonary complications, gastrointestinal bleeding, and the need for emergency surgery negatively impact the outcome of surgery in patients with cirrhosis.

LIVER RESECTION IN PATIENTS WITH CIRRHOSIS

Hepatectomy is a major operation that induces a severe catabolic response and immunosuppression. Cirrhotic patients suffer from underlying catabolism and immunosuppression. Liver resection in patients with underlying liver insufficiency carries the risk of postoperative liver failure. In experienced hands, the mortality rate after hepatectomy ranges from 5–50%.

Other postoperative complications are common, such as development of ascites (5%), encephalopathy (20%), renal failure (15%), and upper gastrointestinal tract bleeding (5%). Factors that contribute to this great variability are the extent of resection and the patient's underlying physiologic status. Preoperative pa-

Table 34–5. Child-Turcotte-Pugh estimate of surgical risk.[1]

Clinical Variable	1 Point	2 Points	3 Points
Encephalopathy	None	Stage 1–2	Stage 3–4
Ascites	Absent	Slight	Moderate
Bilirubin (mg/dL)	< 2	2–3	> 3
Albumin (g/dL)	> 3.5	2.8–3.5	< 2.8
Prothrombin time (seconds prolonged or INR)	< 4 s or INR < 1.7	4–6 s or INR 1.7–2.3	> 6 s or INR > 2.3

Interpretation: Child class A = 5–6 points, Child class B = 7–9 points, Child class C = 10–15 points.

tient selection and perioperative management are critical to successful outcome after liver resection in patients with cirrhosis.

Preoperative Evaluation

Prior to operation, attention is directed to the identification of patients in whom the complication rate or mortality risk is prohibitive. Numerous methods of identification have been proposed. The clinical classification of patients according to their Child score is a time-tested approach and is most commonly used. Patients with Child A liver function have a hospital mortality risk for major hepatectomy of 3–15%. Patients with Child B or C liver function tolerate liver resection poorly, and that procedure should be withheld except in highly selected individuals who require minimal surgery. Others have proposed the use of the indocyanine green clearance test, the lidocaine clearance test, and measuring the degree of fibrosis in the unaffected liver as predictors of morbidity and mortality. Another factor that must be considered in selection of patients is the volume of remaining liver estimated by CT.

As before any other major surgery, a good clinical history and examination should alert the clinician to the presence of any significant pulmonary, cardiac, hematologic, or renal disorders. Screening of hematologic, biochemical, renal, pulmonary, and cardiac function is essential.

Operative Management

Metabolic and hematologic derangements must be corrected prior to surgery. Intraoperative monitoring of blood loss, hemodynamics, and urine output is crucial. Patients with hepatic dysfunction suffer from peripheral vasodilation and are less responsive to catecholamines. It is therefore important to maintain the circulatory volume. Maintaining liver perfusion during surgery is critical to the prevention of any further impairment of hepatic function. Therefore, anesthetic agents that do not impair hepatic perfusion and oxygenation should be selected.

Liver transection must be performed with two issues in mind, minimizing blood loss and having adequate hemostasis and securing biliary radicles to avoid postoperative biliary leakage, which is a cause of postoperative morbidity and sepsis.

Postoperative Care

Postoperative monitoring should include hemodynamics, oxygen saturation, vital signs, fluid balance, electrolytes, and blood glucose. Postoperative pain must be controlled to avoid cardiopulmonary complications. Careful fluid management is a critical component of postoperative care. Maintaining euvolemia is a priority. Due to alterations in the renin-angiotensin-aldosterone axis, cirrhotic patients have a propensity for salt retention and third spacing of extracellular water. This in turn manifests itself as ascites. When salt restriction is required, 0.25% saline solution should be used instead of 0.5%.

Parenteral nutritional support is provided in the form of branched-chain amino acids because it reduces the catabolic response and promotes hepatic protein synthesis and liver regeneration in cirrhosis. Adequate calories and fatty acids are also provided. Perioperative nutritional support reduces overall postoperative morbidity by decreasing septic complications, the incidence of ascites, and deterioration of liver function.

Potassium phosphate is used in the parenteral solution to avoid hypophosphatemia, which occurs commonly after hepatectomy. Phosphate is necessary for production of ATP in the liver.

At least one study supports the use of salt-poor albumin in septic cirrhotic patients as a means of reducing renal complications and mortality.

Hyperbilirubinemia occurs commonly and is generally transient, but progressive hyperbilirubinemia is an ominous sign. Decreased sensorium, hypoglycemia, and acidosis are present in severe hepatic failure and portend a poor prognosis. Hepatic failure is complicated by a noncorrectable coagulopathy and sepsis. Use of the bioartificial liver is potentially a lifesaving measure, but this resource is not yet widely available. Liver transplantation is the only option (see Chapter 35).

REFERENCES

Azoulay D et al: Neoadjuvant transjugular intrahepatic portosystemic shunt: a solution for extrahepatic operation in cirrhotic patients with severe portal hypertension. J Am Coll Surg 2001;193:46–51.

Belghiti J et al: Herniorrhaphy and concomitant peritoneovenous shunting in cirrhotic patients with umbilical hernia. World J. Surg 1990;14:242–6.

Block RS, Allaben RD, Walt AJ: Cholecystectomy in patients with cirrhosis. A surgical challenge. Arch Surg 1985;120:669–72.

Bolder U et al: Preoperative assessment of mortality risk in hepatic resection by clinical variables: a multivariate analysis. Liver Transpl Surg 1999;5:227–37.

Carbo J et al: Liver cirrhosis and mortality by abdominal surgery. A study of risk factors. Rev Esp Enferm Dig 1998;90:105–12.

Conte D et al: Cholelithiasis in cirrhosis: analysis of 500 cases. Am J Gastroenterol 1991;86:1629–32.

Elcheroth J, Vons C, Franco D: Role of surgical therapy in management of intractable ascites. World J Surg 1994;28:240–5.

Ercolani G et al: The lidocaine (MEGX) test as an index of hepatic function: its clinical usefulness in liver surgery. Surgery 2000;127:464–71.

Fan ST et al: Perioperative nutritional support in patients undergoing hepatectomy for hepatocellular carcinoma. N Engl J Med 1994:331:1547–52.

Farges O et al: Risk of major liver resection in patients with underlying chronic liver disease: a reappraisal. Ann Surg 1999; 229:210–5.

Garrison RN et al: Clarification of risk factors for abdominal operations in patients with hepatic cirrhosis. Ann Surg 1984; 199:648–55.

Gopalswamy N, Mehta V, Barde CJ: Risks of intra-abdominal nonshunt surgery in cirrhosis. Dig Dis 1998;16:225–31.

Grace ND: Diagnosis and treatment of gastrointestinal bleeding secondary to portal hypertension. American College of Gastroenterology Practice Parameters Committee. Am J Gastroenterol. 1997;92:1081–91.

Jakab F et al: Complications following major abdominal surgery in cirrhotic patients. Hepatogastroenterology 1993;40:176–9.

Mansour A et al: Abdominal operations in patients with cirrhosis: still a major surgical challenge. Surgery 1997;122:730–5.

Metcalf AM et al: The surgical risk of colectomy in patients with cirrhosis. Dis Colon Rectum 1987;30:529–31.

Sort P et al: Effect of intravenous albumin on renal impairment and mortality in patients with cirrhosis and spontaneous bacterial peritonitis. N Engl J. Med 1999;341:403–9.

Sugiyama M et al: Treatment of choledocholithiasis in patients with liver cirrhosis. Surgical treatment or endoscopic sphincterotomy? Ann Surg 1993;218:68–73.

Wong R et al: Risk of nonshunt abdominal operation in the patient with cirrhosis. J Am Coll Surg 1994;179:412–6.

Wu CC, Huwang CJ, Lui TJ: Definitive surgical treatment of cholelithiasis in selective patients with liver cirrhosis. Int Surg 1993;78:127–30.

Ziser A et al: Morbidity and mortality in cirrhotic patients undergoing anesthesia and surgery. Anesthesiology 1999;90:42–53.

Organ Transplantation 35

Lilly Barba, MD

The intensivist is often actively involved in the postoperative management of patients who have had kidney and pancreas transplants and preoperative and postoperative management of liver transplant patients. Patients awaiting kidney and pancreas transplants usually do not require preoperative ICU care because they are relatively healthy except for the organ failure. If hospitalized prior to transplantation, they are usually not candidates for transplantation until resolution of the acute illness. Transplantation in these patients is elective, and other methods of support (dialysis and insulin) can be used to manage the organ failure. Transplantation does not offer any immediate advantages over these modalities.

The current method of liver distribution within the USA depends to a large extent on how ill the patient is and how long he or she has been in the national organ distribution computer. The highest priority are those who require critical care, such as patients with fulminant liver failure. Expeditious referral to the transplant center will allow the patient to start accruing waiting time. Currently, the average waiting time for patients in the ICU is about 3–4 days. Given the rapid progression of intracranial hypertension once coma occurs, even this interval is too long. As these patients usually do extremely well following transplantation (with 1 year survival rates of 80–90%), it is tragic when a late referral results in a missed opportunity for transplantation.

The exclusion criteria for liver transplantation include irreversible disease in other organ systems, the presence of diseases that would limit survival following transplantation such as HIV infection or malignancy, and assessment of the psychosocial contraindications. This last criterion is usually the most difficult, since the patient is frequently comatose. The decision to proceed with transplantation is frequently made by the relatives and the transplant team without the benefit of interaction with the patient.

POSTOPERATIVE COMPLICATIONS IN TRANSPLANTATION

Complications related to three major aspects of transplantation are important determinants of clinical outcome: (1) technical aspects of graft implantation, (2) the rejection process and concurrent immunosuppression, and (3) infectious complications. In general, technical complications occur early in the postoperative course (0–14 days); rejection primarily occurs later (10–60 days); while most infectious complications (other than bacterial infections) occur 30 days to 6 months after surgery.

EARLY POSTOPERATIVE PERIOD (0–14 Days)

Technical Complications

A. Vascular Thrombosis

A potentially devastating complication in the early postoperative period is vascular thrombosis. Although this is rare in thoracic organ transplantation, it is more common in transplantation of other organs and most common in liver transplantation. The incidence of hepatic arterial thrombosis in adults is 3%. Vascular thrombosis is relatively rare in renal transplantation. This complication is decreasing rapidly in pancreas transplantation for reasons that are not clearly understood but are probably multifactorial.

Early recognition of a vascular thrombosis is difficult, since most patients are asymptomatic. Screening duplex ultrasonography has been used after liver transplantation to document hepatic artery patency. Early diagnosis of occlusion, with thrombectomy of the hepatic artery, has led to salvage of some liver transplants, though late biliary strictures occur frequently. The delay in recognition usually results in irreversible graft loss in kidney and pancreas transplantation.

B. Bleeding

Postoperative bleeding in transplant recipients is dealt with in a manner similar to other postoperative patients. The exception may be liver transplant recipients, since dysfunction of the graft may lead to coagulopathy, which can result in slow continued bleeding. One must decide whether to tolerate six to ten units of blood loss prior to reexploration while the liver recovers and the coagulation parameters are normalized. In general, patients with excellent graft function and bleeding should be reexplored, since there is probably a surgical cause for bleeding. Patients with poor graft function may be best treated by waiting until graft function improves.

Immunosuppression

Because similar immunosuppressive protocols are used in transplantation of most solid organ transplants, the complications related to immunosuppression tend to be similar as well. This is true for both infectious and immunosuppressive complications such as cyclosporine or tacrolimus toxicity. Dysfunction of the implanted organ makes evaluation and diagnosis of complications due to immunosuppressive therapy difficult. For example, renal dysfunction following cardiac transplantation will be due to causes similar to those associated with renal dysfunction following liver transplantation. The major early complications related to the immune system arise from the side effects of immunosuppressive agents: hyperglycemia and mental status changes from corticosteroids, renal and neurologic dysfunction from cyclosporine or tacrolimus, and decreased white blood cell and platelet counts from the antimetabolites or antilymphocyte preparations.

Infection (Figure 35–1)

Infections in the early postoperative period are usually of bacterial origin and take the form of pneumonia, wound infection, abscesses, and infections related to indwelling catheters. These are treated with antibiotics, drainage, and catheter removal. Early infections can be prevented by prophylactic antibiotics, careful hand washing, and limitation of exposure to potential pathogens. Prophylactic antibiotics may lead to the emergence of resistant gram-negative organisms and should be used only in the first 24 hours. Repeated antibiotic treatment results in emergence of resistant organisms and secondary complications of the antibiotics such as *Clostridium difficile* colitis.

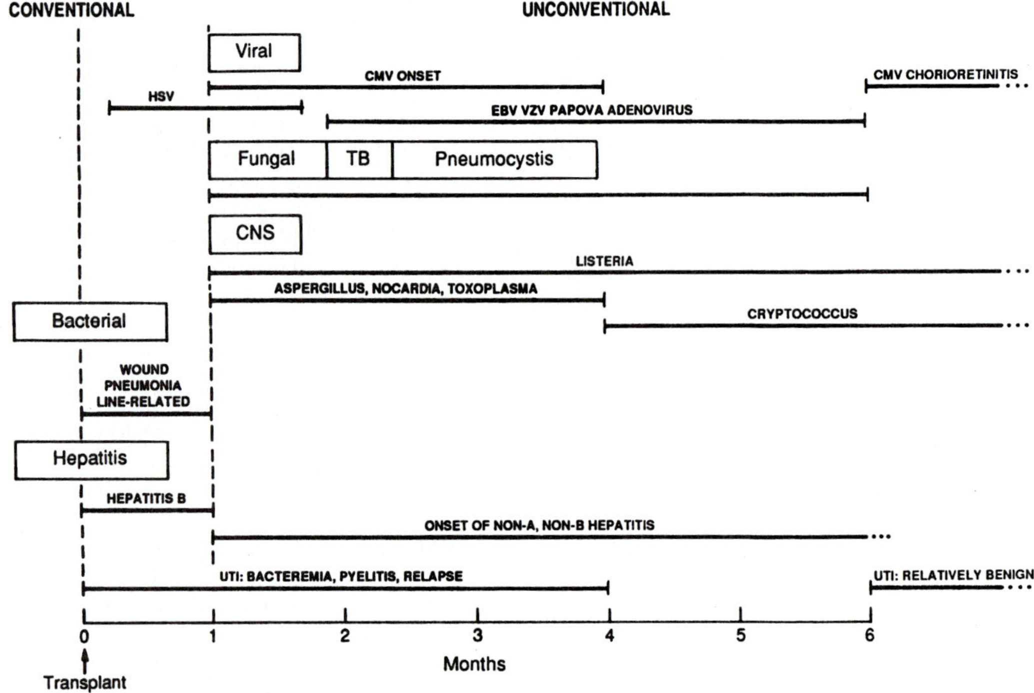

Figure 35–1. Timetable for occurrence of infection in the organ transplant recipient. Exceptions to this timetable should initiate a search for an unusual hazard. (CMV, cytomegalovirus; HSV, herpes simplex virus; EBV, Epstein-Barr virus; VZV, varicella virus; CNS, central nervous system; UTI, urinary tract infection.)

INTERMEDIATE POSTOPERATIVE PERIOD (Days 5–21)

Technical Complications

Complications during this period are frequently related to the epithelial anastomosis, ie, the bile duct anastomosis in liver transplantation, the duodenovesical anastomosis in pancreas transplantation, the ureterovesical anastomosis in renal transplantation, and the tracheal or bronchial anastomosis in lung transplantation. The common underlying cause is probably an inadequate blood supply. Leakage at these anastomoses is generally treated by immediate reexploration. Reexploration can sometimes be postponed or avoided in liver and kidney transplantation by drainage of bile or urine flow proximal to the leak and percutaneous drainage of associated fluid collections.

Immunosuppression & Rejection

The major complication in this period is rejection. It is also one of the major causes of graft dysfunction. However, there are many other causes of graft dysfunction besides rejection. Increased immunosuppressive therapy in response to an unwarranted diagnosis of rejection introduces the probability of unnecessary morbidity as the patient's immune system is further suppressed in the face of a potential undiagnosed technical problem, infection, or preservation injury. A diagnosis of rejection should therefore be made on histologic grounds. This is because the biochemical diagnosis of organ dysfunction, though relatively sensitive, is not very specific during this period. A concept that has been validated in both liver and heart transplantation is that rejection diagnosed on a histologic basis prior to clinical organ dysfunction may lead to improved graft survival. This has led to graft surveillance by means of weekly biopsy in heart, liver, and lung transplantation. Early treatment for rejection results in less damage to the graft, and the rejection can be reversed more easily. Although biopsy of the pancreas has not generally been accepted because of the risk of pancreatitis or leak, combined kidney and pancreas transplantation allows biopsy of the kidney to exclude rejection.

Some evidence indicates that the measurement of urine amylase concentration may be used to make the diagnosis of rejection. A fall in this measurement suggests rejection of the pancreas. In renal transplantation, there is debate about whether biopsy is necessary prior to the first treatment for rejection with corticosteroids, but almost all centers would biopsy the kidney before the second treatment or before antilymphocyte therapy. The other confounding possibility in renal transplantation is that cyclosporine or tacrolimus toxicity can cause renal dysfunction that mimics rejection. This has increased the need for biopsy.

Infection (Figure 35–1)

Prophylactic treatment for the common posttransplant infections appears to improve the therapeutic index of immunosuppressive medications by reducing the incidence of infection. A major cause of morbidity during this period is cytomegalovirus infection. CMV infections may represent reactivation of infection in the recipient or introduction of the virus via the transplanted organ or transfused blood products. Primary CMV infection can be prevented by using seronegative donors of organs and blood products. Matching for serologic status of the organ and blood products is usually precluded by the urgency of heart and liver transplant operations. Despite the shortage of lung donors, many programs will not transplant a lung from a serologically positive donor into a negative recipient because of concern about primary infection complicated by pneumonia in lung recipients.

While almost all transplant patients infected with CMV have only asymptomatic viruria, some develop severe organ dysfunction such as hepatitis, pneumonia, or pancreatitis. Over the last several years, prophylaxis for this infection with ganciclovir or valganciclovir appears to have been effective in decreasing the incidence and severity of CMV infections, particularly in patients at risk for reactivation.

Oral candidiasis may develop secondary to antibiotic administration and immunosuppression and can be prevented with topical antifungal agents. More serious infections, including candidal esophagitis, peritonitis, and complicated urinary tract infections, may develop. Amphotericin B—conventional or lipid-associated—is the antifungal agent of choice. Fluconazole can be considered for candidal esophagitis, but because it is associated with elevation of plasma cyclosporine or tacrolimus levels, careful monitoring levels is important.

Prophylaxis with trimethoprim-sulfamethoxazole should be given to prevent *Pneumocystis carinii* infections.

LATE POSTOPERATIVE PERIOD (1–6 Months)

Infection and rejection dominate the clinical picture during the period of 1–6 months following transplantation. Late infections are usually caused by opportunistic organisms.

Technical Complications

The most common technical problem during this period is stenosis of the epithelial or vascular anastomosis. Treatment (at least temporarily) consists of dilation and stenting, though additional surgery may be required.

Immunosuppression & Rejection

After 6 months, acute rejection is uncommon, though chronic rejection can become a significant problem, usually in patients who have failed treatment for acute rejection. It usually presents as organ dysfunction. After cardiac transplantation, coronary artery disease, a sequela of chronic rejection, may initially present with sudden death. Although a variety of therapies have been attempted for chronic rejection, most patients require retransplantation.

The more chronic complications of immunosuppressive drugs during this period are cyclosporine or tacrolimus nephrotoxicity, hypertension, hyperglycemia, lipid disorders, and malignancies.

Infection (Figure 35–1)

Opportunistic fungal infections may appear during this time. Aspergillus infection in the transplant patient is devastating, and the efficacy of antifungal drugs is poor. As this infection is frequently hospital-acquired, prevention is important. Outbreaks in hospitalized patients occur mainly during periods of construction. It is important that physicians involved with transplantation be alert to unsafe construction practices and make their concerns known to the hospital administrator. Education of building management personnel about the risks of patient dust exposure can be important in saving lives.

Tuberculosis can also complicate the late posttransplant period. It frequently presents as fever of unknown origin and can be difficult to diagnose. The index of suspicion should be high with patients from endemic areas such as Asia. Pleural effusion is a common manifestation, but thoracoscopy may be required to make the diagnosis.

Maddrey W (editor): *Transplantation of the Liver.* Lippincott, 2001.

Pescovitz MD: Oral ganciclovir and pharmacokinetics of valganciclovir in liver transplant recipients. Transpl Infect Dis 19991(Suppl 1):31–4.

Rubin RH et al: The therapeutic prescription for the organ transplant recipient: the linkage of immunosuppression and antimicrobial strategies. Transpl Infect Dis 1999;1:29–39.

Smith SR et al: Viral infections after renal transplantation. Am J Kidney Dis 2001;37:659–76.

IMMUNOLOGY OF ORGAN TRANSPLANTATION

One of the major advances in organ transplantation has been better understanding of the underlying immunology. Although this topic is broad, several points require emphasis.

HLA TYPING

The most important factor in determination of rejection is the difference between the recipient's surface proteins and those of the donor. The proteins primarily responsible for rejection are those coded by location on chromosome 6, the so-called major histocompatibility complex (MHC). The major proteins are classified into two groups: I and II. There are three types of class I antigens expressed on the cell surface: HLA-A, HLA-B, and HLA-C. Similarly, there are three types of class II antigens: DP, DQ, and DR. These proteins are identified on individual cells by serologic typing. This is performed by mixing antibodies of known HLA class with the cells to be tested to allow designation of the individual cells as type HLA-A, HLA-B, or HLA-DR. There are two alleles for each class of antigen, and each individual has one set of HLA-A, HLA-B, and HLA-DR antigens from each parent. Therefore, siblings have a 25% chance of inheriting the same HLA-identical antigens. HLA matching of donors and recipients improves survival results following renal transplantation. This is most important with living related renal transplantation, where a recipient of an HLA-identical kidney from a sibling has a 5-year graft survival rate of 90%, whereas a recipient receiving a nonidentical kidney has a 5-year rate of 65%. The importance of HLA matching in cadaveric renal transplantation is less clear. Matching does appear to provide an advantage for cadaveric kidneys transplanted between patients who have all six HLA antigens in common. Currently, these kidneys are shared across the country on a mandatory basis. The effect in less well matched kidneys is correspondingly less striking. The influence of HLA matching in liver, heart, and pancreas transplantation is much less clear.

CROSS-MATCHING

Cross-matching is used to determine the likelihood of success of transplanting a particular donor organ into a particular recipient. The procedure is necessary because the recipient may have circulating antibodies that react against antigens on the donor graft that can lead to rapid rejection of the organ. The cross-match is performed by mixing cells from the donor with recipient's serum along with complement. Killing of the cells demonstrates the presence of antibody and is called a positive cross-match. These antibodies arise from prior exposure to common HLA antigens in the population by transfusion, pregnancy, and prior organ transplantation. The antibodies appear to be important in determining the outcome following cardiac, renal, and pancreatic transplantation. The effect of a positive cross-match on survival following liver transplantation is unclear.

The presence of antibodies precludes transplantation from that particular donor. Because some patients can have antibodies to many common HLA antigens, they will have antibodies that prevent transplantation from a large number of potential donors. This will result in a prolonged waiting time for transplantation before an acceptable donor can be found. These potential recipients are called "highly sensitized." A patient who has antibodies against 90% of the population will wait about nine times as long as one with antibodies against only 10% of the population.

ABO TYPING

Transplantation is usually performed between ABO-*identical* donors and recipients. ABO-*compatible* donor organs (eg, O blood type to A blood type) should not be used unless the transplant is required on an emergency basis. This leaves the O blood group population at a disadvantage, since these individuals can receive organs only from blood type-identical patients. ABO-incompatible transplants (eg, A to O) are performed only in an extreme emergency or under experimental protocols. Children seem to tolerate ABO-incompatible liver transplants done under special protocols. Adults do less well because of accelerated rejection.

Cacciarelli TV et al: A reassessment of ABO incompatibility in pediatric liver transplantation. Transplantation 1995;60: 757–60.

Terasaki PI: The HLA-matching effect in different cohorts of kidney transplant recipients. Clinic Transpl 2000;497–514.

IMMUNOSUPPRESSION

One of the major factors that has led to the rapid advance of transplantation in the last 10 years has been the development of better immunosuppressive drugs. The mainstay of drug therapy has been the calcineurin inhibitors, cyclosporine and tacrolimus. These drugs are used in combination with prednisone for long-term treatment in many centers. Some institutions add mycophenolate mofetil to the regimen (triple-drug anti-rejection therapy). The idea behind multiple drug regimens is that the complications that arise from any one drug will be minimized, while the drugs may be additive and perhaps synergistic in their immunosuppressive effects.

The intensivist must be aware of the short- and long-term side effects of these drugs. Many can cause chronic disease such as osteoporosis (from corticosteroids) or cancer, which may be a side effect of all immunosuppressive drugs.

Corticosteroids

These agents are used both for the prevention and in the treatment of rejection. A large dose is given at the time of operation (eg, methylprednisolone, 15–20 mg/kg). This is tapered to prednisone (0.1–0.2 mg/kg) by 2 months.

The most troubling early side effects of corticosteroids are hyperglycemia and psychosis. Hyperglycemia is best treated initially with insulin either as a continuous drip or intermittently on a sliding scale basis. The hyperglycemia tends to resolve with a decrease in the steroid dose but will recur with increased steroid therapy during the treatment of rejection. The psychosis observed with steroids frequently results in agitation. Evaluation calls for a head CT scan. The use of antipsychotic medicines is controversial.

The long-term side effects of steroids are growth retardation in children, obesity, hypertension, and osteoporosis. Many clinical centers employ calcitonin or bisphosphonates to prevent early bone loss following transplantation.

Mycophenolate Mofetil

This drug exerts its effects after being hydrolyzed to the active compound mycophenolic acid, which acts by inhibiting DNA synthesis through its effect on purine metabolism. Mycophenolate mofetil has a selective antiproliferative effect on lymphocytes and is more effective in preventing acute rejection than azathioprine, the previously prescribed antimetabolite. Mycophenolate mofetil may also be helpful in treating acute rejection and in the prevention of chronic rejection. Its major toxicity is on the gastrointestinal tract, with diarrhea, bloating, and nausea and vomiting seen frequently. Bone marrow suppression may also occur, necessitating dose adjustment.

Azathioprine

This drug exerts its effect after being metabolized to the active compound 6-mercaptopurine (6-MP). 6-MP acts by inhibiting DNA synthesis through its effects on purine metabolism. It is used for the prevention of rejection and has little role in the treatment of rejection.

The major toxicity of azathioprine is bone marrow suppression. The dose is usually adjusted to maintain the white blood cell count greater than 2000/μL. It also can cause hepatotoxicity and pancreatitis.

The Calcineurin Inhibitors: Cyclosporine & Tacrolimus

The calcineurin inhibitors form the basis of most solid organ transplant immunosuppressive regimens today. Cyclosporine and tacrolimus have a similar mechanism of action, similar clinical efficacy in the prevention of acute rejection, and similar adverse side effect profiles. Transplant programs generally will choose one agent over the other based on their patients' clinical characteristics and adverse side effects. Through inhibition of the phosphatase activity of calcineurin, both cyclosporine and tacrolimus inhibit several cytokine gene expressions, including interleukin-2. As a result of calcineurin inhibition, there is decreased lymphocytic proliferation.

Cyclosporine

Cyclosporine forms the basis of most immunosuppressive regimens in the United States today. The drug is used only to prevent rejection and has little efficacy for treating rejection by itself. It is a lipophilic compound that is administered either orally or intravenously. It is used intravenously primarily in the early postoperative period, when absorption from the gut is uncertain. Intravenous administration of cyclosporine in the early postoperative period can cause problems because the nephrotoxicity of intravenous cyclosporine appears to be worse than that of oral cyclosporine at the same blood level. The drug causes renal vasoconstriction by inhibiting production of intrarenal prostaglandins. Reducing the dosage of the intravenous drug by the use of antilymphocyte preparations in the early transplant period will allow the kidney to recover while preventing rejection (sequential therapy).

Sandimmune, the original oil-based cyclosporine preparation, has generally been replaced by the microemulsified formulation, Neoral. Sandimmune requires the presence of bile salts in the intestine for absorption, whereas Neoral has less dependence on bile salts. The requirement for bile salts can be a problem in the early period following liver transplantation when bile production is impaired or when bile is diverted from the intestine by the presence of a T tube. Absorption in this situation is virtually nil. By refeeding the bile via a nasogastric tube at the time of oral administration of cyclosporine, absorption can be improved dramatically, eliminating the need for intravenous administration.

Cyclosporine is eliminated primarily through the action of the cytochrome P450 system. Its metabolites are excreted into the bile. Drugs such as phenytoin, phenobarbital, rifampin, and warfarin that increase the activity of the P450 system can lead to increased metabolism of cyclosporine and inadequate levels. Conversely, the use of drugs such as ketoconazole, fluconazole, diltiazem, verapamil, or erythromycin can lead to increased levels.

The measurement of cyclosporine is performed either by immunoassay, using a monoclonal antibody to the parent compound, or by HPLC (high-performance liquid chromatography), which measures the parent compound alone. While adequate for most organ transplants, the immunoassay will overestimate the presence of the active parent compound in patients with cholestasis. This is because of the accumulation of metabolites in the blood and the cross-reaction of the assay antibody with the metabolites. The use of immunoassay may therefore be of questionable validity in the jaundiced patient.

Other side effects of cyclosporine are headache, tremors, seizures, myoclonus, gingival hyperplasia, hirsutism, hypertension, and hypercholesterolemia. Most of these side effects respond to dose reduction. Hyperkalemia frequently develops and appears to be caused by hypoaldosteronism. This responds to mineralocorticoid administration.

Tacrolimus

Like cyclosporine, tacrolimus is used to prevent acute rejection. Tacrolimus is highly protein-bound and its absorption is bile-independent. Intravenous administration of tacrolimus is rarely needed, and the drug may be administered through a nasogastric tube in patients unable to take oral medications. Absorption of tacrolimus occurs in the small intestine.

Tacrolimus is also metabolized by the cytochrome P450 enzyme system. Like cyclosporine, its metabolites are excreted in the bile with minimal renal excretion. Dose adjustment for renal insufficiency is not needed. Drug-drug interactions are also important, and care must be taken when starting new medications. As with cyclosporine, medications may increase or decrease tacrolimus levels.

Measurement of tacrolimus is performed using a monoclonal antibody assay. The monoclonal antibody detects the parent compound and metabolites.

Side effects of tacrolimus include nephrotoxicity, tremors, headaches, diarrhea, abdominal pain, and hypertension and glucose intolerance. Less hirsutism and less gingival hyperplasia are reported with tacrolimus.

Antilymphocyte Preparations

These drugs are antibodies to the lymphocytes, whose function is inhibited by removal from the circulation.

Drugs currently available in the United States include the monoclonal preparations (OKT3), the anti-CD25 antibodies (daclizumab and basiliximab), and the polyclonal preparation ATG (antithymocyte globulin), horse or rabbit. While OKT3 and ATG were developed to treat rejection, they have found widespread use in the initial postoperative period in sequential regimens where they can be used to delay the initiation of a calcineurin inhibitor. The decision to employ one or the other is based upon the relative problems in using them. ATG must be given through a central line, while OKT3 can be given peripherally. In general, the immediate side effects of ATG—hypotension, bronchospasm, and fever—appear to be less than those that occur with OKT3. The other problem is that both drugs are foreign proteins, derived from animals; this can lead to the formation of antibodies that can prevent subsequent use.

The rationale for using ATG initially rather than OKT3 in sequential therapy is that OKT3 appears to be more effective for treating rejection, and the ability to give it through a peripheral intravenous line allows easier outpatient therapy. The early use of OKT3 in a sequential regimen may lead to sensitization that would prevent the later use of the drug.

Some transplant centers employ the anti-CD25 monoclonal preparation for induction therapy in a select group of patients. However, the use of a calcineurin inhibitor is recommended.

The antilymphocyte preparations can also be used to treat rejection. These drugs are generally used in patients who have failed prior therapy with steroids. Both preparations are associated with significant side effects related to cytokine release from lymphocyte activation. The effects include hypotension, bronchospasm and respiratory failure, and fever. These side effects appear to be exacerbated by preexisting volume overload, which must be eliminated by either diuretic use or dialysis prior to treatment. The side effects also can be controlled by the use of large doses of steroids (methylprednisolone, 15–20 mg/kg) one-half hour prior to administration. The antibodies in ATG cross-react with other white cells and platelets, leading to leukopenia and thrombocytopenia. The long-term side effects include the development of lymphomas.

Sequential Therapy

Because there have been few trials comparing different immunosuppressive agents or regimens, many different regimens are currently in use. One potential regimen, "sequential therapy," is widely used, but it may not be the only or best regimen.

In sequential therapy, the use of cyclosporine is delayed in the immediate postoperative period, and an antilymphocyte preparation is used in its place. The rationale behind using the drugs in this fashion is that the renal dysfunction that is related to the immediate use of a calcineurin inhibitor can be eliminated until renal function is improved in the postoperative period. The need for a calcineurin inhibitor is delayed by using antilymphocyte preparations that can inhibit lymphocyte function until a calcineurin inhibitor can be added. This regimen was initially used in kidney transplantation after early work with cyclosporine revealed that patients begun initially on the drug had a greater need for dialysis than patients who did not receive it in the initial postoperative period. This finding has led to expansion of the concept to other solid organ transplants where renal dysfunction is also probable as a result of either preexisting dysfunction or intraoperative insults.

Current Controversies & Unresolved Issues

Several new drugs are in clinical trials and will have substantial impacts upon posttransplant immunosuppressive therapy. The newest drug introduced into clinical practice, sirolimus, will undoubtedly have impact in the next few years. It is unclear whether sirolimus will be used as a first-line agent in conjunction with other immunosuppressive medications or be used in those patients with or at high risk for nephrotoxicity from the calcineurin inhibitors, cyclosporine and tacrolimus.

Sirolimus has a distinct mechanism of action and is not considered a calcineurin inhibitor. Early clinical trials in renal transplant recipients showed a decrease in acute rejection when sirolimus was used with cyclosporine and prednisone. Sirolimus has been used in steroid-sparing protocols, without a calcineurin inhibitor, with or without mycophenolate mofetil, and with similar historical graft and patient survival rates.

Sirolimus is absorbed in the gastrointestinal tract, reaching peak serum concentration in 1–2 hours. However, sirolimus has a long half-life of about 60 hours. Metabolism is primarily in the liver, and dose adjustment is required in patients with hepatic dysfunction. Dose adjustment for renal dysfunction is not required. Sirolimus and the calcineurin inhibitors are metabolized by the same enzyme system, and care must be taken when administering other medications that may interfere with the P450 enzyme system.

The main side effects of sirolimus are hypercholesterolemia and hypertriglyceridemia, and many patients will require medical therapy. Thrombocytopenia, leukopenia, and anemia may also be seen with sirolimus. Sirolimus does not appear to be nephrotoxic, as are the calcineurin inhibitors.

Chang GJ et al: Experience with the use of sirolimus in liver transplantation—use in patients for whom calcineurin inhibitors are contraindicated. Liver Transpl 2000;6: 734–40.

Gummert JF et al: Newer immunosuppressive drugs: a review. J Am Soc Nephrol 1999;10:1366–80.

Pascual M et al: Strategies to improve long-term outcomes after renal transplantation. N Engl J Med 2002;346:580–90.

SPECIFIC TRANSPLANT OPERATIONS

RENAL TRANSPLANTATION

Recipient Selection

The recipient of a renal transplant has usually been maintained on chronic dialysis. Although it has been suggested that some patients will do better if they are transplanted prior to requiring dialysis, this is not widely practiced and is generally limited to patients who have a living related donor.

Donor Selection

Because of superior survival results, the best donor for renal transplantation is an HLA-identical sibling. The second choice appears to be a sibling who is a lesser match, and the last choice is a cadaveric donor. It does appear that a transplant from a living unrelated donor provides results superior to those obtained with cadaveric transplantation. Because only a small percentage of patients have a suitable living donor, most patients wait until a cadaveric donor is available. The waiting time depends on the number of other patients waiting, the degree of sensitization of the recipient, and the blood type. Kidneys recovered from cadaveric donors are transplanted within 24–72 hours. Kidneys from living related donors are transplanted immediately after donor nephrectomy and therefore have lower rates of acute tubular necrosis when compared to cadaveric kidneys.

Preoperative Preparation

The recipient usually undergoes dialysis shortly before the transplant to optimize fluid, electrolyte, and acid-base status. For patients who have underlying cardiac disease, preoperative monitoring with a Swan-Ganz catheter and maximization of cardiac output may be warranted. For those maintained on peritoneal dialysis, culture and cell count of the peritoneal fluid is important to eliminate an occult infection.

Operative Procedure

Prior to the operation, a large (20–22F) catheter is placed in the bladder to ensure easy egress of urine and clots. The operation is performed by isolating the iliac artery and vein through an incision over the iliac fossa. The vessels are then clamped, and the renal artery and vein are anastomosed to the corresponding iliac vessels. Prior to vascular unclamping, the patient is volume-loaded and large doses of mannitol and furosemide are given. The kidney frequently produces urine immediately. An anastomosis is then formed between the ureter and the bladder. (See Figures 35–2 and 35–3.)

Postoperative Management

A. Early Postoperative Period

In general, postoperative care following renal transplantation does not require ICU admission. As is true with transplantation of any organ, the postoperative course of these patients is relatively predictable, and complications generally occur in a time-dependent fashion. Monitoring during the first 24 hours may be indicated in the face of hemodynamic instability.

In the first 24 hours posttransplantation, the major concern is urine production. This is the only window that exists through which to examine the function of the transplanted kidney. A significant decrease in hourly urine output can be one of the earliest signs of an untoward event.

Initial urine production following transplant is dependent on several factors. The first is how much urine the patient produced prior to transplantation. Although these patients are dialysis-dependent prior to transplanta-

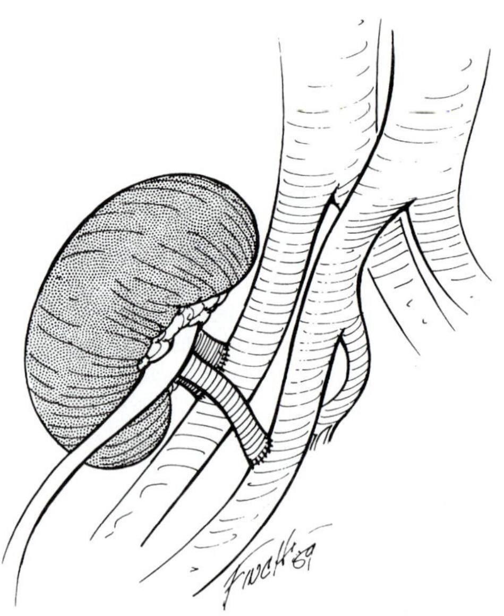

Figure 35–2. Renal transplantation. Anastomosis of renal artery to iliac artery and renal vein to iliac vein.

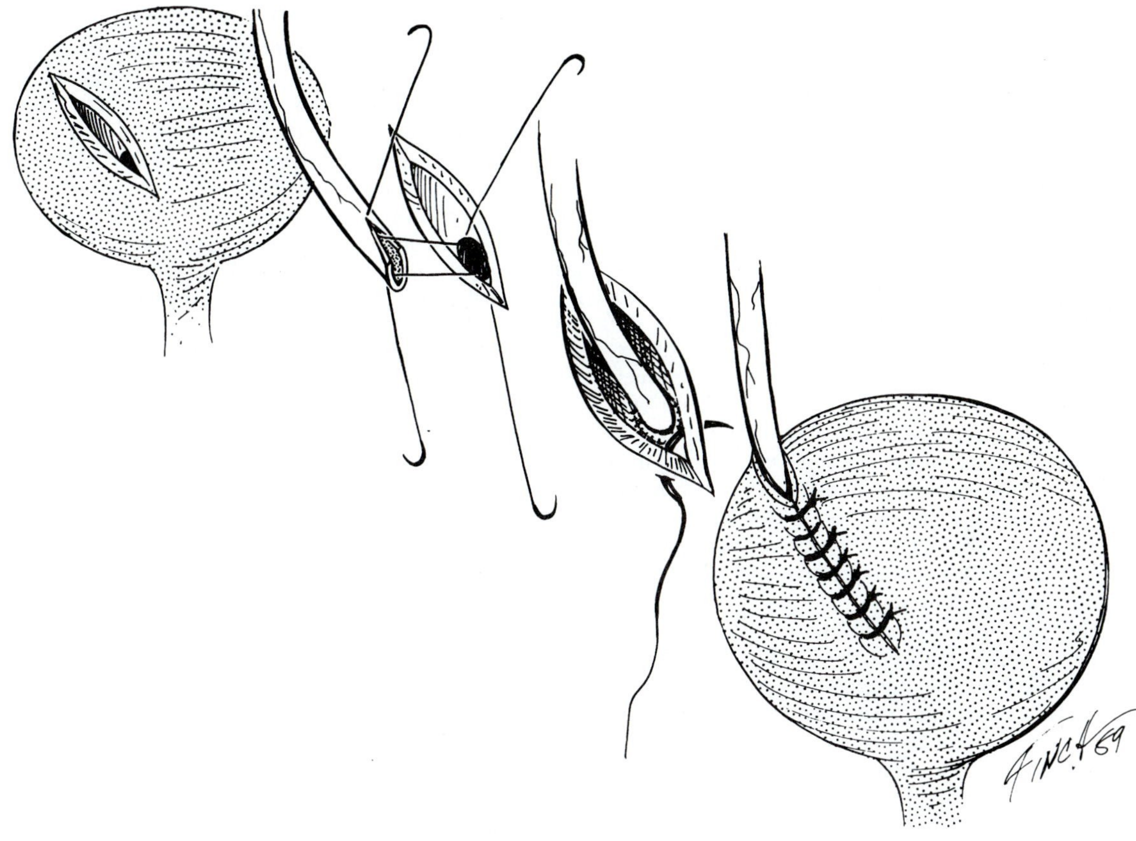

Figure 35–3. Renal transplantation. Creation of ureteroneocystostomy.

tion, they can have significant daily urine output. For example, patients with polycystic renal disease can produce near-normal amounts of urine. Therefore, an important question in the preoperative evaluation of patients is an estimation by the patient of the daily urine output.

The source of the transplanted kidney is important, since in patients receiving an organ from a live donor—either living related or unrelated—significant acute tubular necrosis is rare, and initial urine output tends to be high. In patients who receive a kidney from a cadaveric donor, initial urine output may vary depending upon the degree of acute tubular necrosis. In general, the surgeon who implanted the organ can comment on whether the kidney made urine upon completion of the vascular anastomosis, and this qualitative estimate may be of some value. Further information can be obtained by comparing urine output from the second of the two cadaveric kidneys. Because the initial results of both kidneys are frequently similar, a disparity in urine output may suggest a problem in the oliguric kidney. If both kidneys are oliguric, acute tubular necrosis becomes a likely diagnosis.

The initial evaluation of oliguria following renal transplantation is similar to that of other oliguria in general. Using the model of prerenal, intrarenal, and postrenal causes of oliguria, one of the first possibilities to exclude is a postrenal cause, most commonly a clot in the bladder obstructing the catheter. Although this usually presents with anuria rather than oliguria, it should be excluded either by gentle irrigation of the catheter or by replacement of the catheter with a larger one. If a clot is demonstrated, maximization of urine output may dilute the urine enough to prevent further clot formation. If irrigation demonstrates easy return, catheter obstruction is not the cause. Another postrenal cause of oliguria is obstruction of the transplanted ureter or a leak at the anastomosis of the ureter to the bladder. The question of obstruction can usually be resolved by ultrasound, which reveals hydronephrosis. Demonstration of a leak may require ultrasonography to look for a large fluid collection—or, usually, a radionuclide scan revealing extravasation of the isotope. A common cause of oliguria is volume depletion, which constitutes a prerenal cause of oliguria. This needs to be eliminated by adequate hydration with crystalloid solutions to achieve a central venous pressure within the normal to high range. If there is a question about whether central venous pressure measurements accurately reflect left heart filling pressures, a pulmonary artery flotation catheter should be introduced. Using the information gained from the pressure measurements, a decision can then be made about whether more volume support is necessary. If central venous or left heart pressure is high, a trial of diuretics should be initiated; if there is no response, oliguria is probably due to an intrarenal problem. In patients who show evidence of cardiac dysfunction, cardiac output should be optimized to provide adequate perfusion of the kidney. Volume infusions must be used judiciously during this period to prevent fluid overload and the need for dialysis. The insult of hypoperfusion and hypovolemia during dialysis is not tolerated by the kidney with acute tubular necrosis.

Of the intrarenal causes of low urine output, the most common is acute tubular necrosis. Almost all kidney transplants exhibit some degree of acute tubular necrosis. It is usually less severe in patients who have received living related transplants because the preservation time is very short and the donor has normal circulatory status prior to organ retrieval. In cadaveric renal transplantation, the degree of acute tubular necrosis appears to increase after 24–36 hours of preservation. The cause is probably multifactorial, including premorbid donor factors, preservation injury, and reperfusion injury in the recipient. The diagnosis that must be excluded is very early rejection. These rejections are usually humorally mediated and should have been excluded by cross-matching. Falsely negative cross-matches occur if older serum is used or if the patient was transfused recently. Transfusion represents an antigenic challenge, and some transfused antigens may be held in common with the donor. Vascular complications—either renal artery or renal vein thrombosis—can usually be eliminated either by ultrasound (showing loss of blood flow) or by renal scan. Acute oliguria may also be caused by cyclosporine in the early posttransplant period. This agent is notorious for producing renal vascular constriction that presents as oliguria and sodium retention. Frequent monitoring of cyclosporine or tacrolimus levels and decreases in dose may be effective in resolving the problem.

In general, cadaveric transplant patients may do better if the calcineurin inhibitors, cyclosporine or tacrolimus, are withheld until adequate renal function has been demonstrated. Antilymphocyte preparations can be used to prevent rejection until the calcineurin inhibitor can be started.

B. Intermediate Postoperative Period

Five to 30 days posttransplant, the most common cause of renal dysfunction is either calcineurin inhibitor toxicity or rejection. Although a patient with rejection may present with the classic signs of fever, tenderness over the graft, and decreased urine output, the introduction of cyclosporine as immunosuppressive therapy seems to be effective in blunting these clinical signs of rejection. Therefore, the patient who presents with elevated creatinine needs an evaluation to exclude technical causes of decreased urine output and rising creatinine, followed by consideration of biopsy prior to treatment.

The common technical problems in this period are obstruction of the ureter or urine leak, which can be diagnosed with ultrasound or renal scan. Prerenal causes also need to be excluded. Volume depletion related to overdiuresis warrants a volume challenge for evaluation. Intrarenal causes are usually related to cyclosporine toxicity, which is implied if the cyclosporine level is very high. Given this situation, a 24-hour trial of dose reduction may be warranted. If the cyclosporine level is normal to low or the dose reduction does not have the expected effect, the patient may have rejection. There is controversy about whether to treat the patient empirically with corticosteroids or to obtain a renal biopsy. The controversy arises out of concern about the relative accuracy of the clinical diagnosis of rejection versus the risk of biopsy. If a diagnosis of rejection is made, a trial of steroids is usually started. If this fails to improve renal function, biopsy is mandatory, and an antilymphocyte preparation is begun if rejection is present.

C. Late Postoperative Period

Late renal dysfunction may be due to a variety of causes, including rejection, cyclosporine toxicity, ureteral obstruction, recurrent native renal disease, or lymphocele. The evaluation is similar to that in the early postoperative period. Ultrasound or renal scan is used to make the diagnosis of ureteral obstruction. If obstruction is found, placement of a percutaneous stent with nephrostomy drainage is warranted. A lymphocele is a lymph collection that occurs peritransplant. Lymphoceles often become quite large and can cause ureteral obstruction or a mass effect. Treatment choices are sclerotherapy or drainage into the peritoneal cavity.

Another problem is stenosis of the transplant's renal artery, which usually presents with accelerated hypertension and renal dysfunction. Renal dysfunction in this situation may be exacerbated or induced by the use of ACE inhibitors. A marked decrease in renal function associated with the use of these drugs should arouse suspicion of transplant renal artery stenosis. The diagnosis can be established by arteriography. Angioplasty or surgical repair may be warranted.

Postoperative Immunosuppression

Immunosuppressive management in the recipient of a cadaveric kidney may differ from that of a live donor kidney, since the incidence of acute tubular necrosis is higher with the cadaveric kidney. In general, sequential therapy is used in the recipient to delay the use of cyclosporine until renal function returns to normal. Recipients of live donor kidneys may receive immediate calcineurin inhibitor or be treated with a sequential protocol.

Results of Transplantation

The results of HLA-identical living related transplants are superior to those achieved with nonidentical live donor transplants, which in turn are superior to those achieved with cadaveric transplants. In series reporting the most favorable outcomes, the results of HLA-identical living related transplants are 95% patient and graft survival at 2 years, whereas in cadaveric transplants patient and graft survival was 91% and 77% at 2 years.

Beyga ZT et al: Surgical complications of kidney transplantation. J Nephrol 1998;11:137–45.

Dubovsky EV et al: Radionuclide evaluation of renal transplants. Semin Nucl Med 1995;25:49–59.

PANCREAS TRANSPLANTATION

Recipient Selection

Pancreas transplantation is performed in the hope that physiologic production of insulin by the transplanted pancreas will prevent progression of the complications of diabetes. Although there is some evidence that this may be possible, the patient is exchanging potential diabetic complications for those related to immunosuppression. Because of concern about immunosuppressing a patient without clear demonstration of long-term benefits of pancreas transplantation, this procedure has been limited mainly to patients with diabetic nephropathy and indications for kidney transplantation. Currently, recipients selected for this procedure are in relatively good health. Major cardiovascular disease needs to be excluded, since coronary artery disease in these patients is frequently silent. Patients should understand that the major benefits currently are freedom from administration of exogenous insulin and the possibility of a lower incidence of diabetic nephropathy in the transplanted kidney.

Donor Selection

In general, the pancreas donor is under 50 years of age, without a history of conditions that would predispose to pancreatitis such as heavy alcohol use. Diabetes is an obvious contraindication. A relatively normal serum amylase or serum lipase level is necessary as evidence that there has been no damage to the pancreas itself. Mild hyperglycemia is not a contraindication.

Operative Procedure (Figure 35–4)

As both the kidney and the pancreas are transplanted through one incision, a midline abdominal incision is used. The iliac vessels on both sides are mobilized, and the pancreas is implanted in the right iliac fossa. A graft is used to anastomose both the superior mesenteric artery and the splenic artery of the donor to the iliac artery of the recipient. The portal vein of the donor is anastomosed to the recipient iliac vein. The pancreatic duct is drained via a duodenal segment that is anastomosed to the bladder, allowing the exocrine secretions to be drained into the bladder. The kidney is transplanted in the usual fashion into the left iliac fossa.

Postoperative Management

The postoperative course is similar in many respects of that of kidney transplant recipients. The differential di-

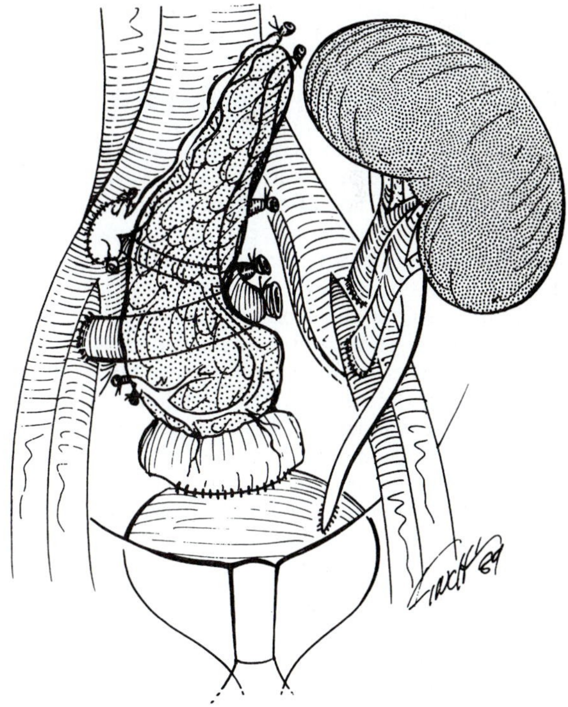

Figure 35–4. Completed combined pancreatic and renal transplantation.

agnosis of decreased urine output is as discussed for kidney transplantation. The pancreas graft usually starts to function immediately, with patients able to be weaned from insulin within 24 hours. Bleeding is a complication that usually requires immediate reexploration.

One of the early problems with pancreas transplantation was the high incidence of vascular thrombosis of the vessels supplying the pancreas. For reasons that are not completely understood, the incidence of this complication has been declining. Part of the explanation may be that dextran and low-dose systemic heparin have been used to prevent thrombosis, although this practice leads to a higher incidence of bleeding complications.

Drainage of exocrine secretions into the bladder leads to a loss of bicarbonate-rich solution into the urine, which produces a severe metabolic acidosis that requires bicarbonate supplementation. The same physiologic result of the procedure allows pancreatic enzymes to become activated, leading to irritation of the bladder and urethra, causing hematuria and urethritis in men. Hematuria may require cystoscopy and electrocoagulation. Urethritis may require urethral catheterization. If these complications become intolerable, conversion of bladder drainage to enteric drainage is performed.

Other complications of pancreas transplantation include leakage at the anastomosis, graft pancreatitis, small bowel obstruction, and recurrent urinary tract infections.

Postoperative Immunosuppression

Because these grafts come from cadaveric donors, a sequential immunosuppressive protocol is used. The primary laboratory sign of rejection is a rise of serum creatinine, calling either for empiric treatment with steroids or kidney biopsy. Biopsy is required prior to the use of antilymphocyte preparations. Transcystoscopic or transabdominal percutaneous biopsy of the pancreas can be performed with a small risk of bleeding. Some centers use the concentration of urine amylase as a marker of rejection, since rejection appears to decrease urinary amylase excretion. Circulating insulin levels are not a good marker for rejection because very severe rejection can be present with no change in these levels. The reemergence of insulin resistance suggests end-stage rejection of the pancreas.

Results of Transplantation

The current results following combined kidney and pancreas transplantation are a 1-year patient survival rate of about 90% with a graft survival rate (survival defined as no insulin requirement) of 80–90%. Survival of the kidney does not appear to be adversely affected by the combined transplant.

Becker BN et al: Simultaneous pancreas-kidney and pancreas transplantation. J Am Soc Nephrol 2001;12:2517–27.

Drachenberg CB et al: Pancreas transplantation: the histologic morphology of graft loss and clinical correlations. Transplantation 2001;71:1784–91.

Krishnamurthi V et al: Pancreas transplantation: contemporary surgical techniques. Urol Clin North Am 2001;28:833–8.

Paty BW et al: Restored hypoglycemic counterregulation is stable in successful pancreas transplant recipients for up to 19 years after transplantation. Transplantation 2001;72:1103–7.

LIVER TRANSPLANTATION

Recipient Selection & Indications

Current criteria for liver transplantation include both acute and chronic disease. The leading indications for transplantation for chronic hepatic disease are cholestatic liver disease (primary biliary cirrhosis, biliary atresia, and sclerosing cholangitis), postnecrotic cirrhosis from viral diseases (hepatitis B and C), and alcoholic liver disease. Transplantation is usually reserved for patients who have developed complications of liver disease such as ascites, variceal hemorrhage, and cholangitis.

Preoperative Management

The physician caring for the pretransplant patient with liver disease is in most cases merely trying to sustain the patient until an organ for transplantation becomes available. Patients with chronic liver failure tend to be admitted for complications related to portal hypertension, including ascites and variceal hemorrhage, exacerbation of encephalopathy, spontaneous bacterial peritonitis, and hepatorenal syndrome. Patients with acute liver failure do not have portal hypertension but have the unique complication of increased intracranial pressure as the major immediate threat to life. The mechanism of this process is unclear.

A. Variceal Hemorrhage

1. Airway—Initial management of patients bleeding from varices is the same as that of patients with massive gastrointestinal hemorrhage from any other cause. Attention should be directed first at management of the airway, with consideration given to intubation for airway protection. The patient with liver disease who bleeds massively often has altered mental status due to exacerbation of encephalopathy, which puts the patient at risk for aspiration. The risk is increased by bedside procedures (eg, endoscopy with sclerotherapy, placement of a Sengstaken-Blakemore tube) and by the sedation required to facilitate them.

2. Fluid resuscitation—After appropriate management of the airway, volume resuscitation is performed with appropriate hemodynamic monitoring. In providing for vascular access and blood bank support, it is important to remember that variceal hemorrhage may be massive, and exsanguination can occur in minutes.

3. Endoscopy—After stabilization of the patient, the next appropriate step is endoscopic confirmation of the diagnosis. Other possible causes, including gastric and duodenal ulcers and Mallory-Weiss tears, can be eliminated. When the bleeding is from esophageal varices, endoscopy should also serve as the initial therapeutic step, since sclerotherapy of the esophageal varices can be performed simultaneously. (Sclerotherapy of gastric varices is usually ineffective.) If sclerotherapy is ineffective or if the patient cannot be stabilized to allow endoscopy, temporization with a Sengstaken-Blakemore or Minnesota tube is appropriate.

4. Portasystemic shunt procedures—For patients who rebleed following these measures, the choices are primarily surgically or radiologically created portasystemic shunts.

In the patient who is a candidate for transplantation and who has liver dysfunction of Child class B or class C, a radiologically placed portacaval shunt (transjugular intrahepatic portasystemic shunt, or "TIPS") is probably the procedure of choice. Under local anesthesia through a transjugular approach, a puncture is made through the wall of the hepatic vein, across the liver parenchyma, and into the portal vein. The liver parenchyma is balloon-dilated and then bridged with an expandable metal stent, creating a tunnel through the liver and allowing portal blood to flow into the vena cava via the hepatic vein. Portal decompression is thus achieved without the stress of a major operation. The stent is removed with the liver during transplantation. This relatively new procedure may become the technique of choice in the acutely bleeding patient who will require transplantation. The rates of liver failure and encephalopathy appear to be similar to those associated with surgically created shunts. Both care of the patient and the subsequent transplant procedure are simplified. The long-term patency rate of these shunts is unknown but is probably less than the patency rate of surgically created shunts.

The decision regarding the type of shunt used in the Child class A patient is more difficult. These patients appear to have excellent survival rates with surgically created portasystemic shunts and can be rescued by transplantation for shunt failure. This philosophy is probably best followed in patients with nonprogressive causes such as alcoholic liver disease in persons who have quit drinking. The outlook is less sanguine for patients with processes such as chronic hepatitis in whom disease progression can be anticipated.

B. Spontaneous Bacterial Peritonitis

The cirrhotic patient with ascites frequently develops spontaneous bacterial peritonitis. Clinical manifestations range from a complex of fever, shaking chills, and abdominal pain to only the more subtle findings of increasing ascites or worsening encephalopathy. The diagnosis is primarily based upon the finding of an absolute polymorphonuclear cell count of >250 cells/mL in an aspirate of ascitic fluid. The most common organisms are *Escherichia coli,* group D streptococci, *Klebsiella pneumoniae,* and *Streptococcus pneumoniae.* Antibiotic therapy is with a third-generation cephalosporin such as ceftizoxime. Treatment is usually provided for 5-7 days or until the cell count in the ascitic fluid becomes normal. It appears that the incidence of recurrence can be significantly diminished by the administration of chronic oral prophylactic antibiotics such as a fluoroquinolone.

C. Hepatorenal Syndrome

The diagnosis of hepatorenal syndrome is based upon the finding of severe liver disease, the demonstration of adequate plasma volume, and a low urine sodium concentration in the presence of a normal urine sediment. Differential diagnosis calls for demonstration of an adequate plasma volume and elimination of other causes of renal failure. This syndrome carries an extremely poor prognosis, and there are few therapeutic options other than liver transplantation. The use of liver transplantation in this situation can lead to rapid resolution of renal failure, particularly if the urine sodium remains low immediately prior to transplantation. If the urine sodium has risen and the patient remains oliguric, combined liver and kidney transplantation should be considered, since acute tubular necrosis may be present. Renal biopsy at the time of transplantation may suggest that severe ischemic injury has occurred and would mandate combined transplantation.

D. Acute Liver Failure

The definition of acute liver failure is somewhat nebulous. In general, it can be defined as liver failure developing over a brief period in a patient who previously was in good health. The clinical definition of fulminant liver failure has been the appearance of encephalopathy within 8 weeks after the onset of liver illness, whereas subfulminant liver failure is the occurrence of encephalopathy within the first 2–3 months. These definitions are useful for patients who present with de novo liver disease. Patients who receive transplants for chronic liver disease whose new liver never functioned properly (primary nonfunction) also have acute liver failure. These patients frequently have a hospital course similar to those with acute liver failure unless retransplantation can be performed.

The most common cause of acute liver failure is viral infection. Both hepatitis A and hepatitis B can cause fulminant liver failure. It appears that hepatitis C rarely if ever causes acute liver failure. Another major causes of liver failure is seen among individuals who deliberately or accidentally ingest a toxin such as acetaminophen or mushrooms. A third group consists of patients with primary nonfunction following transplantation, though these represent fewer than 5% of all patients receiving transplants.

The cause of the disease is a major determining factor in evaluating the necessity for organ transplantation. Patients with acetaminophen-induced liver failure (but not other toxin-induced failure) do significantly better than patients with liver failure due to viral hepatitis. Prognostic indicators have been developed for patients with fulminant liver disease. In patients with acetaminophen toxicity, these indicators include an arterial pH below 7.3, prothrombin time greater than an international normalized ratio (INR) of 6.5, and a serum creatinine greater than 3.4 mg/dL. It has been suggested that for these patients, liver transplantation should considered if the arterial pH is less than 7.3; for patients with encephalopathy, transplantation should be considered if the prothrombin time or serum creatinine meets the above criteria.

For patients who have liver disease due to a cause other than acetaminophen, the risk factors are ages less than 10 or greater than 40, duration of jaundice greater than 1 week prior to encephalopathy; a bilirubin greater than 18 mg/dL; and prothrombin time greater than an INR of 3.5. The presence of one or more poor prognostic indicators in a patient with encephalopathy is associated with a mortality rate of 80–95%. The patient who develops acute liver disease is therefore at great risk of dying, and transfer to a transplant center should be arranged as quickly as possible.

The management of patients with prognostic indicators suggesting a high mortality risk is directed primarily toward rapid evaluation for transplantation, management of intracranial hypertension, and general support until a liver becomes available.

1. Cerebral edema—Pretransplant management of the patient with fulminant liver disease is primarily geared toward diagnosis, prevention, and treatment of acute cerebral edema. The measures taken to prevent cerebral edema should include elevation of the head of the bed, careful management of fluid status, and administration of mannitol. In these patients, lactulose usually does not prevent encephalopathy. The diarrhea lactulose causes may lead to electrolyte imbalances (especially hypernatremia) that can make management more difficult. Serial neurologic examinations will disclose progression of intracranial changes. Therefore, the examination should not be hampered by the use of agents such as benzodiazepines that alter mental status and are poorly eliminated because of liver failure. It is probably best for intubated patients to be given opioids (which are reversible) or, in the case of combative patients, neuromuscular blocking agents.

When a patient has progressed to stage 3 or 4 coma, it is important to obtain a CT scan as a baseline study. A CT scan of the head is not accurate for diagnosis of intracranial hypertension, but it is helpful in documenting the presence or absence of intracranial abnormalities prior to placement of an intracranial pressure monitor. Monitor placement is associated with a substantial risk of intracranial hemorrhage, since a coagulopathy may be present. Correction of the coagulation system to near normal is necessary for safe placement. Epidural monitors used in this situation provide invaluable information that permits ongoing assessment of the adequacy of maneuvers such as administration of mannitol, hyperventilation, and pentobarbital coma to decrease intracranial hypertension. Monitoring allows calculation of cerebral perfusion pressure (CPP). It is important to maintain an adequate CPP by manipulation of the mean arterial pressure (MAP) and the intracranial pressure (ICP):

$$CPP = MAP - ICP$$

Maintenance of CPP at > 50 mm Hg is achieved by lowering intracranial pressure (using the measures noted above) and maintaining the mean arterial pressure with vasopressor agents. If intracranial pressure cannot be controlled, these patients should be excluded from transplantation.

Postoperatively, neurologic recovery is slow. The increased intracranial pressure usually resolves within 24–48 hours. The pressure monitor should be removed within 48 hours to eliminate possible complications. CT scan following removal of the monitor will identify bleeding and other complications.

2. Infection—The second major cause of death in this group of patients is infection, mainly pneumonia, often related to aspiration. Prevention is by early intubation before the patient slips into coma or prior to transportation.

Fungal infections are a threat in patients who have received high-dose corticosteroid therapy to prevent progression of fulminant liver disease. Steroids do not appear to be beneficial for this purpose or as protection against intracranial hypertension. They may increase morbidity and mortality following transplantation.

3. Other measures—Other important preoperative requirements include protection of the gastric mucosa with antacids or H_2 blockers and continuous arteriovenous hemofiltration, when needed, for renal failure. Hemofiltration provides better physiologic control of intravascular volume because it eliminates the hypotensive episodes associated with intermittent hemodialysis. It is quite helpful during the administration of fresh frozen plasma to prevent fluid overload.

Donor Selection

The requirements for a potential liver donor are similar to those for other organ donors. Recent improvements in preservation solutions have allowed extension of preservation times to as long as 24 hours, though most surgeons would prefer to keep the time under 12 hours. There are no absolute biochemical parameters that exclude organ donation, though a large continued increase in aminotransferases in the cadaveric donor suggests that ongoing liver injury is occurring. Recently, the use of partial or split livers has made possible the transplantation of more patients. Another potential source of organs for liver transplantation is living related donors. These donors are used almost exclusively in Japan, where cadaveric donation is rare.

Operative Procedure (Figure 35–5)

The liver transplant operation has been improved over the last several years to the point that it is frequently performed in less than 5 hours. Blood product consumption has been minimized. Both operative time and blood utilization are increased in recipients who have had extensive prior surgery or who exhibit portal hypertension.

The operation consists of mobilization of the native liver with isolation of the vena cava above and below the liver, division of the common bile duct, and isolation of the portal vein and hepatic artery. The native liver is then excised, and the vascular connections are recreated. The biliary reconstruction is performed by recreating the original biliary anatomy by anastomosing the donor duct to the recipient duct over a T tube or by altering the anatomy to create a choledochojejunostomy, usually over a stent.

Postoperative Management

Involvement of critical care specialists in the management of post-liver transplant recipients occurs mainly within the first 2–3 days following transplantation. The average recipient is discharged from the ICU within 48 hours. A number of problems may develop during this period which may require urgent attention.

A. Early Postoperative Period

During the first 48 hours, there are three major concerns: (1) Graft dysfunction may occur and must be diagnosed promptly, (2) postoperative bleeding may require reexploration (10–20% of patients), and (3) respiratory support requires mechanical ventilation. Aggressive critical care management is important in obtaining a good outcome and controlling costs.

In the past, as many as 20–25% of patients required retransplantation. Many require urgent retransplantation secondary to primary nonfunction, in which the transplanted liver simply never functions. This condition is usually manifested by acidosis, hyperkalemia, and severe coagulopathy. It subsequently progresses to hepatic coma and converts a patient with chronic liver disease into one with acute liver failure. The only treatment is urgent retransplantation. Primary nonfunction has become less common with use of new liver preservation solutions.

Many patients still develop poor function initially, which is manifested by marked jaundice and a modest coagulopathy. These patients usually do not become acidemic or develop hyperkalemia. The challenge is to determine which patients will need retransplantation and which will ultimately have good graft function. Decisions about marginally functioning grafts generally do not have to be made within the first 2 or 3 days posttransplant and are delayed to the end of the second week.

The differential diagnosis of early graft failure include primary nonfunction and hepatic artery thrombosis (which can present in a similar way). Because of the lack of arterial collaterals to the transplanted liver, hepatic artery thrombosis results in total loss of arterial blood flow followed by hepatic necrosis and biliary complications. The incidence of hepatic thrombosis is about 3–25%. Hepatic artery thrombosis can be evaluated with Doppler ultrasound examination, performed within the first 24 hours after transplantation.

The second major early complication is bleeding. Most bleeding is related to the surgical procedure itself. Clinical manifestations of bleeding are relatively straightforward, with changes in vital signs and a falling hematocrit. However, occasionally it can be heralded simply by a fall in urine output or increasing abdominal girth. The challenge is to determine which patients can be managed with supportive care and which must be returned to the operating room. Most centers try to prevent postoperative bleeding with the use of fresh frozen plasma and platelet infusions. Imaging studies tend not to be helpful in localizing the bleeding, since hematomas commonly form around the liver even in patients without postoperative hemorrhage. The decision is probably best made by immediately reexploring all actively bleeding patients. Patients who are stable and who have a coagulopathy will benefit from correction of the coagulopathy before the decision is made to reoperate.

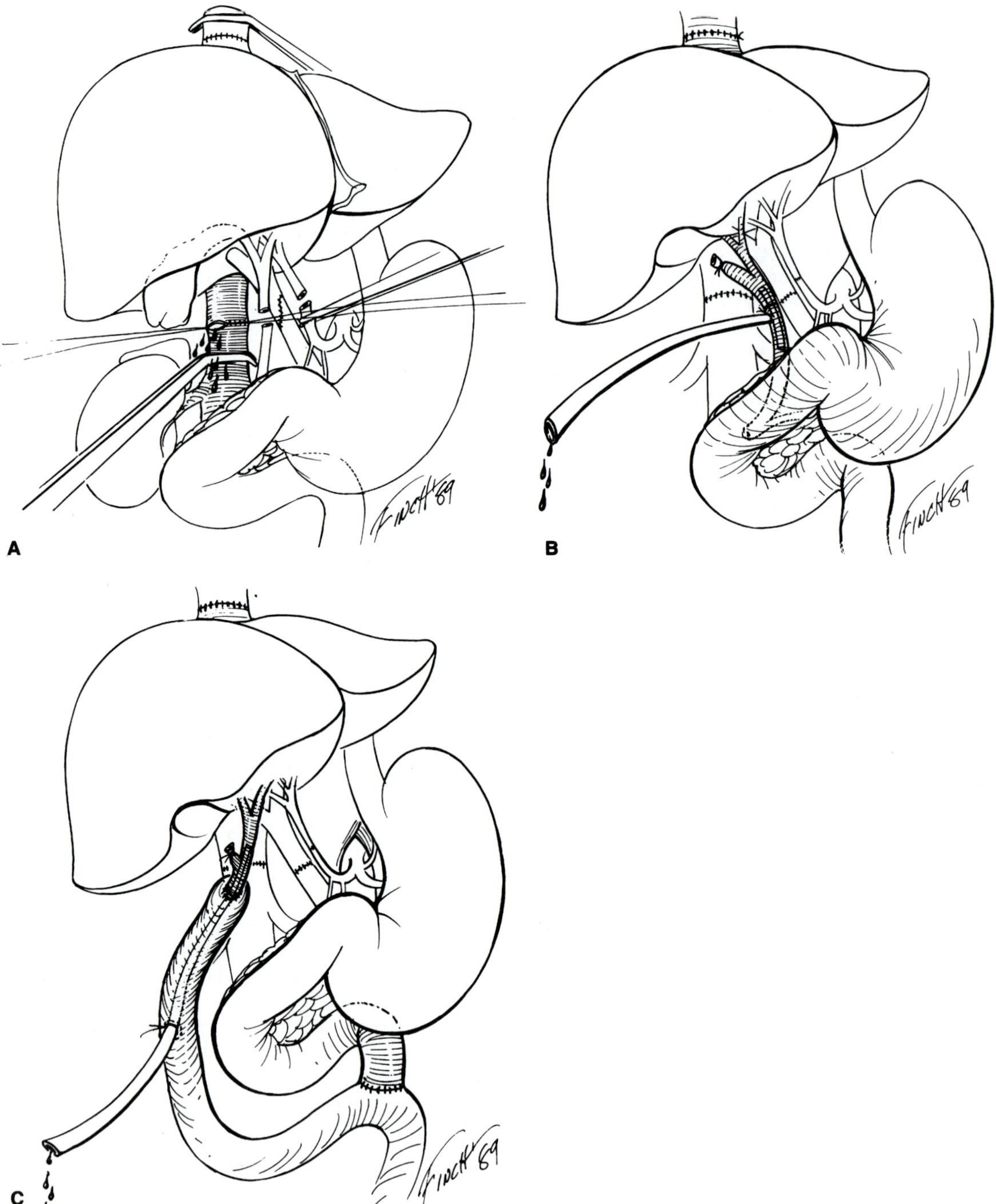

Figure 35–5. Liver transplantation. ***A:*** Completion of portal vein and caval anastomoses. ***B:*** Completed liver transplantation with bile duct to bile duct anastomosis over a T tube. ***C:*** Completed liver transplantation with bile duct anastomosed as duct to Roux-en-Y jejunal loop.

Virtually all patients return to the ICU intubated and have volume overload secondary to the large amounts of blood products received during the procedure. Aggressive diuresis is in order before early extubation can occur. Large doses of diuretics in association with renal-dose dopamine may be used to eliminate the fluid overload. Most patients have pulmonary artery flotation catheters in place to assist with monitoring the volume status. Because patients with cirrhosis may have pulmonary hypertension, measurements of pulmonary artery pressure may not accurately reflect volume status. The cirrhotic patient frequently has a hyperdynamic cardiovascular state, and a cardiac output in the range of 8–15 L/min may be their baseline. Measurements based on preoperative weights are also prone to error given the fact that these patients often have ascites and edema prior to transplantation. Electrolyte abnormalities may also occur during this period, with the most common being changes in serum sodium and potassium concentrations. Hypernatremia may occasionally be a result of fresh frozen plasma infusion.

Patients commonly develop minor gastrointestinal bleeding during the transplant procedure. They are also prone to develop gastritis. Patients with cirrhosis have a high incidence of peptic ulcer disease. Endoscopy can be helpful in the evaluation of marked gastrointestinal bleeding. In the vast majority of cases the bleeding will stop spontaneously without specific treatment. Therapy directed toward gastric cytoprotection is mandatory.

B. Intermediate Postoperative Period

If graft function is adequate, the patient probably will not require retransplantation during the first 2 weeks unless hepatic artery thrombosis occurs. Most patients are extubated by this time. If reoperation has not been required, it becomes less likely that the patient will need to return to the operating room for control of bleeding. The issues during this period relate to biliary tract complications, ongoing assessment of graft function, and metabolic complications that can occur during the first 5 days posttransplant. Early complications largely relate to bile leaks, which usually present with fever, abdominal pain, or increasing ascites. Bile leaks can be treated in a number of ways. One is to simply open the T tube to allow drainage of bile away from the leak. Transhepatic tubes can also be effective in managing small leaks. Patients may need to return to the operating room for repair of the anastomosis. The presence of a biliary tract complication should suggest hepatic artery thrombosis, since the bile duct is damaged immediately by the loss of arterial flow. Stricture formation or leakage of bile should suggest this complication.

Postoperative Immunosuppression

The immunosuppression protocol used during the first 48 hours varies in different centers. Many use sequential immunosuppression therapy, which consists of an antilymphocyte preparation in the early postoperative period followed by the introduction of a calcineurin inhibitor—cyclosporine or tacrolimus—at a later time. Both are nephrotoxic.

The most common time for allograft rejection to occur is 7 days following transplantation. Patients may occasionally present prior to this time with rising liver function test parameters. Laboratory features of rejection are nonspecific and include elevation of serum aminotransferases, bilirubin, and alkaline phosphatase. The differential diagnosis of rising liver function test values includes preservation injury, bile duct obstruction, and allograft rejection. The change in liver tests thus cannot distinguish acute rejection from other causes of graft dysfunction. This is best determined by imaging studies such as cholangiography, ultrasonography, and liver biopsy. Patients with histologic evidence of acute rejection may have normal or unchanged liver tests. For this reason, histologic study has become the most specific indicator of rejection. Treatment of rejection is initially with steroids followed by an antilymphocyte preparation for patients who have recurrent rejection.

A common approach to the diagnosis of rejection following transplantation involves the use of liver biopsies at 1 week posttransplant to make an early diagnosis. Biopsies are continued until two successive reports have offered no evidence of rejection.

Results of Transplantation

Current results following liver transplantation are 1-year patient and graft survivals of 86% and 80%, respectively.

Levy MF et al: Readmission to the intensive care unit after liver transplantation. Crit Care Med 2001;29:207–8.

Lidofsky SD et al: Intracranial pressure monitoring and liver transplantation for fulminant hepatic failure. Hepatology 1992; 16:1–7.

Ozaki CF et al: Surgical complications of liver transplantation. Surg Clin North Am 1994;74:1155–67.

Saab S et al: Liver transplantation. Selection, listing criteria, and preoperative management. Clin Liver Dis 2000;4:513–32.

HEART TRANSPLANTATION

Recipient Selection & Indications

The current indications for heart transplantation are cardiomyopathy in a patient who has failed medical therapy, severe coronary artery disease with loss of myocardial mass, or otherwise unreconstructible disease. The patients who appear to benefit most from cardiac transplantation are those who have ejection fractions below 20%, since the mortality rate in such cases is very high without transplantation.

Patients selected for cardiac transplantation usually have organ failure restricted to the heart, though combined heart and kidney transplantation has been performed successfully. Insulin-dependent diabetes may also be a contraindication depending on the transplant center.

An important postoperative concern is right-sided heart failure in patients with elevated pulmonary vascular resistance preoperatively. These patients have high postoperative mortality rates and should be considered for combined heart-lung transplantation. Therefore, right heart catheterization is important in determining whether there is a contraindication to transplantation. Patients with a high fixed pulmonary vascular resistance are excluded from isolated cardiac transplantation.

Donor Selection

Selection of the cardiac donor has become more liberal as the disparity between the number of potential donors and recipients has grown. The donor is matched with the recipient by ABO blood type, organ size, and the presence of a negative cross-match for sensitized recipients. A normal echocardiogram is necessary, and in patients over the age of 40, coronary catheterization is necessary to exclude coronary artery disease. The ECG may be abnormal in the brain-dead patient, but pathologic Q waves suggesting myocardial infarction is a contraindication. Other criteria for the donor are the same as for other solid organ transplants. The heart has the shortest preservation time for solid organs (about 4–8 hours).

Operative Procedure (Figure 35–6)

The operation is performed via a median sternotomy, using cardiopulmonary bypass. The recipient heart is removed by dividing the atria, aorta, and pulmonary artery. The donor heart is implanted by anastomosing the atria, aorta, and pulmonary artery. This leaves the donor heart with a normal intrinsic conduction system postoperatively.

Postoperative Management

Early postoperative care is similar to that of patients undergoing other major cardiac surgery. The primary risks are bleeding and tamponade. Primary nonfunction of the heart graft is uncommon, though the myocardium frequently does not function normally and requires inotropic support. Other complications following cardiac transplantation are similar for other solid organ transplants. Infection (with CMV and opportunistic organisms) is the leading cause of death. Prophylaxis with ganciclovir and trimethoprim-sulfamethoxazole is important in preventing serious infection.

A severe complication is coronary artery disease in the transplanted heart. This is probably related to chronic rejection and usually presents as sudden death or cardiac failure. The lesion is usually diffuse and is not amenable to standard therapy for coronary artery disease. Retransplantation is the only recourse.

Postoperative Immunosuppression

A variety of immunosuppressive protocols have been developed for use following heart transplantation. Many centers use a sequential protocol to avoid giving cyclosporine or tacrolimus until renal function has recovered. Because there is no clinical evidence for rejection until fairly severe rejection has already occurred, the diagnosis of rejection is through right heart catheterization and biopsy of the myocardium. Histologic examination of the biopsy specimen can confirm early diagnosis of rejection before severe myocardial injury occurs.

Rejection is treated initially with high-dose steroids. For patients who fail this therapy, antilymphocyte preparations are used.

Results of Transplantation

Results following cardiac transplantation are a 1-year patient survival of approximately 85% with a similar graft survival. Retransplantation is rare.

Miniati DN et al: Heart transplantation: a thirty year perspective. Annu Rev Med 2002;53:189–205.

HEART-LUNG & LUNG TRANSPLANTATION

Recipient Selection & Indications

Many of the indications for heart-lung and lung transplantation are the same. Patients with elevated pulmonary vascular resistance from diseases such as Eisenmenger's syndrome and primary pulmonary hypertension are candidates for either heart-lung or lung transplantation. In general, if cardiac function is normal, these patients may benefit from lung transplantation alone, since the procedure is technically easier. Only patients with severe heart failure or cystic fibrosis would be considered for combined heart-lung transplantation. Cystic fibrosis is considered an indication for combined heart-

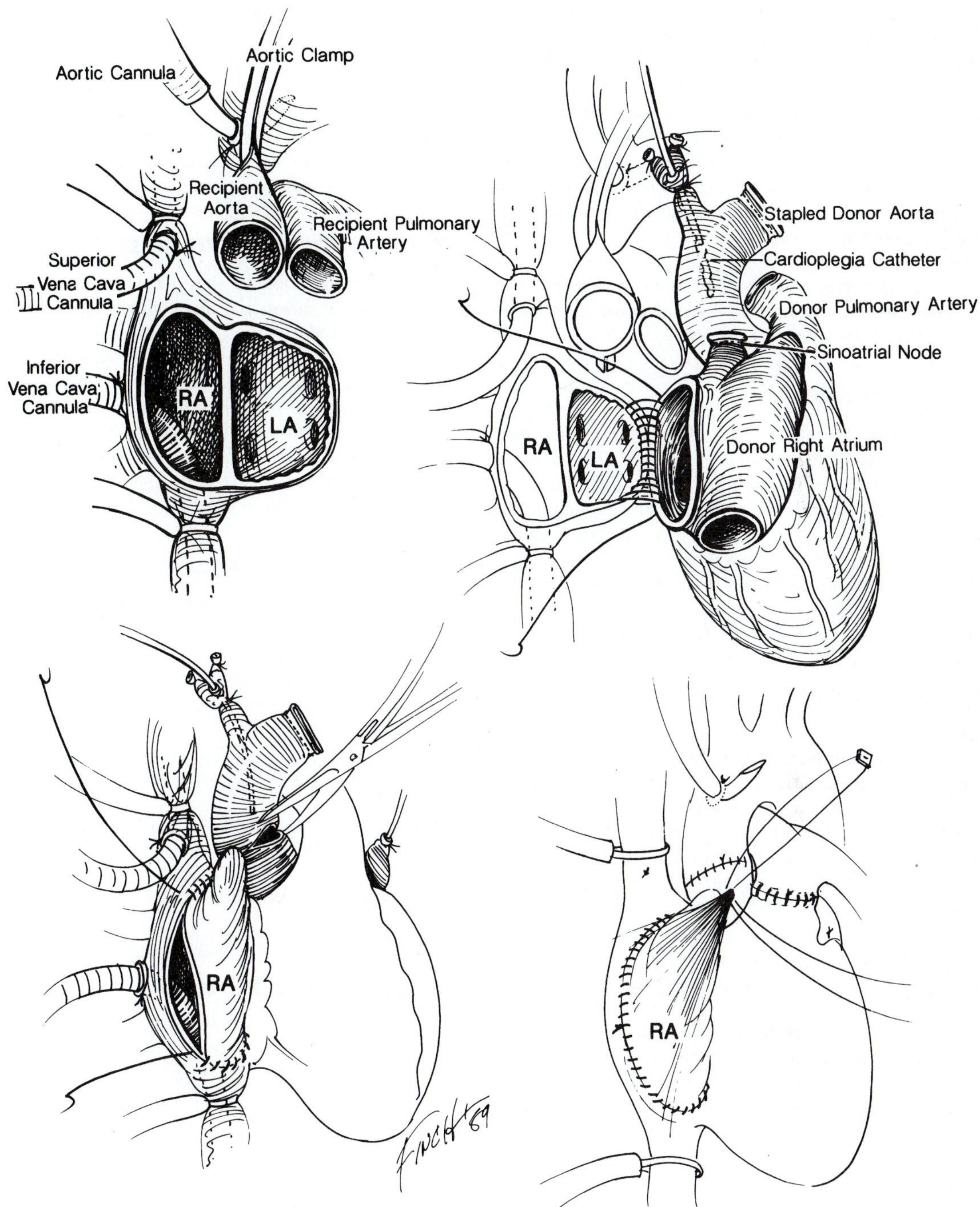

Figure 35–6. Heart transplantation.

lung transplantation because if a single lung transplant were performed, infection in the remaining lung could infect the new graft. Bilateral lung transplantation has been performed for this indication. Some patients who have relatively normal cardiac function and who undergo heart-lung transplantation can serve as cardiac donors for patients who need heart transplantation alone. In this situation, the heart is removed from the heart-lung recipient and implanted into the patient requiring only the heart transplant.

The major benefit to using lung rather than heart-lung transplantation is that the opposite donor lung and the heart can be used in other patients, thus benefiting three patients rather than only one.

Donor Selection

The donor for both heart-lung and lung transplantation must have excellent pulmonary function with an essentially normal chest x-ray. Sputum culture and Gram stain must show no evidence of bacterial or fungal pneumonia. Bronchoscopy is performed at the time of organ recovery to further evaluate the potential for infection. The PaO_2/FIO_2 ratio should be at least 300. In general, the donor is matched by both size and blood type. A negative cross-match is usually required in the sensitized recipient.

Operative Procedure

In the combined heart-lung procedure, a median sternotomy is used through which the heart and lungs are removed. The dissection must avoid the recurrent laryngeal, vagus, and phrenic nerves. The donor organ block is implanted with the anastomosis of the trachea, right atrium, and aorta. Problems with the bronchial anastomosis include stricture and dehiscence. Currently, an omental wrap is performed around the trachea to provide better healing through improved circulation.

In lung transplantation, the procedure is performed via a unilateral thoracotomy. Following removal of the diseased lung, a cuff of atrium surrounding the donor pulmonary artery is anastomosed to the recipient's left atrium, followed by the bronchial and pulmonary anastomosis. Bilateral lung transplantation is usually performed through bilateral thoracotomies.

Postoperative Management

Postoperative care includes the usual measures to identify and deal with bleeding and infections. CMV infections appear to be more severe in lung transplantation, particularly in seronegative recipients at risk for primary infection after having received an organ from a seropositive donor. Prophylactic therapy with ganciclovir and CMV hyperimmune globulin is used in these patients.

The major technical problem with heart-lung and lung transplantation is healing of the bronchial anastomosis. This can be complicated by dehiscence and stricture formation. Strictures are best managed with dilation and stenting of the airway.

Late complications include progressive pulmonary disease and bronchiolitis obliterans secondary to rejection, which occurs in approximately 30% of patients.

Postoperative Immunosuppression

Steroids are avoided in these patients to allow better healing of the bronchial anastomosis. A modified sequential protocol is used consisting of antilymphocyte globulin, a calcineurin inhibitor, and an antimetabolite, with steroids added later. Rejection is suggested by a change in pulmonary function tests with a fall in both flow rates and volumes. These tests can be performed at home by the patient. In general, bronchoscopy and transbronchial biopsy are performed prior to initiation of therapy.

Results of Transplantation

The results of lung and heart-lung transplantation are less favorable than those of cardiac transplantation. The 1-year patient and graft survival rate is 60–75%, though this is expected to increase as operative techniques improve.

King Biggs MB: Acute pulmonary allograft rejection. Mechanisms, diagnosis, and management. Clin Chest Med 1997;18:301–10.

Meyers BF et al: Lung transplantation: a decade of experience. Ann Surg 1999;230:363–70.

Midthun DE et al: Medical management and complications in the lung transplant recipient. Mayo Clin Proc 1997;72:175–84.

ORGAN DONATION

One of the greatest contributions an intensive care physician can make to the process of organ transplantation is the identification, management, and referral of potential organ donors. In this process, it is important to realize that one of the problems with obtaining a high organ donation rate is that many patients' families refuse the request for organ donation. The request for donation must be approached in a standardized fashion in order to obtain the highest possible consent rates. There is a learning curve for doing this, and experienced transplant coordinators have a much higher success rate than inexperienced medical personnel. The approach to the family should be a two-step process. It is important to explain that the patient is brain dead and allow the family to come to terms with this devastating news before making the organ donation request. If the request is made at the same time as the disclosure of brain death, only 18% of families agree to donation. The temporal separation of the two discussions, making sure the family understands the concept of brain death prior to the request for organ donation, has resulted in a 57% incidence of consent.

It is estimated that every year there are 12,000 potential organ donors in the United States but the number of actual donations is only about 5900. Perhaps one-third of potential donors are lost because of failure of the medical personnel caring for the patient to recognize that donation is a possibility.

The current number of patients waiting for organs in the United States is approximately 80,000. It is therefore imperative that potential donors be recognized. The multiorgan donor can provide transplants to individual recipients of each of the two lungs, the two kidneys, the heart, the liver, and the pancreas. This would mean that as many as six or seven patients could be helped just by transplantation of the solid organs without including the benefit of tissue donation.

In general, the potential donor comes from two major pools of patients: (1) those suffering traumatic injuries to the head and (2) those suffering cerebrovascular injuries. The major exclusion criteria for organ donation include diseases that could be transmitted with the organ (HIV, HBsAg positivity, and most malignancies). One major problem is identification of patients at risk for transmission of HIV. This is done by obtaining the social history of the donor from the next of kin and by serologic tests for evidence of past viral exposure. Social behaviors that suggest exclusion from organ donation are any male homosexual activity, the exchange of sex for drugs or money, and intravenous drug use. Relative exclusion criteria include organ dysfunction, the age of the patient, and the degree of hemodynamic instability. A history of cardiac arrest is not a contraindication to donation. As the need for organs has increased with the expansion of patient waiting lists, the relative contraindications to organ donation have decreased. This is particularly true for age. Livers have now been recovered and transplanted from patients 80 years old. If any possibility of organ donation exists, the patient should be referred for consideration as a donor. The process consists of calling the local organ procurement organization. A coordinator will be able to help with questions regarding donation and can come to the ICU to manage the patient if necessary once the declaration of brain death is made. This can relieve medical personnel of the burden of taking care of the donor, and the coordinator can make the request to the family. The expenses of donor evaluation become the responsibility of the procurement organization after brain death is declared.

Brain Death

There currently is no national standard for brain death. In general, a written statement by two physicians (usually a neurologist or neurosurgeon) is necessary. The use of ancillary tests such as electroencephalography, apnea trials, and brain blood flow studies are left to the discretion of physicians and local standards. One absolute requirement is that the physicians involved with the declaration of brain death have no potential conflict of interest with regard to organ recovery.

Management of the Brain-Dead Patient

Several major physiologic events occur with the onset of brain death. The first is that the central nervous system control of cardiovascular function is lost. This can result in hemodynamic instability, which is exacerbated by the volume restriction instituted to prevent cerebral edema. Frequently after brain death, diabetes insipidus develops secondary to loss of antidiuretic hormone production by the brain. This results in the production of large quantities of dilute urine that further exacerbates volume loss.

The initial challenge in management of the donor is to stabilize the cardiovascular system. Although pressor support with drugs such as dopamine is an important temporizing measure, the primary therapy should be aggressive volume resuscitation. This is best done with measurement of central venous pressures to prevent overresuscitation and resultant pulmonary edema that may preclude lung donation. Replacement of urine losses with D_5W or $D_5 1/4NS$ should be instituted. Desmopressin (0.3 μg/kg intravenously) should be administered to prevent excessive urinary losses. The goals of therapy should be to obtain a normal central venous pressure (8–10 mm Hg), a systolic pressure of 100–120 mm Hg, and a decrease in the amount of pressor support to 10 μg/kg/min or less of dopamine. Other problems that frequently need correction are hypernatremia, hypophosphatemia, hypomagnesemia, and hypokalemia from excessive urine losses; hypothermia from loss of thermoregulation; and coagulopathy from severe head trauma. Hypertension can occur in some donors and is best controlled with nitroprusside or esmolol. Neurogenic pulmonary edema should be managed in the usual fashion with increased ventilatory support. Placement of a nasogastric tube with suction is necessary to prevent aspiration. The use of levothyroxine in the hemodynamically unstable donor may decrease vasopressor requirements and prevent cardiovascular collapse.

Evaluation of Organs for Transplantation

Specific tests performed for the evaluation of organ function include urinalysis, urine culture, and serial creatinine measurements for evaluation of the kidney; electrocardiography, echocardiography, and perhaps coronary angiography for evaluation of the heart; serial liver function tests for the evaluation of the liver; chest x-ray, sputum culture and Gram stain, and bronchoscopy for evaluation of the lungs; and serum amylase and lipase for evaluation of the pancreas.

Novitzky D: Donor management: state of the art. Transplant Proc 1997;29:3773–5.

Razek T et al: Issues in potential organ donor management. Surg Clin North Am 2000;80:1021–32.

Salim A et al: The role of thyroid hormone administration in potential organ donors. Arch Surg 2001;136:1377–80.

CURRENT CONTROVERSIES & UNRESOLVED ISSUES

The number of patients awaiting transplantation of any organ now approximates 80,000. A major unresolved question is how to allocate organs to those who are waiting for them. There are two schools of thought—to allocate organs to the sickest patients or to those who will have the best survival rate. Favoring the sickest patients will rescue them in their time of greatest need. But, as can be seen with liver transplantation, use of the organs in patients on life support—particularly those with chronic liver disease—will result in about a 50% 1-year patient survival rate versus a rate of about 80-90% when organs are made available electively. It is also clear that the policy of transplanting the sickest patients will result in much longer ICU stays and greater hospital costs. But failure to immediately transplant these patients will result in death and may lead to increased costs as medical resources are expended for patients who cannot be helped without a transplant. If a policy is developed that restricts the access of these ICU-bound patients to organs, other policies to rationalize their continued medical care seem warranted.

Burns

36

*David W. Mozingo, MD, William G. Cioffi, Jr., MD, & Basil A. Pruitt, Jr., MD**

Burns represent particularly challenging and difficult management problems. This chapter addresses the most common causes, including thermal, electrical, and chemical burns. Because of the far-reaching implications for care, additional aspects of electrical injuries such as lightning strikes and electrocution are discussed further with environmental injuries in Chapter 38.

I. THERMAL BURN INJURY

Approximately 1.25 million burn injuries occur each year in the United States. House and structure fires account for 81% of the 3600 burn- and fire-related deaths that occur each year. Flame injury following a house fire or ignition of clothing is the most common burn injury in patients admitted to burn centers. Scald burns, the most common burn injury in children, are responsible for about 30% of cases requiring hospitalization for burns. Most burn injuries are adequately treated on an outpatient basis; however, approximately 60,000 patients per year require hospital care because of the extent of their injury, the presence of comorbid factors, or extremes of age. Approximately 20,000 patients have injuries of such significance that care is best undertaken in a designated burn care facility. The American Burn Association has developed criteria to identify those patients who require treatment in a burn center. These criteria assess the severity of injury and the need for specialized burn center treatment based upon the age of the patient; the extent, depth, and location of the burn; the type of injury; and the presence of preexisting comorbid factors or associated injuries (Table 36–1).

Thermal burn injury initiates a deleterious pathophysiologic response in every organ system, with the extent and duration of organ dysfunction proportionate to the size of the burn. Direct cellular damage is manifested by coagulation necrosis, with the magnitude of tissue destruction determined by the temperature to which the tissue is exposed and the duration of contact.

HISTOPATHOLOGIC CHARACTERISTICS OF BURNED TISSUE

Following thermal injury, the region of the burn in which protein coagulation and cell death has occurred has been referred to as the zone of necrosis. In full-thickness injury, all dermal elements are destroyed, whereas partial thickness burns are characterized by a variable and incomplete dermal necrosis. Extending radially from the zone of necrosis are areas of cellular damage referred to as the zones of stasis and hyperemia. The zone of stasis is characterized by a decreased microvascular blood flow, which may be restored to normal with successful resuscitation or converted to necrosis following inadequate perfusion, desiccation, or infection. Minimal thermal injury induces a zone of hyperemia characterized by an immediate inflammatory response and increased microvascular blood flow. These early histopathologic changes are depicted as concentric tissue zones about the point of thermal contact. Coagulation necrosis of the skin and skin appendages results in loss of normal skin functions; the antimicrobial barrier is destroyed, control of water evaporation is lost, and regulation of body temperature is impaired.

MECHANISMS OF EDEMA FORMATION

Following thermal injury, edema formation in the burn wound and in unburned tissues is greatest in the first 6 hours following injury and continues to a lesser extent for the first 24 hours postburn. Postcapillary venular constriction results in a marked increase in capillary hydrostatic pressure and the production of interstitial edema in the early postinjury phase. In an animal model of burn injury, a strongly negative interstitial fluid hydrostatic pressure has been shown to occur within 30 minutes following injury. The duration and magnitude of the negative hydrostatic pressure change was proportionate to the size of the burn. An early increase in the interstitial fluid colloid osmotic pressure following burn injury resulting in a reversal of the transcapillary osmotic pressure gradient has also been reported. Following initial changes in the physical characteristics of burn tissue, subsequent edema formation has been generally attributed to an increase in microvascular permeability due to the effects of humoral factors liberated from burned tissue and cytokines produced by activated leukocytes. The plasma concentration of histamine, a potent regulator of

* The views of the authors do not purport to reflect the position of the Department of the Army and the Department of Defense.

Table 36–1. American Burn Association burn center referral guidelines.

Any burn > 10% of TBSA in patients ages < 10 years or > 50 years.
Burns involving > 20% of TBSA, any age.
Full-thickness burns involving > 5% of TBSA.
Burns of hands, face, feet, genitalia, perineum, or major joints.
Significant electrical burn injury.
Significant chemical burn injury.
Inhalation injury, concomitant mechanical trauma, significant preexisting medical disorders.

TBSA = total body surface area.

vascular permeability present in abundance in mast cells, rises in proportion to burn size immediately following injury. Many inflammatory mediators, including activated proteases, prostaglandins, leukotrienes, fibrin degradation products, and substance P have been reported to increase microvascular permeability following burn injury. Specific antagonists to these agents have been shown to decrease but not eliminate edema formation when administered prior to burn injury. The efficacy of inflammatory mediator antagonists in decreasing microvascular permeability when administered following burn injury has not been demonstrated conclusively.

Leukocyte activation results in the production of cytokines and other factors capable of increasing microvascular permeability. Lysosomal enzymes, increased xanthine oxidase activity, products of complement activation, and oxygen radicals are generated following thermal injury and are capable of increasing microvascular permeability and burn wound edema. Interleukin-2-activated human killer lymphocytes have been shown to increase albumin flux across monolayers of cultured endothelial cells in vitro. Even though neutrophil depletion has been reported to protect against postburn lung injury, it did not reduce burn wound edema formation. The response of the leukocyte appears to depend on the agent of injury, the proximity to the site of injury, and exposure to humoral mediators.

Edema formation also occurs in unburned tissues following a major burn. Conflicting reports exist concerning the mechanism of this edema formation. In animal studies, an increase in the ratio of lymph to plasma protein measured in uninjured extremities following burn injury, as well as an increase in extravasation of radiolabeled albumin into uninjured tissue, has been described. Others were unable to demonstrate a change in ratios of lymph to serum protein from an uninjured sheep extremity following burn injury, implying that no change in vascular permeability in the uninjured extremity had occurred. Edema accumulation may be massive in unburned tissue following thermal injury, and despite the conflicting reports, it is most likely due to changes in oncotic pressure and the dilutional effects resulting from the infusion of large volumes of crystalloid fluid required for burn resuscitation. Edema formation is characterized by a shift of fluid and protein from the intravascular into the extravascular compartment. Volume shifts occur in proportion to the extent of burn, resulting in decreased blood volume and decreased cardiac output, which, if untreated, progress to hypovolemic shock.

ORGAN SYSTEM RESPONSES TO BURN INJURY

The magnitude and duration of the prototype organ response to thermal injury of early hypofunction and later hyperfunction is dependent upon the extent of injury.

Cardiovascular System

During the resuscitative phase, the initial cardiovascular response to thermal injury is manifested by decreased cardiac output and increased peripheral vascular resistance followed by a progressive increase in cardiac output and decrease in peripheral vascular resistance during the hypermetabolic flow phase. The fall in cardiac output is proportionate to the size of the burn and attributable to the loss of fluid and protein from the intravascular into the extravascular compartment. There is a corresponding reflex increase in peripheral vascular resistance as a consequence of the neurohumoral response to hypovolemia. A myocardial depressive factor has been implicated as the cause of initial impaired myocardial performance; however, this factor has not been identified. Clinical studies have demonstrated that in the absence of heart disease, the ventricular ejection fraction and velocity of myocardial fiber shortening were increased following thermal injury and that hypovolemia, as measured by decreased left ventricular end-diastolic volume, was the cause of depressed cardiac output. Fluid resuscitation following burn injury improves cardiac performance as hypovolemia is corrected. As microvascular permeability decreases, the plasma volume deficit is replenished in the second 24 hours, and cardiac output increases to supranormal levels. Peripheral vascular resistance decreases below normal, and the postburn hypermetabolic state, which peaks in the second postburn week and slowly recedes thereafter, is established. Studies have demonstrated that the postresuscitation increase in cardiac output is primarily directed toward the burn wound, ie, the blood flow to a burned extremity is significantly increased compared to an unburned extremity in the same patient, and the increase is proportionate to the extent of burn on the involved extremity. As a consequence, a decrease in cardiac output secondary to hypovolemia or pharmacologic intervention may reduce the flow of oxygen and nutrients to the wound and impair wound healing.

Lungs

Following thermal injury, even in the absence of associated smoke inhalation, physiologic changes in pulmonary function occur. Immediately postburn, minute ventilation is unchanged or slightly increased as a result of anxiety- and pain-induced hyperventilation. With the initiation of fluid resuscitation, respiratory rate and tidal volume progressively increase, resulting in a minute ventilation which may be two to two and one-half times normal. The magnitude of this increase is proportionate to the extent of burn and is considered to reflect postinjury hypermetabolism. In patients with circumferential burns of the thorax, the unyielding eschar and underlying edema may restrict ventilation to the point of requiring escharotomy incisions to relieve the restrictive ventilatory defect.

Pulmonary vascular resistance increases immediately following thermal injury, and that increase is more prolonged than the increase in peripheral vascular resistance. The release of vasoactive amines and other mediators following thermal injury may be responsible for the increased pulmonary vascular resistance, and this process may exert a protective effect during fluid resuscitation by decreasing pulmonary capillary hydrostatic pressure and thus prevent pulmonary edema. Lung lymph flow studies have demonstrated no change in pulmonary capillary permeability following cutaneous thermal injury. Complement activation and generation of the chemotactic peptide C5A have been shown to be temporally related to neutropenia, aggregation of leukocytes in pulmonary capillaries, and intra-alveolar hemorrhages. In other laboratory studies, preburn depletion of complement, neutrophils, and platelets was protective of postinjury lung dysfunction. Preinjury treatment with catalase and superoxide dismutase also improve postburn pulmonary function, implicating toxic oxygen products produced by activated neutrophils as mediators of the postburn pulmonary dysfunction.

Whether or not the infusion of large volumes of crystalloid solutions associated with burn resuscitation causes postburn pulmonary changes remains controversial. The accumulation of chest wall edema, exacerbated by infusion of large volumes of resuscitation fluid, decreases total lung compliance and promotes atelectasis and hypoxemia. Furthermore, overzealous initial fluid resuscitation may result in florid pulmonary edema as the edema fluid is resorbed during the third to fifth days postburn. Consequently, the smallest volume of resuscitation fluid which maintains adequate organ perfusion should be administered to avoid secondary pulmonary complications.

Kidneys

The renal response following thermal injury parallels that of the cardiovascular response. In the immediate postburn period, renal blood flow and the glomerular filtration rate are reduced in proportion to the size of the burn and the magnitude of the intravascular volume deficit. Delayed or inadequate fluid resuscitation may cause inadequate renal perfusion and lead to acute tubular necrosis and renal failure. Following a successful resuscitation phase, cardiac output and renal blood flow are increased as edema fluid is resorbed. A diuretic response is observed during the period of edema resorption; however, this response may be modified by a large evaporative loss of fluids through the wound surface and slow rates of edema resorption in patients with large surface area burns. Despite the markedly increased cardiac output and renal plasma flow seen in the flow phase of burn injury, the blood volume of patients measured by ^{51}Cr red blood cell labeling was only 81% of predicted values. Plasma renin activity and antidiuretic hormone levels are elevated as predicted by the decreased blood volume despite the findings of increased blood flow to the kidney. This may explain in part the propensity for sodium retention to occur during the course of treatment for thermal injury. As in other organ systems, the duration of changes in renal physiology is related to the timing of wound closure by primary healing or autografting. Owing to the increased renal blood flow, drugs excreted by the kidneys tend to have markedly shortened half-lives, and appropriate dosing adjustments of these drugs are necessary.

Gastrointestinal Tract & Liver

Gastrointestinal and hepatic dysfunction are also related to the magnitude of thermal injury. In patients with burns of more than 25% of the total body surface, ileus, resulting from the combined effects of hypovolemia and neurohumoral changes, is a prominent feature. Nasogastric intubation for gastric decompression is usually required. Following resuscitation, normal gastrointestinal motility commonly returns by the third to fifth postburn day. Focal ischemic mucosal lesions of the stomach and duodenum may be observed as early as 3–5 hours following burn injury, and in the absence of stress ulcer prophylaxis these early lesions may progress to frank ulceration. Intestinal bacterial translocation following thermal injury has been extensively studied in the laboratory, and increased intestinal permeability to low-molecular-weight sugars has been identified as a prodrome to the onset of infection in thermally injured patients. However, the clinical significance and therapeutic implications of these findings are yet to be fully elucidated.

As the magnitude of a burn increases, so does the likelihood of early postburn hepatic dysfunction. An initial increase in the hepatic aminotransferase is common following burns of more than 50% of the body surface area. This is most likely due to the acute reduction in cardiac output, increased blood viscosity, and associated splanchnic vasoconstriction that occur immediately following thermal injury. Following successful fluid resuscitation, the hepatic enzymes promptly return to normal in most patients. The magnitude of initial enzyme derangements has not been predictive of outcome; however, the early onset of jaundice following thermal injury is associated with a poor prognosis, probably indicating preinjury hepatic dysfunction or severely compromised hepatic perfusion during the resuscitative phase. The onset of hepatic dysfunction later in the postburn period is usually manifested by hyperbilirubinemia and elevation of liver enzymes in a cholestatic pattern. These changes are most often associated with sepsis or multiple organ failure.

Nervous System

Nonspecific neurologic changes such as increased anxiety and disorientation are commonly observed in patients with extensive thermal injury and are most likely due to the neurohumoral stress response and intensive care unit isolation. Specific neurologic changes are more commonly observed in patients with high-voltage electrical injury or mechanical trauma. Changing neurologic symptoms and signs, manifested by increasing disorientation, obtundation, or seizures, may be the earliest indications of hypoxemia, electrolyte or fluid imbalance, sepsis, or the toxic effects of medications. Changes in neurologic findings require prompt intervention to identify and correct such abnormalities.

Endocrine System

The metabolic response to thermal injury is also proportionate to the extent of burn and follows the typical biphasic response documented in other organ systems. Immediately following burn injury, during the period of hypovolemia, the metabolic rate decreases; however, as resuscitation progresses, a catabolic or hypermetabolic hormonal pattern emerges. Serum levels of catecholamines, glucagon, and cortisol increase, whereas insulin and triiodothyronine levels are decreased. There is an increase in net glucose flow, with relative peripheral insulin resistance and a markedly negative nitrogen balance. As the burn wounds heal or are closed by autografting, the catabolic hormone response dissipates; an anabolic state is eventually attained; and restoration of lean body mass ensues. Septic complications superimposed on thermal injury initially exaggerate the hypermetabolic response, but if the septic state persists, progressive deterioration and multisystem organ failure, characterized by hypometabolism, may occur.

Hematopoietic System

Destruction of red blood cells following thermal injury occurs to an extent proportion to the size and depth of burn. In areas of full-thickness burn, red cells are immediately coagulated in the involved microvasculature. There is a continuing red cell loss in patients with extensive burns of 8–12% of the red cell mass per day caused by the continued lysis of cells damaged by heat, microvascular thrombosis in zones of ischemia that subsequently become necrotic, and repeated blood sampling. In the early postburn period, platelet number and fibrinogen levels are depressed, with a corresponding rise in fibrin split products. Following resuscitation, platelets and serum levels of fibrinogen and factors V and VIII rapidly increase to supranormal levels. Erythropoietin levels are increased coincident with the anemia following thermal injury. Recent studies have suggested that the rate of erythropoiesis may be further increased by the administration of recombinant erythropoietin and iron. However, a decrease in transfusion requirements has yet to be demonstrated.

Immunologic Response

Infection remains the major cause of death among burn patients. Following injury, dysfunction of the cellular and humoral immune response occurs which is related to the extent of injury. Destruction of the normal skin barrier results in loss of mechanical protection from microbial proliferation and allows microbial invasion into normal tissues. Modern burn care—with emphasis on effective topical antimicrobial agents, infection control policies, and timely excision with autograft closure of burn wounds—has significantly decreased the incidence of burn wound infection. Other infectious complications, principally pneumonia, remain the major source of morbidity and mortality, and treatment may be made difficult by the generalized immune system dysfunction following thermal injury.

During the first week postburn, the total white blood cell count is elevated, though peripheral blood lymphocyte counts are reduced. Burn injury also causes apoptosis of lymphocytes in various solid organs following burn injury. This process is glucocorticoid-mediated and can be blocked experimentally by the administration of glucocorticoid receptor antagonists. This process is not TNF-α- or Fas ligand-dependent and may represent a counterregulatory mechanism to reduce inflammatory stimuli. Delayed hypersensitivity reactions and peripheral blood lymphocyte proliferation in the mixed lymphocyte reaction are both inhibited following thermal injury. Alterations in lymphocyte subpopulations have been described which normalize over the second postburn week in patients whose course is uncomplicated. Further alterations occur prior to and during the onset of septic complications. Alterations in IL-2 production and IL-2 receptor expression by lymphocytes have been measured following burn injury, and direct correlation has been established between the extent of burn and the decrease of IL-2 production by peripheral blood lymphocytes. Septic complications result in a further decrement in IL-2 production.

Serum IgG levels are decreased following burn injury and gradually return to normal over 2–4 weeks as the patient recovers. Restoration of IgG levels to normal by exogenous administration has not been shown to affect morbidity or mortality. Many investigators, using a number of experimental approaches, have demonstrated immunosuppressive factors present in the serum of thermally injured patients. Similar immunosuppressive properties have been detected in burn blister fluid. Immunosuppressive polypeptides have been the most commonly invoked agents; however, other factors, including complement degradation products, immunoglobulin fragments, prostaglandins, and endocrine secretions, occur in the serum following thermal injury.

Alterations in granulocyte chemotaxis, degranulation, adherence, oxygen radical production, and complement receptor expression have been observed following thermal injury. Granulocytes from burned patients exhibit an increase in cytosolic oxidase activity, suggesting in vivo activation. They also exhibit greater than normal oxidase activity after in vitro stimulation. This increase suggests that neutrophils from burned patients have an increased oxidative burst potential which, if activated, could cause increased tissue and organ injury. A marked and sustained increase in neutrophil expression of the complement opsonin receptors CRT and CR3 have been described following burn injury. The increase in receptor expression correlated with decreased chemotaxis in response to zymosan-activated serum, suggesting that C5A was responsible for inducing systemic neutrophil activation. Recent investigations have demonstrated significant elevation of F-actin content and decreased ability to polymerize and depolymerize F-actin in the granulocytes of burn patients when compared with controls. These alterations may be partly responsible for the observed changes in chemotaxis and migration following thermal injury.

Almost every aspect of immunoregulation is affected following burn injury. At present, no effective immunomodulatory treatment has been identified; however, the development of new immunomodulatory drugs and recombinant lymphokines and their antagonists may prove beneficial in correcting immune dysfunction following burn injury.

Aulick LH et al: Influence of the burn wound on peripheral circulation in thermally injured patients. Am J Physiol 1977; 233:H520.

Bowen BD et al: Microvascular exchange during burn injury: III. Implications of the model. Circ Shock 1989; 28:221–33.

Burleson DG et al: Flow cytometric measurement of rat lymphocyte subpopulations after burn injury and burn injury with infection. Arch Surg 1987;122:216–20.

Cioffi WG et al: Dissociation of blood volume and flow in regulation of salt and water balance in burn patients. Ann Surg 1991;214:213–8.

Cioffi WG et al: Granulocyte oxidative activity after thermal injury. Surgery 1992;112:860–5.

Demling RH et al: Early lung dysfunction after major burns: Role of edema and vasoactive mediators. J Trauma 1985;25: 959–66.

Demling RH, Kramer G, Harms B: Role of thermal injury-induced hypoproteinemia on fluid flux and protein permeability in burned and non-burned tissue. Surgery 1984;95:136–44.

Ferrara JJ et al: The suppressive effect of subeschar tissue fluid upon in vitro cell-mediated immunologic function. J Burn Care Rehabil 1988;9:584–8.

Fleming RY et al: The effect of erythropoietin in normal healthy volunteers and pediatric patients with burn injuries. Surgery 1992;112:424–31.

Fukuzuka K et al: Glucocorticoid-induced, caspase-dependent organ apoptosis early after burn injury. Am J Physiol Regul Integr Comp Physiol 2000;278:R1005–18.

Gadd MA et al: Defective T-cell surface antigen expression after mitogen stimulation: An index of lymphocyte dysfunction after controlled murine injury. Ann Surg 1989;209:112–18.

Harms BA et al: Microvascular fluid and protein flux in pulmonary and systemic circulations after thermal injury. Microvasc Res 1982;23:77–86.

Jones WG II et al: Differential pathophysiology of bacterial translocation after thermal injury and sepsis. Ann Surg 1991;214:24–30.

LeVoyer T et al: Alterations in intestinal permeability after thermal injury. Arch Surg 1992;127:26–9.

Lund T, Reed RK: Microvascular fluid exchange following thermal skin injury in the rat: Changes in extravascular colloid osmotic pressure, albumin mass, and water content. Circ Shock 1986;20:91–104.

Ozkan AN, Hoyt DB, Ninnemann JL: Generation and activity of suppressor peptides following traumatic injury. J Burn Care Rehabil 1987;8:527–30.

Pruitt BA Jr, Goodwin CW, Mason AD Jr: Epidemiological, demographic, and outcome characteristics of burn injury in. In: *Total Burn Care,* 2nd ed. Herndon DN (editor). Saunders, 2002.

Pruitt BA Jr, Mason AD Jr, Moncrief JA: Hemodynamic changes in the early postburn patient: The influence of fluid administration and of a vasodilator (hydralazine). J Trauma 1971; 11:36–46.

Pruitt BA Jr: The universal trauma model. Bull Am Coll Surg 1985;70:2. Solomkin JS: Neutrophil disorders in burn injury: complement, cytokines, and organ injury. J Trauma 1990; 30(12 Suppl):S80–85.

Till GO et al: Oxygen radical dependent lung damage following thermal injury of rat skin. J Trauma 1983;23:269–77.

INITIAL CARE OF THE BURN PATIENT

PREHOSPITAL TREATMENT

The primary concern at the accident scene is to stop the burning process. Burning and smoldering clothing should be extinguished. Patients with electrical injury should be separated from points of electric contact, taking all necessary care to avoid injuring oneself. If the burn was caused by a chemical agent, all contaminated clothing should be removed and copious water lavage initiated.

As with all trauma patients, the primary concern during initial assessment is maintenance of cardiopulmonary function. Airway patency and adequacy of ventilation must be maintained and supplemental oxygen administered as necessary. In the absence of associated mechanical trauma or need for cardiopulmonary resuscitation, placement of an intravenous cannula is not necessary if transport to a treatment facility can be accomplished in less than 45 minutes. The application of ice or cold water soaks will relieve pain in areas of second-degree burn. If the cold therapy is initiated within ten minutes after burning, tissue heat content is also reduced and the depth of thermal injury may be lessened. If cold therapy is used, care must be taken to avoid causing hypothermia. Cold soaks or ice should only be used on patients with burns of less than 10% of the body surface and only for the time required to produce analgesia. After the ice or cold soak is removed, the patient should be covered with a clean sheet and blanket to conserve body heat and minimize contamination of the burn wounds during transport to the hospital.

EMERGENCY MANAGEMENT

Upon arrival at the hospital, the patency of the airway and the adequacy of breathing should be reassessed and endotracheal intubation performed if necessary. Intravenous fluid resuscitation is initiated by infusing a physiologic salt solution, eg, lactated Ringer's solution, through a large-bore intravenous cannula. The order of preference for the site of intravenous cannulation is a peripheral vein underlying unburned skin, a peripheral vein underlying burned skin, and, lastly, a central vein.

A history should be obtained, paying special attention to the circumstances of the injury, the presence of preexisting disease, allergies and medications, and the use of illicit drugs or alcohol prior to injury. A complete physical examination should be performed and associated injuries identified. Baseline laboratory data should include an arterial blood gas and pH analysis, serum electrolytes, urea nitrogen, creatinine, and glucose and a complete blood count. If available, continuous transcutaneous pulse oximetry determination of oxygen saturation should be initiated in patients with suspected inhalation injury or extensive burns.

Since all currently used resuscitation formulas are based upon body weight and the percentage of total body surface area burned (TBSB), the patient should be weighed and the depth and extent of burn estimated. The extent of body surface area burned can easily be estimated using the "rule of nines," which recognizes that specific anatomic regions represent 9% or 18% of the total body surface area (Figure 36–1). Since the area of one surface of the patient's hand (palm and digits) represents 1% of that person's total body surface, one can use that relationship in estimating the extent of irregularly distributed burns. Infants and children have a different body surface area distribution, with relatively larger heads and smaller lower extremities. When estimating the body surface burn area for children under age 10, the Lund and Browder burn diagram (Figure 36–2) or other similar diagram should be used to determine the body surface area burned with greater precision.

The depth of burn is classified as partial-thickness or full-thickness with respect to the extent of dermal destruction by coagulation necrosis (Figure 36–3). First- and second-degree burns are considered partial-thickness injuries and third-degree burns full-thickness

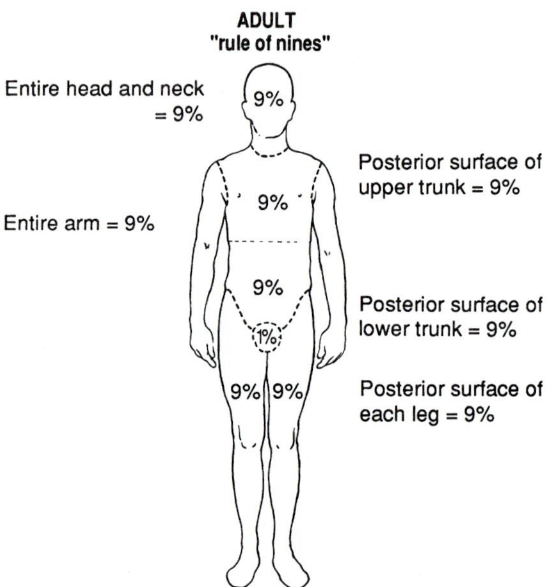

Figure 36–1. Rule of nines, showing distribution of body surface area by anatomic parts in the adult.

BURN ESTIMATE AND DIAGRAM

AGE vs. AREA

Area	Birth 1 yr	1–4 yr	5–9 yr	10–14 yr	15 yr	Adult	2°	3°	Total	Donor Areas
Head	19	17	13	11	9	7				
Neck	2	2	2	2	2	2				
Ant Trunk	13	13	13	13	13	13				
Post Trunk	13	13	13	13	13	13				
R Buttock	2½	2½	2½	2½	2½	2½				
L. Buttock	2½	2½	2½	2½	2½	2½				
Genitalia	1	1	1	1	1	1				
R U Arm	4	4	4	4	4	4				
L.U. Arm	4	4	4	4	4	4				
R L Arm	3	3	3	3	3	3				
L L Arm	3	3	3	3	3	3				
R Hand	2½	2½	2½	2½	2½	2½				
L Hand	2½	2½	2½	2½	2½	2½				
R Thigh	5½	6½	8	8½	9	9½				
L. Thigh	5½	6½	8	8½	9	9½				
R. Leg	5	5	5½	6	6½	7				
L. Leg	5	5	5½	6	6½	7				
R. Foot	3½	3½	3½	3½	3½	3½				
L. Foot	3½	3½	3½	3½	3½	3½				
						TOTAL				

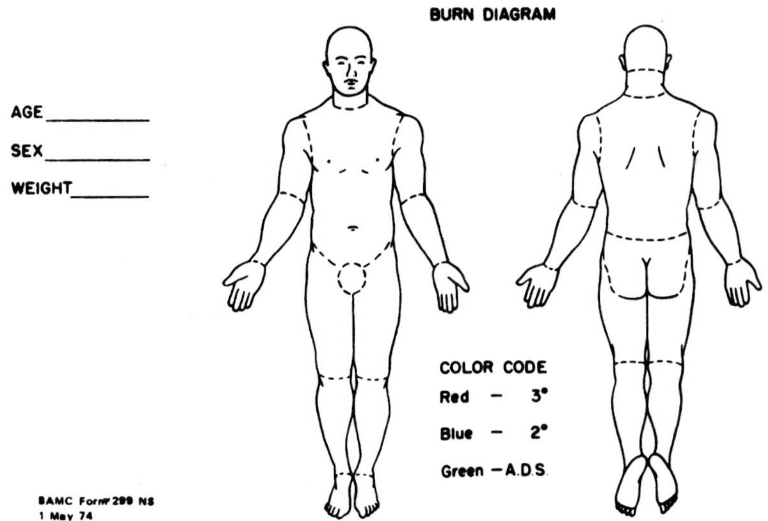

Figure 36–2. The use of a burn diagram permits a more exact estimation of the extent of burn. Note that the surface areas of the head and lower extremities change significantly with age.

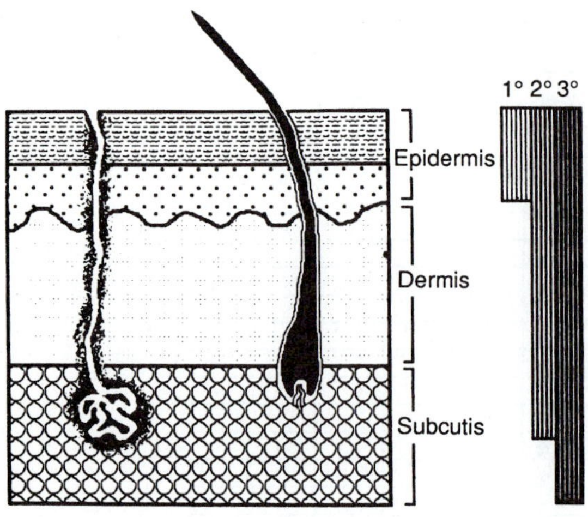

Figure 36–3. Diagram of the skin and subcutaneous tissues demonstrating the depth of burn and relationship to the location of the cutaneous adnexa. First-degree and second-degree burns are considered partial-thickness. Preservation of the hair follicles and sweat glands permits spontaneous healing by epithelial cell migration. Full-thickness (third-degree) burns will not reepithelialize and require skin grafting for closure.

injuries. Superficial partial-thickness burns heal spontaneously by epithelial migration from preserved dermal appendages. Full-thickness injuries have complete destruction of all epithelial elements and require skin grafting for wound closure. Deep partial-thickness burns may heal over a long period of time, but grafting is frequently performed to decrease time to wound closure, reduce scar formation, improve functional outcome, and shorten the hospital stay. The clinical criteria in Table 36–2 permit initial differentiation between the different depths of burn injury. Only the total percentage of skin surface area involved in second- and third-degree burns is calculated or estimated for resuscitation purposes. First-degree burns do not cause significant edema formation or metabolic alteration and are not considered in the calculation of burn size for estimation of resuscitation requirements. Differentiation between second-degree and third-degree burns is more important in the later postburn course, since it has implications for the duration of hypermetabolism, the need for autograft closure of the burn wound, and the anticipated functional result.

The presence of associated mechanical trauma may affect the resuscitation requirements of the thermally injured patient. Soft tissue trauma and bleeding from any injury will increase the fluid required to establish adequate urine output. The presence of thermal injury should not delay or alter the evaluation and subsequent treatment, including operative intervention, of mechanical trauma. An indwelling urethral catheter should be inserted in all patients requiring intravenous fluid therapy, and the urinary output should be measured and recorded hourly. Vital signs and the patient's general condition should be frequently monitored and recorded on a flow sheet. The rectal temperature should be measured hourly, providing a guide for maintenance of core temperature. In patients with high-voltage electrical injury, electrocardiographic monitoring should be initiated in the emergency department.

The tetanus immunization status of the patient should be determined in the emergency department. The burn patient who has been previously immunized against tetanus should be given a booster dose of tetanus toxoid if the last dose was administered more than 5 years previously. Patients with no history of active immunization should receive tetanus immune globulin in addition to an initial dose of tetanus toxoid. Active immunization is subsequently completed according to the routine dosage schedule.

Table 36–2. Characteristics of first-, second-, and third-degree burns.

	First-Degree	Second-Degree	Third-Degree
Cause	Exposure to sunlight, very brief exposure to hot liquid, flash, flame, or chemical agent.	Limited exposure to hot liquid, flash, flame, or chemical agent.	Prolonged exposure to flame, hot object, or chemical agent. Contact with high-voltage electricity.
Color	Red	Pink or mottled red	Pearly white, charred, translucent, or parchment-like. Thrombosed vessels may be visible.
Surface	Dry or very small blisters	Bullae or moist, weeping surface	Dry and inelastic
Sensation	Painful	Painful	Insensate surface

PRINCIPLES OF BURN TREATMENT

FLUID RESUSCITATION

Fluid resuscitation should be started as soon as possible following thermal injury. Generally, burns involving more than 25% of the body surface area require intravenous fluid resuscitation because ileus precludes oral resuscitation. Patients with smaller burns in whom ileus does not develop should have liberal access to electrolyte-containing fluids such as fruit juices or milk, but excessive intake of electrolyte free water should be avoided to prevent hyponatremia. Many formulas have been proposed for calculation of intravenous fluid resuscitation of thermally injured patients (Table 36–3). The central theme is that the volume of fluid required is dependent upon the patient's weight and the extent of burn. Most often, it is recommended that half of the calculated requirement be infused over the first 8 hours following injury, ie, at the time of maximal vascular permeability; the remainder of the first 24-hour resuscitation volume is delivered over the next 16 hours. Certain subgroups of patients require a significantly greater resuscitation volume than that estimated by the formulas. A delay in starting fluid resuscitation, inhalation injury, and ethanol intoxication are frequently associated with greater than predicted fluid requirements. Patients with high-voltage electrical injuries frequently require more resuscitation fluid than that predicted based on the extent of cutaneous injury. One must recognize that any resuscitation formula serves only to guide the initiation of fluid therapy. The actual amount of resuscitation fluid is tailored to each patient's physiologic responses, with frequent reassessment and adjustment of infusion rates as needed to preserve vital organ perfusion.

The various burn formulas in Table 36–3 differ considerably with respect to the volume and composition of the resuscitation fluids; however, each formula has been found to be clinically effective. The general use of burn formulas has decreased the frequency of burn-induced hypovolemic shock and organ dysfunction, which were secondary to inadequate resuscitation. Failure to reevaluate the patient's response to resuscitation frequently on a scheduled basis may lead to over- or underresuscitation. This is frequently observed when the volume of fluid administered is based solely on the initial estimate. With overzealous administration of intravenous fluids, pulmonary, cerebral, and excessive burn wound edema may result. These complications are most evident from the third to sixth postburn days, when vascular permeability has returned to "normal,"

Table 36–3. Commonly used resuscitation formulas.

Formula	Electrolyte-Containing Solution	Colloid-Containing Solution	5% Glucose in Water
FIRST 24 HOURS POSTBURN			
Parkland	Lactated Ringer's, 4 mL/kg per % burn.		
Hypertonic sodium resuscitation	Volume of fluid containing 250 meq of sodium/L to maintain hourly urinary output of 30 mL.		
Modified Brooke	Lactated Ringer's, 2 mL/kg per % burn.		
Consensus[1]	Lactated Ringer's, 2–4 mL/kg per % burn.		
SECOND 24 HOURS POSTBURN			
Parkland		20–60% of calculated plasma volume.	As necessary to maintain urinary output.
Hypertonic sodium resuscitation	33% isotonic salt solution up to 3500 mL limit.		
Modified Brooke		0.3–0.5 mL/kg per % burn[2]	As necessary to maintain urinary output.
Consensus[1]		0.3–0.5 mL/kg per % burn[2]	As necessary to maintain urinary output.

[1]American Burn Association: Advanced Burn Life Support Course.
[2]Administered as a plasma equivalent (eg, 5% albumin in 0.9% sodium chloride solution.)

vascular resistance has decreased, and burn wound edema is being resorbed.

Laboratory and clinical studies evaluating transcapillary fluid movement and the physiologic response to resuscitation have failed to demonstrate a benefit from the use of colloid-containing solutions during the first 24 hours of resuscitation. Extravascular lung water has been shown to remain essentially unchanged during the first week postburn in patients who received only crystalloid-containing fluids in the first 24 hours following injury. However, extravascular lung water increased progressively in patients who received colloid-containing fluids as part of the initial resuscitation. During the latter half of the first week following injury, capillary permeability normalizes and fluid requirements decrease. As this occurs, the use of colloid-containing fluids repletes the intravascular volume deficit more efficiently and with a lesser volume than with crystalloid fluids alone.

The use of hypertonic saline has been proposed as a means of reducing resuscitation fluid volume requirements. Although the initial volume of fluid administered when using hypertonic fluid is clearly less, the proposed benefits of a decreased need for escharotomy, decreased incidence and duration of ileus, and decreased fractional sodium retention have not been found in all studies. Potential problems with hypertonic saline resuscitation include hypernatremia, which, if of sufficient magnitude to require infusion of hypotonic fluid, negates the potential benefits of this resuscitation strategy. The cellular dehydration induced by hypertonic saline infusion of sufficient magnitude (15%) may cause cellular and organ dysfunction necessitating correction with hypotonic fluid administration. Subsequent evaporative water loss from the burn wound may worsen the expected hypernatremia from hypertonic saline resuscitation requiring additional hypotonic fluid infusion. Occasionally, some patients with markedly reduced cardiac reserve may benefit from resuscitation protocols employing hypertonic saline; however, isotonic fluid resuscitation formulas provide adequate resuscitation in the majority of patients. Caution should be observed when implementing hypertonic saline resuscitation, as increases in early acute renal failure and mortality have been reported.

The modified Brooke formula (Table 36–3), which is recommended by the authors, employs a physiologic salt solution during the first 24 hours without the addition of colloid or electrolyte-free crystalloid solutions. Lactated Ringer's is the preferred solution because of its more nearly physiologic concentration of chloride ions compared with normal saline. Fluid needs are estimated as 3 mL (children) or 2 mL (adults) per kilogram body weight per percent TBSB of lactated Ringer's solution. Children have a greater body surface area per unit of body mass and require more resuscitation fluid relative to adults. One-half of the calculated estimate is administered in the first 8 hours and the second half over the subsequent 16 hours postburn. If initiation of fluid resuscitation is delayed, that amount of fluid calculated to be administered in the first 8 hours should be infused at a rate such that half of the estimated 24-hour fluid requirement will be delivered by 8 hours postburn.

In the second 24 hours following burn injury, 5% albumin solution in physiologic saline is administered in an amount proportionate to body weight and the extent of burn to aid in correction of the plasma volume deficit (Table 36–4). During the second 24 hours, lactated Ringer's infusion is stopped and 5% dextrose and water is delivered to maintain adequate urine output.

Monitoring Resuscitation

The objective of fluid resuscitation following thermal injury is maintenance of organ perfusion and function. The adequacy of resuscitation may be assessed by the hemodynamic response, the status of mental function indicating the adequacy of cerebral perfusion, and the volume of urine output, indicating effective renal perfusion.

Patient disorientation, anxiety, and restlessness may be early signs of hypovolemia or hypoxemia that require immediate assessment and correction. Sphygmomanometric monitoring of blood pressure in patients with extensive burns can be misleading. In a burned limb—or in an unburned extremity in which massive edema develops—Korotkoff sounds may be progressively attenuated, falsely implying hypoperfusion. Blood pressure measurements, even when obtained by use of an indwelling peripheral arterial cannula, may not reflect true hydration status because markedly elevated circulating levels of catecholamines and other vasoactive materials may cause severe vasospasm. A resting tachycardia between 100 beats and 120 beats/min is common following thermal injury. Rates above this level may reflect inadequate pain control or inadequate fluid resuscitation. A more objective indication of the adequacy of resuscitation is the rate of production of urine, which reflects the adequacy of renal perfusion. In the absence of osmotically driven diuresis, a urinary output of 30–50 mL/h indicates adequate resuscitation in most adult patients, and 1 mL/kg/h indicates adequate resuscitation in patients weighing less than 30 kg.

Table 36–4. Estimation of colloid replacement during second 24 hours postburn.

30–50% burn: 0.3 mL/kg body weight per % burn
50–70% burn: 0.4 mL/kg body weight per % burn
> 70% burn: 0.5 mL/kg body weight per % burn

Routine use of flow-directed pulmonary artery catheters during burn resuscitation is unnecessary. Even with extensive injury, healthy young adults usually respond to fluid resuscitation in a predictable manner. The previously discussed indicators of adequacy of resuscitation may be used to guide fluid infusion rates. Fluid infusion rates should be adjusted if the hourly urine output is below or above the desired urinary output by more than 33% for 2 consecutive hours. Only those patients who do not respond to fluid resuscitation as expected—or whose fluid administration in the first 6 hours exceeds that volume which will result in a 6 mL/kg per % burn resuscitation—should be monitored with a flow-directed pulmonary artery catheter. If the pulmonary artery occlusion pressure or measurements of right ventricular end-diastolic volume indicate an adequate intravascular volume, this type of patient may benefit from the use of a cardiac inotropic agent to augment cardiac output.

Occasionally, patients manifest a diminished cardiac output with a markedly elevated systemic vascular resistance when pulmonary artery wedge pressures indicate adequate fluid resuscitation. In these patients, administration of a short-acting afterload reducing agent may result in a decrease in the systemic vascular resistance and an increase in the hourly urinary output. Administration of small doses of hydralazine (0.5 mg/kg) has been shown to be effective when used in this manner. In animal models of burn injury, sodium nitroprusside and verapamil administered during the resuscitation period reduced peripheral vascular resistance and increased cardiac output. This therapy should be administered cautiously and only to patients who have received adequate fluid loading. If used inappropriately, the resulting vasodilation will exacerbate the hypovolemia and further depress cardiac output and organ perfusion.

Excessive fluid administration during resuscitation may result in pulmonary edema, increased need for escharotomy, and even the need for fasciotomy in unburned limbs. Recently, the occurrence of intra-abdominal compartment syndrome has been recognized as a complication of excessive fluid resuscitation. An increase in intra-abdominal pressure to greater than 25 mm Hg may impair venous return and decrease cardiac output. This is often associated with elevated peak and mean airway pressures and high pulmonary artery wedge and central venous pressures. It is prudent to monitor intra-abdominal pressure routinely using an indwelling bladder catheter, in patients with extensive burns who receive fluid volumes of more than 25% of preburn total body weight during the resuscitation phase. More importantly, strict attention to the rate of fluid administration and reduction of excessive resuscitation fluid volumes should be emphasized.

Continuous monitoring of arterial blood pressure with indwelling arterial cannulas is not required in uncomplicated burn resuscitations. In patients with inhalation injury or those who do not respond as expected to fluid resuscitation, frequent monitoring of arterial blood gases should be performed and a distal extremity artery should be cannulated to decrease the risk of complications associated with repetitive arterial puncture. Femoral arterial cannulation also has a low complication rate and may be employed if distal arterial cannulation is not possible.

Other measures of perfusion such as serum lactate, base deficit, and intramucosal pH, commonly followed during resuscitation of various shock states, may be difficult to interpret when used to monitor burn resuscitation. An elevation of plasma lactate concentration is frequently observed in severely burned patients and may in part reflect increased circulating levels of catecholamines. Glucose administration increases the rate of glucose oxidation with subsequent increase in plasma lactate and pyruvate concentrations following thermal injury. Thus, caution must be used in interpreting elevated serum lactate levels as related to the adequacy of burn resuscitation and systemic oxygen delivery. Similarly, measurement of the arterial base deficit during burn resuscitation will often yield values as low as −6 even though other measures of resuscitation, such as urinary output, are at normal levels. This may reflect a relative deficit in systemic oxygen delivery; however, the excessive fluid administration required to reverse the base deficit will result in complications of overresuscitation. Measurement of gastric intramucosal P_{CO_2} changes using a gastric tonometer may be used to detect intestinal ischemia during burn resuscitation. Patients with significant gastric acidosis have a mortality rate twice that of patients without acidosis. The deaths in this group were predominantly from multiple organ dysfunction, occurring several weeks after injury. This suggests that intestinal ischemia may still occur in some patients despite apparently adequate fluid resuscitation after thermal injury, inflicting persistent deleterious effects on distant organ function. Conversely, Venkatesh et al have reported depression of gastric mucosal pH in the presence of "normal" indices of systemic circulation and attributed that disparity to selective gastrointestinal vasoconstriction and the development of tissue edema.

At the beginning of the second postburn day, when colloid replacement is initiated and infusion of lactated Ringer's solution is discontinued, the volume of 5% dextrose in water infused per hour should be equal to 25–50% of the preceding hour's volume of lactated Ringer's solution. If the urinary output remains greater than 30 mL/h, that infusion rate should be maintained for the next 3 hours, at which time the rate of infusion of 5% dextrose in water should be further reduced in a similar manner.

Pulmonary function must be continually reassessed throughout the resuscitative phase. Tachypnea may indicate metabolic acidosis from under-resuscitation, hypoxemia, or restriction of chest wall motion due to circumferential burns or massive edema. Evaluation must include auscultation, chest x-rays, and arterial blood gas analysis if a significant tachypnea occurs. Thermally injured patients in the ICU should be monitored with a pulse oximeter. In most patients, hemoglobin saturation by arterial blood gas analysis matches that obtained by pulse oximetry; however, patients with severely burned digits may be difficult to monitor using this method. In addition, a decrease in intensity of the pulsed signal detected in an extremity monitored by pulse oximetry may reflect inadequate distal perfusion from under-resuscitation, constricting circumferential burn wounds, or arterial spasm due to high levels of circulating catecholamines. Low oxygen saturation, as measured by pulse oximetry, may also indicate circulating levels of carboxyhemoglobin or methemoglobin as a consequence of the inhalation of carbon monoxide or cyanide, respectively.

In thermally injured patients requiring endotracheal intubation and mechanical ventilation, end-tidal CO_2 monitoring should be used to detect early changes in ventilation due to inhalation injury or restriction of chest wall motion. This method of monitoring is particularly useful in pressure-controlled modes of mechanical ventilation. Chest radiographs should be obtained at least daily during resuscitation and the period of edema absorption. Subsequent x-rays are ordered as clinically indicated.

Serum chemistry profiles, complete blood count, arterial blood gases, and other baseline blood studies are obtained upon admission, with further tests depending upon the clinical situation. The patient's weight should be measured upon admission and followed daily as an indicator of fluid balance.

Evaporative water loss from the wound typically peaks on the third postburn day and persists until the burn wound is healed or grafted. Insensible water losses may be estimated according to the following formula:

$$\text{Insensible water loss (mL/h)} = (25 + \%\ \text{BSA burned}) \times \text{Total BSA}\ (\text{m}^2)$$

This formula, like the initial resuscitation formulas, is only an estimate, and replacement of evaporative water loss should be guided by assessing the adequacy of hydration by monitoring the patient's weight, serum osmolality, and serum sodium concentrations. Following elimination of the resuscitation-related salt and water load, salt-containing fluids should be administered in the amount needed to maintain a normal serum sodium concentration.

Goodwin CW et al: Randomized trial of efficacy of crystalloid and colloid resuscitation on hemodynamic response and lung water following thermal injury. Ann Surg 1983; 197:520–31.

Gore DC et al: Influence of glucose kinetics on plasma lactate concentrations and energy expenditure in severely burned patients. J Trauma Inj Infect Crit Care 2000;49:673–8.

Gunn ML et al: Prospective randomized trial of hypertonic sodium lactate versus lactated Ringer's solution for burn shock resuscitation. J Trauma 1989;29:1261–7.

Huang PP et al: Hypertonic sodium resuscitation is associated with renal failure and death. Ann Surg 1995;221:543–54.

Ivy ME et al. Intra-abdominal hypertension and abdominal compartment syndrome in burn patients. J Trauma Inj Infect Crit Care 2000;49:387–91.

Lorente JA et al: Systemic hemodynamics, gastric intramucosal P_{CO_2} changes and outcome in critically ill burn patients. Crit Care Med 2000;28:1728–35.

Onarheim H et al: Effectiveness of hypertonic saline-dextran 70 for initial fluid resuscitation of major burns. J Trauma 1990;30: 597–603.

Pruitt BA Jr, Mason AD Jr, Moncrief JA: Hemodynamic changes in the early postburn patient: The influence of fluid administration and of a vasodilator (hydralazine). J Trauma 1971; 11:36–46.

Pruitt BA Jr: Discussion of Caldwell FT and Bowser BH: Critical evaluation of hypertonic and hypotonic solutions to resuscitate severely burned children: A prospective study. Ann Surg 1979;189:551–2.

Venkatesh B et al: Monitoring tissue oxygenation during resuscitation of major burns. J Trauma 2001;50:485–94.

ESCHAROTOMY & FASCIOTOMY

Edema formation beneath the inelastic eschar of circumferential full-thickness burns of the extremities may impair the circulation to the distal and underlying tissues. To prevent secondary ischemic necrosis of those tissues, an escharotomy may be necessary to reduce the elevated tissue pressure. To identify the need for escharotomy, the adequacy of circulation must be assessed at no less than hourly intervals. The most reliable determination is made with a Doppler flowmeter to detect pulsatile blood flow in the palmar arch, digital vessels in the upper limbs, and pedal vessels in the lower limbs. Absence or progressive decrease of pulsatile flow on sequential examination is an indication for escharotomy. Clinical indicators of impaired extremity perfusion, including distal cyanosis, impaired capillary refilling, neurologic deficits, and deep tissue pain, are less precise in determining true impairment of blood flow and should be used only as indications for escharotomy when a Doppler flowmeter is unavailable. Fascial compartment pressure monitoring has also been described following thermal injury. Fascial compartment pressures often exceed 30 mm Hg following circumferential extremity burns, and escharotomy based on compartment pressures has been proposed. A greater sensitivity of direct compartment pressure measurements in detecting critically low flow states and preserving threatened tissues has not been confirmed by direct comparison with Doppler flowmeter assessments. This technique is associated with a risk of infection arising in the pressure cannula tract, but the magnitude of the risk is undefined.

The escharotomy procedure may be performed in the ICU without the use of general or local anesthesia. Since only insensate, full-thickness burn is incised, the use of anesthetic agents is unnecessary. The first escharotomy incision is placed in the midlateral line of the involved extremity. If this does not improve distal blood flow, a second escharotomy incision is made in the mid-medial line of that limb (Figure 36–4). The escharotomy incision should be performed along the entire length of the full-thickness burn to ensure adequate release of vascular and neural compression. The incision must cross involved joints, since the relative lack of subcutaneous tissue in these areas permits ready compression of vessels and nerves. The escharotomy incision should only penetrate the eschar and immediately subjacent thin connective tissue to permit expansion of the edematous subcutis. When performed at this level, loss of blood from the escharotomy incision is minimal and readily controlled by electrocoagulation or application of pressure. When incisions are carried into the subcutaneous tissues, excessive bleeding often occurs. The consumptive coagulopathy that may occur in the early postburn period may contribute to excessive blood loss when escharotomy incisions are made too deep.

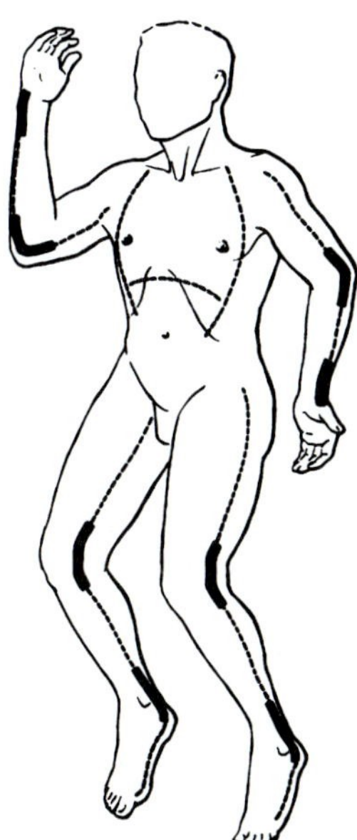

Figure 36–4. The dashed lines show the preferred sites for escharotomy incisions. The solid segments of the lines demonstrate the importance of extending the incisions across joints with full thickness burns.

Fasciotomy is rarely required to restore circulation in a thermally injured limb. However, in patients with high-voltage electrical injury, fasciotomy is often necessary. Patients with very deep burns involving fascia and muscle or patients with associated traumatic injuries may require fasciotomies to restore adequate limb circulation.

Escharotomies may also be required in patients with circumferential truncal burns to relieve restriction of chest wall movement by the unyielding eschar and restore more effective ventilation. The escharotomy incision is made in the anterior axillary line in the area of full-thickness burn. An incision along the lower margin of the rib cage may be necessary in patients with deep burns extending onto the upper abdominal wall (Figure 36–4). Patients may become restless, agitated, and tachypneic despite having an adequate airway, indicating the need for chest escharotomy. In mechanically ventilated patients, the need for escharotomy is manifested by a progressive increase in peak inspiratory pressure, decreased tidal volumes in pressure-controlled ventilation, and an increase in the end-tidal CO_2 fraction. Once chest escharotomy is performed, these changes promptly revert toward normal.

Saffle JR, Zeluff GR, Warden GD: Intramuscular pressure in the burned arm: Measurement and response to escharotomy. Am J Surg 1980;140:825–31.

CARE OF THE BURN WOUND

DEBRIDEMENT

Only after respiratory and hemodynamic stability have been achieved should care of the burn wound be addressed. During transport of the patient from the accident scene or from the initial care facility to a burn center, the burns should be covered with clean sheets or blankets and no attempt made to debride or dress them. In the absence of gross contamination, burn wounds may be safely managed without topical antimicrobial agents for the first 24–48 hours. When the patient arrives at the definitive care facility, general anesthesia is not necessary for initial burn wound debridement; intravenous analgesia is sufficient for pain control during this procedure. The burns are gently cleansed with a surgical soap solution, and nonviable epidermis is debrided. Bullae are excised, and body hair is shaved from the area of thermal injury beyond the margin of normal skin. The patient is placed in a clean bed, and bulky dressings may be placed beneath the burned parts to absorb the serous exudate. These dressings should be changed as they become saturated. Patients should be turned frequently to prevent maceration of burned and unburned skin.

TOPICAL ANTIMICROBIAL THERAPY

The development and clinical use of effective topical antimicrobial agents has significantly decreased the incidence of invasive burn wound infection and subsequent sepsis. This has been associated with improved survival of burn patients and nearly eliminated invasive bacterial burn wound infection as a cause of death. Mafenide (Sulfamylon), silver sulfadiazine (Silvadene), and silver nitrate are the three topical antimicrobial agents most commonly employed for burn wound care. Each agent has specific advantages and limitations with which the physician must be familiar to ensure optimal benefit and patient safety. Mafenide acetate and silver sulfadiazine are available as topical creams to be applied directly to the burn wound. Silver nitrate is applied as a 0.5% solution in occlusive dressings.

Mafenide burn cream is an 8.5% by weight suspension of mafenide acetate in a water-soluble base. Mafenide is very water-soluble and diffuses freely into the eschar. Mafenide is the preferred agent if the patient has heavily contaminated burn wounds or has had burn wound care delayed by several days. Mafenide has the added advantage of being highly effective against gram-negative organisms. The limitations of mafenide burn cream include hypersensitivity reactions in 7% of patients, pain or discomfort of 20–30 minutes' duration when applied to partial-thickness burns, and carbonic anhydrase inhibition. The latter may produce an early bicarbonate diuresis and increase postburn hyperventilation. This metabolic acidosis may develop into significant acidemia if respiratory complications occur and the compensatory hyperventilation is impaired. Carbonic anhydrase inhibition rarely persists for more than 7–10 days, and the severity of acidosis can be minimized if Mafenide is applied once per day followed by an application of silver sulfadiazine cream 12 hours later.

Silver sulfadiazine burn cream is a 1% suspension of silver sulfadiazine in a water-miscible base. Unlike mafenide acetate, silver sulfadiazine has limited solubility in water and thus limited penetration into the eschar. The agent is most effective when applied to burns immediately after injury to minimize bacterial proliferation on the wound's surface. This agent has the advantage of being painless upon application and has no effect on serum electrolytes or acid-base balance. Silver sulfadiazine burn cream may induce neutropenia, which usually subsides after discontinuation of the agent. Hypersensitivity is uncommon and is manifested by an erythematous maculopapular rash on unburned skin. The sulfadiazine component of silver sulfadiazine is ineffective against certain strains of pseudomonas and virtually all enterobacter species; however, the sensitivity of microorganisms colonizing burn wounds to the silver ion of this compound maintains its effectiveness as a topical antimicrobial agent.

Either cream is applied in an ⅛-inch layer to the entire burn wound in an aseptic manner following initial debridement and reapplied at 12-hour intervals to ensure continuous topical chemotherapy. Once each day, all of the topical agent should be cleansed from the patient using a surgical detergent or disinfectant solution and the wounds inspected by the attending physician.

Silver nitrate solution (0.5%) delivered in multilayered occlusive gauze dressings may provide an effective antimicrobial barrier to the burn wound surface. This agent is most commonly employed when a history of allergy to sulfonamide drugs is elicited or when the patient develops a hypersensitivity reaction to one of the burn creams. The dressings are changed two or three times daily and moistened every 2 hours to prevent evaporation from increasing the silver nitrate concentration to cytotoxic levels within the dressings. Transeschar leaching of sodium, potassium, chloride, and calcium should be anticipated and appropriately replaced. Because silver nitrate precipitates upon contact with the proteinaceous exudate of the burn wound and does not penetrate the eschar, it is not effective for treatment of burn wound infection or for prophylactic treatment of heavily contaminated wounds. A common use of silver nitrate is for topical antimicrobial prophylaxis in patients with toxic epidermal necrolysis syndrome, a disorder caused by idiosyncratic drug reactions resulting in significant epidermal sloughing. Hypersensitivity to silver nitrate has not been described.

Acticoat is a new burn wound dressing. It consists of a urethane film onto which nanocrystalline elemental silver is deposited. When moistened, application of this dressing to the wound results in a sustained release of elemental silver, which is bactericidal and fungicidal. The mechanism of action is probably much like that of silver nitrate dressings; however, Acticoat does not cause transeschar leaching of electrolytes. The silver does not penetrate the eschar, limiting its use on infected or heavily contaminated wounds. Transient mild pain may be noted occasionally after application. The use of Acticoat is currently limited to partial-thickness burns.

All of these agents are effective in the prevention of invasive burn wound infection. However, because of their lack of eschar penetration, silver nitrate soaks and silver sulfadiazine burn cream are most effective in the treatment of full-thickness burns when applied immediately following burn injury.

BURN WOUND INFECTION (Figure 36–5)

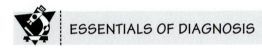

ESSENTIALS OF DIAGNOSIS

- *Hypo- or hyperthermia.*
- *Tachycardia and tachypnea.*
- *Glucose intolerance.*
- *Disorientation.*
- *Ileus.*
- *Change in appearance of the burn wound.*

General Considerations

Inherent characteristics of the microorganisms and the burn wound they colonize influence the rate of microbial penetration of and proliferation in the eschar. The moist, protein-rich, avascular eschar serves as an excellent culture medium from which white blood cells and systemically administered antibiotics are excluded. The density of bacterial colonization of the eschar influences the likelihood of burn wound infection. Bacterial invasion is uncommon unless the number of microorganisms exceeds 10^5 per gram of tissue. Bacterial strain-specific factors such as enzyme production (collagenase, protease, etc), bacterial motility, and antibiotic resistance may be important in the pathogenesis of eschar penetration and invasion of viable tissues.

Although the use of topical chemotherapeutic agents and the timely excision and grafting of the burn wound have decreased the incidence of invasive burn wound infection in most United States burn centers, this problem has not been entirely eliminated. Invasive burn wound infection is uncommon in second-degree burns and in patients with burns of less than 30% of the body surface. Extremes of age and increasing size of burn strongly influence the risk of developing invasive burn wound infection.

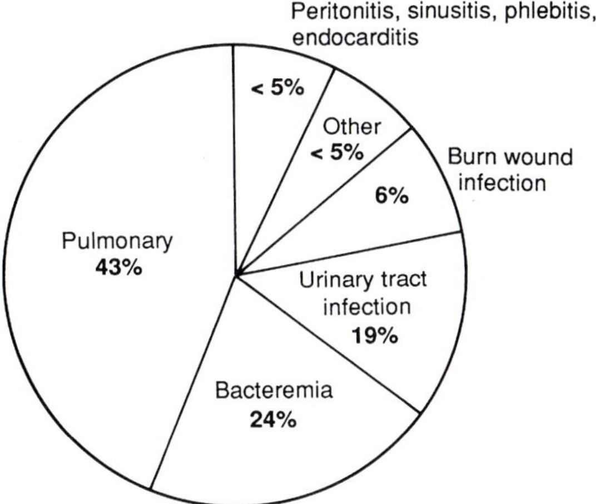

Figure 36–5. The frequency of infection by site expressed as a percentage of all infections complicating thermal injury.

Clinical Features

A. Symptoms and Signs

Clinical signs of invasive burn wound infection are often indistinguishable from those observed in uninfected hypermetabolic burn patients or burn patients with other sources of sepsis and include hyper- or hypothermia, tachycardia, tachypnea, ileus, glucose intolerance, and disorientation. Tinctorial and physical changes in the appearance of the burn wound are more reliable signs of invasive burn wound infection (Table 36–5). The development of clinical signs and symptoms of sepsis in the thermally injured patient should prompt a thorough examination of the burn wound to identify areas suspicious for invasive infection.

B. Laboratory Findings

Surface cultures of the eschar cannot distinguish colonization from invasive infection. Quantitative bacteriologic cultures of burn wound tissue correlate poorly with the presence of invasive burn wound infection. Quantitative bacteriologic counts less than 10^5 per gram of biopsy tissue correlate with absence of invasive burn wound infection; however, even when quantitative counts exceed 10^5 organisms per gram of biopsy tissue, histologic examination confirms invasive infection in less than half of biopsy specimens.

Histologic examination of a biopsy of the burn wound and underlying viable tissue is the most rapid

Table 36–5. Clinical signs of burn wound infection.

Conversion of second-degree burn to full-thickness necrosis
Focal dark brown or black discoloration of wound
Degeneration of wound with "neoeschar" formation
Unexpectedly rapid eschar separation
Hemorrhagic discoloration of subeschar fat
Erythematous or violaceous, edematous wound margin
Metastatic septic lesions in unburned tissue

and reliable method for differentiating microbial colonization of nonviable eschar from microbial invasion of viable subeschar tissue. The latter defines invasive burn wound infection. A burn wound biopsy is performed as an ICU procedure. A 500-mg elliptical biopsy (0.5 × 1.0 cm) including subjacent unburned tissue is obtained by scalpel dissection from the area of the burn wound identified as suspicious for infection. Hemostasis is achieved by application of direct pressure or by electrocoagulation. One half of the specimen is cultured for organism identification and antibiotic sensitivities, and the other half is submitted for histologic analysis. The presence of microorganisms in viable tissue confirms the diagnosis of invasive burn wound infection. The histologic staging scheme for burn wound colonization and infection is presented in Table 36–6. If only colonization (stage 1A to stage 1C) is present, no specific change in antimicrobial therapy is indicated unless serially obtained specimens document a progression of colonization stage. If stage 2 (invasion) is reported, prompt treatment for invasive burn wound infection should begin.

Treatment

When the diagnosis of invasive burn wound infection is made, local and systemic antimicrobial therapy is initiated. In the case of bacterial burn wound invasion, topical chemotherapy should be in the form of twice-daily applications of mafenide acetate because of its superior eschar penetration. Systemic antibiotic therapy is initiated based on prior surface cultures or burn center organism prevalence. Further refinements in therapy are based on biopsy, culture, and sensitivity results. Customary critical care supportive measures are employed to maintain hemodynamic and respiratory stability.

Table 36–6. Histologic staging of burn wound infection.

Stage I: Colonization
- **A. Superficial:** Sparse microbial population on burn wound surface.
- **B. Penetration:** Microorganisms present in variable thickness of eschar.
- **C. Proliferation:** Dense population of microorganisms at interface of nonviable and viable tissue.

Stage II: Invasion
- **A. Microinvasion:** Microscopic foci of microorganisms in viable tissue immediately subjacent to subeschar space.
- **B. Generalized:** Widespread penetration of microorganisms deep into viable subcutaneous tissues.
- **C. Microvascular:** Involvement of lymphatics and microvasculature.

Subeschar antibiotic clysis of the infected area with a broad-spectrum penicillin is recommended at 12 hours and immediately prior to operation to minimize the risk of hematogenous seeding and florid septic shock at the time of eschar excision. Half of the daily dose of a broad-spectrum penicillin (piperacillin, ticarcillin) delivered in 1 L of normal saline is infused into the subeschar tissues by means of a No. 20 spinal needle. Excision of the burn wound to the level of the investing fascia is employed to ensure removal of all nonviable tissue. The wound is usually treated with moist dressings of 5% mafenide acetate, 0.5% silver nitrate, or a biologic dressing. The patient is returned to the operating room in 24–48 hours for wound inspection and redebridement or split-thickness skin grafting as needed.

In addition to bacteria, fungi and yeasts also cause invasive burn wound infection and have become the predominant organisms causing burn wound infection as topical therapy and early excision have reduced the incidence of bacterial infection. Candida species commonly colonize wounds but rarely cause invasive burn wound infection. Aspergillus, the most common filamentous fungus that causes invasive burn wound infection, usually remains confined to subcutaneous tissues and seldom transverses fascial planes. Wounds colonized by candida or aspergillus can be treated with topical application of clotrimazole, but histologic evidence of invasion requires surgical burn wound excision and initiation of systemic amphotericin B therapy. The phycomycetes often behave in a manner similar to aspergillus; however, these organisms may spread rapidly along tissue plains, invade blood vessels, and penetrate fascia. Aggressive wide debridement, including amputation, may be necessary to control these infections.

Becker WK et al: Fungal burn wound infection: A 10-year experience. Arch Surg 1991;126:44–8.

McManus AT: *Pseudomonas aeruginosa:* A controlled burn pathogen? Antibiot Chemother 1989;42:103–8.

McManus WF, Goodwin CW Jr, Pruitt BA Jr: Subeschar treatment of burn-wound infection. Arch Surg 1983;118:291–4.

Pruitt BA Jr: The diagnosis and treatment of infection in the burn patient. Burns 1984;11:79–91.

Waymack J, Pruitt BA Jr: Burn wound care. Adv Surg 1990; 23:261–89.

BURN WOUND EXCISION & GRAFTING

Technique

The current operative management of burns employs tangential excision of eschar to viable dermis or fat and scalpel excision to the level of the investing fascia for burn wound removal. Burn wound excision may be performed early in the postburn course once the patient is hemodynamically stable and resuscitation is complete.

The operative procedure should be limited to excision of 20% of the body surface area, an area of excision producing a blood loss equal to the patient's blood volume, or 2 hours of operative time. Careful anesthetic management is imperative to avoid hypotension and hypothermia. Hypotension may impair blood flow to areas of second-degree burn, resulting in ischemia of the wound and conversion to full-thickness injury. The depth of excision in tangential and sequential burn wound removal is governed by the appearance of healthy tissue and punctate bleeding from dermal beds. Scalpel excision of burns involves removal of the wound and underlying subcutaneous tissue to the level of the investing muscle fascia. This may be accomplished more rapidly and with significantly less blood loss than tangential or sequential wound excisions. Once a viable wound surface is obtained, wound coverage is accomplished with autograft or biologic dressings.

Conventional skin grafting is achieved with cutaneous autografts 0.008–0.012 inches thick. These grafts may be employed as a sheet graft or meshed to provide expansion ratios ranging from 1.5:1 to 9:1. Expansion ratios of 4:1 or greater require a prolonged time for interstitial closure, have a greater propensity for scar formation, and are only utilized in patients with massive burns and limited donor sites. Following grafting, occlusive dressings moistened with topical antibiotic agents are applied. The wounds are kept moist to prevent desiccation until the interstices of the graft have epithelialized.

Skin Substitutes & Biologic Dressings

In massively burned patients, the disparity between donor site area and burn wound area requires the use of temporary skin substitutes or biologic dressings to effect wound closure while awaiting donor site availability. Biologic dressings prevent desiccation of the wound bed, decrease protein and fluid losses, promote angiogenesis of granulation tissue, and reduce pain. Viable cadaver allograft currently provides the best temporary wound coverage. Allograft becomes vascularized from the underlying wound bed and usually remains adherent until surgically excised or immunologically rejected by the patient. As a result of the immunosuppression associated with thermal injury, the allograft may remain intact, vascularized, and viable for several weeks following application. The same theoretical risks of disease transmission (hepatitis, HIV infection, etc) associated with organ donation apply to the use of cadaveric allografts. Appropriate tissue banking measures are imperative. In addition to fresh cadaver allograft, frozen and lyophilized allograft is available from many sources.

Porcine xenograft is also available as a fresh, frozen, or lyophilized preparation. Advantages include an abundant supply and lower cost. This biologic dressing, however, does not become vascularized and adheres to the wound bed by fibrin bonding. The underside of the graft is nourished by the plasma circulation, and desiccation and necrosis of the outer surface usually occur within 1 week. Application of porcine cutaneous xenografts to superficial partial-thickness wounds facilitates healing and decreases pain. Porcine xenografts are of limited usefulness in the coverage of excised wounds because of their lack of vascularization and the limited time until desiccation and necrosis occur.

Several synthetic skin substitutes have been developed in an attempt to avoid the problems of disease transmission and storage requirements common to biologic dressings. The most successful materials have been of a bilaminated configuration with an outer layer mimicking epidermis, which allows water vapor transmission and prevents bacterial contamination. The inner dermal layer is designed to promote adherence and fibrovascular ingrowth from the wound bed. Biobrane is currently the most commonly used synthetic skin substitute. The epidermal layer is composed of pliable Silastic, and the dermal component is derived from porcine collagen. This product is available with a variety of pore sizes, and its elastic nature allows freedom of motion and is well adapted to body contours. Biobrane promotes healing of second-degree burns and usually provides adequate short-term coverage for excised wounds, though submembrane suppuration and lack of adherence cause difficulties. Integra is a synthetic dermal substitute which is unique in that a neodermis is formed by fibrovascular ingrowth into a glycosaminoglycan matrix dermal analogue. The epidermal component is Silastic and is removed once the dermal analogue is vascularized, allowing definitive closure of the wound with ultrathin split-thickness autografts. This permits more rapid healing of donor sites for repeated autograft harvesting. Incomplete adherence, submembrane suppuration, and technical problems with the application of ultrathin autografts have been observed.

TransCyte is a bilaminated biosynthetic skin substitute used as a temporary dressing on second-degree burns or excised full-thickness burns. This product is composed of Biobrane on which human foreskin-derived neonatal dermal fibroblasts are seeded and grown to confluence in culture. The fibroblasts secrete matrix proteins and growth factors that remain active after the product is frozen. Application of TransCyte to the wound surface is similar to that of Biobrane. It also carries the same limitations.

The availability of commercial laboratories capable of carrying out skin culture techniques has led to the recent evaluation of cultured autologous keratinocytes for coverage of wounds in massively burned patients. Current culture techniques require 3 or more weeks of preparation for a product six to eight epidermal cells in thickness. These grafts are quite fragile and susceptible to bacterial colonization of the recipient wound bed and minimal shear forces. The use of cultured autologous keratinocytes effect wound closure in massively burned patients was recently studied. In a series of 16 patients with an average burn size greater than 60% of BSA, definitive final engraftment covered only 4.7% of the body surface area at a cost of over $9000 per percent of BSA closed. Wound bed microbial colonization, lack of dermal elements, and patient age may be significant factors relating to the failure of culture-derived cells as a definitive form of burn wound coverage. This technology has the potential for providing timely coverage of large surface areas but is presently limited by the aforementioned problems.

Hansbrough JF: Current status of skin replacements for coverage of extensive burn wounds. J Trauma 1990;30(12 Suppl): S155–60.

Hansbrough JF et al: Burn wound closure with cultured autologous keratinocytes and fibroblasts attached to a collagen-glycosaminoglycan substrate. JAMA 1989;262:2125–30.

Heimbach D et al: Artificial dermis for major burns: A multicenter randomized clinical trial. Ann Surg 1988;208:313–20.

Pruitt BA Jr, Levine NS: Characteristics and uses of biologic dressings and skin substitutes. Arch Surg 1984;119:312–22.

Pruitt BA Jr, McManus WF, McDougal WS: Surgical management of burns. In: *Operative Surgery: Principles and Techniques.* Nora FP (editor). Saunders, 1990.

INHALATION INJURY

ESSENTIALS OF DIAGNOSIS

- *Facial burns.*
- *Intraoral burns or carbonaceous sputum.*
- *Edema, erythema, mucosal ulcerations on laryngoscopy.*
- *Increased ^{133}Xe retention.*
- *Decreased Pao_2 and expiratory flow rates.*

General Considerations

Pulmonary injury from smoke inhalation is frequently observed in patients with thermal injury who require admission to a burn center. In a recent series, 33% of patients had concomitant inhalation injury. The injury caused by the inhalation of smoke or toxic gases may include chemical damage to the respiratory system, carbon monoxide toxicity, and, infrequently, direct thermal injury to the tracheobronchial tree. Patients most likely to have inhalation injury are those with burns sustained in a closed space and those who were burned during a period of depressed consciousness secondary to head trauma or drug intoxication.

Direct thermal injury to the airway is rarely encountered in patients who survive a fire and are hospitalized for treatment. However, autopsy series of patients dying at the scene of the fire frequently reveal devastating direct thermal injury to the airways. The effective cooling capabilities of the nasopharynx and oropharynx prevent significant heat exposure of the lower respiratory system; however, direct thermal injury to the supraglottic airway does occur and may lead to upper airway obstruction. An exception is burns caused by exposure to steam, since water has a heat-carrying capacity 4000 times greater than that of air.

Smoke inhalation—particularly when the injury occurred in a closed space—may be associated with carbon monoxide poisoning, which may impair tissue oxygenation. The presence of carboxyhemoglobin or the chemical alteration of the cytochrome system by carbon monoxide does not affect the amount of dissolved oxygen in the blood; thus, the Pao_2 will remain normal. However, saturation of hemoglobin by oxygen may be markedly reduced, impairing oxygen delivery.

The inhalation of smoke (incomplete products of combustion) is manifest by deleterious effects on both the airway and the pulmonary vasculature. The anatomic location of pulmonary injury is dependent on the size of the inhaled particle. When the particle diameter is less than 0.05 μm, the larger, endoscopically visible airways may appear normal in the presence of severe alveolar and terminal bronchiolar inflammatory damage. Alternatively, the larger airways may be severely inflamed, leading to mucosal ulceration or necrosis in the presence of relatively normal gas exchange and alveolar function.

In various animal models of inhalation injury, increased pulmonary microvascular permeability and peribronchial edema have been reproduced. Thromboxane A_2 levels have been found to increase within 5 minutes of inhalation injury, with levels correlating with increases in lung lymph flow and extravascular lung water. The role of the neutrophil in the pathophysiology of smoke inhalation is currently under investigation. Both the preinjury induction of a neutropenic state by administration of mechlorethamine and postinjury treatment with pentoxifylline have been reported to attenuate pulmonary artery hypertension, reduce pulmonary vascular resistance, and decrease the severity of pulmonary insufficiency following smoke exposure in animals. Although alterations in surfactant function have been described following smoke inhalation, surfactant replacement has not been shown to improve pulmonary function in animal models of inhalation injury.

Clinical Features

A. Symptoms and Signs

Smoke inhalation should be suspected in patients with facial burns, singed facial hair and nasal fibrissae, intraoral burns or carbonaceous deposits in the oropharynx, or a history of being burned in a closed space.

B. Bronchoscopy

The diagnosis of inhalation injury is made by examination of the upper airway and tracheobronchial tree by fiberoptic bronchoscopy. Direct laryngoscopy may also be used to visualize the upper airway. The presence of carbonaceous material, edema, erythema, or mucosal ulcerations below the vocal cords confirms the diagnosis. An endotracheal tube of appropriate size should be placed over the fiberoptic bronchoscope before the examination so that intubation may be readily achieved if the appearance of upper airway edema threatens airway patency. False-negative bronchoscopic examinations occasionally occur and are usually secondary to the failure to observe inflammation and erythema in the hypovolemic patient with impaired tracheal mucosa perfusion.

C. Radionuclide Studies

^{133}Xe ventilation-perfusion lung scans may be performed in patients in whom the clinical suspicion of inhalation injury is high yet the bronchoscopic examination appears relatively normal. After intravenous injection of 10 μCi of ^{133}Xe, serial chest scintigraphs are obtained. Retention of the gas in the lungs for over 90 seconds following injection or an unequal distribution of radiation density is considered diagnostic of inhalation injury. The false-negative and false-positive rates from this study are 5% and 8%, respectively. False-negatives result from marked hyperventilation and false-positives from preexisting chronic obstructive pulmonary disease, bronchitis, or atelectasis.

D. Respiratory Function Studies

Measurements of pulmonary function may also be helpful in establishing the diagnosis of inhalation injury. Burn patients with inhalation injury may have a decreased arterial $Pa{CO_2}$ and peak expiratory flow and an increased ventilation-perfusion gradient, airway resistance, and nitrogen washout slope. Static and dynamic compliance tend to be normal in the early phase of inhalation injury. The complexity of some pulmonary function tests and the requirement for full patient cooperation often limit their clinical usefulness as aids to the early diagnosis of inhalation injury.

The diagnosis of inhalation injury can be made with 96% accuracy when the results of fiberoptic bronchoscopy, ventilation-perfusion scanning, and pulmonary function testing are combined. Overdiagnosis of inhalation injury accounts for the 4% error.

Treatment

A. General Measures

The current treatment of inhalation injury is primarily supportive, since no specific agent has been identified that minimizes the severity of the insult. The aim of treatment, therefore, is to correct the underlying pulmonary insufficiency while minimizing further iatrogenic pulmonary insults. The amount of intervention required is guided by the severity of pulmonary insufficiency.

B. Respiratory Support

Patients with mild disease require only administration of humidified oxygen-enriched air (usually 40%) and noninvasive pulmonary physiotherapy. Severe injury may require maximal mechanical ventilatory support and frequent flexible fiberoptic or rigid bronchoscopy to clear the airways of sloughed mucosal debris and secretions. Small airway disease may produce significant atelectasis requiring increased oxygen administration and institution of positive end-expiratory pressure. Systemic administration of steroids has not decreased morbidity or mortality rates in patients with inhalation injury, and such treatment has been reported to increase infectious complications.

A recent clinical trial of the prophylactic use of high-frequency percussive ventilation in patients with inhalation injury demonstrated significant improvements in morbidity and mortality rates compared with conventional volume ventilation. Fifty-four burn patients with documented inhalation injury were managed by this type of ventilation within 24 hours after intubation. Fourteen patients (25.9%) developed pneumonia, compared with a predicted historic frequency of 45.8%. The observed mortality rate was 18.5% compared with a historic frequency of 35%. Only four of the ten deaths were attributable to pulmonary failure. Though the exact mechanism by which high-frequency percussive ventilation improves outcome is not known, the ability to maintain ventilation and oxygenation at lower peak airway pressures and inspired oxygen concentrations may reduce the iatrogenic injury associated with the use of volume-controlled ventilators. The high frequency percussive breaths also improve clearance of secretions—similar to results obtained with high-frequency oscillators and jet ventilators.

C. Antimicrobial Therapy

Bronchopneumonia is the most common cause of morbidity and death in patients with inhalation injury. The daily chest roentgenograph should be carefully examined. Appropriate antimicrobial therapy is initiated based on the presence of pulmonary infiltrates and sputum leukocytosis. Pneumonia occurring after inhalation injury is usually caused by gram-positive organisms. Gram-negative pneumonias, which now occur infrequently, usually develop later in the hospital course. Therapy is initiated based on the results of the sputum Gram stain, with refinements of antibiotic choice dependent upon endobronchial culture and microbial sensitivity testing.

Prognosis

Smoke inhalation, in the absence of cutaneous thermal injury, is almost always successfully treated by supportive measures. The tracheobronchial mucosa typically heals completely in 2–3 weeks. However, when smoke inhalation occurs in the presence of moderate to severe cutaneous burn, mortality rates are increased by as much as 20% over that predicted by the age of the patient and the extent of injury. When pneumonia complicates inhalation, the mortality rate may rise to 60% above the predicted level.

Cioffi WG et al: High-frequency percussive ventilation in patients with inhalation injury. J Trauma 1989;29:350–4.

Cioffi WG et al: Prophylactic use of high-frequency percussive ventilation in patients with inhalation injury. Ann Surg 1991; 213:575–80.

Huang Y, Li A, Yang Z: Effect of smoke inhalation injury on thromboxane levels and platelet counts. Burns 1988;14: 440–6.

Pruitt BA Jr et al: Evaluation and management of patients with inhalation injury. J Trauma 1990;30(12 Suppl): S63–8.

Shirani KZ, Moylan JA Jr, Pruitt BA Jr: Diagnosis and treatment of inhalation injury. In: *Pathophysiology and Treatment of Inhalation Injuries.* Loke J (editor). Marcel Dekker, 1988.

Shirani KZ, Pruitt BA Jr, Mason AD Jr: The influence of inhalation injury and pneumonia in burn mortality. Ann Surg 1987;205:82–7.

POSTRESUSCITATION PERIOD

PREVENTION & TREATMENT OF COMPLICATIONS

1. Infection Control

Infectious complications have always been the predominant determinant of outcome in thermally injured patients. Improved care of critically ill patients and the control of burn wound sepsis through effective topical antimicrobial agents and timely excision and grafting has resulted in the salvage of more burn patients who would previously have died in the early postburn period. The hospital course of nonsurvivors has also been prolonged. Since infection continues as the leading cause of morbidity and death in burn patients, prolonged hospitalization increases the risk of colonization and infection by nosocomial organisms which are predominantly true fungi, yeasts, and multiply antibiotic-resistant bacteria.

A strict infection control program can minimize the clinical impact of exposure to nosocomial pathogens during a prolonged hospital stay in an immunocompromised patient. Such a program might employ scheduled microbial surveillance, an actively functioning infection control committee, environmental monitoring procedures, biopsy monitoring of the burn wound, and cohort patient care as deemed necessary. The surveillance program includes thrice-weekly cultures of sputum and the burn wound surface and twice-weekly culturing of urine and stool. Multiple antibiotic sensitivities are determined for all staphylococci as well as all pseudomonas species and other gram-negative organisms recovered from routine cultures. Reports are provided on a daily basis, enabling initial empirical selection of antibiotics to be made more precisely should an infection be diagnosed.

Cohort patient care is initiated if a patient is admitted and found to be colonized or infected with an organism of broad antibiotic resistance or if this resistance pattern develops during broad-spectrum antibiotic therapy.

Cross-contamination is minimized by strict enforcement of hand washing, gowning, and gloving policies. The establishment of patient care teams to provide care for only one specific patient or a limited number of patients and restriction of the traffic of convalescing patients (often colonized with resistant organisms) are imperative in reducing cross-contamination and eradicating endemic microorganisms.

The infection control committee monitors infections occurring in the burn unit to identify changes in microbial prevalence, the incidence of infection, and evidence of cross-contamination. Strict criteria for the definition and identification of infections that occur in burn patients are necessary to avoid unnecessary and inappropriate antibiotic administration. Antibiotics are used only for specific indications to minimize the emergence of microbial resistance. Effective infection control policies require continual reevaluation of surveillance culture results and correlation with the sites and treatment of infections.

2. Infectious Complications: Prevention, Diagnosis, & Treatment

With the decrease in fatal burn wound sepsis and improved survival of patients with massive burns, infections in other sites have shown a relative increase as principal causes of death. Dense bacterial colonization of the burn wound and the presence of immunosuppression associated with burn injury increase the likelihood of development of infectious complications.

Pneumonia

Pneumonia is the most frequent septic complication following thermal injury. As the occurrence of invasive burn wound infection has decreased, bronchopneumonia has surpassed hematogenous pneumonia as the predominant form. The increase in airborne pneumonia may also be attributable to improved survival in patients with severe inhalation injury. Atelectasis is often present prior to the development of infection. The appearance of an ill-defined irregular infiltrate on chest x-ray mandates Gram stain, culture, and sensitivity testing of endobronchial secretions. Empiric antibiotic treatment is begun as determined by microbiologic surveillance and Gram stain of the secretions. Subsequent antibiotic therapy is adjusted on the basis of sensitivity testing.

Compared with bronchopneumonia, hematogenous pneumonia usually occurs later in the hospital course. Remote septic foci such as invasive wound infection, endocarditis, or suppurative thrombophlebitis are common causes. The radiographic hallmark is a solitary nodular pulmonary infiltrate, but progression to multiple nodular infiltrates throughout the lungs may occur. All possible sites of infection must be evaluated if a characteristic nodular pulmonary infiltrate appears. The primary infection must be identified and treated. The pneumonic process is treated by systemic administration of antibiotics directed against the causative organism and ventilatory support as needed. Aggressive pulmonary toilet to prevent atelectasis may help decrease the occurrence of pneumonia, though most routine measures have little proved benefit.

Suppurative Thrombophlebitis

The loss of skin integrity, the presence of dense bacterial colonization of the burn wound, and the frequent need for long-term venous access increase the likelihood that suppurative thrombophlebitis will develop in burn patients. Limiting the duration of cannulation of a vein to 3 days or less in patients with thermal injury has reduced the incidence of this complication from 4.3% to less than 1.4% in recent years. Local signs of thrombophlebitis are present in less than half of patients with this complication because of the presence of overlying burn wound and the systemic immunosuppression accompanying burn injury. With the increased use of central venous cannulation, these patients are also at risk for development of central vein suppurative thrombophlebitis.

The diagnosis of peripheral vein suppurative thrombophlebitis is made by operative exploration, excision, histologic analysis, and culture of the suspected phlebitic vein. Identification of bacteria within the vein necessitates excision of the entire length of involved vein to a level of patent normal vein and the administration of systemic antibiotics to which the causative microorganism is sensitive. The diagnosis of central venous thrombophlebitis is more difficult. Indium, in 111-labeled leukocyte scanning, computed tomography, and contrast venography may help establish the diagnosis. This rare complication is treated with systemic antibiotics directed against the organism isolated by blood culture and anticoagulation with heparin. The efficacy of thrombolytic therapy in the treatment of central venous thrombosis is unclear. The failure of antibiotics and anticoagulation to eradicate the infectious focus mandates surgical exploration and vein excision.

The true incidence of intravascular catheter-related bacteremia in thermally injured patients is unknown. Vascular access through a densely colonized wound in those with extensive surface area burns limits the use and effectiveness of standard catheter care policies employed for other critically ill patients. Presumably, as a result of contamination by removal through colonized eschar and skin, catheter tip cultures are frequently positive even in the absence of sepsis or bacteremia. Exchanging catheters over guidewires, an accepted practice in most critical care units, is discouraged since the catheters and guidewires often transverse heavily contaminated open wounds or intact eschar. Consequently, central venous and pulmonary artery catheters are removed and a new catheter inserted at a different site every 3 days. This policy has resulted in a low incidence of bacteremia and sepsis clinically attributable to catheter-related infections.

Endocarditis

Acute infective endocarditis is an infrequent but consistent source of morbidity and mortality in burn patients (1.3%) due to the bacteremias associated with wound manipulation, prolonged intravenous cannulation, and septic thrombophlebitis. Preventive measures include effective topical antimicrobial therapy, timely excision and closure of the burn wound, and early discontinuation or frequent replacement of intravenous cannulae.

Staphylococcus aureus is the most common causative organism, and the right side of the heart is most frequently affected. Recurrent staphylococcal bacteremia in a burn patient with sepsis and no other apparent identifiable source of infection should suggest the diagnosis. Heart murmurs are difficult to detect in hyperdynamic, tachycardiac patients. Transesophageal echocardiography is the preferred examination to detect valvular lesions, but small vegetations may remain undetected. On occasion, cardiac catheterization—to identify valvular vegetations or valvular incompetence—may be required for definitive diagnosis if echocardiographic findings are equivocal. Systemic maximal-dose antibiotic therapy is directed against the causative organism. Antibiotic therapy is continued for 6 weeks after the last positive blood culture.

Sinusitis

The true incidence of sinusitis in burn patients is unclear, but patients requiring prolonged transnasal intubation of both the airway and stomach are at increased risk. One study reported an incidence of 36% in transnasally intubated ICU burn patients. Sinusitis is most often clinically undetectable and requires radiographic examination by plain films or computed tomography to establish the diagnosis. These studies help to direct sinus aspiration to differentiate between congestion and infection. Treatment involves topical mucosal vasoconstrictors to improve patency of the sinus ostia and removal of transnasal tubes. Appropriate systemic antibiotic therapy should be initiated. Surgical drainage is required in cases not responsive to these procedures. Tracheostomy or gastrostomy may be necessary if prolonged ventilatory support and enteral nutrition are required.

Other Complications

A. Ocular

Thermal injury of the ocular adnexa is common in patients sustaining facial burns, but actual injury to the cornea and globe is uncommon because of the blepharospasm induced by heat, noxious gases, and smoke. Exceptions occur in patients with altered sensoria at the time of burning and incomplete protection of the globe. Shortly after admission, fluorescein staining of the cornea and examination with Wood's lamp should be performed to detect loss of epithelial integrity. If epithelial defects are noted, prophylactic topical antibiotic therapy, eg, bacitracin zinc-neomycin sulfate-polymyxin B sulfate ophthalmic ointment, should be initiated. Ophthalmologic consultation should be obtained and the defects examined daily to document resolution or progression of the epithelial defects, the major hazard of which is bacterial infection. Minor corneal abrasions that become infected may rapidly progress to corneal ulceration and globe perforation. Infections caused by pseudomonas species are particularly prone to this complication.

Frequent ocular examination, adequate eye lubrication, prophylactic and therapeutic use of topical antibiotics, and timely performance of eyelid releases are paramount in the prevention of ocular complications. With severe burns of the eyelids, ectropion or loss of lid margin may occur. If the cornea is no longer protected, operation is indicated in the form of an eyelid release with split-thickness skin grafting. Release of one or both lids may be required, and in severe cases, repeated release of the same lid may be made necessary by progressive skin graft contracture. A temporary tarsorrhaphy is sometimes useful to protect the cornea from exposure, but severe ectropion or loss of the lid margin limits the usefulness of this technique.

B. Gastrointestinal

Many gastrointestinal complications have been documented following thermal injury and include pancreatitis, acalculous cholecystitis, gastroduodenal stress ulceration, and Ogilvie's syndrome. Stress ulceration of the upper gastrointestinal tract has been effectively controlled by prophylactic antacid or H_2 histamine receptor antagonist therapy. Hemorrhage or perforation requiring operative management occurred in only five patients, or 0.1%, during a 14-year series. In a recent study, the prophylactic administration of sucralfate has been found equally effective in stress ulcer prevention. Gastric colonization with gram-negative organisms occurred later among patients receiving sucralfate compared to those receiving antacids, but this did not change the incidence or type of pneumonia occurring following burn injury.

Superior mesenteric artery syndrome may occur in patients who sustain profound weight loss during their hospital course. This condition results in compression and obstruction of the transverse duodenum by the superior mesenteric artery from weight loss-induced changes in the anatomic position of this vessel. Current nutritional practices have nearly eliminated this complication. If diagnosed, initial management should be directed towards nutritional repletion and nasogastric decompression. Naso-enteral feeding tubes may be guided past the obstruction under fluoroscopic guidance and are preferred over parenteral alimentation. Operation is rarely necessary.

The management of gastrointestinal complications in thermally injured patients is the same as in other critically ill patients. If operation is required, retention sutures should be used in closing any abdominal incision in burn patients due to the increased risk of postoperative wound infection and fascial dehiscence.

Bowers BL, Purdue GF, Hunt JL: Paranasal sinusitis in burn patients following nasotracheal intubation. Arch Surg 1991;126:1411–12.

Pruitt BA Jr: The diagnosis and treatment of infection in the burn patient. Burns 1984;11:79–91.

Pruitt BA Jr, McManus AT, Kim SH: Burns. In: *Infectious Diseases in Medicine and Surgery.* Gorbach SL, Bartlet JG, Blacklow HR (editors). Saunders, 1992.

Shirani KZ et al: Effects of environment on infection in burn patients. Arch Surg 1986;121:31–36.

NUTRITION

POSTBURN HYPERMETABOLISM

Extensive thermal injury may cause metabolic rates to rise to levels one and one-half to two times normal, far exceeding the hypermetabolism observed in other critically ill patients. The hypermetabolic response is linearly related to the extent of burn, and the actual physiologic response is influenced by environmental temperature, the patient's age, physical activity, pain and anxiety, and the presence of infection. The hypermetabolic response to burn injury, common to other forms of critical illness and trauma, is partially driven by the neurohumoral milieu produced by the hypothalamic-pituitary and autonomic nervous system response. Activation of the former results in increased release of antidiuretic hormone, ACTH, and beta-endorphins, whereas stimulation of the latter results in the release of catecholamines, glucagon, and cortisol. Postburn hypermetabolism is manifested by increased oxygen consumption, a hyperdynamic circulation, increased core temperature, wasting of lean body mass, and increased urinary nitrogen excretion. An increase in CO_2 production follows that parallels oxygen consumption. Hypermetabolism is temperature-sensitive in patients with burns involving over 50% of the body surface, and a 10% decrease in metabolic rate may be achieved by maintaining ambient temperatures above 30 °C. Blood flow to the burn wound is markedly increased when compared with the blood flow to other organs and tissues. This explains to some extent the relationship of extent of burn to hypermetabolism.

SUBSTRATE UTILIZATION

Glucose metabolism is altered following thermal injury. Hepatic gluconeogenesis and total glucose flow increase. However, owing to relative insulin insensitivity, glucose uptake by insulin dependent tissues is decreased. An exaggerated fraction of nutrient flow is directed to the burn wound. Through anaerobic, insulin-independent means, large quantities of glucose are required to support the immune cellular functions of necrotic tissue removal and microbial containment and destruction. Cellular proliferation and wound healing are also glucose-dependent. The predominance of anaerobic metabolism in the burn wound results in increased lactate production with subsequent hepatic conversion of lactate to glucose via the Cori cycle.

Marked catabolism resulting in muscle protein breakdown and loss of lean body mass is observed following thermal injury. Catabolism of muscle protein provides amino acid gluconeogenic precursors (converted to glucose by liver and gut) and supplies amino acid substrates for synthesis of acute phase proteins. Significant nitrogen loss occurs, with 80–90% excreted as urea. The metabolism of glutamine, a preferred substrate for gut metabolism and a precursor for renal ammonia production, is also increased during the hypermetabolic phase. Glutamine is converted by the gut into alanine, which subsequently enters the gluconeogenic pathway.

The ability to oxidize fat as a source of nonprotein calories is dependent on the extent of injury and the degree of hypermetabolism. In patients with relatively small burns, carbohydrate and fat may be used interchangeably as effective nonprotein calorie sources. In patients with larger burns, carbohydrate is more effective than fat in maintaining body protein stores when each is used as a sole energy source.

ESTIMATION OF CALORIC NEEDS

Many formulas exist for the estimation of caloric needs in thermally injured patients. Some of the more common ones based on body size, age, and sex are presented in Table 36–7. The increase in calories required to support the metabolic demand following burn injury is computed by either adding predetermined stress or injury factors to standard formulas or by incorporating the measured extent of burn into those formulas specifically derived for burn patients. The use of formulas to predict caloric requirements in individual patients may result in overestimation or underestimation of caloric needs. Since most formulas are derived by patient measurements in the resting state, activity factors are customarily applied and range from 10%–50%. Serial measurements by indirect calorimetry provide the most accurate determination of energy requirements for patients with major burns; however, there is no current consensus regarding the most appropriate formula to use when requirements must be estimated.

The best method to calculate the protein requirements of thermally injured patients remains controversial; however, supplying 12–18 g of nitrogen per square meter of body surface area or 1.5–2 g of protein per kilogram of body weight has been recommended. Nonprotein kilocalorie-to-nitrogen ratios of 100:1 to 150:1 are acceptable. Only enough fat to prevent essential fatty acid deficiency is required. Some burn patients may tolerate up to 9 mg/kg/min of carbohydrate administration. However, carbohydrate delivery exceeding 5 mg/kg/min occasionally results in hepatic fat deposition and excessive CO_2 production. This may cause CO_2 retention in patients unable to compensate by increasing minute ventilation.

Table 36–7. Formulas for estimating energy requirements in thermally injured patients.

Based on Harris-Benedict equation	**Basal metabolic rate × Activity factor × Injury factor** BMR male = 66.47 + 13.75 (kg BW) + 5.00 (cm ht) – 6.76 (age yr) BMR female = 65.51 + 9.56 (kg BW) + 1.85 (cm ht) – 4.68 (age yr) Activity factor = 1.2 bed rest, 1.3 out of bed Injury factor = 2.1 for severe burn
Curreri	(25 kcal × kg BW) + 40 kcal × % burn
Shriner's (Galveston)	1800 kcal/m^2 BSA + 2200 kcal/m^2 of burn
USAISR	Basal in kcal/m^2 BSA per hour x Factor Factor = $2.33764 - (1.33764^{[-0.0286 \times \% \text{ burn}]})$

USAISR = U.S. Army Institute of Surgical Research.

Once the optimal delivery rate of carbohydrates is determined, balancing the remainder of the caloric requirements with fat may be safely achieved if the fraction of calories delivered as fat does not exceed one-third of the total. Triglyceride clearance is usually increased following thermal injury, but triglyceride levels should be followed weekly in patients whose nutritional regimens contain a significant percentage of calories supplied as fat. Hypertriglyceridemia, usually from parenteral infusion of fat emulsions, may result in coagulation abnormalities, hepatic dysfunction, and altered pulmonary diffusion capacity. Triglyceride levels above 200 mg/dL should prompt a decrease in lipid administration. The combination of medium and long chain triglycerides provided in most enteral formulas is the preferred form of dietary fat supplementation and rarely results in hypertriglyceridemia.

DELIVERY OF NUTRITIONAL SUPPORT

Administration of nutrition by the enteral route is preferred to preserve enterohepatic delivery of substrates and maintain mucosal function and integrity. Enteral intake may be safely initiated when the ileus associated with thermal injury has resolved. Patients with burns exceeding 30–40% of the body surface area may not be capable of meeting nutritional goals by oral intake alone, and supplementation with any of the commercially available enteral formulas with an appropriate calorie to nitrogen ratio may be used. Nasogastric and nasojejunal feedings are commonly employed based on institutional preference. Nasojejunal feedings have the added advantage of providing continuous nutrition throughout the perioperative and intraoperative period with a low risk of aspiration.

Parenteral nutrition is reserved for patients with prolonged ileus or conditions prohibiting effective gastrointestinal motility or absorption. Glucose intolerance is a more common complication of parenteral nutrition and necessitates frequent monitoring of blood glucose levels.

MONITORING NUTRITIONAL THERAPY

Careful monitoring of nutritional therapy is imperative if the high metabolic demand associated with thermal injury is to be met and adequate nutrition maintained throughout the hospital course. Useful indices include body weights, calorie counts, nitrogen balance studies, and measurement of respiratory quotients. In other critically ill patients, measurement of serum albumin, transferrin, prealbumin, and retinol binding protein are commonly employed to monitor the adequacy of nutritional support; however, these biochemical markers have been shown to be poor predictors of temporal changes in nitrogen balance in thermally injured patients and their use is not recommended. Nitrogen balance calculations based on urinary urea nitrogen (UUN) excretion measurements should be modified to include wound losses and other nonurea protein losses. Wound losses, in grams per day, may be estimated as 0.1 × body surface area (BSA) in m^2 × percent BSA of unhealed burn wound. Total urinary nitrogen excretion exceeds UUN in thermally injured patients. Increasing the measured 24-hour UUN by 25% will provide an accurate estimate of total urinary nitrogen losses. The daily nitrogen loss is increased by adding 2 g to account for stool and normal integumentary losses. The formula derived for daily nitrogen loss following thermal injury is as follows:

$$\text{Total nitrogen loss (g/d)} = 24\text{-hour UUN} \times 1.25 + [0.1 \times \text{BSA} (m^2)] + 2$$

If indirect calorimetric measurements are available, monitoring the respiratory quotient (RQ) provides useful information regarding substrate utilization. An RQ greater than 1.0 indicates carbohydrate oxidation and overfeeding, which may result in hepatic fat deposition. An RQ of less than 0.7 indicates fat oxidation and is consistent with the delivery of insufficient carbohydrate calories. Routine serum chemistries, liver function tests, serum calcium, phosphorus, magnesium, and triglycerides should be monitored once or twice a week during nutritional therapy. Most metabolic complications can be avoided by appropriate adjustment of the elemental and nutrient composition of the formula administered.

COMPLICATIONS

The mechanical, septic, and metabolic complications associated with enteral and parenteral nutrition in thermally injured patients are the same as those common to all critically ill patients. However, the quantity and duration of nutritional supplementation required in thermally injured patients are such that strict attention to the amount, composition, and safe delivery of nutrition is required to avoid complications.

Burke JF et al: Glucose requirements following burn injury: Parameters of optimal glucose infusion and possible hepatic and respiratory abnormalities following excessive glucose intake. Ann Surg 1979;190:274–85.

Carlson DE, Jordan BS: Implementing nutritional therapy in the thermally injured patient. Crit Care Nurs Clin North Am 1991;3:221–35.

Carlson DE et al: Resting energy expenditure in patients with thermal injuries. Surg Gynecol Obstet 1992;174:270–76.

Demling RH, Lalonde C: Nutritional support. In: *Burn Trauma.* Blaisdell FW, Trunkey DD (editors). Thieme, 1989.

Saffle JR et al: Use of indirect calorimetry in the nutritional management of burned patients. J Trauma 1985;25:32–9.

Waxman K et al: Protein loss across burn wounds. J Trauma 1987; 27:136–40.

Wilmore DW et al: Catecholamines: Mediator of the hypermetabolic response to thermal injury. Ann Surg 1974;180: 653–69.

Wilmore DW: Pathophysiology of the hypermetabolic response to burn injury. J Trauma 1990;30(12 Suppl):S4–6.

Current Controversies & Unresolved Issues

Postburn Hemodynamics

Resuscitation of patients to provide supranormal levels of oxygen delivery in states of severe illness or injury has recently been popularized. At present, this goal is impractical in the acute resuscitation of thermally injured patients. Even though large volumes of fluid may be required to maintain urine output, burned patients have decreased oxygen delivery and consumption during the initial phase of resuscitation. Attempts to improve oxygen delivery would result in massive fluid administration leading to excessive edema formation and subsequent morbidity. The goal of fluid resuscitation in thermally injured patients is to maintain vital organ function at the lowest physiologic cost. A more physiologic restoration of intravascular volume and oxygen delivery would seem beneficial.

Several approaches to reduction of edema formation and restoration of circulatory integrity are under investigation. Early intervention to block production of or to scavenge superoxide and oxygen free radicals, has been shown to decrease edema formation. Administration of a soluble complement receptor that blocks the classic and alternative complement pathways has attenuated postburn edema formation in animals. Fluid resuscitation with deferoxamine has been shown to diminish the systemic effects of burn-induced oxidant injury and an inositol phosphate derivative, 1,2,6-D-myoinositol triphosphate, has been shown to decrease burn wound edema and resuscitation fluid requirements by an unknown mechanism. Vitamin C, which has been shown in various animal models to reduce burn wound edema and resuscitation volume, was administered to burn patients in a prospective, randomized, controlled manner. The patients were resuscitated according to the Parkland formula. The 24-hour total fluid infusion volumes were 5.5 mL/kg per percent burn in the control group and 3.0 mL/kg per percent burn in the vitamin C group. The vitamin C group had an initial weight gain of 9.2% of pretreatment weight compared with a 17.8% weight increase in controls. The results of this initial small study are encouraging. Urinary outputs were maintained between 0.5 and 1.0 mL/kg/h during the first 24 hours postburn, and total 24-hour urine volumes were not different between groups. Inhibition of lipid peroxidation accomplished by antioxidant administration may be an important adjunct in limiting fluid resuscitation volume and edema formation following burn injury.

The inclusion of osmotically active macromolecules, such as pentafraction, which have a decreased propensity for transcapillary leakage during resuscitation, could also improve early circulatory integrity. Until mechanisms of edema formation are better understood and means of limiting transvascular fluid loss are developed, "supranormal" resuscitation is neither appropriate nor feasible for burn patients.

Inhalation Injury

The mechanism by which inhalation of smoke and products of incomplete combustion injure the tracheobronchial mucosa, distal airways, and lung parenchyma is not completely understood. In part, injury is governed by particle size, which determines the anatomic region where injury will occur. Toxicities of noxious gases produced by combustion of synthetic and natural materials also contribute to the tissue injury of smoke inhalation but are at present impossible to quantify in patients following exposure. Most animal models used to study the effects of smoke inhalation fail to reproduce the clinical and histologic changes associated with inhalation injury in humans. Problems with smoke composition, carbon monoxide poisoning, and smoke delivery systems are common. In a recent study of smoke inhalation injury in nonhuman primates, high-frequency percussive ventilation was found to be superior to conventional volume ventilation and high-frequency oscillatory ventilation in decreasing barotrauma and the histopathologic severity of injury.

Pharmacologic intervention to modulate the response to smoke inhalation may prove beneficial in decreasing pulmonary vascular changes and improving lung aeration. Recent studies in sheep have shown improved alveolar ventilation and diminished inflammatory response to smoke inhalation following postexposure treatment with pentoxifylline. The use of inhaled nitric oxide—which does not alter the normal inflammatory response—to ameliorate pulmonary artery hypertension following smoke inhalation is also being studied. Other treatments, including complement depletion and antioxidant therapy, are being investigated and may prove beneficial. Any attempt to modulate the host response to inhalation injury must proceed with caution to avoid impairing the normal mechanisms of cellular repair and immunologic defense.

Infection

The immune dysfunction following burns, for which a specific cause is unknown, may also be a potential site of pharmacologic intervention. Granulocyte-macrophage colony-stimulating factor (GM-CSF; sargramostim), in addition to stimulating proliferation of granulocyte and macrophage progenitor cells, increases macrophage phagocytic and cytocidal activity, granulocyte RNA and protein synthesis, granulocyte oxidative metabolism, and antibody-dependent cytotoxic killing in mature cells in vitro. In a small cohort of burn patients, sargramostim therapy increased granulocyte counts by 50%. Administration of sargramostim reduced granulocyte cytosolic oxidative function and myeloperoxidase activity to control levels without changing superoxide production. However, following cessation of treatment, superoxide activity was subsequently increased compared with untreated burn patients. These findings caution against clinical extrapolation of in vitro results. A reduction in myeloperoxidase activity may actually be detrimental since bactericidal capability may be compromised. Increased superoxide production could potentiate endothelial cell damage leading to increased capillary permeability. The inability of immunomodulatory drugs to significantly alter the postburn changes in immune function may simply represent the inability of single agents to alter the complex cascade of pathophysiologic events occurring in extensively burned patients.

The concept that the gut plays a central role in maintenance of a persistent catabolic state in severely injured patients has gained substantial popularity. Many animal studies support this hypothesis; however, the lack of clinically significant bacteremia and endotoxemia in humans make the meaning of these findings unclear. Intestinal permeability is increased preceding and during episodes of sepsis in burn patients. Whether alterations in intestinal permeability result in infection or represent only an epiphenomenon remain to be proved. In a recent clinical study, the administration of prophylactic enteral polymyxin B to burn patients resulted in a decrease in endotoxemia; however, no correlation to illness severity score or outcome was observed.

Wound Closure

Excision of the burn wound with subsequent split-thickness skin grafting is now common practice in most institutions. Some clinicians advocate complete excision of the burn wound within the first several days of hospitalization. The postulated benefits of this treatment include decreasing the extent and duration of hypermetabolism and immunosuppression, shortening the length of the hospital stay, and improving survival. Prompt excision and closure of the burn wound has been shown to ameliorate the hypermetabolic response in laboratory animals provided the entirety of the excised wound is closed by grafting. Similar reversal of the immunosuppressive effects of burning has also been documented. Such findings have yet to be observed in humans, probably because the entirety of the full-thickness wound is seldom removed, partial-thickness wounds are not excised, and definitive closure of large wounds cannot be accomplished in a single operation. In several reports dealing exclusively with early wound excision in burned children, the duration of hospital stay was clearly shortened, intraoperative blood loss was decreased, and survival was reported to be improved. The duration of hospitalization has decreased for adult burn patients in many centers because excisional therapy is routinely employed, but a favorable impact of early complete excision of the burn wound on pathophysiologic changes and outcome has not been documented. Moreover, the deleterious hemodynamic and pulmonary effects of general anesthesia during the early postburn period speak for cautious use of such procedures during the resuscitation period in the severely burned patient. Such excisions should be performed on carefully selected patients and only by experienced operating teams and anesthesiologists.

The identification and availability of various growth factors has stimulated interest in the potential for accelerating the healing of burns, skin grafts, and skin graft donor sites. An effective agent could produce more rapid healing of burns (hastening return to work), permit more frequent harvesting of donor sites in massive burns, and shorten healing time of skin grafts (reducing periods of immobility). The topical application of epidermal growth factor has been shown to enhance healing of split-thickness skin graft donor sites by reducing the time to complete healing by 1.5 days. Although the decrease in healing time was statistically significant, the clinical benefit would be minimal. A 50% reduction in skin graft donor site healing time would be required to be clinically effective. The systemic administration of human growth hormone has also been reported to decrease the time of skin graft donor site healing in children, but the same effect was not routinely observed in adult patients. The ability of growth factors to improve healing in burn patients continues to be an area of active research and debate.

Hypermetabolism

The hypermetabolic response to thermal injury is well described, and in addition to the classic hormonal mediators, cytokines may play an important role in maintenance of the hyperdynamic state. Circulating levels of tumor necrosis factor, IL-1, and IL-6 are increased at various times following thermal injury and sepsis; however, the effect of pharmacologic or immunologic blockade of these cytokines is not clearly established following burn injury. In a series of extensively burned patients, blood levels of TNF-α, IL-1, and IL-6, though frequently elevated, had no correlation with the patients' clinical courses.

The hypermetabolic response to thermal injury can be attenuated by beta-adrenergic blockade. Administration of propranolol has been effective in decreasing metabolic rate and cardiac work in burned children and adults; however, increased nitrogen loss was induced presumably from peripheral beta-receptor blockade. Cardioselective beta-adrenergic blockers are currently being studied that may circumvent the nitrogen wasting effects of nonselective agents. Attempts to decrease catabolism and protein wasting have also been studied. The selective β_2-adrenergic agonist clenbuterol increased resting energy expenditure and normalized muscle protein content, muscle mass, and body weight gain in burned rats. Administration of insulin-like growth factor-1 (IGF-1) to burn patients, decreased protein oxidation, and protein breakdown only in those patients in whom an insulin-like effect also occurred. Similar responses in burn patients were demonstrated with the administration of low-dose exogenous insulin and glucose. Testosterone analogs have also been used to reduce postinjury catabolism. Oxandrolone, a weakly androgenic testosterone analog, has recently been shown to decrease net daily nitrogen loss and weight loss in seriously burned patients. This study also described a decrease in healing time of standarized donor sites from 13 ± 3 days to 9 ± 2 days. Complications were similar between groups, and no side effects directly attributed to the drug were identified. Herndon and colleagues evaluated the effect of beta-adrenergic blockade using orally administered propranolol on resting energy expenditure and muscle-protein catabolism in severely burned children. After 2 weeks of treatment, a dose sufficient to decrease the resting heart rate by 20% resulted in a 24% decrease in resting energy expenditure in the propranolol group compared with a 5% increase in a matched control group. The net muscle-protein balance increased by 82% over baseline values in the propranolol group, whereas it decreased by 27% in the control group.

Further studies are required to determine if the apparent benefits of blockade of the hypermetabolic response result in decreased morbidity and mortality for the severely burned patient or whether they merely reflect short-term changes in protein metabolism.

Basadre JO et al: The effect of leukocyte depletion on smoke inhalation injury in sheep. Surgery 1988;104: 208–15.

Baxter CR: Future perspectives in trauma and burn care. J Trauma 1990;30(12 Suppl):S208–9.

Brown GL et al: Enhancement of wound healing by topical treatment with epidermal growth factor. N Engl J Med 1989;321:76–9.

Chance WT et al: Clenbuterol decreases catabolism and increases hypermetabolism in burned rats. J Trauma 1991;31:365–70.

Cioffi WG Jr et al: Effects of granulocyte-macrophage colony-stimulating factor in burn patients. Arch Surg 1991;126:74–9.

Davis CF et al: Neutrophil activation after burn injury: Contributions of the classic complement pathway and of endotoxin. Surgery 1987;102:477–84.

Demling RH, Lalonde C: Early burn excision attenuates the postburn lung and systemic response to endotoxin. Surgery 1990;108:28–35.

Demling RH, Lalonde C: Effect of partial burn excision and closure on postburn oxygen consumption. Surgery 1988;104: 846–52.

Demling RH et al: Fluid resuscitation with deferoxamine prevents systemic burn-induced oxidant injury. J Trauma 1991;31: 538–43.

Demling RH, Orgill DP: The anticatabolic and wound healing effects of the testosterone analog oxandrolone after severe burn injury. J Crit Care 2000;15:12–7.

Desai MH et al: Early burn wound excision significantly reduces blood loss. Ann Surg 1990;211:753–9.

Gore DC et al: Effect of exogenous growth hormone on whole-body and isolated-limb protein kinetics in burned patients. Arch Surg 1991;126:38–43.

Herndon DN et al: Determinants of mortality in pediatric patients with greater than 70% full-thickness total body surface area thermal injury treated by early total excision and grafting. J Trauma 1987;27:208–12.

Herndon DN et al: Effect of propranolol administration on hemodynamic and metabolic responses of burned pediatric patients. Ann Surg 1988;208:484–92.

Herndon DN et al: Effects of recombinant human growth hormone on donor-site healing in severely burned children. Ann Surg 1990;212:424–49.

Herndon DN et al: The pathophysiology of smoke inhalation injury in a sheep model. J Trauma 1984;24;1044–51.

Herndon DN et al: Reversal of catabolism by beta-blockade after severe burns. N Engl J Med 2001;345:1223–9.

Ireton-Jones CS, Turner WW Jr, Baxter CR: The effect of burn wound excision on measured energy expenditure and urinary nitrogen excretion. J Trauma 1987;27: 217–20.

Lalonde C, Demling RH: The effect of complete burn wound excision and closure on postburn oxygen consumption. Surgery 1987;102:862–8.

Sartorelli KH, Silver GM, Gamelli RL: The effect of granulocyte colony-stimulating factor (G-CSF) upon burn-induced defective neutrophil chemotaxis. J Trauma 1991;31:523–39.

Schirmer WJ et al: Complement-mediated hemodynamic depression in the early postburn period. J Trauma 1989; 29:932–8.

Strock LL et al: The effect of insulin-like growth factor I on postburn hypermetabolism. Surgery 1990;108:161–4.

Tanaka H et al: Reduction of resuscitation fluid volumes in severely burned patients using ascorbic acid administration. Arch Surg 2000;135:326–31.

Tchervenkov JI et al: Early burn wound excision and skin grafting postburn trauma restores in vivo neutrophil delivery to inflammatory lesions. Arch Surg 1988; 123:1477–81.

Thompson P, et al: Effect of early excision on patients with major thermal injury. J Trauma 1987;27:205–7.

Waxman K et al: Hemodynamic and oxygen transport effects of pentastarch in burn resuscitation. Ann Surg 1989;209:341–5.

II. CHEMICAL BURN INJURY

The severity of injury caused by chemical exposure is related to the amount and concentration of the agent and the duration of contact with the tissues. Strong alkalis and acids found in common household cleaners are responsible for the majority of minor chemical injuries. More extensive injuries often result from industrial and laboratory accidents or from assaults. The amount of tissue damage incurred is also dependent on the nature of the specific agent. Strong alkalis react with tissues to produce saponification and liquefaction necrosis. Acids are water-soluble and penetrate easily into subcutaneous tissue and cause coagulation necrosis soon after contact. The exothermic reaction produced by contact with strong acids or bases also contributes to the depth of injury. Organic solvents and petroleum products, which are highly lipid-soluble, injure tissues by delipidation. Cutaneous absorption of certain chemical agents may cause systemic toxicity, which complicates subsequent therapy and makes identification of the causative agent imperative.

INITIAL CARE OF CHEMICAL BURNS

Chemical injuries, unlike other thermal injuries, require immediate care of the burn wound. The caustic agent must be washed from the skin surface as soon as possible. All clothing, including shoes and gloves, must be removed and the wounds copiously irrigated with water. If possible, lavage of chemical injuries should continue for at least 30 minutes. In the case of alkali burns, this treatment should continue for a minimum of 1 hour. If ocular injury is suspected, prompt and prolonged irrigation with saline or water should begin. A search for specific antidotes is unnecessary and may only delay the initiation of adequate water lavage. Assessing the depth of injury in chemical burns is difficult, since many agents may produce a tanned or bronzed appearance of the skin, which remains pliable to the touch but may represent extensive full-thickness tissue necrosis. With the exception of the initial attention given to the burn wound, the resuscitation and later treatment of skin injury follows that of thermal burns.

SPECIFIC CHEMICAL AGENTS & SYSTEMIC TOXICITIES

In general, the use of antidotes for specific chemicals is condemned and copious water lavage is considered the appropriate form of initial therapy. However, several specific chemical agents exist for which treatment with a specific antidote has proved beneficial. Injury due to hydrofluoric acid exposure is an occupational hazard of petroleum refinery workers, etchers, and those employed in the cleaning of air conditioning equipment. Following contact with this agent, there is usually a pain-free interval followed by pallor in the area of contact in association with severe tissue pain. Fluoride ion continues to penetrate the tissues until inactivated by calcium salt formation. Immediately after exposure, the area should be copiously irrigated with water. Topical treatment with a calcium gluconate gel should be instituted, and if the pain does not subside, local injection of 10% calcium gluconate into the damaged tissue may provide prompt pain relief. Intra-arterial infusion of calcium gluconate has also been used to limit tissue damage and relieve pain, but surgical excision of the damaged tissue may be necessary for complete pain control. Hypocalcemia may occur following extensive hydrofluoric acid burns.

Phenol

Phenol is an aromatic acid alcohol with high lipid solubility. Initial treatment consists of copious water lavage; however, owing to the poor water solubility of phenol, a lipophilic solvent such as polyethylene glycol (50% solution in water) may be more effective at removing the residual agent. Sufficient systemic absorption of phenol produces central nervous system depression, hypothermia, hemolysis, renal failure, and hypotension. Maximal intensive care support may be required. No specific antidote is available.

Hydrocarbons

Cutaneous injury from immersion in gasoline and other hydrocarbons is often overlooked in victims of motor vehicle accidents who sustain prolonged exposure during extrication. Skin necrosis results from lipid dissolution. Partial-thickness and full-thickness injuries have been described, and systemic toxicity, similar to that produced by ingestion or inhalation, may occur. The pulmonary excretion of hydrocarbons may produce chemical pneumonitis and bronchitis. Systemic lead poisoning from cutaneous absorption of leaded gasoline has also been described.

INHALATION OF AEROSOLIZED CHEMICALS

Inhalation of aerosolized chemicals may produce pulmonary injury and systemic toxicity, thus requiring accurate diagnosis and aggressive treatment. Varying degrees of pulmonary insufficiency may be agent-specific and manifested by severe airway edema formation, mucosal sloughing, and bronchospasm. Systemic toxicity through pulmonary absorption may occur; thus, the causative agents must be clearly identified to ensure appropriate diagnostic and treatment strategies. The degree of pulmonary support required is determined by the severity of pulmonary insufficiency.

Ocular Injury

If chemical eye injury is suspected, prompt and prolonged irrigation of the eye with water or saline should ensue. A specially designed scleral contact lens with an irrigating sidearm is useful when prolonged irrigation is necessary. Epithelial defects may be identified by fluorescein stain. Ophthalmology consultation should be obtained on all suspected chemical eye injuries.

Mozingo DW et al: Chemical burns. J Trauma 1988;28: 642–7.

III. ELECTRICAL BURN INJURY*

Tissue damage from electrical injury results from heat generated by the passage of electric current through the body as well as direct thermal injury caused by the ignition of clothing. The severity of the injury is dependent on the voltage, the type of current (alternating or direct), the path of the current through the body, and the duration of contact. High-voltage and low-voltage injuries are arbitrarily defined as those above and below 1000 volts.

Tissue damage from electrical injury may be obvious at the cutaneous contact site or sites but may also involve underlying tissues and organs along the path of the current. The amount of heat generated is proportionate to tissue resistance; however, the differences in tissue resistance (bone, fat, nerve, etc.) are so small that the body acts as a volume conductor. Current density then predominates as the main determinant of tissue damage with severity of injury being inversely proportionate to the cross-sectional area traversed by current. Thus, severe injuries to the extremities are often encountered, and significant injuries to the torso are rare. Superficial tissues in a limb may be normal, whereas tissues near bone may be nonviable due to longer duration of heating because of the slower heat dissipation from bone. Alternating current injuries may initiate ventricular fibrillation, whereas high-voltage injury and lightning injury are associated with asystolic cardiopulmonary arrest.

Treatment

Cardiac arrest often occurs following an electrical contact and requires immediate cardiopulmonary resuscitation. Patients with electric injury are more likely to have associated injuries due to falls or tetanic skeletal muscle contractions from the electric current; therefore, the patient's spine should be immobilized until cervical, thoracic, and lumbar radiographs exclude the presence of spinal fractures. In patients not sustaining an initial cardiac arrest, cardiac dysrhythmias occur in a small percentage of patients. All patients should have continuous electrocardiographic monitoring for at least 24 hours, and functionally significant dysrhythmias should be treated promptly if they occur.

The estimation of resuscitation fluid requirements in patients sustaining electrical injury is difficult due to extensive subcutaneous or deep tissue involvement with only limited areas of cutaneous injury. This "iceberg" effect may require the performance of fasciotomy—rather than escharotomy—to ensure adequate perfusion of the distal extremity and to evaluate the viability of

* See also Chapter 38.

the underlying subcutaneous tissue and muscle. With extensive muscle necrosis, hemochromogens may be liberated, resulting in the appearance of those pigments in the urine. Intravenous fluids are administered to achieve a urine output of 100 mL/h in adults. If the hemochromogenuria does not clear with an adequate urine output, 50 meq of sodium bicarbonate should be added to each liter of intravenous fluid to promote alkalinization of the urine and prevent pigment precipitation in the renal tubules. If after aggressive fluid resuscitation the renal output does not reach 100 mL/h, an osmotic diuretic such as mannitol may also be administered (a bolus dose of 25 g with 12.5 g added to each liter of intravenous fluid until pigment clearing occurs) to force an increased urine output. When urine production is increased by the use of diuretics, invasive hemodynamic monitoring with a pulmonary artery catheter should be considered, since urine output is no longer a reliable measure of intravascular volume and organ perfusion.

Complications

Associated injuries are more common in patients sustaining electrical injury than those injured by thermal burns. Owing to the titanic contractions of the paraspinal musculature induced by the electric current, compression fractures of the lumbar and thoracic spine may occur. Furthermore, many electrical injuries involve workers who fall from heights. Blunt traumatic injuries should be suspected and appropriate diagnostic measures initiated.

A complete neurologic examination must be performed on admission and at scheduled intervals in all patients sustaining electrical injury. Neurologic changes may be of early or late onset. Immediate peripheral deficits due to the damaging effects of electric current may be irreversible; however, early deficits in a distribution where there is no clear tissue damage are likely to resolve. Neurologic symptoms of delayed onset, often mimicking upper motor neuron disease, tend to be progressive and permanent. Progressive thrombosis of nutrient vessels of the spinal cord or nerve trunks may play a role in the pathogenesis of the late occurring upper motor neuron deficits.

Direct electrical injury to the viscera is rare; however, liver necrosis, intestinal perforation, focal pancreatic necrosis, and gallbladder necrosis have been reported in patients with high-voltage electric injury and truncal contact points. An increased occurrence of cholelithiasis has been reported in convalescent patients following electric injury.

Delayed hemorrhage from moderate-sized to large blood vessels has been described following electrical injury and attributed by some to an "arteritis" produced by the electric current. The actual mechanism of this complication is unclear, but inadequate initial wound debridement and subsequent exposure and desiccation of the involved vessel appear to be causative factors.

In patients in whom the electrical contact point involved the head or neck, the development of cataracts up to 3 years or more following injury has been described. Ophthalmologic slitlamp examination should document the presence or absence of cataracts during the initial hospitalization. Additional information on electrical injuries is presented in Chapter 38.

Grube BJ et al: Neurologic consequences of electrical burns. J Trauma 1990;30:254–8.

Pruitt BA Jr, Mason AD: Lightning and electric shock. In: *Oxford Textbook of Medicine,* 2nd ed. Weatherall DJ, Ledinghan JGG, Warrell DA (editors). Oxford Univ Press, 1987.

REFERENCES

Advances in understanding trauma and burn injury. June 21–23, 1990, Washington, DC. J Trauma 1990;30(12 Suppl):S1–211.

Demling RH: Burns. In: *Critical Care.* Vol 1 of: *Care of the Surgical Patient.* Wilmore DW et al (editors). Scientific American, 1991.

McManus WF, Pruitt BA Jr: Thermal Injuries. In: *Trauma.* Mattox KL, Moore EV, Feliciano DV (editors). Appleton & Lange, 1988.

Pruitt BA Jr, Goodwin CW Jr: Burns: Including cold, chemical and electrical injuries. In: *Textbook of Surgery,* 13th ed. Sabiston DC Jr (editor). Saunders, 1986.

Pruitt BA Jr, Goodwin CW: Burn injury. In: *Early Care of the Injured Patient.* Moore EE (editor). BC Decker, 1990.

Pruitt BA Jr: The universal trauma model. Bull Am Coll Surg 1985;70:2.

Poisonings & Ingestions* 37

Diane Birnbaumer, MD

An integral part of the practice of critical care is dealing with the patient who either intentionally or inadvertently ingests or is exposed to a potentially toxic substance. The magnitude of this problem is staggering. In 1997, the American Association of Poison Control Centers documented 2,475,010 episodes of toxin exposure resulting in poison center notification. It is disturbing that 70% of poisoning cases are never reported to poison control centers. Treating these patients requires a working understanding of the principles of stabilization and supportive care, decontamination, drug elimination, use of antidotes, and the pathophysiologic features specific to the poisons involved. This chapter will cover the general principles involved in caring for these patients and will discuss the details of treating the poisons typically encountered in the practice of critical care.

The pathophysiologic consequences following exposure are poison-specific, and adequate treatment requires an understanding of these individual differences. However, there are several general guidelines the physician can use in the evaluation and treatment of the patient with a potential ingestion or toxic exposure.

EVALUATION OF POISONING IN THE ICU

DIAGNOSIS OF POISONING

History

Obtaining a history from a patient with a potential ingestion or toxic exposure may be difficult if the patient is too young to communicate, is obtunded, or is for any reason reluctant to cooperate. It may be helpful to question the patient's relatives or coworkers to obtain additional historical information. When the history can be obtained, several points require particular attention: the drugs or toxins involved, the route of exposure (oral, dermal, inhalation, etc), and the time of exposure or ingestion. It must be remembered, however, that the history may be unreliable in patients who intentionally ingest toxins. Careful physical examination, laboratory evaluation, and close observation are required.

Symptoms & Signs

The physical examination can provide a wealth of information even in patients unable to provide a useful history. An abbreviated physical examination, sometimes referred to as the toxidrome-oriented physical examination, focuses on the physical findings observed in patients exposed to particular types of poisons and offers rapid assessment. This physical examination should include vital signs; a brief neurologic examination emphasizing level of consciousness and pupillary and motor responses; palpation of the skin for moisture and inspection for cyanosis and rashes; auscultation and percussion of the lungs; and auscultation of bowel sounds (Table 37–1). Table 37–2 summarizes the physical findings associated with the major groups of poisons and lists several examples of each.

Laboratory Studies

The serum glucose concentration should be measured in all patients with altered mental status. If appropriate, intravenous glucose should be administered. Electrolytes, BUN, serum creatinine, arterial blood gases, serum osmolality, calculated osmolar gap, and a urinalysis (crystals; myoglobinuria or hemoglobinuria) are recommended as part of the basic laboratory evaluation for routine screening of patients with overdoses (Table 37–3). Other tests (eg, drug levels, methemoglobin level, and carboxyhemoglobin level) may be helpful in specific patients and will be discussed subsequently.

As a general rule, toxicology screens are expensive, time-consuming, and of limited usefulness in evaluation and treatment. In some specific situations, however, screening may be helpful. These tests can be useful in narrowing the differential diagnosis in patients who present with altered mental status or abnormal vital signs; in such cases, a directed toxicology screen should be ordered that tests for agents consistent with the patient's presentation and physical findings. A toxicology screen may be helpful also in patients with mixed drug ingestions or

* Envenomation (snakebite, etc) is discussed in Chapter 38.

Table 37–1. The "toxidrome"-oriented physical examination.

Vital signs
- Temperature
- Blood pressure
- Respiratory rate
- Heart rate

Brief neurologoic examination
- Level of consciousness
- Pupillary examination
- Motor responses

Skin examination: moisture
Lung examination
Auscultation for bowel sounds

Table 37–3. Screening evaluation of the poison-exposed patient.

Electrolytes
Serum glucose and rapid bedside glucose level
Blood urea nitrogen
Serum creatinine
Arterial blood gases
Serum osmolality
Calculated osmolal gap
Urinalysis
Electrocardiogram
Acetaminophen level
Other laboratory test (methemoglobin level, carboxy hemoglobin level, etc) as indicated
Specific drug levels (as indicated)
Abdominal flat plate (as indicated)

Table 37–2. Toxidromes.

Physical Examination	Sedative–Hypnotic	Cholinergic	Anticholinergic	Sympathomimetic	Sympatholytic
Temperature	N/–	N	N/+	N/+/++	N/–
Respiratory rate	N/–/––	+/–	N/–	+/–	–
Heart rate	N/–	+ or –	+/++	++	N/–
Blood pressure	N/–	+	N/+	++	N/–
Level of consciousness	Normal Obtunded Comatose	Normal Confusion Coma	Delirium Coma	Normal Agitated Paranoid, delusional	Normal Lethargy, coma
Pupillary examination	Miosis	Miosis	Mydriasis	Mydriasis	N or miosis
Motor responses	N/–	Weakness Paralysis Fasciculations	N	N	N
Skin, moisture	N	++ Diaphoresis	Dry, hot	Diaphoresis	Dry
Lung examination	N	Bronchospasm Bronchorrhea	N	N	N
Bowel sounds	N/–	++ (SLUD)[1]	––	N/–	N/–
Examples	Opioids Benzodiazepines Alcohols Barbiturates	Organophosphates Carbamates Physostigmine Edrophonium Some mushrooms	Tricyclics Phenothiazines Antihistamines Scopolamine Amantadine	Cocaine Amphetamine Methamphetamines Phenylpropanolamine Ephedrine Caffeine Theophylline Phencyclidine	Clonidine

[1]SLUD = salivation, lacrimation, urination, defecation.

Key: N = no effect; + = increased; ++ = markedly increased; – = decreased; – – = markedly decreased.

those who present with signs of major toxicity. Finally, a sample of blood may be saved for future toxicology evaluation in patients in whom the diagnosis is unclear.

Serum concentrations of some drugs are helpful in guiding management decisions (Table 37–4). Specifically, aspirin, acetaminophen, barbiturates, digoxin, ethanol, methanol, ethylene glycol, iron, isopropyl alcohol, lithium, and theophylline serum levels should be considered. They are available on an urgent basis from most hospital laboratories. Routine evaluation of these drug levels is not necessary unless there is suspicion that the patient may have ingested one of the substances. An important exception, however, is acetaminophen. This drug is found in many prescription and over-the-counter medications, and patients may ingest potentially lethal amounts but still show minimal or nonspecific signs of toxicity. A serum acetaminophen level should be ordered in all patients who present with a suspected drug ingestion.

Electrocardiography

An ECG should be ordered in all patients with potential drug ingestions. The heart rate, evidence of dysrhythmias, vector axes, and interval measurements are helpful in determining the presence or severity of several ingestions, and repeated electrocardiographic evaluation can, in some cases, help follow the progression of toxicity.

Imaging Studies

A plain abdominal film may be helpful in patients who ingest radiopaque medications such as iron tablets or some enteric-coated medications. These films are helpful also in visualizing drug packets in "body-packers"—individuals who ingest wrapped packets of illicit drugs to transport them through customs. Such "packages" are not radiopaque and therefore may not be visualized on x-ray.

DIFFERENTIAL DIAGNOSIS OF POISONING

The differential diagnosis of the poison-exposed patient is extensive and varies with the agent involved. In general, infectious processes (meningitis, encephalitis, sepsis) and metabolic disorders (hypo- or hyperthyroidism, hypo- or hyperglycemia, hypo- or hypercalcemia, and hypo- or hypernatremia) are the most common causes of the syndromes found in toxic exposures. Head trauma or hypoxemia may also cause findings similar to those observed following toxin exposure.

Burkhart KK, Kulig KW: The diagnostic utility of flumazenil (a benzodiazepine antagonist) in coma of unknown etiology. Ann Emerg Med 1990;19:319–21.

Caravati EM, McElwee NE: Use of clinical toxicology resources by emergency physicians and its impact on poison control centers. Ann Emerg Med 1991;20:147–50.

Olson KR, Pental PR, Kelley MT: Physical assessment and differential diagnosis of the poisoned patient. Med Toxicol 1987; 2:52–81.

Powers KS: Diagnosis and management of common toxic ingestions and inhalations. Pediatr Ann 2000;29:330–42.

Yourniss J, Litovitz T, Villanueva P: Characterization of US poison centers: a 1998 survey conducted by the American Association of Poison Control Centers. Vet Hum Toxicol 2000; 42:43–53.

Table 37–4. Drug levels helpful in guiding management.

Salicylates	Ethylene glycol
Acetaminophen	Iron
Barbiturates	Isopropyl alcohol
Digoxin	Lithium
Ethanol	Theophylline
Methanol	

TREATMENT OF POISONING IN THE ICU

General Measures

The first priority in dealing with any patient with a toxic exposure is stabilization. Assessment of the patient's airway, breathing, and circulation are the initial goals. This may require establishing an airway, ventilating the patient, and supporting the circulation by maintaining an adequate heart rate and blood pressure. These measures should be taken regardless of the toxin involved; more specific interventions can be made after stabilization is completed.

All overdose patients should be monitored by electrocardiography and given supplemental oxygen. Intravenous access should be established. Endotracheal or nasotracheal intubation is indicated in all patients who are inadequately ventilating, those who have significant hypoxemia (Pa_{O_2} < 60 mm Hg or pulse oximetry < 90%), or those who cannot protect the airway because of obtundation or a poor gag reflex. One potential exception is the patient with a narcotic or benzodiazepine overdose; administration of naloxone or flumazenil may arouse the patient sufficiently so that emergent intubation is no longer required. Intubation should be considered in patients who are having seizures or have been exposed to a substance that may cause seizures and in patients in whom protection of the airway is prudent before decontamination measures are taken (gastric lavage, administration of charcoal). Those patients should have blood drawn for glucose assessment, and dextrose should be given if indicated. In patients with suspected alcohol abuse, administration of dextrose should be preceded by a 100-mg dose of thiamine intravenously or intramuscularly.

Hemodynamic Support

Hypotension or hypertension, tachycardia or bradycardia, and hypothermia or hyperthermia should be managed in the usual way; more specific interventions or modifications of treatment can be accomplished subsequently when more specific information regarding the poison involved is available.

Control of Seizures

Benzodiazepines should be used initially for the management of seizures; phenytoin or barbiturates may be needed if benzodiazepines are not effective. In cases of refractory seizures, general anesthesia or the use of paralytic agents may be required; in this case, electroencephalographic monitoring should be instituted to determine if the patient continues to have electrical seizure activity. It is important to note that normalization of vital signs and control of seizures may require interventions specific to the toxin involved.

Opioid & Benzodiazepine Antagonists

Comatose patients should be given naloxone, particularly if they are hypoventilating and have miotic pupils. The usual dose is 0.8 mg intravenously in both adults and children; if there is a suspicion that the patient may be narcotic-addicted, the dose should be titrated in doses of 0.2–0.4 mg to prevent abrupt withdrawal symptoms. Certain opioid ingestions, particularly propoxyphene, may require larger doses of naloxone to be effective. If this ingestion is suspected, 2 mg of naloxone should be administered.

Flumazenil—a benzodiazepine antagonist—may be indicated in patients who present with obtundation or coma; careful dosing in this setting lessens the likelihood of potential complications from administration of this agent. An initial dose of 0.2 mg intravenously should be given over 30 seconds; if, after observation for 30 seconds, the patient does not respond, an additional dose of 0.3 mg should be given over 30 seconds. If additional doses are needed, 0.5 mg should be given over 30 seconds at 1-minute intervals to a total dose of 3–5 mg; if a patient does not respond to this maximum dose, the primary cause of altered mental status is unlikely to be due to benzodiazepines. It is important to note that resedation occurs in 50–65% of patients with benzodiazepine overdose. When it occurs, the resedation is usually within 1–3 hours after administration of flumazenil; this necessitates close observation of these patients. It occurs because the half-life of flumazenil is approximately 1 hour, which is shorter than the half-life of all currently available benzodiazepines.

Decontamination

After stabilization and initial basic therapeutic interventions have been completed, decontamination should be addressed.

A. External Exposures

Patients who have dermal exposure to the toxin should be undressed and copiously irrigated with tepid water. Health care personnel must take appropriate measures to ensure that they are not exposed to the agent while caring for the patient. Copious irrigation should also be utilized in patients with eye contamination, particularly with alkali or acid substances.

B. Ingestions

The vast majority of poisonings occur by ingestion. Gastric emptying and gut decontamination, therefore, are critical to management. In the past, syrup of ipecac was used extensively to induce gastric emptying in patients with toxic ingestions, but studies have questioned the role of ipecac in these situations. Ipecac is no longer recommended in the treatment of most ingestions. (See Current Controversies and Unresolved Issues.)

1. Gastric lavage—Gastric lavage is a relatively effective means of accomplishing gastric emptying, but studies of its impact on clinical outcome in poisoned patients have reported conflicting results. Gastric lavage should not be used in all poisoned patients, but it does have an important role in specific clinical situations. There are several indications for gastric lavage. The first is in the patient who presents less than 1 hour after ingesting a substance which is rapidly absorbed from the gastrointestinal tract and which has the potential to cause life-threatening toxicity. Another indication is in poisonings with agents that decrease gastric motility (eg, anticholinergic agents). Other situations include ingestions of agents that bind poorly to activated charcoal and specific life-threatening poisonings with agents such as theophylline, tricyclic antidepressants, and cyanide. Table 37–5 summarizes these indications.

When gastric lavage is performed, the patient should be placed in the head-down lateral position. Owing to the risk of potential aspiration, gastric lavage should *never* be performed with the patient supine, particularly if the patient is in restraints and cannot be turned quickly if emesis occurs. Suction equipment should be available at all times. It is important that a large-bore

Table 37–5. Indications for gastric lavage.

Recent ingestion (< 1 hour) of a potentially life-threatening poison
Ingestion of a substance that slows gastric emptying (eg, anticholinergic medications)
Ingestion of a poison that is slowly absorbed from the gastrointestinal tract
Ingestion of a substance that does not bind well to activated charcoal (eg, iron, lithium)
Ingestion of specific life-threatening poisons (eg, tricyclic antidepressants, theophylline, cyanide)

gavage tube (36–42F in adults, 16–32F in children) be used in order to remove large pill fragments and whole pills. Some authors recommend that extra holes be cut along the sides of the distal end of the tube to facilitate pill removal. Owing to the size of these tubes, they should not be passed through the nose; oral passage is better tolerated and has fewer complications. Once gastric tube position is confirmed, aspiration of the stomach should be performed to remove as much of the poison as possible before irrigation is instituted, as this may increase delivery of the agent to more distal portions of the gastrointestinal tract. Once aspiration is complete, gastric lavage is begun. Tepid tap water is an appropriate lavage solution in all patients except those under age 5; in this age group, normal saline should be used to prevent electrolyte disturbances. Using 150- to 300-mL amounts, the fluid should be alternatively instilled down the tube and then allowed to efflux from the stomach; amounts in excess of 300 mL increase the risk of emesis and aspiration. Lavage should be continued until the effluent fluid is clear of pill fragments. If activated charcoal and a cathartic are to be used, they can be placed down the lavage tube before it is withdrawn.

Several complications are associated with gastric lavage. Aspiration and subsequent pneumonitis can occur; therefore, it is critical that patients who cannot protect their airways be intubated prior to gastric lavage. Esophageal perforation has been reported, as has inadvertent tracheal tube placement with instillation of lavage fluid into the lungs. Children under the age of 5 years may develop electrolyte imbalances if normal saline is not used as the lavage fluid. Laryngospasm and cardiac dysrhythmias have also been described.

Gastric lavage has only one absolute contraindication–it should not be used in caustic ingestions, since it may cause the patient to vomit, leading to more extensive esophageal and oral burns.

2. Charcoal—Activated charcoal is an odorless, tasteless powder that is beneficial in many types of ingestions and is a cornerstone of therapy. In the gut, it binds the toxin and prevents its absorption. Although it binds many compounds, there are several potentially life-threatening poisons that do not bind well to charcoal (Table 37–6). When used in repeated doses, activated charcoal can both interrupt enterohepatic circulation and enhance the elimination of some drugs that have already been absorbed from the gastrointestinal tract (Table 37–7); this is referred to as "gastrointestinal dialysis." When used in this fashion, the dose of activated charcoal should be 25–50 g orally every 2–4 hours; in children, it is 0.25–1 g/kg every 2–4 hours.

Activated charcoal is administered as a slurry of water and charcoal. The initial dose is 50–100 g orally in adults and 1–2 g/kg in children. But when the amount of ingested agent is known, the optimal dosing of activated charcoal is in a ratio of 10:1, charcoal: ingested agent.

The only relative contraindication to giving charcoal is in patients with caustic ingestions; the charcoal accumulates in burned areas of the gastrointestinal tract and interferes with endoscopy. The most common complication of charcoal administration is constipation. This problem can be addressed by adding a cathartic to the charcoal. If repeat-dose activated charcoal therapy is to be used, it should be added to the first dose of charcoal *only* because the every 2–4 hour dosing of the repeat-dose activated charcoal regimen would lead to excessive cathartic administration and possible electrolyte imbalances from the resultant diarrhea. In addition, some children have become hypermagnesemic when magnesium citrate was used as the cathartic. The most common cathartics used in this situation are 70% sorbitol (1 g/kg), magnesium citrate (4 mL/kg), and 10% magnesium sulfate (250 mg/kg).

3. Bowel irrigation—Whole bowel irrigation is a relatively new method of removing ingested toxins from the gut. Indications for whole bowel irrigation are limited; the most common use of this technique is in patients who intentionally ingest up to several hundred packets of illicit compounds such as cocaine or heroin in order

Table 37–6. Poisons not well bound by activated charcoal.

Bromides
Caustics
Cyanide
Ethylene glycol
Heavy metals
Iron
Isopropyl alcohol
Lithium
Methanol

Table 37–7. Some drugs amenable to repeat-dose activated charcoal therapy.

Carbamazepine
Diazepam
Digitalis
Phenobarbital
Phenytoin
Salicylates
Theophylline
Tricyclic antidepressants

to transport them without detection. The other indication for this therapy is in patients who ingest toxins that are difficult to remove from the stomach and do not bind well to charcoal, eg, iron. The technique for whole bowel irrigation involves administration of 1–2 L of polyethylene glycol electrolyte solution per hour, either orally or via a nasogastric tube. In children under the age of 5 years, the solution should be given at a rate of 150–500 mL/h. The goal is to produce a rectal discharge with the same appearance as the administered oral solution, which indicates complete cleansing of the gut. This usually takes 6–12 hours to achieve. The patient must be able to cooperate and sit either on a toilet or a bedside commode during the procedure.

The only contraindications to this procedure are the presence of ileus, gastrointestinal perforation, or bleeding. It should not be used in patients who are uncooperative or combative or in those with central nervous system depression or respiratory distress. The complications associated with whole bowel irrigation are abdominal cramping and vomiting. Emesis can be treated with antiemetics and a slowed administration rate of the solution. Hyperchloremia has been reported and requires repeated serum chloride determinations during the procedure. It is also important to note that activated charcoal, if indicated, should be given before the initiation of whole bowel irrigation. Repeat-dose activated charcoal is not effective when given during whole bowel irrigation.

4. Ion trapping—Once a drug has been absorbed from the gastrointestinal tract, several measures can be taken to enhance its elimination. Ion trapping enhances drug elimination by "trapping" it in the urine. Because acidic drugs ionize in alkaline urine, they cannot be reabsorbed by the kidney and are excreted. This treatment is most helpful in salicylate and phenobarbital ingestions.

The simplest method for ion trapping uses 1 L of 0.45% saline solution to which two ampules of sodium bicarbonate have been added. The solution is infused intravenously at a rate of 150–250 mL/h. Urine pH is monitored, with the goal being a pH of 7.0–8.0. Potassium deficits should be replaced because alkalinization of the urine is difficult to achieve when hypokalemia is present. Complications of urinary alkalinization are volume overload and hypokalemia.

5. Hemodialysis and hemoperfusion—In some situations, hemodialysis or hemoperfusion may be required to enhance elimination of the toxin. Indications for these treatments include those patients refractory to supportive care alone, those who have a potentially toxic drug level or highly toxic dose of the ingestant, and those in whom other routes of elimination are impaired (eg, by renal failure). It is essential that the suspected toxin is amenable to this type of therapy. Ingestants in which hemodialysis or hemoperfusion may be useful are listed in Table 37–8.

CURRENT CONTROVERSIES & UNRESOLVED ISSUES

Ipecac is a central- and peripheral-acting agent that has been used for decades to induce vomiting in patients with toxic ingestions. Studies have shown, however, that ipecac and gastric lavage are equally effective in removing toxins from the gut, thereby preventing their absorption. Several studies have shown that patients managed with ipecac-induced emesis plus activated charcoal administration achieve the same clinical outcome as activated charcoal alone. Furthermore, vomiting after ipecac can persist for several hours, precluding the use of oral activated charcoal. Patients given ipecac who are initially alert will continue to vomit despite subsequent development of altered mental status, seizures, or coma and are thus at risk for aspiration. Finally, ipecac is contraindicated in caustic and some hydrocarbon ingestions and in infants under 6 months of age. Because lavage alone is as effective as the use of ipecac and because ipecac has several disadvantages, it has little if any role in the management of toxic ingestions.

In the past, forced diuresis was recommended in the treatment of several drug ingestions. Studies have shown that forced diuresis does not enhance elimination significantly and that the relatively large volumes of intravenous crystalloid needed can lead to pul-

Table 37–8. Poisons amenable to hemoperfusion or hemodialysis.

Hemoperfusion	Hemodialysis
Digitalis	Ethylene glycol
Carbamazepine	Methanol
Paraquate	Lithium
Phenobarbital	Salicylates
Theophylline	Theophylline

monary edema, particularly in patients with cardiac dysfunction. Forced diuresis is therefore no longer recommended as a modality in treating drug ingestions.

Gastric lavage was once a mainstay for decontamination of the gut and removal of the ingested agent. Recent studies, however, have shown little change in outcome for most patients who undergo gastric lavage. In addition, this method has the potential for causing serious side effects such as aspiration. Gastric lavage should be limited to those patients who ingest a potentially lethal amount of an agent poorly adsorbed to charcoal or those who present less than 1 hour after ingesting a potentially significant amount of a toxic agent. Administration of activated charcoal has become the primary means for decontamination of the gut in most cases of toxic ingestion.

Bateman DN: Gastric decontamination—a view for the millennium. J Accid Emerg Med 1999;16:84–6.

Hall AH: Gastrointestinal decontaminations: Sifting through supportive therapeutic options. Emerg Med Reports 1991;12:171–8.

Krenzelok EP, McGuigan M, Lheur P: Position statement: ipecac syrup. American Academy of Clinical Toxicology; European Association of Poisons Centre and Clinical Toxicologists. J Toxicol Clin Toxicol 1997;35:699–709.

Kulig K: Initial management of ingestions of toxic substances. N Engl J Med 1992;326:1677–81.

Position statement and practice guidelines on the use of multi-dose activated charcoal in the treatment of acute poisoning. American Academy of Clinical Toxicology; European Association of Poisons Centre and Clinical Toxicologists. J Toxicol Clin Toxicol 1997;35:731–51.

Tenenbein M: Position statement: whole bowel irrigation. American Academy of Clinical Toxicology; European Association of Poisons Centre and Clinical Toxicologists. J Toxicol Clin Toxicol 1997;35:753–62.

MANAGEMENT OF SPECIFIC POISONINGS

SEDATIVE-HYPNOTIC OVERDOSE

ESSENTIALS OF DIAGNOSIS

- *Dysarthria.*
- *Ataxia.*
- *Emotional lability.*
- *Altered sensorium.*
- *Horizontal and vertical nystagmus.*
- *Respiratory, cardiovascular, and renal failure.*

General Considerations

Sedative-hypnotic abuse is common among patients who began using the drugs therapeutically for sleep or as anxiolytics. Other patients may use these drugs orally or intravenously because of the disinhibition and euphoria they produce. The shorter-acting barbiturates such as amobarbital, pentobarbital, and secobarbital are the drugs of choice, though these agents are used less frequently because benzodiazepines are now prescribed more commonly. They are frequently combined with other drugs or with alcohol.

Unlike opioid abuse, tolerance to barbiturates does not increase with chronic abuse. Therefore, as ingestion increases to sustain the euphoric effect, the relative window of safety becomes progressively smaller. Continued abuse is also more likely to cause mental and physical impairment when compared with narcotics. When administered intravenously, the alkaline barbiturate solutions cause sclerosis of the veins and may result in profound ischemia if intra-arterial injection occurs.

Withdrawal from sedative-hypnotics produces a characteristic syndrome that may be fatal. Although a period of initial improvement may occur after 8–16 hours of abstinence, rapid deterioration frequently follows. ICU admission is mandatory for any patient suspected of having barbiturate withdrawal symptoms.

Clinical Features

A. Symptoms and Signs

An overdose of these drugs results in findings similar to those of intoxication with alcohol: ataxia, altered sensorium, and dysarthria. Both horizontal and vertical nystagmus may be present. When intoxication is severe, respiratory and cardiovascular compromise may occur. Ventilations are usually slow and shallow, and pulmonary edema or pneumonitis may develop. Centrally mediated vasomotor depression results in a decrease in blood pressure. If perfusion is not maintained, renal failure may follow. Tissue hypoxia may develop as a result of decreased respiratory function and may cause pupillary dilation. Deep tendon reflexes may also be depressed.

B. Laboratory Findings

Routine laboratory studies should include electrolytes and an arterial blood gas determination. A sample of blood should be obtained and sent for barbiturate concentration. A lethal level is 1–3 mg/dL, though this may vary widely depending on patient factors and the presence of coingestants. An acetaminophen level should be determined in case this agent was coingested.

C. Imaging Studies

A chest x-ray is advisable to evaluate the extent of atelectasis and pneumonitis present at the time of admission.

Differential Diagnosis

Ingestions of nonbarbiturate sedatives such as chloral hydrate, ethchlorvynol, glutethimide, methyprylon, and methaqualone are the major differential considerations when treating a barbiturate overdose. Coingestion of alcohol or benzodiazepines must also be considered.

Treatment

A. General Measures

When cardiovascular and respiratory parameters are normal and stable, supportive care is generally all that is required. However, when intoxication is severe, shallow respirations may be noted, along with depressed cough and gag reflexes. This is an indication for intubation to protect the airway, prevent aspiration, and allow for mechanical ventilation as needed.

B. Decontamination

Lavage should generally be performed if ingestion has been within the preceding 45 minutes. Food in the stomach decreases absorption and may prolong the time period during which lavage is useful.

C. Diuresis

Excretion of long-acting barbiturates is somewhat improved with forced diuresis. Mannitol should be infused at a rate of 1 L/h. Supplemental potassium chloride should be given. Sodium bicarbonate to alkalinize the urine prevents tubular reabsorption of the drugs. Careful serum electrolyte monitoring is mandatory.

D. Cardiovascular Support

Hypotension usually responds to the administration of balanced salt solutions such as normal saline or lactated Ringer's solution, though vasopressors may be required. If large amounts of fluid are necessary for resuscitation, fluid administration should be guided by central venous or pulmonary artery catheter monitoring to prevent pulmonary edema.

E. Hemodialysis

When renal failure occurs, hemodialysis may be necessary. Most of the barbiturates are dialyzable, though the short-acting forms have the lowest percentage of removal.

Withdrawal

Withdrawal from sedative-hypnotics may be fatal. Symptoms of withdrawal typically occur after 8–16 hours of abstinence and include anxiety, tremulousness, weakness, and insomnia. Gastrointestinal symptoms include abdominal cramping, anorexia, nausea, and vomiting. As withdrawal progresses, neurologic findings become apparent and are characterized by twitching, coarse tremors, increased startle response, and hyperactive deep tendon reflexes. After 2–3 days, grand mal seizures may occur. As the seizures subside, improvement usually is noted, though some patients develop organic brain syndrome with disorientation, visual and auditory hallucinations, and delusions. Hyperthermia may lead to cardiovascular collapse and death.

When withdrawal is suspected, the patient should be given an intravenous dose of pentobarbital or phenobarbital based on an estimate of the most recent consumption. This dose can then be reduced by about 10% per day until the patient is drug-free. Seizures are not responsive to phenytoin and should be treated with short-acting barbiturates.

NARCOTICS

ESSENTIALS OF DIAGNOSIS

- *Decreased level of consciousness.*
- *Depressed respiration.*
- *Miosis.*
- *Pulmonary edema.*

General Considerations

Narcotic abuse is a major problem worldwide. Although the drugs of choice have traditionally been morphine and heroin, the shorter-acting agents such as fentanyl have recently come into vogue, especially among health care workers. The majority of narcotics are administered intravenously because of the rapid euphoric result they produce. Methadone, a long-acting oral agent, is commonly used as part of maintenance programs. Pentazocine is a synthetic analgesic with both agonist and antagonist properties. When given to a narcotic-dependent patient, pentazocine may cause withdrawal symptoms. In high doses, it can cause visual hallucinations and dysphoria.

Critical care of patients suffering from narcotic overdose and withdrawal is often aimed at the treatment of conditions caused by narcotic use and the sharing of injection needles. These include pulmonary hypertension (presumably from cotton fiber emboli), endocarditis (from bacterial contamination), necrotizing fasciitis, and tetanus. Other reported complications include hepatitis, AIDS, cutaneous abscesses, and Guillain-Barré syndrome. Many patients will coingest other intoxicants such as alcohol, which complicates their care.

Clinical Features

A. Symptoms and Signs

Patients with opioid overdoses most commonly present with a decreased level of consciousness, depressed respiration, and miotic pupils. In severe cases, such as intentional suicide, respiratory depression may be pronounced. Pulmonary edema may be seen. Other common findings include: hypo- or hyperthermia, emesis, hypoxia, hypotension, and depression of deep tendon reflexes.

B. Laboratory Findings

A blood sample should be sent for toxicology screen, alcohol, and other central nervous system depressants. Routine electrolytes, a blood count, and liver function tests should be obtained. An arterial blood gas will help assess the severity of pulmonary edema. In patients with oral opioid ingestions, an acetaminophen level should be determined.

C. Imaging Studies

A chest x-ray should be obtained in all patients to determine the extent of pulmonary involvement. A head CT scan may be useful in patients with depressed level of consciousness to exclude the presence of mass lesions or intracranial bleeds which may confuse the diagnostic picture.

Treatment

A. General Measures

Most patients transferred to the critical care unit will already have a secure airway and intravenous access established. These should be confirmed, however, because patients with narcotic overdose are at high risk for respiratory depression and airway compromise. If indicated by either a low rapid blood glucose determination or when this measurement cannot be made, 50 mL of 50% dextrose should be given intravenously along with 100 mg of thiamine by intramuscular injection.

Mechanical ventilation may be required both for decreased respiratory drive and for management of pulmonary edema. Hypotension usually responds to volume infusion and correction of hypoxia. Pulmonary edema caused by narcotic overdose usually does not respond to the customary regimen of digitalis, diuretics, corticosteroids, or antihistamines.

B. Decontamination

If the use of coingestants is suspected, gastric lavage is advisable after a secure and protected airway is ensured.

C. Narcotic Antagonists

Several narcotic antagonists have been used: naloxone, naltrexone, nalorphine, and levallorphan. Because the latter two also have agonist properties, naloxone is the preferred agent (although nalmefine is now available in the United States for intravenous use). An initial dose of 0.4–0.8 mg should be administered intravenously for heroin and morphine overdoses. Although naltrexone is longer-acting than naloxone, its use in the acute setting has been disappointing and naloxone is the drug of choice in this situation. When the abused drug is codeine, pentazocine, or propoxyphene, an initial dose of up to 2 mg of naloxone may be required. An improvement in respiration typically occurs in less than 2 minutes. Because the half-life of naloxone is substantially shorter than that of the narcotic agents, repeat dosing is required to prevent respiratory depression. If no response is noted, the diagnosis of narcotic overdose should be questioned. Continuous administration of the antagonist may be required over the next day to prevent relapse of respiratory depression.

D. Other Modalities

Because of the complications associated with narcotic abuse, additional therapy in the ICU may be required for pulmonary edema, pneumonitis, cardiac valvular compromise, or infectious complications. Overdosage with meperidine may cause hyperactive reflexes and convulsions, which require treatment. Renal failure from myoglobinuria may also occur, particularly in patients who have been obtunded for a significant amount of time.

Withdrawal

Withdrawal from narcotics produces autonomic disturbances, hyperexcitability, and personality changes characterized by drug-seeking behavior. Within the first 8 hours of withdrawal, lacrimation, rhinorrhea, diaphoresis, and sneezing are common. This is followed by nausea and vomiting, diarrhea, and abdominal cramping. Patients may exhibit tremors and twitching in association with myalgias. Pilomotor erection produces the "cold turkey" appearance of the skin. All of the symptoms are relieved by the administration of narcotic.

Hoffman JR, Schriger DL, Luo JS: The empiric use of naloxone in patients with altered mental status: A reappraisal. Ann Emerg Med 1991;20:246–52.

Kaplan JL, Marx JA: Effectiveness and safety of intravenous nalmefene for emergency department patients with suspected narcotic overdose: A pilot study. Ann Emerg Med 1993;22:187–90.

Ungar JR, Schwartz GR, Levine DG: Drug and substance abuse emergencies. In: *Principles and Practice of Emergency Medicine,* 3rd ed. Schwartz GR et al (editors). Lea & Febiger, 1992.

SYMPATHOMIMETICS

ESSENTIALS OF DIAGNOSIS

- *Agitation, anxiety, hallucinations, psychosis.*
- *Seizures.*
- *Coma, stroke, encephalopathy.*
- *Hypertension, tachycardia.*

General Considerations

Sympathomimetics are a category of drugs that induce a physiologic state similar to that caused by catecholamine release. Many different prescription, over-the-counter, and recreational or abuse drugs fall into this category. Examples include amphetamine and its derivatives, over-the-counter products for appetite control, cold remedies, stimulants (phenylpropanolamine, caffeine, ephedrine, pseudoephedrine), and hallucinogenic amphetamines including methylenedioxy-methamphetamine (MDMA; Ecstasy) and methylenedioxyamphetamine (MDA).

Overuse of sympathomimetics causes toxicity by inducing excessive release of neurotransmitters, including epinephrine and norepinephrine, and the subsequent alpha-adrenergic and beta-adrenergic effects they produce. Alpha-adrenergic effects are primarily vasoconstriction, diaphoresis, and dilated pupils; β_1-adrenergic effects lead to tachycardia; and β_2-adrenergic effects cause bronchodilation and vasodilation. The clinical effects that result from any specific sympathomimetic drug depend on the relative alpha-adrenergic or beta-adrenergic actions of that drug (eg, phenylpropanolamine is an alpha-selective drug that causes hypertension, diaphoresis, and mydriasis).

Duration of toxicity is usually limited. Patients may demonstrate prolonged toxicity if they ingest bags containing the drug for illicit transport or if they use Ice, a long-acting smokable form of methamphetamine.

Clinical Features

A. Symptoms and Signs

Sympathomimetic toxicity causes a toxic syndrome that includes primarily central nervous system and cardiovascular effects (Table 37–2). Both illicit drug users and those who use excessive amounts of over-the-counter medications (diet aids, stimulants, and cold medications) may present with sympathomimetic poisoning.

Central nervous system toxicity is manifested as agitation, anxiety, delusions, hallucinations, paranoia, and seizures. Sympathomimetics may cause a psychotic state indistinguishable from that seen in schizophrenia; although almost always temporary, this psychosis may take weeks to months to resolve. Less common but more severe effects include coma, strokes (ischemic and hemorrhagic), hypertensive encephalopathy, and focal neurologic deficits.

Cardiovascular effects include hypertension and sinus tachycardia. Hypertension may be of rapid onset and severe. Because these patients often do not have underlying hypertension, they have no central nervous system autoregulation at these excessively high blood pressures. As a result, they are much more likely to suffer serious central nervous system sequelae such as strokes or encephalopathy from acute hypertension. Sinus bradycardia or atrioventricular block occurs mainly after ingestion of drugs with primarily alpha agonist properties. Patients may suffer tachydysrhythmias, cardiac ischemia, and rarely infarction.

Other findings include rhabdomyolysis with or without renal failure, diarrhea, intestinal cramping, and hyperthermia.

B. Laboratory Findings

Laboratory abnormalities are variable and not diagnostic. Toxicology screening may reveal a limited number of the sympathomimetic drugs but is by no means comprehensive of the wide array of available agents. A negative screen does not exclude sympathomimetic toxicity. Leukocytosis is common as a result of demargination caused by catecholamine stimulation. Patients should have a CK determination to evaluate for rhabdomyolysis. Serum electrolytes (especially potassium) and blood pH should be tested.

C. Imaging Studies

CT scanning is indicated in patients with altered mental status or seizures.

Differential Diagnosis

Metabolic diseases such as thyrotoxicosis may present in a manner identical to sympathomimetic overdose. A history of thyroid disease is suggestive of the diagnosis, as is the presence of goiter or physical findings suggestive of hyperthyroidism. Central nervous system infections may cause similar clinical findings. Drug withdrawal (ethanol, benzodiazepines) also presents with agitation and cardiovascular abnormalities. Similar clinical findings result from toxic effects of theophylline, tricyclic antidepressants, anticholinergics, isoniazid, phencyclidine, and salicylates and from interaction between monoamine oxidase inhibitors and other drugs.

Treatment

A. General Measures

After initial assessment and stabilization, treatment should be individualized to the drug involved and the toxic clinical effects manifest. If the drug was ingested, gastric lavage should be considered if presentation is within 2 hours after ingestion or if the patient is transporting the drugs as a body-packer. Care must be taken to protect the airway as these patients may seize as a result of their ingestion. Activated charcoal should be administered to all patients with an oral ingestion. Repeat dose activated charcoal is helpful in enhancing caffeine elimination. Forced diuresis, hemodialysis, and hemoperfusion are not helpful in these poisonings.

B. Hypertension

Hypertension is a medical emergency in these patients because of the risk of hemorrhage or encephalopathy. Patients with evidence of end-organ dysfunction from hypertension (headache, renal compromise, cardiac ischemia, heart failure) and those whose blood pressure is over 170/110 mm Hg should be treated with antihypertensive agents. Nitroprusside is a good choice since it is easily titratable and doses can be adjusted rapidly. Phentolamine may be used in patients who overdose on pure alpha-agonists such as phenylpropanolamine. Although nifedipine is a potent antihypertensive agent, it is not easily titrated, and cases of prolonged hypotension have been reported. Labetalol may be a good choice in patients with significant tachycardia. Other beta-blockers should not be used to treat hypertension because worsening hypertension from β_2-adrenergic blockade and unopposed alpha-adrenergic stimulation may occur.

C. Arrhythmias

Sinus tachycardia rarely requires intervention. Supraventricular tachycardia is usually benign; however, when the patient suffers compromise from the ventricular response, verapamil or adenosine may be used to control the rhythm. Esmolol may be used to treat both supraventricular tachycardia and ventricular dysrhythmias. Blood pressure must be closely observed for the development of hypertension due to beta-adrenergic blockade.

D. Seizures

Seizures and agitation should be treated with benzodiazepines. Status epilepticus may develop and require treatment with phenobarbital and phenytoin. If these medications are ineffective, paralysis may be required to prevent rhabdomyolysis, acidosis, and hyperthermia. Continuous electroencephalographic monitoring is required in these patients, since they may continue to have electrical seizure activity despite chemical paralysis.

E. Psychosis

Benzodiazepines may be used to treat psychosis associated with sympathomimetic overdoses. Although neuroleptics have been used in the past, they lower the seizure threshold and alter thermoregulation; they should probably be avoided in this situation.

F. Myocardial Ischemia

Although actual myocardial infarction is rare, patients with angina pectoris should be managed with nitrates and heart rate control. Patients usually respond to this treatment and should be monitored for elevation of cardiac enzymes or changes in the ECG consistent with myocardial infarction.

G. Hyperthermia

Hyperthermia can be severe and life-threatening. Aggressive treatment is warranted. Patients with agitation or seizures should receive benzodiazepines. Antipyretics are rarely helpful. All clothing should be removed and patients sprayed with a mist of water or covered with damp sheets to increase evaporation. A fan is helpful. Those with excessive agitation or seizures who do not respond to benzodiazepines may need paralysis to control heat production.

Aaron CK: Sympathomimetics. Emerg Med Clin North Am 1990:8:513–26.

Derlet RW et al: Amphetamine toxicity: Experience with 127 cases. J Emerg Med 1989;7:157–61.

Derlet RW, Horowitz BZ: Cardiotoxic drugs. Emerg Med Clin North Am 1995;13:771–91.

Guharoy R et al: Methamphetamine overdose: experience with six cases. Vet Hum Toxicol 1999;41:28–30.

Swalwell CI, Davis GG: Methamphetamine as a risk factor for acute aortic dissection. J Forensic Sci. 1999;44:23–6.

PHENCYCLIDINE

ESSENTIALS OF DIAGNOSIS

- *Nystagmus.*
- *Hypertension.*
- *Tachycardia.*
- *Agitation, psychosis, violent behavior.*
- *Seizures.*

General Considerations

Phencyclidine (PCP) is an illicit hallucinogen used as a recreational drug. The usual method of consumption is by smoking cigarettes that have been soaked in a solution of PCP. PCP can also be used via the intranasal route or by ingestion. Some patients have become intoxicated from percutaneous exposure by handling the drug. Absorption is rapid by any route; effects are seen within a few minutes to half an hour. The drug is highly lipid-soluble, and inconstant release from adipose tissue may lead to waxing and waning findings that are predominantly due to central nervous system effects. Metabolism is primarily in the liver. The half-life varies from 7 hours to over 3 days.

Clinical Features

The clinical presentation of PCP intoxication is extremely variable. Alterations in mental status are erratic, and violent behavior often occasions transport to a hospital. Concurrent use of other drugs of abuse is common, and the treating physician must be aware of this possibility when evaluating these patients.

A. Symptoms and Signs

The most common findings (over 50% of patients) are nystagmus (horizontal, vertical, or rotatory) and hypertension. Although hypertension is common, medical complications are rare. Tachycardia is also common, but rates over 130 beats/min are unusual. The level of consciousness may vary from comatose to agitated to fully alert. Mental status may wax and wane, and unpredictable and precipitous violent outbursts may occur. These patients may require physical and chemical restraints to prevent them from hurting themselves or the medical personnel caring for them. Hallucinations, frank psychosis, and seizures are common. Most symptoms resolve spontaneously within hours; however, some patients may remain symptomatic for several days or even a week. The psychosis may last months, and recovery is gradual.

Rhabdomyolysis is a relatively common complication of PCP intoxication and may lead to renal failure in up to 2.5% of cases.

B. Laboratory Findings

Urine for PCP level may be sent to confirm the diagnosis. Quantitative levels are not necessary and do not correlate with clinical effects. If patients who appear to be PCP-intoxicated have negative urine results, they need to be evaluated for other causes of their symptoms (see Differential Diagnosis).

Elevated CK levels are found in up to 70% of cases and can occur even in the absence of excessive muscle activity. All patients with PCP intoxication should have their urine tested for hemoglobin with a dipstick. If positive, a serum sample for CK measurement should be sent. Initial urine dipstick may be negative despite a significant elevation in CK. If the clinical situation suggests PCP intoxication, a serum CK level should be obtained despite the presence of a negative dipstick test.

C. Concealed Injuries

Because PCP has anesthetic properties, patients may suffer significant trauma in the prehospital setting that may not be manifested in the usual ways. All patients should undergo a thorough physical evaluation and be reevaluated several times during the hospital stay.

Differential Diagnosis

Lethargic patients may have consumed other intoxicants, including sedative-hypnotic drugs or barbiturates. Patients who are agitated or violent must be evaluated for possible sympathomimetic use or a withdrawal syndrome. Other causes include head trauma, infection (meningitis or encephalitis), metabolic derangements, and psychiatric disorders.

Treatment

A. Decontamination

Gastric lavage is indicated if the patient has ingested a large amount of the drug within 1 hour prior to presentation or if coingestants are suspected; however, because PCP is typically inhaled, this route of decontamination is rarely indicated. Activated charcoal should also be used on a repeat-dosing regimen if the agent was ingested.

B. Supportive Measures

Patients with hypertension or tachycardia rarely need intervention for these problems. End-organ dysfunction should be managed in the usual manner. Hyperthermia requires treatment with antipyretics and a cooling blanket as necessary. Seizures should be treated with benzodiazepines. If the patient develops refractory seizures, phenytoin may be used, but neuromuscular blockade may be required to prevent acidosis, hyperkalemia, and rhabdomyolysis. Continuous electroencephalographic monitoring is required in this situation.

In the past, urinary acidification was advocated to cause urinary ion trapping of the drug and enhance elimination. Because only a small amount of the drug is excreted unchanged in the urine and because induction of aciduria is difficult to achieve and may lead to renal dysfunction due to rhabdomyolysis, this treatment is no longer recommended.

C. Hydration

If serum CK is elevated, vigorous hydration is required, and intravenous crystalloid is the mainstay of therapy. Normal saline should be used until the patient is volume-repleted; the goal is a urine output of 150 mL/h. This should be followed by intravenous mannitol and bicarbonate to prevent precipitation of myoglobin in the renal tubules, which can lead to acute renal failure. Serial CK levels should be obtained to follow the course of the rhabdomyolysis. Blood urea nitrogen and creatinine levels should be measured to monitor renal function. Potassium levels and blood gases should be followed to evaluate hyperkalemia and acidosis.

D. Restraints and Sedation

Patients who are agitated or violent may require physical or chemical restraints. The use of physical restraints alone may exacerbate rhabdomyolysis as the patient fights against the restraints. Restrained patients should be placed in a quiet room to avoid stimulation. Benzodiazepines or haloperidol may be used for sedation.

Baldridge EB, Bessen HA: Phencyclidine. Emerg Med Clin North Am 1990;8:541–50.

Barton CH, Sterling ML, Vaziri ND: Phencyclidine intoxications: Clinical experience in 27 cases confirmed by urine assay. Ann Emerg Med 1981;10:243–6.

Brust JC: Acute neurologic complications of drug and alcohol abuse. Neurol Clin 1998;16:503–19.

Brust JC: Other agents. Phencyclidine, marijuana, hallucinogens, inhalants, and anticholinergics. Neurol Clin 1993;11:555–61.

McCarron NM et al: Acute phencyclidine intoxication: Clinical patterns, complications, and treatment. Ann Emerg Med 1981;10:290–7.

McCarron NM et al: Acute phencyclidine intoxication: Incidence of clinical findings in 1,000 cases. Ann Emerg Med 1981; 10:237–42.

Young JD, Crapo LM. Protracted phencyclidine coma from an intestinal deposit. Arch Intern Med. 1992;152:859–60.

COCAINE

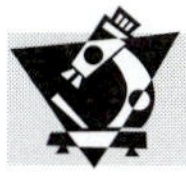

ESSENTIALS OF DIAGNOSIS

- *Hypertension.*
- *Tachycardia and other dysrhythmias.*
- *Headache.*
- *Myocardial infarction.*
- *Transient ischemic attacks, stroke.*
- *Seizures.*

General Considerations

Cocaine is available as cocaine hydrochloride, a water-soluble crystalline salt that can be used intranasally or dissolved and injected intravenously. Cocaine is also available in an alkaloid form that is not water-soluble and can be smoked in a free-base form or mixed with baking soda and water and smoked as the "crack" form. Absorption from all sites is rapid. The half-life varies with the route of administration; intravenous use or smoking leads to a half-life of 60–90 minutes, while intranasal or oral use has a half-life of several hours.

Cocaine has several effects: It causes central nervous system release of neurotransmitters, including dopamine; acts as a local anesthetic; blocks neuronal catecholamine reuptake; and inhibits serotonin reuptake. The end result of these mechanisms is a clinical spectrum of findings primarily in the central nervous and cardiovascular systems. Respiratory and metabolic effects may also be noted.

Clinical Features

A. Symptoms and Signs

Hypertension occurs frequently and can be severe. It can lead to intracranial bleeding, aortic dissection, and cardiac ischemia. Tachycardia is also common, as are dysrhythmias, including atrial fibrillation, atrial tachycardia, ventricular tachycardia, and asystole.

Cocaine is a potent vasoconstrictor that may result in organ ischemia. Myocardial infarction, bowel ischemia, renal infarction, and limb ischemia have all been reported. A combination of vasospasm, enhanced platelet aggregation, and enhanced workload caused by an excessive demand for oxygen produces end-organ dysfunction. In addition to organ ischemia, cocaine can cause a myocarditis manifested by elevated CK-MB enzymes and diffuse ST segment elevations or T wave inversions on the ECG. There are many central nervous system manifestations of cocaine toxicity. Headache is common in chronic abusers. In patients who develop central nervous system complications due to cocaine, cerebral infarction occurs in about one-fourth, subarachnoid hemorrhage in another one-fourth, and intraparenchymal hemorrhage in the remainder.

Patients who abuse cocaine may also present with depressed mental status or frank coma. These patients have characteristically been using large amounts of cocaine for up to a week and present either after a seizure or when they are found obtunded. They may be extremely difficult to arouse, necessitating extensive evaluation of their altered mental status. Typically they awaken after less than 24 hours. This phenomenon is probably due to central nervous system depletion of neurotransmitters. Its presence necessitates evaluation for cerebrovascular accident.

Seizures occur in up to 2% of cocaine abusers and—although they usually occur soon after cocaine use—they may not present until several hours later. Transient ischemic attacks have been described and may lead to stroke. Cocaine use should be considered in the differential diagnosis of a young patient with a stroke. Strokes are independent of the route of administration and may occur as late as 24 hours after use. They can present in first-time users but are more common among chronic abusers due to increased levels of neurotransmitters from sustained abuse.

Pulmonary complications include pneumothorax and pneumomediastinum in patients who smoke or snort cocaine. Pulmonary edema is rare overall but is a common finding in patients who die of cocaine intoxication.

Rhabdomyolysis may occur with excess muscle activity and hyperthermia. Hyperthermia, when present, is often severe.

B. Laboratory Findings

Laboratory evaluation in patients with serious intoxication should include an ECG and measurements of serum electrolytes, CK, and urine myoglobin. Toxicology screens for cocaine may focus the diagnosis.

C. Imaging Studies

CT head scanning should be performed in any patient with a headache or in those with neurologic findings or altered mental status. Plain films of the abdomen may reveal packets in the intestines of patients who swallow containers of the drug for the purpose of transport ("body-packers").

Differential Diagnosis

Other stimulants including sympathomimetics, theophylline, phencyclidine, and anticholinergic drugs can cause a similar clinical picture. Withdrawal from ethanol or benzodiazepines may present similarly, as can thyrotoxicosis and central nervous system infection.

Treatment

A. Supportive Measures

Basic supportive measures should be initiated. In patients who ingest cocaine, lavage should be considered if the patients presents within 1 hour after ingestion. Activated charcoal should be given. Patients who have ingested packets of the drug are candidates for whole bowel irrigation.

B. Hyperthermia

When hyperthermia is present, the patient should be undressed completely and sprayed with a cool mist or draped with a wet sheet. A fan can be used to facilitate evaporation. Ice packs should be placed at the neck, axillas, and groin. Care should be taken not to overcool the patient. Antipyretic agents are not effective.

C. Seizures

Initial treatment of agitation and seizures should be with benzodiazepines. Neuroleptics may be effective, but since they lower the seizure threshold, their use is discouraged. Seizures refractory to benzodiazepines can be treated with phenobarbital or phenytoin. Status epilepticus unresponsive to this therapy should be treated with pharmacologic paralysis and mechanical ventilation.

D. Hypertension

Mild hypertension usually does not require intervention. Nifedipine may be used for moderate hypertension, but severe hypertension or labile hypertension should be treated with intravenous nitroprusside. Labetalol is another alternative, especially in the tachycardiac patient. Tachydysrhythmias that require treatment may respond to beta-blockers such as esmolol or metoprolol, but the patient must be carefully observed for the development of worsening hypertension from the unopposed alpha-adrenergic stimulation and β_2-adrenergic blockade. Concurrent use of nitroprusside with β_2-blockers is often necessary. Patients suspected of having a myocardial infarction should receive standard therapy.

E. Rhabdomyolysis

Rhabdomyolysis should be treated with fluids and alkalinization.

Derlet RW, Horowitz BZ: Cardiotoxic drugs. Emerg Med Clin North Am 1995;13:771–91.

Ghuran A, Nolan J: Recreational drug misuse: issues for the cardiologist. Heart 2000;83:627–33.

June R et al: Medical outcome of cocaine bodystuffers. J Emerg Med 2000;18:221–4.

Olson KR et al: Seizures associated with poisoning and drug overdose. Am J Emerg Med 1994;12:392–5.

Pottieger AE et al: Cocaine use patterns and overdose. J Psychoactive Drugs 1992;24:399–410.

Pudiak CM, Bozarth MA: Cocaine fatalities increased by restraint stress. Life Sci 1994;55:PL379–82.

TRICYCLIC ANTIDEPRESSANTS

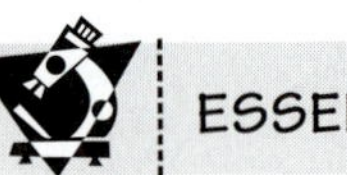

ESSENTIALS OF DIAGNOSIS

- *Sensorium may range from awake and alert to comatose.*
- *Seizures.*

- *Tachycardia, arrhythmias.*
- *Mydriasis.*
- *Dry skin.*
- *Ileus.*
- *Urinary retention.*

General Considerations

Tricyclic antidepressants (TCAs) such as amitriptyline, doxepin, and trimipramine work therapeutically by blocking reuptake of norepinephrine into adrenergic nerves, but they also have significant toxic effects related to their anticholinergic activities, including myocardial depression and peripheral alpha-adrenergic blockade. When ingested, they are rapidly absorbed; in overdose situations, owing to the slowed intestinal motility from the anticholinergic effects, absorption may be prolonged, increasing the half-life to as much as 3–4 days.

Clinical Features

A. Signs and Symptoms

On initial presentation, patients with TCA overdose may range from awake and alert to having seizures to frankly comatose. The potential for rapid deterioration should be remembered. Patients with suspected tricyclic drug ingestion need immediate medical evaluation and close observation. Evaluation often reveals both central and peripheral anticholinergic effects: tachycardia, mydriasis, dry skin, urinary retention, ileus, elevated temperature, altered mental status (agitation, anxiety, delirium, coma), seizures, and occasionally respiratory depression. Cardiovascular effects are usually the cause of death. Findings include sinus tachycardia, dysrhythmias, and atrioventricular blockade with hypotension (decreased contractility and alpha blockade). This ingestion should be suspected in any patient who presents with seizures, anticholinergic signs (including coma), and cardiovascular abnormalities, particularly if the ECG is abnormal.

B. Electrocardiography

The single most valuable test in patients suspected of having a TCA overdose is the ECG. Common findings include sinus tachycardia, PR and QT segment prolongation, and nonspecific ST changes. QRS prolongation suggests a serious overdose. Rightward and superior terminal QRS forces (a wide, prominent S wave in leads I, aVF, and V_6, with a prominent R wave in aVR) are very suggestive of tricyclic overdose.

C. Laboratory Findings

General laboratory evaluation is rarely helpful. Drug levels correlate poorly with toxic effects and can vary widely in an individual patient.

D. Imaging Studies

As some tricyclics are radiopaque, a plain film of the abdomen may show tablets in the stomach or intestines.

Differential Diagnosis

The combination of altered mental status, seizures, and cardiovascular abnormalities suggests several diagnoses. Toxicologic causes include phenothiazines, anticholinergics, and theophylline; less commonly, beta-blockers, calcium channel blockers, and local anesthetic drug overdose (eg, lidocaine) can cause these findings. Nontoxicologic causes include meningitis, sepsis, hypoglycemia (severe), anaphylaxis, and head trauma.

Treatment

A. General Measures

General measures aimed at stabilization, monitoring, and intravenous access should be instituted. A urinary catheter should be placed to monitor urine output and provide easy determination of urine pH. Evacuation of stomach contents should be accomplished by gastric lavage; syrup of ipecac should be avoided because these patients may rapidly deteriorate and become obtunded before vomiting begins, placing them at risk for aspiration. Gastric lavage should be performed, particularly if the patient presents within the first 1–2 hours after ingestion—or even later if they have decreased or absent bowel sounds. Activated charcoal, 100 g, should be placed down the lavage tube or given to the patient via nasogastric tube. There is some evidence that a repeat-dose activated charcoal regimen (every 2–4 hours) may be helpful in significant ingestions.

TCA overdose patients need to be admitted to the ICU if they have any of the following: persistent tachycardia (> 120/min); dysrhythmias, including premature ventricular contractions; QRS > 100 ms; hypotension; or evidence of central nervous system toxicity. Patients who present with none of the above and do not develop any of the listed admission criteria after 6 hours of observation may be discharged; a psychiatric evaluation before discharge is prudent. Patients admitted should be monitored until they are free of toxicity for 24 hours.

B. Bicarbonate Therapy

Alkalinization of the blood is a mainstay in the therapy of TCA ingestion. It effectively treats most of the major adverse effects of the drug, including hypotension, cardiac conduction abnormalities, and dysrhythmias. Alkalinization has varying efficacy in the treatment of seizures and coma. Optimal blood pH is 7.50, which can be achieved by either intravenous sodium bicarbonate therapy or by hyperventilation.

Supportive care and alkalinization therapy are usually adequate to manage patients with TCA overdose. In some cases, additional measures will be needed to stabilize the patient. Those with severe agitation, delirium, or seizures may require benzodiazepines or barbiturates for control. Dysrhythmias refractory to alkalinization can be treated with lidocaine or cardioversion. Class Ia antiarrhythmic agents should be avoided in this patient population. Hypotension that does not respond to alkalinization can be managed with fluid boluses or with pressors. Because the hypotension is often due to alpha-adrenergic blockade, alpha-adrenergic agonists (eg, phenylephrine, methoxamine) are a good choice. Dopamine may be ineffective or may exacerbate hypotension owing to its beta-agonist effects (peripheral β2-adrenergic stimulation produces vasodilation). Hemodialysis and hemoperfusion are relatively ineffective in these patients, as the TCAs are highly protein-bound and not easily removed by these measures.

Current Controversies & Unresolved Issues

In the past, physostigmine was recommended for the treatment of TCA overdose. As an acetylcholinesterase inhibitor, physostigmine increases acetylcholine availability at receptor sites and reverses central and peripheral anticholinergic effects. It has not been proved to be effective in treating hypotension, ventricular dysrhythmias, and conduction disturbances, which are the major causes of fatal toxicity in TCA overdoses. Significant adverse effects such as atrioventricular blockade, bradycardia, and asystole may occur with physostigmine. Therefore, it has no role in the treatment of TCA overdose.

Haddad LM: Managing tricyclic antidepressant overdose. Am Fam Physician 1992;46:153–9.

Kerr GW, McGuffie AC, Wilkie S: Tricyclic antidepressant overdose: a review. Emerg Med J 2001;18:236–41.

Liebelt EL et al: Serial electrocardiogram changes in acute tricyclic antidepressant overdoses. Crit Care Med 1997;25:1721–6.

Niemann JT et al: Electrocardiographic criteria for tricyclic antidepressant cardiotoxicity. Am J Cardiol 1986;57:1154–9.

Smilkstein MJ: Reviewing cyclic antidepressant cardiotoxicity: Wheat and chaff. J Emerg Med 1990;8:645–8.

Vernon DD et al: Efficacy of dopamine and norepinephrine for treatment of hemodynamic compromise in amitriptyline intoxication. Crit Care Med 1991;19:544–9.

ANTIHYPERTENSIVES

ESSENTIALS OF DIAGNOSIS

Beta-blockers:

- *Bradycardia.*
- *Conduction blocks.*
- *Hypotension.*
- *Cardiogenic shock.*
- *Depressed mental status.*

Calcium channel blockers:

- *Bradycardia.*
- *Hypotension.*
- *Heart block.*
- *Drowsiness.*

General Considerations

Although relatively rare, an acute overdose of beta-blockers and calcium channel blockers can be potentially life-threatening and poses significant treatment challenges for the intensivist.

Clinical manifestations of beta-blocker overdose are due to the effects of systemic beta-adrenergic blockade. Toxic effects involve mainly the cardiovascular system, but the severity of symptoms sometimes cannot be fully explained by pure beta blockade alone. Central nervous system effects are common as well. Beta-blockers are rapidly absorbed from the gastrointestinal tract, and clinical effects may appear as rapidly as 20–60 minutes after ingestion. Half-life is dependent upon the specific drug but ranges from 2–12 hours; excessive overdose may prolong this half-life.

Clinical effects of calcium channel blocker overdose are caused by actions on the myocardium and on the smooth muscle of blood vessels. This produces vasodilation and negative inotropic, dromotropic, and chronotropic activity. The most commonly used calcium channel blockers are verapamil, diltiazem, and nifedipine. Each has slightly different effects. All are well-absorbed from the gastrointestinal tract, but diltiazem and verapamil both undergo a significant hepatic first-pass effect. Metabolism is primarily in the liver.

Clinical Features

Patients with significant beta-blockade overdose present with bradycardia, conduction blocks, hypotension, decreased cardiac output, and cardiogenic shock. Bradycardia can be severe and appears to be more common with ingestions of propranolol than with other drugs. Overdose with atenolol, nadolol, carvedilol, and metoprolol tend to present with hypotension and a heart rate within normal limits. Pindolol and practolol overdoses may present with tachycardia owing to their partial agonist activity. First-degree atrioventricular block is common with propranolol overdoses. Junctional rhythms, bundle branch block, complete atrioventricular block, and asystole have all been observed with beta-blocker ingestions. Hypotension is common and may be profound. Depressed mental status is also a common finding and is more common in patients with significant hypotension. Seizures are uncommon but do occur with propranolol ingestion. Significant bronchospasm is surprisingly rare.

Significant calcium channel blocker overdose commonly presents with bradycardia, hypotension, and significant heart block (including third-degree heart block), which can be life-threatening. Hypotension is due to both decreased cardiac output and peripheral vasodilation. These patients may also be somewhat drowsy, though markedly altered mental status is rare.

Differential Diagnosis

Beta-blocker overdoses present with bradycardia and hypotension; these findings can also occur with barbiturate intoxication and in cases of ingestion of some antiarrhythmics such as mexiletine.

Treatment

A. Decontamination

In both beta-blocker and calcium channel blocker overdoses, patients who present within 2–4 hours after ingestion should be considered for gastric lavage. Activated charcoal should be given, and repeat doses are helpful. Patients who are initially stable and who remain so need only be observed and monitored for 12–24 hours.

B. Specific Therapy

1. Beta-blocker overdose—

a. Glucagon—Glucagon has been used with significant success in patients with symptomatic overdoses of beta-blockers and is considered to be the drug of choice. Its effects are independent of beta receptors, and glucagon has both inotropic and chronotropic effects. The dose used is higher than that used for stimulating gluconeogenesis. The recommended initial dose is 0.05 mg/kg intravenously, followed by an infusion of up to 0.07 mg/kg/h as needed. It is important to be certain that the preparation used for these doses does not contain phenol as a diluent, as even small amounts of phenol may be toxic. The most common side effects of this dose of glucagon are nausea and vomiting.

b. Beta agonists—Beta-adrenergic agonists have been used to treat beta-blocker overdoses with varying success. Use of these agents requires quantities sufficient to overcome the competitive blockade at the receptor. These doses may be prohibitively high. Agonists may be tried empirically, but if excessive doses are used with minimal effect, the drug should be discontinued.

c. Atropine—Refractory bradydysrhythmias and heart blockade have been treated with atropine. Little effect may occur, because these rhythms are not vagally mediated. When used, a dose of not more than 1 mg intravenously should be administered. Pacing has been reported, but the heart is often refractory to normal pacing potentials, and the pacemaker may not capture despite the use of high outputs.

2. Calcium channel blocker overdose—

a. Calcium—Calcium channel blocker overdoses have been treated with a variety of medications with varying success. Calcium would intuitively seem to be appropriate therapy, but its use has been disappointing. This result is not surprising, however, as the calcium channels are blocked, and this effect is not easily overcome with additional calcium. Calcium is relatively nontoxic, however, and administration of calcium chloride, 5–10 mL of a 10% solution, is probably indicated.

b. Glucagon—As with beta-blocker overdoses, glucagon is useful in managing patients with calcium channel blocker ingestion, though results have been less impressive. Dosing is the same as that used in treating beta-blocker overdose.

c. Atropine—Atropine has been used to treat bradydysrhythmias and heart blockade but has proved to be relatively ineffective. If the patient does not respond to 1 mg intravenously, use of atropine should be discontinued. Transvenous pacing may be necessary and may require high outputs for capture.

d. Pressors—Dobutamine and dopamine infusions have been used in these ingestions with varying results. These agents may be tried in those patients whose hypotension does not respond to fluid administration and use of glucagon. Norepinephrine may also be used.

Hantson P et al: Carvedilol overdose. Acta Cardiol 1997;52: 369–71.

Kerns W 2nd, Kline J, Ford MD: Beta-blocker and calcium channel blocker toxicity. Emerg Med Clin North Am 1994; 12:365–90.

Love JN et al: Acute beta blocker overdose: factors associated with the development of cardiovascular morbidity. J Toxicol Clin Toxicol 2000;38:275–81.

Love JN: Beta blocker toxicity after overdose: when do symptoms develop in adults? J Emerg Med 1994;12:799–802.

Love JN: Beta-blocker toxicity: a clinical diagnosis. Am J Emerg Med 1994;12:356–7.

Reith DM et al: Relative toxicity of beta blockers in overdose. J Toxicol Clin Toxicol 1996;34:273–8.

Snook CP, Sigvaldason K, Kristinsson J: Severe atenolol and diltiazem overdose. J Toxicol Clin Toxicol 2000;38:661–5.

DIGOXIN

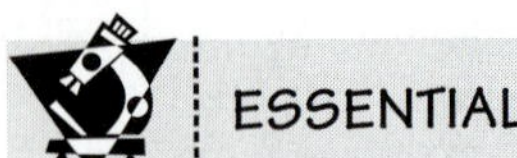

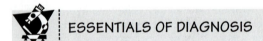

ESSENTIALS OF DIAGNOSIS

- *Weakness, fatigue.*
- *Nausea, anorexia.*
- *Visual complaints.*

General Considerations

Digitalis preparations (digoxin and digitoxin) have two therapeutic effects. The first is to increase vagal tone, which leads to conduction blockade at the atrioventricular node and results in decreased chronotropy. The second is to inhibit the myocardial Na^+–K^+ ATPase pump, which normally pumps calcium and sodium out of the cell and potassium into it. Inhibition causes the intracellular calcium concentration to rise, resulting in increased contractile force (positive inotropic effect). In the patient suffering from digitalis toxicity, inhibition of the pump leads to excessive extracellular potassium and intracellular sodium and calcium, causing exaggerations of the therapeutic effects of the drug. In particular, toxicity is manifested by cardiac, gastrointestinal, neurologic, and electrolyte abnormalities.

Many of the symptoms of digitalis toxicity are nonspecific. Patients may develop digitalis toxicity even when they have normal blood levels of the drug if they have an underlying condition that sensitizes them to its effects. Conversely, patients with elevated levels may show no evidence of toxicity. Making the diagnosis of digitalis toxicity, therefore, often requires that the treating physician know the patient groups at risk and suspect the diagnosis in the appropriate setting. Table 37–9 summarizes the factors that predispose to the development of digitalis toxicity. Patients with any of these factors who are also taking digitalis should be evaluated for possible digitalis toxicity when the clinical setting is suggestive.

Clinical Features

A. Symptoms and Signs

Over 80% of patients with digitalis toxicity will complain of weakness, nausea, anorexia, fatigue, and visual complaints. The visual complaints may be a clue to making this diagnosis. The patient may complain of yellow or green vision or of halos around objects—in addition to other visual disturbances such as photophobia or transient amblyopia. Other complaints include vomiting, headache, diarrhea, and dizziness.

Table 37–9. Predisposing factors in digitalis toxicity.

Increased Sensitivity	Increased Drug Level
Electrolyte disturbances	Renal disease
Hypokalemia	Drugs
Hypernatremia	Quinidine
Hypercalcemia	Verapamil
Hypomagnesemia	Amiodarone
Cardiac abnormalities	
Ischemia	
Cardiomyopathy	
Conduction abnormalities	
Hypoxemia	
Drugs	
Verapamil	
Beta-blockers	
Diuretics	

B. Electrocardiography

Patients with significant cardiac toxicity may not manifest either gastrointestinal or neurologic effects. Cardiac toxicity is due both to the increased vagal effects of the drug and to the effects on the Na^+–K^+ ATPase pump. In general, cardiac toxicity results from depression of impulse formation or conduction (vagally mediated) and from enhancement of automaticity (caused by blocking the Na^+–K^+ ATPase pump). Virtually any rhythm disturbance can be observed in digitalis-toxic patients.

Effects on the sinus node lead to bradycardia, sinoatrial block, and sinus arrest. Increased irritability and automaticity in the atria cause atrial tachycardia and can produce atrial fibrillation or flutter. The ventricular rate is often normal or slow as a result of the conduction block caused by the drug. Digitalis effect in the atrioventricular node can cause atrioventricular block or junctional rhythm. In fact, patients with digitalis toxicity may show a "regularized" atrial fibrillation—ie, a regular junctional rhythm with a background of atrial fibrillation due to the high degree of AV block. The effect in the ventricles may cause premature ventricular contractions (the most common digitalis toxic rhythm), ventricular tachycardia, and ventricular fibrillation.

C. Laboratory Findings

Hyperkalemia may be observed in acute ingestions due to the effect of digitalis on the Na^+–K^+ ATPase pump and the resultant shift of potassium to the extracellular space. This effect is not prominent in patients who are maintained on digitalis on a chronic basis and develop toxicity.

Evaluation of the patient with suspected digitalis toxicity includes a serum digitalis level, serum electrolytes (including magnesium and calcium), serum urea nitrogen, and serum creatinine. An arterial blood gas analysis or pulse oximetry should be performed to ensure that the patient is not hypoxic. An ECG should also be obtained.

Differential Diagnosis

Symptoms of digitalis intoxication are nonspecific and are not infrequently misdiagnosed as gastroenteritis or a viral syndrome. The bradydysrhythmias may be associated with other medications, including beta-blockers and calcium channel blockers. The observed ectopy can also occur with electrolyte disorders, particularly hypokalemia, and in patients who are hypoxic or in those with cardiac ischemia.

Treatment

A. Decontamination

When approaching the patient with suspected digitalis toxicity, one should determine whether the toxicity is acute or chronic. Although both receive the same general care, patients with an acute overdose may need several additional measures, including gastric emptying, which should be undertaken if the patient presents within 2 hours after the ingestion. This should be done carefully, as all gastric emptying techniques cause increased vagal tone and may lead to worsening of any bradydysrhythmias or blocks. Pretreatment with atropine may be considered but may have minimal effect. Charcoal, 50–100 g orally, should then be given to adsorb any digitalis remaining in the gastrointestinal tract. Repeat-dose activated charcoal may be effective in enhancing elimination of the drug. Cholestyramine, which binds digitalis in the gut, has also been used for this purpose in doses of 4–8 g orally, but it has no particular advantages over the use of charcoal. Drug levels should not be drawn until at least 6 hours after the ingestion, as it takes that long for the drug level to equilibrate and levels obtained sooner may be misleadingly high.

In most cases of chronic toxicity, withdrawal of the drug and a period of observation are all that is required for treatment. In cases of both acute and chronic toxicity, forced diuresis, hemoperfusion, and hemodialysis have been shown to be ineffective in removing digitalis owing to its high degree of protein binding.

B. Management of Electrolyte Abnormalities

Patients who develop hyperkalemia should be treated with the standard treatment regimens for this problem. It is important to note, however, that some of these measures may be ineffective with digitalis toxicity. Use of bicarbonate and the administration of glucose and insulin intravenously require an intact Na^+–K^+ ATPase pump in order to reduce the elevated potassium and may not produce the desired effect of lowering the potassium level. Intravenous calcium is contraindicated because it sensitizes the patient further to the toxic effects of the digitalis. Sodium-potassium exchange resins are effective and probably constitute the first choice in treating hyperkalemia from digitalis toxicity (polystyrene sulfonate, 15 g in 20–100 mL of syrup orally one to four times daily, or 30–50 g in 100 mL of water per rectum every 6 hours). Dialysis is also effective and can be used if hyperkalemia is life-threatening or refractory to exchange resin treatment. Digitalis antibodies (see below) are also effective in treating hyperkalemia. A serum potassium level over 5 meq/L in the setting of an acute overdose is an indication for treatment with antidigitalis antibodies.

C. Treatment of Arrhythmias

The major and most life-threatening toxicity associated with digitalis is cardiotoxicity. Bradydysrhythmias, due to the increased vagal tone, are treated with atropine. Starting with doses of 0.5 mg intravenously and repeated at 5-minute intervals as necessary, this drug can be used to a total dose of about 2 mg (0.3 mg/kg). If the bradydysrhythmias are refractory to atropine, electrical pacing may be necessary.

Tachydysrhythmias or rhythms resulting from increased automaticity should be treated in a stepwise approach. First, if the patient is hypokalemic (serum potassium < 3.5 meq/L), particularly if the patient is suffering from chronic toxicity, potassium should be gently replenished, with frequent monitoring of the serum potassium level. Magnesium should be given to virtually all patients with tachydysrhythmias except those with elevated magnesium levels or those with renal failure. The optimal dose is unknown, but 2 g intravenously over 20–30 minutes appears effective. In patients whose tachydysrhythmia does not respond to electrolyte replacement or who have contraindications to electrolyte replacement, lidocaine should be used. If the patient's tachydysrhythmias persist despite adequate lidocaine dosing, phenytoin forms an effective alternative. The therapeutic level is 10–20 μg/mL. Cardioversion is safe when used in patients who have normal digitalis levels and no evidence of toxicity. However, cardioversion in patients with digitalis toxicity can lead to refractory ventricular tachycardia, ventricular fibrillation, or asystole. It should be avoided if possible in this group of patients and dysrhythmias treated medically. However, in some cases, cardioversion may be necessary to regain a perfusing rhythm. If needed, it is critical that the lowest possible energy level be used to achieve cardioversion. If possible, pretreatment with lidocaine may be prudent.

D. Antibodies

Digoxin-specific antibodies (digoxin immune Fab [ovine]) are an important addition to the armamentarium in treating digitalis toxicity, but their use should be limited to very specific situations. These antibodies are sheep serum Fab fragments that have a high affinity for digoxin—higher than the affinity of digoxin for Na^+–K^+ ATPase. They circulate in the intravascular space and diffuse into the extracellular space, where they bind to free digoxin. The complex formed has no biologic activity and is excreted in the urine. The intracellular to extracellular gradient produced by the binding of extracellular free digoxin causes intracellular digoxin to diffuse from within the cells to be bound to the antibody and subsequently excreted. Indications to use these antibodies are listed in Table 37–10. In general, digitalis-specific antibody should be used when there are life-threatening dysrhythmias that do not respond to conventional therapy; in patients with an initial potassium level of > 5 meq/L (particularly in acute ingestions); in patients who have ingested more than 10 mg of digoxin (4 mg in children); and in those who have a steady-state digoxin level > 10 ng/mL. Dosing of digoxin antibodies is based on the fact that each vial contains 40 mg of antibody and will bind 0.6 mg of digoxin or digitoxin. The formula for calculating the dose of antibody in a particular patient is shown below:

CALCULATION OF DOSE OF DIGOXIN ANTIBODY

1. Calculation of body load of digoxin:
   a. Based on amount ingested:
      Digoxin tablets: Amount ingested (mg) × 0.8
      Digoxin elixir or capsules: Amount ingested (mg) × 1.0
   b. Based on serum level (measure 6–8 hours after ingestion)

$$\frac{\text{Serum concentration (ng / mL)} \times 5.6 \times \text{weight (kg)}}{1000}$$

2. Calculation of dose of digoxin antibodies:

$$\frac{\text{Body load of digoxin (mg)}}{0.6\text{mg / vial}} = \text{Number of vials of antibody}$$

3. If ingested amount is unknown or the level not available and the patient has indications for antibody use:
   Administer 20 vials (800 mg)

Table 37–10. Indications for therapy with digoxin antibodies.

Life-threatening dysrhythmias
Serum potassium > 5 meq/L
Acute ingestion of > 10 mg of digoxin (> 4 mg in children)
Steady-state digoxin level > 10 ng/mL

A dose of 20 vials (800 mg) is recommended in patients with life-threatening complications if the amount of ingestion is unknown or if the blood level is unavailable. Dysrhythmias are successfully treated with these antibodies in about 70% of patients. The rhythms usually respond within 20–60 minutes after administration of the antibody. Side effects are generally mild. Up to 15% of patients may develop minor allergic reactions, and some patients with preexisting congestive heart failure may have an exacerbation due to the volume of fluid used to infuse the antibodies. It is important to note that measuring digoxin levels after giving antibodies is unreliable for up to 7 days after their administration. Levels tend to rise to alarming levels because so much of the drug ends up in the circulation bound as the inactive antibody complex.

Current Controversies & Unresolved Issues

The treating physician must understand the indications for digoxin antibodies and use them appropriately. Patients who have minor manifestations of digitalis toxicity such as gastrointestinal complaints or visual changes and those with evidence of cardiac toxicity that does not need intervention or responds to conventional therapy do not need this treatment. In addition, patients with elevated levels but without evidence of toxicity do not need treatment unless their levels measure over 10 ng/mL at steady state. The levels should be measured at least 6–8 hours after the ingestion or the last dose of the medication.

Bosse GM, Pope TM: Recurrent digoxin overdose and treatment with digoxin-specific Fab antibody fragments. J Emerg Med 1994;12:179–85.

Carlebach M et al: Vomiting, hyperkalaemia and cardiac rhythm disturbances. Nephrol Dial Transplant 2001;16:169–70.

Clark RF, Barton ED: Pitfalls in the administration of digoxin-specific Fab fragments. J Emerg Med 1994;12:233–4.

Critchley JA, Critchley LA: Digoxin toxicity in chronic renal failure: treatment by multiple dose activated charcoal intestinal dialysis. Hum Exp Toxicol 1997;16:733–5.

Dawson AH, Whyte IM: Therapeutic drug monitoring in drug overdose. Br J Clin Pharmacol 1999;48:278–3.

Derlet RW, Horowitz BZ: Cardiotoxic drugs. Emerg Med Clin North Am 1995;13:771–91.

Jortani SA et al: Validity of unbound digoxin measurements by immunoassays in presence of antidote (Digibind). Clin Chim Acta 1999;283:159–69.

Klein-Schwartz W, Oderda GM. Poisoning in the elderly. Epidemiological, clinical and management considerations. Drugs Aging 1991;1:67–89.

Rawashdeh NM et al: Gastrointestinal dialysis of digoxin using cholestyramine. Pharmacol Toxicol 1993;72:245–8.

Taboulet P et al: Acute digitalis intoxication—is pacing still appropriate? J Toxicol Clin Toxicol 1993;31:261–73.

ACETAMINOPHEN

ESSENTIALS OF DIAGNOSIS

- *Nausea and vomiting.*
- *Jaundice.*
- *Right upper quadrant pain.*
- *Asterixis.*
- *Lethargy and coma.*
- *Bleeding.*
- *Hypoglycemia.*

General Considerations

Acetaminophen is an antipyretic and analgesic medication available over-the-counter in several brand name preparations. It is also commonly used in combination medications, both over-the-counter and available by prescription. Overdose may occur inadvertently or intentionally. Patients may ingest excessive doses of acetaminophen in an attempt to treat their own pain, being unaware of the potential for toxicity. In the intentional overdose, it must be remembered that many medications contain acetaminophen as a component of a combination preparation, and what might otherwise be a relatively benign ingestion from the other active ingredients in the medication becomes a potentially lethal one in light of the amount of acetaminophen consumed.

Toxicity results from the metabolism of acetaminophen, which occurs in the liver via the cytochrome P450 oxidase system. Intermediate metabolites are then detoxified by glutathione. Excessive amounts of acetaminophen deplete glutathione stores, leading to accumulation of high levels of these toxic metabolites. The major toxicity is hepatotoxicity, with hepatocyte necrosis and, in severe cases, frank liver failure. Acetylcysteine, the antidote for this toxicity, acts by enhancing glutathione stores and providing a glutathione substitute to allow for detoxification of the toxic metabolites.

Susceptibility to toxicity is variable. Patients with liver disease are more sensitive, while children under 9–12 years of age are more resistant than their adult counterparts. Toxic doses vary; in adults doses of less than 125 mg/kg are rarely toxic unless the patient has preexisting liver disease. Doses of 125–250 mg/kg produce variable toxicity, with some patients developing significant liver damage at these levels. Doses over 250 mg/kg commonly place the patient at risk to develop massive hepatic necrosis and liver failure. Patients with severe hepatotoxicity eventually die from massive liver failure 4–18 days after ingestion.

Among patients who recover, liver enzymes begin to normalize 5 days after ingestion, and full recovery occurs within 3 months. Chronic liver disease is extremely rare in patients who were healthy prior to ingestion.

Clinical Features

A. History

It is important that the treating physician be aware that the potential for acetaminophen toxicity is present in virtually all patients with intentional overdoses because of the widespread availability of this compound in combination preparations. Patients may unintentionally take excessive amounts of acetaminophen to treat themselves for painful conditions, not knowing that this drug may be toxic.

B. Symptoms and Signs

Patients with acetaminophen overdose are often asymptomatic or minimally symptomatic in the first 24 hours and may present with minimal clinical symptoms despite having ingested potentially lethal amounts of this medication. Gastrointestinal complaints such as nausea and vomiting are common. Patients may also be somewhat lethargic and diaphoretic. Twenty-four to 48 hours after ingestion, the patient feels well; however, hepatotoxicity begins during this time, and levels of hepatic enzymes begin to rise. Three to 4 days after ingestion, the patient presents with progressive hepatic damage, nausea, vomiting, jaundice, right upper quadrant pain, asterixis, lethargy, coma, and bleeding. Hypoglycemia may develop.

C. Laboratory Findings

The single most important laboratory test in patients who present after acetaminophen ingestion is the acetaminophen level. A serum sample should be drawn at least 4 hours after an acute single ingestion; levels drawn before this 4-hour time delay are unreliable in predicting toxicity. The acetaminophen treatment protocol nomogram (Figure 37–1) is used to ascertain patient risk. In general, patients who have a 4-hour level over 150 μg/mL should be regarded as toxic and treated accordingly.

Patients with hepatotoxicity should have their liver enzymes and coagulation studies checked at least once every 12–24 hours. Patients should be closely monitored for hypoglycemia, which is common among those with hepatotoxicity.

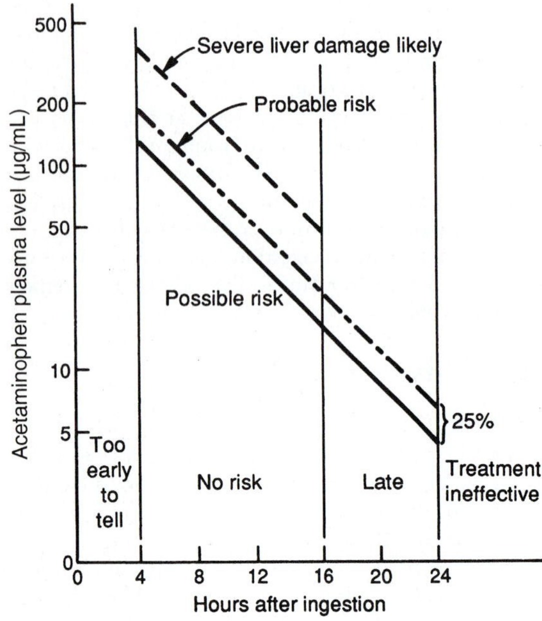

Figure 37–1. Acetaminophen treatment protocol. (Adapted from Rumack BH et al: Acetaminophen overdose: 662 cases with evaluation of oral acetylcysteine treatment. Arch Intern Med 1981;141:382.)

Differential Diagnosis

Liver failure may be caused by a number of other toxins. Cyclopeptide toxicity following mushroom ingestion is an example. Shock liver and massive hepatic necrosis from hepatitis may also cause a similar clinical picture.

Treatment

A. Decontamination

All patients who present within 2–4 hours after ingesting potentially lethal amounts of acetaminophen-containing medications require gastric emptying. Use of activated charcoal is controversial. Activated charcoal binds and prevents the absorption of both acetaminophen and its antidote, acetylcysteine (*N*-acetylcysteine). The charcoal may bind up to 40% of the acetylcysteine. However, increasing the acetylcysteine dose can provide adequate absorption despite the use of charcoal. Therefore, charcoal should be used in patients who present up to 4 hours after ingestion in order to bind any acetaminophen remaining in the gut and prevent its absorption. The acetylcysteine dose, if needed, should be adjusted accordingly.

Patients who present more than 4–6 hours after ingestion have already absorbed the acetaminophen, making gastric decontamination and charcoal administration relatively ineffective. It should be noted, however, that patients may have ingested other medications along with the acetaminophen that may respond to repeat-dose charcoal treatment if the ingested agent is one that can be recovered in this way.

B. Acetylcysteine

To date, there are no reliably effective methods for enhancing the elimination of acetaminophen already absorbed from the gut. Therefore, antidote therapy is the mainstay of treatment for patients with potentially toxic ingestions. Acetylcysteine is indicated in any patient who may have ingested toxic amounts of acetaminophen or in patients who have toxic levels as determined by the treatment nomogram (Figures 37–1 and 37–2). Acetylcysteine is most effective when given within the first 8 hours after ingestion; after this time, efficacy decreases with increasing delay. There is no benefit to giving acetylcysteine in the first 4 hours after ingestion. As a result, treating the patient with acetylcysteine can wait until the acetaminophen level is known if this information will be available within 8 hours after ingestion. If the result will be delayed beyond the 8-hour window and the patient ingested a significant amount of acetaminophen, acetylcysteine therapy should be started empirically and can be discontinued if the level obtained falls in the nontoxic range.

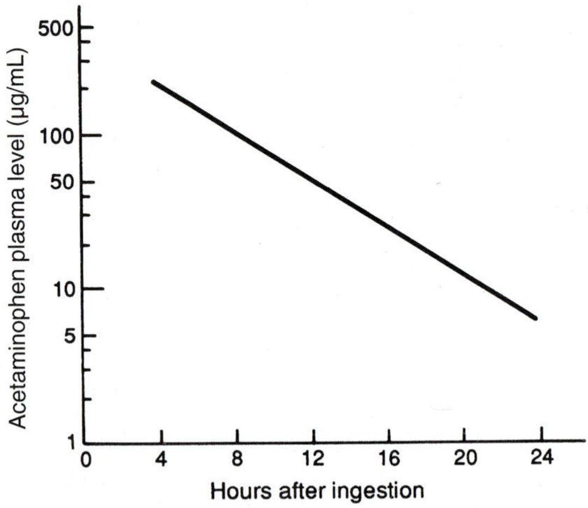

Figure 37–2. Plot of plasma acetaminophen levels versus time. Area above line indicates probable hepatotoxic reaction; area below line, no reaction. (From Rumack BH, Matthew H: Acetaminophen poisoning and toxicity. Pediatrics 1975;55:871–76.)

Acetylcysteine is usually given orally. The loading dose is 140 mg/kg, and subsequent doses of 70 mg/kg are then given every 4 hours for 17 doses. A 2-day regimen has also been used successfully in selected patients. Patients with acetaminophen toxicity may have significant nausea and vomiting, which may make oral administration of acetylcysteine difficult. As a rule, patients who vomit within 1 hour after receiving their oral acetylcysteine dose should have that dose repeated. In addition, several measures can be taken to minimize this difficulty. Antiemetics (prochlorperazine or metaclopramide) should be used. If they prove inadequate, the acetylcysteine may be administered via a nasogastric tube.

Some patients with toxic acetaminophen levels may have persistent vomiting despite the above measures precluding enteric administration of acetylcysteine. In this situation, intravenous acetylcysteine is indicated and can be lifesaving. Currently, intravenous acetylcysteine is not approved for use in the United States, though it has been used safely and successfully for years in Europe and Canada. The oral preparation may be used for intravenous administration, though it is not pyrogen-free. Use of a blood filter removes most of these pyrogens. Dosing is the same as for the oral route. Common complications of intravenous acetylcysteine treatment are rashes and urticaria. Serious reactions are rare. Complications are minimized when acetylcysteine is delivered in at least 250 mL of diluent and infused over 1 hour.

C. Other Measures

Supportive care, including administration of vitamin K and lactulose, is indicated in patients with coagulopathy or encephalopathy, respectively. In severe cases refractory to supportive care, liver transplantation may be necessary.

Current Controversies & Unresolved Issues

Administration of acetylcysteine beyond 24 hours after acetaminophen ingestion has been shown to have little effect. Despite this information and because there are few treatment options other than supportive care and liver transplantation in severely toxic cases, acetylcysteine should probably be used in these situations. The duration of treatment is also controversial. Currently, a 72-hour course is considered the standard of care, but studies have shown that a 48-hour course may be just as effective. Until more studies confirm these data, the 72-hour course should be used. Finally, although intravenous acetylcysteine is not approved for use in the United States, this route of delivery may be life-saving in certain situations, and, when indicated, the treating physician should not hesitate to use this route. Consultation with a local poison control center may aid in making this treatment decision.

Broughan TA, Soloway RD: Acetaminophen hematoxicity. Dig Dis Sci 2000;45:1553–8.

Buckley NA et al: Activated charcoal reduces the need for *N*-acetylcysteine treatment after acetaminophen (paracetamol) overdose. J Toxicol Clin Toxicol 1999;37:753–7.

Clark J: Acetaminophen poisoning and the use of intravenous *N*-acetylcysteine. Air Med J 2001;20:16–7.

Clark RF et al: Safety of childhood acetaminophen overdose. Ann Emerg Med 2001;37:115–6.

Dawson AH, Whyte IM: Therapeutic drug monitoring in drug overdose. Br J Clin Pharmacol 2001;52(Suppl 1):97S–102S.

Gunn VL et al: Toxicity of over-the-counter cough and cold medications. Pediatrics 2001;108:E52.

Isbister G, Whyte I, Dawson A: Pediatric acetaminophen overdose. J Toxicol Clin Toxicol 2001;39:169–72.

Isbister G, Whyte I, Dawson A: Pediatric acetaminophen poisoning. Arch Pediatr Adolesc Med 200;155:417–9.

Kozer E, Koren G: Management of paracetamol overdose: current controversies. Drug Saf 2001;24:503–12.

McClain CJ et al: Acetaminophen hepatotoxicity: An update. Curr Gastroenterol Rep 1999;1:42–9.

Prescott LR: Treatment of severe acetaminophen poisoning with intravenous acetylcysteine. Arch Intern Med 1981;141:386–9.

Richell-Herren K, Harrison M: Towards evidence based emergency medicine: best BETs from the Manchester Royal Infirmary. Activated charcoal in paracetamol overdose. J Accid Emerg Med 2000;17:284.

Whittle J, McGucken B: Paracetamol overdosage. Arch Dis Child 2000;82:428.

Woo OF et al: Shorter duration of oral *N*-acetylcysteine therapy for acute acetaminophen overdose. Ann Emerg Med 2000; 35:363–8.

SALICYLATES

ESSENTIALS OF DIAGNOSIS

- *Nausea and vomiting.*
- *Tinnitus.*
- *Diaphoresis.*
- *Hyperventilation.*
- *Confusion and lethargy.*
- *Convulsions and coma.*
- *Cardiovascular failure.*

General Considerations

Salicylates are widely used as antipyretics, analgesics, for their antiplatelet properties, and as anti-inflammatory agents. They are available not only as aspirin preparations but also constitute a common component of other combination medications readily available over-the-counter. Another important source of salicylates is as oil of wintergreen; this formulation contains very large amounts of the drug, with concentrations as high as 7 g per teaspoon (compared to 325–650 mg per tablet in most aspirin preparations).

When taken orally, salicylates are rapidly absorbed from both the stomach and the small bowel. Peak blood levels occur 2 hours after ingestion of a normal dose. In therapeutic doses, salicylates undergo hepatic metabolism and renal excretion with a half-life of 4–6 hours. In the event of an overdose, the hepatic enzymes become saturated and metabolism changes from first-order (concentration-dependent) to zero-order (concentration-independent) kinetics. Under these circumstances, the drug's half-life increases dramatically to 18–36 hours. In the event of an overdose, renal excretion of the unchanged salicylate becomes the major pathway of drug's elimination.

Salicylates produce respiratory alkalosis by directly stimulating the central nervous system respiratory center and by increasing its sensitivity to changes in CO_2 and oxygen concentrations. Salicylates uncouple oxidative phosphorylation, which leads to an increased metabolic rate with a resultant increase in glucose utilization, oxygen consumption, and heat production. Clinical effects include hypoglycemia and fever. Inhibition of enzymatic components of the Krebs cycle occurs, leading to an increase in pyruvate and lactate that causes a high anion gap metabolic acidosis. As a result of their stimulatory effects on lipid metabolism, salicylates increase ketone formation.

Clinically, it is important to divide patients with salicylate toxicity into two groups: those who take the medication on a chronic basis and those who have taken an acute overdose. Patients who use aspirin chronically, such as the elderly or patients with arthritis, may present subtly and are often misdiagnosed. Their overdose is often unintentional. As the diagnosis is often missed in this group, serious sequelae may develop such as pulmonary and central nervous system complications, with a mortality rate that approaches 25%. The acute overdose group, on the other hand, ingest this drug intentionally. Acute ingestions of over 150 mg/kg are commonly associated with symptoms of toxicity. Pulmonary and neurologic complications are less common in this group, and the mortality rate is only 2%.

Clinical Features

A. Symptoms and Signs

Patients with mild to moderate salicylate toxicity present with nausea, vomiting, tinnitus, diaphoresis, and hyperventilation (hyperpnea, tachypnea), confusion, and lethargy. In cases of severe poisoning, convulsions, coma, and respiratory or cardiovascular failure may occur. These symptoms of coma, seizures, hyperventilation, and dehydration are more common in patients with chronic poisoning and are observed at lower salicylate levels (35–50 mg/dL). Pulmonary edema, cerebral edema, gastritis with hematemesis, and hyperpyrexia are occasionally observed.

B. Laboratory Findings

Salicylate levels are important in the management of these patients. Peak levels after overdose occur 4–6 hours after ingestion. This peak may be delayed or prolonged if the patient ingested enteric-coated preparations or if the patient develops gastric concretions of aspirin after a massive ingestion. The Done nomogram (Figure 37–3) estimates the severity of *acute* salicylate toxicity. It does not apply in the patient with chronic toxicity. Levels obtained 6 hours or more after an acute ingestion can be plotted on the nomogram and extrapolated to obtain the level of severity.

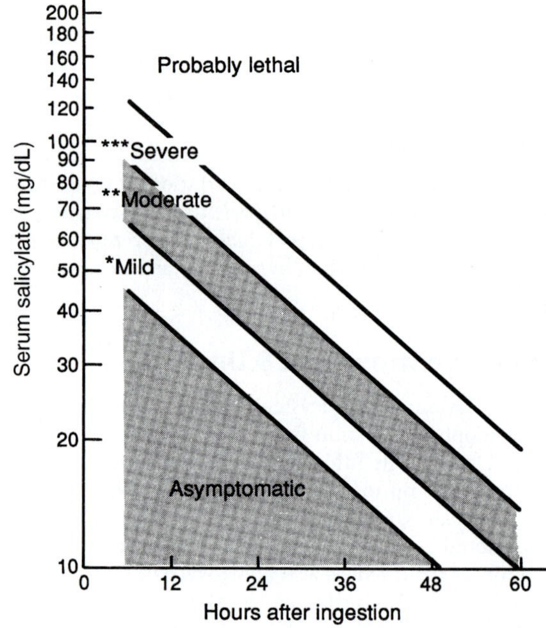

Figure 37–3. Nomogram for determining severity of salicylate intoxication. Absorption kinetics assume acute (one-time) ingestion of non-enteric-coated preparation. (Redrawn and reproduced, with permission, from Done AK: Salicylate intoxication: Significance of measurement of salicylate in blood in cases of acute ingestion. Pediatrics 1960;26:800.)

Common laboratory findings in a patient suffering from salicylism are an elevated anion gap metabolic acidosis and respiratory alkalosis. Other laboratory abnormalities include a prolonged prothrombin time, thrombocytosis, hypernatremia, hyper- or hypoglycemia, ketonemia, lactic acidemia, hypokalemia, and elevated liver transaminases. A urine Phenistix test is usually positive, as is the ferric chloride test (5–10 drops of 10% ferric chloride solution added to urine which has been boiled for 1–2 minutes will turn the solution a burgundy color).

Differential Diagnosis

Because salicylism often presents with altered mental status and an increased metabolic state, other entities that cause this combination should be considered in the differential diagnosis. Stimulants are the primary toxicologic cause, and meningitis, sepsis, or encephalitis are possible infectious sources. Pneumonia, renal failure, diabetic ketoacidosis, and alcoholic ketoacidosis should also be considered.

Treatment

A. Decontamination

Gastric lavage should be performed in any patient with an ingestion of over 100 mg/kg within 2–4 hours before presentation. Gastric lavage should also be considered in patients who have ingested enteric-coated preparations or massive amounts of salicylates, because they are prone to develop intragastric or intraintestinal concretions. Lavage may be helpful as late as 12–24 hours after ingestion in these cases. Activated charcoal should be given to all patients with salicylate ingestion. Repeat-dose activated charcoal administration should be considered in patients with a significant exposure.

B. Alkaline Therapy

Alkalinization is the mainstay of therapy for salicylate poisoning. It is indicated for patients with significant acidemia and for those with blood salicylate levels of over 35 mg/dL. In an alkaline environment, salicylates remain in an ionized form and do not easily diffuse into tissues. Alkalinization of the urine leads to trapping of the salicylates in the renal tubules and facilitates excretion. The goal of treatment is to achieve and maintain the urine pH at 8.0 or above. An adequate serum potassium level is required before urinary alkalinization can be achieved. Patients receiving bicarbonate therapy should be evaluated serially for the possible development of cerebral or pulmonary edema.

C. Hemoperfusion and Hemodialysis

Hemoperfusion and hemodialysis effectively remove salicylates from the blood (Table 37–11). Hemodialysis may be preferable as it can also be used to manage fluid and electrolyte imbalances. Hemodialysis is specifically indicated for patients who are deteriorating despite supportive and conventional therapy; those with acute levels over 120 mg/dL if drawn less than 6 hours after ingestion or 100 mg/dL if drawn at 6 hours postingestion despite the clinical presentation; those with chronic toxicity and levels of 60–70 mg/dL; those with rising salicylate levels despite attempts at elimination; those with significant central nervous system effects; and those with pulmonary edema or renal or hepatic failure.

Table 37–11. Indications for hemodialysis in salicylate therapy.

Acute ingestion with levels of 120 mg/dL if drawn < 6 hours after ingestion, or 100 mg/dL if drawn ≥ 6 hours after ingestion
Chronic toxicity with a salicylate level of 60–70 mg/dL
Deterioration despite conventional therapy
Significant central nervous system toxicity
Renal failure
Hepatic failure
Pulmonary edema
Rising salicylate levels despite attempts at decontamination and elimination

D. Other Measures

Patients who develop seizures should be treated with benzodiazepines or phenobarbital. Hypotension should be treated with fluids and vasopressors. Pulmonary edema may develop as a result of capillary damage from salicylates and can be exacerbated by aggressive fluid therapy. Development of pulmonary edema may require intubation and mechanical ventilation with positive end-expiratory pressures. Hemodialysis is frequently required in these instances.

Higgins RM, Connolly JO, Hendry BM: Alkalinization and hemodialysis in severe salicylate poisoning: comparison of elimination techniques in the same patient. Clin Nephrol 1998; 50:178–83.

Hofman M, Diaz JE, Martella C: Oil of wintergreen overdose. Ann Emerg Med 1998;31:793–4.

Krause DS, Wolf BA, Shaw LM: Acute aspirin overdose: mechanisms of toxicity. Ther Drug Monit 1992;14:441–51.

Malek N: Acute salicylate overdose. Hosp Pract (Off Ed) 1998;33:46.

Skelton H et al: Drug screening of patients who deliberately harm themselves admitted to the emergency department. Ther Drug Monit 1998;20:98–103.

Sporer KA, Khayam-Bashi H: Acetaminophen and salicylate serum levels in patients with suicidal ingestion or altered mental status. Am J Emerg Med 1996;14:443–6.

White S, Wong SH: Standards of laboratory practice: analgesic drug monitoring. National Academy of Clinical Biochemistry. Clin Chem 1998;44:1110–23.

Wrathall G et al: Three case reports of the use of haemodiafiltration in the treatment of salicylate overdose. Hum Exp Toxicol 2001;20:491–5.

THEOPHYLLINE

ESSENTIALS OF DIAGNOSIS

- *Nausea and vomiting.*
- *Tachycardia with atrial or ventricular dysrhythmias.*
- *Hypotension.*
- *Agitation, hyperreflexia, seizures.*
- *Hypokalemia.*

General Considerations

Theophylline is a phosphodiesterase inhibitor which has been used for decades in the treatment of reactive airway disease. It comes in several forms, including an elixir and tablets which are rapidly absorbed. Drug levels usually peak 2–4 hours after ingestion. Theophylline is also available as a sustained-release preparation whose serum level peaks anywhere from 6–24 hours after ingestion. With inhaled agents now first-line, use of this agent has decreased significantly in the last decade.

As a phosphodiesterase inhibitor, theophylline produces an increase in intracellular cAMP, a mediator of beta-adrenergic effects. In addition, at toxic levels, theophylline causes catecholamine release from the adrenal medulla. The result of toxic levels of theophylline, therefore, is excessive beta stimulation, and most of the toxic effects are a result of this excessive catecholamine activity. Theophylline toxicity also causes central nervous system effects, the mechanism of which is unclear.

Theophylline toxicity, like that of salicylates, causes two distinct clinical entities depending on whether the toxicity results from acute ingestion or from chronic intake. Acute toxicity usually results from an intentional overdose in a patient not already taking the medication. Chronic toxicity is usually an inadvertent overmedication in a patient already maintained on this drug. Patients with acute intoxications more commonly have metabolic abnormalities and tolerate higher levels of the drug, often not demonstrating serious toxic effects until the levels reach 80–100 g/dL. Patients with chronic toxicity, on the other hand, often do not demonstrate metabolic abnormalities but may manifest serious toxicity at levels as low as 40 g/dL. It is also important to note that in the patient with chronic toxicity, the serum levels often do not correlate with the severity of toxicity–ie, the patient with what may appear to be a mildly elevated drug level may have life-threatening toxic effects. This is particularly true in elderly patients with chronic theophylline toxicity.

Clinical Features

A. Symptoms and Signs

Theophylline toxicity causes gastrointestinal, cardiovascular, central nervous system, and metabolic abnormalities. As a result of local gastric irritation and central effects, patients often complain of nausea and vomiting. This is not universal, however, and patients may have other life-threatening toxic effects without gastrointestinal complaints.

Owing to the excessive beta stimulation, patients are often tachycardiac and prone to ventricular tachydysrhythmias. Atrial dysrhythmias, including atrial fibrillation and multifocal atrial tachycardia, are also seen. As a result of the stimulation of peripheral β_2-adrenergic receptors and vasodilation, these patients may develop hypotension. Decreased diastolic pressure may be a warning sign that severe vasodilation is developing.

Patients with theophylline toxicity demonstrate agitation, hyperreflexia, and tremulousness. Seizures may develop and are often the first central nervous system sign of toxicity. This is frequently the case in patients with chronic toxicity. Seizures may be focal or generalized and are often prolonged; status epilepticus is not uncommon. Seizures may be refractory to anticonvulsant therapy and can result in permanent brain damage or death.

B. Laboratory Findings

Hypokalemia is common with acute ingestions; it occurs as a result of a theophylline-induced intracellular shift of potassium. Theophylline toxicity also causes hyperglycemia, metabolic acidosis, respiratory alkalosis, and leukocytosis.

Differential Diagnosis

In addition to theophylline, toxic causes of altered mental status, seizures, and cardiovascular abnormalities include tricyclic antidepressants, anticholinergic agents, and phenothiazines. Rarely, calcium channel blockers, beta-blockers, and overdoses of local anesthetic agents cause these findings. Nontoxic causes include meningitis, sepsis, anaphylaxis, head trauma, and hypoglycemia.

Treatment

A. General Measures

Basic supportive measures such as intravenous access, hemodynamic monitoring, oxygen administration, and airway management (as needed) should be the first priority.

B. Correction of Hypotension

Hypotension should initially be treated with infusion of crystalloid as a bolus of 250–500 mL over several minutes. If infusions of balanced salt solution do not correct the hypotension or if the patient cannot tolerate the volume, pressors may be necessary. Pure alpha agonists such as methoxamine or phenylephrine are preferable to pressors with beta effects that may exacerbate theophylline toxicity. Propranolol may also be used to treat the hypotension in patients who do not have contraindications to using this drug. The mechanism for the efficacy of propranolol lies in the fact that it blocks the peripheral β_2-adrenergic receptors that participate in the peripheral vasodilation of theophylline toxicity.

C. Antiarrhythmics

Patients who have severe supraventricular dysrhythmias from theophylline toxicity (severe sinus tachycardia, supraventricular tachycardia, or multifocal atrial tachycardia) may be treated with verapamil or beta-blockers if there are no contraindications to using these drugs. Ventricular dysrhythmias should be treated by correcting hypokalemia and administering lidocaine.

D. Anticonvulsants

Seizures should be treated with benzodiazepines, phenobarbital, or phenytoin, singly or in combination. Seizures accompanying theophylline toxicity are frequently refractory to treatment. It may be necessary to either place the patient under general anesthesia or to use neuromuscular blockade in patients who continue to have seizures in order to prevent acidosis and rhabdomyolysis and to facilitate ventilation. Patients may still have electrical seizure activity despite being anesthetized or paralyzed. Electroencephalographic monitoring should be used to make this determination.

E. Decontamination

Once the patient is stabilized hemodynamically, prevention of further absorption of the drug is the next goal. Patients who present within the first hour after ingestion should have gastric lavage performed. Intubation should be accomplished prior to lavage if the patient is unable to protect the airway. If the patient ingested a sustained-release form of theophylline, lavage should be considered as long as 3–4 hours after ingestion.

Charcoal administration is pivotal in treating patients with theophylline toxicity. All patients, regardless of the time since ingestion, should receive activated charcoal, 1–2 g/kg. This can be given orally or via the lavage tube. For patients who cannot drink the charcoal slurry, a nasogastric tube should be placed and the charcoal delivered directly into the stomach. Serial charcoal dosing is a mainstay in the treatment of theophylline toxicity. Charcoal avidly binds theophylline, making this treatment akin to "gastrointestinal dialysis." Doses of 0.5–1 g/kg of charcoal every 2 hours dramatically decrease the half-life of theophylline. It is essential *not* to give cathartics with each dose of the charcoal. Cathartics should be given with the first dose of charcoal only, and subsequent doses should be a slurry of the charcoal only. If the serial charcoal needs to be continued for more than 24 hours, cathartics can be given once or twice daily as needed. If the patient has persistent vomiting that precludes charcoal administration, metoclopramide can be given intravenously. In these patients, the charcoal may be better tolerated when given as a continuous administration of 0.25–0.5 g/kg/h via a nasogastric tube.

Despite appropriate treatment, some patients with theophylline toxicity continue to have dysrhythmias, hypotension, and seizures. Following an acute ingestion, serum levels of > 90–100 μg/dL are associated with more serious toxic effects. After chronic intoxication, this level is approximately 60 μg/dL. When drug concentrations reach these levels, hemoperfusion or hemodialysis may be indicated. Table 37–12 lists the major indications for initiating hemodialysis or hemoperfusion therapy in patients with theophylline toxicity. Of the two procedures, hemoperfusion is the method of choice. It is important to initiate these procedures early, because if hemodynamic instability develops, hemodialysis may not be possible.

Burgess E, Sargious P: Charcoal hemoperfusion for theophylline overdose: case report and proposal for predicting treatment time. Pharmacotherapy 1995;15:621–4.

Cantrell FL: Treatment of theophylline overdose. Am J Emerg Med 1997;15:547.

Table 37–12. Indications for hemoperfusion or hemodialysis in theophylline toxicity.

Refractory dysrhythmias, hypotension, or seizures
Acute ingestion with level > 90–100 μg/dL
Chronic ingestion with—
Level 60–90 μg/dL
Level 40–60 μg/dL and—
Age < 6 months or > 60 years
Congestive heart failure
Liver disease
Unable to tolerate oral charcoal
Patient not tolerating current level

Chyka PA et al: Prophylaxis of seizures after theophylline overdose. Pharmacotherapy 1997;17:1044–5.

Kempf J et al: Haemodynamic study as guideline for the use of beta blockers in acute theophylline poisoning. Intensive Care Med 1996;22:585–7.

Minton NA, Henry JA: Treatment of theophylline overdose. Am J Emerg Med 1996;14:606–12.

Okada S, Teramoto S, Matsuoka R: Recovery from theophylline toxicity by continuous hemodialysis with filtration. Ann Intern Med 2000;133:922.

Shannon M: Life-threatening events after theophylline overdose: a 10-year prospective analysis. Arch Intern Med 1999; 159:989–94.

Shannon MW: Comparative efficacy of hemodialysis and hemoperfusion in severe theophylline intoxication. Acad Emerg Med 1997;4:674–8.

METHANOL & ETHYLENE GLYCOL

ESSENTIALS OF DIAGNOSIS

Methanol:

- *Visual disturbances.*
- *Nausea, vomiting, abdominal pain.*
- *Lethargy and confusion.*
- *Seizures and coma.*
- *Abdominal tenderness.*

Ethylene glycol:

- *Stage I: Intoxication, slurred speech, ataxia, stupor, hallucinations, seizures, coma.*
- *Stage II: Hypertension, tachycardia, high-output renal failure, myositis.*
- *Stage III: Costovertebral angle tenderness; oliguria or anuria.*

General Considerations

Methanol and ethylene glycol are central nervous system depressants that are found most commonly in antifreeze and deicing products. Ingestions of these compounds occur sporadically in alcoholic patients seeking an ethanol substitute, as an accidental ingestion, or epidemically in groups of patients seeking central nervous system effects. Both methanol and ethylene glycol are rapidly absorbed from the gastrointestinal tract. Methanol blood levels peak 30–90 minutes after ingestion, while ethylene glycol levels peak 1–4 hours after ingestion. Both are metabolized in the liver to toxic metabolites. Alcohol dehydrogenase plays a significant role in their metabolism. Formic acid is the major toxic metabolite of methanol; oxalic acid is the predominant metabolite of ethylene glycol. The half-lives of methanol and ethylene glycol are 14–18 hours and 3–8 hours, respectively. When ethanol is ingested at the same time, the half-lives can more than double. Ingestions as small as 30–60 mL of these compounds have been fatal in adults. Even very small amounts may cause significant morbidity.

Clinical Features

A. Symptoms and Signs

If presentation is soon after ingestion, apparent intoxication may be the only finding. Because toxicity is from metabolites rather than from the parent compound, specific clinical effects may not be noted for many hours after ingestion. The delay is increased when ethanol is ingested at the same time.

1. Methanol—The latent period from ingestion of methanol to manifestations of toxicity is 12–24 hours. At that time about half of the patients will complain of visual disturbances, which include cloudy, blurred, or misty vision. Scotomas are common. The patient typically appears intoxicated and often complains of a headache. Nausea, vomiting, and abdominal pain are common. Ophthalmologic examination may reveal multiple eye abnormalities, including dilated and fixed pupils, constricted visual fields, retinal edema, and hyperemia of the optic disk. However, some patients may have a completely normal eye examination despite having subjective visual complaints. Patients may be lethargic or confused. Seizures and coma may occur. Abdominal tenderness is common. Death may follow abrupt respiratory arrest without warning, so that careful monitoring is mandatory.

2. Ethylene glycol—Ethylene glycol ingestion presents in three stages. Stage I, known as the central nervous system stage, occurs 30 minutes to 12 hours after ingestion. It is characterized by intoxication, slurred speech, ataxia, stupor, hallucinations, seizures, and coma. The patient may complain of nausea and vomiting and may be mildly hypertensive and tachycardiac. Stage II, the cardiopulmonary stage, manifests 12–24 hours after ingestion. Patients become significantly hypertensive and tachycardiac and may develop high-output cardiac failure. Some patients also develop diffuse myositis with muscle tenderness. Stage III, the renal stage, occurs 24–72 hours after ingestion. Patients complain of flank pain and costovertebral angle tenderness. Oliguria, frank renal failure, and anuria develop.

B. Laboratory Findings

Laboratory evaluation of these patients is notable for an elevated anion gap metabolic acidosis (see Table 37–13). Most patients with ethylene glycol ingestion have crystalluria at presentation. The crystals can be either envelope-shaped calcium oxalate crystals or needle-

Table 37–13. Use of the osmolar gap in toxicology.[1]

The osmolar gap (Δosm) is determined by subtracting the calculated serum osmolality from the measured serum osmolality.

$$\text{Calculated osmolality (osm)} = 2[\text{Na}^+(\text{meq/L})] + \frac{\text{Glucose (mg/dL)}}{18} + \frac{\text{BUN (mg/dL)}}{2.8}$$

$$\Delta\text{osm} = \text{Measured osmolality} - \text{Calculated osmolality}$$

Serum osmolality may be increased by contributions of circulating alcohols and other low-molecular-weight substances. Since these substances are not included in the calculated osmolality, there will be a gap proportionate to their serum concentration and inversely proportionate to their molecular weight:

$$\text{Serum concentration (mg/dL)} = \Delta\text{osm} \times \frac{\text{Molecular weight}}{10}$$

	Molecular Weight	Toxic Concentration	Approximate Corresponding Δosm (mosm/L)
Ethanol	46	300	65
Methanol	32	50	16
Ethylene glycol	60	100	16
Isopropanol	60	150	25

[1]Modified from Saunders CE, Ho MT (editors): *Current Emergency Diagnosis & Treatment*, 4th ed. Originally published by Appleton & Lange.

Note: Most laboratories use the freezing point method for calculating osmolality. If the vaporization point method is used, alcohols are driven off and their contribution to osmolality is lost.

Note: A normal osmolar gap may be present in the face of a potentially lethal methanol or ethylene glycol ingestion.

shaped calcium oxalate monohydrate crystals. Leukocytosis and hypocalcemia occur in up to 85% of patients who ingest ethylene glycol.

Treatment

A. General Measures

Supportive care should be initiated as elsewhere described. Gastric lavage is only effective if performed within 1–2 hours after ingestion.

B. Specific Treatment

Specific treatment of these intoxications is the mainstay of therapy and is similar for both methanol and ethylene glycol.

Any patient with a history, clinical presentation, or laboratory findings suggestive of methanol or ethylene glycol ingestion should be treated. There are three major goals: (1) to correct the metabolic acidosis, (2) to block the production of metabolites, and (3) to remove the parent compound and toxic metabolites.

1. Acidosis—Acidosis is treated with intravenous sodium bicarbonate. Bicarbonate therapy should be initiated when the pH drops below 7.2, with therapy directed at maintaining the pH above that level. Massive doses of bicarbonate may be required because the toxic metabolites are inorganic acids that are being produced continuously. Blood pH should be measured frequently. Iatrogenic hypernatremia may develop if large doses of bicarbonate are needed.

2. Metabolites—Production of toxic metabolites can be blocked with the administration of ethanol, either orally or intravenously. The loading dose of ethanol for an average adult is 70 g/kg (2 mL/kg of 50% ethanol orally, or 7 mL/kg of 10% ethanol intravenously). Intravenous solutions should be at concentrations of 10% or less to decrease toxicity. Infusion should provide blood ethanol levels of 100–150 mg/dL. Alcohol dehydrogenase is an important enzyme in the metabolism of methanol and ethylene glycol to toxic metabolites. This enzyme has a higher affinity for ethanol and will preferentially metabolize ethanol rather than the toxic alcohols. The goal is to maintain a blood ethanol level of 100–150 mg/dL, which saturates the enzyme (Table 37–14).

The FDA recently approved fomepizole for the treatment of methanol and ethylene glycol ingestions. This agent works like ethanol by blocking the metabolism of the toxic alcohols at the enzyme alcohol dehydrogenase. Fomepizole is extremely effective, but dialysis remains necessary to definitively remove the alcohols and their metabolites. Cost of this agent may be prohibitive.

3. Decontamination—Once bicarbonate and ethanol therapy have been instituted, hemodialysis is begun to remove the parent compound and toxic metabolites. This has the additional benefit of correcting severe acidosis refractory to intravenous bicarbonate therapy. Patients with methanol ingestion should also receive folic acid, 50 mg intravenously every 4 hours. Those with ethylene glycol ingestion should be given thiamine, 100 mg intramuscularly, and pyridoxine, 100 mg orally.

Brent J et al: Fomepizole for the treatment of methanol poisoning. N Engl J Med 2001;344:424–9.

Burns MJ et al: Treatment of methanol poisoning with intravenous 4-methylpyrazole. Ann Emerg Med 1997;30:829–32.

Jacobsen D, McMartin KE: Methanol and ethylene glycol poisonings: Mechanism of toxicity, clinical course, diagnosis and treatment. Med Toxicol 1986;1:309–34.

Sivilotti ML et al: Reversal of severe methanol-induced visual impairment: no evidence of retinal toxicity due to fomepizole. J Toxicol Clin Toxicol 2001;39:627–31.

ISOPROPYL ALCOHOL

ESSENTIALS OF DIAGNOSIS

- *Headache, dizziness, confusion.*
- *Intoxication with poor coordination.*
- *Abdominal pain, nausea, vomiting.*
- *Tachycardia.*
- *Miosis and nystagmus.*

General Considerations

Isopropyl alcohol is a clear and colorless liquid found in rubbing alcohol, skin and hair products, and antifreeze. It is occasionally ingested by alcoholics who use it as a substitute for ethanol. Up to 80% of the volume ingested is absorbed from the gastrointestinal tract within 30 minutes. Half of the isopropyl alcohol is excreted unchanged by the kidney, with the remainder metabolized in the liver to acetone. Both isopropyl alcohol and acetone are central nervous system depressants. Isopropyl alcohol ingestion is usually relatively benign,

Table 37–14. Ethanol doses[1] for treatment of methanol poisoning in a 70-kg adult.[2]

		Loading Dose	Infusion Rate During Dialysis	Infusion Rate After Dialysis	Total Over 36 Hours
Amount of ethanol	Chronic drinker[3]	42 g	18.0 g/h	10.8 g/h	474 g
	Nondrinker[4]	42 g	11.8 g/h	4.6 g/h	251 g
Volume of IV 10% ethanol	Chronic drinker	530 mL	228 mL/h	137 mL/h	6010 mL
	Nondrinker	530 mL	149 mL/h	58 mL/h	3010 mL
Volume of oral 43% ethanol	Chronic drinker	125 mL	54 mL/h	32 mL/h	1410 mL
	Nondrinker	125 mL	35 mL/h	14 mL/h	749 mL
Volume of oral 90% ethanol	Chronic drinker	60 mL	26 mL/h	15 mL/h	666 mL
	Nondrinker	60 mL	17 mL/h	7 mL/h	359 mL

[1]Calculated to achieve and maintain blood ehtanol concentration of 100 mg/dL, assuming ethanol dialysance of 120 mL/min and a 6-hour dialysis period.

[2]From McCoy HG et al: Severe methanol poisoning: An application of a pharmacokinetic model for ethanol therapy and hemodialysis. Am J Med 1979;67:806.

[3]Assuming V_d = 175 mg/kg/h, K_m = 13.8 mg/dL.

[4]Assuming V_d = 75 mg/kg/h, K_m = 13.8 mg/dL.

with patients surviving after ingestions of up to 1 L. Some develop serious toxicity with doses as low as 2–4 mL/kg. Although uncommon, dermal exposure can cause toxicity.

Clinical Features

A. Symptoms and Signs

Gastrointestinal and central nervous system effects predominate. Patients often complain of headache, dizziness, confusion, intoxication, and poor coordination. Abdominal pain and nausea and vomiting are also common. Because isopropyl alcohol is a gastric irritant, it may cause gastritis, which results in hematemesis. Massive upper gastrointestinal bleeding from hemorrhagic gastritis is a rare but potentially fatal complication of this ingestion.

Examination of these patients is usually normal except for evidence of intoxication. Mild sinus tachycardia may be seen. Hypotension can occur following severe ingestions. Patients may have miosis, nystagmus, and decreased deep tendon reflexes.

B. Laboratory Findings

Serum ketosis without acidosis is the hallmark of isopropyl alcohol ingestion. The metabolism of isopropyl alcohol produces acetone, which is a ketone without acidic properties. An osmolal gap may also be present. For every 1 mg/dL of isopropyl alcohol in the blood, there is a rise in serum osmolality of 0.18 mosm/kg. Hypoglycemia is frequently present.

Differential Diagnosis

Patients who appear intoxicated may have ingested ethanol, methanol, ethylene glycol, or isopropanol. All of these alcohols can cause an elevated osmolal gap, but ethylene glycol and methanol also cause a metabolic acidosis not observed with isopropyl alcohol ingestions. Other causes of metabolic abnormalities such as hyperglycemia, hyperosmolar states, infections (sepsis and meningitis), and head trauma should also be considered.

Treatment

A. General Measures

Intravenous fluid resuscitation, oxygen administration, and hemodynamic monitoring should be initiated. If the patient presents more than 2 hours after ingestion, gastric decontamination is not effective. Activated charcoal does not bind alcohols well and should only be given if coingestion of another substance is suspected.

Patients with hematemesis should have blood sent for typing in case bleeding becomes clinically significant and the patient requires transfusion. Hypotension should be managed with crystalloid infusion; if necessary, vasopressors may be added.

B. Glucose Supplementation

Frequent evaluation of the blood glucose with administration of supplemental intravenous glucose as needed is mandatory. Hourly rapid glucose determinations should be followed with more frequent monitoring if patients have symptoms typical of hypoglycemia.

C. Dialysis

Dialysis is rarely necessary following isopropyl alcohol ingestion. The only indication for hemodialysis is for the patient who remains hypotensive despite crystalloid and vasopressor administration.

Gaudet MP, Fraser GL: Isopropanol ingestion: Case report with pharmacokinetic analysis. Am J Emerg Med 1989;7:297–99.

LaCouture PG: Acute isopropyl alcohol intoxication: Diagnosis and management. Am J Med 1983;75:680–86.

Litovitz T: The alcohols: Ethanol, methanol, isopropanol, ethylene glycol. Pediatr Clin North Am 1986;33:311–23.

MUSHROOM POISONING

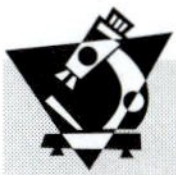

ESSENTIALS OF DIAGNOSIS: CYCLOPEPTIDES

Early:

- *Colicky abdominal pain.*
- *Watery diarrhea, nausea, vomiting.*

Late:

- *Right upper quadrant pain.*
- *Hepatomegaly, asterixis, jaundice, encephalopathy.*

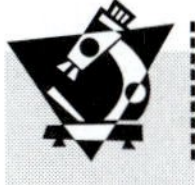

ESSENTIALS OF DIAGNOSIS: GYROMITRIN

Early:

- *Dizziness, bloating, nausea, vomiting.*
- *Headache.*

Late:

- *Hepatic failure.*
- *Seizures and coma.*

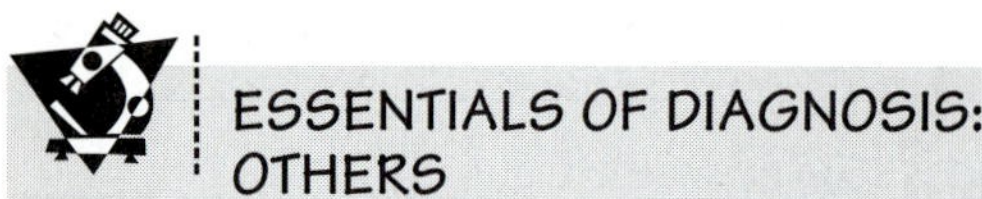

ESSENTIALS OF DIAGNOSIS: OTHERS

- *Findings related to specific ingestion.*

General Considerations

Severe mushroom poisoning is rare in the United States, with only 200–350 cases and 50 deaths reported each year. Children account for half of these ingestions, which occur most commonly in the spring, summer, and fall. Of the 500 species of mushrooms in the United States, 100 are toxic and only ten are potentially fatal when ingested. The toxicity of any particular mushroom is variable and depends on the climate, the amount of rainfall, and the maturity of the plant.

Toxic mushrooms are divided into eight categories grouped by the effects of the toxin and the time to manifestation of effects. Table 37–15 summarizes these categories. Half of the reported mushroom ingestions, and 95% of the fatal cases, result from the cyclopeptide group. Mushrooms harboring this toxin are found chiefly along the northwest Pacific Coast region of North America, including California. Ingestions occur most commonly in the summer and fall. Toxicity is due to gastrointestinal irritation and hepatic failure. Mortality rates are as high as 50%, with death often due to hepatorenal syndrome, which occurs 6–16 days after ingestion. The remainder of the fatal ingestions result from consumption of mushrooms in the gyromitrin group, also known as "false morels." Found in California woodlands, these poisonings most commonly occur in the early spring. Gyromitrins are hydrolyzed in the liver to monomethylhydrazine, which probably causes toxicity by inactivating pyridoxal phosphate. Both of these toxins have delayed symptom onset; this characteristic serves as a clue that the patient may have ingested a potentially lethal mushroom.

Mushrooms that contain toxins which affect the autonomic nervous system are found virtually everywhere, often growing alongside other nontoxic mushrooms. Two types of autonomic syndromes occur in this category. Ingestion of mushrooms that contain significant amounts of muscarine produces stimulation of postganglionic parasympathetic muscarinic effectors, causing a choliner-

Table 37–15. Classification of mushroom toxicity.

Poison	Symptons	Onset	Examples
RAPID-ONSET TOXICITY			
Poisons affecting the autonomic nervous system			
Muscarine	Cholinergic toxidrome	1–2 hours	*Clitocybe* species
Coprine	"Nature's disulfiram": flushing, nausea, vomiting, diaphoresis	30 minutes after ethanol	*Coprinus* species
Poisons affecting the central nervous system			
Ibotenic acid, muscimol	Dizziness, incoordination, myotonic jerks, spasms, hallucinations	30 minutes to 2 hours	*Amanita muscaria*
Psilocybin, psilocin	Euphoria or dysphoria, lethargy, deep sleep, hallucinations (visual)	30 minutes to 1 hour	*Psilocybe* species
Poisons affecting the gastrointestinal system			
Multiple	Nausea, vomiting, diarrhea, abdominal pain	30 minutes to 2 hours	"Little brown mushrooms," widespread
DELAYED-ONSET TOXICITY			
Poisons causing cellular destruction			
Cyclopeptides	Abdominal pain, nausea, vomiting, diarrhea, delayed jaundice, coma	6–24 hours	*Amanita phalloides*, *Galerina marginata*
Gyromitrin, monomethylhydrazine	Nausea, vomiting, diarrhea, incoordination, seizures, coma	6–12 hours	*Gyromitra* species
Poisons affecting the renal system			
Orelline, orellanien	Gastritis, delayed renal failure	3–14 days	*Cortinarius* species (especially Japan, Europe)

gic toxidrome. Ingestion of the coprine group of mushrooms ("inky caps") is usually nontoxic, and these mushrooms are often considered a delicacy. Coingestion of ethanol with these mushrooms, however, leads to a disulfiram-like reaction, probably due to blocking of aldehyde dehydrogenase in the liver. If the ethanol is ingested before or concurrently with the mushrooms, this toxicity does not occur. Instead, sensitivity to ethanol begins 2 hours after ingestion of the mushrooms and lasts up to 5 days.

Ingestion of mushrooms that affect the central nervous system often constitutes a form of recreational drug use. Inadvertent consumption of mushrooms in this category also occurs, as they are often found along the Pacific Coast in the spring, summer, and fall. Although these mushrooms rarely produce serious toxicity in adults, children may develop lethal complications.

Clinical Features

A. History

Mushroom toxicity presents with a wide array of symptoms, depending on the type of mushroom ingested. Patients who present with mushroom toxicity may or may not relate a history of ingestion. They may not connect their consumption of the mushrooms with their illness, or, if they are using mushrooms for recreational purposes, may be hesitant to give medical personnel this information. In clinical settings suggestive of mushroom ingestion, clinicians should ask specifically about this possibility. One of the most important historical pieces of information that should be sought from the patient is the time from ingestion to the onset of symptoms; mushrooms which are potentially lethal have a time delay of at least 4–6 hours from ingestion to symptoms. It should be kept in mind, however, that patients may coingest several different types of toxic mushrooms, and a rapid onset of symptoms does not exclude concurrent ingestion of a potentially lethal one.

The potentially lethal mushroom toxins, cyclopeptides and gyromitrin, are characterized by delayed onset of symptoms. This is an extremely important clinical clue. Any patient who presents with symptoms that occur more than 6 hours after ingesting a potentially toxic mushroom should be considered to have a possibly fatal ingestion.

B. Symptoms and Signs

Cyclopeptides, the most common lethal mushroom toxin, cause a three-phase illness. The gastrointestinal phase begins abruptly 6–12 hours after ingestion and is characterized by severe colicky abdominal pain, profuse watery diarrhea, nausea, and vomiting. These symptoms last up to 24 hours and then resolve. The patient feels well during a latent phase of 3–5 days, but hepatic toxicity then begins. At the end of this phase, the patient presents with findings typical of liver failure, including right upper quadrant pain, hepatomegaly, asterixis, jaundice, or frank encephalopathy.

Gyromitrin-containing mushrooms cause gastritis with onset 6–12 hours after ingestion. The patient complains of dizziness, bloating, nausea, vomiting, and severe headache. Hepatic failure may occur in severe cases, usually 3–4 days after ingestion. Seizures and coma are also described.

The *Cortinarius* species of mushrooms, found most commonly in Japan and Europe, contains orelline, which results in a delayed presentation 24–36 hours after ingestion with a self-limited gastritis-like illness. Three to 14 days after ingestion, the patient presents with night sweats, anorexia, headache, chills, and a severe burning thirst. Oliguria and flank pain may also be present.

The remainder of the toxic mushrooms cause symptoms soon after ingestion. Toxins that affect the autonomic nervous system include muscarine and coprine. Fifteen minutes to 1 hour after ingestion of muscarine-containing mushrooms, the patients will complain of headache, nausea, vomiting, and abdominal pain, and may develop cholinergic symptoms of salivation, lacrimation, urination, defecation, and diaphoresis. In severe cases, bronchospasm, bronchorrhea, bradycardia, and shock may occur. In most cases, however, symptoms are usually mild and resolve in 2–6 hours. Coprine-containing mushrooms alone do not cause toxicity; however, when ethanol is ingested 2 hours to 5 days after ingestion of these mushrooms, the patient may develop a disulfiram-like syndrome. Fifteen to 20 minutes after drinking ethanol, the patient complains of a severe headache, facial flushing, paresthesias, lightheadedness, orthostatic hypotension, vomiting, palpitations, and tachycardia. Although the patient feels ill, these symptoms rarely cause significant compromise and abate after several hours.

Mushrooms that affect the central nervous system contain one of several toxins, including ibotenic acid, muscimol, and psilocybin. Symptoms usually begin 30 minutes to 4 hours after ingestion. Patients complain of drowsiness, incoordination, waxing and waning mental status, and formed or unformed visual hallucinations. Psilocybins are renowned for causing alterations in perceptions of shapes, sounds, and colors. Ibotenic acid and muscimol may cause anticholinergic effects which are rarely severe except in children; these effects are seizures, coma, tachycardia, and hypertension. Most of these patients resolve their symptoms within several hours without sequelae.

The final group of toxic mushrooms are those known as "little brown mushrooms" and cause primarily a self-limited gastrointestinal illness characterized by rapid onset of malaise, nausea, vomiting, and diarrhea within 1–3 hours after ingestion. These symptoms usually resolve within 24–48 hours.

C. Laboratory Findings

Laboratory results are related specifically to the type of ingestion.

1. Cyclopeptides—Laboratory evaluation reveals hypoglycemia, elevated aminotransferases, metabolic acidosis, and coagulopathy.

2. Gyromitirin—Laboratory evaluation shows elevated liver function tests and coagulopathy; these patients may also have methemoglobinemia.

3. Orelline—Laboratory evaluation reveals red blood cell casts, elevated BUN, serum creatinine, proteinuria, and hematuria.

Differential Diagnosis

Owing to the wide range of symptoms caused by toxic mushrooms, the differential diagnosis depends on the type of mushroom ingested. Most of the toxic mushrooms cause a gastrointestinal syndrome that may be confused with gastroenteritis, infectious diarrhea, or other gastrointestinal diseases. Liver failure (associated with the cyclopeptides and gyromitrins) can be caused by other toxins, particularly acetaminophen, as well as entities such shock liver, severe hepatitis, and alcoholism. Central nervous system effects of mushroom toxicity can also be observed in patients who ingest anticholinergics, LSD, peyote, and other hallucinogens. The cholinergic syndrome that occurs with muscarine-containing mushrooms is also found in organophosphate poisoning.

Treatment

Treatment of patients with toxic mushroom ingestions depends on the type of mushroom ingested and the symptoms. If there is any possibility that the patient may have ingested a potentially lethal mushroom—even if it cannot be confirmed—the patient should be treated aggressively.

A. Decontamination

In general, all patients who may have ingested potentially lethal mushrooms should have gastric emptying if they present within 4 hours after ingestion. Repeat-dose activated charcoal should be given after lavage and if the patient presents after this 4-hour time period.

B. Antidotes

Although several potential antidotes have been used to treat patients who may have ingested cyclopeptide-containing mushrooms, none have been proved to be effective. These patients need supportive care and may ultimately need liver transplantation if liver failure becomes severe.

C. Renal Dialysis

Cortinarius mushroom toxicity that results in renal failure should be managed with dialysis as needed. These patients may need dialysis for weeks to months but usually will eventually recover renal function.

D. Other Measures

If significant methemoglobinemia (metHb > 30% or symptomatic hypoxia or ischemia and a metHb < 30%) develops in a patient who ingests gyromitrin-containing mushrooms, one should give methylene blue, 0.1–0.2 mL/kg of a 1% solution intravenously over 5 minutes. Such patients who develop intractable seizures refractory to standard therapy may respond to pyridoxine, 25 mg/kg intravenously given over 25–30 minutes.

Patients with cholinergic symptoms from muscarine-containing mushrooms usually need observation only. However, if they develop bronchospasm, bronchorrhea, bradycardia, or shock, they should be treated with atropine, 0.5–1 mg intravenously. This dose should be repeated every 10–20 minutes until the symptoms resolve.

Patients who ingest hallucinogenic mushrooms do not need specific medical interventions. They should be placed in a dark, quiet room and observed until the effects subside. If patients manifest significant anticholinergic signs, they should be monitored closely and receive specific treatment for anticholinergic toxicity if indicated.

Current Controversies & Unresolved Issues

Several antidotes have been used to treat cyclopeptide toxicity. Thioctic acid, a coenzyme in the Krebs cycle, has been used in a dose of 50–150 mg intravenously every 6 hours with variable results. Its only major side effect is hypoglycemia, which requires close monitoring. Since this poisoning can be life-threatening, use of thioctic acid should be considered with the understanding that its effects have not been validated. Other treatments, including high-dose penicillin, silibinin, high-dose steroids, hyperbaric oxygenation, and pyridoxine, have been used with inconclusive results.

Broussard CN et al: Mushroom poisoning–from diarrhea to liver transplantation. Am J Gastroenterol 2001;96:3195–8.

Bedry R et al: Wild-mushroom intoxication as a cause of rhabdomyolysis. N Engl J Med 2001;345:798–802.

Kaneko H et al: Amatoxin poisoning from ingestion of Japanese *Galerina* mushrooms. J Toxicol Clin Toxicol 2001;39:413–6.

Wellington K, Jarvis B: Silymarin: a review of its clinical properties in the management of hepatic disorders. BioDrugs 2001;15:465–89.

Danel VC, Saviuc PF, Garon D: Main features of *Cortinarius* spp. poisoning: a literature review. Toxicon 2001;39:1053–60.

Alves A et al: Mushroom poisoning with *Amanita phalloides*—a report of four cases. Eur J Intern Med 2001;12:64–6.

Nordt SP, Manoguerra A, Clark RF: 5-Year analysis of mushroom exposures in California. West J Med 2000;173:314–7.

ORGANOPHOSPHATES

ESSENTIALS OF DIAGNOSIS

Muscarinic effects:

- *Bronchospasm, bronchorrhea.*
- *Salivation, lacrimation, urination, defecation (SLUD syndrome).*
- *Blurred vision.*

Nicotinic effects:

- *Muscle fasciculations, weakness, paralysis.*
- *Ataxia.*

General Considerations

Organophosphates are found most commonly in herbicides and insecticides and are in the form of organophosphates or carbamates. They act by causing irreversible inactivation of acetylcholinesterase, resulting in an accumulation of acetylcholine at cholinergic receptors. The toxicity results from excessive muscarinic, nicotinic, and central nervous system effects of the excess acetylcholine. Toxicity may develop after oral or dermal exposure.

Patients with organophosphate toxicity may be exposed accidentally at work, often by dermal exposure. Alternatively, patients may accidentally or intentionally ingest these compounds. The diagnosis is often made clinically, as there are no laboratory tests immediately available to detect these compounds.

Clinical Features

A. Symptoms and Signs

Patients present with a myriad of symptoms. Peripheral muscarinic effects include bronchospasm, bronchorrhea, nausea, vomiting, diarrhea, miosis, blurred vision, urinary incontinence, salivation, diaphoresis, and lacrimation. The combination of salivation, lacrimation, urination, and defecation is known as the SLUD syndrome, and is very suggestive of organophosphate poisoning. Nicotinic effects consist primarily of skeletal muscle symptoms, particularly muscle fasciculations, weakness, ataxia, and frank paralysis. Blood pressure and heart rate effects vary depending on whether muscarinic or nicotinic effects predominate. Patients may be tachycardiac or bradycardiac and hypertensive or hypotensive. Elevated central nervous system acetylcholine concentrations cause headache, slurred speech, confusion, seizures, and coma as well as depression of the respiratory centers. Respiratory failure is the usual cause of death, often due to a combination of central respiratory depression, respiratory muscle weakness, bronchospasm, and increased bronchial secretions.

B. Laboratory Findings

There are no laboratory tests immediately available that characterize this ingestion, and the diagnosis is often made on the basis of a potential for exposure to the toxin combined with a suggestive clinical presentation. Laboratory testing for cholinesterase activity will show decreased activity of this enzyme and often confirms the diagnosis. However, this test is usually not performed on an emergent basis, and several days may pass before results become available. Definitive diagnosis is made by appropriate response to treatment (atropine, pralidoxime) and decreased cholinesterase activity in the blood.

Differential Diagnosis

The combination of salivation, lacrimation, urination, and defecation strongly suggests organophosphate poisoning. This diagnosis is of particular importance if the patient is diaphoretic and bronchospastic, with excessive pulmonary secretions and muscle weakness. Patients with myasthenia gravis in cholinergic crisis present with a similar clinical picture.

Treatment

A. Decontamination

Medical personnel should wear gowns and gloves when treating patients with organophosphate poisoning, since they may become contaminated and symptomatic from either the patient's clothing or secretions and body fluids. Patients with dermal exposure need copious irrigation in a protected area. Gastric lavage should be attempted if the ingestion was less than 1 hour before presentation and the patient is not already vomiting. After lavage, activated charcoal should be given through the nasogastric tube before it is removed. Intubation and ventilatory support should be considered early.

B. Atropine

Atropine antagonizes the peripheral muscarinic effects of the excess acetylcholine and may moderate some of the central nervous system effects, but it does nothing to alter the skeletal muscle nicotinic effects nor does it restore acetylcholinesterase to an active state. Indications for the use of atropine are suspected organophosphate poisoning in a patient who has muscarinic symptoms and signs. The drug can be used both diagnostically and therapeutically. Diagnostically, a dose of 1 mg (or 0.015 mg/kg) intravenously should dilate the pupils and increase the heart rate within 10 minutes. If there is no response to this dose, cholinergic toxicity is suggested. At that point, 2–4 mg (or 0.02–0.05 mg/kg) of atropine should be given intravenously every 10–15 minutes, with the end point being a drying of secretions, particularly bronchial secretions. Pupillary dilation and tachycardia should not be used as end points, since these effects may be seen before drying of bronchial secretions is achieved. Massive doses of atropine may be needed to achieve full effect.

C. Pralidoxime

Pralidoxime reverses phosphorylation of acetylcholinesterase and therefore restores its activity. This drug will reverse the nicotinic effects of muscle weakness and also reverses some of the central nervous system effects of the poison. Because pralidoxime is more effective in reversing the nicotinic than the muscarinic effects, it should be used in conjunction with atropine. Indications for pralidoxime include the nicotinic effects of organophosphate poisoning (fasciculations, weakness) or central nervous system effects (altered mental status). Blood should be drawn and sent for cholinesterase activity before the drug is administered. The dose is 1–2 g (or 25–50 mg/kg) intravenously over 5–15 minutes. End-organ effects are seen in 15–45 minutes and are manifested by increased muscle strength. Dosing can be repeated in 1–2 hours if weakness and fasciculations persist. Pralidoxime can be repeated every 4–12 hours as needed. Its side effects (nausea, headache, tachycardia) rarely occur and usually result from too rapid injection.

In moderate to severe poisoning, atropine and pralidoxime should be continued for at least 24 hours; in severe poisonings, therapy may need to be continued for days to weeks. Treatment with antidotes can be discontinued when clinical response indicates that they are no longer needed, ie, when there is an absence of clinical improvement with therapy and a lack of recurrence of signs and symptoms of toxicity when the antidotes are withheld.

Hsieh BH et al: Acetylcholinesterase inhibition and the extrapyramidal syndrome: a review of the neurotoxicity of organophosphate. Neurotoxicology 2001;22:423–7.

Lee P, Tai DY: Clinical features of patients with acute organophosphate poisoning requiring intensive care. Intensive Care Med 2001;27:694–9.

Lessenger JE, Reese BE: Rational use of cholinesterase activity testing in pesticide poisoning. J Am Board Fam Pract 1999;12:307–14.

Thiermann H et al: Modern strategies in therapy of organophosphate poisoning. Toxicol Lett 1999;107:233–9.

Care of Patients with Environmental Injuries

38

James R. Macho, MD, & William P. Schecter, MD

Patients with injuries due to environmental hazards and toxic exposure may require admission to a critical care unit for resuscitation, stabilization, and definitive treatment. This chapter reviews the essentials of diagnosis and treatment of heat stroke, hypothermia, frostbite, near drowning, envenomation, electric shock (and lightning injury), and radiation injury.

HEAT STROKE

ESSENTIALS OF DIAGNOSIS

- *Core body temperature approaching 41 °C.*
- *Confusion, stupor, coma.*
- *Hypotension and tachycardia.*
- *Muscle stiffness.*
- *Hot, dry skin.*
- *Elevated hematocrit and hyperkalemia.*

General Considerations

The three major manifestations of heat illness are heat cramps, heat exhaustion, and heat stroke. The syndromes usually occur in warm, humid environments after strenuous physical exertion. However, elderly persons with medical problems or infants may be affected under less severe conditions.

Heat cramps and **heat exhaustion** result from the depletion of fluid and electrolytes. Complete recovery occurs after removal of the patient from the stressful environment and the institution of replacement therapy. **Heat stroke** results from the failure of thermoregulatory mechanisms. *It is a medical emergency,* and prompt reduction of body temperature is necessary to prevent morbidity and mortality.

To maintain a constant body temperature, heat loss must equal heat production. Cutaneous vasodilation allows for heat loss through the processes of radiation, conduction, and convection. Evaporative heat loss occurs from sweating and to a lesser extent from the airway. When the environmental temperature exceeds body temperature, the only effective means of heat loss is through sweating. Although significant amounts of heat can be dissipated through this mechanism, sweating becomes less efficient under conditions of high humidity.

Heat stress syndromes develop as a result of processes that attempt to maintain normal body temperature. Heat stroke results from failure of thermoregulatory mechanisms. Heat cramps and heat exhaustion commonly occur after excessive sweating in a hot environment. Heat cramps are painful spasms of voluntary muscles that occur as a result of electrolyte depletion. Depletion of fluid and electrolytes contributes to the weakness and mental status changes associated with heat exhaustion.

Heat stroke occurs when the core body temperature exceeds 41 °C. Heat stroke may occur in otherwise healthy people after extreme exertion in a hot climate, particularly in unacclimatized individuals. In this setting, heat production exceeds heat loss, resulting in failure of thermoregulatory mechanisms. Once these mechanisms have failed, body temperature may rise quite rapidly. Signs and symptoms can develop suddenly. A rise in core body temperature above 42 °C is associated with protein denaturation and cellular lipid membrane dissolution. Hypovolemia due to dehydration may exacerbate the direct organ injury. Nonexertional heat stroke is often called "classic" heat stroke and commonly affects elderly or debilitated individuals with impaired thermoregulation due to disease or medications. The volume status of a patient with nonexertional heat stroke is unpredictable. In both exertional and nonexertional heat stroke, myocardial dysfunction may occur as a result of direct damage to the myocytes.

The neurologic abnormalities associated with heat stroke range from confusion and stupor to coma and seizure disorders. Cerebral and cerebellar neurons may be destroyed by the increased temperature. Brain hemorrhages and cerebral edema can occur in severe cases. Although many patients recover without neurologic sequelae, residual cerebellar symptoms, quadriparesis, hemiparesis, and memory loss may be present.

Hypovolemia results from dehydration, intracellular volume shifts, decreased peripheral vascular resistance, or poor myocardial function. Myocardial depression follows heat-induced myocardial necrosis.

Disseminated intravascular coagulation can result from heat stroke. Denaturation of the proteins involved in the coagulation cascade may produce prolongation of the prothrombin time and partial thromboplastin time. Direct thermal injury may result in platelet dysfunction. Megakaryocytes in the bone marrow may also show thermal damage. Abnormal bleeding develops in numerous sites and results in secondary neurologic deterioration.

Thermal injury results in direct muscle damage and necrosis. It may occur in nonexertional heat stroke as well as in heat stroke associated with exertion. Rhabdomyolysis results in the release of large amounts of myoglobin and muscle enzymes.

Renal failure may result from direct thermal damage to the tubules. Hypoperfusion of the kidneys results in acute tubular necrosis. Myoglobinuria may exacerbate renal failure due to direct toxic effects.

Death in heat stroke can occur from direct heat injury to the brain. Other causes of death and morbidity include cerebral hemorrhage, aspiration pneumonia, cardiac failure, renal failure, and hepatic failure.

Clinical Features of Heat Stroke

A. Symptoms and Signs

Heat stroke can develop suddenly, with loss of consciousness and need not be preceded by prodromal symptoms such as headache, dizziness, muscle cramps, nausea, and fainting. Although hot, flushed skin is associated with heat stroke, about half of patients exhibit sweating. Depression of neurologic status is present in nearly all cases, and most patients are unconscious at presentation. Signs of cerebellar dysfunction and seizures may also occur. Sinus tachycardia and hypotension are common in patients with heat stroke. Hypovolemia with dehydration causes these changes in most cases, but cardiac dysfunction may also occur as a result of direct injury or acidosis. In the later stages of heat stroke, acute respiratory failure, renal failure, and severe coagulation disorders may develop.

B. Laboratory Findings

Serum concentrations of sodium, potassium, phosphate, calcium, and magnesium are usually low during the early stages of heat stroke. Hematocrit is usually elevated as a result of hemoconcentration. In the later stages of heat stroke, hyperkalemia may develop as a result of rhabdomyolysis. This also results in serum enzyme elevations of CK, LDH, and AST. Coagulation studies may be abnormal in the later stages of the syndrome. Elevation of fibrin split products suggests disseminated intravascular coagulation and is associated with a poor prognosis. Arterial blood gases usually reveal a mixed disorder, with respiratory alkalosis due to hyperventilation and a profound metabolic acidosis. Arterial blood gases should be interpreted without temperature correction to avoid misinterpretation.

Differential Diagnosis

The diagnosis of exertional heat stroke is usually straightforward and based on a history of strenuous physical activity in a hot environment. In the elderly patient presenting with fever, hypotension, tachycardia, and mental status changes, sepsis must be considered. A thorough physical examination should be performed and appropriate cultures obtained to exclude this possibility. Heat stroke must also be differentiated from neuroleptic malignant syndrome. In this syndrome, hyperthermia is triggered by major antipsychotic medications such as phenothiazines, thioxanthenes, and the butyrophenones. Neuroleptic malignant syndrome occurs in as many as 1% of patients receiving these medications, and its recognition is important since effective treatment is available with the nondepolarizing muscle relaxants and dantrolene.

It is important to differentiate between fever and the hyperthermia of heat stroke. In the febrile patient, the regulatory set point is increased due to endogenous or exogenous pyrogens and body temperature is balanced at a new set point. Heat stroke represents a failure of thermoregulatory mechanisms. Therefore, antipyretics are ineffective in patients with heat stroke, and the peripheral cooling used to lower body temperature in these patients is generally not effective in treating patients with fever.

Treatment of Heat Stroke

A. Prompt Lowering of Body Temperature

The patient should be placed in a cool environment. If the patient is unconscious, endotracheal intubation should be performed and mechanical ventilation with supplemental oxygen instituted to maintain adequate gas exchange. Fluid resuscitation is required to reverse hypovolemia. In almost all cases, central venous pressure monitoring will be necessary to evaluate fluid status. In the elderly patient with evidence of cardiac dysfunction, pulmonary artery catheterization may be required. After rapid resuscitation, the rapid reduction of body temperature is the major priority. The optimal method for cooling the patient remains controversial. Immediate treatment usually consists of surface cooling with immersion in ice water or cold water or the use of cooling blankets. Cold water immersion has been shown to be as effective as ice water immersion and may be less uncomfortable for the patient. The disadvantages of ice water immersion include peripheral vasoconstriction and shivering. Shivering is undesirable because of increased heat production and metabolic demand. In this setting, shivering can be abolished by the administration of nondepolarizing muscle relaxants. The use of phenothiazines should be avoided because of the risk of toxicity and the possibility of a decrease in the seizure threshold. Other techniques for cooling include cold intravenous fluids, cold-water gastric or rectal lavage, peritoneal dialysis with cold fluids, or the use of external cooling with circulatory bypass. Once the temperature has been reduced to 39 °C, cooling efforts should be discontinued to prevent the development of hypothermia. The use of antipyretics such as aspirin or acetaminophen is ineffective for the reasons previously stated, and their use is contraindicated because they may worsen an existing coagulopathy or exacerbate hepatic injury. The use of alcohol sponge baths is also contraindicated because of the risk of systemic absorption and resulting toxicity.

B. Physiologic Monitoring

Continued monitoring in the intensive care unit is essential, since many of the complications of hyperthermia such as pulmonary failure, renal failure, and coagulation disorders may take 24–48 hours to develop. Electrolytes should be monitored frequently to detect life-threatening electrolyte disorders. If rhabdomyolysis develops, osmotic diuresis and alkalinization of the urine may help to prevent renal damage from myoglobinuria. Organ system dysfunction may necessitate continued mechanical ventilation or hemodialysis.

Current Controversies & Unresolved Issues

Investigations continue to focus on the relationship of heat stroke and malignant hyperthermia and on the role of inflammatory mediators in the pathogenesis of heat stroke. Clinical heat stroke may be associated with an underlying inherited abnormality of skeletal muscle similar to that of malignant hyperthermia. Skeletal muscle biopsies performed in patients who developed heat stroke have shown abnormal responses similar to those seen in malignant hyperthermia. Such an association might suggest that certain patients are more susceptible to heat stroke than others. Several authors have suggested that dantrolene may be effective in the treatment of heat stroke patients. However, the scant data available are still inconclusive.

There is evidence that inflammatory mediators may have a role in the pathogenesis of heat stroke and subsequent organ system dysfunction. Patients with heat stroke have been found to have elevated levels of tumor necrosis factor and interleukin-1α. These elevated levels persisted even after cooling was completed. Heat stroke has also been associated with excessive nitric oxide (NO) production, the magnitude of which is proportionate to the severity of illness. It has been suggested that NO may be an important mediator and integral part of the pathophysiologic processes resulting in heat stroke and may be a central factor linking the observed neurologic and cardiovascular abnormalities. If a role is established for these mediators, new management strategies may be possible by modulation of the inflammatory response or specific blocking agents.

Alzeer AH et al: Nitric oxide production is enhanced in patients with heat stroke. Intensive Care Med 1999;25:58–62.

Bendahan D et al: A noninvasive investigation of muscle energetics supports similarities between exertional heat stroke and malignant hyperthermia. Anesth Analg 2001;93:683–9.

Bouchama A et al: Endotoxemia and release of tumor necrosis factor and interleukin-1 alpha in acute heat stroke. J Appl Physiol 1991;70:2640–44.

Hall DM et al: Mechanisms of circulatory and intestinal barrier dysfunction during whole body hyperthermia. Am J Physiol Heart Circ Physiol 2001;280:509–21.

Hopkins PM et al: Evidence for related myopathies in exertional heat stroke and malignant hyperthermia. Lancet 1991;338:1491–2.

Khosla R et al: Heat-related illnesses. Crit Care Clin 1999;15: 251–63.

Moran D et al: Dantrolene and recovery from heat stroke. Aviat Space Environ Med 1999;70:987–9.

HYPOTHERMIA

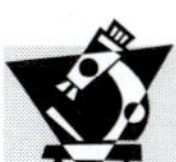

ESSENTIALS OF DIAGNOSIS

- *History of events.*
- *Early hypothermia (35–37 °C): Shivering, cool cyanotic extremities, tachycardia.*
- *Mild hypothermia (32.2–35 °C): Confusion, disorientation, hyperventilation.*
- *Moderate hypothermia (28–32.2 °C): Amnesia, lethargy, "J-wave" on ECG, atrial fibrillation.*
- *Severe hypothermia (< 28 °C): Coma, dilated pupils and absent tendon reflexes, absence of shivering, ventricular fibrillation, asystole, apnea.*

General Considerations

Hypothermia is defined as an unintentional decline in the core body temperature. Below 35 °C, the systems responsible for thermoregulation begin to fail because the compensatory physiologic responses to minimize heat loss are ineffective. Hypothermia may occur as a result of environmental exposure or during prolonged surgical procedures. Prompt diagnosis and treatment are necessary in severe cases to reverse organ dysfunction and to prevent death. Frostbite results from local cold injury and threatens mainly function. Cold injuries are being encountered with increasing frequency in the elderly, in the homeless, and in individuals participating in winter sports without proper protective clothing.

Hypothermia develops because of an imbalance between body heat generation and environmental losses. Body heat is generated as a by-product of metabolic processes and as a result of muscular contraction. Heat is lost from the body by radiation, convection, conduction, and evaporation. Immersion injuries result in rapid conductive heat loss to the cold water. Radiation and evaporation are the mechanisms by which heat is lost during prolonged open-cavity surgical procedures. Hypothermia may occur in individuals with normal thermoregulation following prolonged exposure to extreme cold. Neurologic disorders, drug intoxication, myxedema, and malnutrition may cause thermoregulatory malfunction, and hypothermia may occur after only mild to moderate cold exposure in individuals with these conditions. Hypothermia may be classified as acute if the patient has been hypothermic for less than 6 hours and chronic if for more than 6 hours. Dehydration and electrolyte imbalance are more likely to occur in patients with chronic hypothermia.

When the core body temperature falls below 36 °C, increased sympathetic activity, shivering, and peripheral vasoconstriction develop. These mechanisms have the effect of increasing heat production and preventing further heat loss. Shivering may result in a profound increase in metabolic rate with a sixfold increase in oxygen consumption.

The principal defense against cold is peripheral vasoconstriction. Cold-induced vasoconstriction may lead to an initial rise in central venous pressure from redistribution of blood to the central circulation. Patients with severely compromised cardiac function may develop pulmonary edema as a result of this central circulatory overload. Limb ischemia may develop, and the resulting anaerobic metabolism may contribute to metabolic acidosis. As the core body temperature falls below 35 °C, many patients no longer complain of being cold. When the core body temperature falls below 32 °C, shivering ceases. The metabolic rate falls rapidly, and the muscles become rigid. With profound hypothermia, the metabolic rate is reduced to less than 50% of the basal level. Amnesia and lethargy develop, progressing to coma. Bradycardia is prominent, and cardiac output falls. The respiratory rate decreases, but a relative alkalosis is maintained. This alkalosis may be protective of protein and enzyme function, myocardial function, and cerebral autoregulation. The cerebral ischemic tolerance during hypothermia is considerably increased as compared with the normothermic state. This may, in some cases, contribute to full neurologic recovery. For this reason, most patients with hypothermia should be rewarmed and reevaluated before a diagnosis of brain death is made. An additional consequence of the altered level of consciousness is that normal protective airway reflexes are abolished. This probably accounts for the high incidence of aspiration pneumonia in hypothermic patients. Atrial fibrillation, heart block, ventricular fibrillation, or asystole may develop when the core body temperature falls below 28 °C. Ventricular fibrillation may occur spontaneously or may be induced by line placement or other therapeutic maneuvers. When ventricular fibrillation develops in this setting, it is difficult to convert by countershock or pharmacologic agents without further rewarming.

As the core body temperature falls below 26 °C, hypotension and decreased systemic vascular resistance develop. An additional factor contributing to hypotension may be the hypovolemia that is commonly observed in accidental hypothermia victims. The hypovolemia is frequently related to a preexisting medical condition and may be exacerbated by hypothermia-induced diuresis. Although renal blood flow and the glomerular filtration rate decrease with hypothermia, cold diuresis usually results from the redistribution of blood to the central circulation and from a decreased response of the renal tubule to antidiuretic hormone. With profound hypothermia, severe oliguria develops as a result of generalized hypoperfusion and may also be related to acute tubular necrosis secondary to rhabdomyolysis.

Hypothermia has profound effects on the hematologic and coagulation systems. The hematocrit and the viscosity of the blood increase due to hemoconcentration, and viscosity is further increased by the fall in temperature. Coagulation is impaired as a result of platelet dysfunction and decreased enzymatic protein activity. These coagulation disorders are usually reversed upon rewarming.

Hypothermia may result in severe gastrointestinal complications, including ileus, pancreatitis, and gastric stress ulcers. Depressed hepatic function may result in alterations in the pharmacokinetics of many drugs and reduced clearance of toxins.

As core body temperature falls below 26 °C, spontaneous respirations cease, asystole develops, and electrocerebral silence occurs.

Clinical Features

A. Symptoms and Signs

The history of the events prior to presentation is essential for the diagnosis of hypothermia. In cases such as cold water immersion or prolonged exposure to winter temperatures, the diagnosis will be obvious. The diagnosis may be less obvious in a patient with associated injuries or in the elderly patient with multiple medical problems. Suspicion of hypothermia is particularly relevant when the history suggests that an injury or disease has resulted in a prolonged period of immobility with or without the association of a cold environment.

Patients experiencing early hypothermia (35–37 °C) usually present with shivering. The extremities are cool and cyanotic as a result of reflex vasoconstriction. Tachycardia results from increased sympathetic activity. In patients with mild hypothermia (33–35 °C), confusion and disorientation are common. Hyperventilation may develop in response to increased metabolic activity. Patients with moderate hypothermia (30–33 °C) are amnesic, obtunded, and often progress to coma. When the core temperature falls below 32 °C, shivering ceases and bradycardia develops. Terminal additions to the QRS complex known as Osborne waves or J waves develop in the ECG, and the PR and QT intervals may be prolonged. Atrioventricular block or atrial fibrillation can develop. Patients with severe hypothermia (< 30 °C) present with coma, dilated pupils, and absent tendon reflexes. Life-threatening cardiac arrhythmias or asystole may be present.

B. Temperature Monitoring

Body temperatures should be accurately measured in all patients suspected of being hypothermic. Standard clinical thermometers have a low temperature limit of 32–33 °C and should not be used. Electronic temperature-sensing systems accurate down to 25 °C are desirable, and many of these systems provide for continuous temperature monitoring. If electronic equipment is not available, standard glass laboratory thermometers can be used to monitor temperature. In addition to sublingual, axillary, and rectal sites, specialized electronic systems allow for temperature monitoring in the esophagus, pulmonary artery, bladder, and tympanic membrane. Monitoring temperature at the tympanic membrane may offer some advantage since this area is warmed by cerebral blood flow, but temperature should always be recorded at several sites to ensure accuracy.

C. Laboratory Findings

A complete blood count, arterial blood gas measurements, and blood cultures should be obtained in all patients with hypothermia. The arterial blood gas should be interpreted with and without temperature correction to avoid misinterpretation. Coagulation studies are not usually of benefit, since the blood sample is heated to physiologic temperature prior to testing and the results thus do not correlate with the clinical situation.

D. Electrocardiography

Continuous electrocardiographic monitoring should be established immediately. In cases of moderate hypothermia, a complete ECG should be obtained to determine intervals and to check for the presence of J waves.

Differential Diagnosis

The signs and symptoms of early hypothermia are nonspecific. Accurate temperature determination is essential to establish or exclude the diagnosis. Hypothermia may complicate other disorders, including drug or alcohol intoxication and endocrinopathies—ie, hypoglycemia, hyperosmolar coma, diabetic ketoacidosis, and myxedema. Hypothermia may also occur as a complication of sepsis. Patients with severe trauma or burns are particularly at risk for the development of hypothermia.

Treatment

A. Airway

Orotracheal intubation is indicated for all hypothermic patients with altered mental status. Nasotracheal intubation should be avoided, since nasal bleeding can be a significant problem in the patient with a coagulation disorder. Cricothyroid pressure should be maintained during intubation attempts to prevent aspiration. It should be recognized that even a cuffed endotracheal tube will not offer complete protection against aspiration, and an orogastric tube should be passed and placed on continuous suction to evacuate the stomach contents. During the rewarming process, endotracheal tube cuff pressures must be monitored frequently to avoid tracheal injury because the volume and pressure in the cuff will increase.

B. Breathing

Patients with moderate to severe hypothermia require mechanical ventilation. Warm humidified gases should be used to prevent further heat loss, but they will not play a major role in rewarming due to the small amount of heat they convey. Adjustment of mechanical ventilation should be guided by non-temperature-corrected blood gas values for pH and $Pa{CO_2}$. However, temperature correction is required for accurate determination of $Pa{O_2}$ and hemoglobin saturation.

C. Circulation

Most patients with moderate to severe hypothermia will also be hypovolemic. These patients may require as many as 10 L of crystalloid during rewarming. Ideally, all intravenous fluids should be warmed to 39 °C. This can be accomplished in a number of ways, including use of microwave ovens, but care must be taken to avoid overheating, which can lead to hemolysis. Heating units allow for rapid fluid administration with precise temperature control and should be used if available. Central venous pressure or pulmonary artery pressure monitoring may be necessary in patients who do not respond to aggressive volume administration. Inotropic and vasoconstrictive agents such as dopamine should be avoided, since they are usually ineffective and may result in cardiac arrhythmias.

D. Rewarming

The faster the patient is warmed, the better the prognosis. Once the diagnosis of hypothermia is suspected, all efforts should be directed toward reducing further heat loss and rewarming the patient. In addition to the use of warm intravenous fluids and heated respiratory gases, warm blankets should be applied to prevent radiant heat loss during resuscitation and evaluation. There are three options for rewarming: (1) passive rewarming, (2) active external rewarming, and (3) active internal rewarming. The overall condition of the patient will determine the most appropriate method.

Most patients with mild to moderate hypothermia will be able to rewarm themselves, and passive external measures to prevent further heat loss will be all that are necessary. Active external rewarming, achieved by conductive surface warming with methods such as warm water immersion or heating blankets, is often ineffective in adults because of the low body surface to body volume ratio. The vasodilation resulting from these methods may also worsen hypotension. In addition, the reestablishment of flow in peripheral circulatory beds may lead to increased transport of colder peripheral blood to the central core resulting, in a paradoxic decrease in core temperature. To effect external rewarming, air circulating systems may prove to be more effective because they provide for additional heat exchange by convection. These devices are usually readily available in the operating room or recovery area. To minimize adverse circulatory effects, these systems can be applied initially only to the trunk. In most cases of moderate to severe hypothermia, active external rewarming will need to be combined with active internal rewarming.

Active internal rewarming is achieved by gastric, colonic, or bladder lavage with heated saline, pleural lavage, peritoneal lavage, and cardiopulmonary bypass. Gastric, colonic, and bladder lavage can be easily performed without specialized equipment or facilities. Although rewarming is relatively slow by these methods because of limited surface area, it may be enough to make the difference in cases of moderate hypothermia. Lavage fluid temperatures should not exceed 40.5 °C in order to avoid mucosal injury. With gastric lavage, care should be taken to minimize the risk of aspiration. Gastric lavage should not be performed on a patient receiving chest compressions for cardiopulmonary resuscitation. Although more invasive, peritoneal lavage will result in more rapid warming. Lavage fluid up to 43 °C can be used, and the placement of two catheters will provide for a continuous flow rate up to 6 L/h. An intact cardiovascular status is necessary to provide adequate perfusion so that heat exchange can take place. If the patient has severe hypothermia and cardiac arrest, open cardiac massage and mediastinal and pleural lavage with warm saline are indicated.

The methods available for extracorporeal blood rewarming include hemodialysis, arteriovenous rewarming, venovenous rewarming, and cardiopulmonary bypass. Hemodialysis offers the advantage of requiring only a single venous cannulation with a two-way flow catheter. The femoral approach is preferred to avoid cardiac irritation. Hemodialysis may offer additional advantages in patients with renal failure and drug or other toxicity.

In addition to providing circulatory support for the patient with cardiac arrest or arrhythmia, cardiopulmonary bypass will allow for rapid rewarming. A major drawback of cardiopulmonary bypass is that systemic heparinization is required. Therefore, the technique may be contraindicated in patients who have sustained severe trauma. The use of systems with heparin-bonded tubing may overcome some of these problems. Standard cannulation techniques may be used in the patient with a thoracotomy for open cardiac massage. Alternatively, femoral veno-arterial bypass can be instituted by cutdown or by percutaneously placed catheters in the patient with intact cardiovascular function. Portable systems utilizing percutaneous access may allow the institution of bypass warming in the intensive care unit. The long-term outcome of patients with severe hypothermia treated with cardiopulmonary bypass has been favorable.

Prognosis

The outcome depends on a number of factors, including the severity and duration of hypothermia as well as the presence of coexisting medical conditions. Aggressive treatment is indicated because any hypothermic patient has the potential for full recovery despite severely depressed cardiac or respiratory function. Successful resuscitation with full recovery has been reported after documented ice water submersion for as long as 66 minutes in a small child. Success such as this probably depends on rapid symmetric cooling of the entire body, including the brain.

Current Controversies & Unresolved Issues

Techniques such as the use of very high temperature intravenous fluids and diathermy are being explored for the treatment of moderate to severe hypothermia. Intravenous fluids heated to 65 °C have been utilized in animal studies and have resulted in rewarming rates of 2.9–3.7 °C per hour with minimal intimal injuries.

Diathermy involves the conversion of energy waves into heat. Ultrasound or low-frequency microwave radiation can deliver large amounts of heat to deep tissues. Although animal studies have yielded some promising results, further investigation is needed to determine the optimum clinical use of diathermy. There is controversy about when and when not to resuscitate the victim of hypothermia. The techniques necessary to reverse severe hypothermia require a major allocation of personnel and resources. Although it has been stated that no person is dead until "warm and dead," in many cases additional information will establish a definitive diagnosis. Severe hyperkalemia (> 10 mmol/L) suggests that the patient died prior to the development of hypothermia, since the potassium level is usually normal or low in patients with hypothermia. Of course, other causes of hyperkalemia such as renal failure or crush injury must be ruled out.

Once instituted, resuscitation should proceed until a core temperature of 30 °C is achieved. At this temperature, some signs of life should be evident, and successful cardioversion is usually possible.

Auerbach PS: Some people are dead when they are cold and dead. JAMA 1990;264:1856–7.

Brauer A et al: Severe accidental hypothermia: rewarming strategy using a veno-venous bypass system and a convective air warmer. Intensive Care Med 1999;25:520–3.

Eddy VA et al: Hypothermia, coagulopathy, and acidosis. Surg Clin North Am 2000;80:845–54.

Fildes J et al: Very hot intravenous fluid in the treatment of hypothermia. J Trauma 1993;35:683–6.

Giesbrecht GG et al: Cold stress, near drowning and accidental hypothermia: a review. Aviat Space Environ Med 2000;71: 733–52.

Hanania NA et al: Accidental hypothermia. Crit Care Clin 1999;15:235–49.

Megarbane B et al: Hypothermia with indoor occurrence is associated with a worse outcome. Intensive Care Med 200;26:1843–9.

Mizushima Y et al: Should normothermia be restored and maintained during resuscitation after trauma and hemorrhage? J Trauma 2000;48:58–65.

Owda A, Osama S: Hemodialysis in management of hypothermia. Am J Kidney Dis 2001;38:E8.

Peng RY et al: Hypothermia in trauma patients. J Am Coll Surg 1999;188:685–96.

Sheaff CM et al: Safety of 65 degrees C intravenous fluid for the treatment of hypothermia. Am J Surg 1996;172:52–5.

Ujhelyi MR et al: Defibrillation energy requirements and electrical heterogeneity during total body hypothermia. Crit Care Med 2001;29:1006–11.

Vassal T et al: Severe accidental hypothermia treated in an ICU: prognosis and outcome. Chest 2001;120:1998–2003.

Voelckel WG et al: Intraosseous blood gases during hypothermia: correlation with arterial, mixed venous, and sagittal sinus blood. Crit Care Med 200;28:2915–20.

Walpoth BH et al: Outcome of survivors of accidental deep hypothermia and circulatory arrest treated with extracorporeal blood warming. N Engl J Med 1997;337:1500–5.

FROSTBITE

ESSENTIALS OF DIAGNOSIS

- *First degree: Hyperemia and edema after rewarming. No blister formation.*
- *Second degree: Hyperemia, edema, and serous blister formation. Severe pain during rewarming.*
- *Third degree: Full-thickness skin injury resulting in skin necrosis, black eschars, and hemorrhagic blister formation.*
- *Fourth degree: Complete necrosis of soft tissue, muscle, and bone. After rewarming, the tissue is cyanotic and ischemic. Mummification with minimal edema.*

General Considerations

Local injuries due to cold include chilblains, immersion foot, and frostbite. Chilblains and immersion foot result from prolonged exposure of the extremities in wet conditions to temperatures above freezing. Severe neurovascular damage may result, and ulcerations with chronic infections may be incapacitating.

Frostbite occurs when the tissues are actually frozen. Edema and blister formation develop after thawing or partial thawing. These areas may progress to gangrene.

There are two phases of injury that occur with frostbite:

(1) **Phase 1—direct cellular cryotoxicity:** As ice crystals form within the affected area, cell death occurs as a result of both dehydration and mechanical disruption due to expanding ice crystals. The most severe injuries occur after partial thawing and refreezing of tissues.

(2) **Phase 2—progressive vascular thrombosis:** Cold exposure results in reflex arterial vasoconstriction and freezing of the tissues that result in capillary injuries. In addition, cold increases blood viscosity. When thawing occurs, the circulatory stasis and tissue swelling result in intravascular thrombosis. Tissue necrosis will occur when reperfusion cannot be sustained following rewarming.

Clinical Features

Freezing begins distally and progresses centrally. Therefore, the fingers and toes are most susceptible to severe injury. There is usually a line of demarcation between the frozen and unfrozen areas. However, the severity of injury and the extent of nonviable tissue will not become apparent until several days after thawing. In classifying frostbite, it is most important to differentiate between superficial frostbite with skin injury only and deep frostbite with injury to deeper structures of the extremities. Frostbite has been traditionally classified in somewhat the same way as burns.

Frostbitten extremities are painless, numb, and have a blanched, waxy appearance. Superficial frostbite involves only the skin and subcutaneous tissues. Deep frostbite extends deeper and produces a woody consistency. However, a wide range of frostbite injuries may appear similar at the time of the initial evaluation. Therefore, classification of frostbite should be applied after rewarming.

Treatment

The injury associated with freezing is progressive, and exposure should be limited as soon as possible. However, thawing should be avoided if refreezing is likely, since this will increase the severity of injury.

A. Rapid Rewarming

Extremities can be rewarmed most effectively by immersion in a warm water bath with a mild antibacterial agent such as povidone-iodine at a temperature between 40 °C and 42 °C. Lower temperatures may compromise tissue survival. Higher temperatures should be avoided because of the risk of thermal injury. Thawing should continue until all the blanched tissues of the injured extremity are perfused with blood. A red to purple color and pliability of the tissues will indicate that warming is complete. Active motion during thawing may be beneficial, but it is important to avoid rubbing the affected area since this may worsen the injury. Severe pain is likely to develop during the warming process, and opioid analgesics are usually required. Unfortunately, the high opioid doses often required lead to side effects such as heavy sedation, respiratory depression, and nausea that may become a serious problem. In cases of frostbite injury of the lower extremities, epidural blockade has been demonstrated to provide good pain relief with fewer of these complications.

Epidural opioid administration has the advantage of providing analgesia without sympathetic blockade. The latter has been shown to decrease the pain and edema associated with deep frostbite, but it has not been shown to decrease the extent of tissue loss. A potential problem is that sympathetic blockade may also cause vasodilation, which can result in increased local edema, leading to decreased perfusion and increased tissue loss.

B. Post-Thaw Care

The affected area must be carefully protected after rewarming. White blisters should be debrided and hemorrhagic ones left intact. Aloe vera (available in generic preparations), a topical inhibitor of thromboxane, should be applied topically every 6 hours. The extremity can be splinted in a position of function with elevation, both for protection and to provide a degree of comfort. Tetanus prophylaxis should be administered if required. The use of aspirin as a systemic antithromboxane agent has been superseded by ibuprofen because aspirin has been shown to also inhibit prostaglandins beneficial to wound healing. Ibuprofen 400 mg should be given orally every 6 hours. Penicillin, with excellent coverage of streptococcus, is the antibiotic of choice for prophylaxis and is usually continued for 48–72 hours. Daily hydrotherapy at 40 °C for 30–45 minutes aids debridement of devitalized tissue. Range-of-motion exercises are essential for preservation of function. Adequate analgesia will be necessary to permit effective physical therapy.

C. Avoid Early or Inappropriately High Amputation

Amputation should not be performed until the degree of tissue loss is clearly determined. This may not be possible until weeks or months after injury. In most cases, skin necrosis will not be associated with deep tissue loss. Occasionally, digital escharotomy or fasciotomy is necessary because a compartment syndrome develops or because the range of motion becomes severely limited. Preliminary studies have suggested that imaging studies such as technetium scanning and magnetic resonance imaging may allow for precise determination of viable tissue and earlier debridement and reconstruction with no loss in stump length. In some cases, the survival of deeper structures may be improved by coverage with vascularized tissue.

Prognosis

Patients who sustain superficial frostbite usually achieve complete recovery with minimal loss of tissue and no loss of function. Complete recovery is unlikely for patients with more severe degrees of frostbite injury. Amputation may result in loss of function and severe cosmetic defects. Patients may be incapacitated by the development of reflex sympathetic dystrophy. Numbness, hypertrophic skin changes, chronic pain, hyperhidrosis, stiffness, and cold intolerance are all potential sequelae of frostbite. Regional sympathectomy may improve some of the symptoms of vasospasticity related to sympathetic hyperactivity.

Children exposed to extreme cold may develop early epiphysial closure as a result of injury to the growth plate. This injury results in shortened phalanges. Hand function usually remains excellent, and reconstructive surgery is rarely required.

Current Controversies & Unresolved Issues

Current interest in frostbite management centers around heparin anticoagulation, low-molecular-weight dextran administration, and the role of early sympathectomy.

Frostbite necrosis develops when reperfusion cannot be sustained following rewarming. This has led to the development of experimental treatments designed to maintain blood flow in the microcirculation during the period of reperfusion. However, none of these treatments has been proved to be effective in controlled trials.

Low-molecular-weight dextran may improve circulation by decreasing blood viscosity and red cell clumping. Animal experiments have demonstrated a decrease in tissue loss, but this has yet to be established in a clinical trial. Clinical studies on the use of heparin anticoagulation have been inconclusive. Thrombolytic agents have resulted in significant improvement in tissue survival in animal models of frostbite. These studies have yet to be validated in human trials.

Murphy JV et al: Frostbite: pathogenesis and treatment. J Trauma 2000;48:171–8.

Ozyazgan I et al: Defibrotide activity in experimental frostbite injury. Br J Plast Surg 1998;51:450–4.

Punja K et al: Continuous infusion of epidural morphine in frostbite. J Burn Care Rehabil 1998;19:142–5.

Zook N et al: Microcirculatory studies of frostbite injury. Ann Plast Surg 1998;40:246–53.

NEAR DROWNING

ESSENTIALS OF DIAGNOSIS

- *History.*
- *Hypoxemia.*
- *Metabolic or mixed acidosis.*
- *Hypovolemia.*
- *Profound electrolyte abnormalities.*
- *Hypothermia.*
- *Associated injuries.*

General Considerations

Drowning is death from asphyxia while submerged. The near-drowning victim, having survived the acute episode, is at major risk of developing severe organ dysfunction and of subsequent mortality.

Pathogenic mechanisms of near drowning are related to hypoxemia and aspiration. The physiologic effects of aspiration differ depending on whether the drowning medium is fresh or salt water. Compared with plasma, these fluids are hypo- and hypertonic, respectively. Although it is possible for a drowning victim to die of hypoxemia without aspiration, this rarely occurs. When fresh water is aspirated, the fluid is rapidly absorbed from the alveoli, producing intravascular hypervolemia, hypotonicity, dilution of serum electrolytes, and intravascular hemolysis. Saltwater aspiration produces the opposite effects as water is drawn into the alveoli from the vascular space, producing hypovolemia, hemoconcentration, and hypertonicity. Hemolysis is not a major problem after saltwater drowning.

The initial contact of water with the upper respiratory tract usually stimulates severe laryngospasm. This occasionally results in hypoxia without significant aspiration of water. Aspiration of water into the trachea and bronchi can result in airway obstruction. Additional effects of water aspiration include bronchoconstriction, loss of surfactant, damage to alveolar and capillary endothelium, and direct alveolar flooding. Aspiration of gastric contents is common in near-drowning victims and dramatically increases the severity of the direct injury.

Hypoxemia most often occurs as a result of intrapulmonary shunting. Approximately 50% of near-drowning victims develop ARDS, in most cases reversible.

The pathophysiology of brain injury is directly related to hypoxia and diffuse neuronal damage. The resulting brain edema may increase intracranial pressure, which may further compromise cerebral perfusion. In children, the diving reflex may play a protective role in cases of cold water submersion. Owing to a high surface-to-volume ratio, prompt hypothermia results in decreased cerebral metabolism, with shunting of the circulation to the cerebral and coronary circulations.

Atrial and ventricular arrhythmias occur in the near-drowning victim due to hypoxia, metabolic and respiratory acidosis, and catecholamine excess. Vagally mediated cardiac arrhythmias can develop as well. Electrolyte disturbances contribute to the generation of cardiac arrhythmias.

Acute tubular necrosis in the drowning victim develops as a result of hypotension and hypoxemia. Renal failure is exacerbated by rhabdomyolysis and hemolysis associated with disseminated intravascular coagulation.

Clinical Features

The diagnosis of near drowning is necessarily based on the history. In the surviving victim, the severity of injury is determined by evaluation of the level of pulmonary and neurologic function, metabolic and respiratory acidosis, electrolyte abnormalities, and hypovolemia. Victims should be examined carefully to exclude associated injuries that may require additional management decisions.

Differential Diagnosis

When a history of diving with compressed gas is obtained, several additional diagnoses must be considered. Pulmonary barotrauma occurs when expanding gases are unable to escape from the alveoli during ascent from a dive. Pneumothorax with arterial gas embolization may then occur. Arterial gas embolization may result in neurologic dysfunction and cardiovascular collapse. These diagnoses should be suspected in any case of near drowning associated with compressed air diving.

The use of compressed air while diving may cause other problems due to the release of excess gas from tissues on ascent. Severe pain is the usual clinical manifestation of decompression sickness and is due to the presence of gas bubbles in body tissues. Gas bubble formation may also result in spinal cord injury or central nervous system dysfunction. In some cases, this may have precipitated the drowning episode.

A blood alcohol level and a drug screen should be obtained in all adolescent and adult victims of near drowning, since intoxication is a factor in more than half of the cases.

Treatment

A. Airway

Since a successful outcome in the near-drowning victim is dependent upon early correction of hypoxia, endotracheal intubation should be performed early if there is any evidence of pulmonary dysfunction. Prior to intubation, it is important to clear the airway of vomitus or debris. Cervical spine precautions should be maintained in any victim who suffers a near-drowning episode after diving.

B. Breathing

The arterial oxygen saturation should be maintained at a level greater than 90%. If this level cannot be maintained with high concentrations of inspired oxygen or with continuous positive airway pressure, mechanical ventilation with positive end-expiratory pressure should be instituted. Alveolar flooding, with loss of surfactant and direct capillary injury, results in atelectasis and pulmonary edema. Aspiration injury may result from vomiting and aspiration of gastric contents. Aspiration of polluted water and foreign materials can result in additional lung injury. Early chest radiographs may be normal, with pulmonary infiltrates becoming evident 48–72 hours after injury. Late pulmonary complications include ARDS and aspiration pneumonia.

C. Circulation

The hypotensive near-drowning victim requires vigorous fluid resuscitation. Central venous pressure monitoring is instituted in patients who do not respond to volume resuscitation and in those with hypoperfusion despite fluid challenges.

D. Acid-Base Status

Metabolic acidosis is best managed by optimization of fluid status. In most cases, bicarbonate should not be administered. Mechanical hyperventilation may be used to establish a compensatory respiratory alkalosis in victims with severe metabolic acidosis.

E. Correction of Electrolyte Abnormalities

Electrolyte abnormalities are usually not significant in victims of freshwater near drowning. In the case of saltwater victims, critical elevations of sodium and chloride may occur. Treatment requires aggressive diuresis, adjustment of intravenous fluids, and, in some cases, hemodialysis. Hypermagnesemia and hypercalcemia may also develop in victims of saltwater drowning and require hemodialysis.

The kidney may be adversely affected if significant intravascular hemolysis has occurred. Hemoglobinuria is treated initially by establishing an osmotic diuresis and by alkalinization of the urine. Despite these measures, acute tubular necrosis can develop and require dialysis.

Prognosis

The outcome depends on a number of factors, including the length of submersion, water temperature, time to first breath, initial pH, and the initial neurologic evaluation. A recent review reported 58% survival, with no neurologic deficit, in a group of pediatric victims of near drowning. The major factors that improved outcome were the presence of a detectable heartbeat and hypothermia on admission to the hospital. Neurologic outcome in adults is also improved in cases of cold water near drowning.

Current Controversies & Unresolved Issues

Emergency cardiopulmonary bypass may have a role in the resuscitation of the profoundly hypothermic near-drowning victim. Survival with subsequent normal neurologic function has been reported in victims with severe hypothermia and no vital signs on admission. An obvious limitation of this technique is the necessity for immediate availability of equipment and personnel to institute bypass and the need for systemic anticoagulation. However, it is unlikely that any other method of resuscitation would prove successful in this select group of patients.

Concern regarding the sequelae of cerebral edema in the near-drowning victim has prompted the consideration of various therapeutic interventions to prevent cerebral injury. Unfortunately, the use of steroids, intracerebral monitoring, hypothermia, and controlled hyperventilation have not resulted in improved outcomes in controlled clinical trials.

The potential benefits of calcium channel blockers, prostaglandin inhibitors, free radical inhibition, and hemodilution to decrease tissue injury remain unproved.

Cummings P et al: Trends in unintentional drowning: the role of alcohol and medical care. JAMA 1999;281:2198–202.

De Nicola LK et al: Submersion injuries in children and adults. Crit Care Clin 1997;13:477–502.

Gheen KM: Near-drowning and cold water submersion. Semin Pediatr Surg 2001;10:26–7.

Giesbrecht GG: Cold stress, near drowning and accidental hypothermia: a review. Aviat Space Environ Med 2000;71:733–52.

Graf WD et al: Outcome of children after near drowning. Pediatrics 1998;101:160–1.

O'Flaherty JE, Pine PL: Prevention of pediatric drowning and near-drowning: a survey of members of the American Academy of Pediatrics. Pediatrics 1997;99:169–74.

Tipton MJ et al: Human initial responses to immersion in cold water at three temperatures and after hyperventilation. J Appl Physiol 1991;70:317–22.

Weinstein MD et al.: Near-drowning: epidemiology, pathophysiology, and initial treatment. J Emerg Med 1996;14:461–7.

ENVENOMATION

1. Snakebite

ESSENTIALS OF DIAGNOSIS

Crotalidae:

- *Swelling, erythema, ecchymosis.*
- *Coagulopathy.*
- *Metallic taste, perioral paresthesias.*
- *Hypotension.*
- *Tachypnea.*
- *Respiratory compromise.*

Elapidae:

- *Respiratory compromise, generalized paralysis.*

General Considerations

It is estimated that 1500 snakebites are inflicted annually in the United States by 19 species of venomous snakes. Depending upon the degree of envenomation, significant morbidity and potential mortality can result. Ninety-five percent of poisonous snakebites in the United States are caused by pit vipers (Crotalidae), which include rattlesnakes, cottonmouths and copperheads; only 4–5% of bites are inflicted by coral snakes (Elapidae).

The main functions of crotalid venom are immobilization, death, and digestion of prey. These venoms are complex mixtures of enzymes and toxic proteins. Other components include metalloproteins, glycoproteins, lipids, and biogenic amines. Crotalid venom causes local tissue injury, coagulopathy, and systemic manifestations. The local injury is due to a combination of direct toxic damage to tissue as well as to ischemic damage from compartmental pressure, which results from local tissue edema. The coagulopathy is caused by procoagulant esterases that act on fibrinogen and split off fibrinopeptides. This results in depletion of fibrinogen and elevation of the prothrombin and partial thromboplastin times. The platelet count usually remains normal. Bradykinin is released by the action of arginine ester hydroxylase on plasma kininogen and may cause vasodilation and pooling of blood in the pulmonary and splanchnic beds, resulting in decreased venous return, hypotension, and shock. Interstitial loss of intravascular fluid further worsens the hypotension. Myocardial ischemia and depression of muscular contraction have also been associated with other factors in pit viper venom. Renal failure probably results from hypotension, from the direct effects of the venom, and from myoglobinuria. Disseminated intravascular coagulation further contributes to the development of renal failure.

The Mojave rattlesnake has a different type of venom and represents an important exception to the above. The Mojave venom includes a toxin that immobilizes prey by neuromuscular blockade. This toxin is present to some extent in other crotalid species, but in Mojave rattlesnake venom the higher concentration significantly increases the risk of airway and breathing complications. For these reasons, Mojave rattlesnake venom has the lowest median lethal dose level of any North American crotalid venom.

Venom from the Elapidae causes symptoms that are primarily neurologic in nature, with little or no local tissue toxicity. The neurotoxic elements are polypeptides that bind postsynaptically and effect nondepolarizing blockade of the acetylcholine receptors. Generalized paralysis, bulbar paralysis, and respiratory arrest may occur. The neurotoxic effects of these venoms are severe and in some cases irreversible. The signs and symptoms of envenomation can be delayed for more than 12 hours and often occur precipitously.

Clinical Features

A. Signs and Symptoms

The symptoms in each individual case of snakebite vary depending on the degree of envenomation. It is estimated that approximately 3% of snakebites are "dry," with no evidence of venom injection. In the case of crotalid bites, the degree of envenomation can be estimated by the presence and progression of signs and symptoms. The bites of elapid snakes usually cause minimal early symptoms—it is only after 1–12 hours that severe systemic symptoms suddenly appear.

Minimal envenomation is characterized by the presence of local findings with slow progression and the absence of systemic signs and symptoms. In the case of severe envenomation, local findings will progress rapidly while systemic complications appear early and are particularly severe.

B. Laboratory Findings

Determination of coagulation parameters helps to evaluate the degree of envenomation in crotalid bites. Prothrombin time, partial thromboplastin time, platelet count, fibrinogen levels, and fibrin degradation products should be determined initially and repeated at regular intervals to estimate the severity and monitor the progression of coagulopathy. Serial red blood cell counts should be obtained to evaluate for the development of hemoconcentration caused by third spacing of fluid or to detect anemia due to bleeding or hemolysis. Urinary myoglobin indicates myonecrosis. Laboratory data should be obtained on admission, again after the administration of antivenin, and then every 4 hours until the data have returned to near normal levels.

Differential Diagnosis

Identification of the type of snake is necessary in order to secure the appropriate antivenin. In cases where the snake has not been identified, the diagnosis of venomous snakebite can often be made by examination of the fang marks. Crotalid bites are characterized by two such marks. It must be remembered that elapid bites may not result in local signs or symptoms despite envenomation.

Treatment

A. Resuscitation

The adequacy of the airway and ventilation should be verified. The primary survey and resuscitation should follow standard protocols available from the American College of Surgeons Advanced Trauma Life Support Course. The airway should be secured promptly in patients with envenomation to the head or neck. Subsequent swelling could make endotracheal intubation difficult or impossible. Hypotension is best treated with rapid crystalloid infusion. Fluid resuscitation should be aggressive to preserve organ function. Prophylactic antibiotics are not recommended.

B. Antivenin

In the patient with major systemic signs and symptoms due to severe envenomation, antivenin should be administered as quickly as possible. Antivenin is recommended for moderate to severe envenomation and for any envenomation with symptoms of progression—particularly worsening local injury, progressive coagulopathy, and hemolysis. A skin test is performed with the antivenin prior to administration in an attempt to predict the likelihood of an allergic reaction. The test is performed by intradermal injection of 0.2 mL of antivenin diluted 1:10 with normal saline. Erythema and a wheal reaction within 30 minutes is a positive reaction indicating the need for treatment. Antivenin should only be given by slow intravenous infusion. The use of antivenin should be considered early, since it may have to be obtained from a distance and because the time required to mix the preparation will result in an additional delay. Patients may require additional doses of antivenin if their symptoms progress after the initial administration.

Moderate to severe antivenin reactions occur in 15–20% of patients who receive antivenin. Mild reactions can be treated with intravenous diphenhydramine and epinephrine; severe reactions require increased doses. H_2 receptor blockers should be administered also in severe cases.

In cases of severe envenomation, further antivenin therapy should be strongly considered after treatment of a reaction. In less severe cases, antivenin should be withheld if possible after a reaction since there have been cases of death due to anaphylaxis.

Antivenin information can be obtained from local poison control centers or from a national service by calling 1–800–222–1222.

Exotic envenomations may occur occasionally in the USA from foreign snakes or lizards kept in zoos or private collections. The principles of management are the same: supportive care and administration of appropriate antivenin. Most exotic antivenins are available at the institutions that maintain the snakes. The availability of these antivenins can also be determined through the Antivenin Index.

C. Local Treatment

Local therapy consists of elevation and immobilization of the affected area until swelling recedes. Extremities should be observed for the development of compartment syndrome. If muscle compartments become firm or if pain increases, compartment pressure should be measured. In some cases, fasciotomy may be required to prevent ischemic necrosis. Cruciate incisions should not be performed in an attempt to extract venom.

D. Tetanus Prophylaxis

Tetanus prophylaxis should be administered if the patient's immunization status is not current or not known.

Current Controversies & Unresolved Issues

Immediate excision of the bite down to fascia and including damaged fascia and muscle has been advocated to reduce the incidence of local necrosis and to reduce systemic symptoms. This therapy can only be effective in cases of recent envenomation and in the absence of local diffusion of venom or systemic symptoms. It cannot be recommended for a number of reasons: Most victims of snakebite do not reach medical care for several hours and are therefore beyond the point when local excision would be expected to have any benefit. In addition, this radical therapy can increase morbidity in cases of minimal envenomation without offering any benefit.

A new polyvalent antivenin, CroTAb, has recently been approved for clinical use. This antivenin is sheep-derived and produced by immunizing sheep with venom from the eastern and western diamondback rattlesnakes, the Mojave rattlesnake, and the eastern cottonmouth. In a randomized trial in the United States, CroTAb was demonstrated to effectively terminate venom effects. In another study, CroTAb was successful in immediately and completely reversing neurotoxicity resulting from Mojave rattlesnake envenomation. Conventional polyvalent antivenin is often ineffective in the treatment of venom-induced neurotoxicity.

2. Spider & Scorpion Bites

ESSENTIALS OF DIAGNOSIS

Black widow spider:

- *Numbing pain at the site of the bite.*
- *Muscle cramps and low back pain.*
- *Severe abdominal pain.*
- *Respiratory insufficiency.*
- *Cardiac conduction abnormalities.*

Brown recluse spider:

- *Pain beginning 1–4 hours after bite.*
- *Erythema, central pustule, bull's-eye lesion.*
- *Fever, malaise, arthralgias, rash, hemolysis.*

Scorpions:

- *Pain with little erythema or swelling.*
- *Generalized reactions within 1 hour.*

General Considerations

Spider and scorpion bites are particularly common in the western United States. Only the female black widow spider *(Latrodectus mactans)* is dangerous. Its venom contains a potent neurotoxin that induces neurotransmitter release following interaction with a specific cell surface receptor. This action affects mainly the neuromuscular junction and results in unrestrained muscle contraction and severe cramping. The local reaction at the site of envenomation is usually mild.

Venom from the brown recluse spider *(Loxosceles reclusa)* contains sphingomyelinase D. It is primarily cytotoxic and causes local tissue destruction. Hemolysis is the principal systemic effect, and it is usually minor.

Most scorpion bites are harmless and produce only local reactions. However, venom from *Centruroides exilicauda* contains a neurotoxin that may cause severe systemic reactions.

Clinical Features

A. Symptoms and Signs

Initially, a black widow spider bite is painless. Symptoms begin within 10–60 minutes and include severe pain and muscle spasms of the abdomen and trunk. Headache, nausea, vomiting, and hyperactive deep tendon reflexes may be present. Spasms give way to agonizing pain. Rigidity of the abdominal wall may be confused with an intra-abdominal catastrophe. Hypertension with or without seizures develops uncommonly. Symptoms are maximum at 2–3 hours after the bite and may persist for up to 24 hours.

Brown recluse spider bites produce pain after 1–4 hours. Initially, an erythematous area with a central pustule or hemorrhagic area appears. A bull's-eye appearance of the lesion may be noted because of an ischemic halo surrounded by extravasated blood. Over several days, an ulcer may form, which if extensive requires excision and skin grafting. Systemic reactions are infrequent but may occur 1–2 days after the bite and include massive hemolysis, hemoglobinuria, jaundice, renal failure, pulmonary edema, and disseminated intravascular coagulation.

Scorpion bites are extremely painful but often exhibit no erythema or swelling. Light palpation of the area causes extreme pain. Generalized reactions are not common but may develop within 60 minutes: restlessness, jerking, nystagmus, hypertension, diplopia, confusion, and rarely seizures. Death is uncommon.

Differential Diagnosis

The signs and symptoms of black widow spider envenomation can be easily confused with other common conditions, particularly those cases with minimal bite-related symptoms. In some cases, the abdominal pain may mimic an acute abdomen. Black widow spider envenomation should be considered in patients presenting with the acute onset of severe pain and muscle cramps, particularly if the history is consistent with spider bite.

Brown recluse spider bites are occasionally confused with those of other insects. It should be remembered that spiders usually bite only once, while other insects produce multiple bites.

Treatment

A. Black Widow Spider Bites

The most effective treatment options include specific antivenin alone or with a combination of intravenous opioids and muscle relaxants. Although calcium gluconate administration has been recommended, it has not been shown to be effective. Intravenous morphine and benzodiazepines are helpful in achieving relief of symptoms. Antivenin should be considered in moderate to severe cases but should be used with caution because it has been associated with fatal reactions. Advanced life support measures may be required for patients who develop cardiovascular collapse or respiratory failure.

B. Brown Recluse Spider Bites

Most patients can be treated with supportive measures. Ice may be beneficial. Exercise of the limb or application of heat will potentiate the actions of the venom. Patients requiring admission to the ICU are usually older, with systemic symptoms. Dapsone (50–100 mg orally twice daily for 10 days) has been used in patients who do not have glucose-6-phosphate dehydrogenase deficiency. Some authorities use oral erythromycin (250 mg four times daily for 10 days) to control skin infection.

C. Scorpion Bites

Children and older adults must be admitted to the ICU for observation. The affected part should be immobilized and ice applied. A tourniquet must not be used. Respiratory depression may result from the use of tranquilizers. Opioid analgesics are particularly dangerous, since they seem to potentiate the toxicity of the venom. Seizures, when present, can usually be controlled with intravenous diazepam or phenobarbital. Hypertension may require the use of sympatholytic agents.

3. MARINE LIFE ENVENOMATIONS

ESSENTIALS OF DIAGNOSIS

- *Pain at the site of envenomation.*
- *Systemic symptoms subsequently.*
- *Multiple wounds may be present.*

General Considerations

Marine life envenomations are most commonly caused by stingrays, jellyfish (Portuguese man-of-wars), scorpion fish, and sea urchins. Although many victims can be treated in the emergency department and released, critical care may be required for hemodynamic and respiratory complications.

Clinical Features

A. Stingray

Multiple sites may be present, with pain and swelling occurring immediately. Local hemorrhage may also be present. Systemic symptoms, when present, include nausea, vomiting, weakness, vertigo, tachycardia, and muscle cramps. Syncope, paralysis, hypotension, and tachycardia may occur with extensive envenomations.

B. Scorpion Fish

Central radiation of pain from the wound may cause extreme discomfort requiring ICU admission for control. Systemic symptoms are manifested within the first few hours after envenomation and include vomiting, weakness, diarrhea, paresthesias, seizures, fever, hypertension, cardiac arrhythmias, and respiratory failure.

C. Sea Urchins

Sea urchin venoms contain several toxins, including cholinergic compounds and neurotoxins. Multiple spines are usually present in the skin and indicate the nature of the contact. Systemic reactions include nausea and vomiting, intense pain, paralysis, aphonia, and respiratory distress.

Treatment

A. Stingray

Wounds can be treated with local measures, including warm soaks and lidocaine. Ice should not be applied. Operative debridement may be required. Supportive therapy is usually all that is required. Infection prophylaxis should be instituted with trimethoprim-sulfamethoxazole or tetracycline.

B. Scorpion Fish

Care is similar to that outlined for stingray contact. Infection prophylaxis should be instituted in a similar fashion. Seizures can be treated with phenobarbital, phenytoin, or diazepam.

C. Sea Urchins

Although pain can subside within a few hours, paralysis may last for 6–8 hours and require intubation and mechanical ventilation until the patient has regained sufficient strength.

Bey TA et al: Exotic snakebite: envenomation by an African puff adder *(Bitis arietans)*. J Emerg Med 1997;15:827–31.

Bogdan GM et al: Recurrent coagulopathy after antivenom treatment of crotalid snakebite. South Med J 2000;93:562–6.

Clark RF et al: Successful treatment of crotalid-induced neurotoxicity with a new polyspecific crotalid Fab antivenom. Ann Emerg Med 1997;30:54–7.

Dart RC et al: A randomized multicenter trial of crotalinae polyvalent immune Fab (ovine) antivenom for the treatment for crotaline snakebite in the United States. Arch Intern Med 2001;161:2030–6.

Dart RC et al: Efficacy, safety, and use of snake antivenoms in the United States. Ann Emerg Med 2001;37:181–8.

Forks TP: Brown recluse spider bites. J Am Board Fam Pract 2000;13:415–23.

Hall EL: Role of surgical intervention in the management of crotaline snake envenomation. Ann Emerg Med 2001;37: 175–80.

Jasper EH et al: Venomous snakebites in an urban area: what are the possibilities? Wilderness Environ Med 2000;11:168–71.

Kemp ED: Bites and stings of the arthropod kind. Treating reactions that can range from annoying to menacing. Postgrad Med 1998;103:88–90.

Koh WL: When to worry about spider bites. Inaccurate diagnosis can have serious, even fatal, consequences. Postgrad Med 1998;103:235–6.

Majeski J: Necrotizing fasciitis developing from a brown recluse spider bite. Am Surg 2001;67:188–90.

Moss ST et al: Association of rattlesnake bite location with severity of clinical manifestations. Ann Emerg Med 1997;30:58–61.

Offerman SR et al: Does the aggressive use of polyvalent antivenin for rattlesnake bites result in serious acute side effects? West J Med 2001;175:88–91.

Scharman EJ et al: Copperhead snakebites: clinical severity of local effects. Ann Emerg Med 2001;38:55–61.

Schwartz S et al: Venomous marine animals of Florida: morphology, behavior, health hazards. J Fla Med Assoc 1997;84: 433–40.

Walter FG et al: Envenomations. Crit Care Clin 1999;15:353–86.

Wright SW et al: Clinical presentation and outcome of brown recluse spider bite. Ann Emerg Med 1997;30:28–32.

ELECTRIC SHOCK & LIGHTNING INJURY

ESSENTIALS OF DIAGNOSIS

- *Momentary or prolonged unconsciousness.*
- *Cardiac arrhythmias.*
- *Muscular pain, fatigue, headache.*
- *Rhabdomyolysis and renal failure.*

General Considerations

Electrical injuries account for more than 500 fatalities each year in the United States. One-fifth of these deaths are due to lightning. The number of nonfatal injuries may be three or four times this number. Patients who have sustained electrical injury or a lightning strike exhibit a number of signs depending upon the energy of the current conducted. Most household electrical injuries are produced by alternating current (50–60 Hz) in the 110- to 220-volt range. Direct current usually produces less severe injuries for the same amount of voltage. Electricity can cause partial-thickness or full-thickness burns with injury to the deeper tissues of the body. In some cases, the burn injury at the entry and exit points may correlate directly with the extent of underlying muscle injury, but extensive deep injuries may be present with only minimal superficial findings. Myonecrosis and rhabdomyolysis are frequently present with higher-energy exposures. Rhabdomyolysis may lead to renal failure if not recognized and treated promptly. Compartment syndrome can occur in extremities with resultant circulatory compromise. Ventricular fibrillation may be present if the current pathway has included the heart.

A potential difference of more than 440 V is considered high voltage. At greater than 1000 V, severe tissue destruction occurs as a result of electrical energy being converted to heat. Electrocution may be accompanied by arc and flash burns (Chapter 36). Associated injuries are a result of falls due to tetany of the major muscles.

Lightning strikes impart huge amounts of energy to their victims. Cardiac and respiratory failure are responsible for immediate deaths. Those surviving the immediate period are at risk for delayed neurologic, visual, and otologic as well as musculoskeletal complications. Although neurologic sequelae were previously thought to be transient, recent investigations have demonstrated permanent injury in one-half of the victims.

Clinical Features

A. Electric Shock

Shock from household current commonly produces transient loss of consciousness, though this may be prolonged. Patients have frequently regained normal function by the time they arrive in the emergency room, at which time they complain of headache, muscle cramps, and fatigue. Nervous irritability and a sensation of anxiety are other common findings. Patients with prolonged unconsciousness should undergo CT scanning to rule out an associated cerebral injury from a fall or direct injury. Cardiac arrhythmias typically are tachyarrhythmias, with atrial and ventricular fibrillation being the most common. Difficulty in breathing with varying degrees of respiratory paresis or complete paralysis requires immediate attention. Damage to skeletal muscles may produce a spurious rise in the CK-MB fraction, leading to the erroneous diagnosis of myocardial infarction.

Burn wounds often accompany electrocution victims. These injuries are of three types: (1) direct burn, (2) arc injury, or (3) flame burn from an associated ignition source. Burn wounds are more common with higher voltage injuries. All patients with burn wounds should receive tetanus prophylaxis. Patients with more severe burns should be considered for transfer after stabilization to a specialized burn center. Additional management is discussed in Chapter 36.

B. Lightning Strike

Patients who require critical care after a lightning strike are usually admitted for complications or simply for cardiac monitoring. Lightning victims may present with paraplegia or quadriplegia that resolves over several hours. This may be accompanied by autonomic instability. In cases of prolonged paresis, imaging studies should be obtained to rule out a spinal injury. Electrocardiographic changes include nonspecific ST-T segment changes that may be accompanied by elevation of cardiac enzymes. Initial hypertension usually resolves spontaneously and does not require treatment.

Lightning victims may have a number of associated findings related to blunt trauma sustained at the time of impact. Rib and long bone fractures in the extremities are particularly common. Burns may be present but are superficial in most patients and often require only superficial wound care. Unlike those who have sustained electrical injuries, patients with lightning injuries rarely develop myoglobinuria.

Treatment: Electric Shock

Patients suffering from electrical injuries should be admitted to the critical care unit when the conditions outlined in Table 38–1 are present.

Table 38–1. Criteria for ICU admission following electrical injury.

High-voltage electrocution
Burns > 20% of BSA
Evidence of entrance and exit burns
Cardiac arrhythmias
Unconsciousness
Respiratory or motor paralysis
Multiple associated injuries
Prior medical compromise

A. General Measures

Most electrocution patients admitted to the ICU will already have had the airway secured (if necessary) and large-bore intravenous catheters inserted for resuscitation and fluid management. Adequate urine output must be ensured to prevent renal failure from myoglobinuria. The goal is to maintain a urine output of 75–100 mL/h. Mannitol may be give as a bolus (1 g/kg) and then as an infusion to maintain an osmotic diuresis as long as the urine contains myoglobin (positive hemoglobin nitrotoluidine test). Sodium bicarbonate may be added to alkalinize the urine and prevent the precipitation of acid hematin. The calculated fluid requirement is approximately 1.7 times the standard fluid calculation based on the total body surface area burned. Electrolytes should be monitored frequently during the resuscitation period.

B. Arrhythmias

After initial stabilization, the most immediate risk is from cardiac arrhythmia, particularly when the electrical current has passed through the thorax. Antiarrhythmics and inotropic support should be instituted when appropriate. However, most arrhythmias are self-limited and infrequently cause hemodynamic abnormalities. Atrial fibrillation occurs occasionally and will usually convert without treatment. Electrocardiographic changes are present in 10–30% of cases. The most common abnormality is nonspecific ST-T wave changes. Myocardial infarction is unusual, but patients with high-voltage injuries may sustain direct myocardial damage. In these patients, close monitoring of fluid therapy may be necessary to prevent pulmonary edema.

C. Neurologic Sequelae

More than half of patients with severe electrical injury develop loss of consciousness, but full recovery usually ensues. Neurologic sequelae are sometimes delayed and may develop days to years after the injury. Deterioration of neurologic status may be of three types: (1) ascending paralysis, (2) amyotrophic lateral sclerosis, or (3) transverse myelitis. Peripheral nerve injuries and motor neuropathies result from demyelinization, vacuolization, gliosis, and perivascular hemorrhage. The prognosis for recovery of useful function is poor.

D. Burns

Most critical care required by victims of electrical injury relates to burns. This subject is discussed in Chapter 36.

Treatment: Lightning Strikes

The most severe complication of lightning injury is respiratory arrest caused by depression of the respiratory control center. This can result in secondary cardiac arrest in an otherwise salvageable patient. Surviving victims of lightning strikes tend to have fewer complications than patients with electrical injury. Early emergency resuscitation usually stabilizes these patients to the point that only observation is necessary. The need for cardiac monitoring for more than 24 hours is debatable. Most patients will be confused and have anterograde amnesia covering a period of several days after the incident. If neurologic deterioration is noted, CT scanning or MRI should be obtained to exclude the possibility of intracranial hemorrhage or other injury. In most cases, long-term sequelae from lightning injuries are rare.

Fish RM: Electric injury, Part II: Specific injuries. J Emerg Med 2000;18:27–34.

Jain S et al: Electrical and lightning injuries. Crit Care Clin 1999;15:319–31.

Lee RC: Injury by electrical forces: pathophysiology, manifestations, and therapy. Curr Probl Surg 1997;34:677–764.

Muehlberger T et al: The long-term consequences of lightning injuries. Burns 2001;27:829–33.

Tredget EE et al: Electrical injuries in Canadian burn care. Identification of unsolved problems. Ann N Y Acad Sci 1999;888: 75–87.

RADIATION INJURY

ESSENTIALS OF DIAGNOSIS

- *Nausea and vomiting, diarrhea.*
- *Weakness, dehydration.*
- *Bone marrow depression.*
- *Sepsis.*
- *Severe neurologic changes.*
- *Cardiovascular collapse.*

General Considerations

Acute radiation syndrome consists of characteristic clinical manifestations following accidental or therapeutic exposure to ionizing radiation. In cases of unknown level of exposure, knowledge of the manifestations enables the clinician to estimate the exposure dose and determine appropriate treatment.

Ionizing radiation can be either electromagnetic (x-rays, gamma rays) or particulate (electrons, protons, and neutrons). The power of penetration of these particles is determined by the energy they carry. High-energy particles can travel deep into the body and cause severe damage to tissues.

The principal lethal effect of radiation appears to be the production of chemically active free radicals within cells that damage essential macromolecules such as DNA. Very high radiation doses will disrupt cell metabolism and result in rapid cell death. Moderate radiation doses produce breaks in double-stranded DNA. No visible effects occur until the cell attempts mitosis. At that time, cell division may be arrested, or the daughter cells may lack essential genetic material and become nonfunctional. Small doses of radiation can produce gene mutations. This may result in no observable effect or in subsequent malignant transformation.

Individual tissues vary greatly in their sensitivity to radiation damage. The most sensitive tissues are those that require continued cellular proliferation for proper function, such as the gastrointestinal and hematopoietic systems. Acute radiation syndrome is most pronounced in these systems. With very high levels of exposure, dysfunction of the cardiovascular and central nervous systems is also observed, most likely resulting from direct organ injury.

Radiation Dosimetry

The rad is the unit of absorbed radiation dose. It is defined as that quantity of radiation which deposits 100 ergs of energy per gram of tissue. Clinically, a dose of radiation is often prescribed in grays (Gy) (1 Gy = 100 rads; 1 rad = 1 cGy).

Clinical Features

Radiation injury is characterized by an acute phase, referred to as the prodromal phase; and a subacute phase, characterized by bone marrow and gastrointestinal dysfunction. The phases are separated by a latent period of 1–3 weeks, during which time the patient may be completely asymptomatic. The severity of acute radiation injury is determined by the dose and the time over which the exposure occurs. After exposure to less than 150 cGy, most patients have minimal or no prodromal symptoms. Slight depression of platelets and granulocytes may be observed after a latent period of 30 days. Lymphocytes are most sensitive to radiation and may be decreased.

Patients exposed to 150–400 cGy develop transient nausea and vomiting 1–4 hours following exposure. After a latent period of 1–3 weeks, gastrointestinal symptoms occur: nausea, vomiting, and bloody diarrhea. Bone marrow depression is manifested by anemia, coagulopathy, and depressed immune function. Susceptibility to infection is significantly increased.

An acute whole body exposure of 600–1000 cGy results in an accelerated version of the acute radiation syndrome. Gastrointestinal complications predominate in the early phase of the illness and may be life-threatening. Severe hematologic complications can be expected to develop in survivors.

A fulminating course is seen in patients sustaining acute whole body exposure to higher doses. Vomiting occurs shortly after exposure and is rapidly followed by diarrhea, tenesmus, dehydration, and circulatory collapse. Central nervous system manifestations may include ataxia, incoordination, weakness, confusion, seizures, and coma. Death occurs within 48 hours.

Pericarditis with effusions and constriction are delayed manifestations that develop several months after exposure. Myocarditis can occur but is less common. If injury is mild, full recovery is the rule.

Treatment

In cases of moderate radiation exposure, initial treatment is supportive and uncomplicated. Immediate aggressive therapy is not indicated, since the prodromal symptoms are usually not severe and are self-limited. It is after the latent period of 1–3 weeks that the more severe clinical manifestations of the syndrome develop. In cases in which severe symptoms develop without a latent period, death is inevitable, and only symptomatic care should be provided.

Patients with moderate to severe radiation exposure should be admitted to the hospital and isolated. Care should be exercised to limit patient and personnel movement through the hospital in order to contain the radiation. Many radioactive materials are in particulate form and will not pass through the skin and are removed by washing. To this end, clothes should be removed and stored in specially labeled plastic bags. Showering or washing skin surfaces removes most of the contamination. A Geiger counter should be used to assess the adequacy of decontamination. The process can be aided by hair removal. Undiluted household bleach (5% sodium hypochlorite) can be used after soap and water. A dilute solution (1 part bleach to 5 parts water) should be used around the face and wounds. Wounds should be thoroughly debrided and irrigated to remove radioactive material.

Fluid loss should be corrected with intensive intravenous replacement. The blood count should be carefully monitored. Reverse isolation is required when the white blood cell count falls below 1000/μL. Whole blood and platelet transfusions are nearly always required because of anemia and bleeding. When immunosuppression is apparent, blood products should be irradiated with 5000 cGy before transfusion to decrease the possibility of a graft-versus-host reaction. Intestinal microorganisms are a major source of infection, and prophylactic antibiotics directed against gram-negative organisms should be administered. The appearance of clinical signs of infection should prompt a thorough evaluation. Broad-spectrum antibiotics should be administered until culture results are obtained.

The use of chlorpromazine or promethazine in an attempt to control radiation-induced vomiting should be avoided. These medications depress gastric emptying and may increase the risk of aspiration and subsequent pulmonary infection.

Current Controversies & Unresolved Issues

Antidopaminergic agents appear to prevent radiation-induced vomiting without causing gastroplegia. Clinical trials suggest that domperidone may be effective, but more controlled studies need to be completed.

In most cases of moderate to severe acute radiation injury, exposure of the bone marrow is not uniform, and a return of function can be anticipated. In cases of lethal exposures, the use of bone marrow transplantation as a form of therapy has been suggested. However, based on current experience, the likelihood of success cannot be adequately ensured. Numerous problems exist in the potential application of this type of therapy. It could not be used in a mass casualty situation because of the extensive resources required for the treatment of individual patients. Additional problems can be anticipated in securing suitable HLA-compatible donors and in controlling graft-versus-host disease. This treatment was attempted in 13 victims of the Chernobyl accident. Eleven of these patients died. It is not clear whether the other two patients would have survived with conventional supportive therapy.

A newer mode of treatment of pancytopenia is the stimulation of hematopoietic tissue through the use of cytokines and colony-stimulating factors. This has been demonstrated to decrease the period of leukocyte count depression and to elevate the nadir. Additional studies are required to establish efficacy and optimal dosing regimens.

Gastrointestinal pathogen suppression may be accomplished by the deliberate inoculation of the gut with nonpathogenic bacteria such as lactobacilli. The theory is that this will result in normalization of the intestinal flora that had been altered by antibiotic therapy. Prolonged survival has been demonstrated in animal models, but studies in humans are lacking.

Bice-Stephens WM: Radiation injuries from military and accidental explosions: a brief historical review. Mil Med 2000;165:275–7.

Doll R: Hazards of ionising radiation: 100 years of observations on man. Br J Cancer 1995;72:1339–49.

Reeves GI: Radiation injuries. Crit Care Clin 1999;15:457–73.

Saclarides TJ: Radiation injuries of the gastrointestinal tract. Surg Clin North Am 1997;77:261–8.

Critical Care Issues in Pregnancy 39

Marie Beall, MD, Leonard A. Cedars, MD, & Wilbert Fortson, MD

PHYSIOLOGIC ADAPTATION TO PREGNANCY

The average duration of gestation is 40 weeks from the first day of the last menses, with term defined as being between 37 weeks and 42 weeks. The mother's basic physiology is altered in a number of ways during normal pregnancy. Some of these may alter her baseline state and response to critical illness, but others may predispose to injuries and conditions that require critical care.

CARDIOVASCULAR SYSTEM

Pregnancy causes changes in the appearance and function of the heart and great vessels. Elevation of the hemidiaphragms, which accompanies advancing pregnancy, causes the heart to assume a more horizontal position in the chest, and this results in lateral deviation of the cardiac apex, with larger cardiac silhouette on chest x-ray and a shift in the electrical axis. The heart does increase in size in pregnancy, but only by about 12%. Cardiac output increases by 30–50%, with most of the increase occurring in the first trimester. Both stroke volume and heart rate increase. The heart rate increases by about 17%, with the maximum reached by the middle of the third trimester (32 weeks). Stroke volume increases by 32%, with the maximum reached by mid gestation. After 20 weeks, cardiac output may decrease significantly (25–30%) when the patient lies in the supine position as compared with the left lateral position. This is apparently due to compression of the inferior vena cava by the pregnant uterus, with resultant decreased venous return. The distribution of cardiac output is altered as well. At term, 17% of the cardiac output is directed to the uterus and its contents, and an additional 2% goes to the breasts. The skin and kidneys also receive additional blood flow when compared with the nonpregnant state. Blood flow to the brain and liver may increase. Perfusion of other organs such as the skeletal muscle and gut is unchanged.

Peripheral vascular resistance decreases during pregnancy. A concomitant decrease in systemic blood pressure reaches its nadir at about 24 weeks of gestation. Blood pressure then rises gradually until term but should not exceed nonpregnant levels at any time during pregnancy. Central hemodynamic studies of normal pregnant women demonstrate a significant decrease in both systemic and pulmonary vascular resistance. Mean arterial pressure, pulmonary capillary wedge pressure, central venous pressure, and left ventricular stroke work index are unchanged. Colloid osmotic pressure is decreased.

Labor and delivery are associated with cardiac stress beyond that of late pregnancy. Cardiac output may increase by as much as 40% in patients not receiving adequate pain relief, although those with adequate anesthesia experience much smaller rises. The rise in cardiac output is progressive over the different stages of labor, and there is a further rise of approximately 15% during each uterine contraction resulting from the expression of 300–500 mL of blood from the uterus back into the mother's circulation. Delivery of the fetus is associated with as much as a 59% increase in cardiac output, presumably as a result of autotransfusion of blood contained in the uterus. This increase may be blunted by the blood loss at delivery. In patients with clinically significant mitral stenosis, delivery may be associated with an increase in the pulmonary capillary wedge pressure of up to 16 mm Hg.

RESPIRATORY SYSTEM

During pregnancy, the subcostal angle increases from about 68 degrees to about 103 degrees, with a concomitant increase in the transthoracic diameter. The resting level of the diaphragm is 4 cm higher at term than in the nongravid state. Many authors state that this elevation is a result of pressure from the expanding uterus. However, diaphragmatic excursions are increased by 1–2 cm over nonpregnant values, suggesting that uterine pressure is not the sole cause of the elevation.

Several aspects of pulmonary function change during pregnancy (Figure 39–1). Tidal volume increases by about 40%, and residual volume decreases by about 20%. These changes may make the lung appear denser on x-ray because it is more collapsed during expiration. Data on vital capacity in pregnancy are contradictory, with older studies suggesting that there is no change and some newer ones suggesting that there is a marked increase. During pregnancy, expiratory reserve volume decreases by about 200 mL and inspiratory reserve volume increases by about 300 mL. Forced expiratory volume appears to be unchanged.

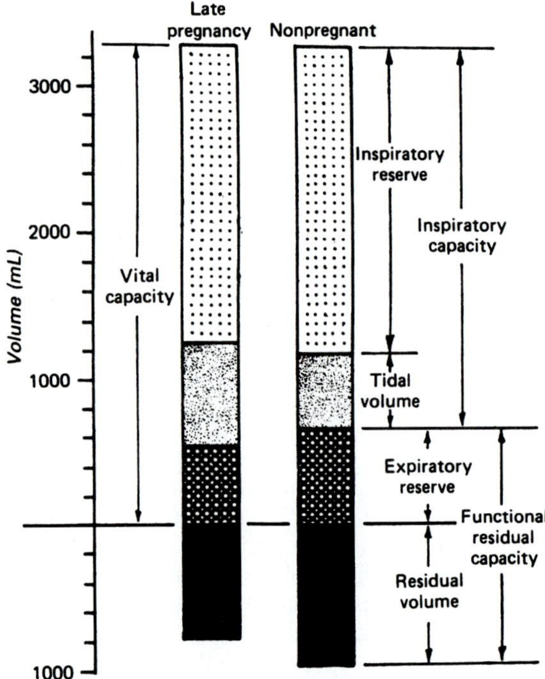

Figure 39–1. The components of lung volume in late pregnancy compared with those in nonpregnant women. (Reproduced, with permission, from Hytten FE, Leitch I: *The Physiology of Human Pregnancy.* Blackwell, 1964.)

Total body oxygen uptake at rest increases by about 30–40 mL/min in pregnancy, or about 12–20%. Most of the oxygen is needed to meet maternal metabolic alterations. The increased oxygen need is met by increased tidal volume alone, as the pulmonary diffusing capacity appears to be decreased in pregnancy and the respiratory rate does not significantly increase. There is a total increase in minute ventilation of 48% at term, which exceeds the need for increased oxygen delivery. This "hyperventilation of pregnancy" appears to be hormonally mediated and results in a decrease in $PaCO_2$ to below 30 mm Hg in normal women. Maternal pH does not change because there is a reciprocal decline in bicarbonate concentration. The net result of these acid-base alterations is facilitation of fetal-maternal CO_2 exchange.

HEMATOLOGIC SYSTEM

Both the volume and the composition of the blood change during pregnancy. Plasma volume increases by 40–60%, the bulk of the increase occurring before the beginning of the third trimester. The red cell mass also expands, with a total increase of 25% at term. This percentage can be maximized (to about 30%) by iron supplementation. An increase in red cell mass occurs throughout pregnancy, but the early—and in some patients disproportionate—increase in plasma volume leads to a dilutional anemia. Normal pregnant women who are not iron-supplemented have hemoglobin concentrations of approximately 11 g/dL at 24 weeks of gestation, with little change until term. Those supplemented with iron have similar hemoglobin concentrations at 24 weeks but manifest an increase in hemoglobin to near-normal at term.

The white blood cell count increases to about 10,000/μL at term. The platelet count may decrease slightly to a mean value of 260,000/μL at 35 weeks of gestation. Platelet levels above 120,000/μL are generally regarded as normal in pregnancy.

Biochemical characteristics of the blood also change. Serum osmolarity decreases by about 10 mosm/L early in pregnancy and remains constant thereafter. Sodium, potassium, calcium, magnesium, and zinc all demonstrate minor decreases in their serum levels. Chloride does not change, though bicarbonate decreases markedly. Serum creatinine decreases early, with a mean creatinine of 0.66 mg/dL at 12 weeks, and this decrease is maintained at least until 32 weeks of gestation. The creatinine clearance in pregnancy is approximately 50% higher than in the nonpregnant state. The plasma concentrations of albumin and total protein decrease in proportion to the plasma volume expansion. Most of the commonly tested serum enzymes do not change in pregnancy, but alkaline phosphatase does increase as a result of the production of a placental form of this enzyme. Creatine kinase decreases in early pregnancy, though the serum levels return to normal by term. Serum lipids increase toward term, with the levels of cholesterol and triglycerides doubling during pregnancy.

The levels of many clotting factors are altered. Fibrinogen increases to levels as high as 600 mg/dL at term, with levels below 400 mg/dL generally being regarded as unusual. The presence of fibrin degradation products in trace amounts is also not unusual at term and depends on the sensitivity of the test being used. Clotting and bleeding times are not increased. The risk of thromboembolism increases, with a relative risk of 1.8 in gestation and 5.5 during the puerperium. The increased risk of thromboembolism may also be due to the increased incidence of venous stasis and vessel wall injury.

IMMUNE SYSTEM

Pregnant women appear to be at increased risk of certain infections, probably due to the same immune alterations that allow tolerance of the antigenically foreign placenta. For this reason, reactivation of viral diseases and tuberculosis are more common during pregnancy. Severe complications of common disorders such as varicella and pyelonephritis are also more frequent. Measurable indices of immune function such as white blood cell counts and immunoglobulin levels do not explain the maternal immune dysfunction. Various theories have been offered to explain these observations but none have achieved general acceptance.

Cruikshank DP, Wigton TR, Hays PM: Maternal physiology in pregnancy. In: *Obstetrics: Normal and Problem Pregnancies,* 4th ed. Gabbe SG, Niebyl JR, Simpson JL (editors). Churchill Livingstone, 1996.

GENERAL CONSIDERATIONS IN THE CARE OF THE PREGNANT PATIENT IN THE ICU

The care of the pregnant patient is necessarily the care of two patients. Although care of the mother is the primary concern in most circumstances, attention must also be paid to fetal health and well-being.

Position

As discussed earlier, a pregnant woman may experience a decrease in cardiac output with associated hypotension when lying in the supine position. For this reason, the pregnant woman who is beyond the 20th week of gestation should avoid lying supine. In the ICU, this means that pregnant women who are bedridden and unable to move by themselves should be positioned with the right hip elevated, usually with an obstetric wedge, to about 4 inches above the plane of the bed. Alternatively, the patient may be positioned in the right lateral decubitus position, taking care that she is tilted adequately to prevent caval compression. This is not necessary in a patient who is in Fowler's position, ie, with the head of the bed elevated. Because of the increased risk of thromboembolism in pregnancy or immediately postpartum, these patients should also receive measures to prevent deep venous thrombosis. Venous compression stockings may be of some benefit, but—especially in the recently delivered patient—heparin in doses adequate to achieve anti-Factor Xa levels 0.05–0.2 units/mL are considered necessary to avoid pelvic or lower extremity venous thrombosis.

Monitoring

When caring for a critically ill pregnant patient, the question of how to monitor the fetus arises frequently. Monitoring by auscultation of fetal heart tones is considered one of the vital signs in any hospitalized pregnant women. However, continuous fetal heart rate monitoring with an electronic monitor may be indicated in the viable or near-viable fetus (23 weeks and beyond), especially if the maternal condition affects pulmonary or hemodynamic function. Use of the continuous fetal monitor requires personnel skilled in its interpretation.

Fetal monitoring may be especially helpful during special procedures or surgery when maternal position, hypotension, or anesthesia can lead to fetal compromise that could be reversed with changes in position or fluid resuscitation. Fetal heart rate monitoring according to a predetermined schedule (nonstress testing) may also be useful in gauging fetal response to the mother's illness and in determining when fetal compromise may necessitate early delivery. This strategy (as opposed to continuous fetal heart rate monitoring) should be reserved for the stable patient, whose underlying condition might result in decreased uteroplacental perfusion or altered placental function. Additional biophysical testing might be deemed necessary by the consulting obstetrician, but that subject is beyond the scope of this chapter.

Teratogenesis & Drugs Used During Pregnancy

Critical care of a pregnant patient necessarily involves the use of drugs and physical agents that may have an effect on the developing fetus. The first concern of the physician is properly with the life and long-term health of the mother. In cases in which alternative therapies or diagnostic modalities are available, the physician must consider their possible fetal effects.

Information regarding the potential risk to the fetus of various agents is available from a number of published sources and from the manufacturer's package inserts. In addition, many areas are served by teratogen "hotline" services. The FDA requires all drug manufacturers to rate their drugs for risk in pregnancy (Table 39–1). Most drugs are not studied in pregnancy during the FDA approval period, and so most new drugs will be placed in category C. For this reason, many drugs routinely used during pregnancy are older ones, with an established record of safe use.

The overriding principal in choice of a therapeutic agent is that the anticipated benefit should outweigh any theoretic risks. Consequently, a potentially teratogenic—but life-sustaining—pharmacologic intervention, for which there is no good alternative would be acceptable, while one with less proven risk but prescribed as a comfort measure only might not be.

Imaging Studies

Ionizing radiation is known to be a human teratogen, and the use of x-ray is appropriately limited in pregnant

Table 39–1. Risk factors for drug use in pregnancy.[1]

Category A	Controlled studies in women fail to demonstrate a risk to the fetus in the first trimester (and there is no evidence of risk in later trimesters), and the possibility of fetal harm appears remote.
Category B	Either animal-reproduction studies have not demonstrated a fetal risk but there are no controlled studies in pregnant women, or animal-reproduction studies have shown an adverse effect (other than a decrease in fertility) that was not confirmed in controlled studies in women in the first trimester (and there is no evidence of a risk in later trimesters).
Category C	Either studies in animals have revealed adverse effects on the fetus (teratogenic or embryocidal or other) and there are no controlled studies in women, or studies in women and animals are not available. Drugs should be given only if the potential benefit justifies the potential risk to the fetus.
Category D	There is positive evidence of human fetal risk, but the benefits from use in pregnant women may be acceptable despite the risk (eg, if the drug is needed in a life-threatening situation or for a serious disease for which safer drugs cannot be used or are ineffective).
Category X	Studies in animals or human beings have demonstrated fetal abnormalities, or there is evidence of fetal risk based on human experience, or both, and the risk of the drug in pregnant women clearly outweighs any possible benefit. The drug is contraindicated in women who are or may become pregnant.

[1]Federal Register 1980;44:31434–67.

women. Persons exposed to high levels of ionizing radiation in utero may exhibit microcephaly, mental retardation, retarded growth, and various structural abnormalities. Some reports have also suggested an increased risk of childhood cancer following prenatal x-ray exposure. Data from atomic bomb survivors suggest that the most vulnerable period for the fetus is from 8–15 weeks of gestation. Fetuses in this gestational age range appear to have a linear increase in mental retardation with increasing x-ray exposure, with an incidence of 0.4% per rad of exposure, though a definite fetal effect may not be seen below 5 cGy. Fetuses at 16–25 weeks were less sensitive to x-rays, and exposure at more than 25 weeks of gestation was not associated with an increased incidence of mental retardation. In one study, the risk of childhood leukemia was estimated to be 1.7 times that of controls in patients exposed to radiation in utero. The risk for childhood cancers also appeared to be higher in fetuses exposed to x-rays in the second as compared with the third trimester. The fetal exposure for different radiologic studies has been calculated and is presented in Table 39–2. As will be apparent, many studies, such as chest films and head and neck studies, entail only slight exposure of the fetus. Nevertheless, the uterus and its contents should be shielded whenever possible.

Iodinated contrast media are not contraindicated in pregnancy and may be used as in nonpregnant patients. These media, may be rated in fetal risk category D because of the risk of fetal goiter when these agents appear in the amniotic fluid; but this issue is probably not a concern with other uses of contrast agents.

Radionuclide scans should be used with caution in pregnancy. Iodine is concentrated in the fetal thyroid after 10 weeks of gestation, and radioactive iodine may cause harm to the fetal thyroid. Other radionuclides may be associated with an increased risk of fetal mutagenesis or teratogenesis if they cross the placenta in large amounts. Agents bound to large protein aggregates do not cross the placenta, and probably represent a negligible risk to the fetus. In particular, the performance of pulmonary ventilation/perfusion scanning for pulmonary emboli has been calculated to result in a fetal dose of only 50 mrem, and this is largely from fetal exposure to the agent in the maternal bladder during urinary excretion of the agent.

Ultrasonography is extensively used in obstetrics. Controlled studies are not available regarding its safety, but numerous observational studies have lead to the conclusion that diagnostic ultrasound is safe for use in pregnancy. However, fetal damage has been demonstrated in animal models using ultrasound power levels sufficient to cause tissue heating. For this reason, the use of therapeutic ultrasound in pregnancy is contraindicated.

Few studies are available concerning the safety of MRI in pregnancy. There is a theoretical concern that the strong magnetic field may affect fetal cell migration in the first trimester, and the use of MRI has been discouraged, although there are no reports of adverse human fetal effects.

Total Parenteral Nutrition

As a consequence of depletion of maternal glucose by the fetoplacental unit, pregnant patients are more sensitive than nonpregnant ones to starvation. Blood sugar is lower by 15–20 mg/dL in a pregnant woman after a 12-hour fast, and starvation ketosis is exaggerated. Undernutrition was associated with increased infant mortality and decreased birth weight in mothers starved

Table 39–2. Embryo (uterine) doses for selected x-ray projections (cGy/R).[1,2]

Projection	View	SID[3] (in)	Image Receptor (in)[4]	Beam Quality (HVL, mm al)[5]					
				1.5	2.0	2.5	3.0	3.5	4.0
Pelvic, lumbopelvic	AP	40	17 x 14	0.142	0.212	0.283	0.353	0.421	0.486
	LAT	40	14 x 17	0.013	0.025	0.039	0.056	0.075	0.097
Abdominal[6]	AP	40	14 x 17	0.133	0.199	0.256	0.330	0.392	0.451
	PA	40	14 x 17	0.056	0.090	0.130	0.174	0.222	0.273
	LAT	40	14 x 17	0.013	0.023	0.037	0.053	0.071	0.091
Lumbar spinal	AP	40	14 x 17	0.128	0.189	0.259	0.309	0.366	0.419
	LAT	40	14 x 17	0.009	0.017	0.027	0.039	0.053	0.068
Hip	AP (one)	40	10 x 12	0.105	0.153	0.200	0.244	0.285	0.324
	AP (both)	40	17 x 14	0.136	0.203	0.269	0.333	0.395	0.454
Full spine (chiropractic)	AP	40	14 x 36	0.154	0.231	0.308	0.384	0.457	0.527
Urethrography, cystography	AP	40	10 x 12	0.135	0.200	0.265	0.327	0.386	0.441
Upper gastrointestinal	AP	40	14 x 17	0.0095	0.016	0.035	0.034	0.045	0.056
Femur (one side)	AP	40	7 x 17	0.0016	0.003	0.0048	0.0069	0.0094	0.012
Cholecystography	PA	40	10 x 12	0.0007	0.0015	0.0026	0.0041	0.0060	0.0083
Chest	AP	72	14 x 17	0.0003	0.0007	0.0013	0.002	0.0031	0.0043
	PA	72	14 x 17	0.0003	0.0006	0.0012	0.002	0.0030	0.0045
	LAT	72	14 x 17	0.0001	0.0003	0.0005	0.0008	0.0012	0.0018
Ribs, barium swallow	AP	40	14 x 17	0.0001	0.0003	0.0005	0.0009	0.0014	0.0020
	PA	40	14 X 17	0.0001	0.0003	0.0005	0.0009	0.0015	0.0022
	LAT	40	14 X 17	0.00003	0.00008	0.0002	0.0003	0.0004	0.0006
Thoracic spine	AP	40	14 x 17	0.0002	0.0004	0.0008	0.0014	0.0041	0.003
	LAT	40	14 x 17	0.00004	0.0001	0.0002	0.0004	0.0005	0.0008
Skull, cervical spine, scapula, shoulder, humerus	...	40	...	<0.000001	<0.000001	<0.000001	<0.000001	<0.000001	<0.000001

[1]Modified from Lione A: Ionizing radiation and human reproduction. Reprod Toxicol 1987;1:3–16. (Data from Rosenstein.)
[2]Average dose to the uterus (mrad) for 1 roentgen entrace skin exposure (free-in-air).
[3]Source image distance.
[4]Field size is collimated to the image receptor size.
[5]Half value layer, millimeters of aluminum.
[6]Include retrograde pyelogram, KUB, barium enema, lumbosacral spine, intravenous pyelogram, and renal arteriogram.

during World War II. These facts suggest that nutrition should be addressed early in the course of critical care. Total parenteral nutrition has been used in pregnancy with good fetal outcomes in patients with intractable nausea and vomiting of pregnancy as well as in patients with other chronic diseases. Total parenteral nutrition should be considered in any pregnant patient who is expected to be without oral intake for more than 7 days and in whom enteral (tube) feedings are contraindicated. In cases in which shorter durations of starvation are expected, peripheral nutritional supplementation is essential. At a minimum, when the patient is denied oral intake, enough intravenous glucose should be administered to avoid ketonemia.

Patient Counseling

The fetal organs are essentially fully formed by the end of the first trimester. This is important when considering the teratogenic potential of medications given to the mother. Teratogenic effects are most likely to occur early, when pregnancy may not yet be diagnosed. Central nervous system growth and development, body growth, and sexual organ development occur in the second trimester, with central nervous system development and body growth continuing during the third trimester. Drugs given during the last trimester may impact neurologic development but will not cause significant structural abnormalities other than perhaps impairing fetal growth. A woman in the ICU who is found to be pregnant should be given complete information on the timing and dosages of the drugs and diagnostic agents used in her care. It may be helpful to refer such a patient and her family to a medical geneticist or prenatal diagnostic center for counseling and perhaps for diagnostic procedures. As a medicolegal issue, it may also be advisable to obtain an obstetric ultrasound examination as early as possible during the pregnant patient's stay in the ICU. Fetal abnormalities apparent at that time are probably preexisting conditions and not the result of medications given in the unit. Furthermore, this will document gestational age and establish a baseline from which to assess fetal growth.

Boice JD Jr, Miller RW: Childhood and adult cancer after intrauterine exposure to ionizing radiation. Teratology 1999;59:227–33.

Briggs GG, Freeman RK, Yaffe SJ: *Drugs in Pregnancy and Lactation,* 6th ed. Lippincott Williams & Wilkins, 2001.

Campbell LA, Klocke RA: Implications for the pregnant patient. Am J Respir Crit Care Med 2001;163:1051–4.

Fattibene P et al: Prenatal exposure to ionizing radiation: sources, effects and regulatory aspects. Acta Pediatr 1999;88:693–702.

Guidelines for diagnostic imaging during pregnancy. The American College of Obstetricians and Gynecologists. Int J Gynaecol Obstet 1995;51:288–91.

Lapinsky SE, Kruczynski K, Slutsky AS: Critical care in the pregnant patient. Am J Respir Crit Care Med 1995;152:427–55.

Levine MG, Esser D: Total parenteral nutrition for the treatment of severe hyperemesis gravidarum: maternal nutritional effects and fetal outcome. Obstet Gynecol 1988;72:102–7.

Lione A: Ionizing radiation and human reproduction. Reprod Toxicol 1987;1:3–16.

Rizk NW et al: Obstetric complications in pulmonary and critical care medicine. Chest 1996;110:791–809.

Shepard TH: *Catalog of Teratogenic Agents,* 10th ed. Johns Hopkins Univ Press, 2001.

Strassner HT, Pombar X: Diagnostic procedures. In: *Principles and Practice of Medical Therapy in Pregnancy.* Gleicher N (editor). 3rd ed. Appleton & Lange, 1998.

Cardiopulmonary Resuscitation (CPR) in the Pregnant Woman

The American Heart Association has recommended when cardiac arrest occurs in a pregnant woman, standard resuscitative measures and procedures can and should be taken without modification. In particular, they endorse the use of closed-chest compression, defibrillation, and vasopressors as indicated and emphasize the need to displace the uterus from the abdominal vessels by a right hip wedge or by manual pressure on the fundus. Finally, they endorse the performance of a perimortem cesarean section promptly if routine ACLS protocols are ineffective in restoring circulation (below).

Labor & Delivery in the ICU

The presence of a pregnant woman in the ICU necessitates a plan for delivery of that pregnancy, if necessary. On occasion, spontaneous labor may occur in a patient too unstable to be transferred to the delivery room. In this case, labor and delivery must be undertaken in the ICU. Fetal heart rate monitoring may be useful in advising the pediatricians about the fetus's condition even if cesarean section is not an option. Attention should be paid to achieving adequate maternal analgesia because of the significant maternal cardiac demands imposed by unmedicated labor. In the case of any fetus of 22 weeks or more of gestational age or expected to weigh more than 500 g, a neonatal resuscitation team should be in attendance at delivery. The delivery should be conducted by experienced personnel in an atraumatic manner.

Rarely, it may be necessary to perform perimortem cesarean section in the ICU if the mother has died and an attempt is being made to salvage the fetus. For this reason, in any critically ill hospitalized pregnant patient, a determination should be made as early as possible about the potential viability of the fetus. If perimortem cesarean section is a possibility, necessary instruments should be kept at or near the bedside. In a large series of such procedures, normal infant survival was associated with delivery within 5 minutes after maternal death (from cardiac arrest). Fewer than 15% of infants survived when delivery was performed more than 15 minutes after maternal demise, though fetal survival after a much longer delay has been reported. Given this information and data suggesting that the effectiveness of CPR in the mother may improve with evacuation of the uterus, some authorities, including the American Heart Association, suggest that cesarean section should be started within 4–5 minutes after initiation of CPR.

Several reports have described mothers who met electroencephalographic criteria for death who were maintained for prolonged periods on life support in order to allow growth and maturation of the fetus. In a number of these cases, apparently healthy infants have been delivered, though the outcome of the infant in such cases cannot be guaranteed.

Cardiopulmonary resuscitation in pregnancy. In: *Critical Care Obstetrics,* 3rd ed. Clark SL et al (editors). Blackwell, 1997.

Feldman DM et al: Irreversible maternal brain injury during pregnancy: a case report and review of the literature. Obstet Gynecol Surv 2000;55:708–14.

Guidelines for cardiopulmonary resuscitation and emergency cardiac care. Emergency Cardiac Care Committee and Subcommittees, American Heart Association. Part IV. Special resuscitation situations. JAMA 1992;268:2242–50.

MANAGEMENT OF CRITICAL COMPLICATIONS OF PREGNANCY

PREECLAMPSIA-ECLAMPSIA

ESSENTIALS OF DIAGNOSIS

- *Hypertension.*
- *Proteinuria.*
- *Seizures (eclampsia).*

General Considerations

Preeclampsia is a common disorder with an incidence of 14–20% in women undergoing their first pregnancy and about 6% in multigravidas. It is one of the leading causes of maternal death in the United States. Most preeclamptic patients will be managed in the delivery suite and will not require critical care. Patients with severe disease may, however, have significant complications often warranting ICU care.

Although the mechanisms of preeclampsia are not completely understood, endothelial cell damage and vasospasm appear to be important in the pathophysiology. Preeclamptic women demonstrate an increased vascular smooth muscle response to pressor agents, particularly angiotensin II, which predates the development of overt hypertension. The resulting vasospasm leads to hypertension and contraction of intravascular volume. In more severe cases, this is accompanied by endothelial cell injury with activation of the coagulation system and multi-organ system damage.

Preeclampsia may occur in previously normotensive patients or in patients with preexisting chronic hypertension, who are then said to have superimposed preeclampsia. Indeed, preeclamptic patients with chronic hypertension or with underlying renal or collagen-vascular disease may in fact have more severe disease and a more complicated course. Preeclampsia generally occurs only after the 20th week of gestation but may develop earlier in the woman with multiple fetuses or with hydatidiform mole.

Clinical Features

A. Symptoms and Signs

Preeclampsia is classically defined by the triad of hypertension, proteinuria, and edema. However, because of the frequent occurrence of edema in pregnant without preeclampsia, edema has been omitted as a diagnostic criterion for preeclampsia. Nevertheless, a sudden and dramatic weight gain in late pregnancy often presages the development of overt preeclampsia. For this reason, all patients receiving prenatal care have regular determinations made of their weight, urine protein content, and blood pressure. According to the National High Blood Pressure Education Working Group Report on High Blood Pressure in Pregnancy, the minimum criteria for the diagnosis of preeclampsia are (1) sustained blood pressure elevation of 140 mm Hg systolic or 90 mm Hg diastolic in a previously normotensive woman after 20 weeks gestation, and (2) proteinuria—at least 300 mg of urinary protein in a 24-hour period or at least 30 mg/dL (1+) in a random urine.

Preeclampsia is classified as mild or severe. Severe preeclampsia is characterized by *at least one* of the following additional criteria: (1) blood pressure > 160 mm Hg systolic or > 110 mm Hg diastolic, (2) proteinuria > 5 g in 24 hours, (3) elevated serum creatinine, (4) pulmonary edema, (5) oliguria (< 500 mL/24 h), (6) microangiopathic hemolytic anemia, (7) thrombocytopenia, (8) hepatocellular dysfunction (abnormally elevated AST or ALT), (9) fetal growth restriction, (10) symptoms suggestive of end-organ involvement (head-ache, visual disturbances, epigastric or right upper-quadrant pain), and (11) eclampsia, defined by the presence of seizures in a pregnant patient without other known cause.

B. Laboratory Findings

Preeclampsia is diagnosed primarily by clinical criteria. The major role of the laboratory is identifying and following the course of complications. These include involvement of the renal, hepatic, or hematologic systems. In the care of a severely preeclamptic patient, serial determinations of platelet count, fibrinogen and fibrin degradation products, hemoglobin, liver function tests, and serum creatinine are essential.

Differential Diagnosis

In addition to preeclampsia, the differential diagnosis of hypertension in late gestation includes chronic hypertension, gestational hypertension (pregnancy-induced hypertension without proteinuria), and acute fatty liver of pregnancy. Acute fatty liver, amniotic fluid embolism, and placental abruption may also be associated with coagulopathy. Proteinuria may result from urinary tract infection or from chronic renal disease. Edema is common in pregnancy and not necessarily a sign of preeclampsia, but generalized edema is commonly associated with complicated pregnancy.

Management

A. Delivery

The only definitive treatment for preeclampsia is delivery of the fetus. In the case of severe preeclampsia, this should be undertaken without delay, except in rare cases when the mother is stable and the fetus very immature. Such a delay in delivery in the patient with severe preeclampsia—while antihypertensive therapy is given—remains controversial and should be permitted only when the anticipated benefits to the fetus outweigh the potential risks to both mother and fetus.

B. Seizure Prophylaxis

Seizure prophylaxis should be employed in all severely preeclamptic patients. This is usually begun as soon as the diagnosis is made and continued until the patient is either delivered or until the patient is deemed stable enough to be followed expectantly. Treatment will prevent eclamptic seizures that might occur during a patient's initial hospital evaluation. Once the decision is made to proceed with delivery of the patient with preeclampsia—regardless of its severity—seizure prophylaxis should be initiated and continued throughout labor and delivery and until 24 hours postpartum.

In the United States, magnesium sulfate is the most commonly employed seizure prophylaxis. It is usually administered intravenously, though the intramuscular route can also be employed. The usual regimen includes an intravenous loading dose of 4–6 g given over 20–30 minutes, followed by a continuous infusion of 2 g/h. The infusion rate should be adjusted to achieve serum magnesium levels in the therapeutic range of 4.8–8.4 mg/dL.

C. Control of Hypertension

In general, blood pressures over 180 mm Hg systolic or 110 mm Hg diastolic should be treated acutely with antihypertensives. Hydralazine, 5–20 mg intravenously, according to patient response, is commonly used. An acceptable alternative is labetalol 20 mg, also given by intravenous bolus. If an adequate response is not obtained, the dose should be doubled and repeated at 10-minute intervals up to a maximum single bolus dose of 80 mg and a total maximum dose of 220 mg. Oral or sublingual nifedipine has also been suggested for this situation, but nifedipine should probably not be used as it may result in profound hypotension, particularly when employed concomitantly with magnesium sulfate. Nitroglycerin and sodium nitroprusside may be used if severe hypertension is unresponsive to the above agents, but intra-arterial pressure monitoring is recommended. Owing to the potential for fetal cyanide toxicity, the duration of nitroprusside treatment should be limited.

One should exercise caution in administering any vasodilators to patients with preeclampsia because intravascular volume contraction is often present, making them susceptible to dramatic falls in blood pressure. Excessive and rapid decreases in blood pressure—even to above-normal levels—may be associated with fetal distress secondary to decreased utero-placental perfusion and should therefore be avoided.

D. Hemodynamic Monitoring

A pulmonary artery catheter may be indicated in the presence of oliguria unresponsive to initial fluid boluses, pulmonary edema that does not respond to furosemide diuresis and positioning, or severe hypertension unresponsive to hydralazine or labetalol. Untreated preeclamptic patients without pulmonary edema have been found to have greater systemic vascular resistance, increased cardiac index and hyperdynamic left ventricular function when compared with normal controls. Treatment may modify these findings. The pulmonary artery catheter is essential in differentiating these mechanisms, as central venous pressures have been found not to reliably reflect pulmonary artery pressures in preeclampsia.

E. Pulmonary Edema

Pulmonary edema may be due to left ventricular dysfunction secondary to high systemic vascular resistance, iatrogenic volume overload in the face of contracted intravascular space, decreased plasma colloid oncotic pressure (occurs in normal pregnancy and is exaggerated in preeclampsia), or pulmonary capillary membrane injury. Colloid oncotic pressure may decrease further following intravenous fluid replacement with crystalloids and as a result of rapid intravascular mobilization of edema fluid after delivery. Nevertheless, pulmonary edema remains an uncommon complication of preeclampsia, with an incidence of 2.9% in severe preeclampsia, usually occurring postpartum. Management consists of diuretics and oxygen, with digitalis glycosides reserved for the rare patient with evidence of left ventricular dysfunction.

F. Oliguria

Oliguria—defined as < 30 mL of urine output per hour for 2 hours—in severe preeclampsia seldom progresses to frank renal failure. Oliguria associated with preeclampsia can be due to (1) intravascular volume depletion (most common); (2) oliguria accompanied by normal cardiac function and systemic vascular resistance, probably due to isolated renal arteriolar spasm and perhaps responsive to low-dose dopamine, 1–5 μg/kg/min; and (3) relative volume overload with depressed left ventricular function secondary to high systemic vascular resistance, managed with fluid restriction and afterload reduction.

G. HELLP Syndrome

Preeclampsia may be complicated by the HELLP syndrome (hemolysis, elevated liver enzymes, and low platelets). There is controversy over whether the HELLP syndrome represents a separate clinical entity or is part of the spectrum of preeclampsia. Patients with the HELLP syndrome are older and more frequently multigravidas than other preeclamptic women. The hemolysis observed in these patients is consistent with a microangiopathic hemolytic process and seldom requires specific treatment (other than fetal delivery). Severe thrombocytopenia (platelet count < 30,000/μL) occurs in fewer than 10% of cases. Treatment with platelet transfusion is usually necessary only for cesarean section or other major surgery. The elevated liver enzymes result from hepatocellular injury secondary to vasospasm and may be associated with hepatic infarction, intrahepatic hemorrhage, and subcapsular hematomas. Rarely, a subcapsular hematoma may rupture, precipitating a true surgical emergency. In the absence of liver rupture, treatment of HELLP syndrome is usually supportive, though the laboratory derangements associated with the syndrome may be transiently reversed with steroid treatment. Dexamethasone, 10 mg intravenously every 12 hours, has been shown to result in clinical improvement and reversal of laboratory abnormalities and may allow some delay in delivery in the extremely preterm pregnancy. This regimen has the added advantage of promoting fetal lung maturation, but abnormalities promptly recur if steroids are discontinued. The maternal mortality rate associated with HELLP syndrome has been estimated to be 1–2%.

H. Eclampsia

Eclampsia is defined as the occurrence of grand mal seizures in a woman with preeclampsia in whom the seizures cannot be attributed to some other cause. Eclampsia carries a maternal mortality rate of 1–2% and a fetal mortality rate of approximately 10%. Onset of seizures is often preceded by a severe unrelenting headache. Management of eclampsia consists of control of seizures, pharmacologic control of severe hypertension, and delivery. Seizures can be controlled with a 4 g intravenous bolus of magnesium sulfate (8 g in 50 mL of 0.9% NaCl), given at a rate no more rapid than 1 g/min, followed by a continuous infusion of 2 g/h with monitoring as described above. A 2 g bolus is employed if the patient is already receiving magnesium sulfate prophylaxis or if there is a recurrent seizure after the initial bolus. Magnesium sulfate is the treatment of choice, as studies have demonstrated its superiority to either phenytoin or diazepam and because it has less sedating effect on the fetus. In addition, levels of magnesium are easy to monitor, and magnesium sulfate has a long record of safe use. Once seizures are controlled and the patient is considered stable, efforts should be directed toward accomplishing delivery. In many cases, labor can be safely induced and vaginal delivery achieved. Seizure prophylaxis with magnesium sulfate should be continued until 24 hours postpartum.

I. Other Complications

Disseminated intravascular coagulation, cerebral edema, cerebral bleeding, transient cortical blindness, retinal detachments, placental abruption, fetal growth restriction, and fetal distress may rarely complicate preeclampsia and eclampsia.

ACOG technical bulletin. Hypertension in pregnancy. Number 219–January 1996. Committee on Technical Bulletins of the American College of Obstetricians and Gynecologists. Int J Gynaecol Obstet 1996;53:175–83.

Barton JR, Sibai BM: Acute life-threatening emergencies in preeclampsia-eclampsia. Clin Obstet Gynecol 1992;35:402–13.

Complications of preeclampsia. In: *Critical Care Obstetrics,* 3rd ed. Clark SL et al (editors): Blackwell, 1997.

Isler CM et al: A prospective, randomized trial comparing the efficacy of dexamethasone and betamethasone for the treatment of antepartum HELLP (hemolysis, elevated liver enzymes, and low platelet count) syndrome. Am J Obstet Gynecol 2001;184:1332–7.

Schlembach D, Munz W, Fischer T: Effect of corticosteroids on HELLP syndrome: a case report. J Perinat Med 2000;28:502–5.

Tsukimori K et al: The possible role of endothelial cells in hypertensive disorders during pregnancy. Obstet Gynecol 1992;80: 229–33.

Visser W, Wallenburg HCS: Central hemodynamic observations in untreated preeclamptic patients. Hypertension 1991;17: 1072–7.

ACUTE FATTY LIVER OF PREGNANCY

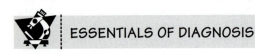

- *Hepatic dysfunction.*
- *Microvesicular fatty infiltration of hepatocytes.*

General Considerations

Acute fatty liver of pregnancy is a rare but potentially catastrophic complication of pregnancy with an incidence of between 1:15,000 and 1:10,000 deliveries. It presents as hepatic dysfunction associated with microvesicular fatty infiltration of hepatocytes occurring during the last trimester of pregnancy or immediately postpartum. Hypertension is commonly present, and some consider the disorder to be a variant of preeclampsia. Indeed, there is an increased incidence of both conditions in first pregnancies and with twin gestation. Although in the past fetal and maternal mortality rates exceeding 70% have been reported, data suggest that fetal and maternal mortality is closer to 20%. This discrepancy is most likely the result of earlier diagnosis and improved management as well as recognition that milder forms of this disorder exist.

The etiology of acute fatty liver of pregnancy remains unknown. Recent reports suggest that it may be much more likely to occur in mothers who are carrying fetuses with a genetic defect of fatty acid beta oxidation. This association is strong enough that infants of affected mothers should be tested.

Clinical Features

A. Symptoms and Signs

Typically, patients present with a history of nausea, vomiting, anorexia, and malaise for 1–2 weeks. Epigastric or right upper quadrant pain may also be present, as may jaundice of varying degrees. Hypertension with or without proteinuria and edema is frequently present, and diabetes insipidus is a common association. In severe acute fatty liver of pregnancy, ascites and progressive hepatic encephalopathy develop along with hypoglycemia, consumptive coagulopathy, metabolic acidosis, and renal failure. Pancreatitis and gastrointestinal bleeding may also occur. Improvement usually follows delivery of the fetus. If delivery has not been performed, fetal death often results, presumably from uteroplacental insufficiency or hypoglycemia.

B. Laboratory Findings

The white blood cell count is usually elevated, often to > 20,000/μL. There may be normochromic, normocytic anemia with fragmented red cells consistent with disseminated intravascular coagulation (DIC) or microangiopathic hemolysis. Prothrombin time and partial thromboplastin time are usually prolonged, and there are decreased fibrinogen and platelets and elevated fibrin degradation products, all indicative of consumptive coagulopathy. Decreased coagulation factors can also result from decreased hepatic synthesis.

AST and ALT are elevated but seldom > 1000 units/L. Alkaline phosphatase and bilirubin are also elevated, and serum albumin is decreased. Hypoglycemia is often present and may be severe. Uric acid is usually high, and BUN and creatinine are elevated if renal impairment is present. Hypernatremia may be present if there is diabetes insipidus, and elevated serum lipase and amylase indicate the presence of pancreatitis.

Diagnosis of acute fatty liver of pregnancy can be made with reasonable certainty from the clinical presentation and the laboratory findings, but confirmation requires the demonstration of microvesicular fat within the hepatocytes on liver biopsy. This is done with either staining a frozen tissue section with oil red O stain or by electron microscopy. Percutaneous liver biopsy should not be attempted if there are significant coagulation abnormalities. Increased echogenicity of the liver on ultrasound examination and decreased attenuation over the liver on CT or MR imaging have been described in cases of the disorder, but these findings are not always present.

Treatment

Management of acute fatty liver of pregnancy can be divided into four categories: monitoring, stabilization, delivery, and support. Monitoring should apply to both the patient and her fetus. Because the fetal condition can deteriorate rapidly, continuous monitoring of the fetal heart rate should be performed until delivery can be accomplished. Fetal biophysical profiles can sometimes aid in the diagnosis of fetal compromise. In severe acute fatty liver of pregnancy, the patient should be managed in the ICU and may require invasive hemodynamic monitoring. Laboratory parameters should be followed at frequent intervals.

Stabilization involves maintenance of a patent airway and adequate ventilation if mental obtundation exists; normalization of intravascular volume; correction of electrolyte disturbances; treatment of hypoglycemia with intravenous glucose; and correction of hematologic and coagulation abnormalities with transfusions of red blood cells, platelets, and fresh frozen plasma. Intravenous magnesium sulfate and, less frequently, hydralazine may be required if there is concomitant preeclampsia. Maintenance magnesium sulfate dosage should be decreased if there is significant renal impairment.

Once the patient has been stabilized, delivery should be accomplished as soon as possible, for this is what will ultimately lead to improvement. Delivery is usually by cesarean section, as this is often the most expeditious method and permits correction of coagulation defects just prior to surgery. However, if the cervix is favorable for labor induction and there is no evidence of fetal compromise, vaginal delivery can be attempted. This avoids the risks of abdominal surgery in the face of coagulopathy and ascites and decreases the need for anesthesia. The choice of anesthetic for cesarean section is controversial. Conduction anesthesia can be used if coagulation abnormalities are corrected. General anesthesia is otherwise used, with care taken to avoid agents that are hepatotoxic or which require metabolism in the liver.

Following delivery, the patient will require supportive management until she recovers from her multiple organ system failure. Protein intake should be avoided, and nutritional maintenance should be primarily in the form of glucose to decrease the load of nitrogenous waste until hepatic function improves. This can be administered intravenously or by nasogastric tube, and blood glucose should be monitored every 1–2 hours to prevent hypoglycemia. To decrease production of ammonia by intestinal bacteria, oral lactulose, 20–30 g (30–45 mL) every 1–2 hours to induce diarrhea, then enough to produce two to four soft stools per day, can be administered. Alternatively, oral neomycin, 0.5–1 g every 6 hours, can be used. Although poorly absorbed, small amounts of neomycin may reach the bloodstream, and care should be taken to avoid levels that might cause nephrotoxicity. Magnesium citrate administered orally will decrease intestinal transit time, further decreasing ammonia absorption.

Optimal fluid and electrolyte management is critical, particularly if there is significant renal impairment, diabetes insipidus, or ascites. Diabetes insipidus can be managed with desmopressin acetate until this phase of the disease resolves. Vitamin K should be administered to aid restoration of coagulation, and further transfusions of fresh frozen plasma or platelets should only be necessary in the face of clinical bleeding or if a surgical procedure is anticipated. Care should be taken to avoid nosocomial infection in this already compromised patient. Some patients have been successfully treated with liver transplantation after delivery for acute fatty liver of pregnancy.

Acute fatty liver. In: *Critical Care Obstetrics,* 3rd ed. Clark SL et al (editors): Blackwell, 1997.

Bacq Y: Acute fatty liver of pregnancy. Semin Perinatol 1998;22: 134–40.

Ibdah JA et al: A fetal fatty-acid oxidation disorder as a cause of liver disease in pregnant women. N Engl J Med 1999;340, 1723–31.

AMNIOTIC FLUID EMBOLISM

ESSENTIALS OF DIAGNOSIS

- *Hypotension, hypoxia, coagulopathy.*
- *Frequently seizures, pulmonary edema, cardiac arrest.*

General Considerations

Amniotic fluid embolism is a rare but catastrophic complication of pregnancy. Its incidence is unknown but is thought to be between 1:80,000 and 1:8000 pregnancies. It appears to be triggered by the release of amniotic fluid, which contains fetal squamous cells, into the maternal pulmonary circulation. It is characterized by hypotension, hypoxia, and coagulopathy. Cardiac arrest is common, and up to 80% of cases may end in maternal demise. There is significant controversy about the pathophysiology of the condition, and treatment is therefore empiric and supportive.

Amniotic fluid embolism has been reported as a complication of first- and second-trimester pregnancy termination, and during otherwise normal pregnancy and the puerperium. The time of greatest risk is during labor. Placental abruption and fetal death are commonly associated with amniotic fluid embolism. Although links with hypertonic uterine contractions, augmented labor, and meconium-stained amniotic fluid have also been reported, a national registry of amniotic fluid embolism did not confirm these associations.

Clinical Features

A. Symptoms and Signs

The patient with amniotic fluid embolism presents with dyspnea and hypotension, which may rapidly deteriorate to cardiac arrest. Half of all patients will die within an hour after developing symptoms. An alternative presentation is as a severe coagulopathy. Up to one-third of patients have seizures, and nearly 75% exhibit pulmonary edema.

Although animal studies demonstrate a rise in pulmonary artery pressure at the time of embolism, with resolution within 30 minutes, no human patient has ever had an amniotic fluid embolus with a pulmonary artery catheter in place. Reports of patients who have had a pulmonary artery catheter placed hours to days after the acute event show no clear pattern of pulmonary artery pressures. Patients surviving the initial phase of the disorder may exhibit left heart failure with elevated pulmonary capillary wedge pressures and decreased systemic vascular resistance. Acute respiratory distress syndrome is common, and 40–50% may have DIC with hemorrhage. The bleeding picture may be further complicated by uterine atony, which appears also to be a result of the amniotic fluid embolism.

B. Laboratory Findings

The classic laboratory finding of amniotic fluid embolism has been fetal squamous cells in the maternal pulmonary circulation at autopsy. Some authors have reported finding such cells in blood from a pulmonary artery catheter in patients suspected of having the diagnosis, but these appear to come from the maternal skin as an artifact from insertion of the catheter. The presence of squamous cells in the pulmonary circulation is of uncertain significance.

Treatment

Amniotic fluid embolism is a rare and unpredictable disorder. Few practitioners have seen more than a handful of cases, and published data are subject to arguable interpretation. Treatment is supportive. The most common manifestation of the disorder in the ICU is acute respiratory distress syndrome, which should be managed in the same way as for other patients. The severe uterine atony associated with amniotic fluid embolism may necessitate hysterectomy to control uterine bleeding.

Locksmith GJ: Amniotic fluid embolism. Obstet Gynecol Clin North Am 1999;26:435–44.

PYELONEPHRITIS IN PREGNANCY

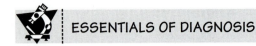

ESSENTIALS OF DIAGNOSIS

- *Fever, flank pain.*
- *Dysuria, pyuria.*

General Considerations

Pyelonephritis occurs in 1–2% of pregnancies. In pregnancy, progesterone mediates ureteral relaxation, predisposing to urinary stasis. In this context, bacteria from lower urinary tract infections can more easily ascend to the kidney. Most obstetricians now aggressively treat even asymptomatic lower tract infections in order to prevent pyelonephritis. The most frequent etiologic organism in pregnant women is *E coli.* Pregnant women with pyelonephritis are usually treated as inpatients because of the greater incidence of severe complications of this disease in pregnancy. In one series, 3% of pregnant women with pyelonephritis developed septic shock, and up to 8.5% of these patients will develop acute respiratory distress syndrome, which can occur 24–48 hours after starting antibiotic therapy and is presumably due to release of bacterial endotoxin.

Clinical Features

A. Symptoms and Signs

The typical patient presents with flank pain and fever of recent origin, often with rigors or chills. There may be a history of lower urinary tract infection, and many patients complain of concurrent lower tract symptoms such as dysuria and frequency. Some patients also have nausea and vomiting and anorexia. On physical examination, flank tenderness is usually present, more frequently on the right. There is usually fever, occasionally > 40 °C. Tachycardia of both mother and fetus may be present due to fever and volume depletion. Uterine contractions may also be present. The presence of hypotension, tachypnea, extremely high fever, or marked tachycardia is ominous.

B. Laboratory Findings

The urine nearly always contains white blood cells and bacteria, and red blood cells and casts are also frequently seen. The urine should be sent for culture to confirm the diagnosis and to check for antibiotic resistance.

Differential Diagnosis

In any febrile pregnant patient, it is critical to exclude the diagnosis of intra-amniotic infection. If any doubt exists, consideration should be given to performing amniocentesis to exclude this possibility. Amniocentesis is usually performed after the administration of antibiotics in order to avoid injecting bacteria into a sterile uterus. Amniotic fluid should be sent for cell count, glucose, Gram stain, and cultures. A leukocyte count > 30/μL (especially polymorphonuclear cells) or glucose < 18 mg/dL should be considered suspicious for infection. Similarly, a Gram stain showing increased PMNs—even in the absence of organisms—suggests bacterial infection. Any organisms seen on Gram stain should be considered significant and are probably an indication for delivery.

The pregnant patient may also have a renal stone, and one should be sought especially in patients in whom the febrile course does not respond to antibiotics. This diagnosis can be made by ultrasound in most cases, though an intravenous urogram (single film to minimize radiation exposure) is still sometimes necessary.

Also included in the differential are appendicitis, cholecystitis, and viral gastroenteritis. Appendicitis in the pregnant patient often presents with tenderness higher in the abdomen than at McBurney's point, and in many cases there are less remarkable peritoneal signs.

Treatment

The mainstay of treatment is intravenous antibiotics, with an antimicrobial agent empirically chosen to cover the majority of community-acquired urinary pathogens. As nausea and vomiting and anorexia frequently accompany pyelonephritis, volume depletion and dehydration are common and should be promptly corrected with intravenous crystalloid. The fever and dehydration of pyelonephritis frequently lead to premature uterine contractions. In addition, high maternal fevers have been shown to be associated with fetal neurologic harm. For this reason, fever should be brought down below 38.3°C with acetaminophen or a cooling blanket. Because of the high risk of pulmonary damage in these patients, fluid overload should be avoided, and tocolytic drugs should be reserved for patients who demonstrate clear cervical changes.

Even with adequate treatment, the typical patient with pyelonephritis demonstrates a hectic fever course, though uncomplicated patients become afebrile after 48 hours. Effective treatment of pyelonephritis often results in the liberation of bacterial endotoxins, which may be associated with hypotension, hypothermia, pulmonary infiltrates, and, rarely, ARDS. Patients who develop pulmonary edema or respiratory distress syndrome do so 24–48 hours after hospital admission. Transient impairment of renal function is also common. One group found that essentially all patients with pyelonephritis demonstrated evidence of hemolysis, sometimes leading to anemia and associated with bacterial endotoxins. Finally, the number of uterine contractions increases after the initiation of antibiotic therapy in some patients; this effect has also been attributed to the release of bacterial endotoxin. Treatment for endotoxin-mediated complications is symptomatic and supportive, while antibiotics are continued. Pyelonephritis-induced ARDS has been treated with the fetus in utero, with subsequent good fetal outcome.

The possibility of endotoxin-mediated complications mandates close observation of pregnant patients with pyelonephritis even after antibiotics have been begun. This should routinely include continuous fetal heart rate monitoring in all pregnancies beyond 22 weeks gestation. Even prior to this gestational age, maternal hypotension and hypoxemia should be detected and corrected before fetal injury can result.

Pregnant patients with pyelonephritis are typically treated for 10 days with antibiotics. These antibiotics can be administered orally on an outpatient basis after the patient becomes afebrile. After an episode of pyelonephritis, the pregnant patient is at increased risk for a recurrence. Often, these patients are given antibiotic prophylaxis for the duration of the pregnancy and for 6 weeks postpartum. Serial urine cultures are also an acceptable management scheme.

Wing DA: Pyelonephritis. Clin Obstet Gynecol 1998;41:515–26.

SEPTIC ABORTION

ESSENTIALS OF DIAGNOSIS

- *Fever.*
- *Uterine or pelvic tenderness.*
- *Recent history of uterine instrumentation with pregnancy.*

General Considerations

Septic abortion is defined as sepsis in association with a recent pregnancy termination, (spontaneous or induced). This complication was much more common when abortion was illegal. Abortion-induced sepsis can progress rapidly to septic shock with an incidence of 2–10%. Data from the 1960s suggests that 300 of 100,000 illegal abortion procedures resulted in the death of the mother. The current maternal mortality related to abortion is about one death in 200,000, but infection still accounts for a significant percentage of these deaths. The likelihood of complications increases in patients who have later abortions and in those having dilation and evacuation procedures. Clostridial infection was a feared complication of illegal abortions and remains a factor in septic abortions today.

Clinical Features

A. Symptoms and Signs

Patients will present with pelvic pain and a serosanguineous to purulent discharge. Some patients will complain more of vaginal bleeding, while others will emphasize their crampy pain. All should have a history of recent (within a week) pregnancy termination, spontaneous or induced, or other intrauterine instrumentation in pregnancy. Hematuria and shock may develop rapidly.

B. Laboratory Findings

Blood, urine, and cervical specimens should be obtained for culture. Gram stain of potentially infected material is useful for initial therapy. The diagnosis of clostridial infection *(Clostridium perfringens)* is suggested by the presence of large gram-positive rods on Gram stain of the cervical secretions or tissue obtained by curetting. The white blood count is usually elevated but may be low in patients with severe disease. Studies of renal and coagulation function and blood gas analyses may be helpful to predict the more severe complications of the infection. Abdominal x-rays may be helpful in the diagnosis of uterine or bowel perforation (which can be a complication of the original procedure) or in the diagnosis of clostridial infection. The presence of gas in the myometrium is consistent with clostridial infection and is a grave prognostic sign. Finally, ultrasound may be helpful in assessing the presence of retained products of conception and in detecting possible pelvic abscesses.

Treatment

The sepsis is treated with high-dose antibiotics followed promptly by uterine evacuation. In clostridial infections, which are more than superficial, prompt hysterectomy may be lifesaving. Pelvic surgery may also be required to drain hematomas or abscesses. These may also be approached by guided needle aspiration. Other aspects of septic shock, including hypotension, anemia, and ARDS, are treated supportively.

Stubblefield PG, Grimes DA: Septic abortion. N Engl J Med 1994;331:310–4.

PULMONARY EDEMA

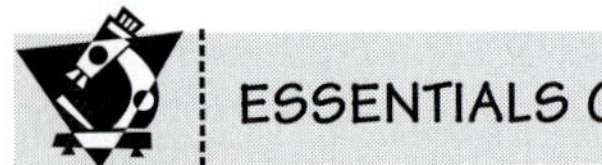

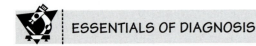

ESSENTIALS OF DIAGNOSIS

- *Dyspnea, hypoxemia, cough.*
- *Chest x-ray showing pulmonary edema with usually bilateral diffuse interstitial and alveolar infiltrates and perihilar congestion.*

General Considerations

Women without known predisposing conditions may develop pulmonary edema during the course of pregnancy, especially at the time of delivery. Common obstetric conditions responsible for this complication are: (1) hypertensive disorders of pregnancy; (2) undiagnosed underlying heart disease, especially mitral stenosis; (3) use of tocolytic drugs, especially beta-adrenergic agonists; (4) iatrogenic fluid overload; (5) systemic infection, especially pyelonephritis or amniotic fluid infection; and, more rarely, (6) peripartum cardiomyopathy.

Hypertensive disorders of pregnancy are discussed above. These patients are particularly disposed to pulmonary edema because of contracted intravascular volume and decreased plasma oncotic pressure. Pulmonary edema may also supervene in these patients if left ventricular function is compromised or in cases of pulmonary capillary or epithelial injury. In other patients, the rapid mobilization of edema fluid that follows delivery may result in transient pulmonary edema. Patients with flow-restricting cardiac lesions (eg, mitral stenosis) may be intolerant of the autotransfusion that accompanies delivery. In some women, the first symptom of cardiac disease is pulmonary edema after delivery.

Pulmonary edema associated with the use of beta-adrenergic agonists appears to be unique to pregnancy. There is no association of pulmonary edema with these drugs in nonpregnant patients despite considerable experience with beta-adrenergic agonists as bronchodilators. The incidence of pulmonary edema as a complication of tocolytic therapy with these drugs has been estimated to be between 0.15% and 4% in different studies. This risk may be increased to more than 20% in the face of intra-amniotic infection. Pulmonary edema has been reported after treatment with terbutaline, isoxsuprine, ritodrine, and albuterol. Intravenous beta-adrenergic agonists are much less commonly used now than formerly because of the number and severity of complications experienced with these agents. Pulmonary edema may also complicate subcutaneous use of beta-adrenergic agonists, but the risk appears to be much less. Pulmonary edema has also been described with all other tocolytic agents, with an incidence of 1:300 in one study of magnesium sulfate.

Patients in labor may receive large volumes of intravenous crystalloid fluids. It is common practice to give laboring women a 1000 mL bolus before administering epidural anesthesia, and most women receive a minimum of 125 mL/h at other times. The majority of laboring patients do not have difficulties related to their fluid management. In patients with pyelonephritis or who are undergoing tocolysis, however, careful fluid management can make the difference between developing pulmonary edema or not.

Peripartum cardiomyopathy is a rare complication of pregnancy, occurring in about 1:15,000 pregnancies in developed countries. It appears to be much more common in less developed countries. It is characterized by a dilated cardiomyopathy and is frequently associated with systemic and pulmonary emboli. About half of patients with peripartum cardiomyopathy have complete resolution after delivery, with return of normal heart size and cardiac function. The remainder have continued cardiac dilation. These patients tolerate future pregnancies poorly, and some have required cardiac transplantation. The cause of this condition is unknown, but at least some of the affected patients have evidence of viral myocarditis.

The mechanism for the increased susceptibility to pulmonary edema in pregnancy is not clear. Fluid overload has been suggested as a cause because of the known increase in extracellular fluid volume during pregnancy, decreased excretion of sodium and water in pregnant patients when supine, and concomitant administration of large amounts of intravenous fluids in many cases. However, there is no convincing evidence of increased pulmonary artery wedge pressure to identify either fluid overload or left ventricular failure as the sole cause of pulmonary edema in many cases. The finding of a low pulmonary artery wedge pressure in the face of pulmonary edema would normally be indicative of increased capillary permeability pulmonary edema, but evidence against this mechanism is the usually rapid resolution of edema with treatment in the case of tocolytic use or in many cases of preeclampsia. Hypoalbuminemia and decreased plasma oncotic pressure of pregnancy may also play a role in the etiology of pulmonary edema.

Clinical Features

A. Symptoms and Signs

Patients present with dyspnea, cough, chest discomfort, and frothy sputum. Findings include bilateral rales, but most patients lack other signs of heart failure such as a third heart sound. Review of the hospital records frequently documents administration of large amounts of intravenous fluids, sometimes for treatment of tachycardia or mild hypotension. Patients may have fever or other symptoms of infection.

B. Laboratory Findings

The chest x-ray shows bilateral interstitial or alveolar infiltrates consistent with pulmonary edema. Occasionally, findings are unilateral. The cardiac size may not be greatly enlarged, but it has been pointed out that there is an apparent increase in heart size during normal pregnancy. Pleural effusions are rare. Arterial blood gases show hypoxemia with respiratory alkalosis in most patients. Fetal heart monitoring will often reveal late decelerations and loss of variability of the fetal heart rate, consistent with fetal hypoxia and acidemia.

Ventilation-perfusion lung scans may be useful in excluding pulmonary thromboembolism in selected patients, and some patients will benefit from echocardiography to diagnose cardiomyopathy or valvular heart disease.

Differential Diagnosis

Acute onset of dyspnea during late pregnancy may be due to pulmonary embolism, amniotic fluid embolism, or asthma. Patients with known underlying heart or lung disease should also be suspected of having an exacerbation of these problems if symptoms occur.

Prevention

Patients who have severe underlying heart diseases should not receive beta-adrenergic agonists as tocolytic therapy because of the risk of inducing pulmonary edema. Magnesium sulfate, if necessary, may be considered. There is no place for tocolytic therapy in preeclampsia. Any patient at increased risk of pulmonary edema requires careful attention to fluid status. The presence of an intra-amniotic infection mandates delivery in the great majority of cases, and patients with other infections must be monitored closely while undergoing therapy.

Treatment

Discontinuation of the administration of any tocolytic agent, intravenous furosemide (20–40 mg as needed), and oxygen are generally associated with rapid reversal of symptoms and resolution of pulmonary edema in the absence of structural heart disease or sepsis. Patients with associated infection should be treated with appropriate antibiotics. Continuous fetal heart rate monitoring is essential until normal maternal pulmonary function is restored and hypoxemia corrected.

In patients with slow resolution of pulmonary edema, structural abnormalities should be considered. A pulmonary artery catheter may be helpful in identifying the cause of pulmonary edema and guiding therapy. A normal echocardiogram often predicts rapid resolution, but in patients with abnormal findings long-term treatment is usually needed.

Lamont RF: The pathophysiology of pulmonary oedema with the use of beta agonists. BJOG 2000;107:439–44.

Zlatnik MG: Pulmonary edema: etiology and treatment. Semin Perinatol 1997;21:298–306.

STATUS ASTHMATICUS IN PREGNANCY

Asthma is the most common respiratory disease occurring in conjunction with pregnancy. In general, the influence of pregnancy on lung volumes, tidal volume, minute ventilation, and arterial blood gases has little effect on asthma. About 33–40% of asthmatics that become pregnant have worsening of their asthma; 35–42% have no change in the frequency and duration of symptoms; and 18–28% show an improvement in symptoms. In most patients, the course of asthma during pregnancy is similar in subsequent pregnancies. This constancy of asthmatic outcome may be altered with newer methods of asthma control.

Asthma can have adverse effects on pregnancy, especially when maternal hypoxemia affects oxygenation of the fetus. Premature labor and low birth weight are well-known complications of maternal asthma, and patients with hypoxemia due to asthma are also at increased risk of fetal death. Thus, the central theme in managing the pregnant asthmatic is prevention of maternal asthma exacerbation and hypoxemia.

There is no known association of pregnancy with status asthmaticus (asthma unresponsive to treatment and usually requiring hospitalization) or with severe asthma (daily wheezing and need for medication). On the other hand, pregnant women with asthma may have worsening of asthma or may be reluctant to use prescribed asthma medications, thus increasing the risk of these complications. Patients with a history of asthma requiring hospitalization, mechanical ventilation, and prolonged use of systemic corticosteroids or of asthma complicated by pneumothorax should be watched especially carefully. These patients should be instructed to report any asthmatic exacerbations, upper respiratory infections, increased cough, or other respiratory symptoms. Anemia, because it can adversely affect maternal oxygen transport, should be assessed and treated.

Clinical Features

A. Symptoms and Signs

Pregnant asthmatics present no differently than other patients with asthma. Patients with status asthmaticus complain of dyspnea, wheezing, cough, and failure of response to inhaled bronchodilator drugs. They may note inability to sleep because of dyspnea or cough, and they may report a frank upper airway infection. The time from onset of the attack should be noted because a prolonged duration may be predictive of poor response to treatment. Physical findings include wheezing, use of accessory muscles of respiration, a prolonged expiratory phase, tachypnea, tachycardia, and cyanosis. Patients presenting with acute severe asthma usually have a history of asthma; rarely, asthma will present initially during pregnancy.

B. Laboratory Findings

Arterial blood gases should be interpreted in the light of changes seen in pregnancy. In normal pregnancy, serum bicarbonate is decreased and arterial P_{CO_2} is low. Development of hypercapnia may therefore be subtle, and only a slight elevation of Pa_{CO_2} above 40 mm Hg may be indicative of impending respiratory failure in the pregnant woman. Severe hypoxemia in status asthmaticus is due to ventilation/perfusion mismatching resulting from bronchospasm and plugging of airways with mucus. As in nonpregnant asthmatics, spirometry is useful for assessing severity of asthma and following the response to therapy, especially as the peak expiratory flow rate does not change in pregnancy. Strong consideration should be given to obtaining a chest x-ray in those with unexplained fever, persistent bronchospasm, heavy sputum production, asymmetry on chest examination, severe hypoxemia, or suspicion of heart disease, pleural effusion, or pneumothorax.

Differential Diagnosis

Dyspnea during pregnancy is common, with most patients complaining of some subjective shortness of breath during the last trimester. Patients with acute onset of shortness of breath may have congestive heart failure, pulmonary edema, pulmonary thromboembolism, amniotic fluid embolism, pneumothorax, or sepsis. Valvular heart disease should be considered—especially previously undiagnosed mitral stenosis, mitral valve prolapse, aortic regurgitation, and aortic stenosis. A rare but important problem that should be considered in young women is primary pulmonary hypertension; this disorder can present with new onset of dyspnea and other symptoms in response to the increased cardiac output that occurs with pregnancy.

Treatment

Treatment of status asthmaticus in the pregnant asthmatic should be aggressive and rapid. Fetal oxygenation is highly dependent on adequate maternal arterial blood oxygen content, and delay in treatment is hazardous to the fetus. As with all conditions adversely affecting maternal respiratory function, fetal heart rate should be monitored continuously in potentially viable fetuses. Bronchodilator and anti-inflammatory therapy are directed at reversing airway obstruction; oxygen is given to treat hypoxemia. Pharmacologic therapy of asthma in pregnancy is based on administering drugs with a long history of use with good outcome rather than drugs which have been tested specifically during pregnancy.

A. Bronchodilators

Beta-adrenergic agonists have been used extensively in pregnancy, but there are no controlled experimental studies in pregnant women for any of these agents. Terbutaline, albuterol, and metaproterenol have been administered to pregnant asthmatics with good results. Inhaled terbutaline is an FDA category B drug, while metaproterenol and albuterol are category C drugs. Several clinical studies following pregnant asthmatics have not found any differences in complications of pregnancy or fetal outcome between asthmatics receiving bronchodilators and nonasthmatics who did not receive these drugs. In general, the newer more selective β_2-adrenergic agonist drugs are used more commonly than other agents. Administration of beta-agonists by metered-dose inhalers, as in nonpregnant asthmatics, is probably preferred to nebulizers. The dose and frequency of inhaled bronchodilators should be titrated to the clinical response (see Status Asthmaticus in Chapter 24).

B. Corticosteroids

These drugs play a major role in reversing airway obstruction. Systemic corticosteroids—eg, intravenous methylprednisolone and oral prednisone—are well tolerated in pregnant women and are essential in the management of status asthmaticus. The optimum dose of corticosteroids in status asthmaticus is not known in the nonpregnant patient, but 40–60 mg of methylprednisolone every 6 hours is usually given, and the dose in pregnancy should be similar. Use of corticosteroids should be aimed at achieving control of asthma, followed by rapid tapering and discontinuation over approximately 2 weeks, if possible. In some patients, continued administration of oral prednisone, 15–30 mg/d, is necessary for prevention of asthma attacks. Inhaled corticosteroids may also be used in the treatment of chronic asthma in the pregnant patient.

C. Cromolyn Sodium

Cromolyn sodium in inhaled or nasal spray form has not been associated with any fetal effect in observational studies. In chronic asthma, inhaled cromolyn may be a valuable agent, but cromolyn has no role in status asthmaticus.

D. Oxygen and Other Therapy

Supplemental oxygen should be provided to maintain arterial PO_2, at 85–100 mm Hg at all times to ensure fetal oxygenation.

Antibiotics are not generally warranted in status asthmaticus because infection, when present as a triggering or exacerbating factor, is usually of viral origin. If there is evidence of bacterial infection, broad-spectrum antibiotics can be given. Ampicillin, cephalosporins, and erythromycin are generally considered safe for use during pregnancy. Sulfonamides should not be given—especially during the third trimester—because there is a theoretical risk of kernicterus in the newborn. Erythromycin estolate, tetracycline, chloramphenicol, and quinolones should be avoided.

E. Intubation and Mechanical Ventilation

If the patient fails to respond to the foregoing measures and exhibits a normal or increased arterial PCO_2, she should be admitted to an ICU. If the fetus is potentially viable, fetal monitoring should be instituted. Intubation and mechanical ventilation are indicated for a PaO_2 of 70 mm Hg or less, significant mental status changes, respiratory acidosis, cardiac arrhythmias, or evidence of myocardial ischemia. If mechanical ventilation does not correct the hypoxemia and the fetus is potentially viable, delivery by cesarean section should be considered for fetal reasons.

ACOG technical bulletin. Pulmonary disease in pregnancy. Number 224–June 1996. American College of Obstetricians and Gynecologists. Int J Gynaecol Obstet 1996;54:187–96.

The use of newer asthma and allergy medications during pregnancy. The American College of Obstetricians and Gynecologists (ACOG) and The American College of Allergy, Asthma and Immunology (ACAAI). Ann Allergy Asthma Immunol 2000;84:475–80.

Greenberger PA: Asthma in pregnancy. Clin Chest Med 1992;13: 597–605.

Mabie WC: Asthma in pregnancy. Clin Obstet Gynecol 1996;39: 56–69.

Schatz M et al: Perinatal outcomes in the pregnancies of asthmatic women: a prospective controlled analysis. Am J Respir Crit Care Med 1995;151:1170–4.

POSTPARTUM HEMORRHAGE

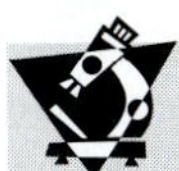

ESSENTIALS OF DIAGNOSIS

- *Rapid loss of 500–1000 mL or more of blood after delivery.*

General Considerations

Postpartum hemorrhage has classically been defined as an estimated blood loss of more than 500 mL after delivery. Investigations have shown, however, that the average blood loss after vaginal delivery is near 500 mL, while that following cesarean section is in excess of 1 L. The working definition of postpartum hemorrhage is, therefore, relative. Most would acknowledge the presence of postpartum hemorrhage when blood loss exceeds 1 L, when there is a 10% change in the hematocrit between admission and postpartum determinations, or when transfusion is necessary.

The most common causes of early postpartum hemorrhage (< 24 hours after delivery) are uterine atony, lower genital tract lacerations, retained products of conception or placenta accreta, uterine rupture, inversion of the uterus, and coagulopathies. Uterine atony is by far the most common and may be associated with the antepartum use of oxytocin or with uterine overdistention from multiple gestation or polyhydramnios. Other factors thought to be associated with uterine atony include prolonged labor and cesarean section, precipitous labor, chorioamnionitis, the use of tocolytic agents (including magnesium sulfate), and high parity.

Lower genital tract lacerations occur frequently and usually present with vaginal bleeding immediately after delivery. Uterine lacerations can bleed into the peritoneal cavity and therefore do not always present with vaginal hemorrhage. Factors associated with lower genital tract lacerations are forceps or vacuum delivery, fetal macrosomia or malpresentation, or precipitate delivery.

Failure of the placenta to completely separate is a risk factor for the development of both uterine atony and postpartum hemorrhage, presumably due to the placental fragments interfering with the normal contraction of the uterus that is necessary for hemostasis. Retention of a succenturiate lobe (accessory lobe of the placenta) may present with postpartum hemorrhage in the early postpartum period. Placenta accreta may also cause life-threatening hemorrhage due to the inability of the placenta to completely separate from the uterine wall. Risk factors for placenta accreta include previous puerperal curettage or previous uterine surgery, including cesarean section.

Uterine rupture is an uncommon but catastrophic cause of postpartum hemorrhage. Because uterine artery blood flow is between 500 mL and 600 mL/min, hemorrhage from this cause can result in rapid exsanguination. Conditions thought to predispose to uterine rupture include previous uterine surgery, breech extraction, obstructed labor, abnormal fetal position, and high parity.

Uterine inversion is also a rare complication of delivery, though it may recur in a patient's subsequent pregnancies. Uterine inversion is most remarkable for the development of shock out of proportion to the amount of blood apparently lost.

Coagulopathies are frequently associated with postpartum hemorrhage. They often occur in association with other complications of pregnancy such as abruptio placentae, retained dead fetus, and amniotic fluid embolism. In addition, preexisting chronic coagulation disorders are significant contributors to postpartum hemorrhage.

Delayed postpartum hemorrhage occurring between 24 hours and 6 weeks after delivery may require admission to the ICU for resuscitation, observation, and perioperative care. Common causes include infection, placental site subinvolution, and retained products of conception as well as underlying coagulopathy.

Clinical Features

Although the initial management of postpartum hemorrhage will be accomplished in the delivery room, the intensive care physician should be familiar with the basic principles of diagnosis and early management.

The first priority is to establish the cause. The relationship between the onset of hemorrhage and the time of delivery is critical in establishing the diagnosis. Bleeding prior to delivery of the placenta often indicates a genital tract laceration, a coagulopathy, or a partial separation of the placenta. When bleeding begins after the placenta is delivered, uterine atony, uterine inversion, retained fragments of the placenta, or placenta accreta may be responsible. The placenta should be inspected to ensure that torn vessels are not present, which might indicate the presence of an accessory lobe; that appropriate contour is observed; and that portions are not missing (suggesting placenta accreta).

Uterine atony requires fundal massage and the administration of ecbolic drugs (see below). Lacerations should be sutured in a manner that allows closure of the wound and compression of the underlying vessels. Hematomas may form as the result of lacerations. Hematomas below the pelvic diaphragm are usually accompanied by severe pain and a palpable mass. Sudden onset of shock without significant apparent blood loss suggests that the bleeding point is above the pelvic diaphragm.

A coagulopathy is suggested by the presence of bleeding from remote locations such as intravenous insertion sites. The diagnosis of coagulopathy may be made rapidly by observing a tube of the patient's blood for clot formation. If a firm clot forms within 5 minutes, it is unlikely that clinically significant hypofibrinogenemia is present.

Treatment

A. General Measures

Postpartum hemorrhage represents a special cause of hemorrhagic (hypovolemic) shock. A stable airway and adequate intravenous access must be assured. Initial resuscitation should be with balanced salt solutions, though blood replacement will be required early if hemorrhage cannot be arrested. Packed red blood cells are usually used. In the event of severe hemorrhage, replacement of clotting factors may also be needed via the use of fresh frozen plasma. Fresh frozen plasma should be given only if laboratory testing shows that the patient has developed a coagulopathy. Blood should be warmed to prevent hypothermia.

Arterial blood gas and hematocrit determinations should be performed regularly during resuscitation and after control of bleeding. Measurements of blood pressure, pulse rate, and urine output will help assess volume status. Pulmonary artery catheters are seldom required, though a central venous catheter may be helpful in actively bleeding patients who require ongoing resuscitation and transfusion.

B. Ecbolic Agents

Hemorrhage from uterine atony should be managed with fundal massage plus an intravenous infusion of oxytocin (10–40 units/L of normal saline). If oxytocin does not arrest the hemorrhage, treatment with either methylergonovine (0.2 mg intramuscularly) or carboprost tromethamine (15-methylprostaglandin $F_{2\alpha}$), 0.25 mg intramuscularly, may be tried. Methylergonovine may be associated with an increase in maternal blood pressure and should not be used in the patient with hypertension. Prostaglandin agents may provoke bronchospasm and should be not be used in patients with significant asthma.

C. Surgery

When postpartum hemorrhage cannot be controlled by massage and ecbolic agents, emergent surgery is usually required. In many cases, these procedures will have been performed before the patient is transferred to the ICU. Occasionally, however, a previously stable patient will require exploration for hemorrhage after it has been controlled. Common surgical procedures include evacuation of hematomas caused by lacerations (combined with suturing of the injury and control of the bleeding vessel), ligation of pelvic arterial vessels, packing, and hysterectomy. Recent reviews of cesarean hysterectomy reveal that the average blood loss for this procedure when done emergently was 3000 mL and the most common antecedent complications were placenta accreta and uterine atony.

D. Angiographic Embolization

When bleeding continues from an identifiable localized area, embolization via a radiographically placed catheter may be extremely helpful. Some authors have described the placement of embolization catheters prophylactically in patients at highest risk of postpartum hemorrhage.

E. Delayed Postpartum Hemorrhage

Fewer than 1% of patients with postpartum hemorrhage present more than 24 hours after delivery. Infection and retained products of conception are the most common causes, with subinvolution of the placental site also being a consideration. Uterine curettage should be performed only when retained products of conception are suspected because of the risk of intrauterine adhesions. Pelvic and uterine ultrasonography are extremely helpful in determining whether retained products are present. Even when there is not retained placental tissue, evacuation of intrauterine clots allows more efficient uterine contraction and often results in hemostasis. Estrogens may be used to improve endometrial regrowth after curettage and hopefully avoid intrauterine adhesions. Ecbolic agents and antibiotics may be given if retained products of conception are not present. If hemorrhage persists more than 12–24 hours, the patient should undergo curettage for presumed retained products, even in the absence of a definite diagnosis.

ACOG technical bulletin. Blood component therapy. Number 199–November 1994 (replaces no. 78, July 1984). Committee on Technical Bulletins of the American College of Obstetricians and Gynecologists. Int J Gynaecol Obstet 1995;48: 233–8.

ACOG technical bulletin. Postpartum hemorrhage. Number 243–January 1998. American College of Obstetricians and Gynecologists. Int J Gynaecol Obstet 1998;61:79-86.

Baker ER, Dalton ME: Cesarean section birth and cesarean hysterectomy. Clin Obstet Gynecol 1994;37:806–15.

Tamizian O, Arulkumaran S: The surgical management of postpartum haemorrhage. Curr Opin Obstet Gynecol 2001;13: 127–31.

TRAUMA DURING PREGNANCY

Accidental injury occurs in approximately one in 12 pregnancies. While many of these incidents are minor, one should bear in mind that two patients are at risk. Serious injuries during pregnancy do not result in a higher maternal mortality rate than do similar injuries in a nongravid patient. Fetal death, however, is common, with fetal loss rates of up to 61% reported in studies of severe trauma. Eighty-five percent of all maternal deaths from trauma are due to closed head injuries and hemorrhagic shock, while fetal deaths result from abruptio placentae as well as maternal death and fetal hypoxia. Because of this combined risk and because of the risk of preterm labor, pregnant patients often require inpatient observation.

The physiologic changes of pregnancy make the patient both more and less susceptible to the effects of trauma. The increased plasma volume and decreased hematocrit further the potential for diminished oxygen delivery following blood loss. Fluid resuscitation requirements after hemorrhage are greater because of the 50% increase in maternal intravascular volume. Conversely, the increased blood volume makes the mother more tolerant of blood loss without change in her vital signs. The increase in maternal heart rate (15–20 beats/min) and the decrease in both systolic and diastolic blood pressures (10–15 mm Hg) may confound attempts to evaluate volume replacement. Furthermore, an elevation of coagulation factors during pregnancy increases the risk for thrombogenesis with surgery or prolonged immobilization.

As pregnancy progresses into the second trimester, fetal growth distends the uterus upward into the abdomen, where it becomes more susceptible to direct injury. The bladder also becomes more prone to injury, especially after the 12th week of gestation. Because blood flow to the uterus is abundant (as much as 600 mL/min), direct injury to the uterus may cause rapid exsanguination. Uterine blood vessels lack autoregulation, so maternal shock causes a substantial decrease in fetal oxygen delivery. Uterine blood flow may fall before maternal shock becomes manifest and may result in fetal hypoxia in the face of normal maternal vital signs. Fetal responses to decreased perfusion and hypoxia include alterations in heart rate (bradycardia or tachycardia), loss of heart rate variability, and repetitive late decelerations.

Motor vehicle accidents are the principal cause of accidental injuries during pregnancy and account for about 50% of all cases of blunt abdominal trauma. Three-point restraint seat belts are preferable for pregnant passengers because the incidence of body flexion and uterine compression is less than that induced by lap belts alone. Placental abruption is the most common cause of fetal demise after blunt abdominal trauma. Abruption is caused by deformation of the elastic uterus around the inelastic placenta. The shearing force thus produced tears the decidua basalis. Current evidence indicates that the position of the placenta does not influence the development of abruption. Uterine rupture is uncommon and probably occurs in less than 0.6% of all traumatic injuries during pregnancy. It carries a maternal death rate of less than 10% but a fetal death rate of nearly 100%. Maternal pelvic fractures occur frequently but do not necessarily preclude subsequent vaginal delivery. Such fractures are of concern when they are comminuted and badly displaced because they carry the potential to injure the uterus and fetus. Placental abruption and pelvic fractures are highly correlated.

Gunshot wounds are the most common type of penetrating injury sustained by pregnant patients. Regrettably, the number of incidents in which there was clear intent to harm the fetus has increased over the past several years. When compared with nonpregnant victims, pregnant patients actually have a lower mortality rate after abdominal gunshot wounds, perhaps because the enlarged uterus and its contents protect the patient by absorbing and dissipating the missile's kinetic energy. Upper abdominal gunshot and stab wounds, however, cause a higher incidence of intestinal injury because of cephalad displacement of the viscera by the uterus. Direct injury of the fetus by a bullet occurs in 70% of cases, with a 65% intrauterine fetal death rate. Maternal death is much less common.

Burns, electrocution, and suicide attempts are less common causes of injury. Unless a burn covers more than 30% of the patient's body surface area, it generally will not affect the pregnancy. Fetal outcome is probably related to gestational age at the time of the burn. The highest mortality rate is recorded during the first trimester. Topical iodine solutions should be avoided, because large amounts may be absorbed through the burn wound. House current electrical injuries occur uncommonly but may be associated with a high fetal mortality rate because of the path of the current through the patient's body. Pregnant victims of electrocution may report a reduction in fetal movements immediately after the incident. Fetal demise or intrauterine growth retardation may follow. Oligohydramnios has been reported at the time of delivery.

Management

A. General Principles

Pregnant patients who require ICU admission following injury will commonly be resuscitated and stabilized in the emergency department. Initial treatment in the ICU may be advisable, however, because of the availability of invasive monitoring.

Upon arrival, initial concern must be directed toward the mother, with attention paid to establishment of an adequate airway, breathing, and circulation. The patient should lie in the left lateral position, if possible, to prevent compression of the vena cava by the gravid uterus. Both maternal hypotension and fetal hypoxia may result from caval compression. If concern about the cervical spine precludes the decubitus position, an assistant should displace the uterus by hand to the left in an attempt to decompress the vena cava. Supplemental oxygen should be given to increase oxygen delivery to the fetus. Upper extremity intravenous catheters should be placed to ensure adequate intravenous access. A nasogastric tube should be inserted during the early stages of resuscitation to allow gastric decompression and prevent aspiration. In the presence of a viable fetus, continuous fetal heart rate monitoring should be instituted as soon as possible.

Blood is preferred as the initial fluid for resuscitation of hypotensive trauma patients. Particular attention must be paid to Rh compatibility. If Rh-incompatible blood is inadvertently given to an RH-negative woman, anti-D antibody should be given in a dose of 300 mg for every 30 mL of whole blood or 15 mL of packed red blood cells transfused. Pregnant patients require more volume replacement than do nonpregnant patients because of their physiologically expanded intravascular space.

A bladder catheter should be placed as soon as possible, both to measure the urine output and to help establish the integrity of the urethra and bladder. Urine so obtained should be inspected for gross blood and tested for microscopic hematuria.

Normal physical signs of abdominal injury such as pain and loss of bowel sounds may be masked by the pregnant uterus. Conversely, all of these findings may be produced by the pregnancy itself. Vaginal bleeding is generally considered an ominous sign because it may signal placental abruption.

B. Laboratory Studies

Studies should include hematocrit, serum electrolytes, coagulation profile, amylase, and blood crossmatch.

Routine arterial blood gases are advisable. When placental separation is suspected because of a pelvic fracture, fetal distress, uterine tetany, or vaginal bleeding, measurement of blood fibrinogen concentration, fibrin degradation products, and platelet count is of particular importance. Additionally, a tube of blood should be obtained and observed for clot formation. Noncoagulable blood indicates probable placental abruption and mandates immediate replacement of fibrinogen with fresh frozen plasma or cryoprecipitate, followed by evacuation of the uterus. The possibility of fetomaternal hemorrhage should be evaluated with a Kleihauer-Betke study. Fetomaternal hemorrhage is most common when the placenta is located anteriorly, when pelvic tenderness is present, and following motor vehicle accidents. If severe, it can result in fetal anemia or fetal death.

C. Imaging Studies

Critical radiographic studies should not be withheld in an attempt to avoid fetal x-ray exposure. The fetal risks from various doses of x-ray and the expected doses from various procedures have been discussed previously. The need for chest and abdominal x-rays should be guided by the nature and severity of the injury. Free air under the diaphragm on an upright chest x-ray is an indication for immediate laparotomy. Traumatic separation of the pubic symphysis in or after the second trimester is difficult to detect on x-ray because of the normal ligamentous laxity that accompanies pregnancy. Maternal and fetal complications are more common after pelvic fractures, and their presence must be identified.

Obstetric ultrasound should be performed in all cases of trauma during pregnancy. It is helpful in diagnosing a retroplacental clot and can aid in estimating gestational age when a history cannot be obtained.

D. Peritoneal Lavage

Open peritoneal lavage through a supraumbilical incision is an excellent technique for diagnosing abdominal injuries. Approximately 1 L of lavage fluid is instilled through the small incision and allowed to return passively to the container. Criteria that constitute a positive lavage include (1) a red cell count > 100,000/μL; (2) a white cell count > 500/μL; (3) the presence of gastrointestinal contents, bile, or bacteria; and (4) increased amylase.

E. Fetal Monitoring

Immediately upon arrival in the ICU, fetal heart monitoring should be instituted. Such monitoring provides information about both the fetus and the mother. The fetus may be compromised by hypoxia before the mother becomes hypotensive. Bradycardia, tachycardia, and loss of beat-to-beat variability are ominous signs. Monitoring in gestations beyond 18–20 weeks may be able to predict abruptio placentae. Although intermittent auscultation is possible, it should not substitute for electronic surveillance. The gestational age at which monitoring is mandatory is controversial, but all authorities would monitor potentially viable fetuses (> 22 weeks) and some would monitor at 20 weeks. Monitoring necessitates the presence in the ICU of personnel experienced in the interpretation of fetal heart rate patterns.

F. Tocodynamometry (Uterine Contraction Monitoring)

Tocodynamometry is of significant importance in predicting early placental abruption. The incidence of abruption increases with frequent uterine activity (more than 8 uterine contractions per hour), and about 25% of trauma patients with at least three uterine contractions in a 20-minute period suffered either abruptio placentae or preterm labor. Another study found that these complications did not occur in patients who were without contractions for the first 4 hours. Monitoring during the first 4–6 hours after admission has therefore been proposed, with additional monitoring only in those patients with contractions on initial monitoring or with a change in maternal condition.

G. Surgery

1. Trauma—Certain kinds of trauma must be managed operatively. Bowel injuries must be repaired, fractures reduced, and wounds closed. Pregnancy should not delay or contraindicate surgical exploration.

2. Abruptio placentae—Evacuation of the uterus is indicated for placental abruption. If gestation has continued for more than 30 weeks, immediate cesarean section may save both the fetus and the mother. In cases of intrauterine fetal demise, labor and spontaneous vaginal delivery may occur. Caution must be exercised to detect disseminated intravascular coagulation, which is more common after extensive abruption. If both the platelet count and the fibrinogen concentration decline, fresh frozen plasma or cryoprecipitate should be given and a cesarean section performed if delivery is not imminent. The coagulopathy usually ceases when the placenta is removed.

3. Uterine rupture—Shock, severe abdominal pain, and lack of fetal heart tones suggest uterine rupture. It may be difficult to localize the top of the uterus, and fetal parts may be easily palpable through the abdominal wall. An abdominal x-ray usually shows that the fetal skeleton is in an unusually high location in the abdomen. Peritoneal lavage is always positive for blood and returns more fluid than was instilled (amniotic fluid). At surgery, massive bleeding may have to be controlled with bilateral internal iliac artery ligation. Supracervical hysterectomy may be required.

4. Cesarean section—Adequate exposure of abdominal injuries can usually be achieved with careful mobilization of the uterus. Cesarean section may be required, however, when the gravid uterus prevents access to deep pelvic injuries. Patients with undisplaced pelvic fractures usually do not require cesarean section.

Premature separation of the placenta and fetal head injuries may both be consequences of maternal trauma during pregnancy. Placental separation coexistent with a living fetus often mandates an emergent cesarean section. In the case of a live fetus undergoing labor after maternal trauma, consideration should be given to fetal ultrasound for evidence of fetal head injury. If such evidence exists, this fetus may also benefit from cesarean delivery.

ACOG technical bulletin. Blood component therapy. Number 199–November 1994. Committee on Technical Bulletins of the American College of Obstetricians and Gynecologists. Int J Gynaecol Obstet 1995;48:233–8.

ACOG technical bulletin. Postpartum hemorrhage. Number 243–January 1998. American College of Obstetricians and Gynecologists. Int J Gynaecol Obstet 1998;61:79–86.

Baker ER, Dalton ME: Cesarean section birth and cesarean hysterectomy. Clin Obstet Gynecol 1994;37:806–15.

Tamizian O, Arulkumaran S: The surgical management of postpartum haemorrhage. Curr Opin Obstet Gynecol 2001;13: 127–31.

Antithrombotic Therapy

40

Elizabeth D. Simmons, MD

Pathologic blood clot formation within blood vessels (thrombosis) and embolization of clots to distant sites results from complex interactions between platelets and coagulation proteins, the fibrinolytic system, and the blood vessel itself. Thrombi are composed of red blood cells, platelets, and fibrin in varying proportions depending upon the conditions present at the site of thrombus formation. Very diverse clinical conditions are associated with increased risks of such pathologic thrombosis and embolization (Table 40–1). Thromboembolic disease is a major cause of morbidity and mortality; 30–40% of all deaths in the United States are attributed to thrombotic events, and nonfatal events occur in hundreds of thousands of people each year.

Antithrombotic therapy consists of strategies (both pharmacologic and physical) to prevent pathologic blood clot formation or to treat established thromboses in order to limit the clinical consequences of such clots. The decision to use antithrombotic therapy in clinical practice is often complicated because of the diversity of the clinical conditions affecting patients, difficulties in establishing accurate diagnoses of thromboembolism, and our still incomplete understanding of the risks and benefits of antithrombotic therapy in prevention and treatment of thromboembolic disease. Numerous new pharmacologic agents have been developed or are under development, and various combinations of antithrombotic agents are being used in diverse settings.

PHYSICAL MEASURES

Venous stasis and damage to blood vessels are the two most important risk factors for the development of venous thromboembolism. Physical measures to decrease venous stasis are quite important in preventing venous clots, particularly in hospitalized patients. Limiting bed rest as much as possible for most medical patients and early mobilization after surgery can decrease the period of risk for venous thrombosis. External pneumatic leg compression (EPLC) is a safe and effective physical method of prevention of deep vein thrombosis in average-risk patients over 40 undergoing general surgery and may be useful in higher-risk patients who cannot tolerate prophylactic anticoagulation. EPLC works largely by preventing venous stasis, though activation of fibrinolysis may also contribute to its antithrombotic effect. EPLC should not be used in the presence of established thrombosis, severe peripheral vascular disease, skin ulcers, or after leg trauma if there is compromised tissue viability. Graduated compression stockings may help control leg edema but are not highly effective for prevention of venous thromboembolism. They are not recommended as an isolated measure for prevention of venous thromboembolism in patients at moderate to high risk.

Interruption of the inferior vena cava using a fluoroscopically placed filter is indicated for treatment of patients with lower extremity venous thrombosis who have a major contraindication to anticoagulant therapy or for patients with recurrent thromboembolism despite adequate anticoagulation. Inferior vena cava filter placement reduces the risk of pulmonary embolization but does not prevent recurrence or extension of lower extremity thromboses.

Surgical or transvenous embolectomy is occasionally performed in selected patients with life-threatening thromboembolic disease, particularly in patients with contraindications to anticoagulation or thrombolysis.

ANTIPLATELET AGENTS

Antiplatelet therapy (alone or in combination with anticoagulants) is most beneficial in prevention or treatment of arterial thrombosis. Arterial thrombi usually develop in abnormal blood vessels and are associated with activation of both blood coagulation and platelets; however, arterial thrombi are composed primarily of platelets held together by fibrin strands. Antiplatelet agents inhibit platelet function through several biochemical pathways or by exerting effects on the platelet membrane.

Antiplatelet agents have been shown to be useful in the management of patients with unstable angina, suspected acute myocardial infarction, a history of myocardial infarction, nonfatal stroke, transient ischemic attacks, peripheral vascular disease, and persons undergoing vascular procedures. Antiplatelet agents are not as useful as other measures for prevention of venous thromboembolism such as anticoagulation, particularly in high-risk surgical patients.

Table 40–1. Conditions associated with pathologic thromboembolism.

Stasis	Immobilization Congestive heart failure Surgery Advanced age Obesity
Blood vessel abnormalities	Trauma, coronary artery disease, peripheral vascular disease, varicosities, vasculitis, artificial surfaces (grafts), diabetes mellitus Homozygous homocystinuria Previous thrombosis
Abnormalities of physiologic antithrombotic mechanisms	Antithrombin deficiency Protein C or S deficiency Hereditary resistance to activated protein C (factor V Leiden and prothrombin gene mutation G20210A) Methylenetetrahydrofolate reductase gene mutation C677T Defective or deficient plasminogen Plasminogen activator deficiency
Abnormalities of coagulation and fibrinolysis	Malignancy Pregnancy Oral contraceptives Hormone replacement therapy Tamoxifen Nephrotic syndrome Lupus anticoagulant Prothrombin complex concentrate solution Dysfibrinogenemia Factor VIII > 150%
Abnormalities of platelets	Myeloproliferative disorders Paroxysmal nocturnal hemoglobinuria Hyperlipidemia Diabetes mellitus Heparin-associated thrombocytopenia Thrombotic thrombocytopenic purpura
Hyperviscosity	Polycythemia Leukemia Sickle cell disease Leukoagglutinin Hypergammaglobulinemia

Inhibitors of Cyclooxygenase (Aspirin, Nonsteroidal Anti-inflammatory Agents)

Cyclooxygenase (COX) is a key enzyme in the prostaglandin pathway within platelets and endothelial cells. The final product of this pathway differs in platelets and endothelial cells. Thromboxane A_2, a potent inducer of platelet aggregation, is produced in platelets, whereas prostacyclin, an inhibitor of platelet aggregation, is produced in endothelial cells. Aspirin irreversibly inhibits cyclooxygenase (COX-1 more so than COX-2), which cannot be resynthesized by platelets (since they have no nucleus). Endothelial cells can resynthesize cyclooxygenase, so aspirin's effect on prostacyclin production is short-lived. Small doses of aspirin have significant antiplatelet effects without interfering with prostacyclin generation, thus making aspirin an ideal pharmacologic agent for treatment and prevention of thromboembolic disease. Several of the nonsteroidal anti-inflammatory drugs (NSAIDs) also inhibit platelet cyclooxygenase, but the inhibition is reversible. NSAIDs may cause clinical bleeding in patients with underlying hemostatic defects or after invasive procedures, but they are generally not used therapeutically for treatment or prevention of thromboembolic disorders.

Three reversible COX inhibitors (indobufen, flurbiprofen, and triflusal) that may have beneficial effects similar to those of aspirin are under investigation to determine what role they may play in treatment or prevention of ischemic vascular disease.

The effect of aspirin on platelet function begins within 1 hour after ingestion and lasts the life of the platelet (8–10 days). Ingestion of aspirin in doses commonly used in clinical practice prolongs the bleeding time in normal subjects somewhat variably, typically by 1–3 minutes, and out of the normal range only in about half of subjects). Aspirin inhibits platelet aggregation in vitro, but these laboratory effects do not correlate well with in vivo hemostasis. In patients with underlying hemostatic defects (such as hemophilia, von Willebrand's disease, uremia, mild preexisting disorders of platelet function, and thrombocytopenia), aspirin may markedly prolong the bleeding time and cause serious bleeding in such patients.

The clinical benefits of aspirin have been established by large clinical trials of patients with various thromboembolic phenomena, with end points including development of thrombosis, death from thrombosis, and bleeding complications. Laboratory tests of platelet function are not useful for monitoring such patients in clinical practice. The measurable antiplatelet effects of aspirin are equivalent over a wide range of daily aspirin dosage (300–3600 mg/d), and the therapeutic benefits have been demonstrated with as little as 75 mg/d (or, in one study, 30 mg/d). Most trials have demonstrated antithrombotic efficacy with aspirin doses between 50 mg/d and 100 mg/d. There is no evidence that high-dose aspirin (eg, 650–1500 mg/d) improves outcome; in fact, in high doses aspirin may be detrimental.

Aspirin is rapidly and completely absorbed from the gastrointestinal tract, metabolized to salicylate, and circulates (as salicylate) primarily bound to albumin. Salicylate is metabolized in the liver and excreted in the urine. The serum half-life of salicylate is dose-dependent (3.5–4.5 hours after a single 650 mg dose; 15–20 hours when taken daily at a dosage of 4.5 g/d). Many forms of aspirin are available ("plain," buffered, enteric-coated, timed-release, and rectal suppositories). Platelet inhibition occurs within 1 hour after ingestion of plain aspirin but may take 3–4 hours after ingestion of enteric-coated preparations. Enteric-coated tablets should be chewed if rapid antiplatelet effect is necessary. Gastric irritation may be reduced with enteric-coated and timed-release forms of aspirin, but absorption may be reduced or delayed. Rectal suppositories have less salicylate bioavailability.

Adverse effects of aspirin include dose-dependent gastrointestinal irritation (dyspepsia, nausea and vomiting, occult blood loss, gastric ulceration), hypersensitivity reactions, abnormal liver function tests (rare), nephrotoxicity (rare), and, at high doses, tinnitus and hearing loss. Concomitant use of NSAIDs may increase the risk of gastrointestinal bleeding. Overdosage of aspirin (salicylate intoxication) may be life-threatening and is manifested by metabolic acidosis and respiratory alkalosis, dehydration, fevers, sweating, vomiting, and severe neurologic symptoms. Reye's syndrome in infants and children appears to be associated with aspirin usage. In patients at risk for major bleeding, the antithrombotic effects of aspirin may result in serious bleeding. High doses of aspirin may result in interference with prothrombin synthesis, prolongation of the prothrombin time, and significant hemorrhagic sequelae.

Currently available data support the use of aspirin in a wide variety of situations: cardiovascular disease prevention, stable and unstable angina, acute myocardial infarction, transient ischemic attacks and incomplete stroke, stroke following carotid artery surgery, and prosthetic heart valves (in combination with oral anticoagulation). The benefits of aspirin following vascular or valve surgery, arterial procedures, or creation of fistulas or shunts are less certain but appear to include a reduction in risk of arterial occlusion compared with no therapy. Aspirin, although more effective than placebo, is less effective than anticoagulation in preventing recurrent stroke associated with nonvalvular atrial fibrillation. Aspirin has not been shown to be effective for treatment of established venous thromboembolism and is inferior to other measures for prevention of venous thromboembolism, especially in high-risk patients. Although one large trial showed a benefit of aspirin—alone or in combination with anticoagulation—for patients undergoing hip surgery, it is less effective than anticoagulation. The safety and efficacy in combination with anticoagulants has not been clearly established. Aspirin is not effective for preventing preeclampsia or for improving perinatal outcomes in women at risk for this complication of pregnancy.

Aspirin resistance (poor clinical response or lack of demonstrable antiplatelet effects in vitro) has been observed in some patients receiving aspirin for treatment of ischemic vascular disease. The mechanisms underlying apparent resistance are not known, and there is currently no reliable platelet function test to predict which patients are unlikely to benefit from aspirin. Patients who develop recurrent ischemic events despite aspirin are candidates for alternative antiplatelet therapy or anticoagulation. Concomitant therapy with other NSAIDs can reduce the antiplatelet effect of aspirin because of competition for binding sites in the platelet.

Inhibitors of ADP Mediated Platelet Aggregation (Ticlopidine, Clopidogrel)

Ticlopidine and clopidogrel are structurally related thienopyridines that inhibit platelet function. Repeated daily dosing results in cumulative inhibition of ADP-induced platelet aggregation and slow recovery of platelet function after stopping the drug. The major properties of ticlopidine and clopidogrel are compared in Table 40–2.

Ticlopidine is well absorbed (80–90%) from the gastrointestinal tract. It is rapidly metabolized, with one active metabolite. Steady state levels are achieved with 250 mg twice daily after 14 days. The onset of antiplatelet effect is delayed (up to 2 weeks), so ticlopidine should not be used when a rapid antiplatelet effect is needed. Ticlopidine is better than placebo in patients with recent stroke for prevention of recurrent stroke, myocardial infarction, and vascular death. It may be slightly better than aspirin for stroke prevention in high-risk patients and appears to be about as effective as aspirin in the management of unstable angina or myocardial infarction. Ticlopidine may improve exercise tolerance in patients with claudication due to peripheral vascular disease. Ticlopidine in combination with aspirin may improve outcome after coronary artery stent placement, but clopidogrel appears to be safer for this indication. The usual dose of ticlopidine is 250 mg orally twice a day.

Ticlopidine may cause neutropenia (2.4%), thrombocytopenia, or pancytopenia (0.04–0.08%), particularly in the first 3 months of therapy, so monitoring of blood counts must be done during that time. Thrombotic thrombocytopenic purpura (TTP) has been reported with ticlopidine therapy (0.02–0.04%), but ticlopidine also has been used successfully in management of TTP. Other adverse effects of ticlopidine include diarrhea (20%), skin rash (2–15%), increase in total cholesterol levels (mean increase of 9%), and reversible liver function test abnormalities (rare). Ticlopidine is used as a second-line antiplatelet agent because

Table 40–2. Comparison of ticlopidine and clopidogrel.

	Ticlopidine	Clopidogrel
Absorption (oral)	90%	Rapid
Half-life	24–36 hours (single dose); 96 hours (> 14 days dose)	Active metabolite SR 26334: 8 hours
Active metabolities	Yes	Requires metabolism to active inhibitor: SR 26334
Onset of antithrombotic action	Delayed up to 2 weeks	2 hours (single 400 mg dose); 1 day (50–100 daily dose)
Recovery of platelet function after discontinuing drug	7 days	7 days
Recommended dose	250 mg orally twice daily	300 mg loading dose; 75 mg orally daily
Clinical use	Cerebral ischemia with aspirin failure or intolerance	Peripheral vascular disease, prevention of recurrent stroke, myocardial infarction. Combined with aspirin after coronary artery stent placement.
Side effects	Neutropenia (2.4%), thrombocytopenia, TTP (0.2%–0.04%), aplastic anemia, rash, diarrhea	Rash, diarrhea, TTP (1/1,000,000), neutropenia (0.8%), gastrointestinal bleeding (2%)
Expense	About $2–3/pill	About $3/pill

TTP = thrombotic thrombocytopenic purpura.

of its side effects and high cost. Ticlopidine is approved for stroke prevention when aspirin has failed or in patients who are cannot tolerate aspirin.

Clopidogrel is rapidly absorbed and metabolized to active metabolites (the main one being SR 26334, a carboxylic acid derivative). The onset of inhibition of platelet aggregation is dose-dependent, occurring 2 hours after a single dose (400 mg) but after 2–7 days with lower daily dosing (50–100 mg daily). Platelet function returns to normal 7 days after stopping the drug, consistent with irreversible inhibition of platelet function. A loading dose of 300 mg followed by 50 mg daily will result in a rapid and sustained antiplatelet effect. Clopidogrel appears to have approximately the same antiplatelet effects as ticlopidine. Its therapeutic efficacy appears to be equivalent to aspirin in most settings except for symptomatic peripheral artery disease, in which it may be superior to aspirin. It is currently approved for use in patients with recent stroke or myocardial infarction or who have peripheral arterial vascular disease. Clopidogrel added to aspirin may decrease ischemic complications in patients with unstable angina, but it also increases the risk of major bleeding compared with aspirin alone. Other trials of clopidogrel and aspirin are ongoing. The most common side effects of clopidogrel are rash and diarrhea. Gastrointestinal bleeding occurs less often than with aspirin (2%). Neutropenia has been reported less often than with ticlopidine (0.8%), as has TTP (reported occurrence, 1:250,000 persons, about the same as the general population), usually within the first 2 weeks of treatment.

Platelet Glycoprotein IIb/IIIa Receptor Inhibitors

Platelet glycoprotein IIb/IIIa (GPIIb/IIIa) inhibitors block the binding of fibrinogen to its receptor on the platelet membrane, preventing platelet aggregation. There are three GPIIb/IIIa inhibitors currently approved for use in the United States: abciximab (recombinant humanized monoclonal antibody), eptifibatide (synthetic heptapeptide similar to that found in snake venom from *Sistrurus m barbouri*), and tirofiban (a nonpeptide mimetic). Prolongation of bleeding time and decreased platelet aggregation in vitro are seen with all of these agents, but—in contrast to aspirin, ticlopidine, and clopidogrel—these effects are rapidly reversible after discontinuation of the drug. Results of six large studies have shown that these agents, in combination with aspirin and heparin, are effective for preventing ischemic complications associated with percutaneous coronary artery interventions. They are also effective in combination with heparin for medical management of patients with unstable angina and acute myocardial infarction and may improve outcome of thrombolytic therapy in acute myocardial infarction.

The three agents currently available are administered intravenously. Orally active agents are under investigation, but increased bleeding and a possible paradoxical prothrombotic effect with excess mortality compared with aspirin have limited development. GPIIb/IIIa inhibitors can cause bleeding similar to that seen with fibrinolytic therapy. They are contraindicated in patients with platelet counts less than 100,000/μL.

Abciximab rapidly binds to the platelet receptors, followed by dose-dependent inhibition of platelet aggregation accompanied by prolongation of the bleeding time. Bleeding time returns gradually to normal by 12 hours after a bolus injection, and platelet aggregation normalizes within 48 hours. A bolus dose of 0.25 mg/kg followed by a 10 μg/min continuous infusion results in sustaining of the antiplatelet effect. This regimen has been used to prevent ischemic events in patients undergoing percutaneous transthoracic coronary angioplasty (PTCA). Major bleeding, especially in combination with full-dose heparin, can occur with abciximab. Reversible thrombocytopenia may occur (1–2%) as soon as 2 hours after starting therapy. Antibodies develop in about 6%. The antiplatelet effects of abciximab may be responsible for its therapeutic benefits, but it also inhibits thrombin formation, which may contribute to its antithrombotic properties.

Eptifibatide may cause less bleeding time prolongation than other GPIIb/IIIa inhibitors while causing equivalent inhibition of platelet aggregation, though this effect may have been related to methods of measurement. Like abciximab, eptifibatide can inhibit thrombin generation. Doses of eptifibatide have ranged from a 90–180 μg/kg bolus, followed by continuous infusion rates between 0.5–1 μg/kg/min for 18–24 hours. Bleeding time returns to normal 1 hour after stopping the infusion; while inhibition of platelet aggregation may last 4 hours or more. Eptifibatide does not appear to increase the overall rate of thrombocytopenia, but it may cause severe thrombocytopenia in a small number of patients.

Tirofiban is a nonpeptide inhibitor of the GPIIb/IIIa receptor that increases bleeding time and inhibits platelet aggregation. Its effects are augmented by simultaneous administration of aspirin. Onset of platelet inhibition is rapid (5 minutes) and returns to normal within 1.5–4 hours after discontinuation. Reported studies use bolus doses of 5–15 μg/kg followed by infusions of 0.05–0.15 μg/kg/min. Severe reversible thrombocytopenia may complicate treatment with tirofiban.

Dextran

Dextran (available in high- and low-molecular-weight formulations) interferes with platelet function and fibrin polymerization and enhances plasmin-mediated fibrinolysis. Although dextran is a volume expander, hemodilution induced by dextran does not appear to influence its antithrombotic effects. Although dextran is more effective than placebo in prevention of venous thromboembolism in postoperative patients, it is less effective than low-dose heparin or low-molecular-weight heparin following general surgery or orthopedic surgery, respectively. Dextran is associated with a slightly higher risk of major hemorrhage than low-dose heparin but less risk of wound hematomas. Dextran has not been established to be effective in the treatment of active thromboembolic disease. Because of its volume-expanding properties, dextran should be avoided in patients at risk for volume overload. Dextran may occasionally cause hypersensitivity reactions.

Phosphodiesterase Inhibitors

Dipyridamole is the only phosphodiesterase inhibitor currently in use in the United States. Dipyridamole does not affect platelet aggregation but prolongs platelet survival time in patients with arterial thrombosis or prosthetic heart valves. Dipyridamole does not appear to be a particularly effective antithrombotic agent on its own, and although a recent consensus panel suggested that there is no added benefit of adding dipyridamole to aspirin, one large study reported a benefit of adding modified-release dipyridamole (200 mg twice daily) to aspirin and demonstrated a significant reduction in recurrent stroke or death in patients with prior strokes or TIAs. The most common side effect of dipyridamole is headache; it does not appear to increase risk of bleeding compared with placebo.

ANTICOAGULANTS

The commonly used anticoagulants interfere with blood clot formation and extension by inhibiting coagulation factors (heparin, unfractionated and low-molecular-weight) or blocking the synthesis of biologically active coagulation factors (warfarin). These anticoagulants have demonstrated efficacy in a wide range of thromboembolic conditions, both venous and arterial. Indications for use of anticoagulants are expanding. The development of several new anticoagulants with different mechanisms of action and more favorable therapeutic indices has expanded the use of anticoagulant therapy and increased the therapeutic options for patients with complicated medical conditions.

Heparin

Heparin is derived from porcine intestine or bovine lung and is a mixture of molecules of heterogeneous size (MW 3000–33,000). Heparin binds to antithrombin (AT, also known as antithrombin III), and accelerates antithrombin's inhibition of activated thrombin and other coagulation factors (particularly activated factor X). Only about one-third of administered heparin contains the specific pentasaccharide sequence that is necessary for binding to AT, and only those molecules have anticoagulant activity. An additional sequence of 13 saccharides is required for the AT-heparin complex to bind with thrombin; however, only the pentasaccharide sequence is required for inactivation of activated factor X. This heparin-AT interaction is the major mechanism for heparin's anticoagulant effect. At high concentrations, heparin can also directly bind to heparin cofactor II and inactivate thrombin. Heparin, particularly the high-molecular-weight fractions, also inhibits platelet function.

Heparin is not well absorbed from the gastrointestinal tract so it must be administered parenterally (subcutaneously or intravenously). Subcutaneous heparin has lower bioavailability and should be accompanied by an intravenous bolus injection if immediate anticoagulation is required.

The pharmacology of heparin is complex. It circulates bound to plasma proteins, binds to endothelial cells where it is neutralized by platelet factor 4, and is taken up by macrophages and desulfated. There is a nonlinear dose-response relation and a dose-dependent biologic half-life. The route of elimination of heparin is not certain; plasma clearance is accelerated by the presence of acute thromboembolism. The rate of clearance of heparin depends on the size of the molecules; larger molecules are cleared more rapidly than low-molecular-weight molecules.

Although there is a relationship between the dose of heparin and its efficacy (as well as safety), the variability of response to heparin requires monitoring and adjustment of heparin dose. Monitoring of heparin activity is based on its biologic effect on in vitro coagulation. Heparin prolongs three important in vitro coagulation parameters: the thrombin time (TT), the prothrombin time (PT), and the activated partial thromboplastin time (aPTT). The TT is the most sensitive indicator of heparin's effect and may be used to detect even small amounts of heparin. The TT is useful to differentiate heparin's effect from that of circulating inhibitors of coagulation, which are phospholipid-dependent and therefore will result in a prolonged aPTT but normal TT. The PT is the least sensitive measure of heparin's effect and is usually normal unless the patient is also receiving oral anticoagulant treatment or is overanticoagulated. The aPTT is intermediate in sensitivity and is the most commonly used test for monitoring heparin. However, recent clinical studies have found that the aPTT does not always reliably predict response to therapy. In addition, commercial reagents used in the aPTT assay have variable sensitivity to heparin, which makes monitoring heparin therapy of uncertain accuracy. Nevertheless, the aPTT is still the most commonly used method for monitoring response to heparin. In most clinical situations, the desired aPTT while receiving heparin is one and one-half to two times the control time. Suggested adjustment of heparin dose based on aPTT results is outlined in Table 40–3. Dose modifications should be made when heparin is used in

Table 40–3. Body weight-based dosing of intravenous heparin.[1]

Initial dosing

Loading: 80 units/kg
Maintenance infusion: 18 units/kg/h using 25,000 units in 250 mL D5W (100 units/mL)
Obtain aPTT before and 6 hours after starting heparin

Subsequent dose adjustments based on aPTT measured at 6-hour intervals[2]

aPTT (s)	Rate Change (units/kg/h)	Additional Action	Next aPTT
< 35 (< 1.2 × normal)	+4	Rebolus with 80 units/kg	6 hours
35–45 (1.2–1.5 × normal)	+2	Rebolus with 40 units/kg	6 hours
46–70 (1.5–2.3 × normal)	0	None	6 hours
71–90 (2.3–3.0 × normal)	−2	None	6 hours
> 80 (> 3 × normal)	−3	Stop infursion after 1 hour	6 hours

[1]Modified from Hyers TM: Venous thromboembolism. Am J Respir Crit Care Med 1999;159:1–14.
[2]During the first 24 hours, repeat aPTT every 6 hours. Thereafter, obtain aPTT every morning unless it is outside the therapeutic range.

combination with thrombolytic therapy or platelet glycoprotein IIb/IIIa antagonists. When heparin is given subcutaneously, peak plasma levels are reached after 3 hours.

Heparin is effective for prevention and treatment of venous thromboembolism (deep vein thrombosis and pulmonary thromboembolism), mural thrombus after myocardial infarction, unstable angina, and acute myocardial infarction. Heparin is usually combined with antiplatelet agents in the treatment of acute ischemic heart disease (aspirin, clopidogrel, and, more recently, GPIIb/IIIa receptor inhibitors). Heparin has been used in conjunction with thrombolysis for coronary artery occlusion; however, recent studies have suggested that heparin may increase the risk of bleeding with little added benefit over thrombolysis, particularly in patients receiving aspirin. Guidelines for use of heparin in coronary artery disease have been proposed (Table 40–4); however, ongoing trials will probably result in modification of these guidelines as results of studies using newer agents and combinations of agents are reported. Heparin is also used during extracorporeal circulation of blood (in cardiovascular surgery and hemodialysis), prior to cardioversion in atrial fibrillation (if no mural thrombus is detected by transesophageal echocardiography), in some cases of disseminated intravascular coagulation, and to treat fetal growth retardation in pregnant women. Heparin is generally the anticoagulant of choice during pregnancy because it does not cross the placenta and is not teratogenic. Heparin is also used when chronic oral anticoagulation (eg, in patients with heart valves, atrial fibrillation, recurrent thromboembolic disease) is interrupted for invasive procedures or when recurrent thromboembolism occurs despite adequate oral anticoagulation.

There is a very wide range of responsiveness to heparin among patients with thromboembolic disease. There are multiple factors that modify the anticoagu-

Table 40–4. Indications and administration of unfractionated heparin.[1]

Prevention of venous thromboembolism	Moderate-risk patients (age > 40, undergoing general surgery or with serious medical disorders): 5000 units SC every 8–12 hours. No aPTT monitoring required. High-risk patients (orthopedic surgery, prior deep vein thrombosis or other factors increasing risk for thromboembolism):[1] Adjust low-dose unfractionated heparin to maintain aPTT at upper limits of normal *or* use LMW heparin.
Treatment of acute venous thromboembolism	Bolus 80 units/kg followed by 18 units/kg/h infusion. Monitor and adjust according to Table 40–3. Begin oral anticoagulation on day 1. Continue unfractionated heparin until fully anticoagulated with oral agent (minimum 5 days).
Coronary artery disease (if no contraindication to anticoagulation)	Unstable angina and non-Q wave myocardial infarction (non-St segment myocardial infarction):[2] Use in combination with aspirin, ticlopidine, or clopidogrel; 80 units/kg intravenous bolus followed by continuous infusion, initial rate 18 units/kg/h; adjust dose to maintain aPTT 1.5–2 times control *or* 7500 units SC twice daily if low risk for systemic emboli. ST segment acute myocardial infarction, or with left bundle branch block: a. Patients undergoing percutaneous or surgical revascularization: Monitor activated clotting time (ACT), maintain 300–350 seconds during procedure. b. Combined with thrombolytic therapy (alteplase, and likely reteplase)[3] 60 units/kg initial intravenous bolus followed by continuous infusion of 12 units/kg/h; adjust does to maintain aPTT 1.5–2 times control. Continue for 48 hours (or longer in patients at high risk for systemic or venous thromboembolism). c. Combined with nonselective thrombolytic agents (streptokinase, anistreplase, urokinase): (1) High risk for systemic emboli: Withhold heparin for 6 hours, monitor aPTT, initiate heparin when aPTT is less than 2 times control, then begin infusion with 1000 units/h; adjust dose to maintain aPTT 1.5–2 times control for 48 hours, then switch to subcutaneous heparin, warfarin, or aspirin. (2) Not high risk: Subcutaneous heparin, 7500–12,500 units twice a day until fully ambulatory.
Chronic outpatient use (pregnancy, warfarin failure)[1]	12,000 units SC twice daily. Monitor aPTT 6 hours after injection. Adjust dose to maintain aPTT 1.5–2 times control.

[1]LMW heparin may be preferred over unfractionated heparin for many indications.
[2]American Heart Association/American College of Cardiology guidelines.
[3]Benefit of adding heparin to thrombolytic therapy is controversial.

lant effects of heparin (Table 40–5), so the precise dose of heparin in a given patient cannot be predicted in advance. When immediate therapeutic anticoagulation is required, an intravenous bolus is given followed by continuous intravenous infusion or intermittent subcutaneous heparin (Table 40–3). Continuous infusion is more often used because of its lower risk of hemorrhage, but intermittent subcutaneous heparin may be preferable in certain situations (eg, during pregnancy or other conditions requiring long-term outpatient heparin therapy). Careful monitoring of the aPTT is essential to ensure adequate anticoagulant effect without undue risk of hemorrhage. The aPTT should be checked 6 hours after initiation of heparin or after any change in dose, and daily thereafter (Table 40–3). Larger doses of heparin are required to treat established thromboembolic disease than for prevention of venous thromboembolism, possibly because thrombin bound to fibrin is much less sensitive to inhibition by heparin compared with circulating thrombin and because of increased plasma reactive proteins, which bind and neutralize heparin. It is not necessary to cause prolongation of the aPTT for prevention of venous thromboembolism in moderate-risk patients, though in very high-risk patients—eg, those undergoing orthopedic surgery—prolongation of the aPTT to the upper end of normal is required in order to prevent thrombosis.

Hemorrhage is the most common complication of heparin therapy. Hemorrhage occurs more frequently with high-dose heparin therapy and when the aPTT is prolonged beyond the therapeutic range (> 2.5 times control). Intermittent bolus heparin results in a higher rate of hemorrhage than continuous-infusion heparin, which may be due to the higher total daily dose required to maintain a therapeutic aPTT with intermittent administration. Concomitant use of aspirin or other antiplatelet drugs increases the risk of hemorrhage, but in patients with coronary thrombosis the risk is felt to be acceptable. The presence of other hemostatic defects, chronic alcoholism, and the overall general condition of the patient also influence the risk of hemorrhage with heparin therapy.

Table 40–5. Endogenous factors modifying the anticoagulant effect of heparin.

Factor	Mechanism
Platelets	Bind and protect factor Xa from heparin. Produce platelet factor 4, neutralize heparin.
Fibrin	Binds thrombin and protects if from heparin.
Endothelial surfaces	Bind thrombin and protects it from heparin. Bind and neutralize heparin via displaced platelet factor 4.
Plasma proteins	Bind and neutralize heparin.
Antithrombin (antithrombin III)	Hereditary or acquired deficiency state results in heparin resistance.

Management of hemorrhage associated with heparin varies depending upon the severity of the bleeding as well as the degree of the anticoagulant effect as measured by the aPTT. If the indication for anticoagulation is strong, continuation of heparin with close monitoring of the aPTT and blood counts may be acceptable for patients with trivial bleeding. If minor bleeding is associated with an aPTT that is markedly prolonged above the therapeutic range, withholding heparin until the aPTT falls into the desired range (usually within a few hours) is recommended if the patient is stable, with clinical evaluation of the patient before resuming heparin for evidence of continued hemorrhage. Serious bleeding requires cessation of heparin therapy, while truly life-threatening bleeding (eg, intracranial hemorrhage or hemorrhage associated with hemodynamic instability) may require immediate reversal of heparin with protamine sulfate. One milligram of protamine sulfate per 100 units of heparin (50 mg protamine sulfate for 5000 unit dose of heparin), given intravenously over 10 minutes (to avoid hypotension) will neutralize heparin given 30 minutes earlier. The dose of protamine sulfate should be reduced depending upon the time interval from heparin administration (eg, give 50% of the dose if 60 minutes have elapsed, 25% if 2 hours have elapsed). Since protamine sulfate has a shorter half-life than heparin, the dose may need to be repeated. Side effects of protamine sulfate include hypotension with rapid administration and prolongation of the aPTT (with possible bleeding) if excess protamine is given. Recombinant platelet factor 4 (2.5–5 mg/kg) has been reported to be effective for reversal of heparin as well.

Heparin-induced thrombocytopenia occurs commonly (5–15%) with therapeutic heparin administration, less commonly with prophylactic heparin, and appears to be more common with heparin derived from bovine lung than porcine intestine. Thrombosis, usually associated with very severe thrombocytopenia, occurs in about 0.4% of patients. The onset of thrombocytopenia is usually between 3 and 15 days after initiation of treatment with heparin (median 10 days), but may be as short as a few hours in a previously sensitized individual, particularly if the prior treatment with heparin was within 3 months of reexposure. Resolution of thrombocytopenia occurs within 4–5 days after discontinuation of heparin.

Thrombocytopenia in this disorder is immunologically mediated. Heparin molecules greater than MW 4000 bind to platelet factor 4, and form complexes to which heparin-induced thrombocytopenia antibodies bind. Platelets are activated, resulting in increased thrombin generation, and thrombosis may subsequently occur. Diagnosis is usually made on clinical grounds, but confirmation requires performing either a platelet release assay (platelet activation assay) or a platelet antigen assay (to detect antibodies against platelet factor 4 bound to a substrate). Prevention of this disorder by shortening the duration of heparin administration is important. Initiation of oral anticoagulants simultaneously with heparin in patients who will require long-term anticoagulation will permit a shorter course of heparin and is highly recommended for patients requiring long-term anticoagulation. Daily monitoring of the platelet count is important for identification of patients before thrombosis occurs. The use of low-molecular-weight heparin (or heparinoids) appears to be associated with a lower risk of heparin-induced thrombocytopenia as well.

Management is outlined in Table 40–6. Stopping heparin is the most common intervention, but there appears to be a marked risk in clinically significant thrombosis in the week after cessation of heparin. Warfarin therapy may aggravate the thrombotic process and should be delayed until the platelet count is over 100,000/μL. There are three anticoagulants currently approved for use in heparin-induced thrombocytopenia: lepirudin (a recombinant hirudin), argatroban, and danaparoid (a heparinoid), which should be considered even without overt thrombosis. Anticoagulation with the alternative agent should be continued until the platelet count has returned to normal. Ancrod has also been used for treatment of heparin-induced thrombocytopenia (Table 40–7).

If anticoagulant therapy is necessary in a patient with a suspected history of heparin-induced thrombocytopenia (without complicating thrombosis), laboratory assessment for heparin-dependent antibodies (platelet activation assay or antigen assay) may help determine the risk of reexposure. If the assessment is negative, short-term treatment with heparin with careful monitoring

Table 40–6. Management of heparin-induced thrombocytopenia.

1 Monitor daily platelet counts during heparin therapy.
2. Exclude other causes of acute thrombocytopenia (other drugs, sepsis, DIC, pseudothrombocytopenia).
3. Evaluate for thrombotic complications (iliofemoral artery occlusion, cerebral infarction, and myocardial infarctions are the most common; other arterial thromboses and venous thromboses occur less commonly).
4. Do not administer platelet tranfusions (increased risk of thrombosis).
5. Discontinue heparin (including heparin flushes) for platelet count below 100,000/uL.
6. Administered alternative anticoagulant until the platelet count has recovered (and oral anticoagulation has taken effect, if long term anticoagulation is required):[1]

Anticoagulant	Dose/Monitoring
Lepirudin (a recombinant hirudin derivative)	0.4 mg/kg IV bolus followed by 15 mg/kg/h. Adjust dose to maintain aPTT 1.5–2.5 times normal range.
Danaparoid (a heparinoid)	2250 units IV bolus followed by 400 units/h for 4 hours, then 300 units/h for 4 hours, then 150–250 units/h. Monitor anti-factor Xa activity (if available), maintain at 0.5–0.8 anti-factor Xa units/mL
Argatroban (a selective thrombin inhibitor)	2 μg/kg/min. Adjust dose to maintain aPTT 1.5–3 times control (but < 100 seconds)
Bivalirudin[2] (an analog of hirudin)	0.2 mg/kg/h. Adjust dose to maintain aPTT twice normal range.
Ancrod[3]	See Table 40–7

[1]Do not administer warfarin in patients with heparin-induced thrombocytopenia and deep venous thrombosis until platelet count is > 100,000 (potential risk for vneous limb gangrene). If anticoagulant therapy is necessary in a patient with a suspected history of heparin-induced thrombocytopenia (without complicating thrombosis), laboratory assessment for heparin-dependent antibodies (platelet activation assay or antigen assay) may help determine risk of reexposure. If negative, short-term treatment with heparin (with careful monitoring) may be acceptable. Patients with a history of hepain-induced thrombocytopenia-associated thrombosis should be considered for alternative anticoagulants.

[2]FDA-approved for other indications (angioplasty).

[3]Not an FDA-approved agent for heparin-induced thrombocytopenia; available on compassionate use basis.

Table 40–7. Dosing guideline for ancrod.

Initial dose: 1 unit/kg IV over 8–12 hours, followed by daily maintenance according to fibrinogen level:

Fibrinogen Level	Ancrod Dosage
0.5–1.0 g/L	1 unit/kg IV over 24 hours
1.0–1.5 g/L	1 unit/kg IV over 18 hours
1.5–2.0 g/L	1 unit/kg IV over 12 hours
> 2.0 g/L	1 unit/kg IV over 8 hours

may be acceptable. Patients with a history of heparin-induced thrombocytopenia-associated thrombosis should be considered for alternative anticoagulants.

Other adverse effects of heparin include transient elevation of liver function tests (particularly alanine aminotransferase [ALT] and aspartate aminotransferase [AST]), osteoporosis (due to heparin binding to osteoblasts that release factors which stimulate osteoclasts; clinically significant with long-term heparin administration), skin necrosis, alopecia, hypersensitivity reactions, and hypoaldosteronism.

Low-Molecular-Weight Heparins

Low-molecular-weight heparins are prepared by depolymerization of unfractionated heparin by chemical or enzymatic means. Like unfractionated heparin, low-molecular-weight (LMW) heparin accelerates antithrombin-mediated inactivation of factor Xa, but unlike unfractionated heparin, LMW heparin does not inactivate thrombin because it lacks the additional 13 saccharides required for AT-heparin to form a complex with activated thrombin. Because it binds less strongly to plasma proteins, cells, and thrombin, LMW heparin has greater bioavailability at low doses, a longer half-life, and a more predictable anticoagulant response at a fixed dose than unfractionated heparin. Low-molecular-weight heparin can be administered subcutaneously at a fixed dose (adjusted for weight) once or twice daily (dosing differs for different preparations) and does not require laboratory monitoring using the aPTT. These two factors make outpatient use of LMW heparin possible in selected situations. LMW heparin preparations are renally excreted, and biologic half-life is prolonged in patients with renal failure. The incidence of heparin-induced thrombocytopenia appears to be lower with LMW heparin than with unfractionated heparin. Low-molecular-weight heparin has been used in some patients with heparin-induced thrombocytopenia, but thrombocytopenia may persist in some.

Several LMW heparin preparations are now approved for use in the United States: enoxaparin, dalteparin, and tinzaparin. Selection of one preparation over another is difficult at present, since few studies comparing different preparations and dosing regimens have been performed. Cost may ultimately be as important as any other factor for choosing which LMW heparin to use. The major advantage of LMW heparin compared with unfractionated heparin relates to its convenience of administration, predictable anticoagulant response at a weight-adjusted fixed dose, and lack of need for laboratory monitoring. A comparison of unfractionated heparin and LMW heparin is presented in Table 40–8.

Low-molecular-weight heparin is effective for prevention of venous thromboembolism in patients undergoing major orthopedic procedures (hip fracture or replacement, knee replacement) or neurosurgery, after major trauma (in patients eligible for anticoagulation), and in high-risk medical patients. Low-molecular-weight heparin is as effective as unfractionated heparin in the treatment of deep vein thrombosis and pulmonary thromboembolism. It can be administered to outpatients with acute deep vein thrombosis, but treatment of pulmonary thromboembolism requires hospitalization. Low-molecular-weight heparin is equivalent in efficacy to warfarin for prevention of recurrent deep vein thrombosis following acute deep vein thrombosis, with a lower incidence of minor bleeding, but it is much more expensive. There may also be a higher rate of rebound thromboembolism after discontinuation of the drug than with warfarin.

The role of LMW heparin in coronary artery disease continues to evolve as studies in various clinical syndromes are completed. LMW heparin is effective in combination with aspirin in the acute treatment of unstable angina and non-Q wave myocardial infarction and may be superior to unfractionated heparin. There does not appear to be any additional benefit from continuing LMW heparin beyond the acute event to prevent recurrent ischemic events. LMW heparin in combination with thrombolytic therapy for acute Q wave myocardial infarction has not been as extensively studied. LMW heparin reduces the risk of left ventricular mural thrombus formation, but in one study it was associated with excessive bleeding and did not appear to decrease recurrent ischemic events or mortality from myocardial infarction. A more recent study found LMW heparin to be as effective as unfractionated heparin when combined with alteplase and aspirin. LMW heparin is not effective for prevention of restenosis after coronary angioplasty. The use of LMW heparin is not recommended for thromboprophylaxis in patients with prosthetic heart valves.

Complications of therapy with LMW heparin are similar to those seen with unfractionated heparin, with

Table 40–8. Comparison of unfractionated heparin and LMW heparin.

	Unfractionated Heparin	Low-Molecular-Weight Heparin
Plasma half-life	Dose-dependent; range 1–2.5 hours	Increased; range 2–6 hours; prolonged in renal failure
Bioavailability	Lower	Better
Molecular weight: range (Mean)	3000–30,000 (15,000)	100–10,000 (4500–5000)
Binding properties: proteins, cells (macrophages, endothelium, osteoblasts)	High	Low
Relative inactivation: Xa/IIa	Lower	Higher (five to six times compared with unfractionated heparin)
aPTT	Prolonged	Not prolonged
Efficacy	Equivalent	Equivalent (most situations)
Major bleeding	Approximately equivalent: 0–7% higher (fatal, 0–2%), higher in acute stroke	Approximately equivalent: 0–3% (fatal, 0–0.8%), higher in acute stroke
Heparin-induced thrombocytopenia	2.5–6%	Decreased
Osteoporosis	30%: decreased bone density; 15%: vertebral fractures 2–3%: vertebral fractures in pregnancy	Decreased 2.5%: vertebral fractures
Cost	$15/d, full dose	> $100/d, full dose

the exceptions of thrombocytopenia and osteoporosis, which occur less often with LMW heparin. There may be less major bleeding in patients treated for deep vein thrombosis with LMW heparin, but in most other situations the risk is approximately equivalent to that seen with unfractionated heparin. The FDA issued an advisory, however, warning that the use of LMW heparin and heparinoids in the setting of spinal or epidural anesthesia—or with spinal puncture—may cause bleeding in the spinal column with subsequent prolonged or permanent paralysis. If excessive bleeding does occur, laboratory assessment with a anti-factor Xa heparin assay can be performed. The usual therapeutic range is between 0.5 and 1.0 unit/mL. When heparin anti-factor Xa is greater than 1.0 unit/mL, the aPTT may also be prolonged.

NEW ANTICOAGULANTS

Direct Thrombin Inhibitors

Recombinant hirudin (lepirudin), bivalirudin (an analog of hirudin), and argatroban are direct thrombin inhibitors that are not dependent on antithrombin to exert their anticoagulant effects. Unlike heparin, these agents bind to free and clot-bound thrombin, do not bind to plasma proteins, and are not neutralized by platelet factor 4. Hirudin and argatroban are approved for use in heparin-induced thrombocytopenia (Table 40–6). Hirudin, unlike heparin, has no natural antidote should bleeding occur, which limits its safety. Bivalirudin is under investigation, and because it has a shorter half-life than hirudin it may be safer than hirudin. Argatroban is a carboxylic acid derivative that interferes with thrombin by binding to its active site. Several other agents in this class are under investigation, some of them well absorbed from the gastrointestinal tract (eg, melagatran) with a predictable anticoagulant response, making laboratory monitoring unnecessary. In addition to their role in the treatment of heparin-induced thrombocytopenia, these agents are under investigation for use in other clinical situations

Indirect Thrombin Inhibitors (Heparinoids)

Heparinoids are low-molecular-weight glycosaminoglycuronans derived from porcine intestinal mucosa. Danaparoid is the only heparinoid currently approved for use in the United States by the FDA. It is a mixture of heparan sulfate, dermatan sulfate, and chondroitin sulfate. The small heparan sulfate portion of this drug

(4% of the total) has a high affinity for antithrombin and is responsible for the major anticoagulant effect of danaparoid. Dermatan sulfate also mediates development of heparin cofactor II-thrombin complexes, and contributes to the anticoagulant effect. Danaparoid has a higher ratio of anti-factor Xa activity compared with anti-factor IIa activity (20:1) compared with unfractionated heparin (1:1) and LMW heparin (2–4:1), and has less effects on platelet function than unfractionated heparin. It is similar to LMW heparin in its anticoagulant effects and has minimal effect on coagulation parameters (aPTT, prothrombin time, and thrombin time), but it has certain structural differences (contains galactosamine, absent in LMW heparin) that distinguish it from LMW heparin. A functional anti-factor Xa assay using danaparoid as the standard can be used to monitor the anticoagulant effect of danaparoid when the agent is given for more than 3 days.

Danaparoid is used for prevention of deep vein thrombosis, especially to prevent clotting during hemodialysis or hemofiltration. Danaparoid appears to be safer than LMW heparin for anticoagulation of patients with heparin-induced thrombocytopenia (Table 40–6).

Defibrinating Agents

Ancrod, an enzyme derived from the Malayan pit viper, is an anticoagulant that cleaves fibrinogen and causes hypofibrinogenemia. Ancrod is licensed for use in Canada and is available for compassionate use by its manufacturer (Knoll Pharmaceutical) in the United States. Ancrod is an effective anticoagulant which apparently causes minimal excess bleeding. It is not associated with the development of thrombocytopenia and is an excellent alternative anticoagulant for patients with heparin-induced thrombocytopenia. An initial dose of 1 unit per kilogram is infused intravenously over 8–12 hours, followed by daily maintenance doses adjusted for the level of fibrinogen (Table 40–7). Neutralizing antibodies develop with long-term use, thus limiting its usefulness to situations in which only short-term anticoagulation is required. An antivenom is available to reverse its effect, and cryoprecipitate may also be required for fibrinogen replacement if excessive bleeding occurs.

ORAL ANTICOAGULANTS

Warfarin

Warfarin (a 4-hydroxycoumarin compound) is the most commonly used oral anticoagulant in North America. Warfarin interferes with the metabolism of vitamin K, inhibiting reduction of vitamin K to its active form, vitamin KH_2, in a two-step process in the liver. Vitamin KH_2 is essential for posttranslational modification (γ-carboxylation) of the vitamin K-dependent coagulation factors and natural anticoagulants (II, VII, IX, X, and proteins C and S). Decreased carboxylation of these important proteins impairs their biologic function (impedes calcium-binding capability) and induces an anticoagulant effect.

Warfarin is absorbed rapidly from the gastrointestinal tract—reaching peak plasma levels in 90 minutes—circulates bound to plasma proteins (97% albumin-bound), is metabolized in the liver, and is excreted in urine and bile. The anticoagulant effect of warfarin is not immediate. Until carboxylated coagulation factors are adequately depleted, blood coagulation is normal. The vitamin K-dependent proteins have plasma half-lives ranging from 6 hours (factor VII) to 72 hours (prothrombin; factor II). Proteins C and S have relatively short half-lives (about 8 hours). Because levels of factor VII, protein C, and protein S levels fall at about the same time—and 1–3 days before depletion of the other coagulation factors—a relative hypercoagulable state may exist in the first 1–2 days after initiation of warfarin. Although an observable anticoagulant effect usually occurs after 2 days, the full anticoagulant effect is delayed for 4–5 days. The delayed effect may be of significant importance for patients with inherited or acquired deficiency of either protein C or protein S, who may be particularly susceptible to warfarin-induced skin necrosis.

Whenever rapid anticoagulation is needed, heparin (unfractionated or low-molecular-weight) should be given for at least 4 days at the start of warfarin therapy until the INR is in the therapeutic range. A loading dose of warfarin, though commonly given, is not necessary. The initial dose is based on clinical criteria, with larger doses given to patients requiring rapid anticoagulation and smaller doses to elderly patients (who have increased sensitivity to warfarin), those with poor nutrition or liver disease, or those at high risk for bleeding. The average dose required to achieve a therapeutic level by 4–5 days is 5 mg daily.

The anticoagulant effect of warfarin is assessed by in vitro coagulation tests, the prothrombin time (PT) and partial thromboplastin time (aPTT). The therapeutic range for warfarin depends upon the indication for which it is used, but at usual doses the aPTT is normal or minimally prolonged while the PT is maintained at 1.3 (low-intensity) to 2.5 (high-intensity) times control (PT ratio). Because of marked interlaboratory variability in the sensitivity of the thromboplastin reagents used in the PT assay, a standardized approach has been adopted internationally. This approach requires calibration of the thromboplastin to a reference preparation using the International Sensitivity Index (ISI). Results are then reported as a ratio (International Normalized

Ratio; INR) based on a formula comparing the PT ratio obtained with the laboratory thromboplastin to that with the reference thromboplastin. The therapeutic range of warfarin for most indications when the INR is used ranges from 2–3 (low intensity) to 2.5–3.5 (high intensity). If the thromboplastin reagent used by a clinical laboratory remains constant, the PT and INR will be predictably related to each other. Substitution of the reagent (with either a more or a less sensitive preparation), however, may dramatically alter the relationship of the PT and INR. The INR is more reliable than the PT and is the preferred method of reporting for warfarin monitoring.

Although there is a direct dose-response relation, there is marked variation in anticoagulant response to warfarin among patients. There is also significant variability of anticoagulant response during long-term therapy in individual patients. This variability results from many factors, including endogenous stores of vitamin K, changes in dietary intake or recent therapeutic administration of vitamin K, genetically determined differences in warfarin sensitivity, use of antibiotics (which may impair synthesis of vitamin K by intestinal flora) or other drugs (may increase or decrease warfarin effect), the presence of liver disease, fat malabsorption (including obstructive jaundice), hypermetabolic states, pregnancy, poor patient compliance, and laboratory inaccuracy. In addition, elderly patients appear to be more sensitive to warfarin, possibly due to decreased clearance of warfarin with age. Because of this marked variability, continued monitoring is required, and most patients require dosage adjustments periodically. Initial monitoring should be performed daily until therapeutic, then two or three times weekly until the INR is stable. When the PT or INR is stable, monitoring every 4 weeks is usually adequate, though more frequent monitoring may increase the amount of time the PT or INR is in the therapeutic range ("time in therapeutic range," or TTR). Intensity of therapy and TTR are important determinants of therapeutic efficacy of warfarin. More frequent monitoring is advisable for elderly patients, those who take multiple medications, or those who are at higher risk for bleeding.

Although patients taking warfarin are commonly instructed to limit their intake of vitamin K-rich vegetables, it is preferable to suggest that the intake of these vegetables remain relatively constant in the diet, since the nutritional benefits of these foods unrelated to vitamin K may be important. Numerous drugs influence the anticoagulant effect of warfarin through multiple mechanisms, and bleeding unrelated to the anticoagulant effect of warfarin may result from effects on other hemostatic pathways (aspirin and other antiplatelet drugs, and heparin) as well as effects on intestinal mucosa (aspirin). Before beginning warfarin therapy—or before adding new medications when a patient is taking warfarin—a review of potential interactions should be undertaken (readily available in pharmaceutical handbooks such as the *Physicians' Desk Reference* or other drug compendiums). The frequency of PT or INR monitoring should be increased in patients taking warfarin whenever new medications are started to allow proper dose adjustments.

The decision to use long-term oral anticoagulation is based upon an assessment of the risk to the patient of bleeding compared with the potential benefits related to its anticoagulant effect. Warfarin is effective for management of multiple thromboembolic conditions and is used when long-term anticoagulation is required. Candidates for long-term anticoagulation include those with artificial heart valves, chronic atrial fibrillation, left ventricular mural thrombus, recurrent cerebrovascular ischemia, and antiphospholipid antibody syndrome.

The role of warfarin is well established and accepted in the prevention and treatment of venous thromboembolic disease. It is generally used for 3–6 months for uncomplicated first events and may be required on a long-term basis for recurrent venous thromboembolism or in patients with multiple thrombophilic conditions such as combined factor V Leiden and prothrombin gene mutation G20210, though ongoing studies are attempting to address the issue of risks of recurrent thrombosis versus risks of bleeding in these patients.

Warfarin is effective for prevention of systemic or cerebral emboli in atrial fibrillation and artificial heart valves. It is also effective for the prevention of acute myocardial infarction in patients with peripheral arterial disease; for prevention of stroke, recurrent infarction, or death in patients with acute myocardial infarction; and for prevention of myocardial infarction in men at high risk. Other antithrombotic agents, particularly antiplatelet agents, are used more often for prevention of coronary and cerebrovascular thrombosis. Warfarin is currently used only in selected patients for this indication (eg, patients with left ventricular mural thrombi or very poor ventricular function). Warfarin is often used for stroke prevention in patients who have had recurrent cerebrovascular ischemia despite antiplatelet agents; however, it has not been proved to be effective for this indication and may be associated with a high risk of major bleeding, particularly if the INR is maintained at a high range (3–4.5). The target INR for most indications is 2–3 (low-intensity) except for prosthetic mechanical heart valves, prophylaxis of recurrent myocardial infarction, and perhaps thrombosis associated with antiphospholipid antibodies, where high-intensity warfarin (INR 2.5–3.5) is recommended. Very low-intensity warfarin (INR 1.3–1.8) combined with aspirin may be effective for primary prevention of ischemic coronary events in patients at high risk.

Bleeding is the most common complication of warfarin and is related to the intensity of the anticoagulation (especially in patients over 75 years of age), concomitant use of aspirin, coexisting hemostatic defects (including renal failure), age over 65 years, history of gastrointestinal bleeding, anemia, presence of anemia, and history of stroke or atrial fibrillation. If bleeding occurs when the INR is less than 3.0, an underlying gastrointestinal or renal lesion should be suspected, though spontaneous bleeding may occur when the INR is in the high-intensity range or above. Prolonged use (lifelong) may also increase the cumulative risk of bleeding. Patients who consume excess alcohol or those who suffer from frequent falls have a much higher risk of serious bleeding. There are rare patients who have been identified to have mutations in factor IX, which causes an unusual susceptibility to bleeding without prolongation of the INR.

Overdosage of warfarin (accidental or intentional) may lead to serious bleeding. Management of hemorrhage associated with warfarin is similar to that encountered with heparin in terms of using clinical criteria to determine the urgency of the situation. Mild excess prolongation of the INR (< 5.0) without hemorrhage should be managed expectantly by withholding warfarin until the INR returns to the desired range, then resuming at a lower dose. Serious bleeding may require immediate reversal with fresh frozen plasma (two to three units) to provide functional vitamin K-dependent factors. Because vitamin K is a fat-soluble vitamin that is stored in the liver, reversal of warfarin effects with vitamin K may result in resistance to subsequent warfarin therapy. Low-dose oral vitamin K_1 (phytonadione, 1–2.5 mg) will lower the INR to < 5 in patients with INR values between 5 and 9, and 5 mg will correct INR values to > 9 in the majority of patients within 24 hours without inducing warfarin resistance. Intravenous vitamin K_1 should be reserved for patients with an urgent need to reverse anticoagulation—particularly those patients with life-threatening hemorrhage not controlled by fresh frozen plasma who will not require subsequent warfarin therapy.

Patients receiving chronic warfarin therapy undergoing invasive procedures likely to cause bleeding may require interruption of warfarin. Depending upon the patient's risk for perioperative thromboembolism, coverage with unfractionated heparin or LMW heparin may be necessary until the patient resumes warfarin. Dental procedures may not require interruption of warfarin; local hemostasis can be achieved with the use of topical agents, such as tranexamic acid or aminocaproic acid mouthwashes. Tables 40–9 and 40–10 summarize guidelines proposed by the American College of Chest Physicians for warfarin therapy (dose, monitoring, adjustment, and perioperative management).

Warfarin skin necrosis is a rare but serious complication of warfarin, usually occurring 2–7 days after initiation of warfarin therapy. Extensive thrombosis of venules and capillaries of subcutaneous fat, particularly in the lower extremities, buttocks, or breast, appears to be most common in patients who have an inherited or acquired deficiency of protein C or protein S. Patients who are known to be deficient in protein C or S should receive warfarin only with simultaneous administration of heparin for at least 5 days to

Table 40–9. Administration and monitoring of warfarin.

Initial dose: 5 mg/d (lower in patients who are elderly, on multiple medications, malnourished, or have liver disease).

Check INR daily until therapeutic, then two or three times per week until stable, then every 4 weeks.

INR	Intervention
Subtherapeutic	Increase dose. Continue frequent monitoring until therapeutic.
Therapeutic (range based on underlying condition requiring anticoagulation)	Continue current dose.
Between therapeutic range and 5	Omit dose. Resume at a lower dose when INR is therapeutic.
5.0–9.0, no bleeding	Omit 1 or 2 doses. Resume at a lower dose when INR is therapeutic *or* give vitamin K_1, 1–2.5 mg orally. Resume warfarin at reduced dose when therapeutic.
> 9.0, no bleeding	Hold warfarin, give vitamin K_1, 3–5 mg orally. Resume warfarin at reduced dose when therapeutic.
> 20.0 *or* serious bleeding	Hold warfarin. Give vitamin K_1, 10 mg by slow intravenous infusion. Supplement with fresh frozen plasma or prothrombin complex concentrate if needed.

Table 40–10. Management of warfarin during invasive procedures.

Low risk for thromboembolism (VTE > 3 months ago or artial fibrillation without stroke)	Stop warfarin 4 days before surgery. Give heparin at prophylactic dose postoperatively; resume warfarin postoperatively.
Intermediate risk for thromboembolism	Stop warfarin 4 days before surgery. Use low-dose unfractionated heparin or LMW heparin starting 2 days before surgery. After surgery, resume warfarin, continue heparin until INR therapeutic.
High risk for thromboembolism (VTE < 3 months ago; multiple VTE; mechanical mitral valve; ball/cage valve)	Stop warfarin 4 days before surgery. Start full-dose intravenous or subcutaneous heparin or LMW heparin 2 days before surgery. Stop before surgery (5 hours for intravenous unfractionated heparin, 12 hours for subcutaneous unfractionated heparin or LMW heparin). Resume warfarin, continue heparin postoperatively until INR therapeutic.
Low risk of bleeding	Continue warfarin at lowered dose (INR 1.3–1.5) for 4–5 days before surgery. Resume full dose postoperatively. Use prophylactic dose of heparin until INR therapeutic.
Dental procedures with low risk of bleeding	Continue warfarin at usual dose and INR.
Dental procedures with higher risk of bleeding	Continue warfarin at usual dose and INR. Use tranexamic acid or aminocaproic acid mouthwash to control bleeding.

VTE = venous thromboembolism.

allow for depletion of all the vitamin K-dependent coagulation proteins to prevent skin necrosis.

Warfarin is teratogenic, resulting in a fetal embryopathy associated with multiple anomalies when warfarin is administered during the first trimester of pregnancy (estimated incidence, 7–28%). Warfarin crosses the placenta and may result in fetal bleeding. Because of these negative fetal effects, warfarin is contraindicated between weeks 6 and 12 of pregnancy, and because it may cause fetal bleeding it should be avoided near term. Women of reproductive age who are taking warfarin should be advised of the teratogenic effects of the drug, and if pregnancy is contemplated, heparin or LMW heparin should be substituted prior to pregnancy (except for women with mechanical heart valves; see Antithrombotic Therapy in Pregnancy, below). Warfarin does not cause anticoagulation in infants who are breast-fed by mothers taking warfarin.

Other infrequent side effects of warfarin include alopecia, gastrointestinal discomfort, rash, and liver dysfunction. In patients with underlying arterial vascular disease, warfarin therapy has been associated rarely with the development of atheroembolic complications, including ischemic toes, livedo reticularis, gangrene, abdominal pain, and renal and other visceral infarctions due to cholesterol emboli.

Anisindione

Patients who cannot tolerate warfarin may be treated with anisindione, an oral anticoagulant that is structurally unrelated to warfarin but works by a similar mechanism, namely, inhibition of γ-carboxylation of the vitamin K-dependent coagulation factors. The drug is well absorbed from the gastrointestinal tract, is highly protein-bound, and is metabolized to inactive metabolites that are excreted in the urine. These metabolites may cause a red-orange discoloration of the urine. The anticoagulant response of anisindione occurs within 20–72 hours, and it is cleared slowly from circulation with a half-life of 3–5 days. Like warfarin, its anticoagulant effect can be reversed by vitamin K and fresh frozen plasma. Anisindione crosses the placenta and causes fetal malformations and fetal bleeding, so it should be avoided during pregnancy.

Anisindione is FDA-approved for use in myocardial infarction and venous thrombosis, but there is a lack of good clinical studies to support its use as a substitute for warfarin except for those patients who are truly intolerant of warfarin. In those patients, a loading dose of 300 mg on day 1, 200 mg on day 2, and 100 mg on day 3 is followed by daily maintenance of 50–250 mg, adjusted according to the INR. Anisindione may cause myelosuppression, dermatitis, jaundice, and renal insufficiency, which have limited its use.

THROMBOLYTIC THERAPY

Thrombolytic (fibrinolytic) agents differ from other antithrombotic agents in that they actually dissolve established clots rather than interfering with initiation and propagation of thrombosis. The mechanism of action of these agents is complex and involves many components of the naturally occurring fibrinolytic system. Activation of plasminogen to plasmin (the major fibrinolytic enzyme) is enhanced by these drugs, accompanied by increased consumption of its inhibitor (α_2-antiplasmin). The net effect is an increase in free plasmin, which results in degradation of fibrin and other coagulation factors.

All of the available agents cause varying degrees of systemic activation of the fibrinolytic mechanism and therefore induce generalized fibrinolysis and fibrinogenolysis and some degree of platelet dysfunction due to proteolysis of key membrane receptors by plasmin, though some are more specific for plasmin bound to clot ("fibrin-specific"). These drugs work best when given soon after onset of symptoms (eg, within 3–4 hours in acute arterial thrombosis, 48 hours for pulmonary thromboembolism, 7 days for deep vein thrombosis), before thrombi are highly cross-linked and more resistant to thrombolysis.

There are five thrombolytic agents that have received FDA approval for use in the United States. Selected features of these agents are outlined in Table 40–11. Thrombolytic therapy is used in the treatment of acute arterial thrombosis, including myocardial infarction and peripheral arterial occlusion, and in the treatment of severe venous thromboembolic disease (massive pulmonary thromboembolism and hemodynamic compromise, massive deep vein thrombosis, or phlegmasia cerulea dolens). Thrombolysis can improve neurologic function in patients with acute nonhemorrhagic stroke if patients at high risk for bleeding are excluded. Thrombolytic agents are also used to reestablish patency of clotted indwelling venous catheters and vascular grafts.

Indications, timing of administration, use of adjunctive antithrombotic agents, and choice of agent for thrombolytic therapy are evolving. Thrombolysis reduces mortality from acute myocardial infarction by

Table 40–11. Comparison of selected fibrinolytic agents.

Drug	$t_{1/2}$ (min)	Fibrin-Specific	Indications (FDA-Approved)	Neutralizing Antibodies[1]	Typical Dose[2]	Estimated Cost
Alteplase	5	Yes	Myocardial infarction, acute cardiovascular accident, pulmonary thromboembolism	No	Myocardial infarction: 100 mg infusion/90 minutes to 3 hours; cardiovascular accident: 0.9 mg/kg (maximum 90 mg)/60 minutes. Part of total dose is given as a bolus	$2750
Anistreplase	70–120	No	Myocardial infarction	Yes	30 units/2–5 minutes	$1950
Reteplase	13–16	Yes (less than alteplase)	Myocardial infarction	No	Two bolus injections, 10 units each, 30 minutes apart	$2750
Streptokinase	20	No	Myocardial infarction (intravenous or intracoronary), deep vein thrombosis, pulmonary thromboembolism, catheter thrombosis, peripheral arterial occlusion	Yes	1.5 million units/30–60 minutes IV or– 140,000 units by intracoronary injection	$500–$700
Urokinase	20	No	Myocardial infarction (intracoronary), pulmonary thromboembolism, catheter thrombosis	No	2 million unit bolus or 3 million units/90 min 5000 units for catheter thrombosis	$4000–$6000 (myocardial infarction, pulmonary embolus) $60 (catheter thrombosis)

[1]Presence of neutralizing antibodies precludes repeat use within 6–24 months, possibly longer, because of allergic reactions and decreased effectiveness of the agent.
[2]Doses may vary depending upon clinical situation.

about 20–50%. In patients not undergoing percutaneous transthoracic coronary angioplasty for acute myocardial infarction, alteplase may be more effective than streptokinase, but further studies need to be done to elucidate the optimal regimen for each specific clinical situation. Although the newer agents are much more expensive than the older drugs (streptokinase and urokinase), the contribution of drug costs to the overall cost of care—particularly for acute myocardial infarction—has not been shown to be significant. When cost effective analyses have been done, streptokinase appears to be marginally more cost-effective compared with other agents.

The principal goal of fibrinolytic therapy is to reestablish patency of an occluded blood vessel (or indwelling catheter). Fibrinolytic therapy for myocardial infarction results in angiographically-confirmed patency about 50% of the time. Additional antithrombotic therapy may be required to improve reperfusion. The role of heparin combined with fibrinolytics for patients with acute myocardial infarction is controversial. Ongoing studies are required to define the optimal use of heparin (unfractionated or low-molecular-weight) or other anticoagulants such as the hirudin derivatives and heparinoids in combination with fibrinolytic therapy. Antiplatelet agents have been shown to be very important as an adjunct to fibrinolytic therapy. Platelets play a key role in the development of coronary thrombosis. Aspirin and platelet glycoprotein IIb/IIIa inhibitors potentiate fibrinolysis and improve coronary artery patency rates, though bleeding complications may also be increased when streptokinase is combined with glycoprotein IIb/IIIa inhibitors. Large trials recently completed will provide additional information about safety and efficacy of various combinations of antiplatelet agents and fibrinolytics in the treatment of acute myocardial infarction. In addition, the combination of reduced-dose fibrinolytic therapy with invasive coronary interventions (eg, angioplasty) may improve outcomes. Further study in this area is needed to define optimal dosing to enhance coronary artery patency while maintaining an acceptable rate of hemorrhage.

Alteplase is approved for use in acute nonhemorrhagic stroke and is effective when administered intravenously within 3 hours after onset of symptoms. The risk of intracerebral hemorrhage is 3%, but because it can lead to improved neurologic function this may be an acceptable risk. An estimated 2% of all stroke patients are able to receive alteplase within the 3-hour time frame, limiting its potential impact on outcomes from stroke. Recently, MRI to locate arterial occlusions, followed by superselective intra-arterial thrombolysis, has been suggested as a potentially beneficial approach for patients with acute stroke who are more than 3 hours from the onset of symptoms. This approach has an even higher risk of hemorrhage (10% overall), but in centers equipped with a stroke center and all necessary personnel and technologic support quickly available it may prove to increase the number of patients who could benefit from thrombolysis for acute stroke.

Each of the fibrinolytic agents is effective in the treatment of pulmonary thromboembolism and deep vein thrombosis, though comparative trials have not been performed, and only streptokinase, alteplase, and urokinase have FDA approval for treatment of pulmonary thromboembolism. (Streptokinase is also approved for use in deep vein thrombosis, peripheral arterial occlusion, and catheter thrombosis.) Patients with massive pulmonary thromboembolism and hemodynamic compromise may experience better overall outcomes with thrombolytic therapy, but hemorrhagic complications are twice that observed with standard anticoagulation. Although lysis of clot can be demonstrated in 50% of patients with deep vein thrombosis after fibrinolytic therapy, the clinical benefit for this condition is less clear. Patients with uncomplicated deep vein thrombosis have a generally favorable prognosis with a very low mortality. The hemorrhagic complications of fibrinolysis are substantial, so fibrinolytic therapy is usually reserved for patients with massive proximal clots or those with compromise of arterial circulation secondary to venous thrombosis. Despite the high rate of clot lysis, there is no good evidence to support the concept that thrombolytic therapy reduces the rate of postphlebitic syndrome after deep vein thrombosis.

Fibrinolytic therapy is effective in the treatment of acute arterial thrombus in medium and large peripheral arteries. A fibrinolytic agent administered through a catheter proximal to the clot dissolves it completely about 75% of the time. Catheter-directed intra-arterial administration appears to be superior to intravenous administration. Thrombolysis should be considered prior to surgery as long as the affected limb is still salvageable. Surgery can be avoided in 35% of these cases, and overall mortality appears to be somewhat better than with immediate surgery.

Urokinase, 5000 units, may be instilled into an occluded venous catheter without excessive pressure, which could dislodge clot or rupture the catheter. Because venous catheters may be occluded by substances other than clots (eg, drug precipitate), urokinase is not always effective.

The most common complication of thrombolytic therapy is hemorrhage (3–40%). Hemorrhagic complications can be minimized if patients are selected properly and monitored carefully. The use of other antithrombotic agents—particularly heparin—increases the risk of bleeding. Contraindications to thrombolytic therapy include active visceral bleeding, aortic dissection, intracranial disease, recent surgery or invasive procedures, head trauma, severe uncontrolled hypertension (> 180/110 mm Hg), pregnancy, recent retinal laser surgery, cardiogenic shock, and the use of oral anticoagulants resulting in an INR > 1.5. Thrombolytic therapy results in decreased plasma fibrinogen concentration and increased fibrin degradation products, but these tests are not predictive of efficacy or clinical bleeding. The bleeding time, if prolonged, may correlate with minor bleeding but is not usually monitored.

The thrombin time is the best laboratory test for monitoring the status of the fibrinolytic system. When thrombin time is prolonged more than five to seven times normal, the incidence of bleeding complications increases significantly. Intracerebral hemorrhage is more common in patients who are elderly or underweight, who have prior neurologic disease, or who are receiving antithrombotic drugs. Women appear to have a higher risk of intracerebral hemorrhage. If major bleeding occurs with thrombolytic therapy, the drug should be stopped immediately. Hypofibrinogenemia can be reversed with cryoprecipitate, and aminocaproic acid can be given to inhibit plasmin activity. If the patient is receiving heparin, protamine sulfate can be used to reverse its effect.

Other potential adverse reactions to certain thrombolytic agents (streptokinase, anistreplase) include allergic reactions and the development of neutralizing antibodies that preclude repeated usage for 6–24 months and perhaps longer. Cholesterol emboli may rarely complicate thrombolytic therapy, resulting in the "purple toe syndrome," and multiorgan failure. Arrhythmias may accompany reperfusion of an ischemic myocardium.

ANTITHROMBOTIC THERAPY IN PREGNANCY

Pregnancy and the postpartum period pose special challenges in the management of thromboembolic disorders. In addition to the apparent increased risk of venous thrombembolic events, certain pregnancy complications (fetal loss, preeclampsia, abruption, fetal growth retardation, and intrauterine death) are associated with maternal thrombophilias (eg, antiphospholipid antibodies, factor V Leiden, prothrombin gene mutation, antithrombin deficiency, hyperhomocysteinemia). In addition, women who are taking warfarin for preexisting conditions (venous thromboembolism, mechanical heart valves) require continued antithrombotic therapy during this higher-risk period. Warfarin is contraindicated between 6 and 12 weeks of pregnancy because of its teratogenicity and because it may increase the risk of fetal bleeding. Unfractionated heparin does not cross the placenta and appears to be safe and effective during pregnancy. LMW heparin and danaparoid have a lower risk of osteoporosis and thrombocytopenia than unfractionated heparin. Dosing may be adjusted for increasing weight, or anti-factor Xa levels (drawn 4 hours after morning dose) can be monitored (target range, 0.5–1.2 units/mL). Because these agents do not cross the placenta, fetal bleeding is not a complication; however, there have been recent reports of congenital anomalies with some of the LMW heparin preparations (enoxaparin, tinzaparin), and there has been insufficient clinical experience with danaparoid during pregnancy to determine its teratogenicity. Maternal bleeding occurs with the same frequency as in other situations requiring anticoagulation (major bleeding, about 2%). Bleeding can complicate delivery. The aPTT may not adequately reflect the anticoagulation effect of unfractionated heparin because of increased factor VIII and fibrinogen. When possible, unfractionated heparin or LMW heparin should be discontinued 24 hours before labor (eg, when electively induced). Unfractionated heparin and LMW heparin are not secreted in breast milk, and warfarin does not appear to cause an anticoagulant effect in babies who are breast-fed by mothers taking warfarin.

The use of heparin during pregnancy appears to be effective for prophylaxis and treatment of venous thromboembolism. In women with mechanical heart valves, heparin is not be as effective as warfarin for prevention of thromboembolic complications, particularly if the aPTT is only moderately elevated. Choices for anticoagulation in these women include using warfarin (target INR 3.0) except for weeks 6 through 12, and near delivery, when unfractionated heparin can be substituted, to prevent fetal embryopathy or bleeding, or to use unfractionated heparin throughout pregnancy. If unfractionated heparin is used, it is imperative that high doses be used and that the aPTT (6 hours after subcutaneous injection) is closely monitored. The addition of low dose aspirin (81 mg daily) may reduce the risk of thrombosis but also increases the risk of bleeding. Maternal and fetal deaths from thrombotic complications have been reported when enoxaparin was used for thromboprophylaxis in pregnant women with prosthetic heart valves; therefore, the use of LMW heparin cannot be recommended for these women. Low dose aspirin appears to be safe when administered in the second and third trimesters to prevent complications such as pregnancy-induced hypertension or intrauterine growth retardation; however, its efficacy for these indications has not been proved. There may be a role for aspirin in the treatment of antiphospholipid antibodies and recurrent fetal loss.

ANTIPHOSPHOLIPID ANTIBODY SYNDROME

Significant thrombotic events in the presence of the antiphospholipid antibody syndrome pose special therapeutic challenges. Acute management with heparin is complicated by the frequent presence of a baseline elevation in the aPTT. Therefore, monitoring should be performed using a specific heparin assay that is dependent upon factor Xa inhibition (therapeutic range, 0.3–0.7). Low-molecular-weight heparin can be used without the need for laboratory monitoring. High intensity warfarin (INR at least 3) is superior to lower-dose warfarin. Long term anticoagulation (eg, lifelong) is necessary because of the unusually high rate of recurrent thrombotic events after discontinuance (50% after 2 years; 80% after 8 years). Low-dose aspirin (81 mg) should be added to oral anticoagulation for arterial thrombosis or for recurrent venous thromboembolism despite adequate oral anticoagulation. Some patients also have hypoprothrombinemia, with baseline prolongation of the prothrombin time, which makes monitoring with INR unreliable. Coagulation tests that are insensitive to the lupus anticoagulant may be required in these patients (prothrombin-proconvertin test, chromogenic factor X level). Corticosteroids and immunosuppressive agents may improve coagulation abnormalities, but the benefits are usually short-lived. If patients have multisystem involvement, corticosteroids, immunosuppressives, and plasmapheresis may be beneficial; however, ongoing treatment of the thrombotic diathesis is advisable.

The optimal therapeutic approach for women with antiphospholipid antibody syndrome and recurrent fetal loss is not clear. Aspirin, with or without corticosteroids, high dose immune globulin, and anticoagulants have all been tried, with variable results. Thrombocytopenia, immunologically mediated, is common in antiphospholipid antibody syndrome but is generally mild and does not require treatment. With severe thrombocytopenia (< 20,000/μL), it may increase bleeding during anticoagulation. Treatment as for other immune thrombocytopenias should be given to achieve a reasonable platelet count to decrease the risk of serious hemorrhage with concomitant anticoagulation. Catastrophic antiphospholipid antibody syndrome (multiorgan and bowel thrombosis, gangrene, livedo reticularis, and strokes) requires aggressive therapy with anticoagulation, plasmapheresis, and aggressive immunosuppressive therapy.

FUTURE DIRECTIONS

There are several exciting active areas of research in the field of antithrombotic therapy. Many new agents are in various stages of development. Modifications of existing antithrombotic agents may serve to increase the predictability of anticoagulant effect, improve bioavailability and convenience, and decrease complications. Combinations of various antithrombotic agents are under investigation in an attempt to improve efficacy while maintaining an acceptable risk for hemorrhage.

A specific pentasaccharide on heparin is responsible for binding to antithrombin and subsequently exerting antithrombotic effects by inhibition of factor Xa. One of the more promising new agents, Org31540/SR90107A, a synthetic pentasaccharide, is a selective indirect inhibitor of activated factor X (via antithrombin). It has been shown to be more effective than enoxaparin for preventing venous thromboembolism after hip replacement, with a lower risk of hemorrhage. It does not interact with platelets, is not neutralized by platelet factor 4, and is unlikely to cause thrombocytopenia. There are other natural and synthetic compounds under investigation that bind directly to factor Xa and inactivate it. Tick anticoagulant peptide and antistasin (from *Haementeria officinalis,* the Mexican leech) are now available in recombinant form.

The development of orally active agents with a more predictable anticoagulant response would be a major development for the outpatient management of thromboembolic disease. Oral delivery systems to allow heparin or LMW heparin to be absorbed from the gastrointestinal tract are undergoing trials for thromboprophylaxis after major orthopedic surgery. Several thrombin inhibitors that appear to be orally bioavailable are under development (eg, melagatran, efegatran).

Many other classes of agents are under active investigation as well. In addition to new anticoagulants, attempts to augment the naturally occurring anticoagulant pathway of protein C and the fibrinolytic system may prove useful. Recombinant activated protein C has been tested in patients with sepsis and has been shown to decrease mortality; however, it may increase the risk of bleeding. New antiplatelet agents, including additional platelet glycoprotein IIb/IIIa receptor inhibitors, are also being studied.

While endeavoring to improve the benefit-risk ratio of antithrombotic therapy, cost-effectiveness holds major importance in the future of antithrombotic therapy. The indications for antithrombotic therapy are continuously expanding, and the cost of many new agents is very high. It is important that any new antithrombotic drug be compared with older, established therapies, with demonstration of definite advantage, before changing the standard of care for patients with or at risk for thromboembolic disease.

REFERENCES

Ansell J et al: Managing oral anticoagulant therapy. Chest 2001;119:22S-38S.

Armstrong PW, Collen D: Fibrinolysis for acute myocardial infarction, Parts 1 and 2. Circulation 2001;103:2862–6 and 2987–92.

Attia J et al: Deep vein thrombosis and its prevention in critically ill adults. Arch Intern Med 2001;161:1268–79.

Hirsh J et al: The sixth (2000) ACCP guidelines for antithrombotic therapy for prevention and treatment of thrombosis. Chest 2001;119:1S–2S.

Hirsh J et al: Guide to anticoagulant therapy: Heparin. A statement for healthcare professionals from the American Heart Association. Circulation 2001;103:2994–3018.

Hirsh J et al: Oral anticoagulant: mechanism of action, clinical effectiveness, and optimal therapeutic range. Chest 2001;119: 8S–21S.

Ginsberg JS, Greer I, Hirsh J: Use of antithrombotic agents during pregnancy. Chest 2001;119: 122S–131S.

Levine GN, Ali MA, Schafer AI: Antithrombotic therapy in patients with acute coronary syndromes. Arch Intern Med 2001;161:937–48.

Marchetti M et al: Low-molecular-weight heparin versus warfarin for secondary prophylaxis of venous thromboembolism: a cost-effectiveness analysis. Am J Med 2001;111:130–9.

Patrono C et al: Platelet-active drugs: The relationships among dose, effectiveness, and side effects. Chest 2001;119:39S-63S.

Ross AM et al: Randomized comparison of enoxaparin, a low-molecular-weight heparin, with unfractionated heparin adjunctive to recombinant tissue plasminogen activator thrombolysis and aspirin: second trial of heparin and aspirin reperfusion therapy (Part II). Circulation 2001;104:648–52.

Ryan TJ et al: 1999 update. ACC/AHA guidelines for the management of patients with acute myocardial infarction: a report of the American College of Cardiology/American Heart Association Task Force on Practice Guidelines (committee on Management of Acute Myocardial Infarction). J Am Coll Cardiol 1999;34:890–911.

Seligsohn U, Lubetsky MD: Genetic susceptibility to venous thromboembolism. N Engl J Med 2001;344:1222–31.

Turpie GG, Gallus AS, Hoek JA: A synthetic pentasaccharide for the prevention of deep-vein thrombosis after total hip replacement. N Engl J Med 2001;344:619–25.

Warkentin TE, Kelton JG: Temporal aspects of heparin-induced thrombocytopenia. N Engl J Med 2001;344:1286–92.

Weitz JI, Hirsh J: New anticoagulant drugs. Chest 2001;119: 95S–107S.

Yusuf S et al: Effects of clopidogrel in addition to aspirin in patients with acute coronary syndromes without ST-segment elevation. N Engl J Med 2001;345:494–502.

Index

Note: Page numbers followed by *t* and *f* indicate tables and figures, respectively.